Textbook of

Paediatric Anaesthesia

Textbook of Paediatric Anaesthesia

Editors

Namita Padvi
MBBS, MD, DNB, Fellowship in Paediatric Anaesthesiology

Assistant Professor, Department of Anaesthesia
Topiwala National Medical College and BYL Nair Charitable Hospital
Mumbai

Amit Padvi
MBBS, MD, Fellowship in Paediatric Anaesthesiology

Assistant Professor, Department of Anaesthesia
Faculty Member of Department of Paediatric Anaesthesia
Seth GS Medical College and KEM Hospital
Mumbai

Varsha Gupta
MBBS MD

Faculty
Government Medical College
Kota

Mahesh Baldwa
MBBS MD (Paediatrics) DCH LLB LLM PhD (Law) MBA FIAP

Consultant Paediatrician
Baldwa Hospital, Mumbai
Ex-Assistant Professor of Paediatrics
TN Medical College and Nair Hospital, Mumbai
Ex-Assistant Professor, JJ Hosp, Grant Medical College, Mumbai
Ex-Visiting Professor, Paper Setter and Examiner
Department of Law, University of Mumbai

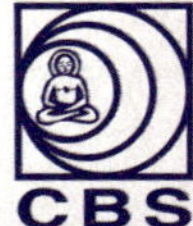

CBS Publishers & Distributors Pvt Ltd

New Delhi • Bengaluru • Chennai • Kochi • Mumbai • Pune
Hyderabad • Kolkata • Nagpur • Patna • Vijayawada

Disclaimer

Medical field is always in a dynamic state, with continuous influx of new knowledge and practices. Everyday results of new researches broaden our understanding of the subject, improve our medical practices and change the research methods.

Clinicians and researchers should use their own clinical acumen, experience, skill and knowledge in evaluating and using any information, drugs, techniques, procedures, equipment or experiments described herein. In clinically applying such knowledge or methods they should be careful of their own safety as well as that of others, including parties for whom they have a professional liability.

When using any drug described herewith, readers are advised to check the most current information provided by the manufacturer. They should verify the recommended dose or formula, the method, route and duration of administration, side effects and contraindications. Clinician should assess each patient individually and use their own knowledge, skill and experience to make diagnosis and determine the best perioperative or procedural anaesthetic regime for each patient.

Contributors are individually responsible for their respective opinions, views, information and figures assimilated in their respective chapters and are hereof individually responsible for the source of such information.

To the fullest extent of the law neither the publisher, nor the authors, contributors nor editors assume any liability for any injury and / or damage to persons or property as a matter of product liability, negligence or otherwise, or from any use or operation of any methods, products, instructions, or ideas contained in the material herein.

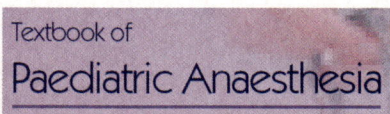

ISBN: 978-81-239-2589-9

First Edition: 2015

Published by Satish Kumar Jain and Produced by Varun Jain for
CBS Publishers & Distributors Pvt Ltd
4819/XI Prahlad Street, 24 Ansari Road, Daryaganj, New Delhi 110 002, India.
Ph: 23289259, 23266861, 23266867 Fax: 011-23243014 Website: www.cbspd.com
e-mail: delhi@cbspd.com; cbspubs@airtelmail.in.

Corporate Office: 204 FIE, Industrial Area, Patparganj, Delhi 110 092
Ph: 4934 4934 Fax: 4934 4935 e-mail: publishing@cbspd.com; publicity@cbspd.com

Branches

- **Bengaluru:** Seema House 2975, 17th Cross, K.R. Road, Banasankari 2nd Stage, Bengaluru 560 070, Karnataka
  Ph: +91-80-26771678/79 Fax: +91-80-26771680 e-mail: bangalore@cbspd.com
- **Chennai:** No. 7, Subbaraya Street, Shenoy Nagar, Chennai 600 030, Tamil Nadu
  Ph: +91-44-26260666, 26208620 Fax: +91-44-42032115 e-mail: chennai@cbspd.com
- **Kochi:** 36/14 Kalluvilakam, Lissie Hospital Road, Kochi 682 018, Kerala
  Ph: +91-484-4059061-65 Fax: +91-484-4059065 e-mail: kochi@cbspd.com
- **Mumbai:** 83-C, Dr E Moses Road, Worli, Mumbai-400018, Maharashtra
  Ph: +91-22-24902340/41 Fax: +91-22-24902342 e-mail: mumbai@cbspd.com
- **Pune:** Bhuruk Prestige, Sr. No. 52/12/2+1+3/2 Narhe, Haveli (Near Katraj-Dehu Road Bypass), Pune 411 041, Maharashtra
  Ph: +91-20-64704058, 64704059, 32392277 Fax: +91-20-24300160 e-mail: pune@cbspd.com

Representatives

- **Hyderabad** 0-9885175004
- **Kolkata** 0-9831437309, 0-9051152362
- **Nagpur** 0-9021734563
- **Patna** 0-9334159340
- **Vijayawada** 0-9000660880

Printed at: Paras Offset Pvt. Ltd., New Delhi

With love

To

Baby Parneeka

who spreads smiles on all faces

which makes life worth living

Foreword

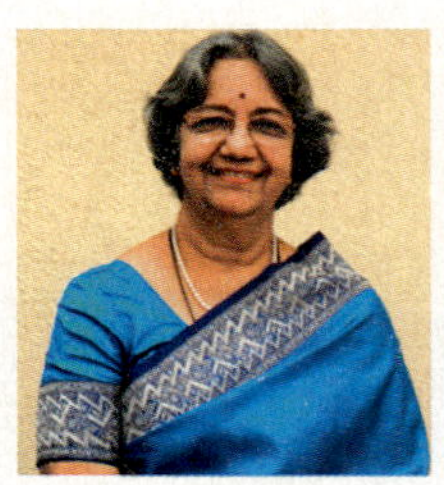

It is a great pleasure and honour for me to be asked to write Foreword to this new *Textbook of Paediatric Anaesthesia*. This book is edited by young, enthusiastic and energetic paediatric anaesthesiologists with the help of well-known contributing authors.

The editors have divided their text into four sections, each devoted to an area of special importance which will be immensely useful for practising paediatric anaesthesiologists as well as to the fellows pursuing DM in paediatric anaesthesiology. The topics are judiciously chosen and are widely applicable to perioperative paediatric patient care both inside and outside the operating room and at remote locations. The contributing authors in this well-written textbook comprise over forty paediatric anaesthesiologists, paediatricians, paediatric intensivists and cardiac anaesthesiologists from all over India. The widening role of paediatric anaesthesiologist has been well identified. Many techniques including new methods of monitoring and measurement are performed in their role as intensivist, emergency practitioner and proponent of innovative life support techniques. The *key points* and *take home messages* outlined at the end of each chapter are appropriate and informative and are welcome addition for quick reference.

The editors are to be congratulated for making this textbook excellent compilation of all aspects of paediatric anaesthesia from basics to principles and anaesthesia for surgical procedures from head to toe along with special consideration that encompasses ethical, medicolegal aspects and evidence based guidelines. Paediatric anaesthesia has become so complex and some of the children are so sick and some presenting with various syndromes are at high risk, that success will only be achieved if there is complete understanding between the anaesthesiologist and his or her surgical and medical colleagues. So it is a team work.

I strongly recommend this book to all residents aspiring to be paediatric anaesthesiologist and also all members of our fraternity. It is a valuable addition to every medical library and departments of anaesthesia in all medical institutions.

Snehalata H Dhayagude
DA (London) FRCA (England)

Founder President of Indian Association of Paediatric Anaesthesiologists
Consultant Paediatric Anaesthesiologist
Bombay Hospital and Medical Research Centre
Mumbai, Maharashtra

Contributors

Bhvya Baldwa MBBS, Resident in MD Chest medicine
Department of Chest Medicine
Seth G.S. Medical College and K.E.M. Hospital
Parel, Mumbai

Mahesh Baldwa MBBS MD (Paediatrics) DCH LLB LLM PhD (Law) MBA
Consultant Paediatrician
Baldwa Hospital, Borivali West, Mumbai
Ex-Assistant Professor of Paediatrics,
Topiwala National Medical College and
B.Y.L. Nair Charitable Hospital, Mumbai
Ex-Assistant Professor J.J. Hospital, Grant Medical College, Mumbai
Ex-Visiting Professor, Paper Setter and Examiner
Department of Law, University of Mumbai, Mumbai

Sushila Baldwa MBBS MD
Senior Consultant
Apollo Clinic, Kandivali West, Mumbai

Rochana Bakhshi MBBS DNB DA MNAMS PG DHHM PGDMLS
Professor
Department of Anaesthesiology
D.Y. Patil Medical College and Hospital
Navi Mumbai

Rakesh Bhadade MD
Assistant Professor
Department of Medicine
Topiwala National Medical College and
B.Y.L. Nair Charitable Hospital
Mumbai Central, Mumbai

Pradnya Bhalerao MBBS MD
Associate Professor
Department of Anaesthesiology and Critical Care
B.J. Government Medical College and Sassoon General Hospitals, Pune

Rahul Bhamkar MBBS DCH DNB MNAMS, Fellowship in Paediatric Critical Care
Associate Consultant
Department of Paediatrics
Sir H.N. Reliance Foundation Hospital, Mumbai

Niraja Bhardwaj MBBS MD
Professor
Department of Anaesthesia and Intensive Care
Postgraduate Institute of Medical Education and Research
Chandigarh

Gayathri Bhat MBBS MD
Professor, Department of Anaesthesiology and Critical Care
K.S. Hegde Medical Academy
Mangalore

Pallavi Butiyani MBBS MD
Consultant Anaesthesiologist
Noble Hospital, Pune

Vaishali Chaskar MBBS DA DNB Fellowship Paediatric Anaesthesiology
Assistant Professor
Department of Anaesthesia
Seth G.S. Medical College and K.E.M. Hospital
Parel, Mumbai

Indrani Hemantkumar Chincoli MBBS MD DA DNB
Professor
Department of Anaesthesia
Topiwala National Medical College and
B.Y.L. Nair Charitable Hospital
Mumbai Central, Mumbai

Rachana Chhabria MBBS MD Anaesthesia, Fellowship in Paediatric Anaesthesia
Assistant Professor in Anaesthesia at
Seth G.S. Medical College and K.E.M. Hospital
Parel, Mumbai

Rajen Daftary MBBS DA MD
Consultant Anaesthesiologist
BIDS, Global Hospital and Research Centre
Parel, Mumbai

Swati Daftary MBBS DA MD
Consultant Anaesthesiologist
Jaslok Hospital and Research Centre, Mumbai
Ex-Associate Professor of Anaesthesia
LTM Gen Hospital and Medical College
Mumbai

Sona Dave MBBS MD DNB
Professor
Department of Anaesthesia
Topiwala National Medical College and
B.Y.L. Nair Charitable Hospital
Mumbai Central, Mumbai

Vidhya Deshmukh MBBS DA FCPS DNB (Anaesthesiology), Fellowship in Paediatric Anaesthesiology
Senior Assistant Professor
Department of Anaesthesiology
Topiwala National Medical College and B.Y.L. Nair Charitable Hospital, Mumbai

Rakesh Garg MD DNB PGCCHM MNAMS FCCS
Assistant Professor of Dr BRAIRCH
Anaesthesiology, Intensive Care, Pain and Palliative Care
All India Institute of Medical Sciences
New Delhi

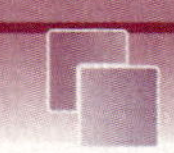

Varsha Gupta MBBS MD
Government Medical College
Kota

Minal Harde MD DNB
Associate Professor
Department of Anaesthesia
Topiwala National Medical College and
B.Y.L. Nair Charitable Hospital
Mumbai Central, Mumbai

Uma Hariharan MBBS MD
Consultant Anaesthesiology
Department of Anaesthesia
Rajiv Gandhi Cancer Institute and Research Centre
New Delhi

Ruchi Jain MBBS MD DNB (Anaesthesiology), Fellowship in Neuroanaesthesia
Assistant Professor
LTMC and Sion Hospital
Mumbai

Jimmy John MBBS
Resident in Anaesthesia
Seth G.S. Medical college and K.E.M. Hospital
Parel, Mumbai

Preetha Joshi MBBS DNB (Paediatrics) FCCM (Australia, Canada)
Senior Paediatrician
Neonatal and Cardiac Intensivist, Department of Paediatric, Neonatal and Cardiac Intensive Care, Kokilaben Hospital
Mumbai

Vinay Joshi MBBS MD DM (Neonatology) FCCM (Australia and Canada)
Senior Neonatal
Paediatric and Cardiac Intensivist, Department of Paediatric, Neonatal and Cardiac Intensive Care, Kokilaben Hospital
Mumbai

Prashant Kamdi MD (Anaes) Fellowship in Paediatric Anaesthesia
Assistant Professor
Seth G.S. Medical College and K.E.M. Hospital
Parel, Mumbai

Shruti Kamdi MD (Transfusion Medicine)
Seth G.S. Medical College and K.E.M. Hospital
Parel, Mumbai

Deepa Kane MBBS MD (Anaesthesiology)
Professor
Seth G.S. Medical College and K.E.M. Hospital
Parel, Mumbai

Jalpa Kate MBBS DA DNB (Gold Medalist)
Consultant Anaesthesiologist
BARC Hospital
Anushakti Nagar
Mumbai

Manish Kela MBBS DNB MD (Anaesthesiology) Fellowship in Cardiac Anaesthesia
Assistant Professor
Seth G.S. Medical College and K.E.M. Hospital
Parel, Mumbai

Nirav Kotak MBBS MD (Anaesthesiology)
Associate Professor
Seth G.S. Medical College and K.E.M. Hospital
Parel, Mumbai

Archna Koul MD
Consultant
Department of Anaesthesiology
Pain and Perioperative Medicine, Sir Ganga Ram Hospital
New Delhi

Hemlata DNB PDCC
Senior Resident
Department of Anaesthesiology
Sanjay Gandhi Postgraduate Institute of Medical Sciences
Lucknow

Indu Lata MD MNAMS FICMCH MICOG
Associate Professor
Department of Maternal and Reproductive Health
Sanjay Gandhi Postgraduate Institute of Medical Sciences
Lucknow

Ashish Mali MBBS MD
Senior Assistant Professor
Department of Anaesthesia
Topiwala National Medical College and
B.Y.L. Nair Charitable Hospital
Mumbai Central, Mumbai

Anita Malik MBBS MD FICA
Professor
Department of Anaesthesiology and Critical Care
King George's Medical University, Lucknow

Namisha Malik MBBS DA

Vibhavari Naik MBBS MD DNB (Anaesthesiology)
Senior Consultant
Department of Anaesthesia and Surgical Critical Care
Basavatarakam Indo-American Cancer Hospital and
Research Institute
Hyderabad, Telangana

Shrikanta Oak MBBS DA DNB
Associate Professor
Department of Anaesthesia
Seth G.S. Medical College and K.E.M. Hospital
Parel, Mumbai

Amit Padvi MBBS MD Fellowship in Paediatric Anaesthesiology
Assistant Professor
Department of Anaesthesia,
Faculty member of Department of Paediatric Anaesthesia
Seth G.S. Medical College and K.E.M. Hospital
Parel, Mumbai

Namita Padvi MBBS, MD (University topper), DNB, Fellowship in Paediatric Anaesthesiology
Assistant Professor
Department of Anaesthesia
Topiwala National Medical College and
B.Y.L. Nair Charitable Hospital
Mumbai Central, Mumbai

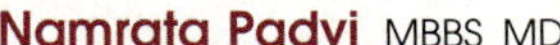

Namrata Padvi MBBS MD
Assistant Professor
Government Medical College
Dhule

Nitin Padvi MBBS
Medical Officer, Gondia

Deepanjali Pant MD
Senior Consultant
Department of Anaesthesiology
Pain and Perioperative Medicine
Sir Ganga Ram Hospital, New Delhi

RD Patel MBBS DA MD
Professor
Department of Anaesthesia
Seth G.S. Medical College and K.E.M. Hospital
Parel, Mumbai

Tushar Patel MBBS MD
Senior Resident
Department of Anaesthesiology and Critical Care
K.S. Hegde Medical Academy
Mangalore

Chinmayi Patkar MBBS MD DNB
Assistant Professor
Department of Anaesthesia
Topiwala National Medical College and
B.Y.L. Nair Charitable Hospital
Mumbai Central, Mumbai

Archana Prabhu MBBS MD
Consultant Anaesthesiologist
Sahyadri Specialty Hospitals, Pune

Ekta Rai MBBS MD MRCA
Professor
Department of Anaesthesia, Christian Medical College
Vellore, Tamil Nadu

Anjana Sahu MBBS MD
Senior Assistant Professor
Department of Anaesthesia
Topiwala National Medical College and B.Y.L. Nair Charitable Hospital, Mumbai Central, Mumbai

Dinesh Kumar Sahu MD (Anaesthesiology), Fellowship in Pain Management (ISSP)
Consultant
Jagjivanram Railway Hospital
Mumbai Central, Mumbai

Sandeep Sahu MD PDCC MNAMS FICCM FACEE
Associate Professor
Department of Anaesthesiology
Sanjay Gandhi PG Institute of Medical Sciences
Lucknow

Prasanna Salvi MBBS, MD, FNB in Cardiac Anaesthesia
Consultant
Paediatric Cardiac Anaesthesiologist and
intensivist Wockhardt Hospital, Mumbai

Pradnya Sawant MBBS DA MD, Fellowship in Paediatric Anaesthesia
Chief of Department
Wadia Children Hospital
Parel, Mumbai

Anita Shetty MBBS DA MD (Anaesthesiology)
Professor, Seth G.S. Medical College and K.E.M. Hospital
Parel, Mumbai

SK Shrivastav MBBS MS (ortho)
Professor
Department of Orthopaedics
Seth G.S. Medical College and K.E.M. Hospital
Parel, Mumbai

Prem Raj Singh MD
Senior Resident
Department of Anaesthesiology
Sanjay Gandhi Postgraduate Institute of Medical Sciences
Lucknow

Jayashree Sood MD FFARCS PGDHHM FICA
Senior Consultant and Chairperson
Department of Anaesthesiology, Pain and Perioperative Medicine
Sir Ganga Ram Hospital, New Delhi

Sushama Tandale MBBS MD, Fellowship in Paediatric Anaesthesiology
Assistant Professor
Department of Anaesthesia
Rajeev Gandhi Medical College and Chatrapati Shivaji Maharaj Hospital
Thane, Mumbai

Roopali Telang MBBS MD, Fellowship in Paediatric Anaesthesiology
Associate Consultant
Department of Anaesthesiology
P.D. Hinduja National Hospital
Mumbai

Harshwardhan Tikle MBBS MD
Associate Professor
Department of Anaesthesia
Topiwala National Medical College and B.Y.L. Nair Charitable Hospital
Mumbai Central, Mumbai

Raveendra US MBBS MD DNB (Anaesthesiology)
Specialist and Head Intensive Care
Department of Anaesthesia and Suri Seri Begawan Hospital
Kuala Belait
Brunei Darussalam

Anjana Wajekar MBBS DNB Fellowship in Neuroanaesthesia
Assistant Professor, Department of Anaesthesia
Seth G.S. Medical College and K.E.M. Hospital
Parel, Mumbai

Naveen Yadav MBBS MD
Assistant Professor
JPNATC and AIIMS
New Delhi

Preface

Motivation is like fire—unless you keep adding fuel to it, it dies. Your fuel is your belief in your inner values
—Shiv Khera
You Can Win: A step by step tool for top achievers.

With continuous motivation from God, family, teachers, friends, students we have come out with our first textbook. We will never forget the intellectual joys we had during our contact with various enlightened and accomplished contributors and once again we thank one and all from the bottom of our heart.

Contributors have duly filled copyright forms and have tried their best, to give due credit to the source of various information, securing intellectual's right of property. For all copyrighted authors' works, books, information sources which are not acknowledged in this book, firstly we seek their forgiveness and secondly, we overtly apologize for not doing so. We assure them of doing so in the next edition of this book.

Paediatric Anaesthesia is now becoming a fast growing super-specialized branch of medical science in India. Several institutes have started fellowship programmes in Paediatric Anaesthesiology. For the first time in India, a DM superspecialty degree is granted and recognized by MUHS and MCI at GS Medical College and KEM Hospital, Mumbai. At present a few Indian standard textbooks are available, addressing the superspecialty of Paediatric Anaesthesiology. Hence this book was written with the aim to occupy the existing vacuum and to take the knowledge and skills of Paediatric Anaesthesiology to newer heights.

How will the new topics help the reader?

It will provide new insight for postgraduates pursuing MD and DM in paediatric anaesthesia and clinicians practicing paediatric anaesthesia. The entire practice of paediatric anaesthesia from anatomy, physiology, regional and general anaesthesia, various paediatric surgical disciplines, and special situations to medicolegal and ethical aspects has been compiled in various sections of this book.

What is special about the style of presentation in the proposed book?

It has the usual textbook style of presentation but it has been made reader friendly by adding *summary*, *key points*, *take home messages*, *FAQs*, *one fact to remember*, and *Paediatric Anaesthesia Pearls*. Summary is given at the end of each topic for better understanding and to provide a bird eye view of the topic.

The book delivers the knowledge essential to the safe practice of paediatric anaesthesia. It covers everything from paediatric anatomy, physiology and pharmacology principles through important paediatric diseases; preoperative, intraoperative, and postoperative care; anaesthesia for a full range of specific surgical procedures; and critical care. Geared primarily for learners of paediatric anaesthesia, these tightly focused, user-friendly chapters make it ideal for general anaesthesiologists as well as postgraduate students.

There is ample literature generated from the West which analyses the issues related to paediatric anaethesiology thoroughly. There is scanty literature on this subject in India where the volume of patients surpasses many times over most of the western countries. We should have our own literature, written in simple English suited to our milieu. With the phenomenal increase in the patient volume in India, the need for indigenous literature related to paediatric anaesthesiology is going to be even greater in the future.

The editors sincerely hope that this book will serve to fill the void effectively. This book looks beyond the problems and moves on to solutions. It comprehensively provides solutions to almost all vulnerable areas of this super-/sub-specialty. Paediatric Anaesthesia has now become a well-recognized superspecialty branch of anaesthesia. Let us welcome this change and brace ourselves with the knowledge to cope with the change. A few years back a book was published "Who moved my cheese". It is a wonderful book which easily teaches us about how to cope with changes in life.

Namita Padvi
Amit Padvi
Varsha Gupta
Mahesh Baldwa

Acknowledgements

The editors wish to acknowledge the hard work of all those, who have made this book a reality, especially the contributors. Without the expertise of the contributors, the book would not have seen the light of the day.

We would also like to acknowledge all our teachers, who have taught and mentored us throughout our lives. We acknowledge the role of one and all, who have enlightened and motivated us to write the book, especially our families, friends, teachers, students, patients and God, the Almighty. Finally, we are grateful to the outstanding staff of CBS Medical Publishers and Distributors, especially Mr Ramesh Krishnamachari, RM, Mumbai branch.

We are thankful to Mr SK Jain (Matta), CMD, Mr YN Arjuna, Sr Vice President—Publishing, Editorial and Publicity. We are also thankful to Mr Ankit Gupta, Software Engineer, for his personal help to us.

We invite appreciations, suggestions and criticisms at 2014tpa@gmail.com. It is a well-known fact that ignorance breeds and feeds uncertainty. Uncertainty breeds and feeds unfounded fears, which leads to inaction. Let us learn and drive away ignorance.

Happy reading!!!

Namita Padvi
Amit Padvi
Varsha Gupta
Mahesh Baldwa

Contents

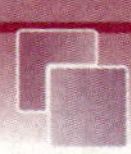

SECTION 2: Scientific Basis for Practice of Paediatric Anaesthesia

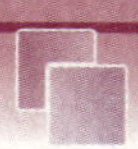

SECTION 4: Special Considerations: Complications of Anaesthesia, Medicolegal, Ethical Aspects of Paediatric Anaesthesia

Section

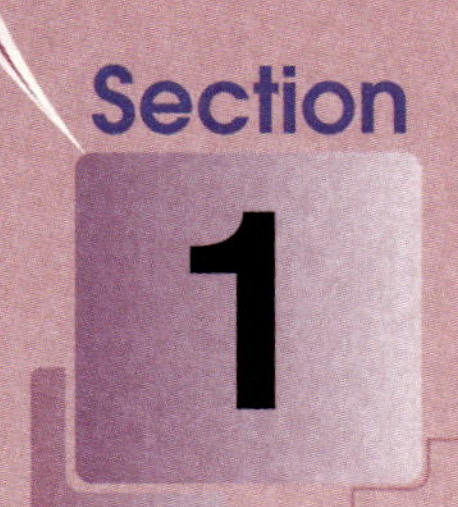

Principles in Paediatric Anaesthesia

1

History of Paediatric Anaesthesiology

Namita Padvi, Varsha Gupta and Mahesh Baldwa

History of paediatric anaesthesiology cannot be dissected from general historic development in anaesthesiology, historic developments in paediatrics, historic development of general surgery, historic development of paediatric surgery, historic developments in pharmacology and general historic developments and increased understanding of medical science and technology.

History in General

Many surgeons had strong notions that average men should tolerate pain caused by surgery and thus kept patients away from administering anaesthesia during surgery. Humans have inhabited the Earth for 200,000 years, yet the public demonstration of surgical general anaesthesia happened in 1846. The conviction that small infants did not need anaesthesia. The "whiskey nipple" had been used widely as a sedative supplement to local anaesthesia in infants undergoing abdominal procedures. Giving wine for pain relief became a ritual for doing circumcision surgery for millennia.

History in Specific

Among advances in medicine during the past more than 170 years, certainly the introduction of surgical anaesthesia must be considered the greatest gifts of medical profession to mankind, especially to children. Anaesthesia for children was considered a bit risky endeavour, in India as well as abroad before 1980. Before 1980s, anaesthesiologists preferred open drop ether method for anaesthesia in children in India. Soon later intravenous sodium pentothal was used for short procedures for children. In a short span of less than a quarter of century, paediatric anaesthesiology which started as a subspecialty branch of anaesthesiology has become a superspecialty branch of medicine. Millions of *paediatric* patients receive *anaesthetics* every *year*, (Gregory's Paediatric Anaesthesia by George A Gregory, Dean B. Andropoulos, 5th edn., 2012) but it has been established that those under one year of age require higher standard of care. It is now clear that paediatric anaesthesiology is a well-established and well-recognized subspecialty in its own right.

HISTORY OF PAEDIATRIC ANAESTHESIOLOGY IN INDIA

Overview

In the year 1944, the anaesthesiologists attending a surgical conference at Mumbai (Bombay) thought of forming a common platform for exchange of scientific views, which was consolidated in 1946 following "Ether Day" celebrations in October of that year. With the continued efforts of leading anaesthesiologists of India, the Indian Society of Anaesthesiologists was born on 30th December 1947 with its logo (www.isa.web.in).

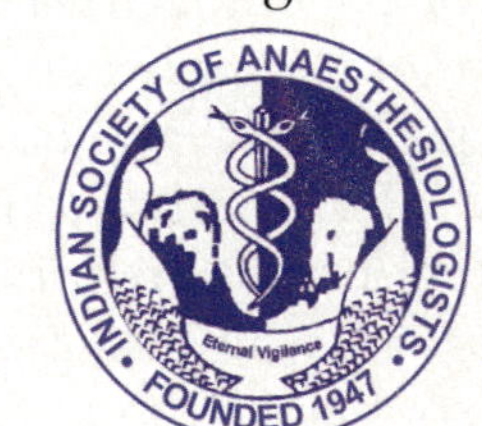

In India, paediatric anaesthesiology has evolved slowly over the past 20 years, as both a viable clinical and academic subspecialty of anaesthesiology in medical colleges, where paediatric surgery is done on a large scale and dedicated basis.

PERIOD BEFORE 2005

Anaesthesiologists, who would administer anaesthesia to adult patients, would generally take roles of paediatric anaesthesiologists in various medical colleges. Paediatric anaesthesia has advanced enormously from the days when anaesthesiologists and surgeons adapted adult techniques and equipment to small children.

In the city of Mumbai paediatric anaesthesia was practiced mainly at teaching institutes like BJ Wadia Children's Hospital and Research Centre, GS Medical College and TN Medical College, where paediatric surgery departments were set. Hence it was found necessary to create a platform to share, discuss and do constructive work in paediatric anaesthesia.

PERIOD AFTER 2005

The Indian Association of Paediatric Anaesthesiologists (IAPA) (http://www.iapa-india.org) was formed in March 2006 by a small group of Mumbai based paediatric anaesthesiologists. Constitution of IAPA was formed, approved and was officially registered in March 2006. Its main aim was to promote safety and higher standard of care in the specialty through education and research. It also advises other professional bodies on anaesthesia for children. It has completed six successful national conferences on paediatric anaesthesia. It is one of the most popular fields to pursue for further training after the basic anaesthesia residency, and its practitioners are desired by surgeons, paediatricians, and parents alike. Hence Paediatric Anaesthesia is fast getting recognition as a superspeciality branch in India. Several institutes have started fellowship programmes of Paediatric Anaesthesia. The paediatric anaesthesiologist must be facile in providing empathetic, efficient care for a wide gamut of special paediatric procedures. There are a tremendous number of technical skills and a body of knowledge to be mastered about the totality of paediatric anaesthesia. Challenges are ongoing as more complex surgical and diagnostic techniques are performed on younger and younger patients.

This maturation of the superspecialty includes better understanding of clinical care in line with advances in paediatrics and paediatric surgery along with increased sophistication in anaesthesia automation and clinical research. DM course in the branch of paediatric anaesthesia has been for the first time granted and recognized in India by Maharashtra University of Health Sciences (MUHS), Nashik and Medical Council of India (MCI) at Seth, GS Medical College and KEM Hospital, Mumbai in the year 2014.

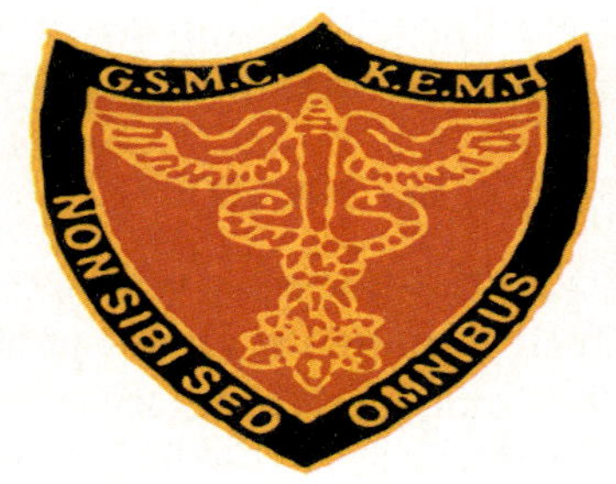

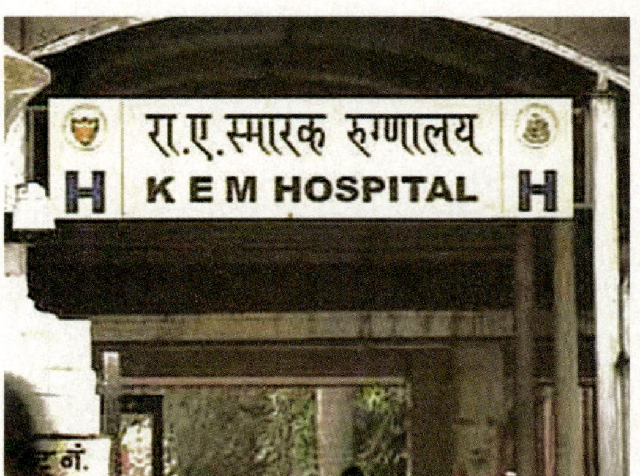

HISTORY OF PAEDIATRIC ANAESTHESIOLOGY IN ASIA

The main aim of Asian Society of Paediatric Anaesthesiologists (ASPA) is to create a platform for interaction between anaesthesiologists from different Asian countries with different health care needs and capabilities. Its official website: http://www.aspa-2000.com.

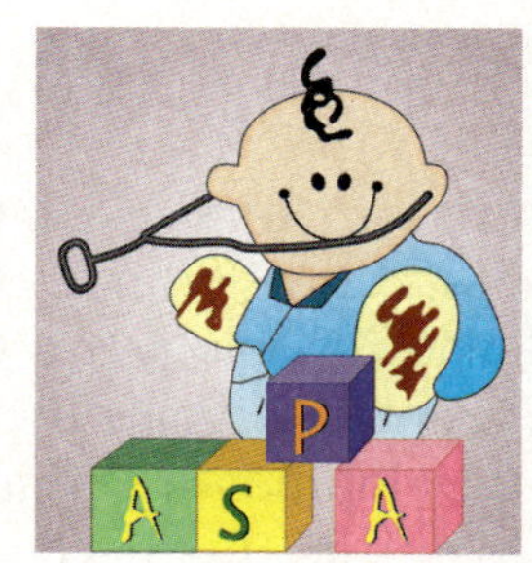

ASPA was launched in 1999 at the KK Women's and Children's Hospital in Singapore with the goal to foster the growth of safe and quality paediatric anaesthetic care and assist with professional development of its members through high quality academic meetings.

ASPA meetings have now been held in Singapore, Cebu—Philippines, New Delhi—India, Vellore—India, Pattaya—Thailand and Ho Chi Min City—Vietnam. Apart from providing state of the art knowledge on current developments in paediatric anaesthesia the ASPA meetings are also a forum to share experience in providing anaesthesia to children under diverse circumstances that are unique to Asia.

PRIMITIVE PERIOD OF PAEDIATRIC ANAESTHESIA ACROSS THE WORLD

Before the era of ether, circumcisions, amputations, excisions of tumors, cleft lip/harelip repair and correction of gross deformities performed on infants and children without any relief of pain for hundreds of years. Child crying and struggling with pain was controlled manual force. Pain was accepted and unavoidable part of surgery on children. In Japan, general anaesthesia with the herb mixture *tsu san sen* was used in 1837 by Gancho Homma for children over 5 years of age for harelip repair but withheld it from use in younger patients because of its toxicity (Iwai and Satoyoshi, 1992).

PHASE I: INTRODUCTION OF ETHER AS ANAESTHETIC AGENT IN THE USA AND PROGRESS OF PAEDIATRIC ANAESTHESIA UP TO 1940

Early successful experiments with ether

1. **Dr Crawford Williamson Long** (November 3, 1815–1878) on March 30, 1842, when he extirpated a small glandular tumour out of the two from the neck of James M Venable, a boy in Jefferson, Georgia. Next on July 3, 1842, in the amputation of the toe of a negro boy belonging to Mrs Hemphill, of Jackson, Ga. Later on Sept. 9, 1843, did extirpation of a tumour from the head of Mary Vincent, of Jackson, Ga. Followed by on January 8, 1845, in the amputation of a finger of a Negro boy belonging to Ralph Bailey, of Jackson, Ga (Long, 1849).[1]

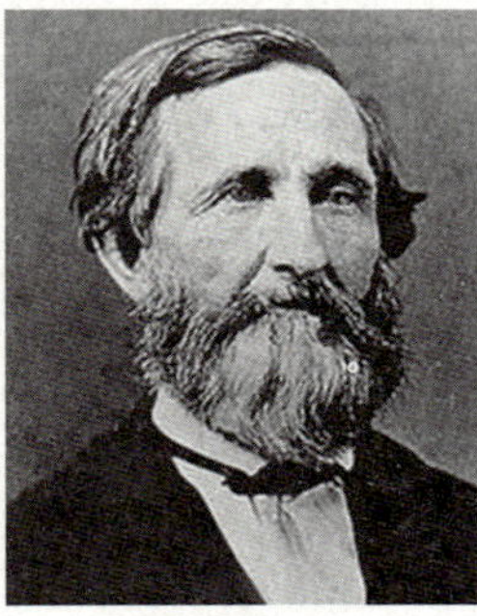

Dr Crawford W Long

2. **William Thomas Green Morton** (August 9, 1819–July 15, 1868), Morton was an USA dentist who first publicly demonstrated the use of inhaled ether as a surgical anaesthetic in Massachusetts General Hospital in Boston in 1846.[2,3]

   Children and women were considered to be **more sensitive to pain** hence anaesthesia was considered appropriate.[4,5] Morton was reluctant to administer ether anaesthesia to children because of the high incidence of nausea and vomiting.[6]

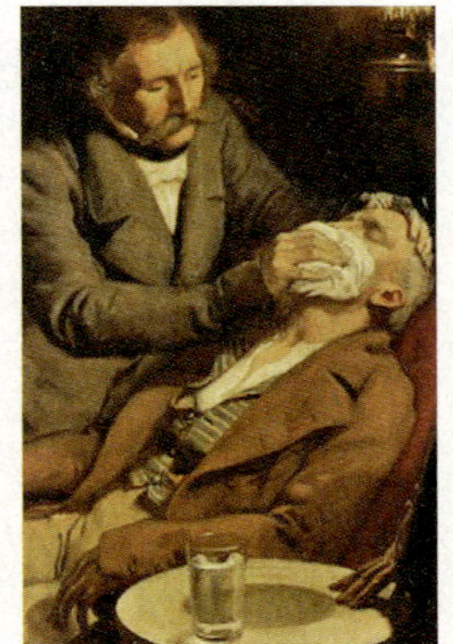

William Thomas G Morton

Initial short general anaesthesia with ether

The introduction of ether was the first giant step in the history of anaesthesia. Ether drenched small cloth was applied to the child patient's face until the child was quiet and limp. The surgeon could get 3 or 4 minutes to operate on such patient as the child regained consciousness after that.

Initial use of ether as continuous method of anaesthesia

The use of continuous administration of ether was slowly learnt over a period of time and soon use of ether for anaesthesia became a trivial routine that it was relegated to any inexperienced (non-medical) person by surgeon, while performing surgery.

Nurse anaesthetists

The administration of anaesthesia with ether was such a trivial medical activity; hence qualified physicians never took any special interest in the field of anaesthesia. For patients safety reasons nurses eventually began to assume increasing responsibilities for providing anaesthesia care. In the USA, as late as 1940, a physician, in the lead article published in the first edition of the new journal Anaesthesiology, commented, "During my internship I was trained by a nurse. I was given a cone, a can of ether and a few empirical tricks".[7]

Stagnancy in field of anaesthesia in the USA

Because of anaesthesia was considered a trivial procedure adjunct to surgery, hence the medical field of anaesthesia could not develop in the USA for several decades harming development of anaesthesia in the USA, leave aside development of paediatric anaesthesia.

Surgeons did not differentiate between adult and child in the USA

For many years in the USA, the child was treated as "a little man," surgeons operated with large instruments, and all equipment which was adult sized. Ether remained the principal agent. Use of chloroform was criticized in children.[8] Use of chloroform was advocated in the USA in 1957.[9] Progress was by trial and error. Before 1900, most of the medical literature in the USA related to anaesthesia for children was authored by surgeons.

Increase in initial interest in child anaesthesia

Interest grew in child anaesthesia slowly. Children were given anaesthesia for longer period and for more difficult procedures. Tonsillectomy operation grew to thousands in number between 1887 and 1900. Although often considered dangerous appendectomy surgery slowly became an accepted surgical procedure. The most common type of paediatric surgery done under ether anaesthesia was orthopedic surgery from year 1900 onwards.

Beginning of recognition of preoperative anxiety

One of the first signs of concern for the child's anxiety when undergoing anaesthesia was voiced by James Gwathmey (1907).[10] When he recommended that one should "add a few drops of the mother's cologne to the ether mask and induce the child in the mother's arms." Another step toward easing induction came in 1928 with the entry of tribromoethanol, the German Avertin, which was used widely as a rectal agent. It provided almost certain sleep in 7 to 8 minutes and was of special value prior to ether induction because, unlike the barbiturates used later, it had a bronchodilating effect and facilitated rather than retarded induction.

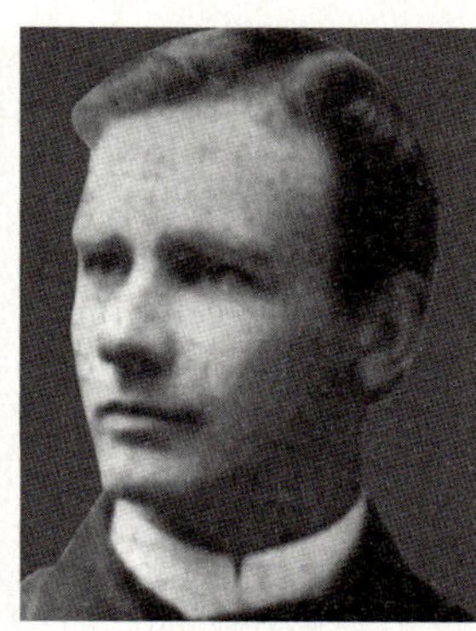

James Gwathmey

Development of paediatric surgery and anaesthesia

William Ladd, whose interest stemmed from his experience in caring for children injured in a massive explosion in Halifax, Nova Scotia in 1917, led the development of paediatric surgery in the USA.[11,12] Between 1925 and 1940, activity in both paediatric surgery and anaesthesia began to accelerate. Ladd at Children's Hospital Boston corrected harelip and other neonatal defects under ether anaesthesia. Both Leven and Ladd performed secondary multi-procedure repair of trecho-oesophageal fistula in 1939.

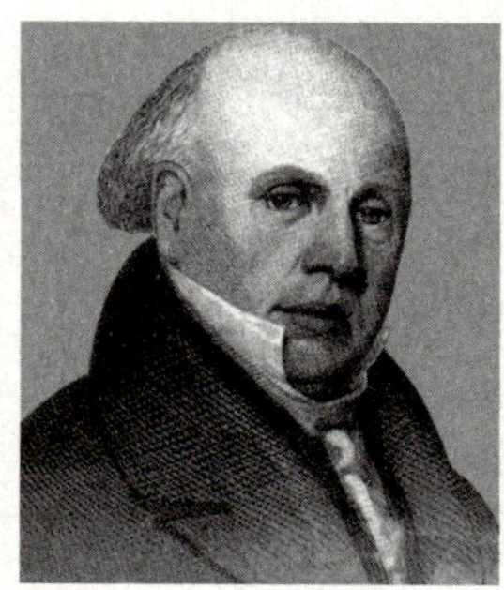

William Ladd

Cyclopropane in 1930 for cardiovascular surgery

In 1930 cyclopropane by closed-system apparatus proved particularly helpful for paediatric anaesthetists Lamont and Harmel developed a miniaturization of the to-and-fro canisters. Waters described in Wisconsin and used this technique for Blalock's "blue baby" (tetralogy of Fallot) operations at Johns Hopkins Hospital. Betty Lank, nurse anaesthetist provided anaesthesia, relaxation, and controlled respiration for Ladd's infants as well as for Robert Gross for surgery of patent ductus arteriosus in 1938 without using endotracheal intubation. She used miniature to-and-fro apparatus with less dead space by using infant size masks.

Fresh initial beginnings in paediatric anaesthesia

By 1940, considerable progress had been made in the ability of minimally trained anaesthetists to provide quite satisfactory operating conditions for the surgeons of that time. By 1940, Ladd with great difficulty corrected the established dictum of "the child is not a little man" He also emphasized on supportive warming, preoperative correction of electrolyte balance, and intraoperative charting of Clinical signs of anaesthetic depth of anaesthesia described by Guedel in 1937. Ladd had used local infiltration for abdominal procedures in premature infants in the late 1930s, and Leigh wrote of spinal anaesthesia for open chest work in the 1940s, but improved inhalation anaesthesia methods phased out both. Robson of Toronto had described intubation of children using digital guidance rather than a laryngoscope[13] did not receive much attention.

Introduction of Chloroform in UK and Progress of Paediatric Anaesthesia up to 1940 of PHASE I

Initial use of chloroform for general anaesthesia

Chloroform was used in England because of smoother and more rapid action. The incidence of deaths after chloroform was very high hence specialized care was recommended. Hence in the UK only physicians were allowed to administer anaesthesia.[14] Hence throughout the UK Empire including India anaesthesiology became a medical specialty, its physicians trained in anaesthesia got equal status with other physicians, and establishing early leadership in this field of anaesthesia for several decades. This helped in early development of paediatric anaesthesia in the UK.

John Snow era of experimentation with chloroform

John Snow (1813–1858), kept notes on hundreds of anaesthetic experiences and research experiments, between the period of 1846 to1958.[15] Snow formulated the first description of signs by which one could monitor and control the depth of anaesthesia in patients of all ages.[16] Guedel's guide to Inhalation Anaesthesia (A Fundamental Guide to Inhalation Anaesthesia by Arthur E. Guedel published in 1937) was used by Snow to describe five stages of anaesthesia, based on excitement, loss of consciousness, relaxation, eye movement, and depth of respiration, served as guidelines throughout the remainder of the century. Snow experimented with ether and chloroform for giving anaesthesia in children. Snow preferred chloroform for infants and children. He warned of its danger with excessive depth in children.[17] His record of successfully anaesthetizing 147 infants for harelip repair in light of high mortality during this operation in that era and later on also, is considered a great paediatric anaesthesia feat.

Era of chloroform mixtures with ether and alcohol

Despite recognized dangers, for next 20 years, chloroform and ether remained the only anaesthetic agents after the remarkable progress made in anaesthesia in England and throughout Europe by Snow. Chloroform remained the principal agent in England and Europe and efforts were made to reduce the complications of chloroform by diluting it with ether [Chloroform + Ether (CE)] and with alcohol and ether [Alcohol + Chloroform + Ether (ACE)].

Initial use of nitrous oxide

The introductions of nitrous oxide into general use by 1870 and ethyl chloride shortly after 1900 were important advances, reducing or replacing the use of chloroform in many operations not requiring muscular relaxation. They were nonirritating made them particularly acceptable for induction. Between 1888 and 1912, the UK physician anaesthetists Buxton alone published five consecutive editions of Anaesthetics: Their Uses and Administration by Dudley Wilmot Buxton. More anaesthetists contributed more number of articles and texts to medical journals. The first text on paediatric anaesthesia was published in 1923 by C Langton Hewer in "The Lancet" about Anaesthesia for Children.

Following World War I, Magill and Rowbotham popularized tracheal intubation for adult procedures, and in 1937, Philip Ayre of Newcastle-Upon-Tyne reported endotracheal intubation with a T-tube device for harelip repair in neonates (Ayre, 1937). In England, there had been more progress in airway control during anaesthesia.

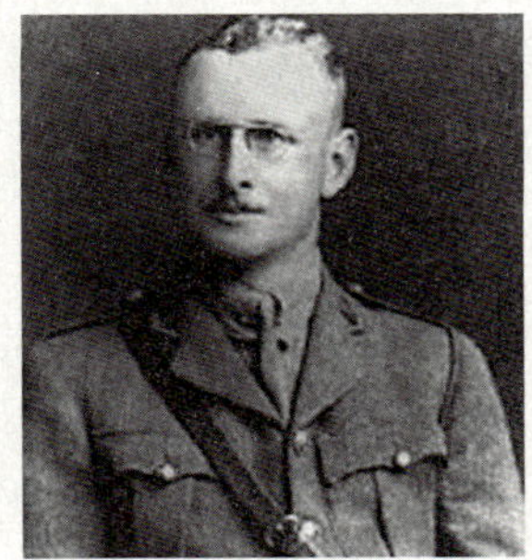

Magill

PHASE II: EMERGENCE OF PAEDIATRIC ANAESTHESIA (1940–1960)

The practice of adult anaesthesia become established. It expanded by understanding children through Textbook of Paediatrics. Clement Smith's *The Physiology of the Newborn Infant* (1945), Taussig's *Congenital Malformations of the Heart* (1947), and Nelson's *Textbook of Paediatrics* (1950) defined normal and abnormal infants. Charles Robson, in Toronto used fresh information on new agents and techniques adaptable to children and established paediatric anaesthesiology in USA. Robert Cope, at London's Hospital for sick children established paediatric anaesthesiology in England.

M Digby Leigh

First USA Canadian author M Digby Leigh authored *Paediatric Anaesthesia* (1948). He was trained by Waters in Wisconsin. He was appointed head of anaesthesia at Montreal Children's Hospital, where he taught and innovated with Kathleen Belton. They described the use of spinal anaesthesia for intrathoracic procedures. They innovated original paediatric circle absorption apparatus, and a non-re-breathing valve. Leigh moved to Vancouver, UK Columbia in 1947 and to Los Angeles in 1954, where he started the yearly paediatric anaesthesia teaching conference in the USA. He attempted to monitor exhaled carbon dioxide in 1952.

G Jackson Rees

G Jackson Rees anaesthetist at the Alder Hey Children's Hospital Liverpool, worked with mentor and teacher Cecil Grey. Together, they conceived the idea that practically all surgery could be performed under the simple and non-explosive combination of nitrous oxide and curare. Rees, adapting the Ayre T-tube system by adding an expiratory limb and breathing bag (the well-known Jackson Rees system), proceeded to carry-out this concept with astounding success. Rees' foresighted that respiration be controlled in infants with reduced tidal volumes and rates of 60 to 80 times per minute were widely criticized but proved to be rational when increased tidal volumes were found to cause surfactant washout and barotrauma.

> **Historical Pearl**
>
> Children were rarely intubated before 1940 because Jackson Rees ruled intubation in children to be avoided. In the subsequent 30 years saw a proliferation of paediatric laryngoscopes a change in airway management philosophy slowly happened.

New field of paediatric anaesthesia

The new field of paediatric anaesthesia got established by:

1. McQuiston of Children's Hospitals in Chicago
2. Smith of Children's Hospitals Boston
3. Rackow worked at Columbia Presbyterian Hospital in New York.

Foundations of Clinical Control and Support

Progress in Neonatal Surgery and Anaesthesia

1. Primary surgical repair was a challenge but achievable with progress in neonatal surgery and anaesthesia for three difficult congenital defects:
   a. Tracheoesophageal fistula (TEF),
   b. Omphalocele, and
   c. Congenital diaphragmatic hernia (CDH).[3]
2. Open-drop divinyl ether (Vinethene)—ether was preferable over local anaesthesia by the average surgeon for herniorrhaphy and pyloromyotomy

3. Before 1912, pyloric stenosis operation by gastroenterostomy resulted in 50% mortality. Pyloromyotomy replaced gastroenterostomy by Ramstedt where prevention of aspiration during anaesthesia was main aim to reduce mortality to near zero if diagnosed early.

Early attempts to control fear

Fear of needles and the horrors of anaesthetic induction was voiced by psychologists,[20] paediatricians[21] and anaesthesiologists.[22]

Premedication

Morphine, scopolamine, atropine and barbiturates

In this article recommended[23] morphine and promoted[24] the combination of morphine and scopolamine premedication. Intramuscular barbiturates plus morphine mixed with either atropine or scopolamine resulted in severe horror of needles, an uncomfortable dry mouth, and an unpredictable degree of sedation. With the repeated failure of sedative agents, greater skills were developed by caring anaesthetists to gain the confidence of children in preoperative visits and then to divert their attention at induction by telling them stories or by simply lulling them to sleep.

Hypnosis

Limited acceptance could not make hypnosis routine procedure for induction. It was used by Betcher (1958)[25] and Marmer (1959)[26] also favoured hypnosis. Hypnosis used for repair of facial lacerations in small children who were full stomach.

Methods of Induction

Thiopental replaced rectal Avertin, providing greater ease of administration via either the intravenous or the rectal route.[27] Nitrous oxide, cyclopropane, or divinyl ether eliminated use of the dreaded ether.

Control of the Airway

Tongue fall

Simple blockage by the tongue has been an ever-present danger. To prevent obstruction by the tongue, metal and rubber oral airways, often fitted with a metal nipple for insufflation of vaporized ether.

Hypoxia due to secretions

In harelip procedures and tonsillectomy, the complications of hypoxia and death were due to laryngospasm caused by oral secretions, blood, drained pus, aspiration of vomitus. To prevent this suction apparatus was first available in the form of bulb syringes used alone or fitted with rubber catheters and then later as portable motorized pumps

Endotracheal Intubation

Tracheal intubation was outstanding advance in paediatric anaesthesia between 1940 and 1960 to control the airway. It was the efforts of Rees in England and Leigh. Similar efforts were made by various people in Canada, UK, USA (Gillespie, 1939)[28]; Zindler and Deming (1953)[29] and Pender (1954)[30] helped acceptance of tracheal intubation of infants and children in the USA in the 1940s and 1950s.The ongoing development of tracheal intubation led to an increased understanding of laryngeal anatomy.[31]

1. Replacement of the "classic" hyperextension of the head by use of the "sniffing" position for intubation in children.
2. Different types of tracheal tubes made of different materials.
3. Laryngoscopes of several types and sizes.

Medical literature on complications of tracheal intubation,[32] included subglottic stenosis[33] laryngeal irritation from large tubes,[34] and tracheitis caused by contamination.[35]

"Total Control" of Respiration: The Muscle Relaxants

Griffith and Mitchell in Canada in 1942 clinically first used *d*-tubocurarine. Canadians and UK readily accepted it for both children and adults.[36–39] Use of *d*-tubocurarine in the USA had much opposition to "controlled" respiration. But by 1960, the terms "controlled" and "assisted" respiration had gained widespread use in the USA.

Paediatric Breathing Systems: Assisted and Controlled Respiration

With the stimulating effect of ether on respiration in light surgical planes, assisted respiration was not needed. Open chest surgery with cyclopropane and muscle relaxants definitely changed this picture. Special interest was taken in infant circle absorption systems to eliminate problems of carbon dioxide accumulation, several non-rebreathing valves were designed by Leigh and Belton, 1948.[40,41] Over a period of 30 years, apparatus variously called re-breathing (UK), non-re-breathing (USA), and partial re-breathing (general) involved numerous studies and modifications of the basic Ayre T-system.[42] Rees added expiratory limb by attaching breathing bag. At exhaust valves were placed. Valves proximal to face (Mapleson A). Exhaust Valves distal to face (Mapleson D).

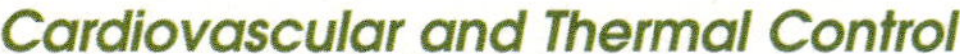

Cardiovascular and Thermal Control

Intentional reduction of arterial blood pressure

Reduced blood pressure is reasonably safe and used as initial step for "induced hypotension" to reduce surgical blood loss in major paediatric surgery and to prevent excessive loss due to blood pressure elevation during correction of coarctation of the aorta.

Controlled Reduction of Body Temperature and Cardiopulmonary Arrest

In 1938 following 'Gross' ligation patent ductus arteriosus, did correction of coarctation of the aorta, did repair of vascular rings, and shunt procedures for tetralogy of Fallot under closed or semi-closed inhalation anaesthesia, usually with cyclopropane.[43–45] Introduction of hypothermic control of body metabolism into paediatric anaesthesia to reduce the oxygen requirement by cooling to 3–4°C by simple ice-water mattress[46] for intracardiac aortic or pulmonary valvotomy[47] and Virtue RW: *Hypothermic anaesthesia*, Springfield, IL, Charles C Thomas, 1955. The drive to bypass both heart and lungs initiated by Gibbon in 1937 became exciting in the early years of 1950s, with competing surgeons Lillihei, Kirklin, and Kay and their respective anaesthesiologists.[48–50] All of them contributing toward the first practical use of the pump oxygenator in 1955, 2 years before publication of the articles cited. Mild and moderate hypothermia techniques were also used in this period for neurosurgery, orthopedic surgery, and harelip repair.[51]

Control during Maintenance of Anaesthesia

Surgeons preferred accuracy rather than speed. The methods of maintenance and support of anaesthesia became more demanding. A precordial or esophageal stethoscope[52] served, first, to keep the anaesthetist in direct contact of strength of breath sounds and the rate, rhythm, and strength of heart sounds. Strength of heart sounds was an important guide to the degree of blood loss at that time. Arterial blood pressure obtained by BP apparatus specially constructed Smith cuff or latex cuff for infants. The electrocardiographs machine was occasionally brought into operating rooms. Body temperature measured intermittently at oral, nasal, or rectal sites. The anaesthesia chart gained importance when legal suits became more frequent.

Control of Blood Loss

Methods of estimating blood loss consisted of assessing blanching of conjunctivae, evaluating the strength of heart sounds, measuring arterial blood pressure, and weighing blood soaked sponges. While speed was still considered essential in paediatric surgery during the excision of Wilms' tumour surgery, it may cause massive hemorrhage and may exsanguinate small infants. Attempts were made to restore the loss with cold, acidified blood brought failing hearts to irreversible arrest. The cautery soon reduced blood loss drastically but inflammable inhalational anaesthetics prevented their use.

Poor Progress in Local Anaesthesia

Local anaesthesia worked well in brachial plexus block[53,54] a little attention was paid to local anaesthesia in the USA. In many other countries, however, where inhalation anaesthesia was less advanced stages, there was routine use of regional and spinal anaesthesia for both infants and children.

Halothane paves way for cautery to control blood loss and electrical gadgets for monitoring in OT

Nitrous oxide anaesthesia with relaxants allowed use of electrical instruments in the operating room. Halothane slowly replaced popular explosive gases used as anaesthetics. Johnstone in 1956 in England first used in Halothane in 10% concentration (nonflammable, nonirritating, and potent anaesthetic agent),which was described by Junkin et al (1957).[55]

Immediately thereafter used in Canada and Stephen, Lawrence, Fabian (1958) in the USA. Flammable anaesthetic agents were replaced by Halothane in the USA allowing cautery to control loss of blood loss. Halothane paved way for development of electronic devices for monitoring and physiologic control of patient during anaesthesia.

Supportive Care

Oxygen Therapy

All pros and cons evaluated for oxygen therapy concentration, pressure and duration.

Fluid Therapy

The time-honored rule developed by Holliday et al (1957)[56] was used for paediatric fluid administration based on metabolic requirements is used even today.

Antibiotic Therapy

Antibiotic agents reduced the morbidity and mortality of small infants by control of infection perioperatively.

Baby Incubators for Temperature Control

Development of enclosed incubators with regulated oxygen, warmth, and humidification for infants with respiratory distress syndrome along with improved oxygen tents were developed for older children including those with cystic fibrosis to help survival.

Teamwork

Paediatric anaesthesiologists and paediatricians along with paediatric surgeon shared responsibility for perioperative care.

Paediatric Intensive Care Unit

The first paediatric intensive care unit was established in Goteburg, Sweden, in 1955. Similar paediatric intensive units were established in Stockholm (Hans Feychtung), Liverpool (Rees), and Melbourne (MacDonald and Stocks) between 1960 and 1964. In USA, the first paediatric intensive care unit was established by John J. Downes at the Children's Hospital of Philadelphia in 1967, followed by Children's Hospital of Pittsburgh (Kampschulte), Yale—New Haven Hospital (Gilman), Massachusetts General Hospital (Todres and Shannon), and the Hospital for Sick Children in Toronto (Conn) in next 4 years.[57]

PHASE III: ERA OF NONFLAMMABLE ANAESTHETICS (1960–1980)

With elimination of flammable agents eliminated, the way was cleared for rapid and extensive advances in each and every areas of paediatric anaesthesia ketamine (Ketalar) by Domino et al (1965)[58] They found a place in paediatric use for uncontrollable patients and to accomplish minor but painful procedures. A major change in the methods for controlling fear in children and their parents was in giving permission to parents, admission next to the child's bedside at all times, including "sleep-in" privileges, and later, to pre-induction and induction areas. While many parents felt the unpleasant feeling of ordeal by these human moves were comforting but statistics failed to show that it helped the children undergoing surgical procedure.[59]

Increasing Clinical Precision

Airway Systems

Major evolution of airway systems for paediatric anaesthesia was done by Bain et al (1972).[60] In this article, they modified the partial re-breathing systems. They made exhalation tube pass inside the inhalation arm. This provided for scavenging expired gases.

Monitoring

"Control by the numbers" gained predominance over the unreliable art of anaesthesia. Greater precision in monitoring were taken in the measurement of infant blood pressure by Doppler sonography and by oscillotonometry (Dinamap).[61] The transcutaneous electrode (ear oximetry) for determination of arterial oxygen saturation with limited success.[62]

Serial ABG and Electrolytes

Led by Downes of Philadelphia, arterial blood gas determinations, blood sugar, haemoglobin, electrolytes, and other measurements were serially evaluated intraoperatively in adjacent laboratories.

Catheters

Insertion of arterial and central venous catheters became commonplace, and urinary catheterization became an important guide to fluid and electrolyte replacement. Progress in controlling fluid balance included the recognition of the importance of electrolytes in all intravenous solutions.[63,64]

Blood Replacement

New concepts concerning blood replacement included Davenport's practical recommendation to give blood when loss reached 10% of blood volume,[65] followed later by Furman's more precise suggestion to maintain the haematocrit level above 28 to 30% in children and 40% in the newborn.[66]

Prevention of Food Aspiration

The Sellick maneuver[67] and Salem's many warnings about "the full stomach"[68] were forever fixed in the mind of each new resident doctor. Great emphasis was placed on the prevention of food aspiration and the damaging effects of hypoxia.

Postoperative Patient Management: Ventilation, Resuscitation and Intensive Care

Apart from preoperative and operative anaesthesia techniques a third dimension was added with advent of extensive operation where survival of patients depended on their supportive control during recovery room period. Recovery rooms or post-anaesthesia care units (PACUs) for routine postoperative care had been established in many hospitals over previous decades.

"Cardiac arrest"

When it became evident that the patients occasionally did not survive both the original insult and the therapeutic assault, the term "cardiac arrest" was coined.[69] Because the exact cause of these mishaps frequently was uncertain, each was considered "an act of God" and successful resuscitation was considered a feather in the cap of any anaesthesiologist who had been associated with one. Intelligent procedures of ventilation and closed-chest cardiac compression, combined with electric and pharmacologic stimulation, brought far greater reason, order, and success.

Twin tenets of anaesthesia

Among many well-known tenets established, two more tenets were added. ***First*** was the danger of succinylcholine in patients with elevated serum potassium levels[70] and ***second*** was poor tolerance to anaesthesia in patients with haemoglobin levels as lower than as 6 g/dL.

Organized Teaching

Accreditation for residency training in paediatric centres was established in Boston in 1970, followed by several other hospitals by 1980. This period marked the definite establishment of teaching facilities for the specialized training of paediatric anaesthesiologists. With markedly enlarged departmental staffs, didactic and clinical instruction became available in numerous institutions. Residents became capable of managing most types of cases and also received instruction in ancillary services. Annual symposia on paediatric anaesthesia initiated by Leigh in 1962 were followed by those organized by Conn in Toronto, Downes in Philadelphia, Salem in Chicago, Ryan in Boston. New texts were written by Davenport (1967) of Canada,[71] Brown et al (1979) in Australia.[72]

International Progress

In France

M. Delegue pioneered the modern paediatric anaesthesia stage, her text *Memento a l 'Uusage de l' Anaesthesiologiste-Reanimateur Paediatrique* celebrated many editions. A marked difference in their approach appeared with their use of combinations of intravenous phenothiazines, antihistamines, and barbiturates in place of inhalation agents, with remarkable success in regional anaesthesia and pharmacology has also been outstanding (Saint Maurice et al. 1986; Murat et al. 1988).

In Europe

Other early leaders in paediatric anaesthesia in Europe include Suuterinen of Finland, Swensson, Feyting, and Ekstrom-Jodal of Sweden, and Rondio and Wezyk of Poland.

In Australia

Douglas Wilson has been called the real pioneer of paediatric anaesthesia in Western Australia, and Margaret McLellan, John Stocks, Ian McDonald, MA Denborough.

In Japan

Japanese interest in paediatric anaesthesia began later but proceeded vigorously beginning in 1958,[73] the publication of *Paediatric Anaesthesia* in 1958 by Onchi and Fujita served as a valuable guide.

In Latin America

Throughout Latin America, Brazilian physicians[74] and others followed USA type of anaesthesia methods to some extent, but in these countries, and especially in Mexico, local and regional anaesthetic techniques were depended on and consequently more highly developed than inhalation anaesthesia.[75]

PHASE IV: PROGRESS AND SOPHISTICATION (1980 TO PRESENT)

Paediatric anaesthesiologists setting computerized monitors and infusion pumps, with syringes loaded and coded with a large cabinet within arm's reach, holding drugs and other equipment for all possible situations. Anaesthesia was induced with minimal resistance from patient. Surgeons waited for fixation of monitors, endotracheal tubes, and catheters. Multiple medications are delivered by the intravenous route, drugs were frequently measured in micrograms per kilogram. The ventilator was set at a prescribed rate and tidal volume. Then surgeons are allowed to drape the patient. Anaesthesiologist uses automated Charting to keep watch on monitors. Now premature infant can receive spinal anaesthesia for herniorrhaphy. Long numbers of hours are required for liver transplantation withstood anaesthesia.

Recognition of Risk

Paediatric anaesthesiologists appreciate that infants and very small children have at increased risk of complications from both anaesthesia and surgery. Previous reports (Salem, 1975) had shown that these were frequently related to cardiovascular factors (including hypovolemia, anaemia), respiratory difficulties (airway obstruction, hypoxia, inadequate ventilation), or electrolyte imbalance (hyperkalemia, hyponatremia, hypoglycemia). In particular, postoperative apnoea, especially in very premature infants, was noted by several doctors[76–78] and overnight hospitalization in these situations was widely recommended. Risk in small children could be decreased if doctors specially trained and experienced in paediatric anaesthesia provided the anaesthesia care.[79–82]

Changing Patterns of Care

Several areas of surgery have shown that corrective procedures performed in infancy, rather than palliative procedures done initially followed by full repair later in life, lead to improved long-term results. The vast majority of paediatric surgical procedures currently are done in ambulatory patients who never remain overnight in the hospital. Paediatric anaesthesiologists have become increasingly involved in caring for children outside the operating rooms for analgesia required for nonsurgical procedures. This has largely occurred in the radiology departments, where increasingly sophisticated equipment and techniques have led to major advances in diagnosis (computed tomography, magnetic resonance imaging, positron emission tomography, etc.) and new, less-invasive treatment options (cardiac catheterization laboratory, radiation therapy). Anaesthesiologists are being requested to provide care for patients in several other areas like gastrointestinal endoscopy, oncology unit for lumbar punctures and bone marrow aspirations. While children clearly benefit from relief of pain and anxiety in these situations, this has greatly increased demands for anaesthesia services.

NEW DEVELOPMENTS IN ANAESTHESIA

The age-old, frequently used restriction of preoperative intake ultimately underwent scrutiny several times which resulted in concept and reduction of fasting time.[83,84] New, potent, inhalational anaesthetic agents have been developed, virtually replacing halothane as the "standard" for the previous generation. To induce anaesthesia via mask, sevoflurane is used almost exclusively because it acts faster and results in less bradycardia and hypotension.[85,86] This has been especially important in infants. Isoflurane is frequently used for maintenance of anaesthesia, in part because it is currently less expensive; desflurane may be used when particularly rapid awaking is desired. None of these newer agents, however, have the smooth induction properties of sevoflurane. Concerns have been raised about breakdown products that may develop when sevoflurane interacts with some carbon dioxide absorbents, especially when dessicated, leading to overheating of the absorbent system, carbon monoxide production, or both.[87] The clinical significance of this remains to be determined. A new, major feature in airway management has been the promotion of the laryngeal mask airway to eliminate tracheal intubation for many simple procedures, as well as provide airway access in emergency situations when intubation is difficult.[88] Mason and Bingham (1990),[89] Pennant and White (1993)[90] endoscopes have also been developed that permit fiberoptic intubation even in small children. Several "descendents" of fentanyl have been developed, with remifentanil capable of providing very potent and transient analgesia when administered via constant intravenous infusion.[91–93] Fentanyl trans-cutaneous "patches" have also been developed, largely to provide analgesia for chronic pain, and fentanyl is sometimes administered trans-nasally or trans-orally.[94,95] Potent opioids have been particularly useful for cardiac procedures when inhaled anaesthetic agents are not well tolerated[96,97] produced evidence of physiologic stress in infants under light anaesthesia. This brought general agreement that all infants should receive anaesthesia during surgery. Propofol has become the most common intravenous induction agent for adults but has not completely replaced thiopental in children because propofol causes some discomfort when injected into small peripheral veins. Midazolam has replaced diazepam as the intravenous benzodiazepine of choice for sedation in children; midazolam is also the most popular oral sedative in the preoperative setting[98] Midazolam can also be administered via several other routes (including intranasal). The use of lidocaine-prilocaine creams[99] for skin desensitization eases the discomfort of venipuncture for intravenous induction but requires advance application to become effective. Intramuscular injections are rarely necessary now in paediatric anaesthesia practice. Several new, non-depolarizing muscle relaxants have replaced curare. Although pancuronium is commonly used for lengthy procedures, several shorter-acting agents (especially cisatracurium and vecuronium) are frequently administered for brief procedures and have fewer side effects. Rocuronium is often used to facilitate emergency endotracheal intubation, and succinylcholine is no longer administered without good cause, because masseter spasm, malignant hyperthermia, or both occasionally develop after its administration, especially in the presence of potent inhaled Halothane.[100] In addition, the Food and Drug Administration (1997)[101] issued a "black box" warning due to serious complications (including cardiac arrest resulting from acute hyperkalemia) associated with its use, particularly in young males with unrecognized muscular dystrophy. Regional anaesthesia has become more commonplace in children, beginning in Europe, with "single-shot" techniques (spinal, caudal, peripheral nerve block) reducing the requirements for general anaesthesia and providing postoperative analgesia.[102,103] Continuous infusions of local anaesthetics with or without fentanyl are often delivered intra-operatively and postoperatively via catheters placed during surgery, especially via the epidural route. This is a reflection of the much greater emphasis being devoted to the need of the reducing pain in the postoperative period. Pain control following surgery has been a major focus of paediatric anaesthesiologists with patient-, parent-, or nurse-controlled analgesia available via computer-controlled infusion pumps for delivery of medications by the intravenous or epidural route. Pain treatment services have become more important aspects of the mission of most departments of paediatric anaesthesia; they provide care for children with medical, as well as surgical, pain.[104,105] Preoperative clinics are used to evaluate many patients in advance of their procedures, and significant attention has been devoted to methods of easing induction of anaesthesia, especially the use of oral premedicants and parental presence during mask induction.[106] In all instances, kindness remains the essential feature in preoperative management.

Progress in Monitoring

Electronic, engineering and technical advances have also greatly enhanced patient monitoring. Smaller equipment are now readily available so that very young patients can be monitored carefully and critically. Percutaneous catheters can be inserted directly into any peripheral vein or artery; the Seldinger technique (if necessary with ultrasound guidance) can be used to insert central catheters. Echocardiography can be performed transthoracically or transesophageally in small children. Its use has greatly facilitated the ability of cardiac surgeons to assess the repair of congenital heart lesions intraoperatively.[107] "Standard" monitoring is now quite extensive and sophisticated as promulgated by the American Society of Anaesthesiologists in 1986 and includes continuous pulse oximetry and capnography.

Advances in Surgery

Laparoscopic techniques, robotics, and intraoperative imaging have progressed so extensively and so rapidly into paediatric practice that anaesthesiologists have had to accommodate the special problems and challenges presented by these situations. In field of foetal surgery, where surgeons, obstetricians, anaesthesiologists, and neonatologists must collaborate to care for mother and foetus simultaneously during surgical repair of prenatal anomalies are developed and assessed.[108–111]

Research Efforts

Physiologic studies of cerebral circulation in the neonate by Rogers et al. (1980),[112] gas exchange in cardiac patients,[113,114] pharmacologic biotransformation of sedatives[115] the infant and the myoneural junction[116] and hypoxia in children following anaesthesia.[117] The report by Lerman et al (1986)[118] which was concerning post-anaesthetic vomiting after strabismus surgery is another illustration of one of the problems of the conscious child that remains particularly difficult to control during anaesthesia.

SUMMARY

Paediatric anaesthesia has advanced enormously. Times of anaesthesiologists adapting adult anaesthesia techniques are things of past. There are dedicated anaesthesia equipment to small children. It is clear that paediatric anaesthesiology is a well-established and well-recognized super specialty at postgraduate level. Anaesthetists accept challenges of undertaking more complex surgical techniques being performed on younger and younger patients for longer and longer duration.

Landmark Years in History of Anaesthesia

1846 The discovery of ether as a general anaesthetic.
1885 The discovery of injectable cocaine and local anaesthesia.
1896 The discovery of the hypodermic needle, the syringe, and the injection of morphine.
1905 Discovery of the measurement of blood pressure by blood pressure cuff.
1913 Discovery of the cuffed endotracheal breathing tube.
1934 The discover of thiopental and injectable barbiturates.
1940 The discovery of curare and injectable muscle relaxants.
1950s The development of the post-anaesthesia care unit (PACU) and the intensive care unit (ICU)
1956 The discovery of halothane, the first modern inhaled anaesthetic.
1983 The discovery of pulse oximetry monitoring.

REFERENCES

1. Long CW. An account of the first use of sulphuric ether by inhalation as an anaesthetic in surgical operations. S Med Surg J 1849; 5:45). (http://archive. org/stream 39002011123289.med.yale.edu 39002011123289.med. yale.edu_djvu.txt).
2. Fenster JM. Ether Day: The Strange Tale of USA 's Greatest Medical Discovery and the Haunted Men Who Made It. New York, NY: Harper Collins (2001) ISBN 978-0-06-019523-6.
3. Morton WTG. Remarks on the proper mode of administering the sulphuric ether by inhalation, Boston, Dutton and Wentworth, Printers. 1847.
4. Warren, Warren JM. Inhalation of ether. Boston Med Surg J. 1847;36:160. (Pernick, 1975).
5. Pernick MS. A calculus of suffering, New York, Columbia University Press. 1975.
6. Bigelow HJ. Insensibility during surgical operations produced by inhalation. Boston Med Surg J. 1846;35:16.
7. Haggard HW. The place of the anesthetist in USA in medicine. Anesthesiology. 1940;1:1.
8. Kopetsky SJ. The selection of anaesthesia in children. Med Rec. 1903;14:534.
9. Schwartz H. Chloroform anaesthesia for ophthalmic examination. Am J Ophthalmol. 1957;43:27.
10. Gwathmey JT. Anesthesiology in infants and children. Pediatrics. 1907;19:734.
11. Goldbloom RB. Halifax and the precipitate birth of pediatric surgery. Pediatrics. 1917;11:164.
12. Gregory GA, Steward DJ. Life-threatening peri-operative apnea in the ex-premie. Anesthesiology. 1983;59:495.
13. Robson CH. Anaesthesia in children. Am J Surg. 1936; 34:468.
14. Eckenhoff JE. Anaesthesia from Colonial times, Philadelphia: JB Lippincott. 1966;27.
15. Griffith HR. John Snow, pioneer specialist in anaesthesia. Anesth Analg. 1934;13:45.
16. Snow J. On the inhalation of the vapour of ether, London, John Churchill. 1847.
17. Snow J. On chloroform and other anesthetics, London, John Churchill. 1858.
18. Conn AW, Montes JE, Barker GA, et al. Cerebral salvage in near-drowning following neurological classification by triage. Can Anaesth Soc J. 1980; 27:201.
19. Conn AW. Origins of paediatric anaesthesia in Canada. Paediatr Anaesth. 1992;2:179.
20. Levy DM. Psychic trauma of operation in children. Am J Dis Child. 1945;69:75.
21. Jackson K. Psychological preparation as a method of reducing the emotional trauma of anaesthesia in children. Anesthesiology. 1951;12:293.
22. Eckenhoff JE. Relationship of anaesthesia to postoperative personality changes in children. Am J Dis Child. 1953; 86:587.
23. Armand-Delille PF. Morphine injection before induction of general anaesthesia in children. Bull Acad Natl Med. 1932;107:890.
24. Waters RM. Pain relief for children. Am J Surg. 1938;39:470.
25. Betcher AM. Hypno-induction techniques in pediatric anaesthesia. Anesthesiology. 1958;19:279.
26. Marmer MJ. Hypnosis as an adjunct to anaesthesia in children. Am J Dis Child. 1959;97:314.
27. Weinstein ML. Rectal pentothal sodium: A new pre- and basal anesthetic drug in the practice of surgery. Anesth Analg. 1939;18:221.
28. Gillespie NA. Endotracheal anaesthesia in infants. Br J Anaesth. 1939;17:2.
29. Zindler M, Deming MV. The anesthetic management of infants for repair of congenital atresia of the esophagus with tracheo-esophageal fistula. Anesth Analg. 1953;32:180.
30. Pender JW. Endotracheal anaesthesia in children. Anesthesiology. 1954;15:495.
31. Eckenhoff JE. Some anatomic considerations of the infant larynx influencing endotracheal intubation. Anesthesiology. 1951;12:401.
32. Flagg PJ. Endotracheal inhalation anaesthesia: Special reference to postoperative reaction and suggestions for their elimination. Laryngoscope. 1951;61:1.
33. Colgan FC, Keats AS. Subglottic stenosis, a cause of difficult intubation. Anesthesiology. 1957;18:265.
34. Baron SH, Kohlmoos HW. Laryngeal sequelae of endotracheal anaesthesia. Ann Otol Rhinol Laryngol. 1951;60:67.
35. Smith RM. The prevention of tracheitis in children following endotracheal anaesthesia. Anesth Analg. 1953;32:102.
36. Anderson SM. Use of depressant and relaxant drugs in infants and children. Lancet. 1951;2:965.
37. Stead AL. The response of the newborn infant to muscle relaxants. Br J Anaesth 1955;27:124.
38. Leigh MD, Jenkins LC, Belton MK, et al. Continuous alveolar carbon dioxide analysis as a monitor of pulmonary blood flow. Anesthesiology. 1957;18(6):878–82.
39. Rees GJ. The child as a subject for anaesthesia. In: Evans FT, Gray TC, (Eds). Modern trends in anaesthesia, New York: Harper & Row Publishers. 1958.
40. Leigh MD, Belton MK. Pediatric anaesthesia, New York, The Macmillan Co. 1948.
41. Stephen CR, Slater HM. A non-rebreathing, non-resisting valve. Anesthesiology. 1948;9:550.
42. Ayre P. Endotracheal anaesthesia for babies with special reference to harelip and cleft lip operations. Anesth Analg. 1937;16:330.
43. Harmel HH, Lamont A. Anaesthesia in the surgical treatment of congenital pulmonary stenosis. Anesthesiology. 1948;7:477.
44. Harris AJ. Management of anaesthesia for congenital heart operation in children. Anesthesiology. 1950;11:328.

45. Smith RM. Circulatory factors affecting anaesthesia in surgery for congenital heart disease. Anesthesiology. 1952;13:38.
46. McQuiston WO. Anesthetic problems in cardiac surgery in children. Anesthesiology. 1949;10:590.
47. Lewis FJ, Taufic M. Closure of atrial septal defect with the aid of hypothermia: Experimental accomplishments and report of one successful case. Surgery. 1953;33:52.
48. Matthews JH, Buckley JJ, Van Bergen FH. Acute effect of low-flow extracorporeal circulation on cerebral circulation. Anesthesiology. 1957;18:169.
49. Patrick RT, Theye RA, Moffitt EA. Studies in extracorporeal circulation: V. Anaesthesia and supportive care during intracardiac surgery with the Gibbon-type pump-oxygenator. Anesthesiology. 1957;18:673.
50. Mendelsohn Jr D, Mackrell TN, Machlan MA, et al. Experiences using the pump-oxygenator for open heart surgery in man. Anesthesiology. 1957;18:223.
51. Kilduff CJ, Wyant GM, Dale RH. Anaesthesia for repair of cleft lip and palate in infants using moderate hypothermia. Can Anaesth Soc J. 1956;3:102.
52. Smith RM. Progress in paediatric anaesthesia in the United States. Paediatr Anaesth. 1991;1:63.
53. Small GA. Brachial plexus block anaesthesia in children. JAMA. 1951;147:1648.
54. Eather KE. Axillary brachial plexus block. Anesthesiology. 1958;19:683.
55. Junkin CL, Smith C, Conn AW. Fluothane for pediatric anaesthesia. Can Anaesth Soc J. 1957;4:259.
56. Holliday MA, Segar WE. The maintenance need for water in parenteral fluid therapy. Pediatrics. 1957; 19:823.
57. Downes JJ. The historical evolution, current status, and prospective development of pediatric critical care. Crit Care Clin. 1992;8:1.
58. Domino EF, Chodoff P, Corssen G. Pharmacologic effects of CI-581, a new dissociative anesthetic in man. Clin Pharm Ther. 1965;6:279.
59. Schulman JL, Foley JM, Vemon DTA, et al. A study of the effect of the mother's presence during anaesthesia induction. Pediatrics. 1967;39:111.
60. Bain JA, Spoerel WE. A streamlined anaesthetic system. Can Anaesth Soc J. 1972;19:426.
61. Cook DR, Marcy JH. Neonatal anaesthesia, Pasadena, CA, Appleton Davies. 1988.
62. Saunders NA, Powles ACP, Rebuck AS. Ear oximetry accuracy practicability in the assessment of arterial oxygenation. Am Rev Respir Dis. 1976;113:745.
63. Bennett EJ, Dougherty MJ, Jenkins MT. Fluid requirements for neonatal anaesthesia and operation. Anesthesiology. 1970;32:343.
64. Herbert WI, Scott EB, Lewis GB. Fluid management of pediatric patients. Anesth Analg. 1971; 50:376.
65. Davenport HT, Barr MN. Blood loss during pediatric operations. Can Med Assoc 1963;789: 1309.
66. Furman EB, Roman DG, Hemmer E, et al. Specific therapy in water, electrolyte and blood volume replacement during pediatric surgery. Anesthesiology. 1975;42:187.
67 Sellick BA. Cricoid pressure to control the regurgitation of stomach contents during induction of anaesthesia. Lancet. 1961;2:204.
68. Salem MR. Anesthetic management of patients with a "full stomach." A critical review. Anesth Analg. 1970;49:47.
69. Singer JJ. Cardiac arrest in children. J Am Coll Emerg Physicians. 1977;6:198.
70. Powell DR, Miller RD. The effect of repeated doses of succinylcholine on serum potassium in patients with renal failure. Anesth Analg. 1975;54:746.
71. Davenport HT. Paediatric anaesthesia, Philadelphia, Lea and Febiger. 1967.
72. Brown TCK, Fisk GC. Anaesthesia for children, Oxford, Blackwell Publishing. 1979.
73. Iwai S, Satoyoshi M. History of paediatric anaesthesia in Japan. Paediatr Anaesth. 1992;2:275.
74. Fortuna A. Caudal analgesia: A simple and safe technique in paediatric surgery. Br J Anaesth. 1967;39:165.
75. Melman E, Pennelas J, Maruffo J. Regional anaesthesia in children. Anaesth Analg. 1975;54:387.
76. Steward DJ. Preterm infants are more prone to complications following minor surgery than are term infants. Anesthesiology. 1982;56:304.
77. Steward DJ. History of pediatric anaesthesia. In: Gregory GA (Ed). Paediatric anaesthesia, New York: Churchill Davidson. 1983.
78. Liu LMP, Coté CJ, Goudsouzian NG, et al. Life-threatening apnea in infants recovering from anaesthesia. Anesthesiology. 1983;59:506.
79. Keenan RL, Shapiro JH, Dawson K. Frequency of anesthetic cardiac arrests in infants: Effect of pediatric anesthesiologists. J Clin Anesth. 1991; 3:433.
80. Morray JP. Implications for subspecialty care of anesthetized children. Anesthesiology. 1994;80:969.
81. Berry FA. The winds of change. Paediatr Anaesth. 1995; 5:279.
82. Downes JJ. What is a paediatric anaesthesiologist? The American perspective. Paediatr Anaesth. 1995;5:277.
83. Coté CJ. NPO after midnight for children: A reappraisal. Anesthesiology. 1990;72:589.
84. Ferrari LR, Rooney FM, Rockoff MA. Preoperative fasting practices in pediatrics. Anesthesiology. 1999;90:978.
85. Sarner JB, Levine M, Davis PJ, et al. Clinical characteristics of sevoflurane in children: A comparison with halothane. Anesthesiology. 1995;82:38.
86. Holzman RS, van der Velde ME, Kaus SJ, et al. Sevoflurane depresses myocardial contractility less than halothane during induction of anaesthesia in children. Anesthesiology. 1996;85:1260.
87. Holak EJ, Mei DA, Dunning MB, et al. Carbon monoxide production from sevoflurane breakdown: Modeling of

exposures under clinical conditions. Anesth Analg. 2003;96:757.

88. Brain AIJ. The laryngeal mask: A new concept in airway management. Br J Anaesth. 1983;55:801.
89. Mason DG, Bingham RM. The laryngeal mask airway in children. Anaesthesia. 1990;45:760.
90. Pennant JH, White PF. Review article: The laryngeal mask airway. Its uses in anesthesiology. Anesthesiology. 1993;79:144.
91. Davis PJ, Galinkin J, McGowan FX, et al. A randomized multicenter study of remifentanil compared with halothane in neonates and infants undergoing pyloromyotomy. Anesth Analg. 2001;93:1380–1387.
92. Galinkin JL, Davis PJ, McGowan FX, et al. A randomized multicenter study of remifentanil compared with halothane in neonates and infants undergoing pyloromyotomy. Anesth Analg. 2001;93:1387.
93. Ross AK, Davis PJ, Dear G, et al. Pharmacokinetics of remifentanil in anesthetized pediatric patients undergoing elective surgery or diagnostic procedures. Anesth Analg. 2001;93:1393.
94. Friesen RH, et al. Oral transmucosal fentanyl citrate for preanaesthetic medication for pediatric cardiac surgery patients. Paediatr Anaesth. 1995;5:29.
95. Viscusi ER, Reynolds L, Chung F, et al. Patient-controlled transdermal fentanyl hydrochloride vs intravenous morphine pump for postoperative pain: A randomized controlled trial. JAMA. 2004;291:1333.
96. Hickey PR, Hansen DD. Fentanyl- and sufentanil-oxygen-pancuronium anaesthesia for cardiac surgery in infants. Anesth Analg. 1984;63:117.
97. Anand KJS, Hickey PR. Pain and its effects in the human neonate and fetus. N Engl J Med. 1987;317: 1321.
98. Kain ZN, Hofstadter MB, Mayes LC, et al. Midazolam: effects on amnesia and anxiety in children. Anesthesiology. 2000;93:676.
99. Freeman JA, Doyle E, Im NG, et al. Topical anaesthesia of the skin. Paediatr Anaesth. 1993;3:129.
100. Schwartz L, Rockoff MA, Koka BV. Masseter spasm with anaesthesia: incidence and implications. Anesthesiology. 1984;61:772.
101. Food and Drug administration, 1997. Dartmouth Pediatric Sedation Project Site: available at http://an.hitchcock.org/Pedi Sedation.
102. Abajian JC, Mellish RW, Browne AF, et al. Spinal anaesthesia for the high-risk infant. Anesth Analg. 1984; 63:359.
103. Yaster M, Maxwell LG. Pediatric regional anaesthesia. Anesthesiology. 1989;70:324.
104. Zeltzer LK, Jay SM, Fisher DM. The management of pain associated with pediatric procedures. Pediatr Clin North Am. 1989;36:941.
105. Schechter NL, Berde CB, Yaster M. Pain in infants, children, and adolescents, 2nd edn. Baltimore, Williams & Wilkins, 2002.
106. Kain ZN, Caldwell-Andrews AA, Wang SM, et al. Parental intervention choices for children undergoing repeated surgeries. Anesth Analg. 2003;96:970.
107. Ungerleider RM, Greeley WJ, Sheikh KH, et al. Routine use of intraoperative epicardial echocardiography and Doppler color flow imaging to guide and evaluate repair of congenital heart lesions: a prospective study. J Thorac Cardiovasc Surg. 1990;100:297.
108. Harrison MR, Adzick NS, Flake AW, et al. Correction of congenital diaphragmatic hernia in utero: VI. Hard lessons learned. J Pediatr Surg. 1993;28:1411.
109. Harrison MR, Adzick NS, Longaker MT, et al. Successful repair in utero of a fetal diaphragmatic hernia after removal of herniated viscera from the left thorax. N Engl J Med. 1990;322:1582.
110. Harrison MR, Golbus MS, Filly RA, et al. Open fetal surgery was performed at UCSF. N Engl J Med. 1982;308:591.
111. Rosen PJ. Bleeding problems in cancer patient. Hematol Oncol Clin North Am. 1992;6(6):315–28.
112. Rogers MC, Nugent S, Traystman RJ. Control of cerebral circulation in the neonate and infant. Crit Care Med 1980;8:570.
113. Lindahl, Lindahl SGE. Oxygen consumption and carbon dioxide elimination in infants and children during anaesthesia and surgery. Br J Anaesth. 1989;62:70.
114. Fletcher R. Gas exchange during anaesthesia and controlled ventilation in children with congenital heart disease. Paediatr Anaesth. 1993;3:5.
115. Saint-Maurice C, Meistelman C, Rey E, et al. The pharmacokinetics of rectal midazolam for premedication in children. Anesthesiology. 1986;65:536.
116. Goudsouzian NG, Standaert FG. The infant and the myoneural junction. Anesth Analg. 1986;65:1208.
117. Motoyama EK, Glazener CH. Hypoxemia after general anaesthesia in children. Anesth Analg. 1986;65:267.
118. Lerman J, Eustis S, Smith DR. Effect of droperidol pretreatment on postanesthetic vomiting in children undergoing strabismus surgery. Anesthesiology. 1986;65:322.

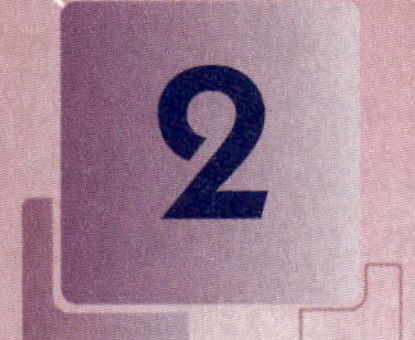

Anatomical Considerations in Paediatric Anaesthesia

Amit Padvi, Namita Padvi and Bhvya Baldwa

INTRODUCTION

For the study of paediatric anaesthesia, a clear understanding of the anatomical, physiological, pharmacological and psychological differences across various age groups is essential. Amongst paediatric patients, neonates and infants require special consideration as they are at higher risk of morbidity and mortality. The risk is generally inversely proportional to age. The most striking contrast between adults and children is obviously the body size. Several anatomical features of the neonatal and infant airway differ from that of adults and are important to the anaesthesiologist. Anatomic relationships and landmarks are constantly changing throughout infancy and childhood, which interferes with regional procedures and requires quite a good knowledge of developmental anatomy.

The key differences between the anatomical features of children and adults are highlighted in the chapter.

BODY SIZE

As previously mentioned, the most obvious difference between children and adults pertains to body size. But

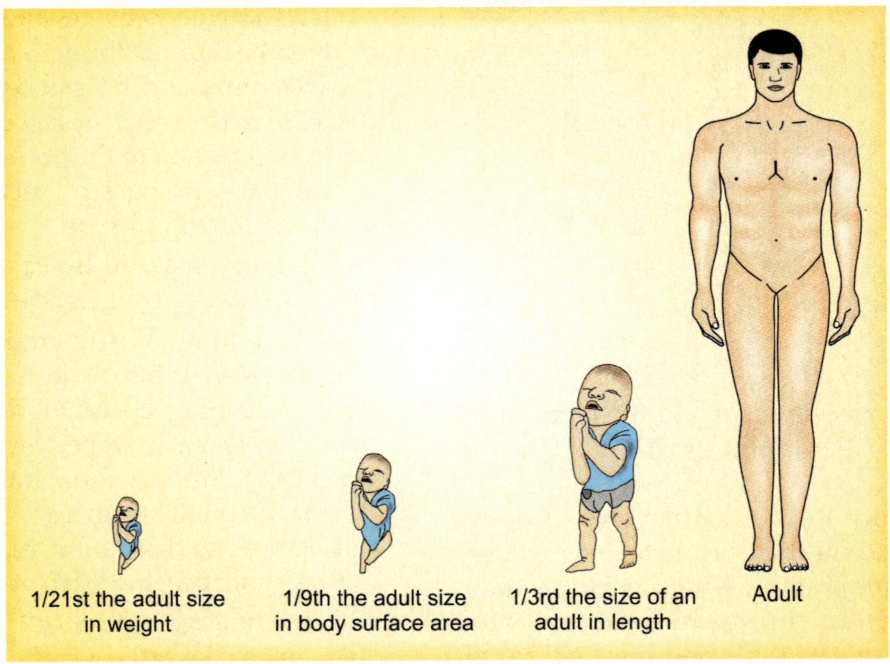

Fig. 2.1 As per Harris (1957), a normal full term, a normal newborn infant weighing 3 kg is 1/3rd the size of an adult in length, but 1/9th the adult size in body surface area and 1/21st the adult size in weight

at the same time, children are not small adults. The paediatric population as per age group can be divided as:

1. Neonates—refers to an infant in the first 28 days after birth.
2. Infants—a child of up to 12 months of age
3. Toddler child—1 to 4 years
4. Schoolgoing child—4 to 12 years
5. Adolescent and teenage—13 to 18 years

"Normal" full-term neonate weighs 3 to 3.5 kg with a height of approximately 50 cm, and within 10 to 15 years they will multiply their weight by more than 12 (>1200%) and their height by more than 3 (>300%).[1]

Amongst these various parameters, body surface area (BSA) is the most important as it closely matches variations in basal metabolic rate measured in kilocalories per hour per square meter. It is for this reason, BSA is considered to be a superior standard than age or weight in judging basal fluid and nutritional requirements. Nomograms, as that of Talbot and associates (1952), are available for clinical calculation of BSA. To calculate BSA, the following formula can be used:

Formula of Gehan and George (1970)

$BSA(m^2) = 0.0235 * Height^{0.42246} * Weight^{0.515456}$.[2]

Table 2.1 Relation of age, height, and weight to body surface area (BSA)

Age (y)	Height (cm)	Weight (kg)	BSA (m^2)
Premature	40	1	0.1
Newborn	50	3	0.2
1	75	10	0.47
2	87	12	0.57
3	96	14	0.63
5	109	18	0.74
10	138	32	1.10
13	157	46	1.42
16 (Female)	163	50	1.59
16 (Male)	173	62	1.74

Based on standard growth chart and the formula of DuBois and DuBois (1916): $BSA\ (m^2) = 0.007184 \times Height^{0.725} \times Weight^{0.425}$.[3]

There is a difference in the relative size of body structures in infants and children. Neonates have a large head (35 cm in circumference), which is larger than chest circumference. Head circumference increases by 10 cm during the first year of life and then 2 to 3 cm during the second year, when it reaches three-fourths the adult size.

AIRWAY

The anatomy of the airway of neonates and infants is different and difficult from that of adults. From about 4 years of age the airway anatomy becomes more like an adult and the airway problems associated with anaesthetizing children become less frequent. The important features of the airway of neonates and infants are listed.

Upper Airway

1. Relatively large head.
2. Prominent occiput.
3. Short neck: In a full-term neonate, the chin often meets the chest at the level of the second rib, making them prone to upper airway obstruction during sleep. In an infant with a tracheostomy, the orifice is often buried under the chin unless the head is extended with a roll under the neck.
4. Relatively small mandible.
5. Relatively large tongue.
   a. The size of the tongue means that there is relatively less space in the infant airway and that they are prone to upper airway obstruction.
   b. The tongue may also complicate direct laryngoscopy. It may be difficult to displace anteriorly with the laryngoscope.
   c. For the first few weeks of life, as a result of the large tongue, neonates and infants preferentially breathe through the nose rather than the mouth. This imposes a resistance to ventilation that is increased in the presence of nasal congestion from infection or the presence of a foreign body such as a nasogastric tube, oxygen prongs, or an endotracheal tube.
6. Abundant lymphoid tissue.
7. The pharynx tends to easily collapse by posterior displacement of the mandible, or external compression of the hyoid. Infants are more prone to upper airway obstruction under anaesthesia or sedation because upper airway muscles, which normally support the airway patency, are extremely sensitive to the depressant effect of anaesthesia and sedation, resulting in pharyngeal airway collapse and obstruction.
8. Relatively large omega or U-shaped epiglottis. It may fall backwards over the laryngeal inlet, if the tip of the laryngoscope blade is in the vallecula. A better view is usually obtained if the tip of the

laryngoscope is positioned on the laryngeal surface of the epiglottis.

9. Larynx is higher up and lies at the level of C_{3-4}.
10. Angled vocal cords: The orientation of the vocal cords directs the tip of an endotracheal tube against the anterior wall of the trachea, where it may hold up and can create the impression that the endotracheal tube is too wide to enter the cricoid ring.
11. Cricoid ring is the narrowest part of the upper airway.
12. Neonates preferentially breathe through the nose. Their narrow nasal passages are easily blocked by secretions and may be damaged by a nasogastric tube or a nasally placed endotracheal tube. Nasal passage contributes to 50% of airway resistance. There might be difficulty in nasal intubation as a "blindly" placed endotracheal tube may easily lodge in anterior commissure of the larynx rather than in trachea.
13. The large head, prominent occiput, and cephalad larynx combine to produce a view of the larynx which is often described as 'anterior' but is actually cephalad compared with adults.[4]
14. The 'sniffing' position does not help in bag mask ventilation or to visualize the glottis. The head needs to be in a neutral position.
15. Endotracheal tube (ETT): The diameter of the ETT must be narrow enough not to exert pressure on the mucosa of the cricoid cartilage. It should also allow a seal adequate for positive pressure ventilation with a minimal leak, at a peak inflation pressure of 20 cm of H_2O.
16. Trauma to the airway can easily result in oedema. One millimetre of oedema can narrow a baby's airway by 60% (Resistance $\propto 1/\text{radius}$). Therefore it is suggested that a leak be present around the endotracheal tube to prevent trauma resulting in subglottic oedema and subsequent post-extubation stridor.
17. Relatively more salivary secretions.

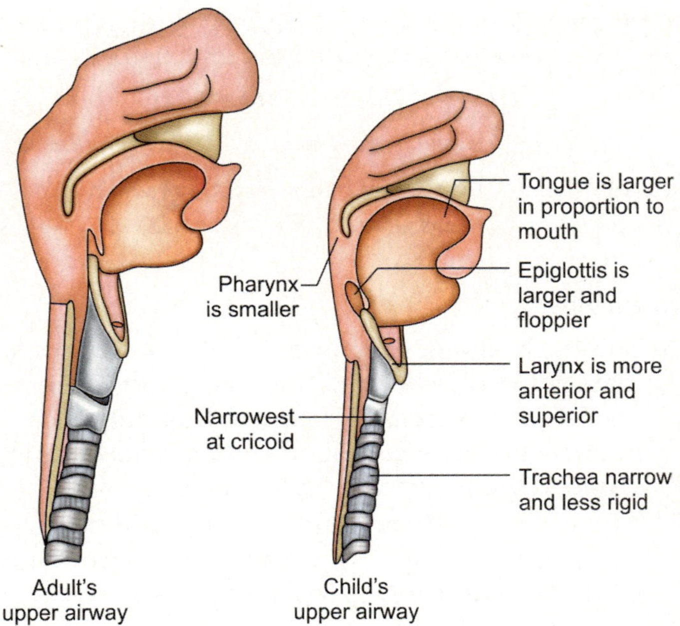

Fig. 2.3 Comparison of upper airway in child and adult

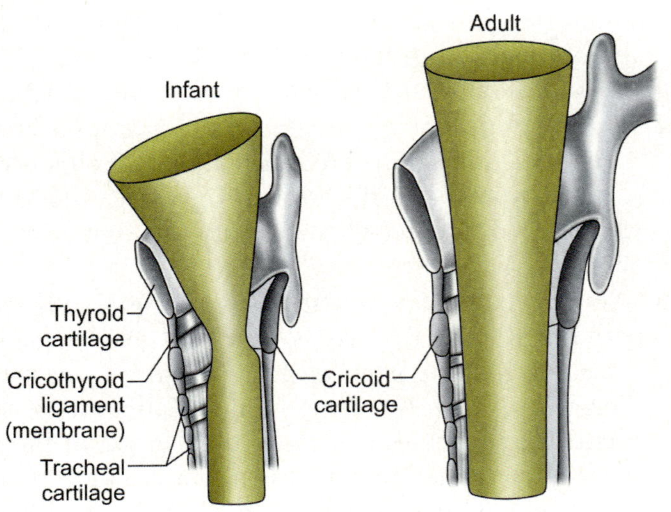

Fig. 2.2 Comparison of infant and adult airway

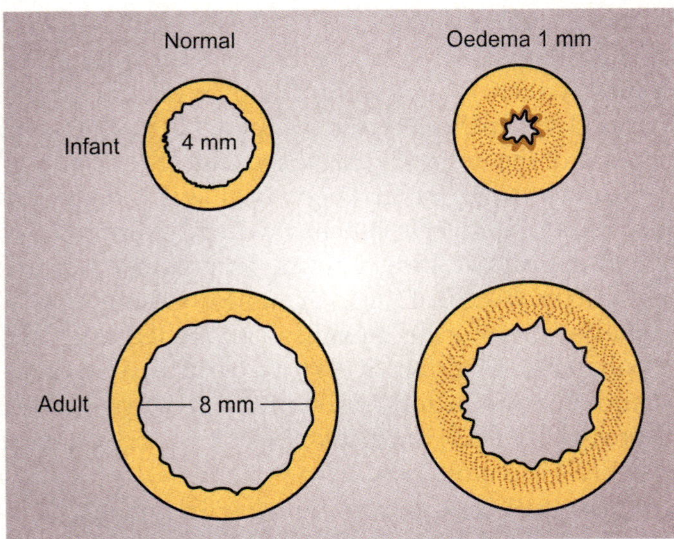

Fig. 2.4 Airway oedema in infant and adult

Table 2.2 Relation of airway oedema, resistance and cross sectional area of infant and adult trachea

	Oedema	
	Resistance ($R \propto 1/r^4$)	Cross section area
Infant	Increase by 16 times	Decreased by 75%
Adult	Increase by 3 times	Decreased by 44%

Lower Airway

1. The tracheal length may be as little as 3 cm and diameter may be 6 mm. Tracheal length is shorter resulting in increased chances of endobronchial intubation. Conversely, short endotracheal tubes are prone to unintentional displacement.
2. At the carina left and right main bronchi bifurcate at the same angle and hence endobronchial intubation is as likely to be left-sided as right-sided.
3. The total number of alveoli is only 10% of that of an adult and is thick-walled. A single terminal bronchiole opens into a single alveolus instead of a fully developed clustering.
4. Horizontal alignment of the soft and pliable ribs prevents the 'bucket-handle' action of the adult thoracic cage. There is less efficient ventilation than in adults because of:
   i. Weak intercostal and diaphragmatic muscles (due to a lack of type I fibres)
   ii. More horizontal attachment of intercostal muscles
   iii. Protuberant abdomen

   Limited respiratory reserve results in earlier onset of fatigue if the work of ventilation increases during anaesthesia or illness.
5. The chest is relatively small in relation to the abdomen, which is protuberant with weak abdominal muscles. The thorax is too compliant to resist inward recoil of the lungs. In the awake state, the chest wall is maintained relatively rigid with sustained inspiratory muscle tension, which maintains the end-expiratory lung volume (functional residual capacity [FRC]). However, under general anaesthesia, the muscle tension is abolished and FRC collapses, resulting in airway closure, atelectasis, and venous admixture unless positive airway pressure (CPAP) or positive end-expiratory pressure (PEEP) is maintained.
6. Chest wall compliance is higher in neonates and infants (0.06 mL/cm H_2O) compared with (0.04 mL/cm H_2O) in adults, because of the cartilaginous ribs and lack of chest wall musculature. This explains why intercostal and sternal retractions occur early in neonates and young infants during respiratory distress and airway obstruction.
7. Upper and lower airways are susceptible to a large increase in airway resistance (and the work of breathing) in the event of laryngeal or bronchial spasm.
8. Muscles of ventilation are easily subject to fatigue due to low percentage of Type I muscle fibres in the diaphragm. This number increases to the adult level over the first year of life.
9. The alveoli are thick walled at birth. There is only 10% of the total number of alveoli found in adults. The alveoli clusters develop over the first 8 years of life.

Toddlers

1. Head is more proportional to body size.
2. Teeth are formed.
3. Jaw becomes larger.
4. Epiglottis becomes less floppy.
5. Diaphragm remains the main muscle of respiration till 7 years of age.
6. Tracheal length on an average in the newborn is 3 cm, in a five year old child 6 cm, at the age of ten 7 cm and at the age of 15 years it is 8.5 cm.[5]

CENTRAL AND AUTONOMIC NERVOUS SYSTEM

1. Neonates have a relatively large brain, weighing about 1/10 of its body weight compared with about 1/50 in the adult. In a child, there is rapid development of the brain; its weight doubles by 6 months of age and triples by 1 year. At birth the brain weighs approximately 330–350 g (10–15% of body weight). Adult proportions (1200–1400 g—2% of body weight) are reached around 12 years of age.
2. The cerebral cortex is not fully developed and synaptic connections are not mature. Myelination and dendritic proliferation progress in the last 3 months of pregnancy and during the first year of life.
3. Approximately one-fourth of the neuronal cells are present at birth. By 1 year of age, the development of cells in the cortex and brain-stem is nearly complete. Myelinization and elaboration of dendritic processes continues till the end of third year. Incomplete myelinization is associated with primitive reflexes, such as the Moro and grasp reflexes, in the neonate.

4. The sutures are open and there is a large anterior fontanelle. Palpation of the anterior fontanelle can be used to evaluate intracranial pressure in neonates and infants. Increasing intracranial pressure is partly relieved by expansion of the fontanelles and separation of the suture lines so that head size increases before intracranial pressure rises.
5. In the preterm neonate cerebral vessels are at risk of rupture especially in the region of the germinal matrix close to the nucleus caudatus. The germinal matrix has a rich blood supply, scarce vascular supporting tissue, and thin vessel walls leading to a high chance of intracerebral and intraventricular haemorrhage. With increasing gestational age the germinal matrix involutes and the risk of bleeding decreases.
6. The volume of CSF is proportionately greater than in adults (4 mL/kg compared with 2 mL/kg) and this partly explains the relatively higher dose requirements for local anaesthetic (LA) solution and shorter duration of subarachnoid analgesia. The sacral hiatus is relatively large compared with later life and is not ossified. For these reasons it provides easy access to the lower epidural space.
7. The blood–brain barrier is not fully developed and it is anatomically and functionally incomplete. Bilirubin, opioids, and barbiturates all cross freely into the CNS through this blood–brain barrier.
8. At birth the spinal cord ends at the third lumbar vertebra. At 1 year of age, the cord assumes its permanent position, ending at the first lumbar vertebra.[6] The spinal cord of the foetus initially occupies the entire length of the spinal canal. Differential growth of the canal and spinal cord causes the termination of the cord to move cephalad relative to the vertebral canal. It is at the level of S1 at 28 weeks' gestation, L3 at term, L2/3 at 1 year, and the adult level of L1/L2 around the age of 8 years. The intercristal line in neonates is at the level of L5–S1 compared with L4 in adults and lumbar puncture is performed below this line. Ossification of the sacral vertebrae is not complete and sacral intervertebral epidural analgesia is feasible.
9. The epidural space in the infant contains fat that is loculated with distinct spaces between individual lobules. This means that a catheter introduced into the epidural space via the sacral hiatus can often be threaded to thoracic level to provide epidural analgesia for thoracic dermatomes.
10. In contrast to the central nervous system, the autonomic nervous system is relatively well developed in the neonate. The parasympathetic components of the cardiovascular system are function optimally at birth. However, the sympathetic components, are not fully developed until 4 to 6 months of age.[7] Baroreflexes to maintain blood pressure and heart rate, which involve medullary vasomotor centres (pressor and depressor areas), are functional at birth in awake newborn infants.[8]

The laryngeal reflex is activated by the stimulation of receptors on the face, nose, and upper airways of the newborn resulting in reflex apnoea, bradycardia, or laryngospasm. Various mechanical and chemical stimuli, like water, foreign bodies, and noxious gases, can trigger this response. This protective response is so potent that it can cause death in the newborn.

RESPIRATORY SYSTEM

At full-term birth, the lungs are still in the stage of active development. The formation of adult-type alveoli begins at 36 weeks post conception but represents only a fraction of the terminal air sacs with thick septa at full-term birth. It takes more than several years for functional and morphologic development to be completed. Similarly, control of breathing during the first several weeks of extrauterine life differs notably from control in older children and adults. Of particular importance is the fact that hypoxemia depresses, rather than stimulates, respiration. The development of the respiratory system and its physiology are detailed in Chapter 4, Essentials of Respiratory System.

CARDIOVASCULAR SYSTEM

During the first minutes after birth, the newborn infant must change his or her circulatory pattern dramatically from foetal to adult type to survive in the extrauterine environment. Even for several months after initial adaptation, the pulmonary vascular bed remains exceptionally reactive to hypoxia and acidosis. The heart remains extremely sensitive to volatile anaesthetics during early infancy, whereas the central nervous system is relatively insensitive to these anaesthetics. Cardiovascular physiology in infants and children is discussed in Chapter 3.

FLUID AND ELECTROLYTE METABOLISM

Like the lungs, the kidneys are not fully mature at birth, although the formation of nephrons is complete by

36 weeks—gestation. Maturation continues for about 6 months after full-term birth. The glomerular filtration rate (GFR) is lower in the neonate because of the high renal vascular resistance associated with the relatively small surface area for filtration. Despite a low GFR and limited tubular function, the full-term newborn can conserve sodium. Premature infants, however, experience prolonged glomerulotubular imbalance, resulting in sodium wastage and hyponatremia (Spitzer, 1982). On the other hand, both full-term and premature infants are limited in their ability to handle excessive sodium loads. Even following water deprivation, concentrating ability is limited at birth, especially in premature infants. After several days, neonates can produce dilute urine; however, diluting capacity does not mature fully until 3 to 5 weeks of life (Spitzer, 1978). The premature infant is prone to hyponatremia when sodium supplementation is inadequate or with overhydration. Furthermore, dehydration is detrimental in the neonate regardless of gestational age.

SUMMARY

1. Neonates have relatively large head and tongue with short neck and small mandible.
2. Neonates are obligate nasal breathers.
3. Epiglottis is large, floppy and omega shaped.
4. Cricoid ring is the narrowest part of the upper airway hence easily prone to.
5. Short length of trachea leads to higher chances of endobronchial intubations.
6. Soft, pliable ribs prevent bucket handle movement of thoracic cage.

Four differences between the adult and paediatric airway

1. Infant tongue is proportionally large.
2. The infants larynx is higher (rostral) in the neck (C3–4) than an adult (C4–5).
3. The infants epiglottis is omega shaped (W) and angled away from the trachea.
4. The narrowest part of the larynx is the cricoid cartilage below the vocal cords.

Positioning

Use of the chin lift and jaw thrust can help restore flow through an obstructed upper airway by separating the tongue from posterior pharyngeal structures.

The goal is to line up three divergent axes: Oral, pharyngeal and tracheal.

1. Aligning the axes (initial)
2. Aligning the axis (occiput roll)
3. Aligning the axis (extension)

REFERENCES

1. Miller RD. Relevant Differences between Children and Adults. In: Miller RD (Ed). Miller's Anaesthesia. 7th edn. Elsevier; Churchill Livingstone, An Imprint of Elsevier.
2. Gehan EA, George SL. Estimation of human body surface area from height and weight. Cancer Chemother Rep. 1970;54:225–35.
3. Smith's Anaesthesia for Infants and Children, 7th edn. Motoyama & Davis 2005.
4. Edward Doyle. Paediatric Anaesthesia, Oxford University Press, 27-Sep-2007.
5. Tahmina B, et al. Cadaveric Length of Trachea in Bangladeshi Adult Male. Bangladesh Journal of Anatomy. January 2009;7(1):42–44.
6. Gray H. Anatomy of Humanbody, 29th edn. Philadelphia: Lea and Febiger, 1973.
7. Friedman WF. The intrinsic physiological properties of the developing heart. Friedman WF, Lesch M, Sonnenblick EH (Eds). Neonatal heart disease. New York: Grune and Stratton. 1973.
8. Moss AJ, Emmanouilides GC, et al. Vascular responses to postural changes in normal newborn infants. Paediatrics. 1968;42:250.

3 Essentials of Cardiovascular System in Infants and Children

Chinmayi S Patkar and Namita Padvi

INTRODUCTION

Paediatric anaesthesia poses a challenge to the anaesthesiologist in view of the ongoing development and maturation of the organ systems, especially the cardiopulmonary system. The stage of organ maturation varies with age in each individual child, thus making it essential for the anaesthesiologist to be familiar with each and every age group ranging from neonates to young adolescents. In addition to age and development, the congenital heart diseases have a profound impact on the pharmacodynamics of anaesthetic agents.

The objective of this discussion is to focus on normal cardiovascular physiology in paediatric population in the context of continual organ maturation, which will aid the anaesthesiologist to deal with any paediatric patient on a routine basis.

FOETAL CIRCULATION (Fig. 3.1)

The chief function of the cardiovascular system is to provide oxygen delivery and metabolic nutrition to all the organ systems of the body. The foetal circulation differs from its adult counterpart in numerous ways. Firstly it encompasses the entire maternal fetoplacental unit comprising of the placenta and umbilical vessels. Secondly unlike in adults, the lungs do not participate in gas exchange but require only nutrient flow. This necessitates the presence of foetal intracardiac and extracardiac shunts to allow minimal blood flow to the lungs while simultaneously ensuring oxygenation to all the tissues. With the first cry at birth, respiratory exchange is initiated in the neonatal lungs and the placenta is soon after eliminated from circulation. The formerly 'shunt dependent' foetal circulation now has to function independently in order to allow a smooth transition to a neonatal circulation. Transitional circulation is an orderly process embracing all adaptive changes in the foetal circulation till it establishes a neonatal circulation. The presence and persistence of transitional circulation can cause adverse effects on the cardiovascular function of the neonate.

Deoxygenated blood is carried down the descending aorta to the umbilical arteries which then enter into the placenta. The umbilical arteries branch out to form the chorionic vessels ultimately ending into an extensive

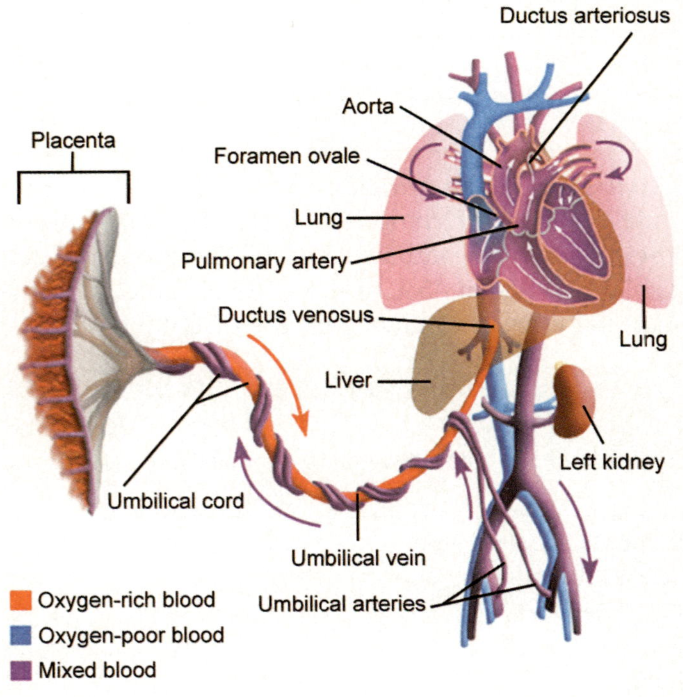

Fig. 3.1 Foetal circulation

arterio-capillary-venous network, namely the intervillous system. This chorionic villus is the site of oxygen and nutrient exchange, thus representing the functional unit of the placenta. Oxygenated blood from the placenta is then carried by the umbilical vein to the foetal organ systems.

50 to 60% of the highly oxygenated umbilical venous blood is bypassed by the ductus venosus to enter the inferior vena cava (IVC) directly. The foramen ovale (FO) preferentially carries the oxygenated blood from the IVC into the left atrium (LA) and left ventricle (LV). The LV carries this relatively highly oxygenated blood to the brain and coronary vessels via the ascending aorta. Also, some portion of blood from the right atrium (RA) coming via the superior vena cava (SVC), coronary sinus and part of IVC enters the right ventricle (RV). Due to high resistance of the pulmonary vasculature and relatively lower systemic vascular resistance of the placental unit, major portion of blood ejected from the RV goes to the descending aorta and placenta via the ductus arteriosus. Thus the foetal blood flow circuit demonstrates that both the ventricles function in 'parallel' to provide a mixed blood supply to the body organs as opposed to that in adults, where we observe the LV and RV working in 'series'. The presence of various intracardiac and extracardiac shunts allows the preferential streaming of oxygenated blood to the vital organs, namely brain and myocardium while bypassing the lungs and liver.

Clinical Pearl

Foetal circulation is shunt dependent and in 'parallel'; adult circulation is in 'series'.

In the foetus, the cardiac output of the left and right ventricles together comprises the total cardiac output, described as the combined ventricular output (CVO) (Table 3.1). About 45% of the CVO is directed to the placental circulation and only 8% of CVO enters the pulmonary circulation.[1] The RV has a cardiac output of approximately 330 mL/kg/min, whereas the LV output measures at about 170 mL/kg/min.[2] At birth, both RV and LV eject an output of 350 mL/kg/min. The reported ratio of right to left cardiac output ranges from 1.0 to 1.5 but most studies have agreed upon the right-sided dominance of foetal cardiac output.[3] Various poorly understood complex mechanisms involving circulating catecholamines and locally mediated vasoactive substances are believed to play a role in the control of foetal circulation.[1]

Clinical Pearl

Cardiac output in foetus is right-sided dominant.

The foetus survives in a relatively hypoxemic environment in-utero and yet has to perform the task of providing optimum oxygenation to the developing organ systems. The highest partial pressure of oxygen (PO_2) in the foetal circulation is observed in the umbilical vein being around 4.7 kPa, i.e. 30–35 mmHg and foetal blood is 80–90% saturated.[1] Optimum tissue oxygen delivery is ensured by adaptive mechanisms such as foetal haemoglobin (HbF) and 2,3-diphosphoglycerate (2,3-DPG). Oxygen delivery to a foetal organ is the product of blood flow to that organ and the oxygen content of foetal arterial blood; which in turn depends upon the haemoglobin (Hb) and its oxygen saturation (SaO_2).[1] Intraerythrocyte 2,3-diphosphoglycerate (DPG) is a product of glycolysis which normally acts to lower oxygen affinity and improve oxygen delivery to tissues. The gamma chains of foetal haemoglobin HbF do not bind as readily to 2,3-DPG thus resulting in higher affinity for oxygen as compared to adult form of haemoglobin (HbA). The high concentration of HbF (~ 80% at term) and low levels of 2,3-DPG permit efficient oxygen uptake in the placenta. Also the P_{50}, i.e. the oxygen tension at which 50% blood is saturated with oxygen is lower in the foetus at 3.6 kPa than in the

Table 3.1 Combined cardiac output and distribution in human foetus during the second half of pregnancy according to Rasanen et al.[4]

% of combined cardiac output at gestational age			
	20 weeks	**30 weeks**	**38 weeks**
Combined cardiac output	210 (mL/min)	960 (mL/min)	1900 (mL/min)
Left ventricle	47	43	40
Right ventricle	53	57	60
Foramen ovale	34	18	19
Lungs	13	25	21
Ductus arteriosus	40	32	39

adult (4.8 kPa). These factors enable to maintain the oxygen saturation in the umbilical venous blood greater than the uterine venous blood.

TRANSITIONAL CIRCULATION

Several changes occur in the foetal circulation at birth to facilitate its efficient transition into neonatal circulation. The separation of placenta, clamping of umbilical vessels and the neonate's respiratory efforts are the initiating events leading to these alterations. The first cry of the baby heralds the entry of blood into the pulmonary circulation with an increase in oxygen saturation. The placenta is eliminated from circulation altogether thus converting the low resistance circulatory system into a high resistance one. The intracardiac and extracardiac shunts cease to function immediately and permanently close over the course of time. Various neurohumoral and chemical mediators such as prostaglandins, kinins and nitric oxide (NO) contribute to these circulatory changes.

At birth, the first breath initiates entry of blood into the pulmonary circulation with reduction in pulmonary vascular resistance (PVR). Thereafter, there is a gradual decline in PVR over the ensuing years due to structural remodeling of the pulmonary vascular musculature. The placenta detaches from the uterine wall to cause constriction of the placental blood vessels. This event combined with clamping of the umbilical vessels leads to a consequent rise in systemic vascular resistance (SVR). With a fall in PVR and rise in SVR, the left atrial pressures increase above that of the right atrium causing the flap valve of the foramen ovale to close functionally. The prostaglandins [prostacyclin (PGI_2) and prostaglandin PGE_2] play a significant role in-utero to maintain the patency of the ductus arteriosus. The reduction in circulating prostaglandin levels with the separation of placenta and increased arterial oxygen tension cause the functional closure of the ductus arteriosus within 24 to 48 hours of birth. The anatomical closure occurs within 2 to 3 weeks by ductal fibrosis to become the vestigial remnant, namely ligamentum arteriosum. The ligation of the umbilical veins leads to a fall in the portal pressure relative to the inferior vena cava pressure which prompts functional obliteration of the ductus venosus within the first week of life. Its anatomical closure follows in the ensuing period to form the ligamentum venosum by the end of three months of birth.

Under certain adverse circumstances, the neonatal circulation can revert back to foetal circulation as the anatomical closure of shunts does not occur immediately after birth. Hypoxemia and acidosis are potent stimuli which are known to cause reversal of shunt patency. Persistence of foetal circulation (PFC) happens when shunting is present in the neonates beyond the transitional period without any evidence of underlying congenital heart disease.

Clinical Pearls

	Functional closure	Anatomical closure	Remnant structure
Foramen ovale	At birth	0–1 week	Fossa ovalis
Ductus arteriosus	24–48 hrs	2–3 weeks	Ligamentum arteriosum
Ductus venosus	0–1 week	2–3 months	Ligamentum venosum

BASIC PRINCIPLES OF CARDIAC FUNCTION

Preload is defined as the ventricular load at the end of diastole and before contraction has begun. In the intact heart, preload represents the diastolic stress caused by distension of the ventricular wall by blood volume. It is a reflection of the atrial filling pressures which then empty into the right ventricle (RV) or left ventricle (LV) during diastole. Clinically, we use indirect measurements of LV volume such as pulmonary wedge pressure or central venous pressure as surrogate markers of preload assessment.

Afterload is defined as systolic load on the LV after contraction has started. In other words, it is the stress developed in the left ventricular wall during ejection. The concept of afterload is more complex as LV ejection is a dynamic process. Preload is considered to be the wall stress at the end of diastole, whereas afterload is the wall stress experienced during LV ejection. To improve our understanding of afterload, we need to elucidate the concept of wall stress. The law of Laplace states that wall stress (σ) is proportional to the product of pressure (P) and radius (R) divided by wall thickness (h) in thin-walled spheres or cylinders:

$$\sigma \propto \frac{P \times R}{2\,h}$$

In accordance with the law of Laplace, wall stress is directly related to intraventricular pressure and inversely related to its wall thickness.

Afterload is often linked to vascular resistance, although impedance offers a more precise measurement. Aortic impedance is described as aortic pressure divided by aortic flow. However, in clinical practice, echocardiography alone can measure aortic impedance noninvasively. Routinely we approximate systolic blood pressure measurement with afterload, provided there is no aortic stenosis.

The sarcomere is the functional unit of the myocardium. The relation between resting sarcomere length and the amount of built-up tension was originally defined in isolated skeletal muscle fibers. The increase in length of the resting sarcomere caused by a rise in venous filling leads to greater force of contraction and ultimately greater stroke volume and cardiac output (Fig. 3.2). This intrinsic ability of the heart to adapt to changing volumes of inflowing blood within physiologic limits is known as the Frank-Starling law.[5] Thus an increased preload initiates myocardial stretching which increases the end-diastolic volume (EDV) generating a positive inotropic effect which translates into a rise in stroke volume.

Contractility represents the intrinsic ability of the myocardium to contract and perform mechanical work at a given preload. Changes in contractility can bear either a positive inotropic effect which enhances cardiac performance or a negative inotropic effect which diminishes performance. Sympathetic input to the heart via $\beta_1$receptors on cardiac membrane increases contractility by release of norepinephrine, thereby exerting positive inotropic effect. Severe hypoxia, acidosis and myocardial depressants like anaesthetic agents are a few examples causing negative inotropic effect.

Stroke volume is the amount of blood ejected by the ventricles per heart beat. This volume is determined by the preload, afterload and myocardial contractility acting in tandem. Cardiac output is the product of stroke volume and heart rate. As the immature myocardium displays limited ability to increase stroke volume in an attempt to improve cardiac performance, the paediatric heart is more dependent on heart rate.

Clinical Pearls
- Frank-Starling mechanism is poorly developed
- Cardiac output is heart rate dependent

STRUCTURAL AND FUNCTIONAL DEVELOPMENT

The cardiovascular system is one of the first organ systems in the foetal body to become operational. As early as five weeks postconception, the basic circulatory parameter, namely heart rate is identifiable. The external heart formation is completed by six weeks of gestation. However, it is still undeveloped in terms of constitution, function and innervation.

Structurally, the neonatal myocardium is immature with lesser proportion of cellular matter (mitochondria, DNA) and lesser contractile proteins, namely actin and

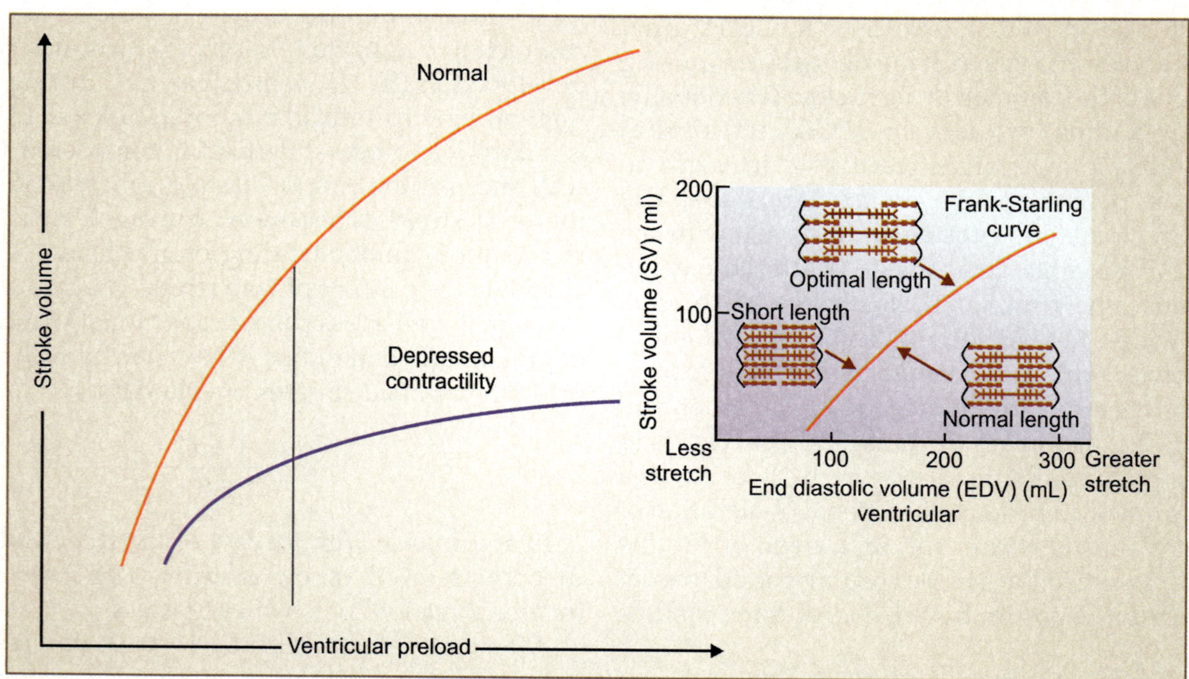

Fig. 3.2 Frank-Starling mechanism and sarcomere length (inset)

myosin. The myofibrils are scanty, poorly defined and aligned peripherally with limited capacity of protein synthesis. The myocardium is composed of higher proportion of non-elastic and non-contractile proteins (60% versus 30% in the adult myocardium) which renders it less compliant as compared to the adult heart. There is a greater extent of Type I collagen in the newborn's myocardium which is more rigid as compared to the adult Type III collagen. The neonatal myocytes contain higher proportion of water than contractile elements accounting for their decreased contractility.

The cell replication process varies in the foetus as compared to the adult. Foetal cardiomyocytes demonstrate the ability to undergo hyperplasia in addition to hypertrophy while the adult mature myocytes can divide only by hypertrophy, i.e. increase in size. The cell dimensions and surface area of the myocytes rapidly increase in the postnatal life.

The functional limitations of the neonatal heart are largely attributed to its structural immaturity. The poor compliance of the myocardium leads to its limited cardiac reserve. The heart is unable to respond to an increase in volume on the Frank-Starling curve to an extent the adult heart would. This results in the cardiac output being dependent upon heart rate more than stroke volume. The adult mechanism of increasing stroke volume to cause a proportionate rise in cardiac output is more resourceful. But infants and children, on the other hand, expend more energy in the process of increasing cardiac output by increasing their heart rate during stressful situations.

The changes in ventricular pressure are more easily transmitted to the opposite ventricle in the immature myocardium. Also, the LV and RV diastolic filling is severely impaired. Limited compliance and equal masses of both the ventricles contribute to their interdependence. The pressure and volume overload experienced by both the ventricles at birth lead to their hypertrophy. The adult ratio of LV to RV mass of 2:1 is attained several months after birth. Also, the biventricular interdependence makes the heart more susceptible to myocardial depression when faced with adverse events such as hypoxia, acidosis or anaesthetic agents. The stiffer nature of the myocardium restricts it potential to respond adequately to fluid overload. Thus, the neonates poorly withstand any increase in preload, afterload or depressed myocardial contractility.

Another important point pertaining to calcium ions is worthy of mention here. Calcium ions are essential for the excitation-contraction coupling resulting in myocardial contraction. These ions diffuse into the t-tubules and are released when required to enhance contractility. The earliest evidence of longitudinal sarcoplasmic reticulum is seen by the beginning of second trimester, but t-tubules are visible only after birth. Due to this underdeveloped sarcoplasmic reticulum in the neonatal heart, there is a limited storage capacity of calcium. Thus the neonatal myocardium is more dependent on sodium calcium channels for calcium influx from the extracellular space. This explains the increased sensitivity of neonatal heart to hypocalcemia and drugs like digitalis, calcium channel blockers, etc. and its dependence on extraneous calcium sources. Also, the reduced Ca-ATPase enzyme activity on the sarcoplasmic reticulum results in a decreased calcium release and reuptake.

Lastly, the source of energy for myocyte metabolism in the neonate is lactate while in adults long chain fatty acids are favored. This difference is due to deficiency of enzyme carnitine palmitoyl transferase-1 which transports long-chain fatty acids into the mitochondria. The relative dependence of the neonatal myocardium on anaerobic metabolism offers a somewhat protective role against hypoxia. The fundamental differences in the cardiovascular functioning of the neonate and adult are summarized in Table 3.2.

AUTONOMIC REGULATION OF CARDIAC FUNCTION

The cardiovascular functioning is regulated by the nervous system so as to ensure its optimum performance under different physiological circumstances. The autonomic system plays a crucial role in the control of cardiovascular homeostasis. During foetal period, this autonomic regulation of the heart is undeveloped

Table 3.2 Functional differences in the neonatal and adult cardiovascular parameters

	Neonate	Adult
Cardiac output	HR dependent	SV and HR dependent
Compliance	Less	Normal
Starling response	Limited	Normal
Preload reserve	Limited	Normal
Afterload compensation	Limited	Effective
Ventricular interdependence	High	Relatively low
Myocardial metabolism	Anaerobic	Aerobic
Chief substrate	Lactate	Long chain fatty acids

and continues to remain immature throughout the neonatal life.

At birth, the heart is innervated by both sympathetic and parasympathetic systems. Both α and β-adrenergic receptors have been detected in the neonatal myocytes. However, it has been demonstrated that the sympathetic nervous system is incomplete at both the postganglionic receptor site and the receptor-effector level.[6] Furthermore, the sympathetic and parasympathetic systems attain maturity at a differential rate; the former being adequately functional by early infancy and the latter in the early neonatal period. This leads to parasympathetic dominance in the neonatal life which is clinically observed as marked bradycardia in response to adverse stimuli such as hypoxia, acidosis or anaesthetic agents.

The two prime functions of the autonomic nervous system are regulation of the distribution of cardiac output to each organ system and maintenance of blood pressure. These functions are determined by equilibrating the arteriolar and venular tone mediated by sympathetic and parasympathetic innervation.

The intrinsic and extrinsic cardiovascular reflexes serve to buffer sudden acute changes in blood pressure. Studies in humans and experimental animals suggest that arterial baroreceptors are present in the foetus, incompletely developed at term and undergo postnatal maturation. The baroreceptor reflex arc consists of an afferent limb located in the carotid body and aortic arch, a central medullary cardiovascular centre and an efferent limb composed of sympathetic and parasympathetic nerves to the heart and blood vessels. The foetal life demonstrates an enhanced sensitivity of the efferent limb of this reflex. In preterm infants, postural changes elicit no change in heart rate, but there is an increase in peripheral vascular resistance, illustrating an incomplete and attenuated baroreceptor response.[7] The chemoreceptor reflex in utero is presumed to be well developed as manifested by foetal bradycardia in response to hypoxia.

The salient features of the major cardiovascular reflexes are presented in Table 3.3.

The autonomic system displays its maximal profound impact on heart rate and contractility. The sympathetic and parasympathetic systems have a complementary action on heart rate. Cardiac output in the paediatric age group is more dependent on heart rate rather than on stroke volume. The resting normal sympathetic tone maintains contractility 20% greater than that in the denervated heart.[7] Heart rate and contractile force both can be raised to about 100% by increasing the sympathetic flow to heart. However, a higher heart rate translates into greater myocardial energy consumption. Thus infants and children tend to expend more energy while increasing their cardiac output especially when subjected to stress.

Circulating catecholamines released from adrenal gland and para-aortic chromaffin tissue also mediate autonomic control over heart much before direct innervation matures completely. An indirect evidence of immature innervation at birth is the lower levels of neurotransmitters as compared to that in adults. Catecholamine secretion is vital at birth to assist the foetus in adapting to the newly acquired external environment.

Clinical Pearls

- Parasympathetic system dominates over sympathetic system in neonates and infants.
- Vagal bradycardia observed in response to hypoxia, acidosis and myocardial depressant anaesthetic agents.

Table 3.3 Major cardiovascular reflexes. The Bainbridge and the "reverse" Bainbridge reflexes: History, physiology, and clinical relevance[8]

Reflex	Receptors and location	Afferent limb	Efferent limb and response
Arterial baroreceptor reflex	Stretch receptors in vessel wall of carotid sinus and aortic arch respond to changes in arterial blood pressure	Fibers in glossopharyngeal and vagus nerves to medulla	Homeostatic control of arterial blood pressure via changes in cardiac output and systemic vascular resistance mediated by the autonomic nervous system
Bezold-Jarisch reflex	Mechanical and chemosensitive receptors in ventricular walls	Nonmyelinated vagal C-fibres to medulla	Inhibition of sympathetic outflow resulting in bradycardia, peripheral vasodilation and hypotension
Bainbridge reflex	Stretch receptors at junction of the vena cava and right atrium and at junction of the pulmonary vein and left atrium respond to changes in volume in central thoracic compartment	Fibers in vagus nerve to medulla	Inhibition of vagal outflow and enhancement of sympathetic outflow to sino-atrial node causing tachycardia

PREOPERATIVE ASSESSMENT OF CARDIOVASCULAR SYSTEM

The cardiovascular system is continually in a state of dynamic transformation as it undergoes physiological development and maturation. The anaesthesiologist should be accustomed to the age related physiological variations while evaluating the patient prior to surgery. The objectives of a scheduled preoperative assessment should be to allay anxiety of parents, establish a friendly rapport with the child and form an individualised plan of anaesthetic management.

History

The skill of eliciting history is an essential prerequisite in the preoperative assessment of paediatric patients posted for surgery. The initial assessment of the cardiovascular system involves the general well-being of the child in terms of ability to 'thrive'. Feeding difficulty is an early indicator of cardiovascular disease in neonates and young infants. Inadequate growth and developmental delays reflect poorly on the overall health of the patient.

It is imperative to review the growth charts in the younger age group to follow the development of the patient over a period of time and compare it with the acceptable standard for age. Acute and chronic illnesses affect growth and development negatively; with loss of weight being the first sign of impairment followed by a lag in height and head circumference. In older age group, we can gauge the child's development by asking the parents to compare his overall growth and activity with that of his peers.

Cardiovascular disease is implied by more specific symptoms such as shortness of breath, cyanotic spells and palpitations. Chest pain and syncope are uncommon in children as compared to adults and signify an underlying cardiac pathology when present. Maternal exposure to drugs such as lithium, phenytoin or alcohol and diseases such as rubella, diabetes mellitus; to name a few are known to be associated with congenital cardiac lesions. Likewise, prematurely born neonates are placed at a higher risk of having patent ductus arteriosus. Hence, prenatal and birth history must be elicited precisely. Family history and enquiry about health of other siblings is also necessary.

Examination

General examination includes a thorough inspection of the child for central cyanosis, clubbing, splinter hemorrhages, pallor or icterus. Features of facial dysmorphism or other associated congenital anomalies such as syndactyly, polydactyly, cleft lip or palate can act as markers of a syndrome and warrant a detailed cardiac examination to rule out heart defects. Assessment of jugular venous pressure is not much relied upon in children less than eight years of age. Inspection of precordium for any obvious bulge or chest deformity like pectus carinatum or excavatum forms an integral part of systemic examination. Palpation of peripheral and central pulses helps to evaluate rate, rhythm, volume status of heart and to identify specific signs such as brachiofemoral delay classically seen in coarctation of aorta. Precordial palpation allows localization of the apex beat which lies in the 4th intercostal space from birth to three years of age and gradually migrates to lie in the 5th intercostal space with increasing age.[9] It also aids in detection of thrills associated with murmurs, if any.

Auscultation of the chest becomes the most significant part of cardiovascular examination. It is mandatory to perform a detailed auscultation of all the components of the cardiac cycle in all the auscultatory areas with both the bell and diaphragm of stethoscope.[10] Innocent, functional or benign murmurs are quite common in childhood and should be distinguished from pathological murmurs which denote an underlying cardiac disease.

These physiological murmurs are soft, systolic in nature and recede with change in position, exercise or hemodynamic status of the child. On the contrary, diastolic or continuous murmurs and those associated with a palpable thrill are always pathological. A notable exception is a venous hum which is a benign continuous murmur best heard at the base of the neck due to turbulent venous flow in the superior vena cava and jugular veins. The benign or innocent murmurs of childhood are enlisted in Box 3.1.[10]

Box 3.1: Innocent murmurs of childhood[10]

Systolic murmurs	Continuous murmurs
Vibratory Still's murmur	Venous hum
Pulmonary flow murmur	Mammary arterial soufflé
Peripheral pulmonary arterial stenosis murmur	
Supraclavicular systolic murmur	
Aortic systolic murmur	

Chest X-ray and ECG

The specific age-related changes in the cardiovascular system add to individual variations in the paediatric chest X-ray and ECG which need to be interpreted correctly.

The heart shadow is relatively large in infants with the cardiac silhouette occupying almost 50–55% of the thoracic width on anteroposterior view. In neonates and infants, the thymus may contribute to apparent cardiomegaly and this should be distinguished by a lateral view X-ray. Apart from size, one should also pay attention to the cardiac shape and pulmonary vasculature for signs suggestive of congenital heart disease.

It is not routine to advise ECG in paediatric patients, except when history and physical examination particularly raise a suspicion of an underlying cardiovascular disorder. Age-specific changes occurring in the cardiovascular system during development are reflected in the ECG. For example, in early neonatal period the right ventricle dominates over the left ventricle in both size and function. This is reflected in the ECG as right ventricular dominance and right QRS axis deviation. Over the early months of postnatal life, the left ventricle grows in size and gradually demonstrates its dominance on ECG. The ECG values which change rapidly in the first year of life evolve more gradually after infancy to mature completely by late adolescence and early adulthood. The normal ranges as per age are represented in Table 3.4 for heart rate, QRS axis, PR and QRS complex intervals and R- and S-wave amplitudes.[11]

Apart from chest X-ray and ECG, 2D-echocardiography forms an important tool of assessment of cardiac function. The non-invasive nature of this investigation goes a long way in predicting the effects of anaesthetic agents in a patient with cardiovascular abnormality. Cardiac catheterization is an invasive method of definitive assessment in paediatric patients having cardiac disorder.

EFFECTS OF ANAESTHETIC AGENTS ON CARDIOVASCULAR SYSTEM

The cardiovascular system is susceptible to the effects of anaesthetic agents in myriad ways depending upon the age-related physiological development. It is necessary to consider physiological evolution while administering anaesthesia to the paediatric patient. One should pay due attention to the type of anaesthetic agent selected for a particular patient as per the nature and duration of surgery. The cardiopulmonary and drug interactions should also be taken into account while applying a tailor-made approach for each individual. The anaesthetic goals relevant to the cardiovascular system are maintenance of optimum oxygen delivery and adequate ventricular output.

Premedication

The need for premedication can be validated by the fact that a calm and composed child offers an opportunity of a smooth and safe induction while maintaining hemodynamic stability. Premedication is unwarranted in the neonates and infants up to eight months age. However, infants start developing stranger anxiety from 8 to 9 months of age, thus necessitating premedication. Elder children above the age of six years can be dealt with reasoning and psychological counseling, again depending upon the emotional and mental make-up of the individual.

Benzodiazepines and opioids administered orally or intravenously are the frequently employed

Table 3.4 ECG variables—normal range values for age[11]

Age	HR (bpm)	QRS axis (degree)	PR interval (sec)	QRS interval (sec)	R in V_1 (mm)	S in V_1 (mm)	R in V_6 (mm)	S in V_6 (mm)
1st week	90–160	60–180	0.08–0.15	0.03–0.08	5–26	0–23	0–12	0–10
1–3 weeks	100–180	45–160	0.08–0.15	0.03–0.08	3–21	0–16	2–16	0–10
1–2 months	120–180	30–135	0.08–0.15	0.03–0.08	3–18	0–15	5–21	0–10
3–5 months	105–185	0–135	0.08–0.15	0.03–0.08	3–20	0–15	6–22	0–10
6–11 months	110–170	0–135	0.07–0.16	0.03–0.08	2–20	0.5–20	6–23	0–7
1–2 years	90–165	0–110	0.08–0.16	0.03–0.08	2–18	0.5–21	6–23	0–7
3–4 years	70–140	0–110	0.09–0.17	0.04–0.08	1–18	0.5–21	4–24	0–5
5–7 years	65–140	0–110	0.09–0.17	0.04–0.08	0.5–14	0.5–24	4–26	0–4
8–11 years	60–130	–15–110	0.09–0.17	0.04–0.09	0–14	0.5–25	4–25	0–4
12–15 years	65–130	–15–110	0.09–0.18	0.04–0.09	0–14	0.5–21	4–25	0–4
>16 years	50–120	–15–110	0.12–0.20	0.05–0.10	0–14	0.5–23	4–21	0–4

premedicants. Alternative routes of drug administration include intramuscular, rectal (methohexital) or intranasal (midazolam) which are less commonly preferred. Sedative doses which can compromise the airway patency should be avoided in patients with decompensated hemodynamics.

1. **Methohexital:** Rectal methohexital 25–30 mg/kg induces sleep in healthy paediatric patients with minimal cardiovascular side effects. The primary effects are increased HR and decreased SV.[12]
2. **Midazolam:** Midazolam is the most widely used benzodiazepine in children for causing amnesia and sedation in short procedures and in the ICU. It has been used as a premedication via intravenous, oral or intranasal route; with the latter two routes being favorable in the paediatric population. It is preferred over diazepam and lorazepam due to its water-soluble properties and faster elimination. Previous studies have confirmed a fall in blood pressure and cardiac output by a bolus dose of midazolam.[13] Continuous infusions have been found to be more cardiostable than intermittent boluses.
3. **Opioids:** Opioids are μ-receptor agonists which attenuate the sympathetic and neuroendocrine response to laryngoscopy and surgical stress. They have a limited direct effect on the hemodynamic stability and are required to be administered with caution in view of major respiratory depression. High-dose opioid induction technique is hence preferred in paediatric patients posted for cardiac surgeries. There exists a wide range of opioids available to select from based on their pharmacological properties such as the long acting (elimination half life 120 minutes), less potent morphine to the ultra-short acting (context sensitivity half-time of 4 min. after 4 hour infusion), highly potent remifentanil (100–200 times more potent than morphine).

Induction Agents

1. **Volatile agents:** Inhalational induction and maintenance holds a pivotal place in paediatric anaesthesia due to numerous reasons. Firstly, the ease of administration by simple mask holding precludes the need of pricking the child, thereby making him uncomfortable or cranky. Secondly, the rapid wash-in and wash-out of the volatile agents guarantee a rapid induction and recovery respectively. All volatile anaesthetics affect the cardiovascular system by their direct myocardial depressive action along with peripheral vasodilation. This is clinically manifested by as a dose-dependent reduction in heart rate, mean arterial pressure, systemic vascular resistance (SVR) and cardiac index. Neonates and infants are more vulnerable to episodes of bradycardia, hypotension, and cardiac arrest than older children when under inhalational anaesthesia.

   Halothane was the inhalational induction agent of choice for paediatric patients in the past decades. Halothane is known to cause dose-dependent direct myocardial depression and sensitization of the heart to the effects of adrenaline. Ever since the introduction of sevoflurane into clinical practice, the use of halothane has considerably declined. Sevoflurane with its low blood gas partition co-efficient and trivial airway irritability, is the inhalational agent of choice for a smooth, stable and rapid induction. It is also preferred for maintenance anaesthesia owing to rapid recovery profile.

   Isoflurane and desflurane both are known to cause a dose-dependent reduction in myocardial contractility and reflex increase in sympathetic tone. However, they do not sensitize the myocardium to effects of adrenaline.

2. **Intravenous drugs**
   a. ***Thiopentone:*** Barbiturates cause a dose-dependent negative inotropic effect on the heart which is mediated through the calcium channels and the medullary vasomotor centre. The recommended dose of thiopentone for induction in children (5–6 mg/kg) and infants (7–8 mg/kg) is higher than that in adults (3–4 mg/kg). In healthy neonates, the dose requirement is 4 to 5 mg/kg which can be explained by a decreased plasma protein binding, underdeveloped blood–brain barrier and higher sensitivity of neonatal receptors.

      Thiopentone causes a reduction in the mean arterial pressure by decreasing the sympathetic tone, preload and cardiac index. Heart rate increases in response to hypotension via baroreceptor reflex mediated sympathetic stimulation. These cardiovascular effects of thiopentone are more prominent with associated hypovolemia, hypertension and sympathetic stimulation as seen in sepsis; and may be exacerbated by accompanying histamine release. Sodium thiopentone being antalgesic, cannot prevent significant hemodynamic responses to noxious stimulation when administered alone.

b. ***Propofol:*** The most profound effect of propofol as an induction agent on the cardiovascular system is a fall in mean arterial pressure by 15–30% in healthy children. This is attributed to a reduction in SVR caused by peripheral smooth muscle relaxation and inhibition of sympathetic activity. Arteriolar smooth muscle relaxation is mediated by closure of voltage gated calcium channels and an enhanced release of local nitric oxide (NO). However, it does not affect the pulmonary vasculature with no reduction of pulmonary vascular resistance (PVR) or mean pulmonary artery pressure. This fact may influence the direction and extent of intracardiac shunting in patients with congential heart defects.

Propofol does not cause a tachycardic response to hypotension on induction by either inhibiting or resetting the baroreflex response. In fact, a fall in heart rate of up to 20% may be observed on induction with propofol. Significant bradycardia can occur in children less than two years age, poor American Society of Anaesthesiologist' Society (ASA) status, strabismus surgery and simultaneous administration of opioid. It may rarely cause rhythm disturbances such as a systole, complete heart block, junctional rhythm and atrial premature beats.

Prolonged infusions of propofol at a dose of more than 4 mg/kg/hour for duration longer than 48 hours are associated with a rare but potentially fatal propofol infusion syndrome. Initially it was reported in critically ill paediatric patients but later was documented in adults as well. It is a constellation of metabolic disturbances such as metabolic acidosis, rhabdomyolysis and hypertriglyceridemia, clinically manifesting as refractory bradydysrhythmias and ultimately resulting in multiorgan failure. The pathophysiological mechanism is propofol mediated impaired mitochondrial fatty acid chain oxidation and respiratory chain inhibition mimicking mitochondrial myopathies.

Previous studies comparing the cardiovascular effects of intravenous induction in children found the reduction in mean arterial pressure to be significantly greater after propofol (28–31%) than after thiopentone (14–21%), whereas the reduction in cardiac index was not significantly different.[14] Baroreflex mediated increases in heart rate and systemic vascular resistance were less after propofol than after thiopentone. The baroreceptor reflex was more attenuated in children aged less than 2 years than in older children.[14] Pain on injection caused by propofol becomes a deterrent for its use in intravenous induction in children.

c. ***Ketamine:*** Ketamine produces dissociative anaesthesia and displays its unique properties in terms of cardiovascular stimulant effects. Routine induction dose of ketamine causes an increase in heart rate, cardiac index, systemic and pulmonary blood pressures as well as SVR and PVR. The increase in these hemodynamic variables translates into a rise in myocardial oxygen consumption and cardiac work. Cardiovascular stimulant actions are probably related to its sympathomimetic effects mediated by the central nervous system and peripheral sympathoneural release of norepinephrine.

Ketamine remains the induction agent of choice in cyanotic congenital heart disease, namely tetralogy of Fallot where maintenance of SVR is of prime importance for the right to left shunt fraction. The incidence of emergence reactions seen after ketamine anaesthesia is lower in the paediatric age group as compared to the adults (10–30%). Another advantage of this drug is the variety of routes of administration such as intravenous, intramuscular, nasal, oral and rectal; making it suitable for use in children.

d. ***Etomidate:*** Among all the intravenous induction agents available, etomidate is the most cardiostable drug with minimal effects on hemodynamics. It has negligible effect on sympathetic stimulation, baroreceptor reflex response and histamine release. However, it is not routinely used in clinical practice due to direct adrenocortical suppression.

The cardiovascular effects of intravenous induction agents are mentioned in Table 3.5.

Table 3.5 Cardiovascular effects of intravenous induction agents

	HR	MAP	CO	Contractility	SVR	Venodilation
Thiopentone	+	–	–	–	±	++
Propofol	–	– –	–	– –	– –	++
Ketamine	++	++	+	±	±	0
Etomidate	0	0	0	0	0	0

Local Anaesthetics

The use of local anaesthetics, namely lignocaine and bupivacaine has been widely practiced in paediatric anaesthesia for topical as well as regional anaesthesia and analgesia. The low levels of pseudocholinesterase in children and limited protein binding alter the pharmacokinetics of these local anaesthetics. Hence the total cumulative dose needs to be taken into consideration while injecting local anaesthetics.

The effect of sympathetic blockade by local anaesthetics on the cardiovascular hemodynamics is minimal in young children. Caudal and epidural anaesthesia have limited hemodynamic alterations and are well tolerated by children of all ages.

FAQs

Q. Describe the foetal circulation in detail and the changes taking place at birth. State the anaesthetic implications of transitional circulation and persistence of foetal circulation.

Q. Describe the physiological differences between the neonatal and adult cardiovascular system.

Q. Describe the anaesthetic management of a 6-year old child with unrepaired and unpalliated Tetralogy of Fallot posted for total intracardiac repair.

Q. Mention the cardiovascular effects of standard intravenous induction agents in paediatric patients. Mention the rationale of using intravenous induction agents in congenital cardiac defect with L $\rightarrow$ R shunt.

SUMMARY

Foetal circulation differs from the adult one in being shunt dependent and in parallel due to the presence of low resistance type placental circuit. At birth, the placenta is eliminated from circulation and SVR increases while PVR falls and pulmonary blood flow rises.

It is vital to understand the basic principles of cardiac physiology as well as the structural and functional immaturities in the paediatric age group. The age related circulatory variables need to be borne in mind while administering anaesthesia to these patients. The parasympathetic overdominance results in a bradycardic response to adverse stimuli such as hypoxia, acidosis and anaesthetic agents. A thorough preoperative assessment and examination of the child enables the anaesthesiologist to formulate a safe and effective plan. A detailed understanding of the clinical pharmacology of anaesthetic agents and their application in the paediatric patients is central to the anaesthetic management.

Take Home Message

A precise knowledge of the cardiovascular physiology, structural and functional development and interactions of anaesthetic agents with the cardiopulmonary system is essential to provide safe and effective anaesthesia to paediatric patients.

REFERENCES

1. Peter John Murphy. The fetal circulation. Continuing Education in Anaesthesia, Critical Care and Pain. 2005; 5(4):140–141.
2. James A DiNardo. Anesthesia for Cardiac Surgery. 2nd edn. Appleton & Lange. 1998.
3. Gunther Mielke, Norbert Benda. Cardiac Output and Central Distribution of Blood Flowin the Human Fetus. Circulation. 2001;103:1662–1668.
4. Torvid Kiserud. Physiology of the fetal circulation. Seminars in Fetal & Neonatal Medicine. 2005;10: 493–503.
5. Arthur C Guyton, John E Hall. Textbook of Medical Physiology. 11th edn. Elsevier Saunders. 2006.
6. Cote, Lerman, Todres. Practice of Anesthesia in Infants and Children. 4th edn. Elsevier Saunders. 2009.
7. John E Jones, Aruna R Natarajan, Pedro A Jose. Cardiovascular and Autonomic Influences on Blood Pressure. Clinical Hypertension and Vascular Disease: Pediatric Hypertension.
8. Hugh C Hemmings (Jr), Talmage D Egan. Pharmacology and Physiology for Anesthesia: foundations and clinical application.
9. Asuquo U Antia, Stefan R Maxwell, Aligh Gough, et al. Position of the Apex Beat in Childhood. Archives of Disease in Childhood. 1978;53:585–589.
10. Andrew N Pelech. The physiology of cardiac auscultation. Pediatr Clin N Am. 2004;51:1515–1535.
11. Ghazala Q Sharieff, Sri O Rao. The Pediatric ECG. Emerg Med Clin N Am. 2006;24:195–208.
12. Audenaert SM, Lock RL, Johnson GL, et al. Cardiovascular effects of rectal methohexital in children. J ClinAnesth. 1992 Mar-Apr;4(2):116–9.
13. Lara Shekerdemian, Andrew Bush, Andrew Redington. Cardiovascular effects of intravenous midazolamafter open heart surgery. Archives of Disease in Childhood. 1997;76:57–61.
14. Aun CST, Sung RYT, O'Meara ME, et al. Cardiovascular Effects of i.v. induction in Children: Comparison between Propofol and Thiopentone. Br. J. Anaesth. 1993;70(6): 647–653.

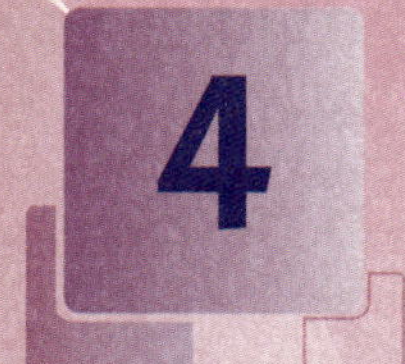

Essentials of Respiratory System in Infants and Children

Vaishali P Chaskar and Jalpa Arvind Kate

INTRODUCTION

The most common critical incidents related to respiratory system are seen in paediatric age group. There are anatomical and physiological differences between neonates, infants and child. Again they differ from adult respiratory system. The knowledge about development in respiratory system helps to provide appropriate anaesthesia to paediatric group and to reduce complication rates. The chapter will provide appropriate informations and also anaesthetic considerations in detail.

Key Points

1. At birth, control of ventilation is immature. This maturity occurs at 3 weeks of age in term baby.
2. Neonates and preterm babies are more prone for post operative apnoea episodes. Risk of postoperative apnoea is less after 1 month of age in term and 60 weeks PCA in preterm babies.
3. In first few weeks, response to hypercapnia is blunted.
4. In hypoxia, neonate responds with hyperventilation followed by apnoea. But the apnoeic response to hypoxia is suggestive of respiratory muscle fatigue or upper airway obstruction.

Developmental Changes

Developmental changes in all systems should be so sufficient to withstand drastic changes at the time of birth. All systems adapt the changes from gestational age and makes foetus to survive in external environment too. Cardiorespiratory adaptation is one of the very crucial adaptations. After the birth, within few minutes, neuronal drive and respiratory muscles must replace all liquid filled in lungs by sufficient amount of air. Therefore, gas exchange will take place. This chapter will provide a clear view of developmental and relevant aspects of respiratory systems and will also discuss about anaesthetic considerations in detail.

DEVELOPMENT OF LUNGS

Development of lungs (Fig. 4.1) starts in prenatal period and changes are as follows:[1,2]

1. Embryonic phase: Groove in ventral foregut, endoderm surrounding mesenchymal tissue to form lung buds.
2. Pseudoglandular phase: [Till 17 weeks of gestation (WOG)]—rapid budding of bronchi and lung growth, preacinar branching is complete. During this phase, any disturbance to free expansion leads to hypoplasia as occurs with *diaphragmatic hernia*.
3. Canalicular phase: (Till 24 WOG), development of respiratory bronchiole, and capillaries surrounding it.
4. Terminal sac period: (After 24 WOG)—appearance of clusters of air spaces (saccules), with thick and irregular septa.
5. (At 26–28 WOG) Capillary proliferation around saccules. In premature infants, it may be seen earlier at 24 WOG, hence they can survive in neonatal intensive care.
6. At 28 WOG: Thinning of saccular walls, lengthening of saccules with additional generation.
7. At 32 WOG: Alveolar formation starts from saccules. Most of alveolar formation occurs in 12–18 months of postnatal life.

However, morphologic and physiologic development of lungs continues during the first decade of life.

1. **Lung volume** in early postnatal period, is disproportionately small compared to body size (Fig. 4.2).

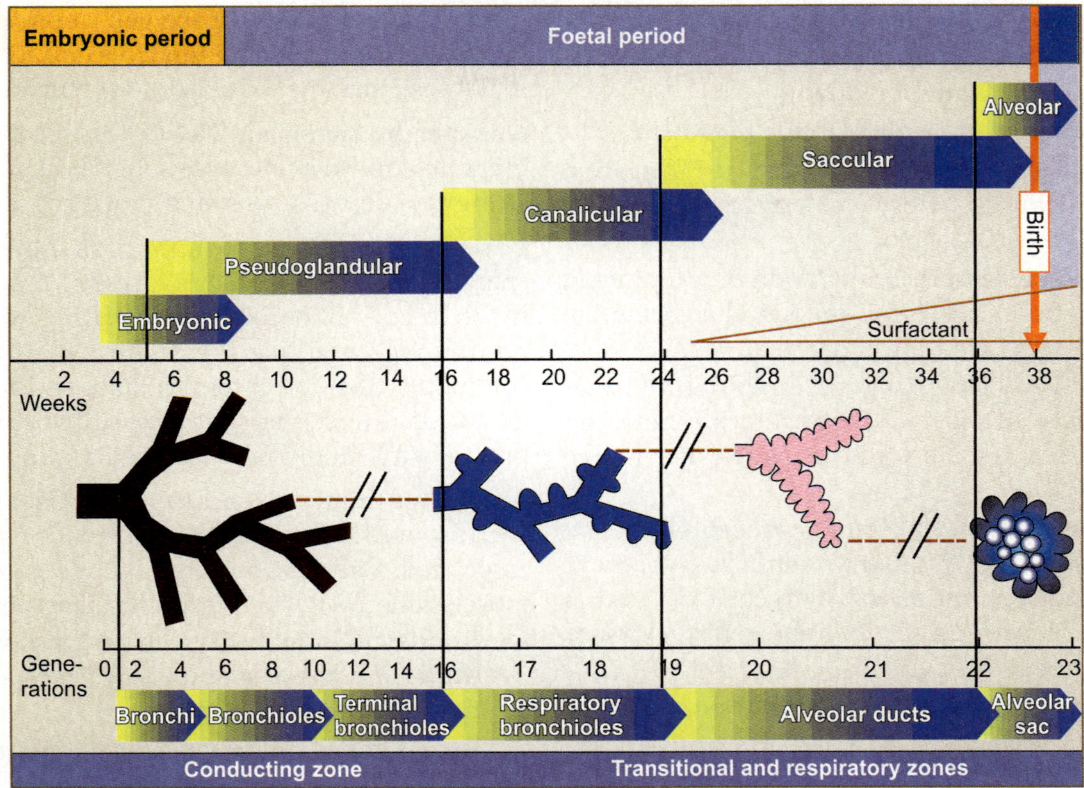

Fig. 4.1 Development of Lungs

High metabolic rate due to higher oxygen consumption markedly increases ventilatory requirement per unit lung volume. Hence infants have less reserve of lung volume and surface area for gas exchange. Therefore, they are prone to **early desaturation** in case of hypoventilation or apnoea for short duration.

2. **Foetal lung fluid**: It is produced in large quantity by lung to expands the airways against closed larynx. This fluid contains growth factor, **human bombesin**, which stimulates lung growth and development. This fluid is periodically expelled into uterine cavity and contributes about one-third of total amniotic fluid. Hence prenatal ligation or occlusion of trachea was tried with some success in **congenital diaphragmatic hernia**, to expand growth of airway and hypoplastic lung.[1,2]
3. **Type II pneumocytes**: It forms alveolar lining and produces pulmonary surfactant. These cells appear as early as 20 WOG or in 24–26 WOG. The pulmonary surfactant helps to reduce surface tension and stabilizes air spaces after air breathing.
4. **IRDS or HMD in premature patients**, leads to immaturity of lungs and hence inefficient production of pulmonary surfactant. Corticosteroids helps to accelerate the growth and maturation of lungs resulting in early appearance of above cells and hence surfactant production. **Prenatal glucocorticoid therapy** has been used widely to induce lung maturation and surfactant synthesis in mothers at risk of premature delivery. It should be given 24–48 hrs before delivery of premature baby.

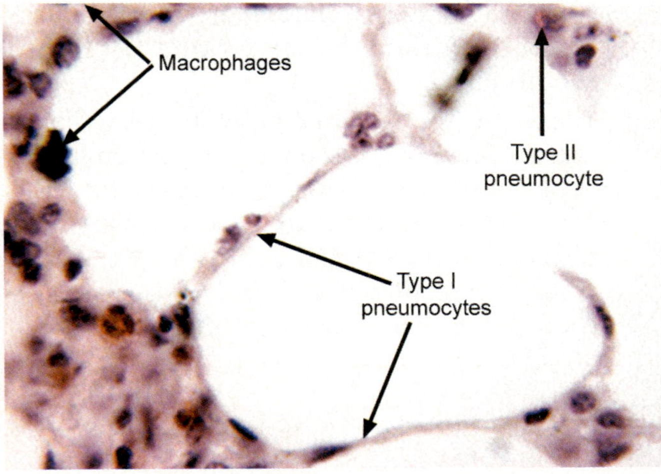

Fig. 4.2 Type II pneumocytes

CONTROL OF BREATHING[2,3]

1. **Central chemoreceptors:** Response depends on changes in H^+ ions conc. in CSF

a. Dorsomedial respiratory group: Inspiratory
b. Ventrolateral respiratory group: Expiratory
c. Pontine group: Rapid breathing
d. PreBotzinger complex: Rhythmic breathing

2. **Peripheral chemoreceptors:** Present at Bifurcation of common carotid artery—response depends on changes in arterial oxygen.
3. **Upper airway receptors:** Stimulation of receptors in the nose produces sneezing, apnoea, changes in the bronchomotor tone and diving reflex.

   During swallowing, there is inhibition of breathing, closure of larynx. Co-ordination between laryngeal and pharyngeal muscles are hence maintained.
4. **Tracheobronchial and pulmonary receptors**
   a. Slowly adapting (pulmonary stretch receptors): Membranous posterior wall of trachea and central airways. Hering-Breuer inflation reflex—apnoea due to inflated ETT cuff.
   b. **Rapidly adapting (irritant or deflation):** Situated in carina and large airways Hering-Breuer deflation reflex—increase in respiratory drive at low lung volumes as in IRDS and pneumothorax. It also mediate paradoxical reflex of Head—deep inspiration instead of inspiratory inhibition and it helps to inflate the unaerated portion of newborn lung.
   c. **C fibre endings:** Near the pulmonary capillaries. It is stimulated by pulmonary congestion, microemboli, pulmonary oedema, anaesthetic gases. Such stimulation leads to apnoea followed by rapid shallow breathing, hypotension and bradycardia. Reflex contraction of the laryngeal muscles responsible for laryngospasm.

Key Points

Maturation of control of breathing depends on postconceptional age than the postnatal age. The hypoxic and hypercapnia response drive is not well developed in newborns and infants. Hence they are more prone to respiratory depression due to immaturity as well as increased respiratory muscle fatigue. This risk is more in preterm infants.

Regulation of Breathing[2,3]

As in adult, infant responds to an increase in **$PaCO_2$** by increasing alveolar ventilation. This strength is totally dependent on gestational age and postnatal age. And hypoxia in infants, may depress the hypercapnic ventilatory response.

High concentration of **oxygen** depresses the respiration in newborn while low concentration stimulates it. But sustained hypoxia leads to ventilatory depression.

Nonspecific factors are blood glucose; anaemia affects breathing due to inadequate substrate availability. Cold stress also depresses ventilator drive.

Periodic breathing common in newborns. It is characterized by recurrent pauses in ventilation lasting more than 5–10 seconds, alternating with bursts of respiratory activity. Periodic breathing is more commonly seen in preterm infants and it is related to gestational age. Periodic breathing and apnoea of prematurity should be diagnosed appropriately.

Apnoea of prematurity may be life threatening event. In this ventilator pauses are prolonged and are associated with desaturation, bradycardia and loss of muscle tone. Factors contributing these events are

i. **Brainstem immaturity:** Blunted response to hypercarbia and hypoxia and **delay** in response conduction through brainstem.
ii. **Respiratory fatigue:** Chest wall deformity.

Treatment: Give tactile stimulation, in mild to moderate cases.

In severe cases:

1. Theophylline or caffeine to increase respiratory drive.
2. Positive pressure ventilation to stabilize respiratory function.

Anaesthesia Pearls

Prematurity is risk factor for postanaesthetic respiratory depression.

This can be life threatening and inversely related to gestational age and postconceptional age at the time of anaesthesia. The greatest risk is up to 60 weeks after conception.

MECHANICS OF BREATHING[1–3]

In infancy, rib grows horizontally from vertebral column and moves a little with inspiration. This anatomic configuration of ribs makes accessory muscles ineffective in infants (Fig. 4.3).

The chest wall consists of mainly cartilages calcification, poorly developed musculature and incomplete calcification of ribs. This results in floppy chest wall. As age grows, chest wall becomes stiff. In preterm, chest wall is more retractile.

The paradoxical chest wall movement commonly occurs in younger children and infancy due to increased

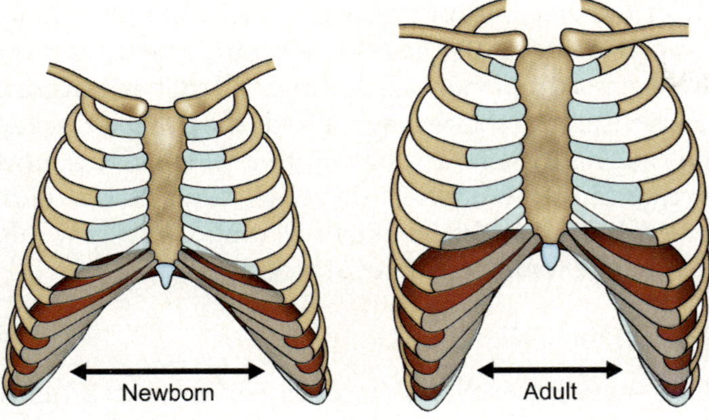

Fig. 4.3 Small lung volume of neonate compared to adult

respiratory effort. It is mainly seen under general anaesthesia with upper airway obstruction or it could be because of decreased intercostals muscles tone. In paradoxical respiration, inward movement of rib cage opposes inspiration of diaphragm. Diaphragmatic displacement may increase as the severity increases to maintain tidal volume. Due to increase workload, there will be respiratory muscle fatigue and hence respiratory failure.

Diaphragmatic fatigue is due to low content of type I muscle fibres. Type I muscle fibre has slow twich and high oxidative capacity. These fatigue resistant fibres make up <10% total muscle fibres before 37 weeks of gestation. A higher content of it confers fatigue resistance as the age advances. In adult diaphragm, Type I fibres is about 50% while those are 25% in term infant.

Lung compliance depends on lung volume which is more in childhood. Specific compliance of the lung does not depend on size. It mainly depends on FRC or TLC. It remains constant while specific compliance of chest declines due to progressive calcification and increasing thoracic muscle mass. Therefore, specific compliance of entire respiratory system declines in the childhood due to changes in the chest wall. Elastic recoil increases as the age advances.

LUNG VOLUME[1,2,4]

Development of airways up to terminal bronchiole completes by 16th weeks of gestation. Full term new born has 20–50 millions terminal primitive air saccules. Later it develops into alveoli. At 12–18 months of age alveoli number reaches to adult value which is 400 million or more.

In early postnatal period, lung volume of infant is disproportionate and smaller in relation to size (Fig. 4.4). Infants metabolic rate is twice as that of the adult. Hence, venitilatory requirement is more in infants. Hence minute ventilation approximately 200 mL/kg/min and oxygen consumption 7 mL/kg/min are twice that of the adult. Less reserve in lung surface area for the gas exchange. Tidal volume remains constant 7–10 mL/kg throughout life. Ventilator need is achieved by increase in respiratory rate in newborns, infants and children. General anaesthesia markedly diminishes FRC, which further reduces oxygen reserve in infants.

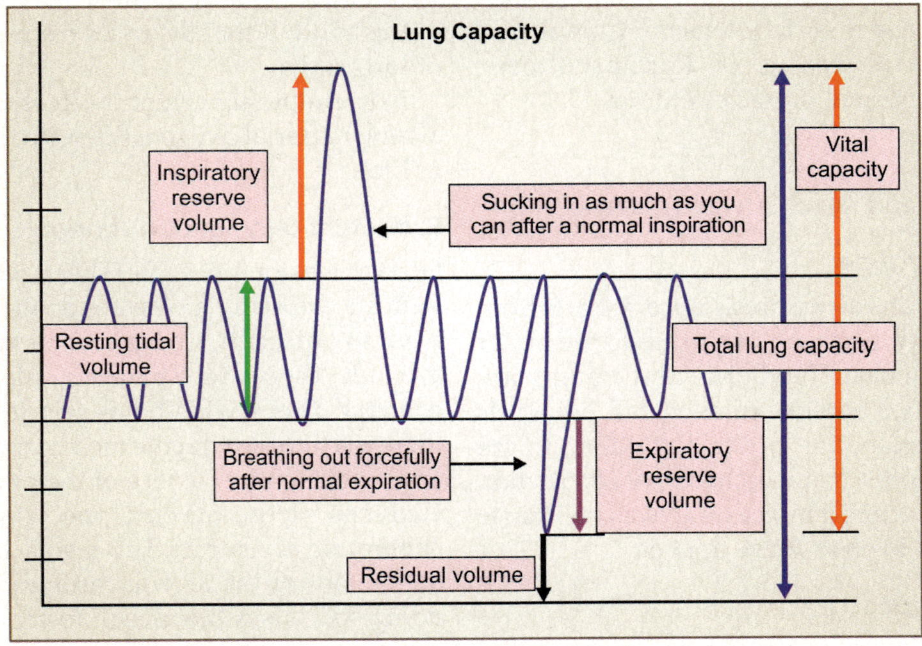

Fig. 4.4 Lung volumes

Total lung capacity: Maximum lung volume allowed by stretching of thorax and lungs. In infant, 60 mL/kg and that in adult 90 mL/kg.

Residual volume: Volume of air remains in lung after deep expiration. It is of 25% of TLC.

Functional residual capacity: It depends on balance between outword stretch of thorax and inward recoil of the lungs. 25% TLC normal in upright position, 40% TLC in supine position. It is 30 mL/kg throughout.

Pleural pressure in older children and adult is –5 cm of water but in neonates and infants, it is slightly negative. In Infants outward recoil of chest wall is very less while lung recoil is slightly less. Hence FRC further reduces 10–15% more in anaesthesia, apnoea and paralysis. In awake patient, FRC is maintained by sustained tonic activity of the inspiratory muscle. In infants, there is no fixed level of FRC.

Closing Capacity [2,3]

$$CC = CV + RV$$

Closing volume: Volume of lung above the RV at which airflow ceases during expiration from dependent lung zones. Closing capacity as percentage of TLC is relatively high in children, while it is very high in infants. The closing capacity is more than the FRC in infants and children leads to early airway closure.

Compliance of the lung decreases in the conditions associated with decreased lung volume such as atelectasis, intrapulmonary tumor. It is also decreased in IRDS due to increased surface tension. Compliance of the chest wall decreases in kyphoscoliosis, scleroderma and abnormal thoracic contour.

Airway Resistance

It consists of upper and lower airway resistance.

Upper Airway Resistance

It consists of 65% of total airway resistance. It starts from the mouth, oral cavity, pharynx, larynx up to the upper thoracic part of trachea. Newborns and infants are obligate nose breather because of cephalad epiglottis and the close approximation of the soft palate to the tongue and the epiglottis. If any occlusion or obstruction to the nasal airway occurs, it increases airway resistance by 50% which leads to obstructive apnoea.

Lower Airway Resistance

It consists of 35% of total airway resistance while smaller peripheral airways consist of 10% of it. This starts from lower thoracic part of trachea, bronchi, bronchioli and alveolar ducts as the gas flows to small airways, flow resistance should increase due to small caliber, but cross sectional area of the airway towards the peripheries and the number of airways are more and hence the flow resistance of the airways decreases towards the periphery. Lung conditions like BPD, cystic fibrosis would not change total airway resistance

GAS DIFFUSION [1-3]

Pulmonary gas exchange occurs by diffusion at all ages. Pulmonary diffusion in childhood is mainly affected by changes in surface area of alveolar capillary membrane.

Total diffusion capacity is similar as that of the adult **with relation to** alveolar ventilation and oxygen consumption. It is more flow limited than the diffusion limited. Total gas exchange surface area is smaller in relation to body size in infancy. This is suggestive of reduce physiological reserve.

As the child grows, diffusion capacity increases linearly with height. This is closely related to lung growth. Thickness of blood gas barrier for diffusion declines in early gestational ages. Therefore, alvoeloar arterial oxygen difference is higher in term neonates and even higher in preterm. Venous admixture is higher in infants than in adult. It is at 10–20% of cardiac output. While in adult, it is 2–5% of cardiac output. Intrapulmonary anatomic shunting is the major factor for venous admixture mainly at the opening of developing alveoli. Ventilation perfusion imbalance is different than that of the adult. It mainly arises from opening and closing of lung units.

Extrapulmonary right to left shunting contributes to alveolar arterial oxygen difference in the first few hours of life.

Surfactant and Surface Tension [5]

Surface tension principle: When water forms a surface with air, the water molecules on the surface of the water have an especially strong attraction for one another. As a result, the water surface is always attempting to contract. This is what holds raindrops together, that is, there is a tight contractile membrane of water molecules around the entire surface of the raindrop. On the inner surfaces of the alveoli, the water surface is also attempting to contract. This results in an attempt to force the air out of the alveoli through the bronchi and, in doing so, causes the alveoli to try to collapse. The net effect is to cause an elastic contractile force of the entire lungs, which is called the surface tension elastic force.

The alveolar surfaces of human lungs are lined with surface active materials with unique properties that are responsible for the stability of air spaces.[6] These materials, which contain specific phospholipids and proteins (discussed later), are collectively called pulmonary surfactant.

Pressure in Occluded Alveoli Caused by Surface Tension[5]

If the air passages leading from the alveoli of the lungs are blocked, the surface tension in the alveoli tends to collapse the alveoli. This creates positive pressure in the alveoli, attempting to push the air out. The amount of pressure generated in this way in an alveolus can be calculated from the following formula:

Pressure = 2 × Surface tension/Radius of alveolus

For the average-sized alveolus with a radius of about 100 μm and lined with *normal surfactant*, this calculates to be about 4 cm of water pressure (3 mmHg). If the alveoli were lined with pure water without any surfactant, the pressure would calculate to be about 18 cm of water pressure, 4.5 times as great. Thus, one sees how important surfactant is in reducing alveolar surface tension and therefore also reducing the effort required by the respiratory muscles to expand the lungs. Note from the preceding formula that the pressure generated as a result of surface tension in the alveoli is *inversely* affected by the radius of the alveolus, which means that the smaller the alveolus, the greater the alveolar pressure caused by the surface tension. Thus, when the alveoli have half the normal radius (50 instead of 100 μm), the pressures noted earlier are doubled. This is especially significant in small premature babies, many of whom have alveoli with radii less than one quarter that of an adult person. Further, surfactant does not normally begin to be secreted into the alveoli until between the sixth and seventh months of gestation, and in some cases, even later than that. Therefore, many premature babies have a little or no surfactant in the alveoli when they are born, and their lungs have an extreme tendency to collapse, sometimes as great as six to eight times that in a normal adult person. This causes the condition called respiratory distress syndrome of the newborn. It is fatal if not treated with strong measures, especially properly applied continuous positive pressure breathing.[5]

The airways contain different types of cells. The walls of the alveoli contain type I cells, which cover 95% of the alveolar surface, and type II cells which produce surfactant.[2] Chemical composition of surfactant is approximately 10% lipoprotein and 90% phospholipid. Of the phospholipid fraction of surfactant, phosphatidylcholine constitutes about 70%, which is mainly surface active.[6] Phosphatidylglycerol, another surface active phospholipid, was subsequently identified in the lung extract and comprises about 10% of surfactant fraction.[7] Phosphatidylglycerol appears late during the development; its appearance or reappearance coincide with the recovery from IRDS and acute respiratory distress syndrome (ARDS) in adults and with the loss of surfactant.[8] Other phospholipids include sphingomyelin (also surface active), phosphatidylethanolamine and phosphatidylinositol, which are not surface active.[9] The production of phosphatidylcholine increases towards term, whereas that of sphingomyelin decreases. The ratio of these phospholipids (L/S ratio) in the amniotic fluid has been used as an index of foetal lung maturity.[10]

There are four surfactant proteins (SP) that have been identified (SP-A, SP-B, SP-C, and SP-D), which comprise about 10% of surfactant on the mature alveolar surface. SP-B and SP-C are intimately linked to the stability of surface active monolayer at the alveolar surface. SP-B is essential for myelin formation of the lamellar inclusions in type II cells and promotes surface adsorption of dipalmitoylphosphatidylcholine in the lipid mixtures and an addition of the mixture of surface active phospholipids, and SP-B restores the normal pressure-volume curves of the lungs in the animal model of IRDS.[11,12] Surfactant proteins SP-A and SP-D are similar in structure, containing proline-rich collagen domain in addition to carbohydrate domain (called collectins). SP-A and SP-D seems to function primarily as innate host defense molecules in the airways and alveoli.[13] A decrease in SP-A is probably common in patients with severe lung injury. Infants born with decreased SP-A/dipalmitoylphosphatidylcholine ratio are at increased risk of developing BPD and dying.[14]

Surfactant phospholipids and proteins are produced within the type II pneumocytes, stored in the osmiophilic lamellar inclusions within these cells, and excreted into the alveolar surface, forming tubular myelins and subsequently spreading to form surface-active alveolar lining layers.[15]

Surfactant replacement therapy using human, bovine, or synthetic surfactant in premature infants with IRDS has been established as an important and essential form of therapy, reducing morbidity and mortality.[16–19]

Surfactant replacement therapy has been extended to cover other clinical conditions with surfactant deficiency or inactivation not only in premature infants but also in full-term infants, children, and adults. These conditions include neonates with persistent pulmonary hypertension (PPHN) in whom surfactant production by type II pneumocytes is depressed because of severe pulmonary hypoperfusion and hypoxia; neonates with severe congenital diaphragmatic hernia (CDH) whose immature lungs are damaged by ventilator-induced lung injury and surfactant inactivation by plasma protein leak on the alveolar surface; meconium aspiration syndrome caused by pulmonary hypoperfusion, inflammation, and inactivation of surfactant by protein leak; and ARDS in children and adults.[20,21]

CILIARY ACTIVITY

The tracheal and bronchial walls have pseudostratified epithelium that consists of ciliated cells, non-ciliated serous and brush cells, and abundant mucus-secreting goblet cells. Goblet cells and mucus-secreting glands diminish in number toward the periphery of the airway system. The mucous of respiratory tract is produced by numerous serous and mucous cell glands present in submucosal area. The mucosal surface is covered by a serous fluid layer, in which the cilia beat. Above this periciliary layer of serous fluid lie discontinuous flakes of mucus which are moved cephalad by the cilia (Fig. 4.5).[22]

Functions of Cilia

The cilia in the respiratory tract play an important role in the removal of mucoid secretions, foreign particles, and cell debris and are an essential defense mechanism of the airway system. These cilia move in a synchronous, whip-like fashion at a rate of 600 to 1300 times per minute. They can move particles toward the mouth at the rate of about 1.5 to 2 cm/min.[19] Ciliary function is influenced by the thickness of the mucous layer and other factors that can occur with dehydration or infection. In tissue culture, some viral infections reduce ciliary motion as much as 50%, and repeated infections in vivo can destroy the cilia completely.[20] Inhalation of warm air with 50% humidity maintains normal ciliary activity, whereas breathing dry air for 3 hours results in a complete cessation of mucus movement. Ciliary activity can be restored by breathing warm, saturated air.[23–25] Breathing 100% oxygen and controlled positive pressure ventilation also affect ciliary function.[26–29]

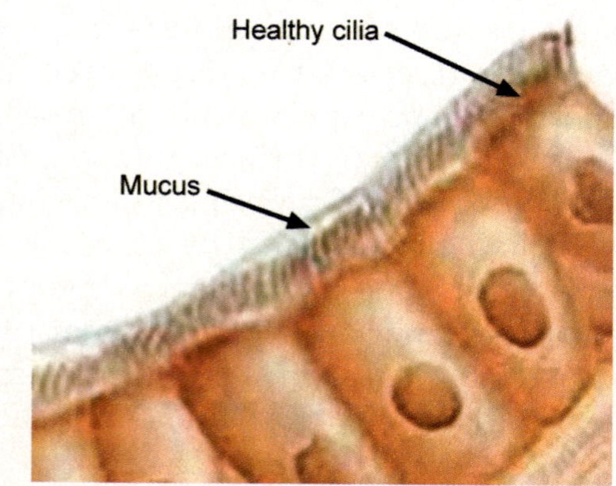

Fig. 4.5 Tracheal epithelium

Inhaled anaesthetics seem to decrease ciliary function in both animals and humans. Forbes and Horrigan observed a dose-related depression of ciliary activity during halothane and enflurane anaesthesia.[30] The same group of investigators found delayed mucus clearance during and 6 hours after discontinuation of halothane or diethyl ether anaesthesia.[29] These findings suggest that inhaled anaesthesia has adverse effects on mucociliary clearance, especially in patients with pulmonary disease. The effect of anaesthetics on mucociliary clearance in infants and children has not been reported.

OXYGEN TRANSPORT

Oxygen is required by almost every tissue metabolism. Continuous supply of oxygen is mainly dependent on three factors—pulmonary ventilation, cardiac output and blood haemoglobin concentration and characteristics. Oxygen is mainly carried in blood in two forms, dissolved in plasma and as oxyhaemoglobin. The amount of oxygen carried by the plasma depends on its solubility and is small (0.31 mL/dL per 100 mmHg). Most oxygen molecules in blood combine reversibly with haemoglobin to form oxyhaemoglobin. Each molecule of haemoglobin combines with four molecules of oxygen; 1 g of oxyhaemoglobin combines with 1.34 mL of oxygen.

Oxygen Haemoglobin Dissociation Curve (Fig. 4.6)

It reflects the affinity of haemoglobin for oxygen. As blood circulates through the normal lungs, oxygen tension increases from the mixed-venous PO_2 of around 40 mmHg to pulmonary capillary PO_2 of above 105 mmHg, and haemoglobin is saturated to about 97% in arterial blood. The shape of the dissociation curve is such that further increase in PO_2 result in a very small increase in oxygen saturation (SO_2) of haemoglobin. The blood of normal adults has SO_2 of 50% when PO_2 is 27 mmHg at 37°C and a pH of 7.4. The P50, which is the PO_2 of whole blood at 50% SO_2, indicates the affinity of haemoglobin for oxygen. An increase in blood pH

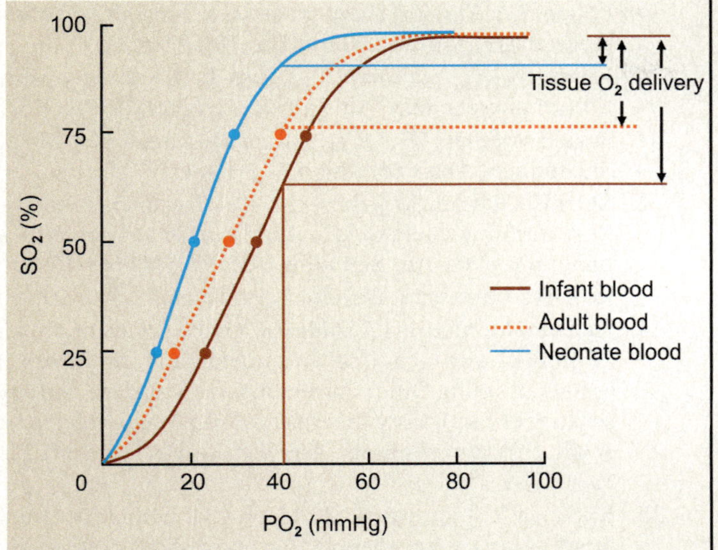

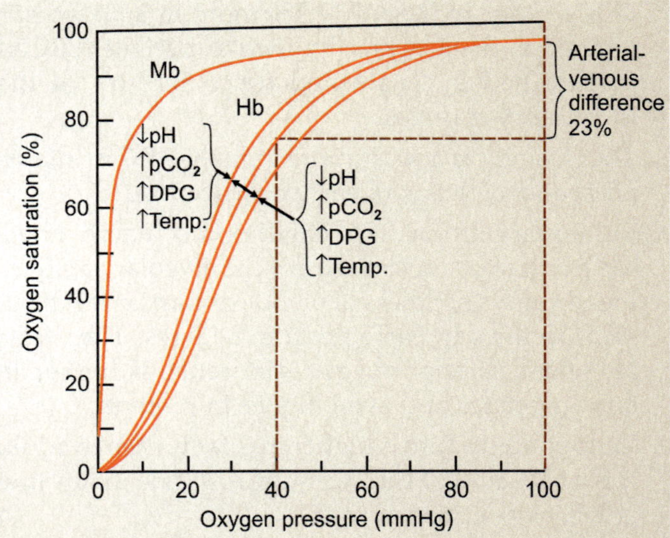

Fig. 4.6 Oxygen haemoglobin dissociation curve

increases the oxygen affinity of haemoglobin (Bohr effect) and shifts the oxygen-haemoglobin (O_2-Hb) dissociation curve to the left. Similarly, a decrease in temperature also increases oxygen affinity and shifts the O_2-Hb dissociation curve to the left; a decrease in pH or an increase in temperature has the opposite effect and the O_2-Hb curve shifts to the right.[33] Human erythrocytes contain an extremely high concentration of 2,3-DPG, averaging about 4.5 mol/mL, compared with ATP (1 mol/mL) and other organic phosphates.[33,34] Thus, an increase in red cell 2,3-DPG decreases the oxygen affinity of haemoglobin, increases P50 (shifts the dissociation curve to the right), and increases the unloading of oxygen at the tissue level. Increase in 2,3-DPG and P50 have been found in chronic hypoxemia.

In the newborn, blood oxygen affinity is extremely high and P50 is low (18 to 19 mmHg), because 2,3-DPG is low and foetal haemoglobin (HbF) reacts poorly with 2,3-DPG. Oxygen delivery at the tissue level is low despite high red blood cell mass and haemoglobin level. After birth, the total haemoglobin level decreases rapidly as the proportion of HbF diminishes, reaching its lowest level by 2 to 3 months of age (physiologic anaemia of infancy). During the same early postnatal period, P50 increases rapidly; it exceeds the normal adult value by 4 to 6 months of age and reaches the highest value (P50 = 30) by 10 months and remains high during the first decade of life.[28–30] This high P50 is associated with a relatively low haemoglobin level (10 to 11 g/dL) and an increased level of 2,3-DPG, probably related to the process of general growth and development and high plasma levels of inorganic phosphate.[34,35] These observations engendered a hypothesis to explain why haemoglobin levels are relatively lower in children than in adults (physiologic "anaemia" of childhood).[35] Because children have a lower oxygen affinity for haemoglobin, oxygen unloading at the tissue level is increased.

SUMMARY

1. Neonates and preterm babies are more prone for postoperative apnoea episodes. Risk of postoperative apnoea is less after 1 month of age in term and 60 weeks PCA in preterm babies.
2. Lung volume in early postnatal period is disproportionately small compared to body size. High metabolic rate due to higher oxygen consumption markedly increases ventilatory requirement per unit lung volume.
3. Type II pnemocytes forms alveolar lining and produces pulmonary surfactant. This cells appear as early as 20 WOG or in 24–26 WOG.
4. Periodic breathing and apnoea of prematurity should be diagnosed appropriately and treat appropriately.
5. Specific compliance of entire respiratory system declines in the childhood due to changes in the chest wall. Elastic recoil increases as the age advances.
6. Upper airway resistance consists of 65% of total airway resistance. If any occlusion or obstruction to the nasal airway increases, airway resistance by 50% leads to obstructive apnoea.

7. FRC further reduces 10–15% more in anaesthesia, apnoea and paralysis. In awake patient, FRC is maintained by sustained tonic activity of the inspiratory muscles.
8. The closing capacity is more than the FRC in infants and children leads to early airway closure.
9. Pulmonary diffusion in childhood is mainly affected by changes in surface area of alveolar capillary membrane. Thickness of blood gas barrier for diffusion declines in early gestational ages. Therefore, alvoeloar arterial oxygen difference is higher in term neonates and even higher in preterm.
10. Venous admixture is higher in infants than in adult. It is at 10–20% of cardiac output. While in adult, it is 2–5% of cardiac output.
11. In the newborn, blood oxygen affinity is extremely high and P50 is low (18 to 19 mmHg), because 2,3-DPG is low and foetal haemoglobin (HbF) reacts poorly with 2,3-DPG. Oxygen delivery at the tissue level is low despite high red blood cell mass and haemoglobin level.
12. Inhalation of warm air with 50% humidity maintains normal ciliary activity, whereas breathing dry air for 3 hours results in a complete cessation of mucus movement.

REFERENCES

1. Robert M Insoft, David I Todres. Growth and development. Charles J Cote, Jernold Lermon, David Todres. A practice of anaesthesia for infants and children. 4th edn. New York. Sounders Elsevier. 2009;27–33.
2. Etsuro K Motoyama, Jonathan D Finder. Respiratory physiology in infants and children. Peter J Davis, Franklyn P Clads, Etsuro Motoyama. Smith's Anaesthesia for infants and children. 8th edn. Philadelphia. Elsevier Mosby.
3. Garry H Mills. Respiratory physiology and anaesthesia. British Journal of anaesthesia. CEPD reviews. 2001;2: 35–39.
4. Fernand, Gregoire. Respiratry physiology in relation to anaesthesia. Canad Anaes Soc J. April 1955; 2(2):142–155.
5. Guyton Arthur C, Hall John E. Textbook of medical physiology, 11th edn.
6. Etsuro K Motoyama, Jonathan D Finder, Smith's Anaesthesia.
7. Rooney SA, Canavan PM, Motoyama EK. The identification of phosphatidyl glycerol in the rat, rabbit, monkey and human lung. Biochem Biophys Acta. 1974;360:56–67.
8. Lewis JF, Jobe AH. Surfactant and the adult respiratory distress syndrome. Am Rev Respir Dis. 1993;147: 218–233.
9. Rooney SA. The surfactant system and lung phospholipid biochemistry. Am Rev Respir Dis. 1985;131:439.
10. Kulovich MV, Hallman M, Cluck L. The lung profile. I. Normal pregnancy. Am J Obstet Gynecol. 1979; 135:57.
11. Suzuki M, Sasaki CT. Laryngeal spasm: a neurophysiologic redefinition. Ann Otol Rhinol Laryngol. 1977;86:150.
12. Rider ED, Ikegami M, Whitset JA, et al. Treatment responses to surfactants containing natural surfactant proteins in preterm rabbits. Am Rev Resir Dis. 1993; 147:669–676.
13. Jobe AH, Weaver TE. Developmental biology of surfactant.
14. Hallman M, Merritt TA, Akino K, et al. Surfactant protein A, phosphatidylcholine and surfactant inhibitors in epithelial lining fluid: correlation with surface activity, severity of respiratory distress syndrome, and outcome in small premature infants. Am Rev Respir Dis. 1991;144: 1376–1384.
15. Kikkawa Y, Motoyama EK, Cook CD. Ultrastructure of lungs of lambs; the relation of osmiophilic inclusions and alveolar lining layer to fetal maturation and experimentally produced respiratory distress. Am J Pathol. 1965;47:877.
16. Merritt TA, Hallman M, Bloom BT, et al. Prophylactic treatment of very premature infants with human surfactant. N Engl J Med 1986;315:785.
17. Hoekstra RE, Jackson JC, Myers TF, et al. Improved neonatal survival following multiple doses of bovine surfactant in very premature neonates at risk for respiratory distress syndrome. Pediatrics 1991;88:10.
18. Long WA, Corbet A, Cotton R, et al. A controlled trial of synthetic surfactant in infants weighing 1250 grams or more with the American Exosurf Neonatal Study Group I and the Canadian Exosurf Neonatal Study Group. N Engl J Med. 1991;325:1696.
19. Holms BA. Surfactant replacement therapy: new levels of understanding. Am Rev Respir Dis. 1993;148:834.
20. Jobe AH. Pulmonary surfactant therapy. N Engl J Med. 1993;328(12):861.
21. Pramanik AK, Holtzman RB, Merritt TA. Surfactant replacement therapy for pulmonary diseases. Pediatr Clin North Am. 1993;40:913.
22. Jeffery PK, Reid LM. The respiratory mucous membrane. In: Brain JD, Proctor DF, Reid LM, (Eds). Respiratory defense mechanisms, New York: Marcel.
23. Lichtiger M, Landa JF, Hirsch JA. Velocity of tracheal mucus in anesthetized women undergoing gynecologic surgery. Anesthesiology. 1975; 41:753.
24. Kilburn KH, Salzano JV, (Eds). Am Rev Respir Dis. 93. Symposium on structure, function and measurement of respiratory cilia, 1966;1.
25. Forbes AR. Temperature, humidity and mucous flow in the intubated trachea. Br J Anaesth. 1974;46:29.
26. Hirsch JA, Tokayer JL, Robinson MJ, et al. Effects of dry air and subsequent humidification on tracheal mucous velocity in dogs. J Appl Physiol. 1975;39:242.
27. Wolfe WG, Ebert PA, Sabiston DC. Effect of high oxygen tension on mucociliary function. Surgery 1972;72:246.

28. Forbes AR. Halothane depresses mucociliary flow in the trachea. Anesthesiology. 1976;45:59.
29. Forbes AR, Gamsu G. Lung mucociliary clearance after anesthesia and spontaneous and controlled ventilation. Am Rev Respir Dis. 1979;120:857.
30. Forbes AR, Horrigan RW. Mucociliary flow in the trachea during anesthesia with enflurane, ether, nitrous oxide, and morphine. Anesthesiology 1977;46:319.
31. Comroe JH. Physiology of respiration: An introductory text, 2nd edn. Chicago, Year Book Medical, 1974.
32. Oski FA, Delivoria-Papadopoulos M. The red cell, 2,3-diphosphoglycerate, and tissue oxygen release. J Pediatr. 1970;77:941.
33. Oski F.A. Designation of anemia on a functional basis. J Pediatr. 1973(a);83:353.
34. Oski FA. The unique fetal red cell and its function. Pediatrics. 1973(b);51:494.
35. Card RT, Brain MC. The "anemia" of childhood: evidence for a physiologic response to hyperphosphatemia. N Engl J Med. 1973;288:388.

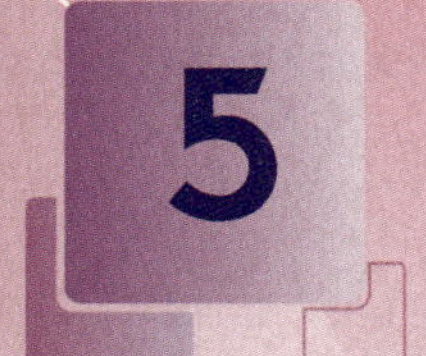

Essentials of Central Nervous System in Infants and Children

Shrikanta P Oak and Anjana S Wajekar

INTRODUCTION

The central nervous system in the infants is immature and differs from older children and adult in several ways. Normal mental development depends on maturation of the central nervous system.

Embrology

Almost the whole of central nervous system is derived from the ectoderm.[1] The neural tube in the foetus has an enlarged cranial part which forms the brain and a narrow caudal part that becomes the spinal cord. The cranial part divides into:

1. Procencephalon (Forebrain): It forms the cerebral cortices, thalamus, hypothalamus and basal ganglia.
2. Mesencephalon (Midbrain): It develops into the midbrain.
3. Rhombencephalon (Hindbrain): It is a precursor of the cerebellum, pons and medulla.

The rest of the neural tube forms the spinal cord. The ventricles arise from the central canal of the neural tube.

Development occurs in three stages: Cytogenesis, histogenesis and organogenesis. The final composition and shape of the nervous system is determined by organogenesis.

Gross Anatomy

Brain weight:

- At birth: 330 to 350 g (10–15% of body weight).
- >12 years–adult: (1200–1400 g approximately 2% of body weight).

The brain doubles in size in the first year and reaches 80% of adult weight by the age of two.[2]

It is encased in a bony cranium.

Proportion of cranial contents in a child:

1. 80% brain parenchyma—It is made up by the neurons, their supporting glia and the interstitium.
2. 10% cerebrospinal fluid
3. 10% blood

The Monro-Kellie hypothesis states that the sum of the intracranial volumes of blood, brain and CSF is constant.

NEURAL DEVELOPMENT

The nervous system develops over a very long period of time extending from the embryonic period through puberty, with some remodelling continuing throughout lifetime.

There are five steps that make up brain development.

1. **Neurogenesis:** It is the process of differentiation of embryonic cells into neurons. It occurs largely in the foetal period.
2. **Neural migration**: The organization of the brain proceeds with migration of these neurons according to their function in particular areas of the brain. It extends from prenatal period to at least 8 to 10 months post-natally.
3. **Myelination**: It involves encasing the axon of the neuron in myelin, which is an electrically insulating material. Schwann cells supply the myelin for peripheral neurons, whereas oligodendrocytes myelinate the axons of the central nervous system. In humans, myelination begins in the 14th week of foetal development, mainly in brainstem and cerebellum, although a little myelin exists in the

brain at the time of birth.[2] During infancy, myelination occurs quickly and continues through the adolescent stages of life. Developmentally it occurs first in the peripheral nervous system spreading centripetally to spinal cord and lastly the brain with some nerves never getting myelinated. It is the major cause of the increase in a child's brain size.

Myelination is generally finished before major neural pathways become completely functional.

Also composition of the myelin in the immature brain is a transitional form differing from the adult myelin.[3] Myelination doesn't entirely encase a nerve leaving nodes of Ranvier at regular intervals which are the site of sodium channels. Breast feeding increases the speed of myelination in the brain.

Functions:

a. Speed of nerve conductions increases with development of nodes of Ranvier. Myelinated fibres succeed in reducing sodium leakage into the extracellular fluid (ECF) helping in agile communication.
b. The myelin sheath provides a track along which regrowth can occur in the event of nerve severance.

Incomplete myelination of nerve tissue in neonates and infants contribute to shorter onset times of local anaesthetics and allows effective blockade with very low concentrations of local anaesthetic solutions.

It is also responsible for variation in waveform morphology during neurophysiologic monitoring.

While **SSEPs** may show blunted peaks with delayed latencies, D waves of MEPs will not be reliable in children <2 years of age.[4] Proper adjustment of stimulus is needed in such cases. Also, MEP monitoring can be done only with TIVA.

4. **Synaptogenesis:** Synapses interconnect the various neurons leading to the functional organisation of the brain. Synapses begin forming prenatally continuing throughout life.
5. **Pruning:** It refines existing useful connections and eliminates unused connections. The most rapid pruning occurs between ages 3 and 16, occurring in different areas of brain.

Pruning helps to play a role in synaptic re-modelling throughout life depending on experience and environmental stimuli.

> **Paediatric Anaesthesia Pearls**
> - Incomplete myelination of nerve tissue in neonates and infants contribute to shorter onset times of local anaesthetics and allows effective blockade with very low concentrations of local anaesthetic solutions.
> - It is also responsible for variation in waveform morphology during neurophysiologic monitoring.

DEVELOPMENT OF BLOOD–BRAIN BARRIER

The blood–brain barrier (BBB) is a highly selective, permeable barrier that separates the circulating blood from the brain extracellular fluid (BECF). Development of blood–brain barrier is incomplete in newborns and infants and continues throughout childhood. It is a functional neurovascular unit composed of the capillary endothelium with basement membrane, astrocytes, pericytes, and extracellular matrix. These are connected by tight junctions (TJ) such as zonula occludens-1 (ZO-1) and claudin-5 (cl 5).

It is deficient in the circumventricular organs, the roof of the third and fourth ventricles, capillaries in the pineal gland, on the roof of the diencephalon and the pineal gland.

Transport Across Blood–brain Barrier[5]

1. Passive diffusion: For example, water, some gases and lipid soluble molecules. Bilirubin, opioids and barbiturates all cross freely into the CNS in infants across blood–brain barrier.
2. Carrier-mediated transporters: e.g. glucose and amino acids.
3. Active efflux transporters such as P-glycoprotein: e.g. some drugs, toxic metabolites, potential neurotoxins
4. Receptor-mediated transcytosis systems.

The blood–brain barrier is unique in that the interstitial osmotic pressure is the determinant of the Starling force in central nervous system.The oncotic pressure is not significant as proteinsand other colloidscannot cross the impermeable blood–brain barrier. According to Pascal's principle, the interstitial fluid pressure in the brain is equal to the intracranial pressure.

Functions of the Blood–brain Barrier

1. To protect the brain from many common bacterial infections
2. Restricts large or hydrophilic molecules into the cerebrospinal fluid (CSF), while allowing the diffusion of small hydrophobic molecules (O_2, CO_2, hormones).

Disruption of the Blood–brain Barrier

A variety of brain insults result in blood–brain barrier disruption including:

1. Traumatic brain injury (TBI),
2. Ischaemic stroke,
3. Intracerebral haemorrhage,
4. Primary and metastatic neoplasms,
5. Infectious diseases (meningitis, ventriculitis, and cerebral abscess),
6. Severe toxic–metabolic derangements (encephalopathy, liver failure).

Although the initial insults to the brain in various pathologies are quite different, there is a common final pathway in the form of disruption of above transport mechanisms resulting in loss of blood–brain barrier integrity.[6]

Pathophysiological Significance of Disruption

1. Blood–brain barrier breakdown endangers the homeostatic control of the cerebral interstitium.
2. Disruption of blood–brain barrier leads to 'vasogenic' oedema in the interstitial space resulting in reduction of the cerebral compliance and increased intracranial pressure.

   This vasogenic oedema from tumour vasculature develops gradually. Tumour oedema leaks from developing vessels that lack some of the typical blood–brain barrier features.
3. With blood–brain barrier disruption, substances present in the plasma come in contact with parenchymal structures. For example, glutamate, a cerebral excitotoxin, has plasma concentration 5–10 times more than found in cerebrospinal fluid. Infusion of amino acid solutions containing glutamate, can double plasma glutamate, and should be used with caution in patients with an open blood–brain barrier.

Almost all general anaesthetic agents can alter the blood–brain barrier function but the degree of the blood–brain barrier disruption is less during isoflurane-anaesthesia as compared to pentobarbital anaesthesia.[5]

Factors Affecting CNS Penetration of Drugs

1. **Lipophilic analogues:** A drug's lipophilicity correlates strongly with BBB permeability. For example, diamorphine, a diacyl derivative of morphine, crosses the blood–brain barrier 100 times more easily than its parent drug just because it is more lipophilic.
2. **Prodrug:** Lipophilic prodrugs may easily cross blood–brain barrier bringing the hydrophilic active form closer to receptor site but it may also increase the systemic tissue absorption, thereby increasing its side effects. For example, steroids and cytotoxic agents.
3. **Carrier and receptor mediated transport:** Non-transportable drugs can be conjugated with carriers for transport across blood–brain barrier by trans-cytosis at the receptor sites. This technology is being used for peptide based pharmaceuticals such as neurotrophins and small molecules incorporated within liposomes. In spite of this, effectiveness of this technique is under investigation.
4. **Transient disruption** with chemical or hyperosmotic agents (egmannitol, etc.) can be used a route for drug delivery like antineoplastic agents as treatment modalities. This treatment is still investigational.

Paediatric Anaesthesia Pearl

- The interstitial osmotic pressure is the determinant of the Starling force in central nervous system.
- Disruption of blood–brain barrier leads to 'vasogenic' oedema in the interstitial space resulting in reduction of the cerebral compliance and increased intracranial pressure.

Cerebral Oedema

Types

1. **Vasogenic oedema:** It is caused by the breakdown of blood–brain barrier or blood–CSF barrier resulting into an exudative oedema in the interstitium. The spread of this can be quite rapid and extensive. Tumour cells can produce vascular endothelial growth factor (VEGF) which can cause disruption of blood–brain barrier. Dexamethasone helps reduce VEGF secretion, thereby reducing cerebral oedema.
2. **Cytotoxic oedema:** This is the intracellular oedema in the neuronal or glial cells occurring secondary to cerebral ischemia or trauma. The blood–brain barrier is intact but the sodium–potassium pump is impaired in the cell membranes leading to retention of sodium and water intracellularly. It is generally focal but if it spreads, the prognosis is very poor.

Generally, both vasogenic and cytotoxic oedema occur together. Cytotoxic oedema occurs initially after the primary insult followed by the vasogenic oedema which may last for days or longer.

Other classification can be according to cause—osmotic, hyperemic, interstitial, etc.

Resolution of Cerebral Oedema

1. Vasogenic oedema resolves partially by drainage of fluid into CSF depending on pressure gradient between brain tissue and CSF.
2. Brain ECF proteins are cleared by glial uptake, thus helping to reduce oedema.

Central Nervous System Physiology

Specific data on cerebral blood flow (CBF) in human infants and children are rare and hence many anaesthetic principles must be inferred from the data in animals and adult humans.

The cerebral blood flow is 10 to 20% of the cardiac output in the first six months of life, increasing up to 55% from 2nd to 4th year and again reaching the adult levels of 15% by 7 to 8 years.[7]

Cerebral Blood Flow (CBF)

- **Adult:** 50 mL/100 g of brain tissue per min—gray matter–80% and white matter–20%.
- **Premature and newborn infants:** 30–40 mL/100 g per min
- **Infants and older children** 65–85 mL/100 g per min.[8,9]

Cerebral Metabolic Rate of Oxygen ($CMRO_2$) Consumption

- **Adult:** 3–4 mL/100 g per min.
- **Child:** 5 mL/100 g per min

CBF and $CMRO_2$ are directly proportional. Increased $CMRO_2$ (seizures or fever) increases CBF and decrease in $CMRO_2$ (hypothermia and barbiturate) decreases CBF.[10]

CBF also depends on[11]

1. **Cerebral perfusion pressure** (CPP)

$$CPP = MAP - \frac{CVP}{ICP}$$

Cerebral blood vessels dilate at lower MAP and constrict at higher MAP, thus maintaining the cerebral perfusion pressure in the range varying between 50 and 150 mmHg in adults. This is autoregulation. This may take up to 2 minutes to occur. Because MAP in infants are often < 60 mmHg, autoregulatory limits are as low as 20 mmHg and upper limit is not known.[7]

Also, this autoregulation is impaired in premature neonates.

Their cerebral blood vessels are at risk of rupture due to varied reasons, increased blood pressure being commonest, especially in the region of the germinal matrix leading to intracerebral and intraventricular haemorrhage. Due to this low autoregulatory reserve, low blood pressure may cause cerebral ischemia. With increasing gestational age, the germinal matrix involutes and the risk of bleeding decreases. Hence maintenance of blood pressure in this narrow range is essential to prevent cerebral ischaemia and intraventricular haemorrhage.

Autoregulation is attenuated by hypercapnia, hypoxia, high concentrations of volatile agents, nitroprusside and trauma. In local areas around brain tumours and focal cerebral ischaemia, autoregulation is lost and perfusion is pressure dependent.

The lower limit of autoregulation is lower with drug induced hypotension than during hypovolemic hypotension.

2. **$PaCO_2$:** Increase in $PaCO_2$ dilates the cerebral vessels linearly and vice versa between 20 and 80 mmHg so that a 4% change in CBF occurs for each 1 mmHg change in $PaCO_2$ in this range. Outside this range, > 80 mmHg vessels are maximally dilated and < 20 mmHg causes ischaemia induced metabolic changes which override the changes to $PaCO_2$. These responses are not completely developed at birth.
3. **PaO_2:** In adults, this is less sensitive. Foetal and neonatal circulation responds to small changes in PaO_2 perhaps due to high O_2 affinity of foetal haemoglobin. The age at which this heightened responsiveness decreases is not known.
4. **Haematocrit:** Adult > 50% increases viscosity and decreases CBF, < 30% increases CBF
5. **Body temperature:** $CMRO_2$ and CBF reduced by hypothermia.

Paediatric Anaesthesia Pearl

- Cerebral perfusion pressure (CPP) = MAP – (Cerebral) CVP/ICP.
- The MAP in infants is often <60 mmHg, autoregulatory limits are as low as 20 mmHg and upper limit is not known.
- The premature neonates are at an increased risk of intracerebral and intraventricular haemorrhage.
- Responsiveness of cerebral circulation to $PaCO_2$ is not developed in infants.

Intracranial Pressure (ICP)

The intracranial pressure is determined by the volume of the intracranial contents. According to the Monro-Kellie doctrine, the intracranial volume remains constant. An increase in volume of any one component will result in a decrease in volume of other two components. CSF and cerebrovascular compartment are the adaptable components. After the intracranial compliance (the change in volume for a given change in pressure) is exhausted, the intracranial pressure (ICP) will rise exponentially. In infants due to open sutures, the rise in intracranial pressure will be further compensated.

Age group	Normal range of ICP (mmHg)
Adult	<10–15
Children	3–7
Term infants	1.5–6

At birth, the sutures are open and there is a large anterior fontanelle, which closes by 9–18 months approximately. Palpation of the anterior fontanelle can be used to evaluate intracranial pressure in neonates and infants. Increasing intracranial pressure is partly relieved by expansion of the fontanelles and separation of the suture lines so that head size increases before intracranial pressure rises. A transducer placed on the anterior fontanelle is a non-invasive technique of intracranial pressure monitoring in infants.

The brain is divided into different compartments by dural projections like falxcerebri and tentorium cerebelli. Rise in intracranial pressure can cause shift in these compartments. The three types of intracranial herniation are transtentorial, tonsillar and subfalcine.[12]

Paediatric Anaesthesia Pearl

Increasing intracranial pressure is partly relieved by expansion of the fontanelles and separation of the suture lines so that head size increases before intracranial pressure rises in infants.

DEVELOPMENT OF CSF CIRCULATION AND VOLUME

Cerebrospinal fluid is an ultrafiltrate of plasma. The choroid plexus epithelial cells constitute the blood—CSF barrier.

Cerebrospinal fluid aspects

CSF pressure [mm of Hg]	
Child	3–7.5
Adult	4.5–13.5
CSF volume [mL]	
Infants	40–60
Young children	60–100
Older children	80–120
Adults	100–160

CSF Formation and Circulation

Production

CSF is formed in the capillary lining of the choroid plexus in the two lateral cerebral ventricles (2/3rd) and also the capillary endothelial cells of the third and fourth ventricles (1/3rd).

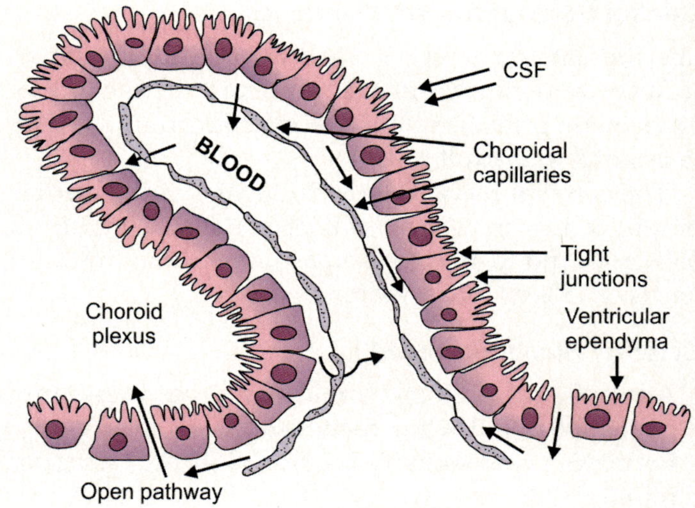

Pathway

The CSF produced in lateral ventricles drains through the two foramen of Munroe into the third ventricle and through the aqueduct of sylvius into the fourth ventricle. Most of the CSF drains through the two lateral Foramen of Luschka and the central foramen of Magendie into the subarachnoid space surrounding the brain and spinal cord. A small proportion of CSF flows from the 4th ventricle into the central canal of the spinal cord.

Absorption

In adults and older children, CSF absorbed by the arachnoid villi in the dural venous sinuses especially the sagittal dural sinus. In neonates the arachnoid villi are not fully developed and absorption also occurs into the paranasal sinuses, lymphatics along the cranial nerves and lymphatics of the nose.[13]

CSF Formation

1. Rate at 0.35–0.40 mL/min or 500–600 mL/day
2. 0.25% of total volume replaced each minute
3. Turn over time for total CSF volume: 5–7 hours = 4 times/day
4. 40–70% enters macroscopic spaces
5. 30–60% enters across ependyma and pia.

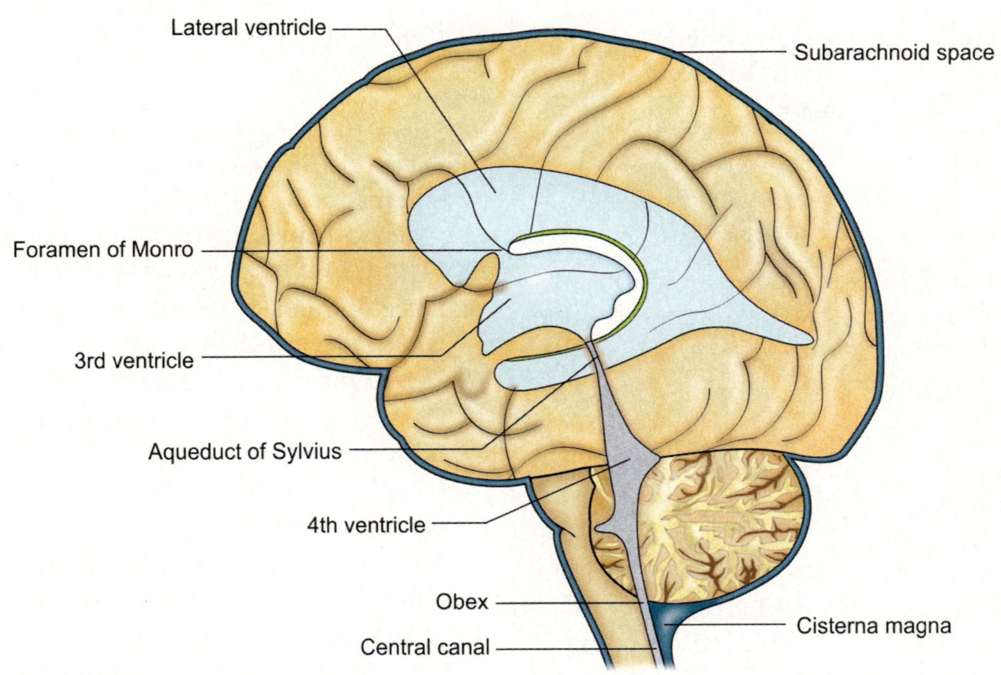

CSF Composition

	Plasma	CSF
Sodium (nM)	140	141
Potassium (nM)	4.6	2.9
Magnesium (nM)	1.7	2.4
Calcium (nM)	5.0	2.5
Chloride (nM)	101	124
Bicarbonate (nM)	23	21
Glucose (nM)	92	61
Amino acids (nM)	2.3	0.8
pH	7.41	7.31
Osmolality (mosm/kg water)	289	289
Protein (mg/dl)	7000	28
Specific gravity	1.025	1.007

Functions of CSF

1. The low specific gravity of CSF (1.007) relative to that of the brain (1.040) reduces the effective mass of a 1400 g brain to only 47 g. It also acts as a shock absorber.
2. It is a source of nutrients, primarily glucose, vitamins, monosaccharides and amino acids.
3. Control of the chemical environment by removal of metabolic products and unwanted drugs.

Paediatric Anaesthesia Pearl

- Rate of CSF production is 0.35–0.40 mL/min or 500–600 mL/day.

Development of Spinal Cord

Anatomic relationships and landmarks are constantly changing throughout infancy and childhood, which requires a good knowledge of developmental anatomy of the spinal cord.[14,15]

Sl. No.	Anatomy and physiology	Anaesthetic implications
1.	Termination of spinal cord. S1 at 28 weeks' gestation, L3 at term, L2/3 at 1 year, and the adult level of L1/L2 around the age of 8 years.	Neuraxial blocks below L3 only in infants.
2.	Dural sac termination S4 at birth and S2 by 12 months	Neuraxial blocks below L3 up to S2 only in infants.
3.	Delayed myelination of nerve fibres	Diluted local anaesthetic to be used. Onset faster but duration shorter.
4.	Curvatures of spinal cord Cervical lordosis: 3–6 months Lumbar lordosis: 6–9 months	Orientation of epidural/spinal needle important

Contd...

Sl. No.	Anatomy and physiology	Anaesthetic implications
5.	Incomplete ossification of sacral vertebra posteriorly	Lower sacral epidural/caudal approaches preferred in children
6.	Intercristal line (line joining two iliac crests) L5–S1 at birth, L5 in young children and L3–4 in adult	Neuraxial blocks below intercristal line in infants.
7.	CSF circulation Volume: 4 mL/kg, double of adult ½ of it in spinal space unlike adult (1/4th)	Pharmacokinetics of intrathecal drugs differ. Short duration of action, e.g. half life of Bupivacaine–45 minutes in neonates and 75–90 minutes till 5 years.
8.	Spinal fluid hydrostatic pressure 30–40 mmH_2O in horizontal position	No need for cervical flexion in lateral position for lumbar puncture. In fact, it may obstruct the airway.
9.	Immature sympathetic system up to 5 years	Fluid preloading and vasopressors drugs unnecessary. Spinal block preferred in critically ill and moribund neonates.
10.	Immature hepatic metabolism and reduced plasma proteins	Increased risk of local anaesthetic toxicity
11.	Loculated epidural fat	Threading of sacral catheter up to thoracic levels difficult.

Paediatric Anaesthesia Pearls

- The spinal cord ends at L3 level at term.
- The volume of cerebrospinal fluid CSF is 4 mL/kg which is double the adult volume.
- In infants half of this volume is in the spinal space, whereas adults have only one-fourth.
- The spinal fluid hydrostatic pressure of 30–40 mm H_2O in horizontal position is much less than that in adults.

Impact of maternal anaesthesia for non-obstetric surgery and foetal surgeries on foetal neurodevelopment.

Substantial foetal neurodevelopment takes place in the second trimester of pregnancy. The foetal neuroendocrine response to noxious stimuli also develops in the second trimester. Certain important developments occurring in the second trimester include:

1. Development of peripheral nerve receptor: 7 to 20 weeks of gestation.
2. Development of C fibres: 8 to 30 weeks of gestation.
3. Development of spinothalamic tract: 16 to 20 weeks of gestation.
4. Development of thalamocortical fibres: 17 to 24 weeks of gestation.
5. Response to pain and foetal stress: In response to painful stimuli, vigorous movements and breathing efforts with increase in levels of cortisol, norepinehrine and beta endorphinsare seen. Also there is no evidence of placental transfer of norepinephrine to foetus, thus proving that independent stress response exists since 18th week of gestation.[16,17]

In this scenario, foetal anaesthesia and analgesia require an independent and important consideration during maternal and foetal surgeries. In the absence of these there may be a significant modulation in development of foetal nervous system leading to altered pain sensitivity such as hyperalgesia.

Paediatric Anaesthesia Pearl

Foetal anaesthesia and analgesia during maternal surgeries is essential since it has been proved that independent stress response develops in foetus in second trimester.

ANAESTHETIC NEUROTOXICITY

Apoptosis is a normal part of the developmental process in the body responsible for remodelling of the architecture of the entire body including the central nervous system.

All commonly used anaesthetic agents like inhalational agents, diazepam, midazolam, pentobarbital, propofol, ketamine, etc. in vivo and in vitro animal studies have found to dramatically accelerate the physiologic apoptosis in the immature brain, altered synapse formation, mitochondrial dysfunction, altered calcium homeostasis leading to neuronal cell death. Immature neurons have GABA and NMDA receptors, which is one of the paths of neurotoxicity in the developing brain. It may be dose and exposure-time related. It is unclear whether this neuro-apoptosis translates into permanent cell loss and dysfunction or is compensated by the developing brain's ability to repair. Various animal studies have found differential effects on the neurocognitive outcomes like impaired learning, memory, behaviour, etc. The possibility of these changes also occurring in humans cannot be ignored and further studies are required for their evaluation. Also, different regions of the immature brain are affected depending on the peak time of neurogenesis in that part. Since apoptosis is a lifelong phenomenon, not only neonates but also older children and adults may show this anaesthetic neurotoxicity leading to increased incidences of postoperative cognitive dysfunction.[16,18]

Paediatric Anaesthesia Pearl

There is growing evidence that exposure of general anaesthetic agents to the growing brain of the child can lead to neuronal apoptosis and long term cognitive impairment.

SUMMARY

The practice of paediatric neuro-anaesthesia encompasses understanding and application of these differences in the anatomic and physiologic mechanisms and their effect on anaesthesia management.

FAQ with Answer

Q. What is the impact of chemical sympathectomy after spinal anaesthesia in children and role of preloading with fluid?

A. The physiological impact of sympathectomy is minimal or none in smaller age groups. The fall in blood pressure and a drop in the heart rate are practically not seen in children less than five years. Therefore there is no role of preloading with fluids before a subarachnoid block.[7]

Key Points

1. Children differ from adults in brain and spinal cord development both anatomically and physiologically. They havedelayed myelination, immature neural pathway development and blood–brain barrier, cerebral blood flow and spinal architecture. These changes affect our anaesthesia management.
2. Delayed myelination in infants contributes to shorter onset times of local anaesthetics and variation in waveform morphology during neurophysiologic monitoring.

Contd...

Key Points *(Contd...)*

3. The premature neonates are at an increased risk of intra-cerebral and intraventricular haemorrhage.
4. Techniques of neuraxial regional anaesthesia in paediatric anaesthesia necessitate understanding the anatomical and physiologic differences between children and adults. The spinal cord ends at L3 at birth.
5. Foetal anaesthesia and analgesia for maternal surgeries for non-obstetric or foetal surgeries are important for foetal neural structural development and cognitive functions.
6. There is a growing evidence that exposure of general anaesthetic agents to the growing brain of the child can lead to neuronal apoptosis and long-term cognitive impairment.

REFERENCES

1. Singh I. Spinal Cord; Cerebellar Cortex. In: Singh I, (Ed). Textbook of Human Histology, 6th edn. New Delhi: Jaypee Brothers Medical Publishers Ltd.; 2011;366–72.
2. Crean P, Peake D. Essentials of neurology and neuromuscular disorders. In: Cote CJ, (Ed). A Practice of Anaesthesia for Infants and Children, 5th edn. Philadelphia: Elsevier Saunders; 2013;475–90.
3. Quarles RH, Macklin WB, Morell P. Myelin formation, structure and biochemistry. In: Siegel G, (Ed): Basic Neurochemistry: Molecular, Cellular and Medical Aspects, 7th edn. California: Elsevier, Inc. 2006;51–72.
4. Glover CD, Carling NP. Neuromonitoring for scoliosis surgery. Anesthesiology Clinics. 2014; 32:101–114.
5. Tanobe K, Nishikawa K, Hinohara H, et al. Blood-brain barrier and general anesthetics. Masui. 2003;52:840–5.
6. Keep RF, Zhou N, Xiang J, et al. Vascular disruption and blood–brain barrier dysfunction in intracerebral hemorrhage. Fluids Barriers CNS. 2014;11:18.
7. Yungfang JH, Krass IS. Physiology and metabolism of brain and spinal cord. In: Newfield P, Cottrell JE, (Eds): Handbook of Neuroanaesthesia. Philadelphia: Lippincott Williams and Wilkins. 2007;120.
8. Vavilala MS, Soriano SG. Anaesthesia for neurosurgery. In: Peter Davis, (Ed). Smith's Anaesthesia for Infants and Children, 8th edn. Philadelphia: Elsevier Saunders. 2011;713–44.
9. Greisen G. Cerebral blood flow in preterm infants during the first week of life. Acta Paediatr Scand 1986;75:43–51.
10. Kennedy C, Sokoloff L. An adaptation of the nitrous oxide method to the study of the cerebral circulation in children; normal values for cerebral blood flow and cerebral metabolic rate in childhood. J Clin Invest. 1957;36:113–7.
11. Chiron C, Raynaud C, Maziére B, et al. Changes in regional cerebral blood flow during brain maturation in children and adolescents. J Nucl Med. 1992;33:696–703.

12. Dunn LT. Raised intracranial pressure. J Neurol Neurosurg Psychiatry. 2002;73(Suppl I):i23–i27.
13. Mack J, Squier W, Eastman JT. Anatomy and development of the meninges: Implications for subdural collections and CSF circulation. Pediatr Radiol. 2009;39:200–10.
14. Dalens BJ. Regional anaesthesia in children. In: Miller RD (Ed). Miller's Anaesthesia, 7th edn. Philadelphia: Churchill Livingstone Elsevier. 2007;p. 2519–21.
15. Goyal R, Jinjil K, Baj B, et al. Paediatric spinal anaesthesia. Indian Journal of Anaesthesia. 2008;52:264–270.
16. Palanisamy A. Maternal anaesthesia and fetal neurodevelopment. Int J Obstet Anesth. 2012;21:152–62.
17. Gupta R, Kilby M, Cooper G. Fetal surgery and anaesthetic implications. Continuing Education in Anaesthesia, Critical Care and Pain. 2008;8(2).
18. Lin EP, Soriano SG, Loepke AW. Anesthetic neurotoxicity. Anesthesiology Clinics. 2014;32:133–156.

6 Essentials of Liver Functions, Kidney Functions and GI and Endocrine System

Ashish Mali

RENAL SYSTEM

The renal system deals with water excretion and reabsorption according to body requirements, meeting severe fluid challenges.

Embryological the urinary and genital systems develop very closely as they both develop from common mesodermal ridge.

During the intrauterine life three overlapping kidney systems are formed in cranial to caudal sequence.

1. Pronephros: First system which is rudimentary and non-functional.
2. Mesonephros: Second system which may be functional for short span during early foetal period.
3. Metanephros: Third system which forms the permanent kidney.

Pronephros: This is represented as seven to ten solid cell groups in the cervical region at the fourth gestational weeks. These are vestigial excretory units called nepherotomes and regress before more caudal ones are formed. The pronephric system disappears by the end of fourth week.

Mesonephros: As the pronephric system regresses early in the fourth week of development, the intermediate mesoderm from the upper thoracic and upper lumbar segments forms the mesonephros and mesonephric duct.

During this time there is appearance of the first excretory tubule of the mesonephros. These tubules then lengthen taking S-shaped loop pattern tuft of capillaries is acquired at their medial extremity forming a

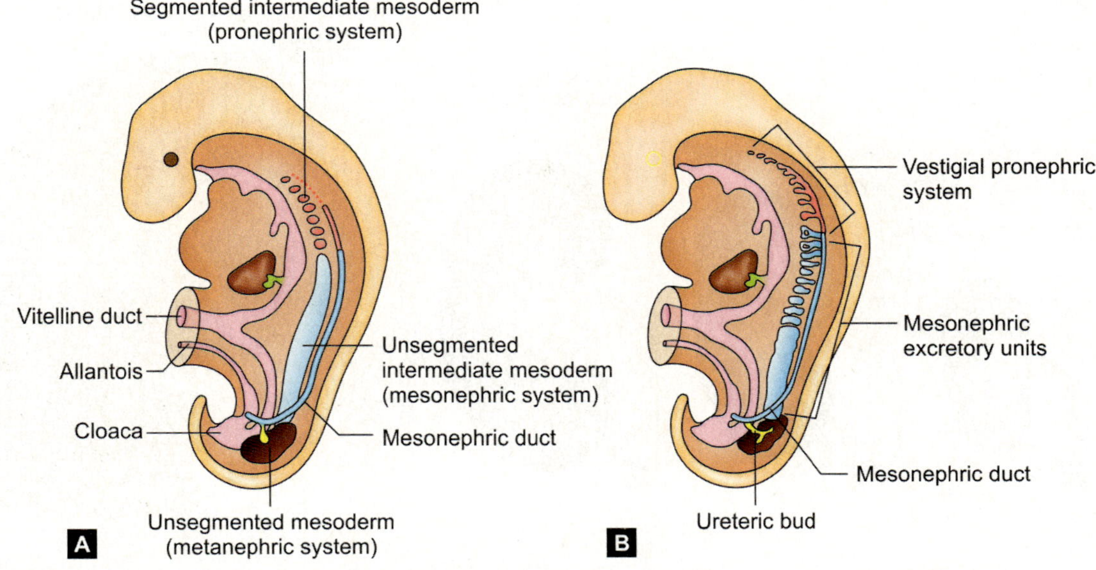

Fig. 6.1A and B Pronephric, Mesonephric and Metanephric system in the initial **(A)** and later stage **(B)**

glomerulus. The tubules then form Bowmen's capsule around the glomerules, these structures collectively constitute the renal corpuscle. The lateral end of the tubule enters the longitudinal collecting ducts called the Wolffian or the Mesonephric duct. Somewhere around the middle of the second month two ovoid shaped organs are developed on each side of the midline by the Mesonephros known as urogenital ridges. As the development proceeds, the differentiation of the tubules start towards the caudal end and degenerative changes starts at the cranial tubules. These changes are so done that by the end of second month majority of these disappears. Some caudal tubules and mesonephric ducts may persists in males but in females they totally disappear.

Metanephros: This is definitive kidney (permanent kidney), which appears in the fifth week. The excretory units of this develop from metanephric mesoderm as it has developed from the mesonephic system.The ureter, pelvic part of ureter and collecting system develops from the ureteric bud as a outgrowth of the mesonephric duct just before it enters the cloacae. The caudal extension of the nephrogenic cords forms the metanephrogenic mass which then forms the excretory system. The ureteric bud penetrates the metanephrogenic tissue that covers the bud as a cap. The ureteric bud differentiates repeatedly to form the ureter, renal pelvis, major calyces, minor calyces, papillary ducts and the collecting tubules which all contribute to make the collecting system.

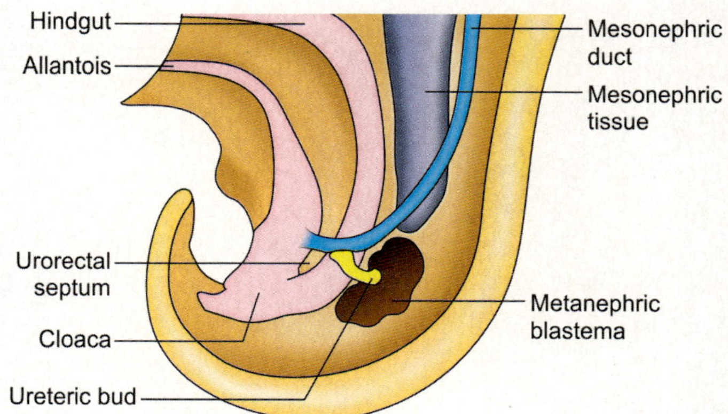

Fig. 6.2 5th week relation of cloaca and hindgut. Note the ureteric bud penetrating the metanephric mesoderm

The collecting tubules induce the metanephic tissue to differentiate and divide so that each tubule is covered by a small tissue of metanephic tissue. This association results in the formation of the renal vesicle which indeed transforms into small tubules that forms the nephon (excreatory unit). The tubule on one end joins a vascular tuft to form the glomerulus, while the other end joins the collecting system.

The end that has the vascular relay forms the Bowman's capsule. The tubule from the Bowman's capsule continues to lengthen and differentiate to form the proximal convoluted tubule, loop of Henle and the distal convoluted tubule. All this continuous till the 34th week of gestation.

The development and distribution is such that the most recently formed nephorns are at the outer cortex

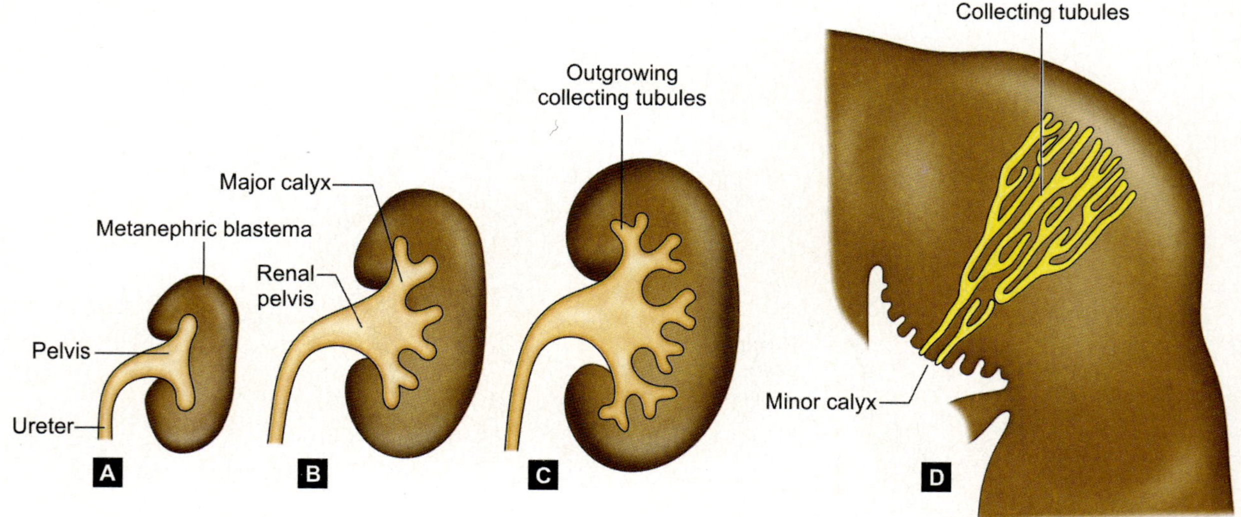

Fig. 6.3A to D Development of pelvic calycial system. (A) 6 weeks, (B) end of 6th weeks, (C) 7th week and (D) newborn

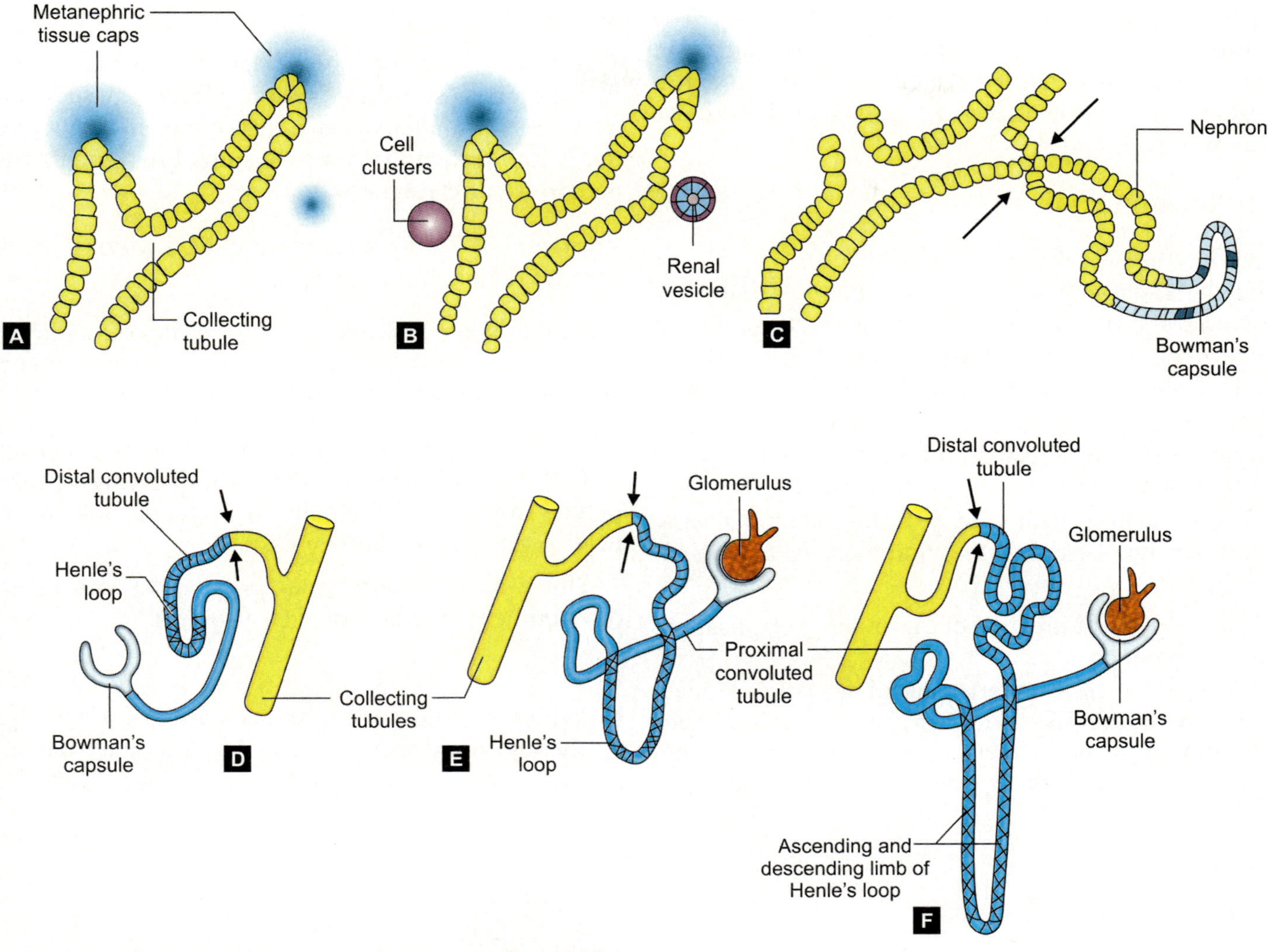

Fig. 6.4A to F Development of excretory unit of the metanephric system

and are called cortical nephorns, while the older nephorns are near the medulla and are called juxtra medullary nephorns, ratio being (8 : 1). In immature newborns (34th weeks) both these are anatomically and functionally different. Regarding the infant status in the uterus, the formation of nephrons does not accerate and is completed at 34th week.

After 34 weeks the increase in the size of the kidney is more due to enlargement and growth of the nephorns rather than formation of new nephorns. Though the renal system develops in cephalo caudal direction, the permanent kidney migrates in the cepaloid direction due to marked growth and development in the lumbar and sacral region and degree of body curvature of the foetus. At 8 weeks it is at the level of 2nd lumbar vertebra. The kidneys also rotate by 90 degrees so that the initially ventrally facing hilum becomes medially placed.

Key Points

Three renal systems come in the development in sequence: Pronephros, mesonephors and metanephros.

Pearls

Metanephros is permanent and definitive kidney.

Foetal Urine

The permanent kidneys produce urine by the ninth week, the time approximately when the ureter opens in the bladder. The development proceeds so that the loop of Henle and tubular re-absorption is started by 14th week. As contrast to adults in foetal life, the placenta does the work of excretion of waste material. The urine contributing to the amniotic fluid acts as a cushion for the foetus and is also necessary for the normal growth and development of the lung. It is a hypotonic solution without sugars and proteins. The foetus starts swallowing the amniotic fluid by 20th week which then is absorbed by the GI tract and through it into the vascular system. It is then filtered by the kidneys and excreted in the urine.

ABNORMALITIES[1]

- Wilms' tumor: Cancer of the kidneys
- Renal dysplasia or agenesis: Transplant or dialysis
- Multicystic dysplasias: Numerous ducts surround undiffentiated cells, nephrons fail to develop, collecting ducts are never formed as ureteric bud fails to branch.
- Renal agenesis: Interaction between metanephric mesoderm and ureteric bud fails to occur.
- Congenital polycystic kidney: Kidney contains many cysts. It may be autosomal dominant or autosomal recessive.

There may be bifurcation of the ureter or duplication, ectopic openings.

Kidneys may have abnormal location—pelvic kidney, near the common iliac artery in the pelvis. The lower pole may be fused to form horseshoe shape kidney. Accessory renal arteries are also not uncommon.

SUMMARY

The development of the urinary system is from the mesodermal tissue. Three systems develop in sequence from cranial to caudal part, out of which 1st two are temporary (**Pronephros and Mesonephros**) and the last is permanent (**Metanephros**).

Pronephros: Comparatively small, develops in the cervical region, but is vestigial.

Mesonephros: Comparatively big, develops in the thoracic and lumbar region, forms a type of excretory system and may function briefly.

Metanephros: Big system, develops from two sources. Collection system from mesonephric duct (ureter, renal pelvis, calyces and the collecting system) and metanephrogenic tissue (kidney tissue).

There may be abnormal position or abnormal development of kidney as well as ureter.

FAQs

Q. Which are the three systems during the development of the urinary system? Mention their parts.

Q. Does any system remain as a vestigial organ?

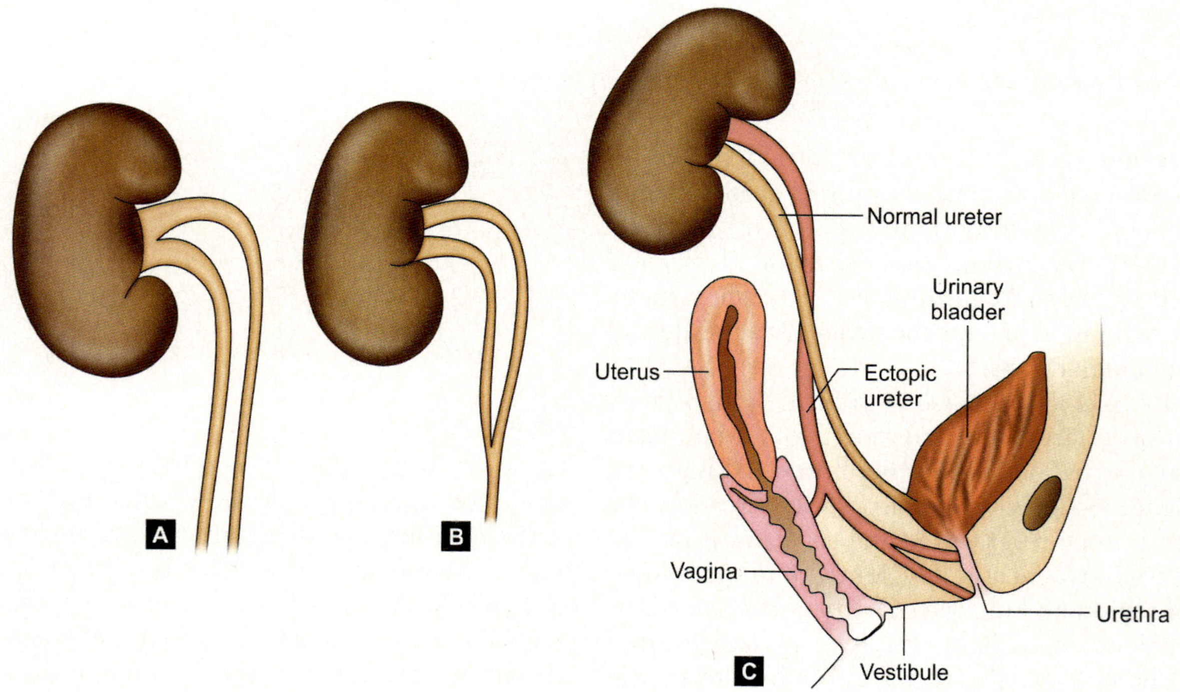

Fig. 6.5A to C Duplication of ureter (A) complete, (B) partial and (C) ectopic openings

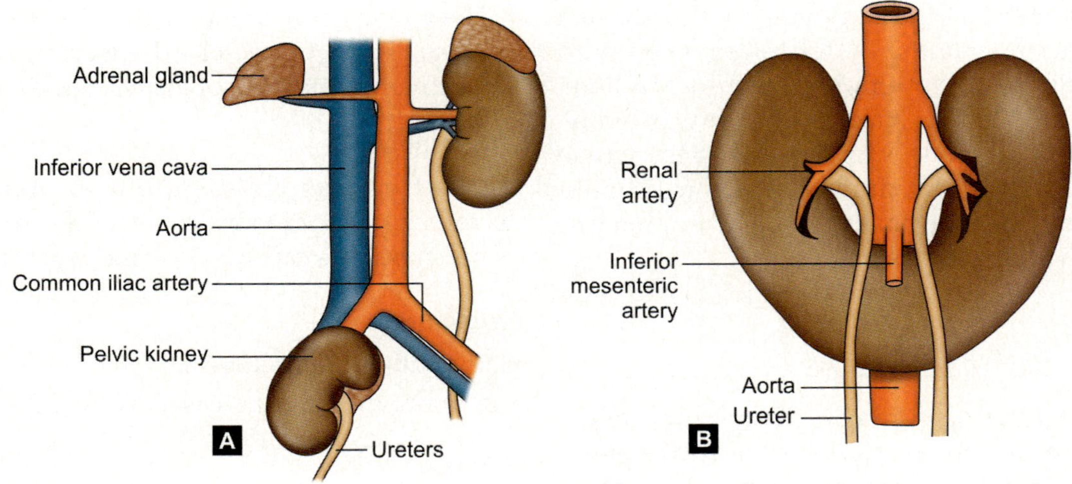

Fig. 6.6A and B Kidneys (A) ectopic (pelvic) kidney and (B) horseshoe kidney

RENAL PHYSIOLOGY

Before birth the kidney is a silent organ as placenta does its work. However, at birth the kidney takes its role which is of excretion of waste products, metabolites, drugs and maintaining volume, osmotic pressure and chemical composition of CSF.

Though being immature at birth the neonate kidneys perform the same function as that of the adult. Some relief is provided to the kidney as 50% of the dietatary nitrogen is incorporated into new tissue, thus decreasing half of the excretory load.

At birth the tubules are not fully grown and also the glomeruli area of filtration is similar in relation to body weight. As already discussed at term nephrogenesis is completed, while in preterm it is still continuous. Urine starts to come from 9 to 12 weeks. At term kidney produces 20–30 mL/ hr of filtrate.

Glomerular Filtration Rate

It is low and slow than adults in term babies (10 mL/ min/1.73 m^2) and even low in preterm. The neonatal GFR increases with fluid challenge or loading but there is a limit to it hence overzealous infusion of fluids can cause oedema.

Renal Blood Flow

Renal perfusion is dependent in neonates on the renal vascular resistance and arterial blood pressure and blood flow. Before and immediately after birth there is high renal vascular resistance and low renal blood flow (6% of circulation). After that the resistance decreases and arterial blood flow and blood pressure increases in the renal vessels causing increase in the GFR. The GFR increases by 2 times in 2 to 4 weeks.

GFR at 2 weeks is 20 to 30 mL/min/1.73 m^2. Adult values are reached at 1 year of age, hence initially the babies have high creatinine values which eventually decrease and come to normal values. Renal blood flow and GFR are decreased by asphyxia and hypoxia due to decrease in arterial blood pressure and renal and cardiac ischaemia.

Tubular Function

Even though the formation of nephrons is completed at term, the functional ability is still limited. The concentrating ability is still less due to urea concentration in the medullary interstitium, the loop of Henle being short and the sensitivity of ADH is still less. The ability to concentrate the urine is quickly develops so that at the age of 2 months it is 1000 mosmols/L.

This becomes important when fluid administration is insufficient due to some reasons (and in case of insensible loss) as it is difficult to handle dietary solutes. Neonates can concentrate urine to half of that of the adult as medullary concentration of urea in immature kidneys is low causing decrease osmotic gradient. In premature babies this ability is further decreased. The conservation of important solutes is also hampered due to marked immaturity of the tubules.

Sodium: An important solute is sodium, the capacity to absorb sodium is very very less, this leads to high renal losses of sodium, hence they are called obligatory sodium loosers.[4] In pre-terms this is still worse, (approximately three times greater) here it is important to mention that the renin–angiotensin aldosterone system is intact in infants. Distal tubule even with increase aldosterone cannot efficiently reabsorb sodium. Slowly, then the tubules start to respond to renin–angiotensin aldosterone system. All these cause hyponaetremia. Hence all fluids of neonates should contain sodium 2–4 mmoles/kg/day and in preterms should contain 5–10 mmoles/kg/day.

Pearls

Neonates are obligatory sodium losers.

Potassium: Kidneys manage potassium levels according to serum aldosterone levels. Aldosterone receptors are present on distal nephrons which cause increase secretion of potassium in urine. In neonates this is less efficient, hence they have hyperkalemia. This hyperkalemia is without ECG changes and is well tolerated by the neonates and does not require treatment.

Key Points

Kidneys are immature in view of excretion absorbtion and handling fluids and electrolytes.

pH balance: The mechanism of acid secretion is mature and efficient at term but not in immature babies. As gestational age increases, the excretion also increases.

The renal threshold for bicarbonates is decreased than adults.

16–20 mmols/L in preterm
19–21 mmols/L in term
24–28 mmols/L in childhood.

The limitation in infant's ability to excrete a hydrogen ion load is due to decreased concentration of buffers like ammonia and phosphates in urine.

Glycosuria

It is not in term children, but in preterm there is decreased tubular re-absorption of glucose. This causes osmotic diuresis causing Na^+ and water losses.

Proteinuria

- Normally no proteinuria.
- In premature it is increased by 16–21%.

Take Home Message

Avoid overzealous hydration.

SUMMARY

Kidneys are immature at birth and find difficult to handle stress. GFR is less in neonates and tubules do not necessarily reabsorb or secrete all the substances presented to them. Tubular re-absorption rate of sodium is reduced and proteins, amino acids are poorly dealt. Also there is limited ability to concentrate the urine and the threshold for bicarbonate is also lowered.

FAQ

Q. What should all IV fluids of neonates contains?

LIVER

- Development of liver and relevant metabolism.
- Anatomy and development.

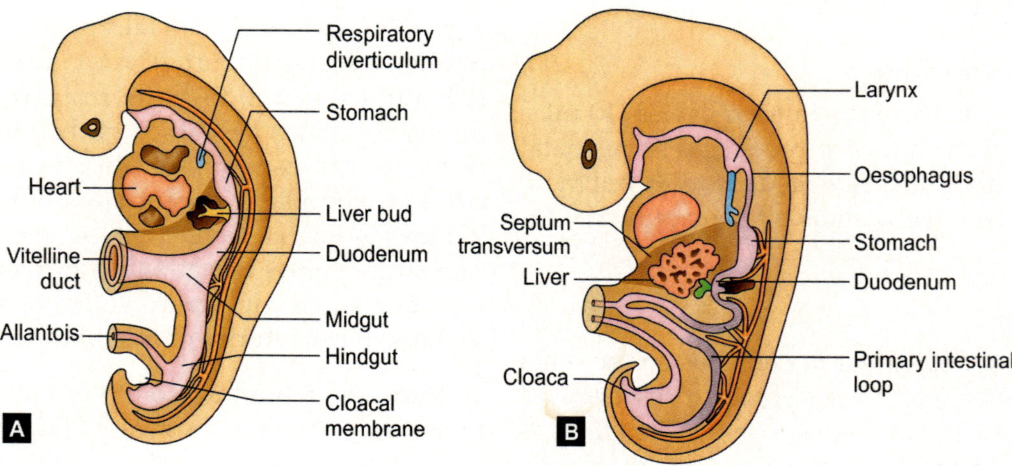

Fig. 6.7A and B (A) 25-day-old embryo showing liver bud formation along with GI in the primitive stage and **(B)** 32-day-old embryo showing epithelial liver cords cells penetrating the mesenchyme of septum transversum

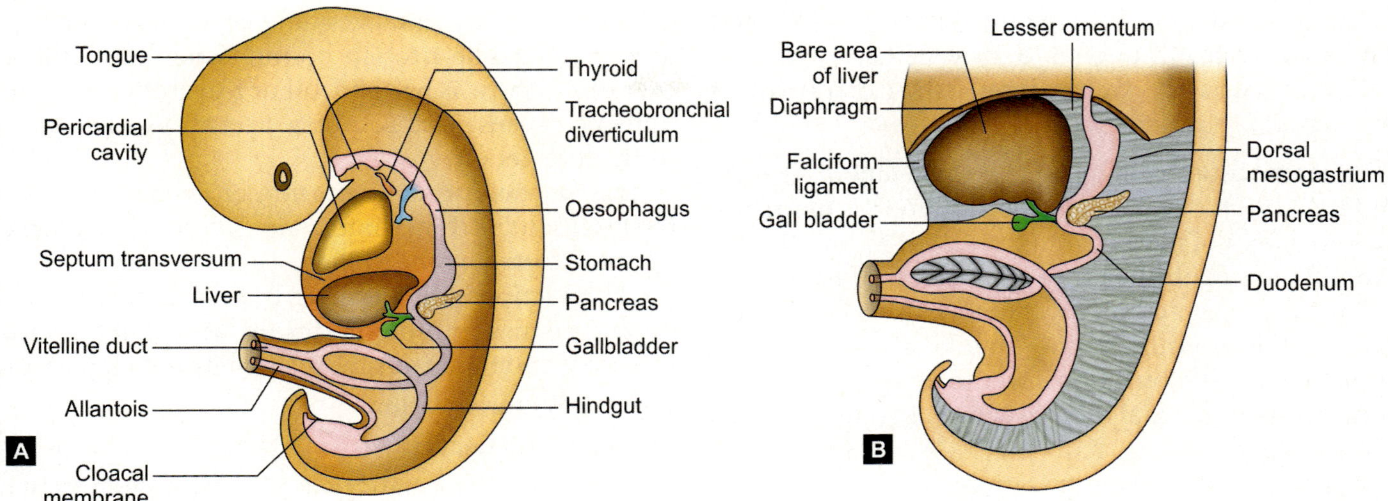

Fig. 6.8A and B Caudally expanding liver pushing the abdominal contents and anterior and posterior attachments of the gut

The liver and biliary tree tract develops in the middle to late of 3rd to 4th week of gestation as a ventral bud from the endodermal epithelium at the distal end of foregut.

The liver bud cells proliferate rapidly which then penetrate the septum transversum (mesoderm connecting pericardial cavity and the stalk of the yolk sac).[1] Three outpouchings then differentiate as liver, gallbladder, and ventral pancreas. By seventh week the morphologic development is completed but not the functional.

At this time bile duct starts to form as the connection between the hepatic diverticuli and the foregut narrows in size.

The bile duct gives small ventral outgrowth which gives rise to the gall bladder and cystic artery. Then the epithelial liver cells intermingle with vitelline and umbilical veins which forms hepatic sinusoids. Later liver cords differentiate into liver cells (parenchyma) and form the lining of the billiary duct. The mesoderm of the septum transversum gives rise to the connective tissue cells, Kupffer cells and haemopoietic cells.

During seventh week only hepatic cannaliculi and the intrahepatic and the extrahepatic bile ducts proliferate. Maternal viruses, drugs and toxins are known to increase the vulnerability of the anomalies at this stage of the hepatic and biliary tract development. Associations include intrahepatic biliary atresia and congenital heart disease.

Weight of the liver at the time of birth is 120–160 gm (nearly 4% of the infant weight). Not yet full structurally mature additional 4 to 8 weeks are required for peripheral branching of intrahepatic biliary tree to develop into proper hepatic portals.

The liver has 2 lobes and 8 structurally independent segments which have hepatic artery, hepatic vein and bile duct.

It has dual blood supply:

1. **Portal vein:** Venous blood from spleen and intestine (70%).
2. **Arterial:** Blood from hepatic artery (30%).

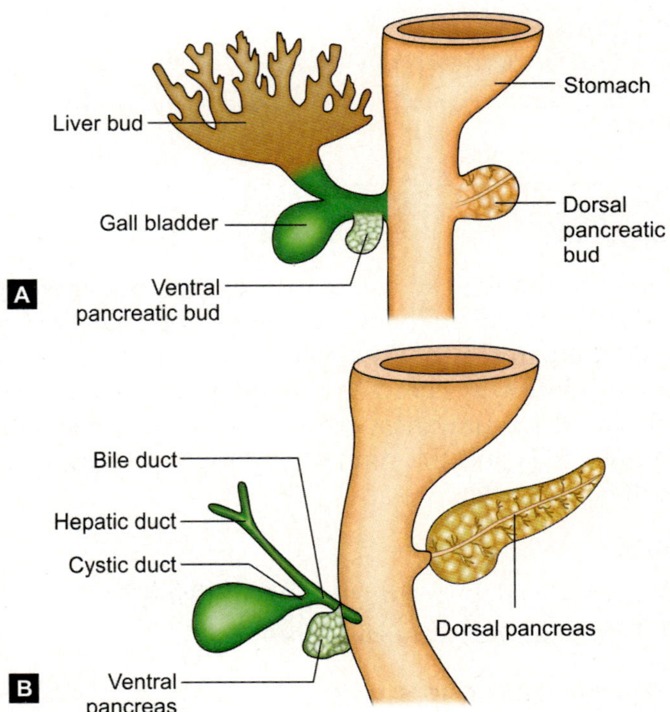

Fig. 6.9A and B Liver, gall bladder, cystic duct, bile duct and pancreatic bud development

Lastly blood from liver goes to heart via right and left hepatic veins through inferior vena cava.

Foetal hepatic circulations differ from adult circulation.

Ductus venosus:[1] Connection between umbilical veins and IVC shunts oxygenated blood around the immature liver to enter the right atrium (an essential shunt). This shunt flow is controlled by a sphincter mechanism.

Ductus venosus closes functionally immediately after birth as the pressure in the umbilical vein decrease immediately after birth. At 2 weeks of age almost 95% of complete functional closure occurs, in others it takes a little longer.

A rare but not a uncommon problem is patent ductus venoses, known as congenital portosystemic venous shunt which may manifest as hepatic dysfunction or encephalopathy. Reversals of the symptoms are seen on closure of the same.

Liver parenchymal structural unit is a lobule,[2] which has central vein at the center of the wheel bordered by portal tracts which has a traid of bile duct, portal vein and hepatic artery, between are the liver cells, kupffer cells, etc. Blood flows from ports towards the central vein bathing the hepatocytes.

Bile has an opposite flow to the portal vein thus forming the hepatic accini to complete.

Key Points
Liver is a mesodermal organ to origin from the foregut.

Pearls
Liver has dual blood supply.

SUMMARY

The liver and the gall bladder develop as out growing of the endoderm epithelium from the upper part of the duodenum (foregut). The parenchyma is formed by the growing biliary system cells and the epithelial liver cord cells in the septum transversum. The hemopoietic cells, Kupffer cells and the connective tissue cells originate in the mesoderm.

FAQs

Q. Liver develops from which primitive gut?

Q. Where do Kupffer cells arise?

LIVER OR HEPATIC PHYSIOLOGY

Lipid solubility is an important factor for passive diffusion across the cellular membrane. These lipid soluble things accumulate in the fat stores of the body and also become protein bound, hence difficult for excretion. Even renal and biliary excretion of these things can cause reabsorption, hence these things are difficult to get off.

The function of major portion of liver is to convert the lipid soluble things into water soluble things which can be excreted by the kidney.

The reactions for the drug biotransformation and metabolism are hydroxylation and conjugation. Hydroxylation prepares the metabolite for conjugation.

Phase 1: Hydroxylation

Phase 2: Conjugation

In neonates the hepatic phase 1 and phase 2 reactions are not fully active and in neonates it is even less causing more problems. They become active at 2 to 3 months of life.

Phase 1 reaction includes:

1. Oxidation
2. Hydrolysis
3. Reduction

Phase 1 reactions[2] are catalyzed by cytochrome P450 enzyme. It is mixed function oxidase system. In neonates its activity is only 28% of that of the adults. Genetic and non genetic factor affect cytochrome P450 activity. The non-genetic factor includes concomitant disease status, diminished nutritional state and exposure to pharmacological and other naturally occurring compounds. Even drugs can inhibit and stimulate the P450 system enzymes.

Stimulants

- Omeprazole
- Phenytoin
- Ethanole
- Carbamazepine

Inhibitors

- Ketaconazole
- Quinidine
- Disulfiran
- Erythromycin

Other system phase 1 reactions such as alcohol dehydrogenase (choral hydrate metabolism), plasma esterase (amino-ester LA metabolism) and N-acetyl transferase (isoniazide and hydralazine metabolism) are also deficient.

Phase 2 reactions[2] is a phase of conjugation to decrease the lipid solubility and increase the water solubility to facilitate excretion by urine or gut. Phase 2 reactions include:

1. Sulfation
2. Glucuronidation
3. Methylation
4. Glutathione
5. Acetylation

Reactions like acetylation, glycination and glucoronidation are very deficient at birth. At the same time sulfation is active which metabolises opiods and in neonate's paracetamol.

During the neonatal period the liver is immature in its ability to metabolise and clear the substance. Size of the liver simply does not matter, as it larger as compared to its body size when compared to adults. Hepatic blood flow, development status of hepatic transport, and enzyme system all affect the drug clearance.

Bilirubin Metabolism

The breakdown of erythrocytes (80%) and ineffective erythropoiesis all together produce bilirubin. Normally this bilirubin is sent to liver where it is conjugated and then excreted.

In neonates the enzyme which catalyzes the transfer of glucuronic acid to bilirubin (urine dephospho-glucuronyl transferase) to form glucuronides and allow the excretion in bile only 1% to that of the adult. It takes 3 to 4 months for it to reach the adult values. Hence increase bilirubin or jaundice is common at term called physiological jaundice. It is more common in pre-term babies due to lower values of the enzyme. This jaundice starts around 2 to 3 days of life and continues till around 10–12 days, when the values of the enzyme start increasing. In adults the production of bilirubin is 50–70 mcg/kg/day but this value is increased to double or triple (100–140 mcg/kg/day) in neonates due to increased production from erythrocyte breakdown, limited metabolism and excretion. In addition there is increased enterohepatic circulation of bilirubin due to limited capacity of urobilinogen and urobilin.

Plasma level of bilirubin can be detrimental when they increase up to or are more than 200 mmmol/L. When level increases it gets deposited and damage basal ganglia, cerebellum and hippocampus. This condition is called kernicterus with elements of cerebral palsy, mental handicap and deafness.

Factors affecting increase serum bilirubin:

1. Decrease albumin concentration
2. Haemolysis
3. Sepsis
4. Gestational diabetes mellitus
5. Delayed passage of meconium
6. Drugs increase binding to proteins.

The commonest treatment for this is phototherapy which converts bilirubin to photoisomer like lumirubin which is excreted in bile and urine.

Vitamin K

Factors like 2, 7, 9, 10 are less at term, all these factors are vitamin K dependant. Hence as a general measure vitamin K is given to all neonates to prevent the haemorrhagic disease of newborn.

Drug metabolism may be affected and in fact prolonged due to certain circulatory shunt bypasses that bypass the hepatic bed which decrease the clearance of drug metabolism in liver. For example, the ductus venosus a connection between IVC, portal vein and umbilical vein remain patent for 7–10 days of birth.

Glycogen Storage

The liver storage capacity of neonate is less and the activity of the rate limiting enzyme in gluconeogenesis is also less (as low as 10% of adult value), hence the neonates are at risk of developing hypoglycemia if not fed frequently. Hence as a precautious method glucose is added to all infusions till feeding is started, with frequent blood sugar monitoring.

Opiod Metabolism

The conduct of anaesthesia is not much affected due to the liver's limited capacity, but we have to be more watchful and careful in the postoperative period when the drugs are going to be metabolized and excreted. Hence modification of dosage, intervals, infusion are required.

Anaesthetic Drugs

Halothane has been associated with development of severe hepatic injury, hence other drugs like sevoflurane, isoflurane should be preferred.

Muscle Relaxants

Scoline metabolizes by plasma cholinesterase, a protein synthesized by liver by only functional hepatocytes.

SUMMARY

Before birth most of the functions of liver are carried by the placenta. Phase 1 and phase 2 reactions of metabolism are not fully developed or some reactions are developed and some are not. Detoxification and carbohydrate metabolism are not nor developed properly at birth and more so in prematurity. The bilirubin load caused by red blood cells breakdown is also not conjugated, hence causes physiological jaundice which regress slowly. Vitamin K dependant coagulation factors are very low, hence vitamin K has to be supplemented.

Gluconeogenesis is also not optimum hence hypoglycemia is common.

Key Points

They do not have a fully mature enzyme and bilirubin handling system.

Pearl

Add glucose to all IV fluids of neonates.

Take Home Message

Avoid starving and giving drugs which are difficult to metabolise in liver.

FAQs

Q. Should all IV fluids of neonates contain glucose?

Q. Why neonates have jaundice?

GASTROINTESTINAL SYSTEM

Structural and Functional Development of Intestine

The primitive gut is formed by the cephalo-caudal and lateral folding of the embryo which causes the endoderm lined yolk sac to incorporate the embryo.[1] During the third week the primitive gut is separated from the notochord and there are two other endoderm lined cavity which remain outside the embryo, the yolk sac and the allantois.

The primitive gut forms a blind ending tube causing foregut at the cephalic end and hind gut at the caudal end. The middle part forms the midgut and this part temporarily remain connected to the yolk sac by means of vitelline duct.

The primitive gut starts from the mouth and ends at the upper end of the anus. Various organs are derived from primitive gut and their derivation is divided into four sections:

1. Pharyngeal gut is the part that starts from the oropharyngeal membrane to the respiratory diverticulum. This part contributes to the formation of head, neck and other important parts.
2. The parts after this till the liver outgrowths form the foregut. It forms the oesophagus, stomach, first part of the duodenum and second part till the liver diverticulum.
3. The midgut is from the second part of the duodenum caudal to liver bud till the right two-thirds (2/3rd) of the transverse colon. It forms the lower duodenum, jejunum, ileum, ceacum, appendix, ascending colon and first 2/3rd of transverse colon.
4. The hindgut starts from distal 1/3rd of left transverse colon. It forms lateral 1/3rd transverse colon, descending colon, rectum and upper part of anal canal.

The endoderm not only gives internal lining to the digestive tract but also forms specific cells of glands (parenchyma) like hepatocytes, exocrine and endocrine cells of pancreas, etc. The connective tissue (stroma) of the gland is derived from the visceral mesoderm. The visceral mesoderm also forms connective tissue and peritoneal components of the wall of the gut.

Each division of the gut is supplied by branches of the primitive aorta. The celiac artery formed by the

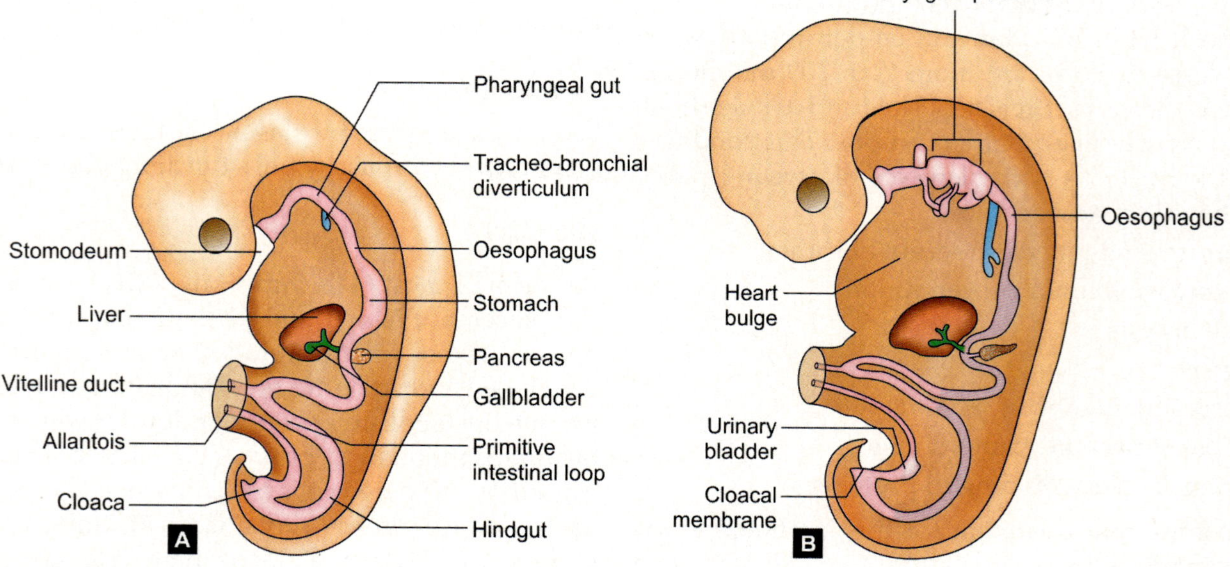

Fig. 6.10A and B (A) 4th week and **(B)** 5th week of development of GI tract along with other derivatives

fusion of paired ventral tributaries of the dorsal aorta supplies the infradiaphragmatic portion of foregut. The superior mesenteric artery supplies the midgut and inferior mesenteric artery supplies the hindgut.

There is a general histology for the gastrointestinal tract in the sequence of mucosa, sub-mucosa, muscular layer and the serosa (from inside to outside in concentric manner). These may vary at various sites for some special purpose.

The Mesenteric Origin

This is a double layer of peritoneum that suspends the gut tube and its various derivatives from the dorsal and ventral body walls. This endorses all organs and the gut and connects them to the body wall. Organs develop inside this are called intraperitoneal organs. There are something called a peritoneal ligaments which are double-layered bands that pass from organ to organ and organ to body wall. The basic intention of the mesentery and ligaments is to provide vascular, neural and lymphatic access to the abdominal viscera.

During the initial phase the mesenchyme of the posterior abdominal wall is connected to foregut, midgut and hindgut with a broad connection. Around the eight week, there is narrowing of the connective tissue bridge such that the latter part of the foregut, midgut and majority of hindgut are suspended from the abdominal wall by the dorsal mesentery.

The mesentery starts from lower end of the oesophagus to the end of hindgut and has various names in various areas, like the region of stomach forms the mesogastrium or greater omentum, the area around duodenum forms dorsal mesoduodenum the colon the dorsal mesocolon. Dorsal mesentery of the jejunum and ileum form the mesentery proper.

The ventral mesentery is not present throughout, it is present only around the terminal oesophagus, stomach, upper duodenum, these are derived from the septum transversum. The liver develops in the septum transversum and divides the ventral mesentery into lesser omentum (extents from the lower portion of the oesophagus, stomach, and upper duodenum to the liver). The falciform ligament extents from the liver to body wall.

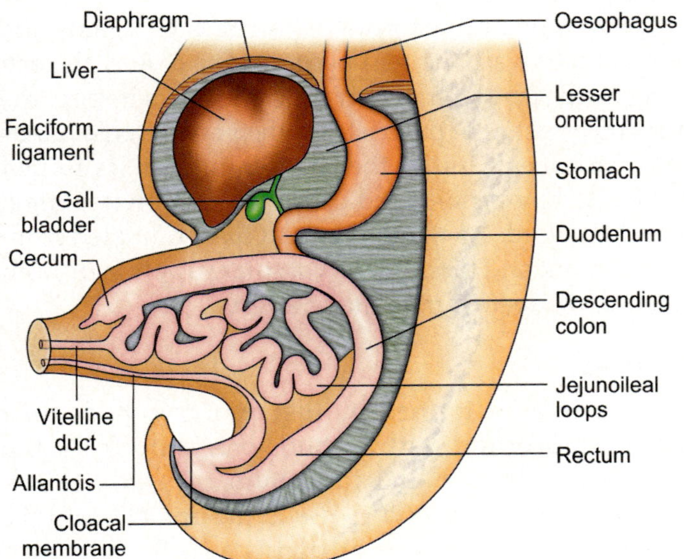

Fig. 6.11 Umbilical herniation of intestinal loops along with formation of caecum. Initially 90 degrees and then 180 degrees

Foregut

Oesophagus

At the 4th week of development of the embryo the respiratory diverticuli develops from the ventral part of the foregut near the pharyngeal gut. Slowly the tracheaoesophageal septum develops from the dorsal part of the foregut, thus separating the respiratory system (anteriorly) and GI system (dorsally) of the oesophagus. Initially the oesophagus is short but then it elongates as the heart and lung descends.

Stomach

Around 4th week a fusiform dilatation occurs of the foregut which develops the stomach later. Following this there is a difference in the growth of various walls of the stomach, which causes change in the shape as well as its relations to other organs.

The stomach rotates by 90° in clockwise direction around its longitudinal axis, as a result its left side faces

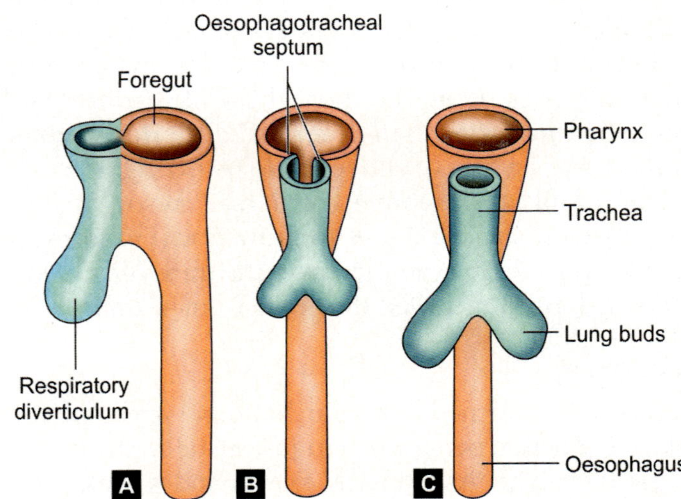

Fig. 6.12A to C Successive development (separation) of respiratory diverticulum and oesophagus from the foregut

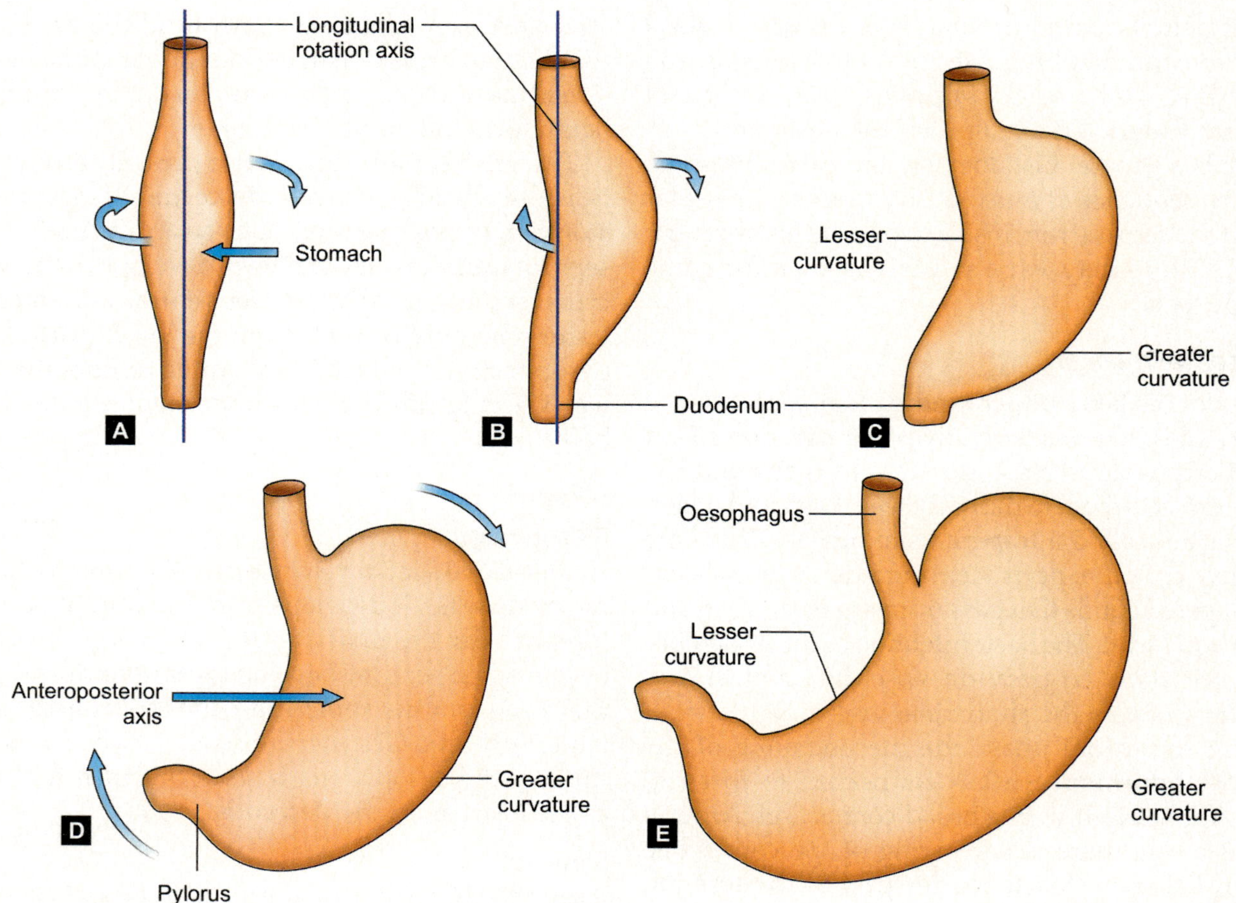

Fig. 6.13A to E Rotation of the stomach in longitudinal and anteroposterior axis

anteriorly and right side faces posteriorly. During this rotation process the original posterior wall of the stomach grows faster than the anterior portion forming greater and lesser curvature.

During the start of the development of stomach the cephalic and caudal end of the stomach are in the midline but due to asymmetrical rotation pyloric part (caudal) moves up and to the right while cardiac part (cephalic) moves to the left and slightly down, thus stomach has an axis of above left to below right.

Due to all of the above the dorsal mesogastrium bulges down and continues to grow down to forms a double layered sac extending over the transverse colon and small intestine called the greater omentum.

Duodenum

Duodenum is formed by terminal foregut and cephalic midgut, junction being the part just distal to the origin of the liver bud. As stomach rotates and shrinks, the duodenum assumes a 'C' shaped loop and rotates to the right. Along with this rotation there is also rapid growth of the head of pancreas, both these factors take the duodenum from the central portion to the right side of the abdominal cavity.

Duodenum and the head of pancreas hit against the dorsal body wall, the two peritoneums fuse with each other so that the later part of the duodenum (except the initial part near the pyloris) and the pancreass becomes retroperitoneal. Initial the duodenum has its lumen obliterated by proliferated cells, but later on its lumen is recannalised. As the duodenum has originated from both foregut and hindgut, its vascular supply is by both celiac and superior mesenteric artery.

Pancreas

The pancreas is formed by fusion of two buds, one dorsal and other ventral; both originate from the endodermal lining of the duodenum.

Dorsal pancreatic bud grows in the dorsal mesentry while the ventral pancreatic bud is near the bile duct. As discussed previously with the rotation of the duodenum and shifting to the right side, there is change

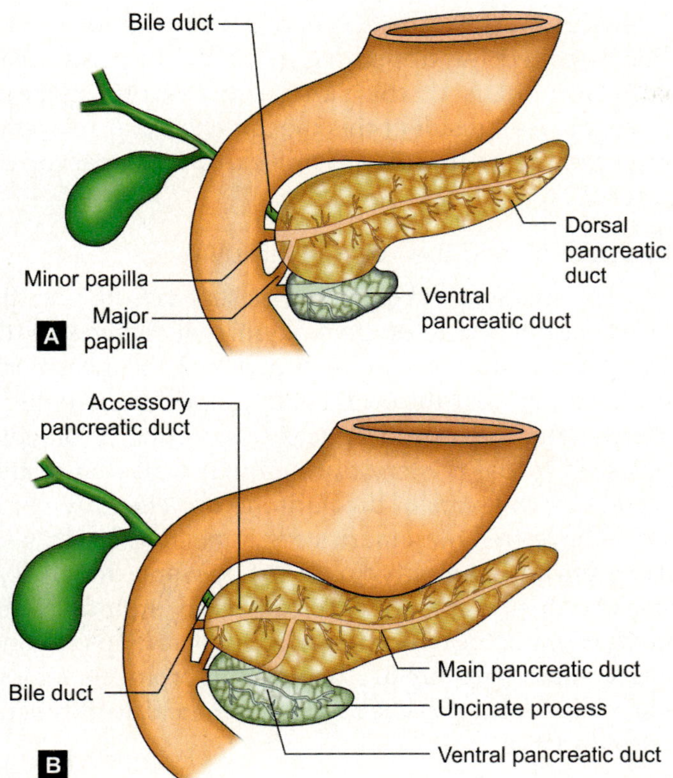

Fig. 6.14A and B Ventral and dorsal pancreatic bud placement and their duct formation

in orientation of the pancreatic ducts such that the ventral bud comes to lie dorsally and immediately below and behind the dorsal bud. Then both these buds fuse to form the parenchyma of the pancreatic tissue. The ventral bud forms the uncinate process and the inferior part of the head of the pancreas. Later the main and the accessory pancreatic duct are formed and open on major and minor papilla on the duodenum respectively.

The 3rd month of the foetal life sees the formation of the islets of the Langerhans from the parenchyma and then distribute in the pancreas. The parenchyma also gives rise to somatostatin and glucagon secreting cells. Insulin secretion starts around 5th month.

Midgut

The midgut in adults starts immediately distal to the bile duct opening into the duodenum and ends at the junction of the proximal 2/3rd and distal 1/3rd of the transverse colon. All the midgut is supplied by superior mesenteric artery as already described.

During the development around the 5th week the midgut is suspended from the dorsal abdominal wall by means of a short mesentry. The midgut at the same time also communicates with the yolk sac by means of vitelline duct or the yolk stalk at the apex. The midgut forms the primary intestine and its development is characterized by rapid elongation of the gut and its mesentries. The midgut is in open connection with the yolk sac by means of the vitelline duct at the apex. The part cephalic to this part develops into duodenum, jejunum and part of ileum, while the caudal part forms the lower ileum, caecum, appendix, ascending colon and part of the transverse colon (2/3rd proximal).

Herniation

As the intestines are developing they have the property of rapid elongation particularly of the cephalic limb. At the same time, the liver is also growing rapidly which accommodates the majority of the abdominal cavity, as a result of this the abdominal cavity becomes small and unable to accommodate all its contents. Hence temporarily all the intestinal loops enter the extra-embryonic cavity in the umbilical cord (approximately 6th week of development). This process is called physiological umbilical herniation.

Rotation of The Midgut

As the length of midgut increases, the primary intestinal loop rotates around an axis formed by superior mesenteric artery. This rotation when viewed from front is anticlockwise.

As rotation is going on, elongation of small intestinal loops continues, causing the jejunum and ileum to form a number of coiled loops. The large intestine on the other side though lengths considerably does not participate in the coiling process.

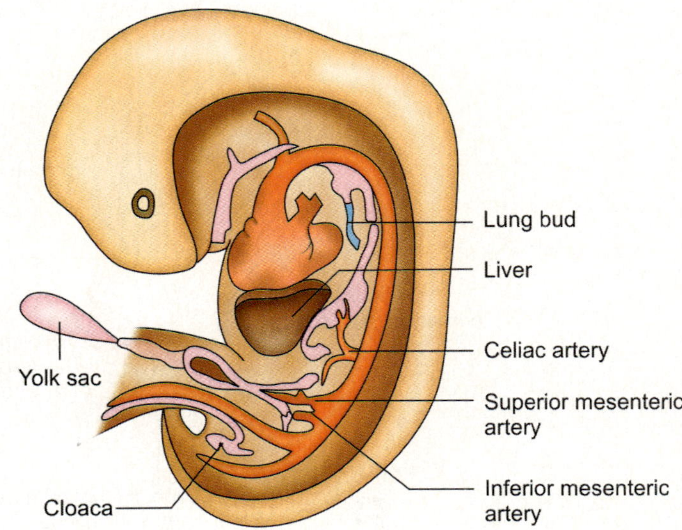

Fig. 6.15 Blood supply to the various developing GI system

Rotation occurs by around 90° during herniation and 180° during return of the intestinal loops back into the abdominal cavity causing a total of 270°.

Retraction of Herniation Loops

The loops of the intestine which have gone out slowly begin to come back to the abdominal cavity, probably due to reduction of the liver size, regression of mesonephric kidney and expansion of the abdominal cavity. The first part to re-enter the abdominal cavity is the proximal portion of the jejunum which occupies the left side. Subsequently the later loops settle more and more to the right side.

During this (6th week) a small conical dilatation of the primary intestinal loop appears which is the caecal bud. This is the last part of the gut to re-enter the abdominal cavity.

At the initial part the caecum lies just below the right lobe of the liver, but slowly then it descends down into the right iliac fossa. Thus the ascending colon and the hepatic flexure comes to lie on the right side of the abdominal cavity. During this time the narrow diverticulum grows at the end of caecal bud, which then is called the appendix. Thus the appendicular development is at the same time as the caecum descends. As a result of this the appendicular relations may change with colon or caecum (retrocaecal or retrocolic).

Mesenteries and The Loop of Intestine

With the rotation of the gut, the mesenteries having the blood supply also undergoes significant changes. With the right side shift of later loops of bowel, the mesentery also twists around the origin of the superior mesenteric artery. Later the ascending and descending colon gets plastered to the posterior abdominal wall due to the fusion of two layers of the peritoneum. The only parts which have free mesenteries are appendix, lower end of caecum and sigmoid colon. The transverse mesocolon fuses with the greater omentum and maintains its mobility. Later the mesentery of jejunoileal loops obtains a new line of attachment that extends from the region where duodenum comes intra peritoneal to the ileo-ceacal junction.

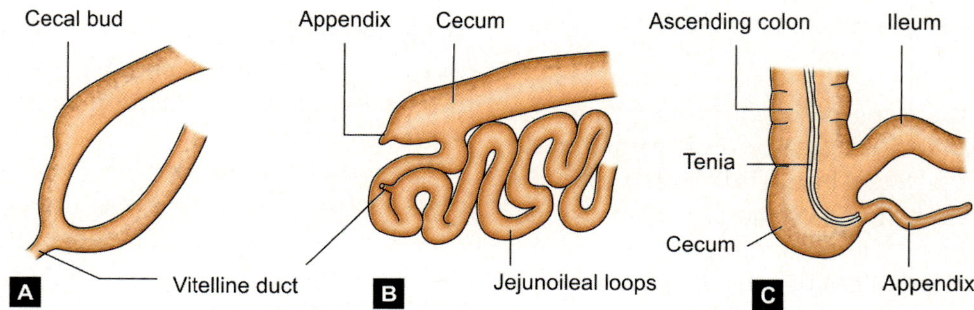

Fig. 6.16A to C Development of caecum and appendix **(A)** 7th week, **(B)** 8th week and **(C)** Newborn

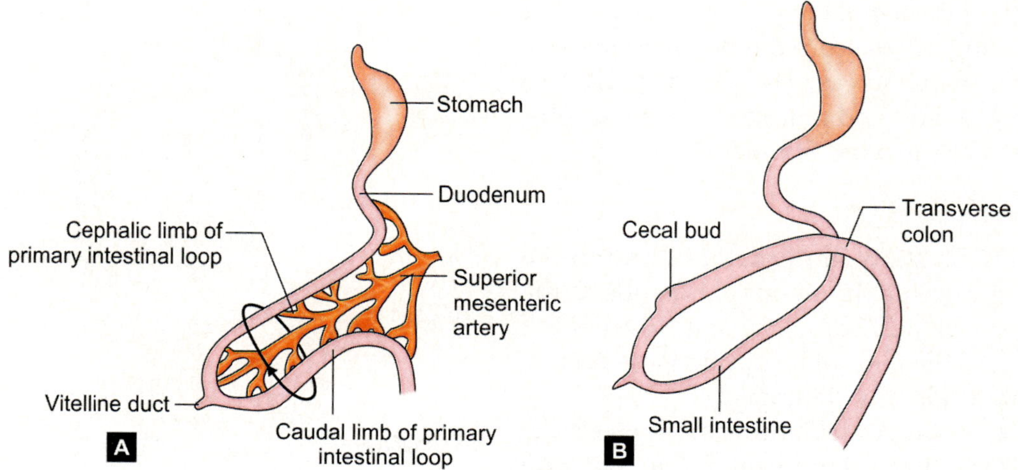

Fig. 6.17A and B Rotation of the intestinal loop along the superior mesenteric artery axis

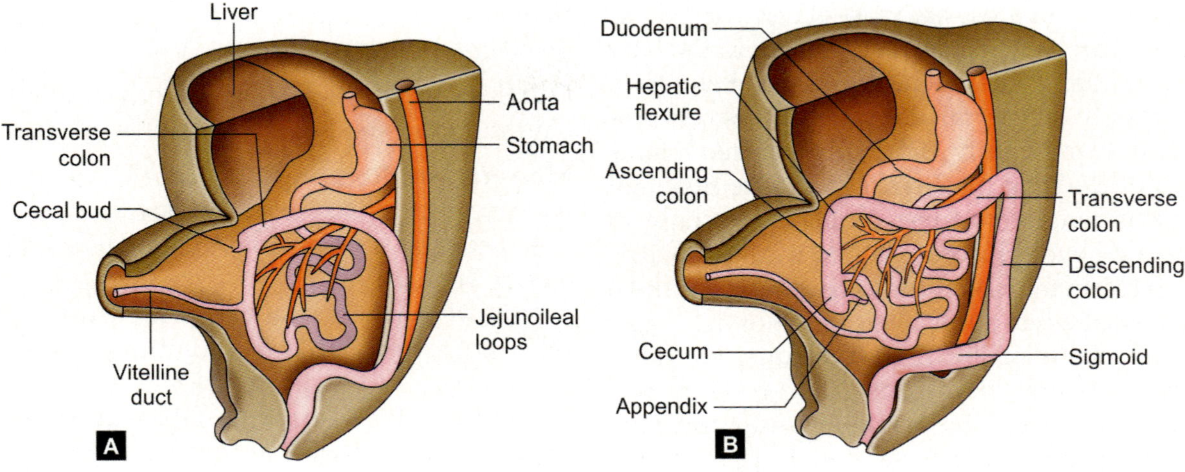

Fig. 6.18A and B Return back of intestinal loops and final position of the intestines in the abdominal cavity

Hindgut

The hindgut forms the later part of colon (distal 1/3rd of the transverse colon), descending colon and upper part of anal canal.

The hindgut in its terminal part slowly starts entering the posterior part of the cloaca that is the primitive ano-rectal canal. At the same time the allantois also enters the anterior part of the primitive uro-genital sinus. The cloaca and endodermal lined cavity is bound at its ventral part by ectoderm, this boundary is the junction of ecto and endoderm which forms the cloacal membrane. From this a mesodermal septum starts developing covering the yolk sac and the allantois, this separates the hindgut and the allantois. Slowly the urorectal septum comes to lie close to the cloacal membrane. The cloacal membrane ruptures at the seventh week creating an anal opening for hindgut and a ventral opening for urogenital sinus.

The upper 2/3rd of the anal canal is formed by hind gut (endoderm), lower 1/3rd by ectoderm, thus the anal opening is formed by the junction of ecto and endoderm (pectinate line). The blood supply of the hindgut is by superior rectal and the ectodermal part by the inferior rectal.

Physiology and Functions

The gastrointestinal system has a general histology with some changes depending on area and functional needs. There are 4 concentric layers—mucosa, submucosa, muscularis and the serosa.

The gastrointestinal tract does the function of ingestion, digestion, selective absorption and excretion. All this start during early foetal life (8th week) and continues slowly till the 40th week. Swallowing starts in the second trimester and co-ordinated intestinal motility in the third trimester. The enzymes required to

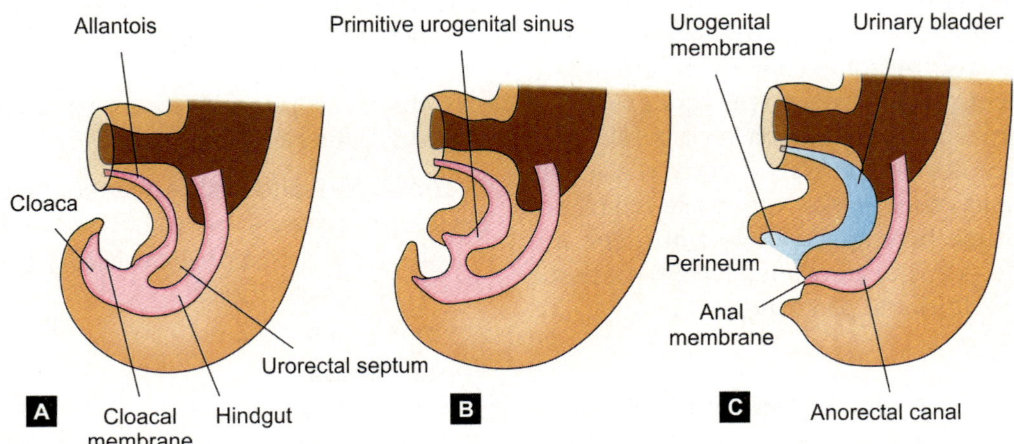

Fig. 6.19A to C Development of the anal canal and cloaca from the hindgut

digest sucrose and maltose are present early and those that digest lactose and proteins are present in the later life. The term infants GI system have a good ability to be managed only on enteral feeds, but this is compromised in cases of premature, IUGR, asphyxiated infants and babies of diabetic mothers, etc. Hence neonatal hypoglycemia is common in neonates especially in premature and hence glucose is added to all paediatric I.V. fluids. At birth the pH of stomach is acidic around 6 which then equalizes to adult levels by 3 months of age. Many normal infants exhibit discordination of swallowing and regurgitation, persistent gastro-oesophageal reflux beyond 6 weeks, this is pathological and may cause laryngospasm, paroxysmal cough, pneumonia, etc. All this is increased in prematurity.

GI Transit

The transit time through the GI tract for food and other ingested material depends on many factors.[4] About 50% of the meals in the stomach empty into intestine in an hour time and total empting takes about 2–3 hours. Subsequently 50% of the small intestine takes 1 to 2 hours to empty. Colon takes 12 to 50 hours for total transit. The gastric transit time is variable in neonates, infants and children. This is also changed by the contents (solids, liquids, etc). In unobstructed patients ½ life of clear isotonic fluids is 10–20 minutes. Pain, fear, anxiety, trauma, sepsis, narcotics all delay the empting.

Immune Function of the Gut

The GI system has very large area and with such a large area it is exposed to various pathogens which have to be prevented from entering the blood and the lymph, thus it provides a very efficient immune system.

To start with it has very low pH in the stomach which kills most of the fatal organisms. In addition the mucus has IgA antibodies which neutralize many toxins and micro-organisms. Still to help are also enzymes in saliva, bile, intestines, etc. The intestines contain bacteria which are health enhancing and these also prevent growth of potentially harmful bacteria. These bacteria breakdown the complex molecules which human body is not able to break. Gases and other wastes are made which are excreted, at the same time absorption of nutrient and water is also made. Also gut associated lymphatic tissue (GALT) provides additional protection.

Gut Anomalies

These are classified according to nature of problem:

Atresia: Interruption in lumen (oesophageal, duodenal, biliary, pyloric).

Stenosis: Narrowing of lumen (oesophagus, duodenal, pyloric).

Duplication: Multiplication due to incomplete recannalisation causing parallel lumen.

Malrotation: Rotation not completed or rotated in wrong direction due to some reason.

In neonates it presents as the bilious vomiting or the bloody stools.

In newborn there is failure to thrive due to infections, recurrent pain, diarrhoea, vomiting, later sepsis and peritonitis.

Ladd bands multiple in nature crossing the duodenum causing duodenal obstruction.

Volvulus

Twisting of the gut causing obstruction to the flow. This may also have compensation of the blood supply causing toxins to accumulate.

Foregut Malformation

Oesophageal atresia, stenosis and tracheo-esophageal fistula:

They may be individual or associated with each other. All these results from either spontaneous posterior deviation of tracheoesophageal septum or may be due to the mechanical factors pushing dorsal wall of the foregut anteriorly causing unequal division of foregut into respiratory and digestive tract.

Its variants are:

1. Proximal part of esophagus forms a blind sac while the distal part is connected to the trachea by the narrow canal above the bifurcation.
2. Oesophagus has 2 blind ends with no traecheal connection (isolated atresia).
3. H-type, without oesophageal atresia.
4. Other variants where upper oesophagus is connected to trachea by narrow channel and lower end is blind.
5. Both oesophageal ends proximal are connected separately to trachea.

Oesophageal and tracheoesophageal abnormalities

These defects may be associated with other abnormalities. Tracheoesophageal fistula is a component of VACTERL association.[1]

V: Vertebral anomalies

A: Anal atresia

C: Cardiac defects

T: Tracheoesophageal fistula

E: Oesophageal atresia

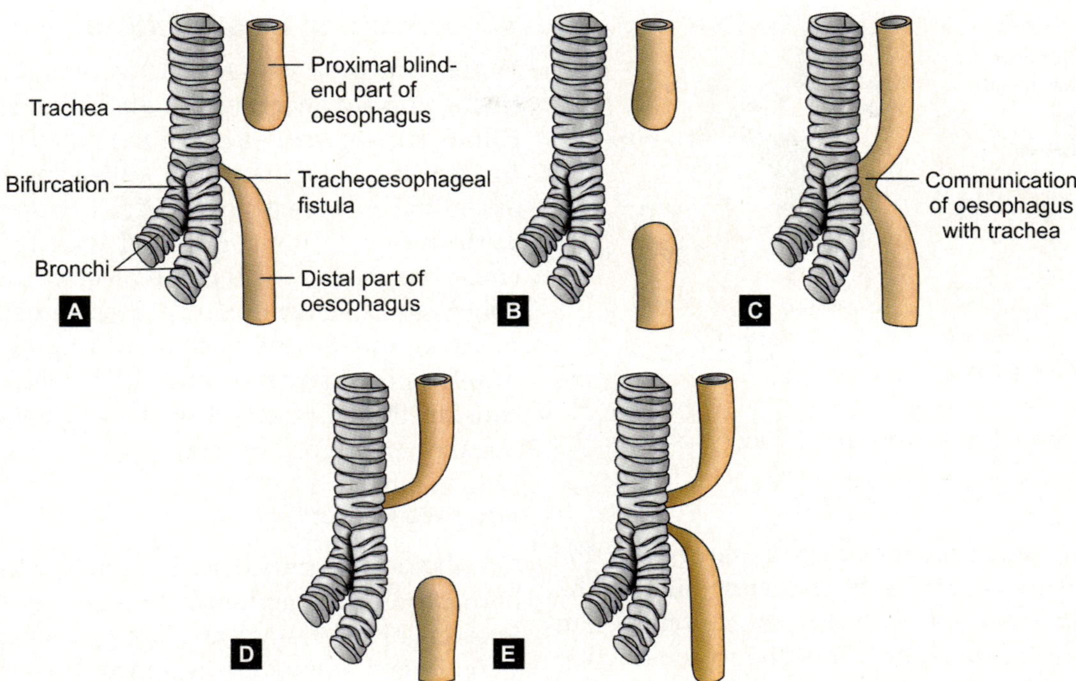

Fig. 6.20A to E Variations of oesophageal atresia and/or tracheoesophageal fistula in order of their frequency of appearance: (A) 90%, (B) 4%, (C) 4%, (D) 1% and (E) 1%

R: Renal anomalies

L: Limb defect

In case of atresia of oesophagus the normal passage of amniotic fluid into the intestinal tract is prevented resulting into poly hydramnious.

Sometimes lumen of the oesophagus may be narrowed, commonly in lower 1/3rd area resulting in oesophageal stenosis.

Occasionally hiatal hernia of congenital origin may be present due to insufficient lengthening of the oesophagus causing pulling up of the stomach through the diaphragmatic opening (congenital hiatal hernia).

Stomach

Pyloric stenosis is the most common of this (1:200 in males and 1:1000 in females) where the circular and longitudinal muscles of the stomach in the pyloric region hypertrophy causing delayed propulsion of the food forwards causing severe vomiting. In rare cases the pylorus may be totally atretic and rarest are stomach duplications and prepyloric septum.

Liver and Biliary System

Variations in liver lobulations are common but they are clinically not significant. Similarly variations (duplications and accessory ducts) of hepatic, common bile ducts and cystic ducts are also common. The more serious among all these (1 : 20000) are the malformations of the extra-hepatic biliary system in the form of atresia of the gall bladder or the bile duct. These may result due to persistence of the solid state of the duct and/or the gall bladder partly or fully. This may result in atretic gall bladder and ducts (in some cases mere cords). Sometimes atresia is limited to a part of the system (part of common bile duct), resulting in distension of the gallbladder and hepatic ducts. Clinically these manifest as increasing jaundice after birth. Duplications, partial subdivisions and diverticuli of the gall bladder are also not uncommon. Occasionally this problem occurs inside the liver causing intrahepatic biliary duct atresia and hypoplasia which is generally lethal.

Pancreas

The accessory pancreatic tissue (other than normal site) may be found anywhere from the distal oesophagus to the tip of the primary intestinal loop. Most frequent site is the wall of the stomach, duodenum, or in the Meckel's diverticulum.

Pancreatic bladder is the condition in which the ventral pancreatic bud grows out with the liver bud and forms the pancreatic nodule.

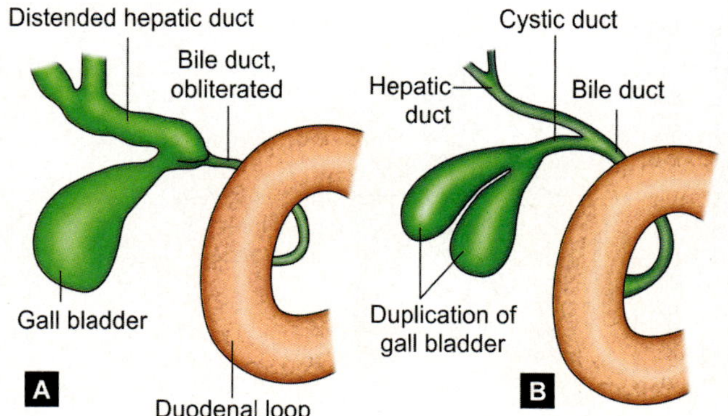

Fig. 6.21A and B Abnormalities of the gall bladder, bile, cystic and hepatic ducts

Annular pancreas is the rare malformation where the pancreatic tissue surrounds the 2nd part of the duodenum like a band. It is mostly asymptomatic but can occasionally cause obstruction due to constriction of duodenum. This is caused by growth of the bipid ventral pancreatic bud around the duodenum which fuses with the dorsal bud to form the ring.

Midgut Malformations

These malformations are common and generally caused by the abnormal digestive tube. development, abnormal and incomplete rotation and/or failure of the fixation and/or location or arrangements by itself or due to the neighbouring viscera during development. The malformations may be single or interconnected making the pathology more complex and less compatible with life.

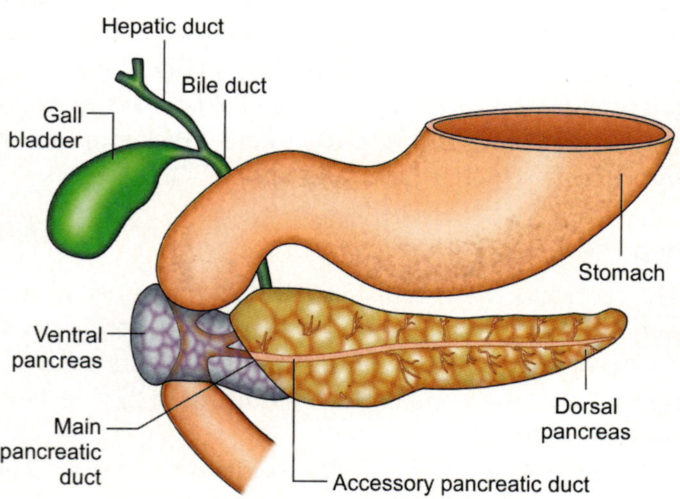

Fig. 6.22 Annular pancreas

Abnormalities of the Mesenteries

When the part of ascending mesocolon persists (mesentery connecting the abdominal wall and the colon), it gives rise to a condition called mobile caecum. In extreme conditions the entire mesentery of the ascending colon may persists due to failure of the fusion with the posterior abdominal wall leading to high chances of the volvulus of the caecum and colon due to abnormal movements. Similar reasons of the incomplete fusion of the mesentery may lead to the development of retrocolic pockets behind the ascending mesocolon causing the entrapment of the portions of the small intestine (retrocolic hernia).

Body Wall Defects

Omphalocoele (incidence 1 in 6500 births): In this there herniation of the abdominal viscera (stomach, spleen, liver, gallbladder, small and large intestine, etc.) through the enlarged umbilical ring and are covered by amnion.

This is caused by failure of the bowel to return to the body cavity from its physiological herniation during its 6th to 10th week, thus causing the abdominal visera to develop outside the embryo in the amniotic sac. Omphalocoele may be associated with severe and several cardiac and neural tube defects or may have association with chromosomal and genetic abnormalities. In rare cases there may be extrophy of the urinary bladder.

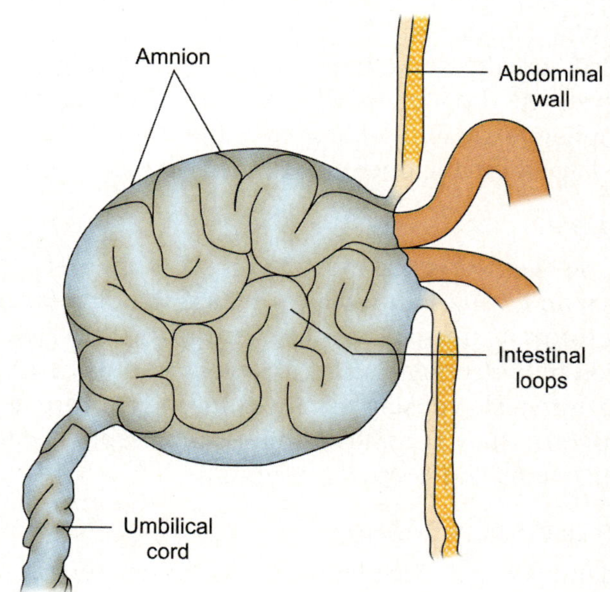

Fig. 6.23 Omphalocele

Gastrochises (Incidence 1 : 10000)

This is a condition where the abdominal contents protrude directly into the amniotic cavity through the defect caused by the abnormal closure of the body wall around the connecting stalk generally from the right side of the umbilicus. In this the viscera is not covered by amnion or by peritoneum, but there may be damage to the intestine as they are directly exposed to the amniotic fluid. No association is found with any chromosomal anomalies or any vital organ defects but volvulus is common due to compromised blood supply.

Vitelline Duct Abnormalities

In very minor percentage of people (2–4%) the entire or part of the vitelline duct remains patent or the band formed by the vitelline duct which connects ileum to the umbilicus (which should disappear) remains. This causes outpouching of the ileum causing a diverticuli called Meckel's diverticulum. This is generally present on the antimesentric border of the ileum 40–60 cm from the I–C junction in adults. It is generally asymptomatic but symptoms occur when the diverticuli contains gastric mucosa or the pancreatic tissue causing ulceration, bleeding or even perforation.

In some cases the vitelline duct gets converted to fibrous band or cord which connects the umbilicus to the ileum. In rare cases middle portion of this cord remains patent forming a cyst called enterocystoma or the vitelline cyst. Intestines may get strangulated, twisted or obstructed causing volvulus due to this band. In extreme cases the entire tract of the vitelline duct is patent forming a fistula called an umbilical fistula or a vitelline fistula which may discharge a faecal matter.

Gut Rotation Abnormalities

An abnormal rotation of the intestinal loop can cause twisting of the intestine which might compromise even the blood supply causing volvulus.

The normal rotation of the primary intestinal loop is 270° counterclockwise, sometimes the rotation is only by 90° resulting in colon and caecum to enter and lie on the left side of the abdominal cavity. The later returning loops settle on the right side, thus a left, sided colon is formed.

Reverse Rotation

In some cases the rotation occurs clockwise by 90°. Due to this the transverse colon passes behind the duodenum and lie behind the superior mesentery artery.

Duplication and Cyst (Overdevelopment)

The intestinal loops may duplicate anywhere along the length of the gut tube and sometimes cyst may also develop with the same (commonest site ileum). There may be associated findings like imperforate anus, gastrochises, omphalocoele, atresia, etc. Commonest cause is failure of normal recannalisation.

The cause of underdevelopment (atresia and stenosis) of the intestine may be due to lack of recannalisation and/or vascular accidents. In case of vascular accidents causing decreased blood supply either a part of the bowel is lost, remains as a fibrous band or bowel narrowing. Most common atresia occurs in duodenum, but even colon, jejunum or ileum is not excluded. Agenesis of the intestinal segment is also common but when extensive is incompatible with the life.

Mucoviscidosis is the adherence of the meconium to the intestinal wall secondary to deficiency of trysin secretion by the pancreas as a result the later being invaded by intestinal fibrosis of unknown origin.

Hindgut Malformations

This is generally caused due to problems of the uro-rectal septum.

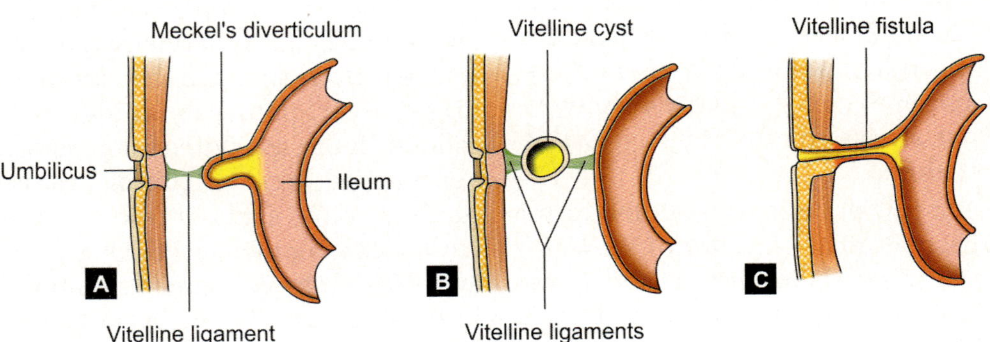

Fig. 6.24A to C Vitelline duct remnants

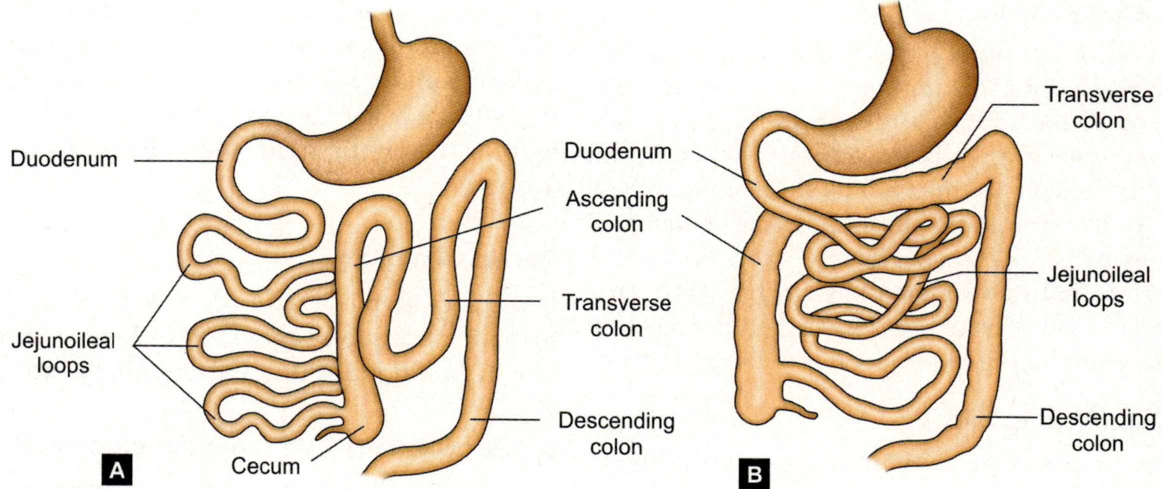

Fig. 6.25A and B Abnormal rotation of the primary intestinal loops. (A) Left sided colon and (B) Transverse colon behind the duodenum

Rectoanal atresia may be present or remain as a fibrous band. Imperforate anus may be present when the membrane fails to breakdown, this is a surgical emergency. Recto-uretral and recto-vaginal fistula are caused by abnormalities of the cloaca and urorectal septum when it is not able to extend till the end. Sometimes there may be absence of parasympathetic ganglia in the bowel wall causing a condition called **Congenital Megacolon (Hirschsprung's disease)**. It may involve rectum (common), sigmoid, transverse, right-sided colon and in rare cases the entire colon.

To concise the above in sequence:

Foetal part: Adult parts margins—organs formed—arterial supply—abnormalities.

1. **Foregut:** Oesophagus to 2nd part of duodenum — oesophagus, stomach, duodenum (1st and 2nd part), liver, gall bladder, pancreas—celiac trunk—oesophageal atresia and fistula, gastrochisis, duodenal atresia, pyloric stenosis.
2. **Midgut:** Lower duodenum to the proximal 2/3rd of the transverse colon—lower duodenum, jejunum, ileum, cecum, appendix, ascending colon and first 2/3rd of the transverse colon—superior mesenteric artery—intestinal atresia, malrotation, volvulus, Meckel's diverticulum.
3. **Hindgut:** Distal 3rd of the transverse colon to the upper part of the anal canal—last 3rd of the transverse colon, descending colon, rectum and upper part of the anal canal—inferior mesenteric artery—Hirschsprung's disease, anorectal malformations like fistula, imperforate anus.
4. **Other anomalies** of the abdominal wall and diaphragm causing abdominal wall defects, omphalocele and diaphragmatic hernia.

Key Point

Three development guts form the adult gut foregut, midgut and hindgut.

Must Remember Fact

Gastric empting is delayed in neonates in stress, pain trauma sepsis.

Take Home Message

Look out for other system abnormalities if one finds some GI system congenital abnormality.

SUMMARY

The endoderm forms the epithelial lining and the parenchymal derivatives of the digestive system. The gut extends from oropharynx to the cloacal membrane and is divided into pharyngeal gut, foregut (esophagus, tracheal bud, stomach duodenum till the bile duct origin, liver, pancreas), midgut (distal duodenum, jejunum, ilium, ascending colon, right 2/3rd of the transverse colon), hindgut (distal 1/3rd of the colon descending colon, sigmoid colon and upper anal canal). During development at 6th week, bowel grows rapidly and causes physiological herniation and then returns in the body by 270 degree rotation counterclockwise. Problems arise if these do not rotate completely or partially.

FAQ

Q. Does polyhydramnios in the antenatal period signify something?

ENDOCRINE SYSTEM

Consists of thyroid, parathyroid, pancreas, pituitary, adrenal, thymus.

Pituitary gland

It develops from two different parts:

1. An ectodermal outpocketing of the stomodium which is immediately in front of the oropharyngeal membrane called the Rathke's pouch.
2. A downward extension of the diencephlon, the infundibulum.

During the 3rd week of gestation the Rathke's pouch appear as an evagination from the oral cavity. Slowly it grows towards the infundibulam and then lose its contact with the oral cavity and come to lie anterior to the infunibulum.

Then later the cells of the Rathke's pouch in the anterior part divide rapidly to form anterior part of adenohypophysis. A small part of this pouch grows along the stalk of infundibulum to form pars tuburalis (stalk). The posterior part forms the pars intermedia. The infundibulum forms the stalk and the posterior lobe called the pars nervosa (neurological).

Congenital Defect

Sometimes Rathke's pouch persists in the roof of pharynx. These may give rise to cranio pharyngioma.

Congenital absence of pituitary gland is possible causing neonatal death.

Suprarenal Gland

The development of the suprarenal gland starts in the 5th week of gestation. The suprarenal gland is made of two parts.

- Cortex: Mesodermal origin
- Medulla: Ectodermal origin

During development the mesothelial cells which lie between the developing gonads and the roof of the mesentery start to divide and proliferate at the same time.[1] They also penetrate the underlying mesenchyme. These then differentiate in cells forming foetal cortex which is composed of large acidophilic organs. After that another set of cells which are smaller in size than the initial cells penetrate the mesenchyme from the mesothelial tissue. These cells surround the initial cells and later form the definitive cortex. After birth the foetal cortex regresses rapidly except for the outermost layer which forms the reticular zone. The adult type of cortex is only achieved at the puberty. During the cortex formation in the foetal life, cells of the sympathetic system origin invade in the medial part and gets arranged in cords and clusters which forms the medulla of the suprarenal gland.

Abnormalities

Adrenals may be absent or ectopic.

Thyroid

Thyroid gland develops as an epithelial proliferating growth from the floor of the pharynx between the tuberculum impar and the foramen ceacum. It then descends in front of the pharynx but at the same time remains connected to the tongue by the stalk called the **Thyroglossal Duct**. Over a period of time the gland losses its connection with the tongue as the duct disappears. The gland still goes downwards and passes the hyoid bone and laryngeal cartilages where it takes the final position (7th week) as a bilobed structure. The thyroid starts functioning in the third month when the follicular cells produce thyroxine and tri-iodothyronine. Parafollicular or C cells are derived from ultimo-branchial body which causes secretion of the calcitonin.

Abnormalities

Congenital hypothyroidism may be seen in thyroid dysgenesis. Thyroid dyshormonogenesis is also not uncommon (Pendral syndrome). Abnormal thyroid tissue may be present along the descent of the thyroid path, but commonest site is at the base of the tongue. The thyroglossal duct may remain in some (part, fully or partly) along the the path, sometimes even forming

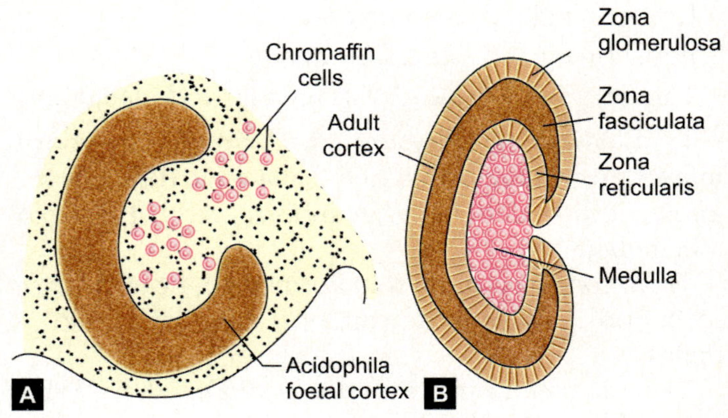

Fig. 6.26A and B Suprarenal gland formation

a cyst (thyroglossal cyst). Characteristics of this is that it is always in midline, and the most common sites is near the hyoid bone and at the base of the tongue. In occasional cases the cyst may communicate with outside causing thyroglossal fistula.

Parathyroid and Thymus Glands

These are paired bodies, one superior and one inferior, both on dorsal surface of the thyroid gland.

The 5th week witnesses the formation of the inferior parathyroid glands which arise from the dorsal region of the 3rd pouch (the ventral region forms the thymus). Both these start moving caudally and lose contact with pharyngeal wall. Actually the thymus pulls the parathyroid glands with it. Later the thymus enters the thoracic cavity and fuses with its part from opposite side completing the gland.[1] During this the parathyroid tissue of the 3rd pouch comes to rest on the dorsal surface of the thyroid gland, then labeled as inferior gland.

The dorsal surface of the 4th pouch forms the superior parathyroid gland. As the development proceeds the parathyroid tissue of the 4th pouch losses its contact with the pharynx and gets rested on the dorsal surface of the thyroid gland then labeled as superior parathyroid glands.

Abnormalities

Congenital absence of the parathyroid gland is not uncommon. There may be migration of the glands along the path of development. The inferior glands are more variable in position than the superior ones and are sometimes found at the bifurcation of the common carotid artery.

Endocrine disorders may be divided into three groups:

- Endocrine gland hyposecretion.
- Endocrine gland hypersecretion
- Tumors of endocrine glands (benign and malignant)

Congenital hypothyroidism (1 in 4000 newborn infants): It can occur due to the anatomic defect in the gland, iodine deficiency or inborn error of thyroid metabolism.

It is a condition of thyroid hormone deficiency since birth and is twice more common in females than in males.

Genetic causes like mutations in DUOX2, TSHR, TPO, TSHB, TG, PAX8, SLC5A5 in genes can cause congenital hypothyroidism.

Congenital hypothyroidism if not treated after birth can lead to growth retardation and intellectual disability of permanent nature. Decreased serum thyroid levels and increased thyroid stimulating hormone levels are the main stay for diagnosis of primary hypothyroidism. All of the developed countries screen the newborns for congenital hypothyroidism in the early weeks of life to prevent the permanent damage. The treatment consists of daily oral thyroxine.

Congenital Hyperthyroidism

It is very uncommon condition, hence details are not known properly but the course and treatment is the same as the adults.

Congenital Adrenal Hyperplasia

This results from the mutations of genes for enzymes mediating the biochemical steps for production of cortisol from cholesterol from adrenal glands (autosomal recessive). There is mutation of genes due to 21-OH deficiencies (found on 6p21.3 a part of HLA complex) which produces active and inactive genes. Mutants are formed due to gene conversion or recombination between the active and inactive genes. These cause hypo or hyper secretion of sex steroids causing alteration in the development of primary or secondary sex characters in infants and children.

Treatment consists of supplying the necessary glucocorticoids and mineralo corticoids according to the need.

Congenital Adrenal Hypoplasia

It is rare as compared to hyperplasia though some cases were found in Japan.

Congenital Diabetes

It is an extremely rare condition and very little is known about its pathogenesis.

Type 1 Diabetes Mellitus

It is a condition in which there is an organ-specific T-cell mediated autoimmune condition where there is cellular inflammation of the pancreatic islets and destruction of insulin producing beta cells.

Parathyroid Diseases

Hyper or Hypoparathyroidism

Congenital hypoparathyroidism is a condition where the babies are born without parathyroid tissue causing calcium deficiencies resulting in fragile bones and developmental problems. Treatment consists of calcium supplementation.

Congenital hyperparathyroidism is secondary to maternal hypoparathyroidism.

Pituitary Gland

Congenital absence of pituitary gland may be present but will result in death in neonatal period.

SUMMARY

Pitutary develops from ectodermal outpouching (Rathke's pouch and extension of the diencephalon). Thyroid develops from epithelium from the floor of the pharynx. Parathyroid develops from 3rd and 4th pharyngeal pouch floor. Development problems occur if there is a remnant part at abnormal sites.

> **Pearl**
> Thyroid function in a newborn becomes important.

FAQ with Answer

Q. Why does thyroglossal cyst occur?

A. Thyroglossal cysts (TGCs) arise from a persistent epithelial tract, the thyroglossal duct, formed with the descent of the thyroid from the foramen caecum to its final position in the front of the neck.

REFERENCES

1. Langman's J. Medical Embryology. 11th edn. Williams & Wilkins, 2009.
2. Cote, Lerman, Todres. A Practice for Anaesthesia for Infants and Children. 4th edn.
3. Frederic A Berry, David J Steward. Paediatrics for Anaesthesiologists.
4. Gregory GA, Edger EJ, Munson ES. Anaesthesiology. 1969.
5. Arnold G. Coran. Paediatric Surgery. 7th edn.
6. Smith CA, Nelson NM. Physiology of the Newborn Infant. 4th edn.

Essentials of Fluids, Electrolytes and Nutrition in Infants and Children

Mahesh Baldwa, Varsha Gupta and Sushila Baldwa

INTRODUCTION

Factors which determine the overall water weight of a human being include sex, age, bones, muscles and body fat percentage. Infants, have low bone mass and low body fat, are 73% water. Due to the high concentration of water, an infant's skin appears "dewy" and soft. Total body water (TBW) slowly becomes less after infancy, and by the time one becomes old age, total body water is only about 45%.[1] Adipose (fat) tissue is the least hydrated tissue in the body (20% hydrated), even bone contains more water compared to fat. By now skeletal muscle contains 75% water.

NORMAL PHYSIOLOGY AND ANATOMY OF THE BODY FLUIDS FOR PAEDIATRIC ANAESTHETIST (PA)

Why Compartments are known as Compartments?

Water constitutes and holds major percentage in each compartment as compared to colloids and crystalloid. Water acts as medium to carry colloids and crystalloid across the semi-permeable membrane. Each compartment operates independently, but interacts with neighboring compartments partitioned by semi-permeable membrane. Each compartment has unique colloid, electrolyte and water level and maintains the mean level by homeostatic mechanism. Only water moves depending on the concentration of crystalloids and collides across semi-permeable membrane of each compartment. Sometime false compartment are created by accumulation of fluids, blood within ventricles of brain, pleura of lungs or peritoneum and lumen of organs like intestine, etc. This fluid can be drained. This may be blood, pus, transudate or exudates. One has to keep in mind hidden nature of such compartments.

a. **Fluid compartments:** There are two main fluid compartments water occupies in the body. About two-thirds (2/3) is in the intracellular fluid (ICF) compartment. The intracellular fluid is the fluid within the cells of the body and is entirely enclosed by cell membranes. The remaining one-third of body water is outside cells, in the extracellular fluid compartment (ECF). The ECF is the body's internal environment and the cells external environment.[2] The ECF includes the interstitial fluid and the plasma. Exchange occurs between the ECF and ICF due to the permeability of cell membranes, but the two fluid compartments retain their distinctive characteristics. Although the ECF and ICF differ in terms of their ionic composition, osmolarities are same and no movement of water occurs between the two compartments. Alterations in the osmolarity of either compartment results in water/fluid shifts that eliminate the differences.[3]

b. **Three fluid compartments of the body:** There is exchange of gases, nutrients, water, and wastes between three above mentioned fluid compartments of the body. In the image below, the ECF compartment is divisible in two compartments: (1) Plasma, the fluid portion of blood which is 10% of TBW, and (2) interstitial fluid (IF) which is 3–4% of TBW, the fluid in the spaces between tissue cells.

Water losses are balanced by gains from eating, drinking, and metabolic generation of water.

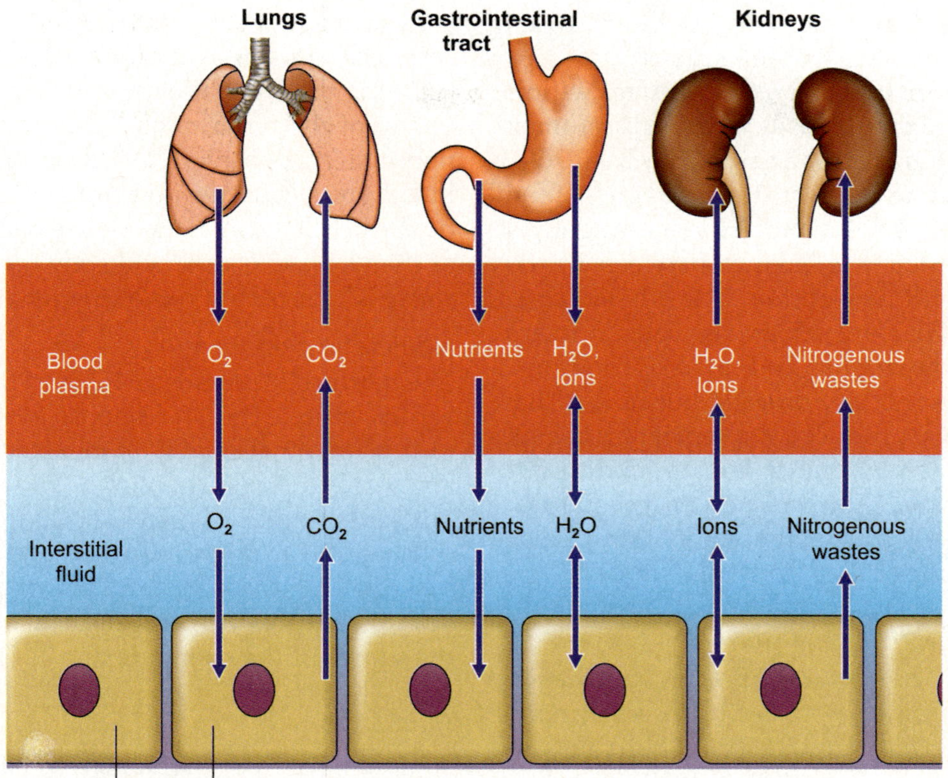

FOUR BASIC PHYSIOLOGICAL PRINCIPLES AND SIMPLE PRINCIPLES IN THE REGULATION OF FLUIDS AND ELECTROLYTES APPLICABLE TO CHILDREN

1. **Homeostatic mechanisms fluids respond to changes in the ECF and not to ICF:** Receptors monitoring the composition of two basic components of the ECF—plasma and cerebrospinal fluid—detect significant changes in their composition or volume and trigger appropriate neural and endocrine releases. This makes functional sense, because a change in one ECF component will spread message rapidly throughout the extracellular compartment and affecting entire mass body's cells. In the striking contrast, the ICF is contained bound within individual cells that are physically and chemically isolated from one another by their cell membranes. Thus, changes in the ICF in one cell have no direct effect on the composition of the ICF in distant and far off cells and tissues, unless these changes create effect in ECF. So changes in ECF are key to homeostatic mechanisms.[4]

2. **No provision of receptors which can directly monitor fluid or electrolyte balance in body.** In other words, body receptors cannot detect how many litres of water or how many grams of sodium, chloride and potassium is contained in the body. Body has no mechanism to measure how many litres of water and how many grams of electrolytes body gains or losses during 24 hours. But body receptors *can* monitor *plasma volume* and *osmotic concentration*. This is because fluid continuously circulates between interstitial fluid and plasma in ECF. This is also true that there is continuous process of exchange between the ECF and the ICF, the plasma volume and osmotic concentration are good indicators of the state of fluid balance and electrolyte balance in body.[4]

3. **Principle of "water follows salt" and cells cannot move water molecules by active transport.** Normally movement of water across cell membranes and epithelia occurs passively. The principle is "*water follows salt*." Osmotic as well as oncotic gradients are generated by the active transport of specific ions, such as sodium and chloride etc. In body sodium and chloride ions (or other solutes) are actively transported across a membrane or epithelium, water follows the rule of osmosis. The principle is "*water follows salt*", accounts for water absorption by digestive system. The principle is

"*water follows salt*" also happens in kidney leading to conservation of water in the kidneys.[4]

4. **The body's content of water or electrolytes will rise if dietary gains exceed losses to the environment, and will fall if losses exceed gains.** This basic rule is important when one considers the mechanics of fluid balance and electrolyte balance. Homeostatic adjustments mainly affect the balance between urinary excretion and gut absorption. The physiological adjustments in renal function are regulated primarily by circulating hormones like aldosterone, antinatriuretic hormone, antidiuretic hormone. These hormones can also produce complementary changes in actual behavior of child. The combination of angiotensin II and aldosterone can give child a sensation of thirst, which stimulates child to drink fluids and develops a taste for salted foods.[4]

The Primary Regulatory Hormones

Major physiological adjustments affecting fluid balance and electrolyte balance are mediated by three hormones: (1) *antidiuretic hormone (ADH)*, (2) *aldosterone*, and (3) the *atrial natriuretic peptides (ANP)* and *brain natriuretic peptide (BNP)*.[4]

Antidiuretic hormone

The hypothalamus contains special cells known as **osmoreceptors**, which monitor the osmotic concentration of the ECF. These cells are sensitive to at least 2 percent change in osmotic concentration (approximately 6 mOsm/L). The rate of ADH release varies directly with osmotic concentration: The higher the osmotic concentration, more ADH is produced. Increased ADH has two important effects: (1) It stimulates water conservation from kidneys, reducing urinary water losses and concentrating the urine; and (2) It stimulates the thirst centre, promoting the intake of fluids.[4]

Aldosterone

The secretion of aldosterone by the adrenal cortex plays a major role in determining the rate of Na^+ absorption and K^+ loss along the distal convoluted tubule (DCT) and collecting system of the kidneys. The higher the plasma concentration of aldosterone, the more efficiently the kidneys conserve Na^+. Because "water follows salt," the conserved Na^+ stimulates water retention: As Na^+ is reabsorbed, and as sodium and chloride ions move out of the tubular fluid, water follows by osmosis. Aldosterone also increases the sensitivity of salt receptors on the tongue promoting consumption of salty foods. Aldosterone is secreted in response to rising K^+ or falling Na^+ levels in the blood reaching the adrenal cortex, or in response to the activation of the renin–angiotensin system. Renin release occurs in response to: (1) a drop in plasma volume or blood pressure at the juxtaglomerular apparatus of the nephron, (2) a decline in filtrate osmotic concentration at the DCT, or, as we will soon see, (3) falling Na^+ or rising K^+ concentrations in the renal circulation.[4]

Natriuretic peptides

The natriuretic peptides ANP and BNP are released by cardiac muscle cells in response to abnormal stretching of the heart walls, leads to elevated blood pressure or an increase in blood volume. This reduces thirst and block the release of ADH and aldosterone that might otherwise lead to the conservation of water and salt. The resulting diuresis (fluid loss at the kidneys) lowers both blood pressure and plasma volume, eliminating the source of the stimulation.

Fluid Shifts

A rapid water movement between the ECF and the ICF in response to an osmotic gradient is called a **fluid shift**. Fluid shifts rapidly happens in response to changes in the osmotic concentration of the ECF and reach equilibrium within minutes to hours.

1. **If the osmotic concentration of the ECF increases, fluid will become hypertonic as compared to the ICF.** Water will move from cells to the ECF until osmotic equilibrium restored. Osmotic concentration of the ECF will increase if one loses water but retain electrolytes.[5]
2. **If the osmotic concentration of the ECF decreases, that fluid will become hypotonic with respect to the ICF.** Water moves from the ECF to cells, hence ICF volume increases. Osmotic concentration of ECF will decrease if one gains water but does not gain electrolytes.[5]
3. **In sum, if the osmotic concentrations of the ECF changes, a fluid shift between the ICF and ECF will tend to oppose the change.** Because the volume of the ICF is much greater than that of the ECF, the ICF acts as water reserve. In effect, instead of a large change in the osmotic concentration of the ECF, smaller changes occur in both the ECF and ICF.[5]

Physiology of Major Electrolytes

Two cations, Na^+ and K^+, merit particular attention, because—(1) they are major contributors to the osmotic concentrations of the ECF and the ICF, respectively, and (2) they directly affect the normal functioning of all cells. Sodium is the dominant cation in the ECF. More than 90 percent of the osmotic concentration of the ECF results from the presence of sodium salts, mainly sodium chloride (NaCl) and sodium bicarbonate ($NaHCO_3$), so changes in the osmotic concentration of body fluids generally reflect changes in Na^+ concentration. Normal Na^+ concentrations in the ECF average about 140 mEq/L, versus 10 mEq/L or less in the ICF. Potassium is the dominant cation in the ICF, where concentrations reach 160 mEq/L. Extracellular K^+ concentrations are generally very low, from 3.8 to 5.0 mEq/L.[6]

RENAL FUNCTIONS IN CHILDREN

Children have immature renal function at birth with reduced GFR by 25% of adult level. Hence concentrating capacity of newborn kidney for term infant is maximum 600–700 mOsm/kg as compared to adult kidney with maximum concentrating ability of 1200 mOsm/kg.[7] By four to five days of age in neonate there is a marked improvement in renal function, and the ability to conserve fluid and excrete an overload. After one month the kidney is approximately 60% mature even though GFR remains low. Fluid and sodium conservation is limited in newborns and infants, while excretion of water and electrolytes is possible even in premature infants. Tubular function is especially limited for special excretion and re-absorption mechanisms. Prematures have limited ability to reabsorb sodium, and will therefore become hyponatremic without adequate replacement. The thresholds for glucose and sodium bicarbonate are lower than in adults. Hyperglycemia may lead to osmolar diuresis with consequent deficits in water and sodium. By 18 months of age renal function is completely matured.

ECF and ICF in Children

The major difference between infants and adults is the fact that 40% of body water in newborns is extracellular fluid (ECF), while in adults, the ECF is 20%. This extracellular water is in the interstitial fluid volume, while plasma volume is proportionate at all ages. The high percentage of ECF causes a high turnover of water and electrolytes, especially sodium. A newborn child may lose 10% of its body weight if it drinks nothing for a day. Hence there has been a change in the recommended time for patients to be fasted. Fat and milk slow gastric emptying time, hence avoided preoperatively. For infants younger than one year, milk should be given up to 6 hours before surgery, and clear liquids up to 3 hours.

FLUID AND ELECTROLYTE HOMEOSTATIC MECHANISMS

1. Homeostatic mechanisms that monitor and adjust the composition of body fluids respond to changes in the ECF, not the ICF. Maintenance of normal fluid volume, composition, and pH in the ICF and ECF occurs due to three integrated processes:
   - fluid balance
   - electrolyte balance
   - acid–base balance.
2. There are receptors which are sensitive to changes in the composition of the plasma and thus give proper homeostatic signal.
3. The body content of water or electrolytes will rise if intake exceeds by dietary absorption and no corresponding physiological increase in outflow through urinary excretion.
4. Three hormones are involved in the regulation of fluid and electrolyte balance are
   - Antidiuretic hormone (ADH): ADH encourages water resorption at the kidneys and creates a desire to drink water.
   - Aldosterone: Aldosterone increases the rates of sodium resorption at the kidneys.
   - Antinatriuretic (ANF): ANF opposes these actions and promotes fluid and electrolyte losses in the urine.
5. Increase in water content without electrolytes will lower the osmolarities of the ECF and ICF.
6. Losing water without electrolytes will increase the osmolarities of both compartments. ADH secretion plays key role in both situations by regulating water intake and loss.

Electrolyte Balance

Sodium Ion Regulation

The rate of sodium absorption by intestine is directly proportional to sodium intake from diet. Sodium losses chiefly occur through urine and perspiration. Sodium filtered by GFR is reabsorbed by distal convoluted tubules and collecting segments of kidney with the help of circulating aldosterone. Sodium re-absorption is tied to absorption of a corresponding anion, which is usually chloride and/or bicarbonate, and the secretion of either hydrogen in exchange of potassium ions. Changes in the rates of sodium uptake or excretion do not alter the sodium concentration of the ECF with help of osmotic movement of water. The volume excess changes in total fluid are regulated by the secretion of ADH and aldosterone and ANF. Identical homeostatic adjustments occur in response to volume depletion caused by blood or tissue fluid losses.

Potassium Ion Regulation

Potassium ion concentrations in the ECF are very low, and they are not as closely regulated by body. Potassium excretion increases as ECF concentrations rise, under aldosterone stimulation, and if pH rises. Potassium retention occurs when the pH falls.[3]

Calcium Ion Regulation

Total serum calcium levels in term infants decline from values of 10–11 mg/dL at birth to 7.5–8.5 mg/dL over the first 2–3 days of life. Approximately 50% of the total calcium biologically available is in the ionized form. Calcium concentrations can be reported either in milligram per deciliter (mg/dL) or in millimolar units (mmol/L). Conversion between the two methods is accomplished by dividing by 4 (e.g. 4 mg/dL of ionized calcium equal to 1 mmol/L). It is regulated by vitamin D, parathormone.

ACID–BASE BALANCE

A neutral solution contains hydrogen and hydroxyl ions in equal concentrations. The pH represents the negative log of the hydrogen ion concentration, and it ranges from 0 to 14. Acids dissociate in water and release hydrogen ions. Bases remove hydrogen ions or introduce hydroxyl ions. Salts dissociate with a little change on hydrogen or hydroxyl ion concentrations. Acids and bases may be categorized as strong or weak depending on their behavior building H ion concentration in solution. Normal body pH ranges from 7.35 to 7.45.Variations outside of this relatively narrow zone produce acidosis or alkalosis.[4]

The Maintenance of Normal pH

Disturbances to pH homeostasis are from ketoacidosis and lactic acid. The regulation of pH occurs through the bicarbonate buffer system operates in ECF. It removes hydrogen ions to stabilize pH. Pulmonary carbon dioxide is a volatile acid because it readily diffuses out of solution into the alveolar air of lungs. The loss of carbon dioxide at the lungs lowers the concentrations of hydrogen ions and bicarbonates in solution. Increase and decrease of the rate of respiration thus has a direct effect on pH. Renal mechanisms operate through kidneys vary their rates of hydrogen ion secretion and bicarbonate ion resorption depending on the pH of the extracellular fluids. In acidosis the rates of H^+ secretion and bicarbonate ion reabsorption and generation increase. Phosphate in ECF and protein buffer systems in both ECF and ICF are less important and less amenable to correction to paediatric anaesthetist. Any deviation from the normal range is extremely dangerous, because changes in H^+ concentrations disrupt the stability of cell membranes, altering structure of proteins, and activities of important enzymes.[4]

Disturbances in Acid–Base Balance

Respiratory acidosis results from the excessive accumulation of carbon dioxide in body fluids. The common cause is hypoventilation, which gets corrected by chemoreceptor reflexes. In the absence of usual homeostatic mechanisms, acute respiratory acidosis develops. Respiratory alkalosis is an uncommon condition associated with hyperventilation. Metabolic acidosis due to lactic acidosis or ketoacidosis results from any condition that depletes the normal reserves of bicarbonate ions. This can result from a loss of bicarbonate ions or their utilization in neutralizing of lactic acid and keto acids. The most frequent cause of metabolic acidosis is an inability to excrete hydrogen ions at the kidneys. It can also result from the bicarbonate loss by intestine in cases of chronic diarrhoea. Metabolic alkalosis occurs when bicarbonate ion concentrations become elevated. In rare cases it may occur following extended periods of vomiting where gastric HCL acid is lost.[4]

Fluid Balance and Fluid Administration

Total body water content is comparatively large in neonates and infants with respect to adult values after the age of 1 year. As age advances the amount of muscle mass increases, intracellular water content rises. Water turnover in the infant is more than double that of an adult. In infants approximately 40% of extracellular water is lost every day as urine, stool, sweat, and insensible losses via skin and airways and lungs. Dehydration can easily follow if reduction of intake (preoperative fasting for 6 hours) or increased loss of fluids occurs (which is most commonly due to vomiting and diarrhoea).

Table 7.1 Body water and blood volume with age

	Water (%) body weight	Extracellular volume (%) body weight	Blood volume (ml/kg)
Premature	90	60	100
Term neonate	80	40–45	90
1 year	60	25–30	80
Adult	55	18	70

1. Clinical assessment of fluid balance in children is aided by recognition of situations where deficits are likely:
   a. Gastrointestinal
   b. Pre- or postoperative ileus
   c. Pre- or postoperative sepsis
   d. Burns
   e. Trauma
   f. Pre- or postoperative bleeding.
2. Hypovolaemia and dehydration or salt and water depletion are diagnosed clinically
   a. Loss of turgor of skin
   b. Sunken eyes
   c. Sunken fontanelle
   d. Capillary refill time prolonged to >2 sec
   e. Tachycardia (rule out if caused by pain, fever, anxiety)
   f. Oliguria
   g. Cool peripheries, cold limbs
   h. Increased core-peripheral temperature gap
   i. Thready fast pulse
   j. Reduced level of consciousness/sensorium or irritable or toxic looking child 'the child that is confused might not be perfused'
   k. Hypotension is a late sign; often occurs only after >30% of blood volume is lost.
3. Shock is the clinical state when demand is higher than delivery of oxygen and nutrition to the cells of body.
4. Preoperative fluids and fluid resuscitation
5. Replace circulating volume with crystalloids (0.9% saline/RL) or colloids (plasma protein solution, or dextran/starch/hemaccele solution). Blood products are given for major or ongoing losses.
6. Extracellular fluid losses are replaced with isotonic crystalloid solution, e.g. 0.9% saline, RL solution.
7. Some situations are managed according to a local institutional protocol, e.g. burns, pyloric stenosis, diabetic ketoacidosis.
8. Blood volume is estimated at 90 mL/kg in neonates, 85 mL/kg in infants and 80 mL/kg in children.
9. In shock give fluid boluses of 20 mL/kg crystalloid or colloid, then re-assess.
10. Even after 40, 60, and 80 mL/kg without stabilization (depends on the dynamics of the clinical situation and expected ongoing losses) consider endo-tracheal intubation, inotropic support, and blood products.
    a. Consider blood after 15–20% of circulating volume is lost.
    b. Consider fresh frozen plasma after 50% of circulating volume is lost after giving blood.
    c. Consider platelets after 100% of circulating volume is lost after giving plasma.
    d. Rapid laboratory testing for specific factors and selective replacement may minimize blood product administration and the associated risks and costs.

INTRAOPERATIVE FLUID ADMINISTRATION

1. Child anaesthetist is required to replace a fluid deficit if any, provide maintenance requirements and replace ongoing intra-operative losses.
2. For elective cases fluid deficits is rarely a problem. Current recommendations about fasting times are relatively short in duration and IV fluids are given to children who are not able to drink fluids. Non-elective cases come to operation theatre with a fluid deficit need extra fluids. In most cases fluids are administered during preoperative resuscitation and preoperative preparation.
3. Maintenance fluids during surgery can be given as dextrose with saline or dextrose-free crystalloid, e.g. RL or 0.9% saline. Giving 0.9% saline is preferred over other fluids expect in newborns.
   a. Dextrose containing fluids are usually unnecessary except in premature babies, neonates, and babies receiving parenteral nutrition.
   b. Hypoglycaemia rarely occurs in healthy children during anaesthesia and surgery. Children show increase in dextrose levels during the perioperative period in response to fasting and stress of surgery.
   c. IV fluids containing 5% dextrose usually cause hyperglycaemia during surgery.
   d. Dextrose containing solutions are isotonic when administered but once the dextrose is metabolized, hence rest of fluid behaves free water leading to

hypotonicity in vascular compartment, hence there is a risk of hyponatraemia. ADH is secreted during the perioperative period (stress, pain, hypovolaemia, drugs) and further reduces plasma sodium concentration and osmolarity.

e. Children develop hyponatraemia readily compared to adults make them susceptible to its effects on the CNS. It is now considered to be a major risk in the perioperative care of children.

4. Fluid losses during surgery are by and large isotonic. Losses are replaced with crystalloid or colloids or blood products.

Maintenance Fluid Regimens

Maintenance fluid at birth to 7 days.

Term babies and babies with birth weight >1500 grams

Day 1: 10% Dextrose

Day 2 to 7: 10% Dextrose and sodium and potassium to be added after 48 hours

Preterm baby weighing 1000–1500 grams

Day 1: 10% Dextrose

Day 2 to 7: 10% Dextrose and sodium and potassium to be added after 48 hours

After day 7: Fluids to be given at 150–160 ml/kg/day and sodium supplementation at 3–5 mEq/kg should continue till 32–34 weeks corrected gestational age.

1. **Neonatal regimens**
   a. *Fluid requirement during the first 5 days in the neonate:*
      i. Day 1: 60 mL/kg/day
      ii. Day 2: 90 mL/kg/day
      iii. Day 3: 120 mL/kg/day
      iv. Day 4: 150 mL/kg/day
      v. Day 5: 150 mL/kg/day.
   b. *Electrolyte requirements:*
      i. Sodium: 2–4 mmol/kg/day (in contrast to fluid requirements, this is relatively stable)
      ii. Potassium: 2–3 mmol/kg/day.
   c. *Dextrose requirements:* Usually provided using a 10% solution for maintenance. A 20% solution is occasionally required in septic or fluid restricted neonates.
2. **Infants and children**
   a. There are several formulae used to calculate maintenance fluid requirements. These are derived from the relationship between body weight and metabolic rate (energy requirements). Infants require 100 kcal/kg/day and children 75 kcal/kg/day. 1 mL of water per kcal is required for metabolism.[8]
   b. A common formula is the 4-2-1 of Holiday segar:
      i. 4 mL/kg for first 10 kg
      ii. plus: 2 mL/kg for next 10 kg
      iii. plus: 1 mL/kg thereafter.
      iv. e.g. a child of 17 kg requires 40 + 14 = 54 mL/hour; a child of 24 kg requires 40 + 20 + 4 = 64 mL/hour.
   c. Electrolyte requirements in kilogram/day:
      i. Sodium 2–4 mmol/(mili Eq)/kg/day
      ii. Potassium 2–3 mmol/(mili Eq)/kg/day
   d. Maintenance electrolyte requirements per 100 calories/day
      i. Sodium 3 mEq (mmol) per 100 kcal/day
      ii. Potassium 2 mEq (mmol) per 100 kcal/day
      iii. Chloride 2 mEq (mmol) per 100 kcal/day
3. Additional losses: Depending on their nature, losses are replaced as appropriate, e.g.:
   a. Nasogastric losses: Volume for volume with Hartmann's solution or 0.9% saline with 10 mmol KCl per 500 mL.
   b. Stoma losses: 50–75% of losses as 0.9% saline with 10 mmol KCl per 500 mL.
4. Fluids should be administered through a volumetric pump with a pressure limit set.
5. Common solutions for maintenance are:
   a. 0.45% saline/5% dextrose
   b. 0.225% sodium/5% dextrose
   c. 10% dextrose is commonly used in premature children and neonates.
6. Monitoring of electrolyte concentrations is required if maintenance fluids are given for more than 24–48 hours. The formulae used are only a guide to estimate fluid requirements. In clinical circumstances, electrolyte derangements can occur. Hyponatraemia is a particular risk and may have devastating effect on brain.
7. Some anaesthetists restrict maintenance fluids to 50–75% of the calculated requirement during the postoperative period to reduce the risk of these problems.

Choice of Resuscitation Fluid upon Cause of the Deficit

Haemorrhage

Loss of RBCs diminishes O_2-carrying capacity, safety margin of about 9 times the resting O_2 requirement. Thus, non-O_2 carrying fluids (e.g. crystalloid or colloid solutions) may be used to restore intravascular volume in mild to moderate blood loss. However, in severe shock, blood products are required.

Crystalloid solutions for intravascular volume replenishment are typically isotonic [e.g. 0.9% saline or Ringer's lactate (RL)]. H_2O freely travels outside the vasculature, so as little as 10% of isotonic fluid remains in the intravascular space. With hypotonic fluid (e.g. 0.45% saline), even less remains in the vasculature, hence this fluid is not used for resuscitation. Both 0.9% saline and RL are equally effective; RL may be preferred in hemorrhagic shock because it somewhat minimizes acidosis and will not cause hyperchloremia. Child patient's having acute brain injury, 0.9% saline is preferred. Hypertonic saline is not recommended for resuscitation because the evidence suggests there is no difference in outcome when compared to isotonic fluids.

Colloid solutions (e.g. hydroxyethyl starch, albumin, dextrans) are also effective for volume replacement during major haemorrhage. Colloid solutions have no advantage over crystalloid and albumin is associated with poorer outcomes in traumatic brain injury. Both dextrans and hydroxyethyl starch may adversely affect coagulation when more than 1.5 L is given.

Blood typically is given as packed RBCs, which should be cross-matched, but in an urgent situation, 1 to 2 units of type O Rh-negative blood are an acceptable alternative. When > 1 to 2 units are transfused (e.g. in major trauma), blood is warmed to 37 °C. Patients receiving > 6 units may require replacement of clotting factors with infusion of fresh frozen plasma or cryoprecipitate and platelet transfusion.

Nonhaemorrhagic hypovolemia

Isotonic crystalloid solutions are typically given for intravascular repletion during shock and hypovolemia. Colloid solutions are generally not used. Patients with dehydration and adequate circulatory volume typically have a free water deficit, and hypotonic solutions (e.g. 5% D/W 0.45% saline) are used.

Common Terminology used for Fluid and Electrolyte Balance

Salt and water depletion

Dehydration or 'salt and water depletion' or 'blood loss' or 'plasma deficit' , the term 'dehydration' strictly means lack of water, which means to laymen lack of salt and water or even more loosely to describe intravascular volume depletion. The terms 'wet' and 'dry' also have imprecise meaning.

Using specific terminologies is better like using 'salt and water depletion' due to diarrhoea and vomiting or DKA or excessive use of diuretics is better instead using words like dehydration. Clinically visualized by dry tongue, loss of skin turgor, sinking of eye balls in children. Also 'blood loss deficit' specifies the cause due to bleeding/haemorrhage, which may be overt or hidden 'plasma protein deficit' specifies the cause which is commonly due to burns or malnutrition like Kwashiorkor or diseases of liver.[10]

Salt and water excess: This is common iatrogenic reason, resulting from excessive administration of saline, but is, of course, a feature of congestive heart failure and other oedema producing conditions. It takes 40–50% (2–3 litres in adults) of salt and water excess before the extracellular fluid is expanded sufficiently for oedema to become clinically apparent.

Solution: Fluid acts as solvent, e.g. dextrose or salt is dissolved.

Crystalloid: A term used commonly to describe all clear glucose and/or salt containing fluids for intravenous use (e.g. 0.9% saline, 5% dextrose, etc.).

Colloid: A fluid consisting of microscopic particles (e.g. starch or protein) suspended in a crystalloid and used for intravascular volume expansion (e.g. 6% hydroxyethyl starch, 4% succinylated gelatin, 20% albumin, etc.).[10]

Balanced crystalloid: A crystalloid containing electrolytes in a concentration as close to plasma as possible (e.g. Ringer's lactate, etc.).

Osmosis: This describes the process by which water moves across a semi-permeable membrane (permeable to water but not to the substances in solution) from a weaker to a stronger solution until the concentration of solutes are equal on the two compartments is termed osmotic pressure or, in the case of colloids, e.g. albumin, oncotic pressure which is proportional to number of atoms/ions/molecules in solution and is expressed as mOsm/litre (osmolarity) or mOsm/kg (osmolality) of solution. In clinical chemistry the term 'osmolality' is the one most often used.[10]

For example, out of approximately 280–290 mOsm/kg in extracellular fluid the largest single contributor is sodium chloride which dissociates in solution as Na^+ and Cl^- exert osmotic pressure independently, i.e. Na^+ (140 mmol/kg), contributes 140 mOsm/kg, and Cl^- (100 mmol/kg) contributes 100 mOsm/kg. Additional balancing negative charges come from bicarbonate (HCO_3^-) and other anions. In the intracellular space K^+ is the predominant cation. Because glucose does not dissociate in solution, each molecule, although molecule is much larger in weight and size than NaCl salt molecule, dextrose behaves as a single entity in solution and at a concentration of 5 mmol/kg, contributes only 5 mOsm/kg to the total osmolality of plasma.[11]

Partially Permeable Membranes

The cell membrane and the capillary membrane are both partially permeable membranes although not strictly semi-permeable in the chemical sense. They act, however, as partial barriers dividing the extracellular (ECF) from the intracellular fluid (ICF) space and the intravascular from the interstitial space. Osmotic or oncotic shifts occur across these membranes, affected by physiological as well as pathological processes.[10]

Hyponatremia

Hyponatremia is defined as a serum sodium level of less than 130 mEq/L. It is not a cause for alarm until the serum sodium has dropped to less than 125 mEq/L.inadequate sodium intake can contribute to the development of hyponatremia, in the extremely premature babies with increased sodium loss.

Hypernatremia

Hypernatremia is defined as a serum sodium level greater than 150 mEq/L. It is not a cause for alarm until the serum sodium level has risen to greater than 155 mEq/L. Hypernatremia is very often seen in the first few days after birth in ELBW preterm infants and most often occurs when free-water intake is inadequate to compensate for very high insensible water loss (IWL).

Hypokalemia

Hypokalemia is defined as a serum potassium level of less than 3.5 mEq/L. Unless the patient is on digoxin therapy, hypokalemia is rarely a cause for alarm until the serum potassium level is less than 3.0 mEq/L.

Hyperkalemia

Hyperkalemia is defined as a serum potassium level of greater than 6 mEq/L measured in a nonhemolyzed sample. Hyperkalemia more alarming than hypokalemia, when serum potassium levels exceed 6.5 mEq/L or alternatively electrocardiographic changes have developed showing high potassium levels. ECG of hyperkalemia shows peaked T waves, as earliest sign, worsening to widened QRS, bradycardia, tachycardia, supraventricular tachycardia (SVT), ventricular tachycardia, and ventricular fibrillation.

Hypercalcemia

Hypercalcemia is rare in neonate. it is defined as a total serum calcium concentration of higher than 11 mg/dL or an ionized calcium concentration of higher than 5 mg/dL (1.25 mmol/L).

Hypocalcemia

Hypocalcemia is defined as calcium concentration of less than 7 mg/dL or an ionized calcium concentration of less than 4 mg/dL (1 mmol/L).[4] Early onset hypocalcemia may occur within the first 3 days of life in premature infants of mothers of poorly controlled diabetes and/or perinatal asphyxia.[4] Close observation of asymptomatic infant who has calcium level of more than 6.5 mg/dL or ionized calcium more than 0.8–0.9 mmol/L, requires calcium if calcium level drops. Late onset hypocalcemia develops after the first week of life is associated with conditions with high serum phosphate levels, which is also seen in hypoparathyroidism, maternal anticonvulsant use.[9] Hypocalcemia due to vitamin D deficiency resolves with D supplementation.

Anion Gap

The difference between plasma concentration of the major cation Na^+ (135–145 mmol/L) and the major anions Cl^- (95–105 mmol/L) and HCO_3^- (22–30 mmol/L), giving a normal anion gap of 5–11 mmol/L.

- Anion gap is enlarged in metabolic acidosis due to organic acids as seen in diabetic ketoacidosis, lactic acidosis, renal failure, and ingested drugs and toxins.
- Anion gap (mmol/L) = $(Na^+) - [(Cl^-) + (HCO_3^-)]$.[10]

Normal Anion Gap

The anion gap is normal in hyperchloraemic acidosis (e.g. after excess 0.9% saline administration). It is useful differential diagnosis of metabolic acidosis.

Strong Ion Difference (SID)

Stewart has described a mathematical approach to acid–base balance in which the strong ion difference $[(Na^+) + (K^+) - (Cl^-)]$ in the body is the major determinant of the H^+ ion concentration. A decrease in the strong ion difference is associated with a metabolic acidosis, and an increase with a metabolic alkalosis.[12] A change in the chloride concentration is the major anionic contributor to the change in H^+ homeostasis. Hyperchloraemia caused by a saline infusion, which will decrease the strong ion difference and result in a metabolic acidosis.

Strong ion difference (mmol/L) = (Na^+) + (K^+) – (Cl^-), e.g. if Na^+ is 140 mmol/L, K^+ is 4 mmol/L and Cl^- is 100 mmol/L, the SID is 44 mmol/L. The normal range is 38–46 mmol/L.

Base excess: Base excess is defined as the amount of strong acid that must be added to each litre of fully oxygenated blood to return the pH to 7.40 at a temperature of 37°C and a pCO_2 of 40 mmHg (5.3 kPa). A base deficit (i.e. a negative base excess) can be correspondingly defined in terms of the amount of strong base that must be added.

Acidaemia: An increase in the H^+ ion concentration or a decrease in the pH is called acidaemia

Acidosis: Processes that tend to raise the H^+ ion concentration or decrease in the pH is called acidosis

Alkalaemia: A decrease in the H ion concentration or an increase in the pH is called alkalaemia.

Alkalosis: Processes that tend to lower the H^+ ion concentration is called alkalosis. These may be metabolic or a combination of both.

Respiratory acidosis

CO_2 retention causing a rise in pCO_2 in respiratory failure leads to respiratory acidosis.

Respiratory alkalosis

Hyperventilation with a consequent lowering of pCO_2 leads to respiratory alkalosis.

Metabolic acidosis

Accumulation of organic acids such as lactate or hydroxybutyrate or of mineral acidic ions such as chloride cause a metabolic acidosis in which arterial pH falls below 7.4, bicarbonate is reduced and pCO_2 falls as the lungs attempt to compensate by blowing out more CO_2. This is known as compensated metabolic acidosis.

Metabolic alkalosis

Ingestion of bicarbonate or loss of gastric acid in vomiting can give rise in pH and a metabolic alkalosis.

Provision of maintenance of fluid and electrolyte requirements is to provide daily physiological fluid and electrolyte requirements.

Replacement: Provide for maintenance requirements and add like for replacement for ongoing fluid and electrolyte losses (e.g. slow blood loss, intestinal fluid loss).

Resuscitation: Administration of fluid and electrolytes to restore intravascular volume (haemorrhage, hidden internal bleeding, etc.).

> **Warning**
>
> Large volume fluid resuscitation is often associated with excessive electrolyte administration and may have physiological consequences (e.g. hyperchloraemic acidosis) or cause complications (e.g. pulmonary oedema, acute kidney injury).[15]

MONITORING OF PARAMETERS OF SIGNIFICANCE FOR ONGOING FLUID LOSSES/EXCESS

1. History sounding new alerts.
2. Fresh vomiting/diarrhoea/haemorrhage or excess (e.g. from intra-operative fluids).
3. Newly appearing autonomic pallor of face, sweating, combined with tachycardia, hypotension and oliguria are indicative of intravascular volume deficit.
4. New blood pressure fall is compatible with intravascular hypovolaemia, particularly when it correlates with other parameters such as pulse rate, urine output, etc. Systolic pressure does not usually fall until 30% of blood volume has been lost.
5. Decreasing skin turgor due to diminished in salt and water depletion.
6. Increase in sunken eyes due to ongoing salt and water depletion.
7. Fresh signs of pulmonary oedema means fluid load
8. Fresh signs of peripheral oedema (pedal scrotal sacral) occurs in volume overload, decreasing albumin.

Parameter significance for usual monitoring

1. Urine output < 30 mL/h (< 0.5 mL/kg/h)
2. Weighing: 24 h change in weight on same weighing scale (best measure of change in water balance which takes account of insensible loss. Simple to carry out by bedside)
3. Input and output charts
4. Haematocrit: Changes in fluid balance cause increase or decrease in the concentration of red cells
5. Serum sodium: Hyponatraemia most commonly caused by water excess.
6. Serum potassium: Hypokalaemia, nearly always indicates the need for potassium supplementation confirm with flat or lowered T waves in ECG.
7. Blood bicarbonate and pH levels for acidosis and alkalosis.

8. Chloride concentrations for iatrogenic hyperchloraemia.
9. The first indication of a falling intravascular volume is a decrease in central venous pressure (CVP).
10. Arterial lines and catheters to measure plumonary artery wedge pressure are useful to help direct fluid therapy in more complex patients.
11. Albumin: Dilution by infused crystalloids is one of the main causes of hypoglbuminaemia in surgical patients.
12. Urea: The rate of increase is of greater importance.

Must Avoid Things

Postoperatively, over hydration occurs in between 17 and 54% of patients and prolongs hospital stay, increases morbidity (e.g. pulmonary oedema)[15] where possible weigh the child before operation and postoperatively to get insight about over hydration.

Must Do Things in Time

Stop intravenous fluids as soon as oral (or nasogastric) intake is possible or when the patient is haemodynamically stable, to reduce associated complications (e.g. line sepsis).

Physiological oliguria

Oliguria occurring soon after uncomplicated surgery is usually part of the normal physiological response to injury, conserving salt and water in an attempt to maintain intravascular volume. Isolated oliguria in the first 48 hours after uncomplicated surgery does not necessarily therefore reflect hypovolaemia, although it if confirmatory features of intravascular hypovolaemia are present, e.g. tachycardia, hypotension, low central venous pressure decreased capillary refill, etc. then oliguria needs to be treated.[12]

Diuretics in fluid overload and pulmonary oedema

Loop diuretics may have a very short-term role in managing fluid overload and pulmonary oedema. In these patients start with very small dose of intravenous loop diuretics cautiously to try and establish a diuresis and treat the pulmonary oedema.

DIABETIC KETOACIDOSIS (DKA), HYPERGLYCAEMIC HYPEROSMOLAR NON-KETOTIC COMA (HONK)

Represent the two extremes of the spectrum of decompensated diabetes, although intermediate cases are not infrequent, depending on the precipitating cause and the percentage loss of insulin secretion. In both situations, hyperglycaemia causes an osmotic diuresis with excessive urinary losses of salt, water, and potassium, leading to ECF and intravascular volume depletion and the risk of prerenal acute kidney injury (AKI). With both types of decompensation, potassium is lost from cells and excreted in the urine causing a deficit, which only becomes apparent as hypokalaemia once insulin treatment is started. In severe cases the rate of K^+ loss from cells, combined with pre-renal AKI, can cause hyperkalaemia (> 5.5 mmol/L) with the risk of cardiac arrest.[77]

Summary of fluid and electrolyte therapy and outcome

Intravenous fluid therapy is an integral component of perioperative care, but its practice has often been based on dogma rather than evidence, and patients have frequently received either too much or too little fluid. There is a relatively narrow margin of safety for perioperative fluid therapy and either too much or too little fluid and electrolyte (particularly sodium chloride) can have a negative effect on physiological processes, and be detrimental to outcome. The goal of perioperative intravenous fluid therapy is, therefore, to maintain tissue perfusion and cellular oxygen delivery, while at the same time keeping the patient in a state of as near neutral fluid and electrolyte balance as possible.[10]

FAQ with Answer

Q. The paediatric anaesthetic is caring for a patient with hyperkalemia. Which investigation would be most important to monitor closely?

A. Continuous ECG monitoring for tall T waves.

TOTAL PARENTERAL NUTRITION (TPN)

If child is unable to get a healthy level of nutrition by taking in food through his or her intestines, then total parenteral nutrition (TPN) is the standard therapy. With total parenteral nutrition, a solution of essential nutrients (which are proteins, fluids, electrolytes, and fat-soluble vitamins) is given intravenously. Because TPN solutions are concentrated and thick, the solutions must be given by catheters that are placed in large veins in neck, chest, or groin. An infusion pump regulates the rate at which the TPN solution is given, so that concentrate does not overload other metabolizing organs.[13] The TPN constitute the following ingredients.

Summary

The main fluid in the body is water. Total body water is 60% of body weight. Distribution of water in three main compartments separated from each other by cell membranes. The intracellular compartment (ICF) is the area within the cell. The extracellular compartment (ECF) consists of the interstitial area (between and around cells) and the inside of the blood vessels (plasma).

Compartments of body and distribution of water by weight

Plasma	5%	**Solids**	40% (fat, protein, carbohydrates and minerals)
Interstitial	15%		
Intracellular	40%		
Total water	**60%**		

Cation Distribution

Electrolyte	*Extracellular meq/liter*	*Intracellular meq/liter*	*Function*
Sodium	142	10	Fluid balance, osmotic pressure
Potassium	5	100	Neuromuscular excitability acid–base balance
Calcium	5	—	Bones, blood clotting
Magnesium	2	123	Enzymes
Total +ve ions	**154**	**205**	

Anion Distribution

Electrolyte	*Extracellular meq/liter*	*Intracellular meq/liter*	*Function*
Chloride	105	2	Fluid balance, osmotic pressure
Bicarbonate	24	8	Acid-base balance
Proteins	16	55	Osmotic pressure
Phosphate	2	149	Energy storage
Sulfate	1	—	Protein metabolism
Total –ve ions	**154**	**205**	

Carbohydrate

IV dextrose provides most of the energy in TPN. The caloric content of aqueous glucose is 14.28 kJ/g of glucose, which is equal to 142.8 kJ/100 mL of 10% glucose. As a result of the high osmolarity of concentrated glucose solutions, the maximum glucose concentration that can be delivered safely through a peripheral vein is 12.5%. With central venous access, a glucose concentration up to 15% is often used, and in special situations (e.g. when fluids need to be restricted), a concentration of as much as 25% may be used.

A glucose infusion rate expressed in milligrams of glucose/kg/min is the most appropriate way to express glucose administration because the rate accounts for the glucose concentration and the rate of infusion.

Very small premature infants who weigh less than 1500 g demonstrate impaired glucose tolerance. For this reason, in infants weighing less than 1 kg start at an infusion rate of 6 mg/kg/min. In infants who weigh 1 to 1.5 kg, start at 8 mg/kg/min. If the glucose infusion rate is in excess, hyperglycemia develops. If blood glucose levels are greater than 150–180 mg/dL, glucosuria can occur, which can lead to osmotic diuresis. This is controlled by either decreasing the glucose infusion rate or treating the baby with insulin. Persistence of hyperglycemia may need a continuous infusion of insulin.[16] Acute increase in the blood glucose concentration when the glucose infusion rate is unchanged are often the first sign of sepsis in the preterm infant.

Fat

At least 3% of the total energy should be supplied as essential fatty acids (EFA). This can be accomplished by providing a fat emulsion (e.g. intralipid, liposyn), 0.5 g/kg/day 3 times a week. Fat emulsions provide 37.8–42 kJ/g.

Parenteral fat emulsion is usually provided as a 20% lipid emulsion made from soybeans (e.g. intralipid). Intralipid is a concentrated source of energy with a caloric density of 8.4 kJ/mL (for 20% intralipid). Lipids play a primary role in supporting gluconeogenesis in parenterally fed preterm infants.[17] Start with 0.5–1.5 g/kg/day on first day and increase to 3–3.5 g/kg/day.

Limiting intralipid infusions in infants with sepsis and severe lung disease is often recommended, although no evidence supports this practice. The use of intralipid (as well as prolonged TPN and use of central venous lines) is a risk factor for candidemia in neonates.[18]

Neonates with hyperbilirubinemia who are on phototherapy often have intralipid intake restricted to less than 2 g/kg/day (especially if bilirubin levels are rising while the infant is on phototherapy) because some evidence suggests that a high lipid emulsion intake may decrease bilirubin binding.[19] Monitor triglyceride levels and adjust infusion rates to maintain triglyceride levels of less than 150 mg/dL.

Infants with cholestasis (increase in conjugated bilirubin >2 mg/dL) due to parenteral nutrition [parenteral nutrition–associated liver disease (PNALD)] should preferably have their intralipid infusion reduced (e.g. to 1 g/kg/day, given over 12 h). Use of lipid infusions with omega-3 fatty acids (e.g. omegaven) may reduce cholestasis.

Protein

Term babies need 1.8–2.2 g/kg/day along with adequate nonprotein energy for growth. Preterm VLBW babies need 3–3.5 g/kg/day along with adequate nonprotein energy for growth. Providing more than 4 g/kg/day of protein is not advisable. Babies under stress or who have cholestasis are given limiting proteins to 2.5 g/kg/day because of severity of TPN-induced cholestasis which depends on the duration of TPN and the amount of amino acids infused.[20,21]

Protein administration should be started on the first day of life or as soon as fluid and electrolyte requirements have stabilized. It is better to maintain nonprotein-to-protein calorie ratio of at least 25–30:1. Role of supplements, such as additional inositol and carnitine, is under research. They have not yet been shown to be of benefit in large, randomized, controlled trials.[22,23] The addition of glutamine has not been shown to improve outcome.[24]

Minerals (Other than Sodium, Potassium, Chloride)

Once protein intake has been started, calcium and phosphorous should be supplemented to TPN. Calcium and phosphorous need to be concurrently administered for proper accretion. Ensure that solubility is not exceeded; if that happens, calcium and phosphorous spontaneously get precipitated. Also magnesium should be added to TPN once protein has been started.

Vitamins and Trace Elements

Vitamins A, D, E, and K are fat soluble. Vitamins B_1, B_2, B_6, B_{12}, C, biotin, niacin, pantothenate, and folic acid are water soluble. Vitamin supplementation should be started moment protein is added to TPN. The commercially available neonatal vitamin preparation provides appropriate quantities of all vitamins, except vitamin A. Vitamin A supplementation in ELBW infants has been shown to reduce death and bronchopulmonary dysplasia.[25] The usual dose of vitamin A is 5000 IU intramuscularly administered 3 times per week for next 4 weeks in ELBW infants who receive respiratory support at age 24 hours.

The trace elements zinc, copper, selenium, chromium, manganese, molybdenum, and iodine also should be added to TPN once protein is started. A commercially available solution containing trace elements can be used.

Complications of Total Parenteral Nutrition

TPN gives many children a chance to live long enough, productive lives. Still, patients receiving TPN are always at risk of complications from the procedure. Complications may include:

- Clotting (thrombosis) in central access veins
- Frequent infections in the central-vein access lines
- Inflammation of the gallbladder (cholecystitis)
- Bone disease (osteoporosis)
- TPN-induced liver damage or liver failure

TPN-induced liver failure occurs more often in children than adults. Some children who receive long-term TPN may develop social problems because TPN can severely limit their everyday activities.

Survival Prospects of Total Parenteral Nutrition

The long-term survival prospects of patients maintained through total parenteral nutrition vary, depending on the problems. Three-year survival of TPN-dependent patients ranges from 65 to 80 percent. 20 to 35 percent of patients fare poorly on TPN.[13]

What are the Risks of Total Parenteral Nutrition?

There are risks associated with TPN. Some of the most common are:

- **Infection.** It is important to be able to recognize the signs and symptoms of infection. Before child leaves the hospital on TPN, parents are counselled about signs and symptoms of infection. The parents must inform doctor immediately if child develops fever or experiences any of the following at their catheter site:
  - a. Tenderness
  - b. Warmth
  - c. Irritation
  - d. Draining
  - e. Swelling
  - f. Redness
  - g. Pain
- **TPN liver disease or damage.** TPN increases the risk of having liver disease as well as damage. Infants on

TPN are more at risk for liver disease than older children and adults. The organs of infants are still developing. They are not as capable of handling the burden and metabolic strain of TPN. Children who are on TPN for longer duration are more at risk than those who are on TPN temporarily or for a short time. Transplant patients may also receive a liver transplant at the same time due to liver disease associated with TPN.[13]

- **Growth and developmental delays.** Although TPN will help your child grow and develop, TPN cannot be given life long since it is not complete nutrition like eating a regular diet. Children on TPN may still be smaller and less developed than other children of their age eating normal food orally.

REFEEDING SYNDROME

Definition

Refeeding syndrome is defined as severe, (and potentially fatal) electrolyte and fluid shifts associated with metabolic abnormalities in malnourished children undergoing refeeding, whether orally, enterally, or parenterally. The cardinal feature is hypophosphataemia, other biochemical derangements are usual including disorder of sodium and fluid balance, changes in glucose, protein and fat metabolism, thiamine deficiency, hypokalaemia and hypomagnesaemia. It is often forgotten.[14]

Pathophysiology

Prolonged Fasting

In early starvation, blood glucose levels decline, resulting in declining insulin and increasing glucagon levels. This stimulates glycogenolysis in the liver and lipolysis of triacetylglycerol in fat reserves producing fatty acids and glycerol which are used by tissues for energy and converted to ketone bodies in the liver. As glycogen reserves get depleted, gluconeogenesis is stimulated in the liver, utilising amino acids (derived from the breakdown of muscle mass), lactate and glycerol leading to synthesis of glucose for use by the brain cells and red blood cells. The main consequence of these changes is that body switches main energy source from carbohydrate to protein and fat. The basal metabolic rate decreases by as much as 20–25%.[13]

As fasting continues, the body aims to conserve muscle mass and protein. The tissues in turn decrease their use of ketone bodies, and use more and more fatty acids as their main energy source. This results in an increase in blood levels of ketone bodies, promoting the brain to switch from dextrose to ketone bodies as its main energy source. The liver decreases its rate of gluconeogenesis due to the reduced need for glucose by the brain thus preserving muscle protein which is its source of amino acids. As a result, several intracellular minerals become completely depleted. The concentrations of minerals like phosphate may remain normal.[13]

Refeeding

The underlying cause of refeeding syndrome is the metabolic and hormonal changes caused by quick and rapid refeeding, be it enteral or parenteral. On refeeding, absorbed glucose leads to increased blood glucose levels, increasing insulin and decreasing glucagon secretion. The net result of all these changes is the synthesis of glycogen, fat and protein. This new anabolic state in child requires minerals such as phosphate and magnesium and cofactors such as thiamine. Insulin stimulates the absorption of potassium into the cells (via the Na-K ATPase symporter), with both magnesium and phosphate also taken up by cells. Water is drawn into the intracellular compartment (ICF) by osmosis. This decline in serum levels of phosphate, potassium and magnesium further, which are responsible for clinical features of refeeding syndrome.[14]

KEY ELEMENTS AND MINERALS

Phosphorus

Phosphorus is a predominantly intracellular anion. It is essential key for almost all intracellular processes and structural integrity of the cell membrane. It is important for energy storage—adenosine triphosphate (ATP), for enzyme/and second messenger activation by phosphate binding, for control of the affinity of the oxygen binding to haemoglobin (via 2,3-diphosphoglycerate (DPG), ATP). It is very important in the regulation of pH by acid–base buffering.

In refeeding syndrome, long-term depletion of phosphorus in the body of child occurs along with a greatly increased use of phosphate in the cells resulting in insulin surge. This leads to all round deficit in intracellular and extracellular levels of phosphorus. In this environment, even small drops in serum levels of phosphorus may lead to widespread dysfunction of the cellular processes.

Potassium

Potassium is the main intracellular cation. This is depleted in undernutrition, whilst its serum concentration usually remains within the normal range. On refeeding, insulin causes potassium to go into the cells. This causes symptomatic as well as real hypokalaemia and as a result, derangements in the electrochemical membrane potential, potentially leading to abnormalities in cardiac rhythm and even cardiac arrest may occur.

Magnesium

Magnesium is an important intracellular cation. It is an essential cofactor in most cellular enzymatic systems including oxidative phosphorylation and ATP production. It is also important for the structural integrity of DNA, RNA and ribosomes. In addition it regulates membrane potential, and deficiency can lead to mainly cardiac dysfunction and neuromuscular dysfunctions. Magnesium and potassium levels are linked, hence severe hypomagnesaemia will lead to hypokalaemia. Therefore, only replacing potassium will not correct potassium deficit, as magnesium replacement has to take place concurrently.

Glucose

After starvation, glucose intake suppresses gluconeogenesis by leading to the release of insulin and the suppression of glycogen. If it is taken in large quantities, glucose intake may therefore result into hyperglycaemia, leading to osmotic diuresis, dehydration, metabolic acidosis and ketoacidosis. Excess glucose also leads to lipogenesis (again result of insulin stimulation). This can lead to fatty liver, increased CO_2 production, hypercapnoea and respiratory failure.

Vitamin Deficiency

Starvation commonly leads to several vitamin deficiencies. The most essential of these with respect to refeeding is thiamine, as it is an essential coenzyme in carbohydrate metabolism. Deficiency in thiamine can result into Korsakoff's syndrome (retrograde and anterograde amnesia, confabulation) and Wernicke's encephalopathy (ocular abnormalities, ataxia, confusional state, hypothermia, coma).

Sodium, Carbohydrate and Fluid

Consumption of carbohydrate result into rapid decrease in renal excretion of sodium and water. If fluids are then given to maintain a normal urine output, patients may quickly become fluid overloaded. Matter becomes worse by the loss of cardiac muscle mass during starvation. This can result into cardiac myopathy and reduced cardiac contractility further leading to resulting in acute congestive cardiac failure.

Management

Treatment of Refeeding Syndrome

The re-introduction of feeding needs to be done with caution. Earlier guidelines have stressed importance of proper replacement of electrolytes, vitamins and minerals before starting of feeding, be that enterally or parenterally. This has potentially risks prolonging the period of malnutrition National Institute for Health and Clinical Excellence (NICE) guidelines says replacement be parallel with feeding.

Vitamin replacement should be started straightaway, with thiamine and other vitamin B to reduce the incidence of Wernicke's encephalopathy or Korsakoff's syndrome, with 200–300 mg oral thiamine daily, and 1–2 tablets vitamin B of high potency 3 times daily, and multivitamin or trace element supplement once daily. This replacement once began should be continued for at least 10 days in a row.[9]

If levels of key electrolytes are measured to be low, they can be supplemented via oral, enteral or intravenous routes depending on how low the levels are and what methods of refeeding are possible a given child patient. There is a little good quality evidence on the best replacement regimes, (where future research needs to be focused) but NICE have made working recommendations, including potassium (2–4 mmol/kg/day), phosphate (0.3–0.6 mmol/kg/day), and magnesium (0.2 mmol/kg/day intravenously or 0.4 mmol/kg/day orally).

The rate of refeeding from these same guidelines depends on the severity of the malnutrition prior to refeeding. In moderate risk child patients (patient who has eaten a little or nothing for more than 5 days), the recommendation is to feed at a rate of no more than 50% of the energy requirements. If after careful monitoring of clinical and biochemical status, all is well this rate can start to be increased carefully but slowly. If the patient falls into one of the high risk categories, replacement of energy should be started slowly with a maximum rate of 10 kcal/kg every 24 hours. It can then be subsequently increased to meet or exceed full needs over the next 4 to 7 days, and as before, particular caution needs to be observed to biochemical indices and fluid balance. In patients who are very malnourished (body mass index $\leq$ 14 or a negligible intake for two weeks or more), the NICE guidelines recommend that refeeding should start at a maximum of 5 kcal/kg/24 hours, with active continuous ECG cardiac monitoring owing to the risk of cardiac arrhythmias. Circulatory volume should also be replaced but care should be taken not to overload child patients.

Why use the NICE guidelines on refeeding syndrome?

1. The guidelines are the most recent comprehensive review of the literature on refeeding syndrome.
2. The guideline developing group was strongly multidisciplinary who had wide ranging consultation with both professional and patient party as stakeholders.
3. The guidelines clearly identified points of good medical practice and suggested areas for further research.
4. The new guidelines give explicit clinical criteria for patients "at risk" and "highly at risk" of developing refeeding syndrome, enabling better identification and prevention of morbidity and mortality.
5. For patients with electrolyte deficits the new guidelines recommend immediate start of nutritional support at a lower rate, rather than waiting till the electrolyte imbalance has been corrected (as was recommended by earlier existing guidelines), thus potentially avoiding further nutritional deterioration in patients. For NICE guidelines visit www.nice.org.uk.

CONCLUSIONS

Refeeding syndrome is an important condition which is often diagnosed late in patients at risk. The key to better patient care in this area is prevention by increased clinician awareness and involvement of specialist dietetic support. If patients are diagnosed or suspected, then there are proper and new guidelines in place to help with management. It must be stressed that many of the recommendations are not based on high quality evidence and this shall help in highlighting areas that need future research.

REFERENCES

1. Anatomy and Physiology: a learning initiative (updated 18 September 2014) available on *http://anatomyand physiologyi.com/body-fluids*.
2. Rhoades RA, Bell DR. Medical Physiology: Principles for Clinical Medicine, 4th edn. Lippincott Williams & Wilkins 2013.
3. Fluid, Electrolyte, and Acid-base Balance (homepage on the Internet). (Updated 18 September 2014). Available from: *http://rmoskowitz.tripod.com/fluids.html.*
4. Fluid, Electrolyte and Acid–Base Balance (updated 18 Sept., 2014). Available on *https://worldtracker.org/media/library/.../27-Chapter.doc.*
5. Martini, Frederic Anatomy and Physiology, 2007 edn. Rex book store inc. 2007 available on books. google.co.in/books?isbn=9712348075.
6. Martin RJ, Fanaroff AA, Walsh MC, Fanaroff and Martin's Neonatal-Perinatal Medicine: Diseases of the Fetus and Infant, 9th edn, Elsevier Inc., 2014.
7. Feld LG, Kaskel FJ, Editors, Fluid and Electrolytes in Pediatrics: A Comprehensive Handbook, Springer Science & Business Media, 2010.
8. Gleason: Avery's Diseases of the Newborn, 9th edn. Saunders, Elsevier 2011.
9. Puri P et al Editors, Pediatric Surgery 2009, pp 75–88 Nutrition Pierro A, Eaton S. e-book available on link.springer.com/book/10.1007%2F978-3-540-69560-8.
10. Lobo DN Lewington AJP , Allison SP, Basic Concepts of Fluid and Electrolyte Therapy, Bibliomed—Medizinische Verlagsgesellschaft mbH, Melsungen 2013 available on *http://www.bbraun.com/documents/Knowledge/Basic_Concepts_of_Fluid_and_Electrolyte_Therapy.pdf.*
11. Basic Concepts of Fluid and Electrolyte Therapy Published by: Judith Pachas Serpa on April 13, 2013 available on *http://www.scribd.com.*
12. Basic Concepts of Fluid and Electrolyte Therapy Published by Jossue Espinoza Figueroa available on July 18, 2014 on *http://www.scribd.com.*
13. Frequently Asked Questions about Total Parenteral Nutrition (TPN) on website of Children's Hospital of Pittsburgh of UPMC, One Children's Hospital Drive available on *http://www.chp.edu/CHP/tpn+intestine* on 18th September 2014.
14. Mehanna H, Nankivell PC, Moledina J, Travis J, Refeeding syndrome—awareness, prevention and management, Head Neck Oncol. 2009;1:4. Published online Jan 26, 2009. doi: 10.1186/1758-3284-1-4 PMCID:PMC2654033.
15. Available on internet on 20-9-20124 at https://www.*rcplondon.ac.uk/sites/default/files/rcp_ten_top_tips_for_intravenous_fluid_administration.pdf.*
16. Ng SM, May JE, Emmerson AJ. Continuous insulin infusion in hyperglycaemic extremely-low-birth-weight neonates. Biol Neonate. 2005;87(4):269–72 (Medline).
17. Sunehag AL. The role of parenteral lipids in supporting gluconeogenesis in very premature infants. Pediatr Res. Oct. 2003;54(4):480–6 (Medline).

18. Saiman L, Ludington E, Pfaller M, et al. Risk factors for candidemia in Neonatal Intensive Care Unit patients. The National Epidemiology of Mycosis Survey study group. Pediatr Infect Dis J. Apr 2000;19(4):319–24 (Medline).

19. Spear ML, Stahl GE, Paul MH, et al. The effect of 15-hour fat infusions of varying dosage on bilirubin binding to albumin. JPEN J Parenter Enteral Nutr. Mar-Apr 1985; 9(2):144–7 (Medline).

20. Sankaran K, Berscheid B, Verma V, et al. An evaluation of total parenteral nutrition using Vamin and Aminosyn as protein base in critically ill preterm infants. JPEN J Parenter Enteral Nutr. Jul-Aug, 1985;9(4):439-42 (Medline).

21. Yip YY, Lim AK, R J, Tan KL. A multivariate analysis of factors predictive of parenteral nutrition—related cholestasis (TPN cholestasis) in VLBW infants. J Singapore Paediatr Soc. 1990;32(3-4):144–8 (Medline).

22. Kumar M, Kabra NS, Paes B. Carnitine supplementation for preterm infants with recurrent apnea. Cochrane Database Syst. Rev. 2004; CD004497. (Medline).

23. Howlett A, Ohlsson A. Inositol for respiratory distress syndrome in preterm infants. Cochrane Database Syst Rev. 2000;CD000366 (Medline).

24. Poindexter BB, Ehrenkranz RA, Stoll BJ, et al. Parenteral glutamine supplementation does not reduce the risk of mortality or late-onset sepsis in extremely low birth weight infants. Pediatrics. May 2004;113(5):1209–15 (Medline).

25. Darlow BA, Graham PJ. Vitamin A supplementation for preventing morbidity and mortality in very low birthweight infants. Cochrane Database Syst Rev. 2002;CD000501 (Medline).

Thermoregulation in Neonates

Rachana Chhabaria

ABSTRACT

Newborns are prone to hypothermia due to immature thermoregulatory system. Heat loss is further exaggerated under anaesthesia for surgery. This chapter highlights the physiology of temperature regulation, various sites used for monitoring temperature, mechanisms by which heat loss occurs and ways to prevent heat loss in newborns. There are mechanisms for heat generation to compensate for heat loss, which are explained, along with effect of anaesthesia on temperature regulation.

Humans are considered as homeothermic organisms as they maintain a constant body core temperature independent of changes in ambient temperature (within a limited range). Body temperature is one of the physiological parameters effectively controlled by the body. Normal body temperature is essential to provide necessary thermal environment for appropriate function of enzymatic systems. Thermodynamically, the human body is considered a three compartment model consisting of a central (core), a peripheral, and a shell compartment. The central compartment consists of the vessel-rich group of organs (brain, heart, lungs, liver, kidneys, and endocrine glands). The core temperature refers to the temperature of the central compartment and under normal conditions it is maintained within ± 0.2°C of its set point of 37.0°C. This is called the interthreshold range, and within this narrow range no thermoregulatory effector responses are triggered to control the body temperature, and the human organism behaves in a poikilothermic manner. The peripheral compartment consists of the musculoskeletal system, which acts as a dynamic buffer between the central and the shell compartment. The shell compartment consists of the skin, which acts as a barrier between the body and the environment.

Thermoregulation refers to the ability to balance between heat production and heat loss in order to maintain body temperature within a certain "normal" range. Temperature control is subjected to a circadian rhythm and the control within these rhythms is very tightly maintained by an effective thermoregulatory system. Extremes of environmental temperature, anaesthesia and surgery can significantly attenuate the normal thermoregulatory system, resulting in cellular and tissue dysfunction. This explains the need for strict temperature control and regulation by monitoring and appropriate measures.

Due to immaturity of thermoregulatory system and sudden change of environment from intrauterine to extra uterine life, neonates, terms and preterms are susceptible to heat loss and experience difficulty in maintaining their temperature than adults.

The definition of hypothermia is variable, although most acceptable is core temperature of less than 36.1°C (97°F) as being hypothermic.

Hypothermia may be graded into three categories according to severity: mild [33.9–36.0°C (93.0–96.8°F)], moderate [32.2–33.8°C (89.9–92.8°F)], or severe [below 32.2°C (89.9°F)].

THERMAL ENVIRONMENT AND BODY TEMPERATURE

Two interrelated concepts regarding thermal care:

1. "Set point" defines the controlled temperature in the thermoregulatory system and is set at 37 ± 0.2°C.
2. "Neutral thermal zone" (or environment) is defined as the ambient temperature at which the oxygen

demand reflected by the metabolic rate is minimal and thermoregulation is achieved through non-evaporative physical processes alone means (that is, by vasomotor control). For unclothed adults, the neutral temperature is about 28 °C; for neonates—32 °C; and for preterm infants—34 °C. Within this range, the infant is in thermal equilibrium (thermo-neutrality) with the environment, the cutaneous arteriovenous shunts are open and skin blood flow is maximal. The lower temperature limit of thermal regulation in adults is 0 °C, whereas that in newborns is 22 °C. In general, maintaining the core temperature in a cool environment leads to increased oxygen consumption and metabolic acidosis may develop. However, oxygen consumption in a full-term neonate does not correlate with a decreased rectal temperature but rather correlates directly with the skin-to-environment temperature gradient. Oxygen consumption is minimal with skin-to-environment temperature gradients of 2 °C to 4 °C. Therefore, at environmental temperatures between 32 °C and 34 °C and an abdominal skin surface temperature of 36 °C, the resting neonate is in a state of minimal oxygen consumption (i.e. the thermoneutral state). Given the significance of the skin-to-environment temperature gradient associated with a state of minimal oxygen consumption, normal rectal temperature does not imply a state of minimal oxygen consumption.

In view of immature thermoregulation in neonate, the head is of special importance because it comprises up to 20% of the total body surface area and forms the source for highest regional heat flux. Furthermore, a large caloric heat loss occurs from the head due to the thin skull bones, often sparse scalp hair, and the close proximity of the highly perfused brain (with core temperature) to the skin surface. Facial cooling may increase oxygen requirements by up to 23% in the full term and 36% in the preterm infant, which indicates the importance of the practice of covering the infant's head to minimize heat loss.

Thermoregulatory vasomotor response causing vasoconstriction and vasodilatation are most likely established during the first day of life in both the preterm (>1 kg) and the full-term neonate. Vasoconstriction leads to decreased cutaneous blood flow and an increased effect of tissue insulation; these results in an overall reduction in conductive and convective heat loss. However, vasoconstriction abilities are outmatched by propensity for heat loss due to limited layer of subcutaneous fat; limited development of muscle and other tissues that provide insulation.

Sweat production is observed in infants of 29 weeks gestational age; maturation of this pseudomotor response is enhanced by extrauterine development. However, the response is slower, less efficient than in older child or adult, and occurs at a higher environmental temperature.

Heat dissipation in the premature or small-for-gestational-age infant represents the extreme of thermal regulation in the neonate, thereby challenging their thermoregulating capacity. In small-for-gestational-age infants, a slightly lower skin surface area-to-volume ratio and an increased motor tone offer some protection when compared with the premature infant for heat loss or transfer. The extended or "spread eagle" posture, for instance, increases heat loss by as much as 35 percent when compared to a flexed (foetal) position. In addition to the physical limitations of heat conservation in infants and children, surgery can further increase heat loss and fluid requirements by exposing the visceral surfaces of the abdomen and thorax, thereby exacerbating evaporative and convective heat and water losses.

Physiology of Thermal Regulation

The human body tolerates cold temperatures with a three-fold greater margin than hot temperatures. Like other control systems in the body, the thermoregulatory system depends on a negative feedback loop to maintain the body temperature within narrow limits.

The body's principle temperature regulation centre is the hypothalamus, which integrates afferent signals from temperature-sensitive cells found in most tissues, including other parts of the brain, spinal cord, central core tissues (i.e. brain, heart, lungs, liver, kidneys, and endocrine glands), respiratory tract, gastrointestinal tract, and the skin surface. The processing of thermoregulatory information occurs in three stages:

1. Afferent thermal sensing
2. Central regulation
3. Efferent response

Afferent Thermal Input

Distinct central and peripheral thermoreceptors sense ambient temperature of the body. Central thermosensitive receptors are located in the brain and the spinal cord and in close proximity to the great vessels, the viscera, and the abdominal wall. Warm and cold receptors in the skin form the peripheral thermoreceptors.

Warm receptors outnumber cold receptors by 10-fold, acknowledging the importance of detecting and correcting an increase in body temperature than a decrease in body temperature. Each receptor type transmits the information through an afferent nerve conduction pathway and the velocity is related to the intensity of the stimulus and the rate of temperature change than to the type of nerve fibre.

Impulses from the cold-sensitive receptors, which have their maximal discharge rate at a temperature of 25°C to 30°C, is transmitted by A delta fibres to the preoptic area of the hypothalamus.

Impulses from the peripheral warm receptors, which have their maximal discharge rate at 45°C to 50°C, is transmitted by unmyelinated C fibres. These C fibres also detect and convey nociceptive impulses, explaining why intense heat cannot be distinguished from severe pain. Most afferent thermal impulses are transmitted along the spinothalamic tracts in the anterior spinal cord.

Central Regulation

Afferent thermal information is integrated in the preoptic area of the anterior hypothalamus, which contains cold- and heat-sensitive neurons. The cold-sensitive neurons predominate the heat-sensitive neurons in the ratio of 4 : 1. This area also receives and processes non-thermic afferent information, which controls the adaptive mechanisms and the behaviour of the organism. The hypothalamus compares the afferent information with the threshold temperatures for heat and cold and then carefully regulates mechanisms for heat generation and dissipation to maintain body temperature within the narrow limits of its set point (interthreshold range). The posterior hypothalamus controls the descending pathways to the effectors.

Under normal conditions, the contribution of the central thermoreceptors to thermal regulation is limited by the marked predominance of the input of peripheral receptors. Central receptors take over thermoregulation if the sensory input from peripheral sensors is disrupted (e.g. central neuraxial anaesthesia or spinal cord transsection), but they are less efficient compared with peripheral thermoreceptors.

The threshold represents the central temperature which initiates a particular regulatory effector response. When the integrated input from all sources exceeds the upper or falls below the lower threshold, efferent responses are initiated from the posterior hypothalamus to maintain normal body temperature. The slope of the response intensity plotted against the difference between the thermal input temperature and the threshold temperature is called the *gain* of that response (i.e. the intensity of the response).

The difference between the lowest temperature at which warm responses are triggered and the highest temperature at which cold responses are triggered is the thermal sensitivity of the system. The interthreshold range, i.e. temperature range over which no regulatory responses occur, changes from approximately 0.4°C in the awake state to approximately 3.5°C during anaesthesia. The interthreshold range is wider in the hypothermic state than in the hyperthermic state as compared with normal human body temperature (37.0 ± 0.2°C). This physiologic system acts as an "all-or-none" phenomenon. Central regulation is fully functional in infancy but may be impaired in the premature.

Efferent Response

Mean body temperature (MBT) is a physiologically weighted average temperature reflecting the thermoregulatory importance of various tissues especially of the central compartment.

In unanaesthetized subjects, the mean body temperature can be calculated as:

$$\text{MBT} = 0.85\ (\text{central T}) + 0.15\ (\text{skin T})$$

where T denotes the temperature measured in °C.

Temperature regulation is a system of thresholds and gains for each particular thermoregulatory response and these responses are actively regulated by the hypothalamus when temperatures exceed the interthreshold range. Efferent responses are behavioural changes or autonomic changes, initiated to either increase or decrease heat loss depending on the central interpretation of the afferent input. Skin temperature is the most vital parameter triggering behavioural changes, but the thermal input from the skin contributes only about 20% for the thermoregulatory autonomic response. The majority of the autonomic response depends on the afferent information from the central core compartment, which includes the brain (parts other than the hypothalamus), the spinal cord, and deep abdominal and thoracic tissues, with each of them contributing about 20% to the central thermoregulatory control.

Efferent Responses to Hypothermia

1. **Behaviour responses:** Quantitatively the most important thermoregulatory effectors in humans (e.g. heating the home, looking for shelter, putting on a jacket, etc.), mainly contribute in decreasing heat loss. These are much more efficient than all of the autonomic responses combined and the newborns are unable themselves and dependent on caretakers to do these.
2. **Autonomic responses:** Cutaneous vasoconstriction, the first and the most consistent one. Total digital skin blood flow can be categorized into a nutritional (capillaries) and a thermoregulatory (arteriovenous shunts) component. Competent abilities to regulate skin blood flow are documented in infants weighing >1 kg. Cutaneous blood flow is drastically reduced in arteriovenous shunts of the hands, feet, ears, lips, and nose (1% of the normal blood flow in an environment with neutral temperature). These shunts are typically 100 µm in diameter, can divert 10,000 times as much blood as a capillary with a 10 µm diameter. Shunt flow is primarily regulated by norepinephrine, by binding to peripheral α_2-receptors which are sensitized by local cooling and inhibited by temperatures equal to or higher than 35°C. In spite of the thermoregulatory vasoconstriction, the resulting reduction of heat loss from the hands and feet decrease by 50%, but only by 17% from the trunk, resulting in an overall heat loss reduction of only 25%. Other responses include non-shivering thermogenesis and shivering which increase metabolic heat production.

The ability to increase metabolic rate in response to cold stress begins around 28–30 weeks post-conceptional age. Post-conceptionally older infants can increase heat production, but the response is weaker than in the adult. Shivering response is not well developed in newborns and they cannot initiate increased tone and shivering to increase heat production. Lower post-conceptional aged and ill infants are prone to decreased motor tone and less activity, resulting in decreased heat production. Infants with poor tone cannot use flexion posture effectively to reduce surface area and hence decrease heat loss. Heat production needs are met primarily through non-shivering thermogenesis. This depends on the amount of brown fat stores which are inversely related to gestational age. Heat production increases oxygen consumption, challenging the immature cardiovascular and pulmonary systems.

Efferent Responses to Hyperthermia

1. **Behaviour responses:** Wearing light clothing, cold sponging.
2. **Autonomic responses:** Sweating, this triggers massive pre-capillary vasodilatation with marked increase in skin blood flow, allowing for huge amounts of heat to be transported to the skin, which then dissipates to the environment, mainly by evaporation due to preconditioning by sweat. Sweat production is observed in infants of 29 weeks gestational age; maturation of response is enhanced by extrauterine development. This response is slower, less efficient than in older child or adult, and occurs at a higher environmental temperature.

Temperature Monitoring

Temperature is most commonly measured in degrees Celsius (or centigrade), or may be measured in degrees Fahrenheit. In the System International the temperature unit used is Kelvin (K), where 0 K = –273.15° C and it includes absolute zero temperature. The following formulas can be used to convert from one unit to the other:

$$°\text{Celsius} = 0.56 \times (°\text{Fahrenheit} - 32)$$

$$°\text{Fahrenheit} = (1.8 \times °\text{Celsius}) + 32 \text{ Kelvin}$$
$$= (273 + °\text{Celsius})$$

The American Society of Anaesthesiologists guidelines state that "every patient receiving anaesthesia shall have temperature monitored when clinically significant changes in body temperature are intended, anticipated or suspected". An appropriate measurement of temperature, at an appropriate site with an accurate sensor to detect perioperative changes is mandatory.

Today, the thermometers used in clinical practice are thermistors and thermocouples. The thermistor type thermometer is based on an exponential, temperature dependent change in the electrical resistance of a semiconductor resistor, which consists of a tiny drop of metal (e.g. copper, nickel, manganese, or cobalt). This change in resistance is used to measure temperature. The thermocouple thermometers consist of two different metals, often copper and constantan (a copper-nickel-manganese-iron alloy), to sense the temperature. The principle behind thermocouples is the Seebeck effect, which states that a small electrical current is generated at the junction between two different metals (of the thermoelectric series) that are exposed to a temperature gradient. The magnitude of this voltage is temperature dependent and is used as a measurement of the temperature. Both, thermocouple and thermistor probes are inexpensive and sufficiently accurate for clinical purposes, explaining their wide usage in daily practice.

Depending on the site of measurement, body temperature varies widely. The central tissues maintain a constant temperature (core temperature) because of their high perfusion. The peripheral tissues usually maintain a significantly reduced homogeneous temperature. Therefore, the temperature in the central and peripheral compartments may differ by several degrees within small measurable distances of each other.

Core temperature is of the greatest clinical interest because it is the most vital thermoregulatory controller in the body. Core temperature may be measured at a number of sites within the body, including tympanic membrane, naso-pharynx, distal oesophagus, the pulmonary artery, and, with some limitations, bladder and rectum. These sites usually provide similar readings in awake as well as anaesthetized humans undergoing non-cardiac surgery, but may actually represent different temperatures under certain conditions whose physiologic and clinical implications may vary.

Body temperature can be monitored at various anatomic sites. The precision and accuracy of measurements at these sites vary and each site has its advantages and disadvantages. The ideal site of temperature monitoring should reflect core temperature, be non-invasive and be associated with none or only minimal morbidity. Various sites include:

1. **Tympanic membrane:** Considered the most ideal site to monitor core temperature. It is not necessary for the temperature probe to directly contact the tympanic membrane to obtain an accurate reading. It can simply be done by sealing the external auditory canal by the probe and allowing the air column trapped between the probe and the tympanic membrane to reach a steady state. The tympanic membrane temperature may not be accurate in some situations. In the initial post-cardiac reconstructive surgery period in infants and children, tympanic membrane temperature does not correlate well with brain temperature and thereby fails to provide an accurate estimate of central body temperature. With difficulties obtaining appropriate-sized thermistors and clinical reports of tympanic membrane perforation, its clinical use is no longer encouraged.
2. **Naso-pharynx:** Nasopharyngeal temperature probes are considered to provide a good estimate of the hypothalamic temperature, thereby accurately reflecting the core temperature, provided the probe is adequately placed (i.e. placing the tip of the temperature probe in the posterior nasopharynx close to the soft palate). However, when used in combination with un-cuffed tubes with a moderate to large air leak, the resulting airflow may lead to inaccurate reading. Slight and self-limiting bleeding from the nose is commonly noticed (especially in children with large adenoids), and its preclusion in mask anaesthesia has limited its routine use.
3. **Oro-pharynx:** Oral temperature is considered less accurate and hence not recommended as an accurate intraoperative temperature-monitoring site.
4. **Oesophagus:** Oesophageal temperature probes when combined with an oesophageal stethoscope decently reflect the core temperature, making this site particularly attractive in the paediatric population. In infants and children, and in cachectic patients, the thermal insulation between the tracheobronchial tree and the oesophagus is minimal due to thin tissue planes. This may result in erroneous temperature readings, especially when the respiratory gas flow is high and there is a significant temperature gradient between the respiratory gases and the body temperature. In order to measure the central temperature the tip of the probe should be properly placed in the distal third of the oesophagus at the point where the heart sounds are the loudest. In children with endotracheal intubation, oesophageal temperature is more reliable than rectal temperature and more practical than tympanic membrane temperature.
5. **Axilla:** It is considered the most convenient site for monitoring temperature in children so most widely used. They are frequently malpositioned and can be unreliable if not adequately placed. The accuracy of the axillary probe depends on careful position of the tip of the probe close to the axillary artery with the arm tightly adducted. Axillary temperature can be as accurate as tympanic membrane, esophageal and rectal temperature sites in measuring core temperature. Maintaining low room temperature or infusing cold solutions at high flow rates in small children in the same extremity as the axillary temperature is monitored may result in falsely low temperature readings. Falsely high readings may be recorded when the tip of the probe senses the hot air from a forced warming air device.
6. **Rectum:** The rectal temperature can provide accurate core temperature measurements, is easy to access

and associated with minimal morbidity. But may impose problems if the probe becomes embedded in faeces, exposure of the probe to cooler blood returning from the legs, the influence of an open abdominal cavity during laparotomy, or bladder irrigations with either cold or warm solutions on the probe proximity. Absolute contraindication to the use of a rectal probe includes imperforate anus, and relative contraindications include inflammatory bowel disease, rectal tumours, neutropenia or thrombocytopenia, coagulopathy, and circumstances in which the bowel or bladder is to be irrigated.

7. **Bladder:** It is considered to be one of the most accurate sites for measuring core temperature; identical to pulmonary artery temperature provided urinary output is high. When urinary output is normal or less than normal, this site fails to reflect the core temperature.
8. **Pulmonary artery:** A pulmonary artery catheter with a distal-tip thermistor can accurately reflect pulmonary blood temperature, but its use is limited, in critically ill children due to its invasive nature.
9. **Skin:** Skin surface is considered the least invasive site and highly unreliable measure of the core temperature. It varies dramatically depending on the part of the body where the skin temperature is measured.

The site or sites of temperature monitoring depends on the operative procedure. For children undergoing cardiac surgery temperature is usually measured at multiple sites (e.g. rectum, bladder, oesophagus, nasopharynx, tympanic membrane).

Heat Loss Mechanisms

Humans are homeothermic, with the ability to dissipate and produce heat in a controlled manner. Heat loss is governed by the physical laws of conduction, radiation, convection, and evaporation and is a two-stage process. The first stage is internal redistribution of heat, in which heat is dissipated from the central core compartment to the periphery and the skin surface. The second stage in the process is the transfer of heat from the skin surface to the environment.

Heat transfer occurs from a warmer to a cooler object, never from a cooler to a warmer object. This means that the warmer object, in the operating room setting, which is exclusively the patient losses heat to the surrounding environment (operating room walls, tables, etc.).

In a thermoneutral environment, total heat loss by the neonate occurs via four mechanisms (Table 8.1).

Table 8.1 Mechanisms (by percent) of heat loss in neutral thermal environments

Radiation	39%
Convection	34%
Evaporation	24%
Conduction	3%

Physiological manipulations in regional blood flow and changes in the thermal conductance properties of the insulating tissue can influence gradients in both stages.

Changes in the operating room environment, e.g. the air and/or room temperature can affect the overall magnitude of the heat loss as well as the relative contributions of each of these mechanisms.

Radiation

It is the mechanism in which there is transfer of heat between two objects of different temperature not in direct contact with each other (e.g. radiation is the mechanism by which the sun warms the earth). The emitted radiation carries energy in the infrared light spectrum from the warmer to the cooler object. This leads to cooling of the warmer object and warming the cooler object.

The following factors affect radiant heat flux:

1. **The emissivity of the radiating surfaces:** It is the power to emit or give off heat by radiation. The emissivity of a neonate's skin is relatively constant. Clothing and blankets reduce emissivity as well as provide insulation. As radiation involves heat exchange between solid surfaces, the surface temperature and emissivity of solid objects surrounding the infant should be considered.
2. **The temperature gradient between the solid surfaces:** Radiant heat transfer is driven by the temperature gradient between the solid surfaces. The infant's skin temperature is typically warmer than other surrounding surfaces, so this leads to heat loss from the infant's surface to surrounding solid surfaces. The infant gains heat via radiation when placed below a radiant heating source, which is warmer than the infant's skin temperature.
3. **The surface area of the solid surfaces:** The infant's large body surface area to body mass potentiates radiant heat loss. Solid surfaces surrounding the infant are enormous in comparison to the infant's surface area, causing more radiant heat loss. For the supine infant, the largest surface areas to which

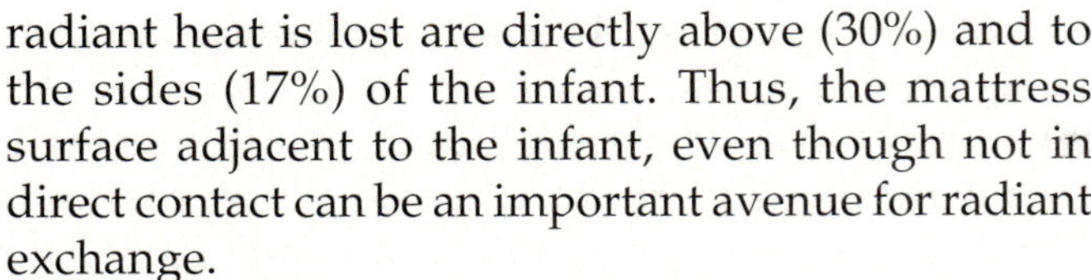

radiant heat is lost are directly above (30%) and to the sides (17%) of the infant. Thus, the mattress surface adjacent to the infant, even though not in direct contact can be an important avenue for radiant exchange.

4. **The distance between the solid surfaces:** The closer the two solid surfaces, the greater the radiant heat flux. In both, the awake and the anaesthetized state, radiation is the most important mechanism of heat loss in the neonate. Heat exchange by radiation is based on the Stefan-Boltzmann law of radiation:

$$H = esA\,(T_1^4 - T_0^4)$$

Where, H is the energy transferred in Joules per second;

e is the emissivity (0–1, human body is approximately 0.7);

s is the Stefan-Boltzmann constant, 5.67×10^{-8} (Joules/s·m^2·k^4);

A is the surface area (m^2); and

T is the temperature of the two bodies (K).

Using this equation with a body surface area for a neonate of 0.25 m^2, increasing the room (wall) temperature from 21° C to 30° C decreases the radiation heat loss by 63%. Thus, the radiant heat loss can be substantively reduced by increasing the ambient room temperature of the operating room, thereby reducing the temperature gradient between the neonates and surrounding. A thin single-layer covering can dramatically reduce the losses by radiation and provide thermal comfort.

Conduction

It is the mechanism in which there is transfer of heat between two surfaces in direct contact. It is the heat flux between the infant's body surface and other solid surfaces.

The following factors influence conduction:

1. The solid surface conductivity coefficient: The greater the conductivity, the greater the heat flux between the infant and the solid surface in contact.
2. The size of the surface area of contact between the infant and the solid surface:

   Larger the surface area in contact with the object, the greater is the heat flux. In the supine position, an infant has approximately 10 percent of his surface area in contact with the mattress. In a prewarmed incubator or under a radiant warmer, in preheated the operating room table/sheets, conductive loss is not significant.
3. **The temperature gradient between surfaces:** Warming pads and similar devices typically reduce heat loss by decreasing gradient between the infant and the solid surface.

The physiologic factors controlling conductive heat loss in newborns are cutaneous blood flow and the thickness of the subcutaneous tissue which provides insulation. This is further poorly developed in preterms.

Measures to prevent conductive heat loss include

- Warming solid surfaces before they come in contact with an infant, ensuring that the infant's skin is not in direct contact with metallic surfaces.
- Warming cool irrigation solutions and intravenous fluids.
- Providing insulation between the infant and the solid surface by covering infants with disposable drapes, this decreases the cutaneous heat loss by 29%.
- Wrapping X-ray plates with warmed blankets, weighing infants with a warmed blanket.

Convection

It is the mechanism in which there is transfer of heat between a solid surface (the infant) and moving molecules such as air or liquid. The thin air layer adjacent to the skin is heated by conduction from the body but the ambient air currents carry heat away from the body. Changes in body posture and minute ventilation may affect convective heat loss. Factors determining convective loss that are relevant to nursing care include the following:

1. **Skin surface area:** The infant's large surface area to body mass results in increased loss by convection. The exposed surface area should be reduced to minimise convective heat loss.
2. **Airflow velocity and turbulence:** These affect the convective heat loss in direct proportion.
3. **Temperature gradient between infant skin and air or liquid:** The larger the gradient between the infant's skin temperature and the surrounding ambient temperature, the greater is the heat loss or gain. Interventions increasing the ambient air temperature reduce the gradient and convective heat loss, e.g. use of incubator decreases the gradient between air and skin temperature. Airflow velocity in a closed incubator is fully consistent, but opening portholes or side panels can alter airflow creating turbulence. Therefore clothing and blankets should be used in incubators to reduce the infant's exposed surface area as well as provide external insulation.

Evaporation

It is the mechanism in which heat is loss through vaporization of water from the body or a mucosal surface. This uses the latent heat of vaporization of water as its source and is an energy-dependent process. This energy for sweat has a value of 2.5×10^6 J/kg, causing its transition from the liquid to the gaseous state. This signifies the power of the human sweating mechanism for dissipating heat. A healthy adult in good physical condition can produce up to 2 L of sweat per hour, dissipating approximately 5×10^6 J/hr or 1.4 kW by sweating mechanism. Under conditions of thermal neutrality, evaporation accounts for 10% to 20% of heat loss.

Evaporative loss occurs by:

1. Sensible water loss by sweating
2. Insensible water loss from the skin, respiratory tract, and open surgical wounds
3. Evaporation of liquids applied to the skin such as antibacterial solutions.

Sensible water loss by sweating depends on the infant's ability to sweat and development of sweat glands. Full-term neonates have mature sweat glands and sweat when rectal temperature is between 37.5°C and 37.9°C and ambient temperature exceeds 35°C. Maximum rate of sweat production is comparable in infants small for gestational age in spite of slower onset of sweat production. Premature neonates with a gestational age of less than 30 weeks do not produce sweat as their sweat glands are not yet fully developed.

Insensible water loss from the skin (transepidermal loss) depends on gestational age and the degree of keratinisation of the epidermal stratum corneum. Mature keratin, which consists of tough fibrous protein is relatively water impermeable and protects the underlying epithelium. Keratin formation is directly related to gestational age, thus premature neonates loose heat through evaporation via the immature permeable skin. In the very low birth weight (VLBW) infant, evaporative loss alone is greater than the heat-producing capabilities. Keratinisation under influence of extrauterine environment increases over the first three to four weeks of postnatal life, decreasing evaporative heat loss. Adhesive dressings which strip the keratin layer increase evaporative loss.

A small amount of heat is lost via evaporation of water from the trachea-bronchial epithelium, which humidifies the dry respiratory gases inspired. Humidification of dry inspired respiratory gases by evaporating water from the trachea-bronchial epithelium results in only a small heat loss. In adults, respiratory losses lead to 5% to 10% of the total heat loss during anaesthesia and surgery and total insensible losses lead to approximately 25% of the total heat dissipated. Children have higher respiratory rate and higher minute ventilation per kilogram, this leads to higher heat loss, approximately up to 33% of the total heat loss. This loss is exaggerated with use of cool, dry gases as compared to warm, moisturized gases. Heat loss by evaporation is maximum from a large surgical incision and may equal all other sources of intraoperative heat loss when combined. Evaporative loss may be increased further when the child is covered with wet drapes or skin is kept wet. Evaporative heat loss may be decreased when neonate is draped with warm gamgees.

Factors affecting evaporative losses include the following:

1. The infant's surface area: Greater the surface area available, greater is the heat loss by evaporation.
2. Vapour pressure, which is governed by air pressure, temperature and humidity.
3. Air velocity: Evaporative heat loss is *potentiated* by the increased speed and turbulence of airflow.

Heat Generation

In order to maintain a constant body temperature, thermal regulation in the homeothermic provides the ability to generate heat in a cool environment along with the ability to dissipate heat in a warm environment.

Heat is generated by increasing the metabolic rate and oxygen consumption.

The three of the four physical mechanisms that account for heat loss (i.e. conduction, radiation and convection) can theoretically also be used to passively warm a child. This passive re-warming helps in increasing the temperature of a neonate postoperatively in a short period due to the same factors which lead to rapid heat loss.

The human body has the ability to actively produce heat and heat generation is achieved by four mechanisms:

1. Voluntary muscle activity
2. Non-shivering thermogenesis
3. Involuntary muscle activity (shivering)
4. Dietary thermogenesis

The behavioural aspect of heat production by voluntary muscle activity has limited importance in infants with low muscle mass and is absent in the perioperative period. Of the remaining, non-shivering thermogenesis is the main mechanism for heat production in the neonate and shivering thermogenesis is the main mechanism for heat production in the adult. The contribution of non-shivering thermogenesis in adults is still debatable. The contribution of non-shivering thermogenesis to maintain the body temperature rapidly decreases after the first year of life along with rapidly increasing the contribution of shivering thermogenesis. The appropriate time and developmental factors which control the switch from non-shivering to shivering thermogenesis in an infant still remain to be elucidated.

Non-shivering Thermogenesis

Non-shivering thermogenesis is defined as an increase in metabolic heat production (above the basal metabolism) which is not associated with muscle activity. It primarily occurs through metabolism of brown fat, but to a lesser extent also occurs in skeletal muscle, liver, brain, and white fat. Brown fat differentiation in the human foetus begins at around 26 to 30 weeks of gestational age, comprising 2% to 6% of the newborn's total body weight. It is located in six main areas: between the scapulae, in small masses around blood vessels in the neck, in large deposits in the axilla, in medium-size masses in the mediastinum, around the internal mammary vessels in the mediastinum, and around the adrenal glands or kidneys.

Brown fat is highly vascularized and richly innervated with primarily β-sympathetic nerve fibres that are responsible for the uncoupling of oxidative phosphorylation. The brown colour is by the abundance of mitochondria in the cytoplasm of its multinucleated cells. These mitochondria are tightly packed with cristae and have a high content of respiratory chain components. They are unique in their ability to uncouple oxidative phosphorylation, resulting in heat production instead of generating adenosine triphosphate. The activation of brown fat metabolism results in an increased proportion of the cardiac output (up to 25%) being diverted through the brown fat, thereby facilitating the direct warming of the blood. Inhalational anaesthetics attenuate non-shivering thermogenesis as soon as 5 minutes after starting halothane, isoflurane, or enflurane or 50% nitrous oxide, but this effect wanes within approximately 15 minutes of discontinuing the anaesthetic agent. During general anaesthesia in children, neither mild core hypothermia nor cold exposure may trigger non-shivering thermogenesis. Non-shivering thermogenesis is also reduced in infants anaesthetized with fentanyl and propofol.

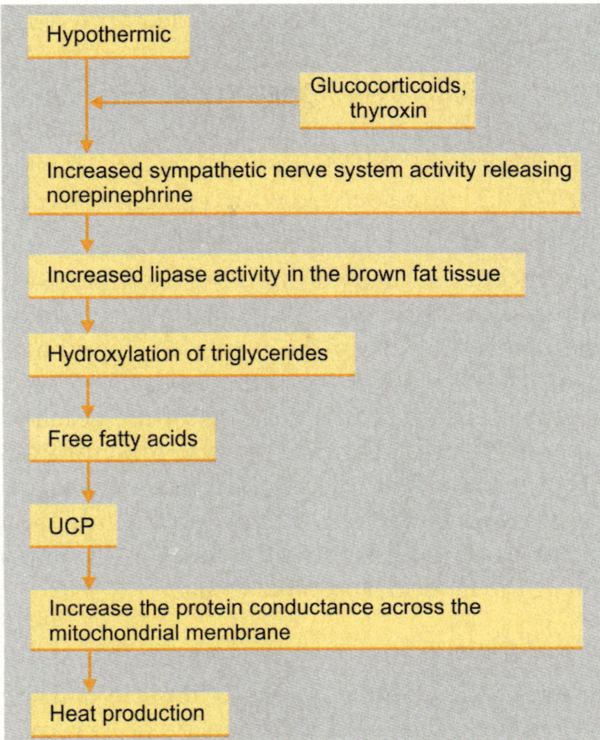

Prematures, full-term neonates, and infants can double their metabolic heat production during cold exposure with non-shivering thermogenesis. This is possible within hours after birth and may persist up to the age of 2 years, but overall has limited ability to compensate for hypothermia.

Shivering Thermogenesis

As the infant and child keep growing, shivering thermogenesis gradually presumes a significant role in thermoregulation. The precise mechanisms and/or factors that lead to this development are still unclear. The role of shivering in thermogenesis gets activated only when all the other mechanisms like the behavioural responses, non-shivering thermogenesis (both ineffective under anaesthesia), and maximal vasoconstriction are unable to maintain body temperature within the interthreshold range. Shivering has limited role in maintaining body temperature in neonates and infants because:

1. The musculoskeletal system is immature
2. Muscle mass is limited

Shivering is characterized by involuntary, irregular muscular activity beginning in the muscles of the upper body, most commonly the masseter. The intensity is greater in central muscles than in peripheral muscles. This leads to metabolic heat production by up to sixfold, which is sustainable by only a twofold.

Shivering occurs in two types of electromyographic patterns:

1. Basal, continuous shivering with a low intensity at a rate of 4 to 8 Hz, associated with type 1 muscle fibres.
2. Superimposed bursts with a high intensity at a rate of 0.1 to 0.2 Hz, associated with type 2 fibres, creating typical "waxing and waning" pattern.

Cold receptors transmit impulses from the skin and the spinal cord to motor centre for shivering, located in the dorsomedial part of the posterior hypothalamus adjacent to the wall of the third ventricle. This then stimulates anterior motor neurons of the spinal cord resulting in increased skeletal muscle tone throughout the body, which when exceeded causes shivering. Under warm conditions, the shivering centre is inhibited by impulses from the heat-sensitive area in the preoptic region of the anterior hypothalamus.

Effects of Shivering

1. In healthy children: Increased muscle activity → oxygen consumption and carbon dioxide production increase → increase in cardiac output (up to 400% to 600% for a brief period)
2. In children with limited haemodynamic or coronary or pulmonary reserves:

   Increase in oxygen consumption → decrease mixed venous oxygen content → decrease arterial oxygen content (due to V/Q mismatch) → decrease tissue oxygen delivery → tissue hypoxia

An inverse ratio exists between intraoperative temperature and postoperative oxygen consumption, as well as between different anaesthetic agents and postoperative oxygen consumption. Shivering is an unpleasant experience for the child as well as the parents in the postoperative period. This can cause increased intraocular and intracranial pressure, wound dehiscence and dental damage. Postoperative shivering has an inverse relation to the core body temperature. But shivering has also been observed in children maintained strictly normothermic during isoflurane or desflurane anaesthesia. This suggests nonthermoregulatory mechanisms also control shivering with pain contributing as a significant factor. Meperidine, clonidine and doxapram have been proven to be effective in attenuating shivering after anaesthesia.

Dietary Thermogenesis

Stimulation of energy expenditure and thermogenesis by certain nutrients (i.e. proteins and amino acids) is a known phenomenon. In spite of muscle paralysis and decreased metabolic rate during general anaesthesia, small amount of infusion of amino acids, fructose may increase heat generation under anaesthesia. The exact mechanisms causing thermogenesis is still not fully understood. Dietary thermogenesis can result in hyperthermia in awake state as well as during anaesthesia with attenuated thermoregulation.

Anaesthesia and Hypothermia

General anaesthesia decreases the temperature threshold at which a thermoregulatory response to cold stress is initiated. Mild intraoperative hypothermia [33.9–36°C (93.0–96.8°F)] which occurs commonly, results from a combination of events:

1. A 30% reduction in the metabolic heat generation during anaesthesia
2. Increased exposure to the environment
3. Anaesthesia-induced central inhibition of thermoregulation
4. Internal redistribution of heat within the body

Hypothermia has a typical profile during general anaesthesia and usually develops in three phases:

1. Internal redistribution of heat,
2. Thermal imbalance, and
3. Thermal steady-state (plateau or re-warming phase).

Internal Redistribution

The concept of internal redistribution of heat refers transfer of heat within the compartments within the body, and not heat loss to the environment. The human body divided into three compartments—the central (or core), peripheral, and skin (or "shell") compartments.

At rest, the central compartment, i.e. vessel-rich group of organs receive approximately 75% of the cardiac output, representing approximately 10% of the body weight in adults and about 22% in neonates. In awake state, the central compartment accounts for approximately 66% of the body mass in an adult, which expands to about 71% during general anaesthesia.

The peripheral compartment consists of the remaining body mass, acting as a dynamic buffer to accommodate any changes in core temperature caused by vasodilatation or vasoconstriction.

Last, the skin compartment acts as a barrier between the first two compartments and the environment.

After induction of anaesthesia, peripheral vasodilatation increases the size of the central compartment, leading to redistribution of its heat over a larger volume.

The core temperature decreases rapidly, by 0.5°C to 1.5°C within the first hour of anaesthesia Furthermore, the decrease in metabolic heat production caused by anaesthesia reduces the amount of energy available to compensate for the enlargement of this compartment. The internal redistribution compresses the peripheral compartment while expanding the central compartment. This explains the decrease in core temperature (the same amount of heat getting distributed to a larger volume), with a corresponding increase in the temperature of the peripheral and skin compartments.

Thermal Imbalance

During this second phase of the hypothermic response, reduced heat production and increased heat loss to the environment leads to thermal imbalance. This lasts for 2 to 3 hours, resulting in a linear decrease in mean body temperature (typically 0.5–1.0°C/hr). Anaesthesia leads to decreased heat production by limiting muscular activity, reducing the metabolic rate, and eliminating the work of breathing. Heat loss occurs by radiation, convection, evaporation, and conduction from the patient to the environment, as a function of the temperature gradient between the skin and ambient structures (i.e. air, walls, and ceiling).

Thermal Steady State (Plateau or Re-warming)

1. **Adults:** The third phase consists of a thermal steady-state plateau, which occurs when metabolic heat dissipation to the environment equals heat production and the core temperature remains constant. This plateau occurs between 34.5°C (94.1°F) and 35.5°C (95.5°F). To maintain the core temperature, heat production must increase and/or heat loss must be decreased to prevent further fall in temperature.
2. **Infants:** The third phase in infants and small children consists of a re-warming phase rather than a plateau phase. Heat production under anaesthesia is decreased by inhibiting muscular activity and non-shivering thermogenesis and reducing metabolic heat generation. This re-warming phase occurs as a result of intense vasoconstriction within the peripheral and central compartments. This compresses the central compartment, and the metabolic heat produced is distributed within this compartment, thus increasing the core temperature. In comparison to adults, the intraoperative thermoregulatory response in infants is not effective enough to increase the core temperature in low ambient temperatures. With either active or passive re-warming, significant physiologic stress response occurs in the infant. Passive surface re-warming (by warm blankets, bundling, or other measures) turns off the skin cold receptors. If the normal core temperature is not reached or maintained by passive surface re-warming, hypothermia may result in hypoventilation or even apnoea, relative anaesthetic overdose (reduced minimal alveolar concentration at lower temperatures), and finally, metabolic acidosis.

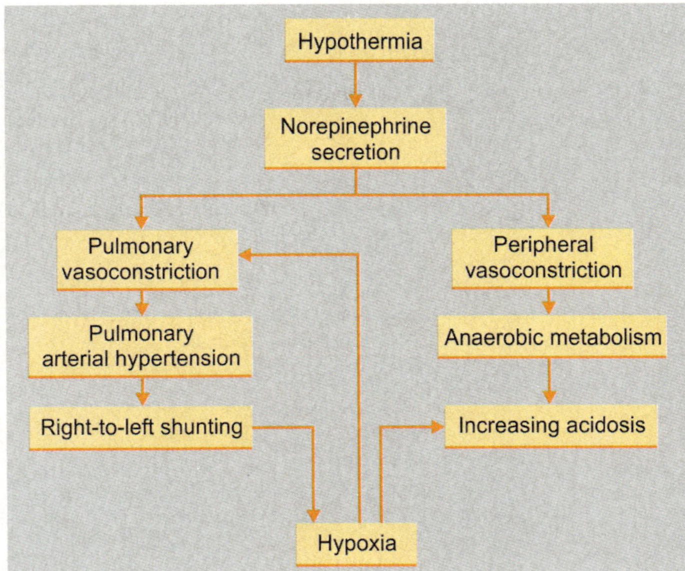

Fig. 8.1 Vicious circle due to prolonged hypothermia[2]

Hypothermia further delays factors of coagulation cascade causing exaggerated blood loss during surgery. Wound healing is also delayed as explained in Fig. 8.2.

SUMMARY

Newborns are susceptible to hypothermia physiological with small size and increased body surface area, immature thermoregulatory system, musculoskeletal system and inadequately developed skin. Hypothermic loss is further exaggerated in preterms and small for gestation. Temperature should be monitored mandatorily in newborns in the intensive care and during surgery under anaesthesia. All measures to prevent heat loss under anaesthesia as well as during transportation should be taken. Measures for passive re-warming should be taken whenever babies become hypothermic. A thorough knowledge of physiology of temperature regulation, its effects under anaesthesia and measures to prevent hypothermia, is essential to provide safe anaesthesia.

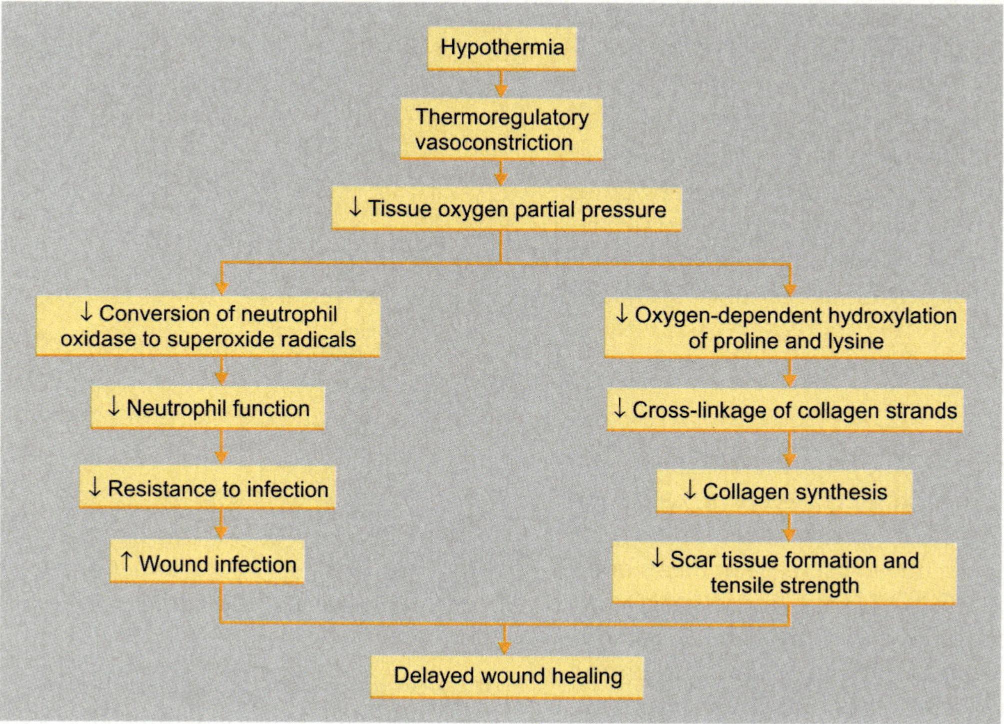

Fig. 8.2 Hypothermia and its effects on wound healing[2]

Key Points

1. Thermoregulation refers to the ability to balance between heat production and heat loss in order to maintain body temperature within a certain "normal" range. In normal conditions it is maintained within ± 0.2° C of its set point of 37.0° C, called the interthreshold range.
2. Thermoregulatory system is immature in neonates. Heat loss occurs with small size and high body surface area, and the head is of special importance because it comprises up to 20% of the total body surface area and forms the source for highest regional heat flux.
3. The thermoregulatory system depends on a negative feedback loop to maintain the body temperature within narrow limits. It includes afferent sensing receptors, the central regulatory hypothamalus and the efferent responses.
4. Temperature monitoring is mandatory as per ASA guidelines and various sites can be used to monitor temperature intraoperatively.
5. The various mechanisms by which heat transfer occur are radiation, evaporation, conduction and convection. These leads to heat loss from neonate to environment and the same can be used to re-warming.
6. The human body has the ability to actively generate heat; non-shivering thermogenesis forms the most important mechanism in neonates.
7. Hypothermia during general anaesthesia develops in three phases in neonates: internal redistribution of heat, thermal imbalance, and thermal steady-state (re-warming phase).
8. Hypothermia in neonates can lead to stress response causing impaired coagulation, apnoea, acidosis, and hypoxia. It can cause delayed wound healing.

FAQs with Answers

Q. What is interthreshold range?

A. The interthreshold range under normal conditions refers to the temperature of the central compartment maintained at set point of 37.0°C ± 0.2°C, and within this narrow range no thermoregulatory effector responses are triggered to control the body temperature, and the human organism behaves in a poikilothermic manner.

Q. When does thermoregulatory vasomotor and pseudomotor response develop in newborns?

A. Thermoregulatory vasomotor response causing vasoconstriction and vasodilatation are most likely established during the first day of life in

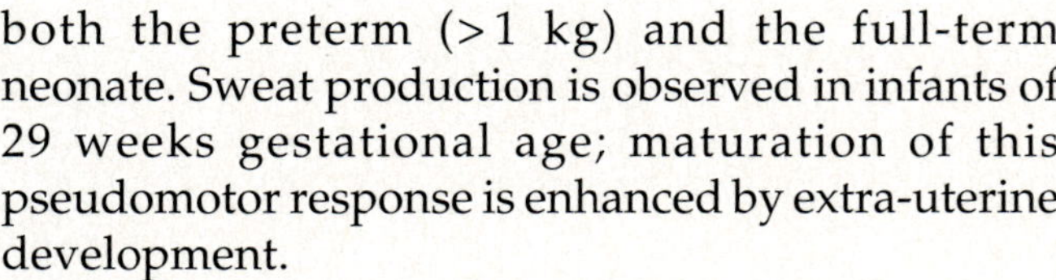

both the preterm (>1 kg) and the full-term neonate. Sweat production is observed in infants of 29 weeks gestational age; maturation of this pseudomotor response is enhanced by extra-uterine development.

Q. What are mechanisms of heat loss under anaesthesia?

A. Radiation, evaporation, conduction and convection.

Q. What are the various ways to prevent heat loss in the operating theatre?

A.
- Transportation of neonate in incubators
- Raising the ambient temperature of OT
- Placing the neonate under radiant warmer during procedure
- Placing the neonate on pre-warmed heating mattress
- Covering the neonate with plastic sheet, warm gamgees
- Using warm solutions to clean surgical parts
- Using warm IV fluids intraoperatively
- Using warmed humidified gases

REFERENCES

1. Luginbuehl I, Bissonnette B. Thermal Regulation In: Cote CJ, Lerman J, Todres ID, (Eds). A Practice of Anesthesia for Infants and Children, 4th edn. Elsevier Saunders; 2009; 559–67.
2. Luginbuehl I, Bissonnette B, Davis PJ. Thermoregulation Physiology and Perioperative Disturbances In: Peter JD, Franklyn PC, Etsuro KM (Eds). Smith's Anaesthesia for Infants and Children, 8th edn. Elsevier Mosby. 2011; 158–78.
3. Thomas K. Thermoregulation in Neonates. Neonatal Network/March 1994;13(2).

9

Essentials of Haematology

Anjana Sahu

ABSTRACT

Paediatric age group is the most vulnerable group for haematological disorders. Haemolytic patients may have multiorgan dysfunction. Therefore, for paediatric anaesthesiologist, it should be of great concern to know the status of the major organs and should be optimising preoperatively. The children with hematological derangement may have repeated infection, severe abdominal and/or bone pain, failure to thrive, poor mental growth, require multiple transfusion and may develop typical haemolytic facies. An anaesthesiologist may encounter the surgical procedure which may be the part of treatment of haemolytic anaemia disease itself such as palliative splenectomy. These children may require some other surgical procedures having origins in haemolytic anaemia to cholelithiasis, dental carries, etc.

INTRODUCTION

Paediatric hematological system is an intricate and complex system of the body. The study of blood and its components is known as haematology. Blood has all the essential cells which help to maintain tissue oxygenation as well as to fight against the infections. The components are red blood cell (RBC) or erythrocytes, white blood cells or leukocytes, platelets and plasma which is rich in coagulation factors. Genetic mutations are common cause of functional derangement of hematological system. Haemolytic anaemia occurs due to ineffective erythropoiesis and lysis RBCs. Neonate and infants have different physiological aspects of haematology as compared to adult, therefore, for better understanding we discuss a little about it before proceeding for anaesthesia consideration in these patients. Earlier morphology and quantitative analysis of blood cells were the available methods of diagnosing bleeding disorder but now in the modern era it has been shifted to higher level with the invention of biochemical and genetic engineering. These methods allow to detect the root cause and to treat more precisely.

PHYSIOLOGY OF ERYTHROCYTE

During foetal life hematopoiesis occurs in three phases: Mesoblastic, hepatic and myeloid. Mesoblastic phase starts in the yolksac from 10 to 14 days of gestation and regresses by 10 weeks. Hepatic phase starts from 5th week and occurs in the placenta till 10–12 weeks and in the liver till the second trimester. Myeloid phase starts from 20 to 24 weeks and remains throughout the life. In the body there is balance in the production and destruction of RBCs. Bone marrow is the main site of synthesis of RBCs and old and defective RBCs are sequestrated through the spleen. Excess but ineffective production leads to enlargement of bone marrow as well as spleen (splenomegaly) owing to defective erythrocyte. Normal survival of a RBC is 90–120 days. In neonate lifespan of RBC is about 80–100 days while 60–80 days in preterm infants.

Haemoglobin

An erythrocyte contains 95% of haemoglobin as major protein. Haemoglobin has two components, the heme particle and four globin chains. The heme has iron content and carries oxygen in the blood and there are two pairs of globin chain, alpha (α) and beta (β). In intrauterine life, the arrangement of globin chains differs with the stages of gestation. There are epsilon ε, gamma γ, theta ζ and delta δ chains apart from α and β chains.

Embryonic stage has the haemoglobins Gower 1 (ε_4 or $\zeta_2\varepsilon_2$), Gower 2 ($\alpha_2\varepsilon_2$), Portland ($\zeta_2\gamma_2$), Foetal ($\zeta_2\gamma_2$), foetal stage has haemoglobins Foetal ($\zeta_2\gamma_2$), haemoglobin A ($\alpha_2\beta_2$) and adult stage has haemoglobin A ($\alpha_2\beta_2$), haemoglobin A_2 ($\alpha_2\delta_2$) and foetal haemoglobin ($\alpha_2\gamma_2$). During intrauterine life the major number of Haemoglobin is foetal haemoglobin (HbF). Normal haemoglobin distribution in extrauterine life is >95% HbA, <3.5% HbA_2 and <2.5% HbF. Their arrangement is controlled by various genes present on different chromosomes. Mutations of genes lead to disorder of particular cell and affect its function.

Erythrocytes cell membrane is made up of various proteins which help to maintain the integrity of the cell. Neonatal RBC membrane is more resistant to osmotic lysis as compared to adult. Deficiency of membrane protein can lead to membrane hereditary spherocytosis. Normally mean corpuscular volume decreases after birth from 100–130 fl to 70–85 fl by the age of one year. Its persistent increased level indicates α thalassemia in newborn. Usually in newborn the appearance of nucleated RBCs and reticulocytosis is normal phenomenon but persistence is suggestive of haemolytic anaemia. The various hematological components level is shown in Table 9.1

ERYTHROCYTE METABOLISM

There are series of enzymes involve in the oxidative energy generating pathways in the metabolism of erythrocyte. Deficiency of any of these enzyme lead to defective formation of erythrocyte such as pyruvate kinase, glucose 6 phosphate dehydrogenase. Foetal and neonatal RBCs utilize more glucose and galactose as compared to adults. ATP generation is also more in preterm and term infants RBC than in adult RBC.

Oxyhaemoglobin dissociation curve

The haemoglobin oxygen saturation is plotted against the different partial pressure of oxygen. P_{50} is the value that the haemoglobin is 50% saturated with oxygen at particular partial pressure (PaO_2). In adult haemoglobin P_{50} is achieved at 26.3 PaO_2 while in foetal haemoglobin it is at 19.4 PaO_2 (Fig. 9.1). This shows the affinity of foetal haemoglobin is higher for oxygen and curve shifts to the left. This is helpful in intrauterine life to extract oxygen from maternal haemoglobin but in extrauterine life it has deleterious effect. Actually this property of foetal haemoglobin helps in diffusing oxygen from maternal haemoglobin at placental level. The 2,3 diphosphate glycerate (2,3-DPG) is produced during glycolysis in RBCs and it is present in higher amount at placenta. The 2,3-DPG interacts with β chain and increases dissociation of oxygen from HbA and shifts the curve to right. The HbF has α and γ subunits instead

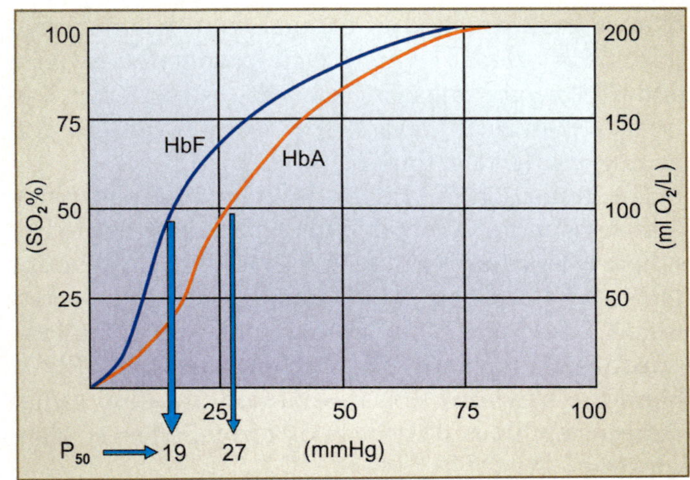

Fig. 9.1 Oxyhaemoglobin dissociation curve for foetal haemoglobin and adult haemoglobin

Table 9.1 Levels of various haematological components

Age	Hb (gm/dL)	HCT (%)	RC(%) (%)	WBC count (/mm³)	PC (/mm³)	PT (sec)	INR	APTT (sec)	Fibrinogen (mg/dL)	BT (min)
Preterm	13.6	43.6	—	7,710	260,000	13	1	53.6	243	3.5
At birth	17	55	5	18,000	300,000	13	1	42.9	283	3.5
1 year	12	36	1	10,000	300,000	11	1	30	276	6
Child	13	38	1	8,000	300,000	11	1	31	279	7
Adult	15	45	1.6	7,500	300,000	12	1	28	278	5

Haemoglobin (Hb), Haematocrit (HCT), Reticulocyte count (RC), Platelet count (PC), Activated partial thromboplastin time (APTT), Bleeding time (BT). The values are expressed as mean.[1]

Source: Modified and adapted from Essential of Haematology, Ch-9 Charles J. Cote. A practice of anaesthesia for infants and children.

of β, therefore it has a poor response to 2, 3-DPG and shows greater affinity for oxygen. The preterm infants contain high concentration of HbF and less of 2, 3-DPG therefore they need more amount of oxygen to prevent hypoxic event. The level of erythropoietin is high in preterm child as a result of decreased oxygen delivery at the tissue level which stimulates the hormone production. Owing to increased affinity for oxygen of HbF, there is difficulty in delivering oxygen at tissue level. To overcome this there is increased production of RBCs per blood volume and also exaggerated Bohr reaction in foetus. Acidic pH shifts the oxy-haemoglobin curve to right and helps in dissociation of oxygen at tissue level. Gradually in the third trimester the level of HbF starts decreasing and HbA increasing. Infant has high haemoglobin concentration at birth which gradually decreases to acquire the adult haemoglobin with increase in age. Concomitantly there is increase in concentration of 2, 3 –DPG. Both 2, 3-DPG and HbA enhance the extraction of oxygen from haemoglobin molecule at cellular level. In well oxygenated preterm child the oxygen releasing capacity is higher at 8 to 9 weeks than birth despite low oxygen content and haemoglobin concentration.

This transition of HbF leads to Pentose phosphate pathway is more vulnerable to oxidant induced injury as there is less number of membrane sulfhydrol groups in RBCs and decrease antioxidant capacity of newborn plasma. Also there is decrease number of Glutathione peroxidase in newborn RBCs as compare to adult RBCs. Therefore, newborn RBCs eventually develop glutathione instability and Heinz body formation on oxidant exposure.

Anaemia

Anaemia is defined as a reduction of haemoglobin concentration or RBC volume below the normal range. There are various causes of anaemia like nutritional, metabolic, environmental, infection, drugs, hereditary, etc. Iron deficiency anaemia is the most common cause of anaemia in children. Symptoms become apparent when haemoglobin level falls below 7–8 gm/dL. Sign and symptoms include sleepiness, pallor, irritability, decrease exercise tolerance, weakness. Gradually symptoms become severe in case of long standing anaemia such as tachypnea, shorteness of breath due to pulmonary hypertension, tachycardia, cardiac dilatation and high output cardiac failure.

Neonatal anaemia may occur due to placenta previa, abruption placenta, placental laceration, fetomateranal blood loss and twin-twin transfusion. The haemoglobin concentration per blood volume is higher therefore small amount of blood loss develops significant anaemia. These neonates present with pallor, hypovolemia, and hypotension. These patients do not show hyperbilirubinaemia as found in haemolytic disorder. The treatment lies with the infusion of crystalloid and blood transfusion in severe cases. At birth the haemoglobin level is 14–20 gm/dL which decreases to approximately 11 gm/dL by the age of 4–5 months. This is known as physiological anaemia of infancy. It is a normal response and adaptation to extra-uterine life.

Transfusion therapy is required to achieve normal level of blood indices and it improves the quality as well as the quantity by infusing the number of blood components. It improves the oxygen carrying capacity, immunological function and hemostatic functions. In children the recommendations for transfusion practice varies and it should be preferred to consult paediatrician before if excessive blood loss and fluid shifts suspected. The blood volume (BV) varies with the age in paediatric group. The preterm has blood volume 90–100 mL/kg which constitutes a greater proportion of body weight in comparison to full term neonate with blood volume 80–90 mL/kg. The infant between 3 months and 1 year has BV of 70–80 mL/kg and old child has 70 mL/kg. Anaemic preterm infants require blood transfusion to prevent apnoeic spell, respiratory and cardiac failure and neurological dysfunction. Fall of the haemotocrit level during intraoperative period define the requirement of blood transfusion. The normal healthy infant does not require blood transfusion until the fall of haemotocrit level 20–25%. The maximum allowable blood loss (MABL) is estimated by the formula of simple proportion:

$$\text{MABL} = \frac{3}{4}\,\frac{\text{EBV} \times \left(\text{Child's haematocrit} - \text{minimum accepted haematocrit}\right)}{\text{Child's haematocrit}}$$

EBV is effective blood volume for the age. The calculation obtained through this formula is only a rough estimation of blood loss because the haemotocrit varies with rapid blood loss and the crystalloid infusion.

> For infants and children that require massive transfusions, hyperkalemia will likely be a result. Be prepared to deal with it.

HAEMOLYTIC ANAEMIA

Haemolytic anaemia is caused by lysis of erythrocytes and ineffective erythrocytosis. Any anatomical,

Table 9.2 Causes of haemolytic anaemia in newborn

Congenital red blood cell disorder	Acquired red blood cell disorder
Red blood cell membrane disorder	Drug induced:
Hereditary spherocytosis	Toxins
Hereditary elliptocytosis	DIC
Red blood cell enzyme defect	Infections:
Glucose 6 phosphodehydrogenase	Thrombocytic thrombocytopenic purpura
Pyruvate kinase	Congenital heart disease
Haemoglobinopathies	Extra corporeal membrane oxygenation:
Sickle cell disease	Hemangioma
Thalassemia	

physiological and biochemical error in the RBC can lead to haemolytic anaemia.

It is classified as disorder of membrane proteins, disorder of enzymes and disorder of haemoglobin. Table 9.2 shows haemolytic anaemia in newborn due to red cell disorder.

How to Detect Bilirubin

Hyperbilirubinaemia with normal hepatic function is the marker of excessive red cell destruction. The occurrence of hyperbilirubinaemia in the first week after birth is known as physiological jaundice and it is a normal phenomenon. In term neonate and preterm neonate it is approximately 12 mg/dL (peak at 4th day) and 15 mg/dL (peak at 7th day) respectively. Normally the hyperbilirubinaemia in neonate occurs due to increase level of circulating red cell mass at birth, decrease life span of RBCs and increase enterohepatic circulation of bilirubin. In case of accelerated hemolysis the hyperbilirubinaemia is found more than this normal physiological value. Mild anaemia and reticulocytosis is normal findings in neonate but excessive hyperbilirubinaemia is the only factor which indicates haemolytic disease of newborn.

Carboxyhaemoglobin

Carbon monoxide has been produced from breakdown of heme group and carried in blood as carboxyhaemoglobin. It is also the marker of exccesive destruction of RBCs. The exhaled carboxyhaemoglobin is measured from lungs.

Hyperbilirubinaemia and carboxyhaemoglobin are the indicator of ongoing hemolysis, therefore, these neonates should be closely monitored and evaluated for cause of hemolysis.

Increased lactic dehydrogenase (LDH) is also a maker of destruction of RBCs which is released from LDH 2 isozyme from RBC.

The haptoglobin interacts with free haemoglobin and forms haptoglobin-haemoglobin complex. The decreased level of haptoglobin is an indicator of intravascular hemolysis.

DISORDER OF ERYTHROCYTE MEMBRANE PROTEIN

Hereditary Spherocytosis

Hereditary spherocytosis (HS) is the most common inherited haemolytic anaemic disorder. The incidence is approximately one in 5000.[2] Most of the HS has autosomal dominant inheritance (> 60%), however, some has sporadic mutation (20%) and remaining has autosomal recessive inheritance. There is defect in RBC membrane protein especially spectrin, ankyrin and band 3. These membrane proteins maintain the integrity of RBC membrane by maintaining surface tension. Defect in these proteins lead to osmotic fragility and hemolysis.

Clinical Manifestation

These patients are usually asymptomatic but may become symptomatic on exposure to bacterial or viral infections.[3] Neonate presents with anaemia and hyperbilirubinemia. Infant and young children present signs of anaemia (pallor, easy fatigability, weakness, exercise intolerance, irritability, palpitation,) and splenomegaly. In severe case jaundice has become the major feature in addition to severe anaemia. Pigmented gall stones are seen in 5% of children less than 10 years of age.[4]

Aplastic crisis is a severe form of HS is seen when these patients suffer from Parvo B19 virus infection.[5] There is fever with chills, lethargy, vomiting, diarrhoea, maculopapular rashes over the face, trunk and extrimities. They may require emergency splenectomy. All patients should be vaccinated against capsular organism before splenectomy.

Splenectomy is considered in case of severe anaemia (Hb < 10 gm%) and reticulocytosis (> 10%), hypoplastic or aplastic crisis, poor growth and cardiomegaly. Splenectomy should be preferred after 4–5 years of age as immunological function is poorly develop in younger children.

Laboratory Investigation

Peripheral blood smear: Increase reticulocytes, polychromatophilic reticulocytes and spherocytes. Spherocytes are dense, round, hyperchromatic cells with lack of central pallor and have decrease mean cell diameter. In severe cases these spherocytes become dense, irregular, contracted or budding spherocytes.

Red blood cell indices: Normal or decrease haemoglobin 4–12 gm/dL, increase mean corpuscular haemoglobin concentration MCHC 36–38 gm% RBCs, Mean corpuscular volume is low shows dehydrated state of red cell.

Osmotic fragility test shows positive result as there is decrease in surface area in relation to cell volume. In this test the RBCs are suspended in the hypotonic buffered sodium chloride solution and membrane protein analysis has been carried out.

Indirect hyperbilirubineamia, increase fecal urobilinogen and erythroid hyperplasia of bone marrow are other markers of HS.

Treatment

Once the diagnosis confirmed, child should be called for regular follow-ups and screening should be done to know the spleen size, growth, iron stores, infection with Parvo virus B19 and presence of gall stones. Usually children are put on folate therapy 25 mg/day till 5 years of age and 5 mg/day thereafter in case of moderate to severe HS. In case of severe HS with splenomegaly, splenectomy should be considered as it checks the ongoing hemolysis, helps in returning of normal haemoglobin level. Splenectomy will be of benefit in all cases with severe HS and some with moderate HS, but is usually not needed in mild cases.[6]

Cholecystectomy can either be done alone in case of cholelithiasis or in combination with splenectomy.[7] After splenectomy patient's condition improves and there is no reported incidence of cholelithiasis.[8]

Anaesthetic Consideration

Preoperative presence of anaemia, thrombocytopenia, jaundice and splenomegaly is of great concern in a child posted for either splenectomy or cholecystectomy. After splenectomy patient improves dramatically, however, in initial period potential thrombocytosis happens but it will be transient.[1] However, Das et al. reported in their study that the risk factor for thromboembolism was increased with c-reactive protein, persistant thrombocytosis and elevated D-dimer following splenectomy in children.[9] Postoperatively there is increased risk of overwhelming infection with encapsulated organisms such as by *Streptococcus pneumoniae, Neisseria meningitidis* and *Haemophilus influenzae* type B. Especially younger children below 5 years of age are vulnerable to these infections, therefore, prophylactic vaccination against capsular organisms should be done before splenectomy. During intraoperative period avoid intramuscular injections and drugs associated with increase bleeding risk. Drugs such as aspirin, other NSAIDs and antiplatelets should be avoided. Splenectomy can be done either through conventional laparotomy or laparoscopic. Nowadays laparoscopic splenectomy is gaining popularity over conventional open splenectomy. Laparoscopic splenectomy decreases morbidity and hospital stay.[10] It is minimally invasive procedure, safe, effective and associated with less pain.[11] Partial splenectomy is done in case of young child below 5 year age. The immune functions not fully developed, therefore, they are more prone to develop postsplenectomy sepsis.

DISORDER OF ENZYMES

Glucose 6 Phosphate Dehydrogenase

Glucose 6 phosphate dehydrogenase deficiency G6PD is the most common hereditary RBC enzymatic disorder. It has been estimated that approximately 400 million peoples are affected with this disease.[12] It is an X-linked disorder affecting male population. G6PD enzyme is one of important enzymes of phosphogluconate pathway in the erythrocyte. G6PD catalyzes the process through which glucose 6 phosphate is converted into phosphogluconate.[13] The nicotinamide adinine dinucleotide phosphate (NADPH) is produced during this process which keeps the glutathione in the reduced state (functional) (Fig. 9.2). This pathway interacts with environmental oxidants and prevents globin denaturation. G6PD deficiency leads to denaturation of Haemoglobin and it gets precipitated inside the RBC known as Heinz bodies. This leads to damage of RBC membrane and the onset of haemolytic anaemia. Whenever patient exposes to certain metabolic disorder, infection, ingestion of certain drugs and fava beans widespread hemolysis occurs (Table 9.4).[14]

Table 9.3 Anaesthesia consideration in hereditary spherocytosis

Preoperative
Haemoglobin, reticulocyte count, platelet count
History of transfusions and special blood requirement such as extended phenotype, matching or leukocyte reduction
History of infections, aplastic crises
Check pre-splenectomy vaccination
Intraoperative
Antibiotic coverage
Blood and blood products if bleed
Avoid intramuscular injections
Avoid platelet inhibitory drugs: NSAIDs
Regional anaesthesia should be used cautiously in case of thrombocytopenia
Nasal intubation, nasogastric tube insertion also be done with care
Postoperative
Potential thrombocytosis but transient
Regular haemoglobin and platelet level
Maintain sterility and hygiene

Source: Modified and adapted from Essential of Haematology, Ch-9 Charles J. Cote. A practice of anaesthesia for infants and children.

It has provided some protection against the malaria especially against the deadliest form plasmodium falciparum.[13]

Clinical Manifestation

Acute neonatal anaemia, jaundice and abdominal or lumbar pain are common manifestations. Two types of clinical syndrome is encountered; chronic nonspherocytic hemolitic anaemia and episodic haemolytic anaemia.

Table 9.4 Drugs triggering hemolysis in glucose-6-phosphate dehydrogenase

Ibuprofen, Aspirin
Chloroquine, Primaquine, Pamaquine, Quinine
Chloramphinicol, Ciprofloxacin, Sulphonamide
Thiazide, Furesamide
Ranitidine, Antiemetics
Nitrates, Dopamine, Beta-Blocker
Barbiturate, Phenytoin, Benzodiazepine, Insulin
Methylene Blue, Local Anaesthetic

Table 9.5 Anaesthesia consideration in G6PD deficiency

Preoperative
History of haemolysis and offending factors
Haemoglobin, reticulocyte count
Intraoperative
Avoid triggering agents
Maintain good hydration, ABG
Cautiously use of triggering agent in infants
Monitor haemoglobin and urine output in high risk cases (on Cardiopulmonary bypass)
Postoperative
Haemoglobin, reticulocyte count, urine output in case of hemolysis

Source: Modified and adapted from Essential of Haematology, Ch-9 Charles J. Cote. A practice of anaesthesia for infants and children.

Laboratory Investigation

It includes complete blood picture, if there is recent history of hemolysis there would be anaemia, reticulocytosis, decrease serum heptoglobin and an

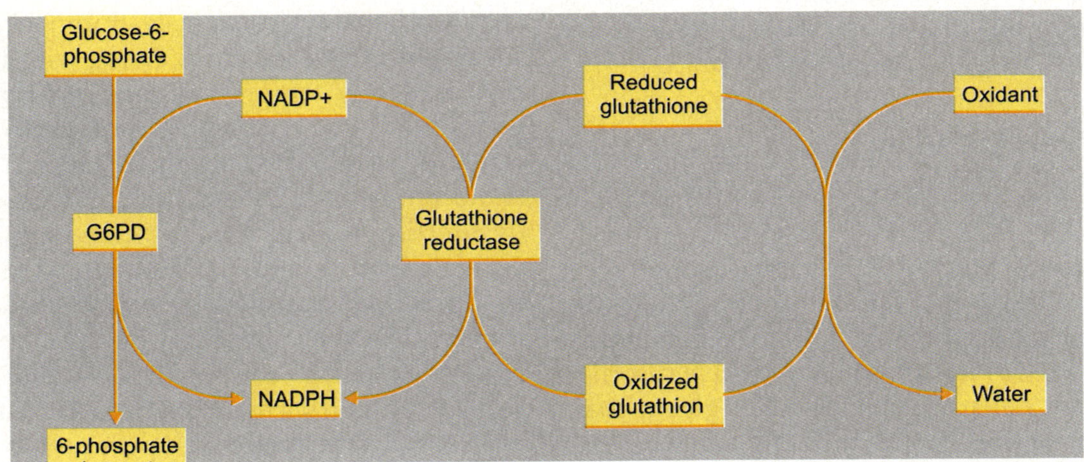

Fig. 9.2 Glucose-6-phosphate

elevated indirect bilirubin. Heinz bodies are seen on peripheral smear. Fluorescent spot test is the specific test to diagnose G6PD.

Anaesthetic Consideration

History of previous episodes of haemolysis, frequency of blood transfusion and exposure to precipitating factors are suggestive of type and severity of disease. Drugs used during anaesthesia should be given with precaution such as thiopentone sodium, non-steroidal antiinflammatory agents, ranitidine, anticonvulsant, certain antibiotics, diuretics, insulin.[15,16] Table 9.4 shows the list of drugs triggering hemolysis in G6PD deficiency. Surgical stress could be a precipitating factor, therefore, proper anxiolysis and good coverage of analgesia is required during perioperative period. Drugs such as benzodiazepins, propofol, ketamine, codein or codein derivative, fentanyl are safe and do not cause any haemolytic crisis in G6PD deficiency.[17] Benzocaine, lidocaine, articaine, prilocaine, silver nitrates should be avoided as they may induce methaemoglobinaemia and methlyne blue is ineffective in these patients.[18,19] Avoid acidosis and hyperglycaemia which are known to cause hemolysis. Postoperatve hypotension may not be a good guide of ongoing haemolysis but hematuria could be a reliable sign. Therefore, these cases require adequate monitoring of urine output. Actual hemolysis starts after 24–48 hours of exposure to triggering agent. Remove the trigger agent, maintain hemodynamics with vaso-pressors and maintain good urine output by infusing crystalloids. Consider blood transfusion in case of low haemoglobin. If patient gets discharge early, family should be informed about the sign and symptoms of acute hemolysis such as pallor, cyanosis, headache, breathlessness, jaundice, yellowish discoloration of sclera, lethargy, weakness, lumbar or substernal pain, dark-coloured urine. So that they should report to the clinician immediately for early intervention.

DISORDER OF HAEMOGLOBIN (HAEMOGLOBINOPATHIES)

Thalassemia

Thalassemia is due to reduced or deficient production of one of the globin chain of haemoglobin. The disease is prevelant in mediterranean, African and southeast Asian ancestors. It is an autosomal recessive disorder. Homozygous or heterozygous for either globin chain is known as a major or minor (trait) disease. Each year approximately 400,000 babies born with serious haemoglobinopathies and carrier frequency is about 270 million.[20] Approximately 32,400 infants in India born with serious haemoglobinopathies per year.[21]

Alpha (α) thalassemia occurs due to decrease production or absence of α chain and excess of β chain. In α-thalassemia mutation occurs at two closely located gene loci on chromosome 16. It means that four globin gene control the globin synthesis. It mainly affects HbA (α_2, β_2) and HbA_2 (α_2, δ_2). There is excess production of beta chain. In case of neonate there is excess production of uncontrolled γ chain as foetal haemoglobin contains γ. Number of mutant gene controlling the formation of globin chain will decide the clinical presentation. Four gene deletions is most serious presentation. These patients die in intrauterine life (hydrops foetalis) or may be stillborn or may die shortly after birth. Three gene deletions or haemoglobin H (HbH) show picture of chronic haemolytic anaemia and have history of multiple transfusion. This hemolysis is triggered by exposure to stress and oxidants. Two gene deletions have mild type of presentation and insignificant microcytic anaemia. Single gene deletion patients are silent carrier with no anaemia.

Beta (β) thalassemia is due to decrease production of beta chain and excess of alpha chain. In β thalassemia there is two globin gene defects on chromosome 11. Approximately 200 mutations found in α gene including substitution, inclusion and deletion. It is rare but carries poor prognosis. Clinical manifestation is of microcytic hypochromic anaemia. β thalassemia is again classified into three classes:

β thalassemia major

β thalassemia major is also known as cooley's anaemia or mediterranean anaemia. It is homozygous for β globin chain. Clinical presentations are of prehepatic jaundice, hepatosplenomegaly, thrombocytopenia, and severe microcytic anaemia. Along with these patients may have bony deformity of skull, vertebrae, facial, long bones and pelvis. Patient may develop high output congestive cardiac failure due to chronic anaemia and hemochromatosis. Patient also has liver and endocrine dysfunction. It is a severe life threatening condition and patient may die if left untreated. Patient requires frequent blood transfusions in first few years of life to combat anaemia. Patient may have recurrent fever and exposed to risk of getting multiple blood transfusion related infection such as HIV, hepatitis B or C. Children have delayed milestones and poor growth and may die in 5–6 years of age.

β thalassemia intermedia

β thalassemia intermedia is not that severe condition as major. Symptoms lie between major and minor state. Patient may have mild microcytic anaemia and may or may not need blood transfusion. Patient has symptoms of pathological fracture especially long bone fracture. Owing to ineffective erythropoiesis patient develops gall stones and splenomegaly. There is increase risk of venous thrombosis, pulmonary embolism, stroke and cardiomyopathy.

β thalassemia minor

β thalassemia minor is also known as thalassemia trait or carrier. It is an asymptomatic condition. Patient of this category has mild microcytic anaemia and does not need blood transfusion.

Sometimes β thalassemia is associated with other haemoglobinopathies like HbE, HbC or HbS.

Pathophysiology

Abnormal globin polymers aggregate and precipitate inside the RBCs known as inclusion bodies and destroy its membrane resulting into formation of abnormal RBCs. These abnormal RBCs are phagocytised inside the bone marrow and some comes out into the circulation leading to haemolytic anaemia. Decreased oxygen carrying capacity of blood owing to low haemoglobin content triggers release of erythropoietin and there are proliferation of premature erythroblasts to form erythrocytes. They are defective with globin precipitate and this results into ineffective erythropoiesis. This also initiates extramedullary erythropoiesis in liver and spleen.

Anaemia is due to ineffective erythropoiesis, increase peripheral hemolysis and overall low haemoglobin synthesis. Haemolytic anaemia leads to increase hemocromatosis. This increases iron load and damages the heart, bones and endocrine organs. Bony cortex becomes brittle and fragile and also gets easily fractured. There is enlargement of bone marrow and widening of bone especially face and skull bone. In severe cases splenomegaly, congestive cardiac failure and arrhythmias occur.

Laboratory Investigation

Peripheral blood smear, haemoglobin electrophoresis, bone marrow aspiration, iron studies, imaging studies such as computed tomography, magnatic resonance imaging, ultrasonography, echocardiography depending on the severity.

Treatment

Patient requires frequent blood transfusion and may undergo palliative splenectomy. Due to increase iron deposits patient requires iron chelation therapy. Currently phenotypic matching and leukocyte depleted blood transfusion; hormone and vitamin D therapy are being used. The bone marrow transplant and peripheral blood stem transplant are advanced therapies to cure haemoglobinopathies. Studies are still going on to find the cure. Gene modulation, erythropoietin, foetal haemoglobin modifier anti-oxidants are under investigation.

Anaesthetic Consideration

Careful evaluation of family history and history of multiple transfusions suggestive of thalassemia should be carried out. Planning of anaesthesia depends on the severity of disease and multiorgan dysfunction. Apart from routine investigations, special investigation should be done depending upon the organ dysfunction. Difficult airway suspected in case of maxillofacial bony deformity. Therefore keep difficult airway cart ready. Assess airway, size of the liver and spleen

Table 9.6 Anaesthesia consideration in thalassemia

Preoperative
Haemoglobin,
Appropriate available crossmatch (antibody-matched, leukocyte depleted)
Endocrine work up for diabetes mellitus, hypopituitarism, etc.
Cardiac evaluation
Liver functions
Airway assessment
Pre-splenectomy immunisation
Intraoperative
Difficult airway preparation
Gentle handling of demineralised extremities and proper padding to pressure points
Monitor cardiovascular function and post-splenectomy hypertension
Physiologic effects of laparoscopy on respiratory and circulatory function
Thromboembolism prophylaxis
Postoperative
Monitoring includes cardiovascular function
Thromboembolism prophylaxis

Source: Modified and adapted from Essential of Haematology, Ch-9 Charles J. Cote. A practice of anaesthesia for infants and children.

preoperatively. Chest X-ray to know the status of lungs as lung congestion might be there due to anaemia and repeated blood transfusion. Preoperative vaccination should be checked. Adequate blood, type specific antibody matched and leukocyte depleted plasma should be arranged before surgical procedure. Regional anaesthesia is safe to avoid systemic complications but may have difficulty in positioning and performing procedure. In severe cases general anaesthesia is safe, however, difficulties can occur in securing of airway due to bony deformity of skull and vertebrae. Apart from splenectomy and cholecystectomy children may come for vascular access placement for frequent blood transfusion. Also, demineralised bones are prone to fracture and older children may come for osteotomies for bony deformities. The sodium nitroprusside should be administered with caution during open heart surgeries or in other cases.

SICKLE CELL ANAEMIA

Sickle cell disease (SCD) is a congenital haemoglobinopathic disorder. Sydenstricker and associates described the first occurrence in children, recognised the association with haemolytic anaemia and introduce the term crisis to describe periodic acute episodes of pain.[22] Haemoglobin comprises active heme group and two globin chain. Mutation occurs at sixth codon of β globin chain and encodes valine instead of glutamate. Sickle cell anaemia is severe and homozygous form of HbS. It has >90% of circulating HbS. Sickle cell trait is mild form with single allele HbS (<50%) and HbA. Compound heterozygous is with HbS and HbC. SCD may be associated with α thalassemia known as sickle β thalessemia (S/β^o or S/β^+). Intrauterine life, the major concentration of Hb is Foetal Haemoglobin HbF, while HbA and HbA_2 are in minor. Normal haemoglobin distribution in extrauterine life is >95% HbA, <3.5% HbA_2 and, <2.5% HbF. In India haplotype is found in Odisha and Pune region. These patients have mild disease and there is increase level of foetal haemoglobin. HbF inhibits HbS polymerisation in sickle cell anaemia and it is considered as powerful modulator of the clinical and hematological features of sickle cell anaemia.[23] Studies found that higher concentration of HbF were associated with reduced rate of acute painful episodes, fewer leg ulcers, less osteonecrosis, less frequent acute chest syndromes and reduced disease severity.[23] Therefore, nowadays increasing the level of HbF is geared up as one of the treatment modality.[24]

With increase in haemolytic episodes 30–50% of children may develop cholelithiasis.[25] Most of the gall stones are pigmented and made up of calcium bilirubinate. Severe right hypochondriac pain and fever of cholelithiasis require cholecystectomy at an early age. Patient develops characteristic haemolytic facies with frontal bossing, wide intercanthal distance, flat nose or depressed nose bridge, malar prominence and muddy sclera along with pallor and icterus. Sickle with thalassemia β^o present with haemoglobin 6–10 gm/dL, vaso-occlusive crises and aseptic necrosis of bone. Sickle with thalassemia α^+ present with haemoglobin 10–14 gm/dL and rarely vaso-occlusive crises and avascular necrosis.

Sickle cell disease or anaemia is also known as vaso occlusive disease. Oxygen is extracted from HbS results in deformation of erythrocyte into sickle shaped. Sickling occurs in case of oxidative stress (PaO_2 <40 mmHg) and it occludes the microvascular circulation leading to tissue ischaemia and infarction. Gradually it involves all the systems leading to multiorgan failure. Deformed red blood cells obstruct the flow leading to severe bone and joint pain, renal insufficiency to concentrate, stroke, acute chest syndrome (ARDS) and heart failure.

Clinical Manifestation

Frequent bacterial infections are common due to abnormal immune function. Recurrent episodes of fever and bone or joint pain (Dactylitis) are common manifestations. The precipitating factors are physical stress, infection, acidosis, dehydration, hypoxia, and exposure to cold or sometime swimming. Newborn with sickle cell anaemia is usually not anaemic and asymptomatic due to presence of HbF.

The most fatal is splenic sequestration or splenic crisis in infant and young children. Patients experience severe form of abdominal pain, anaemia and hypovolumic shock. These patients require aggressive supportive treatment and emergency splenectomy. Sometime patients undergo autosplenectomy due to splenic infarction. Acute splenic sequestration is a life threatening complication in infants. In case of severe anaemia 5 mL/kg packed red blood cell transfusion should be considered and after the acute attack prophylactic splenectomy should be done.

Acute chest syndrome present with fever, dysponea, tachyponea, cough, wheezing, pulmonary hypertension and respiratory failure. Decreased oxygen saturation, acidosis, hypoxia and diffuse lung infiltrations are other characteristic features. Good hydration, antibiotic coverage, oxygenation can improve the lungs but severe cases might require mechanical ventilation.

Treatment

All children should receive oral prophylactic dose of penicillin VK (125 mg twice a day up to 3 years, then 250 mg twice a day) till the age of 5 years. After 5 years of age, the prophylactic dose recommended only for those children who has history of pneumonia. In case of penicillin allergy erythromycin ethyle succinate 10 mg/kg twice a day is recommended. British Journal of Haematology (BJH)[26] has given the guideline for blood transfusion in sickle cell disease is shown in Table 9.7.

Anaesthetic Consideration

History of previous attacks and repeated hospitalization is important part of preanaesthetic checkup. It provides the valuable information about the extent, pattern and severity of the disease. Degree of organ dysfunction should be judged by all essential investigations. Pulse oximetry, chest X-ray, BUN and creatinine, ECG, haemotocrit are routinely advised investigation to know the organ dysfunction. Rarely echocardiography and arterial blood gas is advised. Patients may present with sepsis, renal insufficiency, splenomegaly, pulmonary hypertension, stroke, seizures and cardiac failure. Previous history of blood transfusion will guide us the patient response to the treatment. All patients who are posted for splenectomy should receive vaccination against the capsular organism such as pneumococcus, Streptococcus, *Haemophilus influenzae*. In younger patient sometime partial splenectomy is done to provide immune action against these infections but later life they might require total splenectomy. Goal for prophylactic blood transfusion is to achieve haemoglobin 10 gm/dL as above this limit hyperviscosity syndrome may occur. Exchange transfusion is no longer advised as there is increase risk of red blood cell alloimmunisation. It is indicated in case of severe anaemia and if when phototherapy and other measures fail to control bilirubin load. In this technique antibody coated RBCs are replaced with RBCs negative for antigen to which mother is alloimmunized. In sick or preterm neonate additional platelet therapy should be considered during exchange transfusion. Prophylactic transfusion has controversies like some studies are *pro and say* it is always beneficial to transfuse preoperatively as it is helpful to prevent sickling by maintaining good amount of haemoglobin. Perioperative consultation with haematologists and paediatric intensivists is helpful in treating these patients. Surgical procedures are classified according to the need of blood transfusion. Low risk surgeries are inguinal herniotomy and extrimities, intermediate risk surgeries include intra-abdominal and high risk surgeries are intracranial and intrathoracic. Minor low risk surgeries rarely require transfusion. In sickle cell disease the history of episodes of vaso-occlusive phenomenon tells the severity and pattern of the disease, therefore, as an anaesthesiologist we should check the extent of organs dysfunction preoperatively. All the triggering factors leading to oxidative stress during intraoperative period should be avoided. Factors such as hypothermia, hypoxia, hypercarbia, acidosis and dehydration should be avoided.[27] Keep the operating theatre little warm maintain the temperature around 80–85° F and keep the patient also warm with the help of warming blankets and infusing warm fluids. Maintain good and peaceful environment inside the operation theatre. Give adequate dose of anxiolytic and analgesia with 100% oxygenation. To avoid hypoxic crises administered 100% oxygen a few minute before and after the intubation or extubation. Acute chest syndrome and pain are two most frequently encountered postoperative complications. Along with these fever or infection, vaso-occlusive crisis and transfusion related complications may occur in the perioperative period (Table 9.8).

Anaesthesiologist is often called for pain management in case of acute sickle crisis. Lower extremity pain due to vaso-occlusive crisis can be managed with continuous neuraxial blocks. Analgesia is managed with opiates and NSAIDs should be used with caution in case of renal involvement.

When rapid reduction of level of HbS is necessary, as in CNS crisis exchange transfusion, ET has been preferred. 60–80% decrease in number of circulating sickle cells in 6–12 hrs by exchanging two times the red cell mass (2 × Blood volume × Haematocrit). In determination of the total blood volume or number of units of blood needed for the exchange, one must take into consideration the pack red cell mass in a unit of blood.

Table 9.7 BJH guideline for blood transfusion in SCD

Top-up (Standard) transfusion	Splenic and hepatic sequestration Aplastic crises
Exchange transfusion	Chest syndrome, stroke, priyaprism
Hypertransfusion	Stroke, renal failure (in case of recurrence)

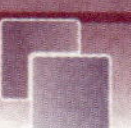

Table 9.8 Anaesthesia consideration in SCD

Preoperative
Screening of at risk children
Consultation with haematologist
History of acute chest syndrome, vaso-occlusive pain crises, hospitalization, transfusions, transfusion reactions
Neurological assessment (stroke, cognitive limitation)
History of analgesic and other medications
Haemoglobin, haematocrit
Oxygen saturation (room air), chest X-ray
Pulmonary function tests (if the history suggestive)
Echocardiography (if the history suggestive)
Neurological imaging (if the history suggestive)
Renal function tests
Transfusion crossmatch (antibody matched, leukocyte depleted, sickle negative)
Transfusion parenteral hydration if nil per oral
Pain management
Bronchodilator
Appropriate antibiotic coverage
Pre-splenectomy immunisation
Intraoperative
Maintenance of oxygenation, perfusion, normal acid–base status, temperature, hydration
Type specific blood for transfusion
Appropriate anaesthesia procedure and postoperative analgesia
Laparoscopic consideration
Appropriate antibiotic therapy
Judicious use of tourniquets, cell saver and cardiopulmonary bypass
Postoperative
Haematologist consultation
Monitoring of complication especially acute chest syndrome and vaso-occlusive crises
Maintenance of oxygen saturation monitoring and supplementation as required including supplemental oxygen in the first 24 hours regardless of oxygen saturation
Good hydration
Antibiotic coverage
Pain management
Early mobilization
Incentive spirometry and bronchodilator therapy

Source: Modified and adapted from Essential of Haematology, Ch-9 Charles J. Cote. A practice of anaesthesia for infants and children

Initially by PCV once HCT reaches 35, PCV diluted with appropriate electrolyte solution or plasma. BJH recommends the haemoglobin level at 8–10 gm/dL in preoperative period which is as effective as ET and safe practice. Minor and straightforward cases such as tonsillectomy and cholecystectomy can be done without transfusion. The major cases such as hip or knee replacement, organ transplantation, eye surgery and major intraabdominal surgeries may require preoperative transfusion. Maintain HbS below 20% by transfusion of RBCs.

Researcher from cooperative study of sickle cell disease found comparable complication rates in both HbSS and HbSC groups and suggested that regional anaesthesia were at higher risk of complications than those undergoing general anaesthesia.[28]

Simple transfusion to raise the Hb levels to 10 gm% in all SS group. The choice should be antigen-matched, leukocyte-depleted packed red cells. All patients, especially those with prior occurrence of pulmonary dysfunction or a history of multiple hospital admission, should receive a minimal 12 hrs of oxygen treatment and maintenance of intravenous fluid to avoid dehydration. High-risk patients should be monitored for oxygenation and regular measurement of input, output and weight.

COAGULATION SYSTEM

Any injury to vessel wall initiates coagulation (clotting) cascade. There are two main pathways and a common pathway involve in clotting mechanism. Intrinsic pathway occurs at sub endothelial wall whenever there is breech in the integrity of vascular wall. Extrinsic pathway occurs at tissue level and it potentiates the intrinsic pathway and common pathway. Three mechanisms occur to reduce the blood loss or to stop further loss.

1. **Vascular spasm:** As soon as there is breech in vessel wall, the vascular smooth muscle contraction occurs immediately to reduce the further blood loss.
2. **Platelet plug:** There is formation of platelet plug as a result of platelet adhesion, platelet release reaction and platelet aggregation, this is known as primary hemostasis. When there is injury to vessel wall, the breeched endothelium is exposed to circulating platelets. Platelets adhere to collagen with the help of collagen glycoprotein surface receptor Ia/IIa. The chemical messangers like adinosine diphosphate (ADP), serotonin, thromboxane A_2 released by these adhere platelets and attract more platelet to stick with them resulting into formation of platelet plug. This process is also strengthen by activation of

von Willebrand factor vWF which is released by endothelium and platelets. It also carries factor VIII.

3. **Blood coagulation mechanism:** Haemostasis is the complex physiological process that ceases the blood loss from the bleeding vessels. The coagulation factors are activated by intrinsic, extrinsic and common pathways to form fibrin clot is known as secondary haemostasis. This occurs simultaneously with primay haemostasis to prevent further blood loss. The fibrin clot is formed over the platelet plugs and seals the broken blood vessel. Intrinsic pathway is initiated when sub-endothelial surface is breeched, also known as contact activation pathway. This involves a series of activation of XII or Hageman factor, XI, prekallikrein and high molecular weight kininogen (HMWK) clotting factors. The factor XII is activated by kallikrein and interacts with HMWK to activate factor XI. Activated XII also activate prekallikrein to convert into kallikrein, which in turn, can convert HMWK into bradykinin. Bradykinin is a potent vasodilator and increases vascular permeability. Activated factor XI further activates factor IX. Now on the platelet surface in presence of factor IXa, factor VIIIa, phospholipid and calcium factor X is activated. Extrinsic pathway is initiated when tissue factor is exposed to factor VII and factor VIIa is formed. Extrinsic pathway plays a major role in the coagulation cascade and it is the primary pathway. Factor VIIa potentiates Xa. From this step the common pathway starts. Xa and Va then catalyze the reaction of conversion of prothrombin (Factor II) into thrombin. This thrombin converts soluble fibrinogen (factor I) into insoluble strands of fibrin. And multiple fibrin fibres join together and form fibrin clot. This thrombin also activates factor IX, factor VIII, factor V and factor XIII. Factor XIII provides stability to the fibrin clot.

In Case of Deficiency of Coagulation Factors the Blood Indices are Affected

Prothrombin time (PT): PT is the time that measures the clotting tendency of blood. It measures the efficacy of extrinsic pathway of coagulation. PT is used to measure the factors I, II, V, VII and X. PT and its derived measures such as prothrombin index and international normalized ratio are also used to measure the extrinsic pathway. Calcium containing thromboplastin reagent is added to citrated plasma sample and time taken to clot formation is noted by using an automated instrument. The reference range varies with the laboratories as type of instruments and amount of thromboplastin reagent differ. However, the normal prothrombin time is 10–11 seconds. It is usually prolong in neonate owing to poor availability of vitamin K. It is increased in case of clotting factor deficiency (level < 30%), liver damage, vitamine K deficiency, anticoagulant therapy warfarin.

Activated partial thromboplastin time (APTT): It measures the intrinsic pathway of coagulation and it has been measured with PT to know the deficiency of other factors. Proteins of intrinsic pathway are present in liquid form. When blood comes in contact with foreign object or damaged endothelial cell initiates clotting cascade. This process is monitored by standard clinical clotting assay known as activated partial thromboplastin time. In this test the partial thromboplastin reagent deficient tissue factor is mixed with citrated plasma sample and in this mixture surface contact agent (celite, kaolin, silica, etc.) is added. This is incubated for 3–5 minutes and calcium chloride is added. Factor XII, prekallikrein or HMWK deficiency results into markedly prolonged APTT without significant clinical bleeding. Isolated prolongation of APTT occurs in case of deficiency of factors VIII, IX or XI with clinical bleeding. Usually the reference level for children and adult is 26–35 seconds, while a little longer 30–54 seconds in term infants and even longer in preterm infants. The sensitivity depends on the specific reagent used. Most of the APTT reagents cause prolongation of APTT in case of deficiency of factor VIII less than 35 percent. It is also a useful method to monitor standard heparin therapy. Sometime contamination of patient sample with heparin may cause prolongation of APTT. Polycythemic infants also show prolonged APTT as citrate to plasma ratio has not been corrected for high haematocrit level.[29]

Thrombin Time (TT)

It measures reduced level and function of fibrinogen. The test is performed by adding bovine thrombin to the citrated plasma sample and time to clot formation is recorded. Time is 16–18 seconds.

Bleeding Time (BT)

Bleeding time originally described by Harker and Slichter. It gives us idea of platelet number and function. The normal bleeding time ranges from 3 to 9 minutes. It is pronged when the platelet count below the 100,000/µL and also in case of deranged platelet function (congenital or acquired), vasculitis, connective tissue disorder, and vWD. In this test a spring loaded blade is used, which makes a linear cut of 1–2 mm depth and bleeding blotted away by using filter paper and time is recorded with stopwatch.

Specific Clotting Factor Assay

This can be carried out by mixing the diluted test plasma with specific factor deficient substrate plasma. Clotting time is measured.

Disorder of Coagulation Factor

Haemophilia

Haemophilia is a hereditary disorder of coagulation factors. Haemophilia A and haemophilia B occur due to deficiency of clotting factor VIII and IX respectively. The incidence of haemophilia is 1 in 5000 males.[30] It is an X-linked recessive disorder, therefore, males are the affecting gender and females act as a carrier. Usually patient presents with bleeding disorder. The extrinsic pathway (tissue factor) requires factor VIII and factor IX for normal thrombin formation and therefore deficiency of either factor leads to impairment in production of thrombin and fibrin. This disruption in hemostasis leads to delay in clot formation and bleeding diathesis occur.

Haemophilia A accounts for 85–90% of total haemophilic disorder and is due to deficiency of factor VIII (antihemophilic factor). Haemophilia B or Christmas disease is due to factor IX (plasma thromboplastin component). Depending upon the factors concentration, patients are classified into three groups: Mild, moderate and severe. Mild group has 5–50% of normal level of clotting factor VIII or IX, moderate group has 1–5% of normal level of clotting factor while in severe group <1% (1 unit/dL) of normal level of clotting factor. Minimal haemostatic level of factor VIII is 0.3–0.5 U/mL and factor IX is 0.2–0.5 U/mL.

The genes for factor VIII and factor IX are present on long arm of X chromosome. Numerous genetic mutations are found in haemophilia but most common genetic mutation is gene inversion in haemophilia A and missense point mutation in haemophilia B.

Clinical Features

The patient of mild group may remain asymptomatic till adulthood or throughout life. Patient of haemophilia presents with unexplained bleeding, easy bruising, painful bleeding joints (hemarthrosis), nose bleed, gum bleed, blood in urine or stool and intramuscular bleed. The hallmark of haemophilia is musculoskeletal haemorrhage. Study shows 40–60% of children with severe haemophilia A are clinically symptomatic as newborn, approximately 40% may become clinically symptomatic by age of one year and approximately 50% show major bleed by the of age one and half year.[31] About 30% of child experience bleeding at the time of circumcision.[32] Along with it 1–2% of neonate may have an intracranial haemorrhage ICH.[33] In children the risk of ICH varies from 2 to 8%. Bleeding joints are common in older infants and children while rare in neonate. Severe factor VIII deficiency is most common hereditary disorder of neonatal age group. Diagnosis can be made when child begins to crawl and walk. Ankle joint haemorrhage is most common presentation when toddler tries to maintain upright posture. Other joints involved are knees and elbows.

Laboratory Investigation

If clinical manifestations and family history are suggestive of disease, then PT, APTT, BT, fibrinogen or TT, platelet count should be carried out. PT is found normal in haemophilia but APTT is prolonged in factor VIII or IX. Identify vWF also.

Anaesthetic consideration

Most of the haemorrhagic disorders have familial inheritance, therefore, family history may give valuable information related to the disease. Children of mild group may have not been experienced of spontaneous bleeding episodes but during surgery they are at risk. Screening of the patient should be carried out for the factor deficiency and clotting factor level should be normalised before taking the patient for surgery. According to The Royal Children's Hospital (RCH)[34] recommendation, the peripheral venous cannulation should be performed very carefully. Distraction, relaxation and sometime mild inhalational sedation technique is required. Invasive procedures such as arterial cannulation and lumbar puncture should only be attempted after appropriate clotting factor replacement.[34] Do not give intramuscular injections. NSAIDs (e.g. Ibuprofen, diclofenac, ketorolac) should be avoided, paracetamol, codein/codein derivative, morphin and tramadol can be given for analgesia.

In case of oral bleeding, torn frenulum or for tooth extraction, the aim of achieving the factor levels is 30–40 units/dL with replacement therapy. The tranexamic acid or e-aminocaproic acid can be used as supplement therapy with replacement therapy to stabilize the clot until healing. In case of oral surgery nasal intubation should be avoided as far as possible as it may cause injury to adenoids and uncontrollable bleeding provoked. Make the endotracheal tube soft with warm water and do careful oral intubation. After oral intubation, fix the tube with adhesive by keeping the mouth probe in place which widens the intraoral space.

In case of severe haemophilia minimum hemostatic level should be achieved 100%, then 50% until wound healing begins, then 30% until wound healing is complete. Start the therapy with 30–50 U/kg, 12 hourly or by continuous infusion.

Desmopressin DDAVP is a synthetic vasopressin analog which significantly increases the level of factor VIII and vWf. It is the treatment of choice in cases of mild and moderate haemophilia A if patient had responded well to the drug during therapeutic trial. It is not effective in case of severe haemophilia A, severe vWd and in any form of haemophilia B.[35] The side effect of desmopressin are headache, flushing, tachycardia, hypotension and rarely hyponatremia. Fluid intake should be limited to the maintenance levels for at least 24 hours. In case of repeated dosing serum sodium level should be checked. Usually DDAVP is not recommended in children less than 3 years as documented studies show hyponatremia and seizures. It is relatively contraindicated in known case of epileptic disorder. RCH recommended dose of intravenous desmopressin is 0.3 µg/kg and should be administered in 25 to 50 mL of normal saline over 20 to 30 minutes. It should be given one hour before the surgery as the maximum response seen at 30 to 60 minutes after the administration.

Choice of replacement therapy (concentrates) depends on the purity and viral inactivation. Fresh frozen plasma contains all the clotting factors and can be used as a replacement therapy in all bleeding disorders. FFP and cryo poor plasma contain factors IX, XI, X, VII and widely used for treating haemophilia B. Cryoprecipitate which is obtained by slow thrawing of FFP at 4°C for 12–24 hrs is used to treat of haemophilia A as it contains factor VIII, vWF, XII and fibrinogen. World Federation of Haemophilia (WFH) has given the guideline over treatment preference for bleeding disorder. They have advised to use factor concentrates instead of giving FFP. Commercially available lyophilized FVIII is preferred in case of haemophilia A. it is given by calculating the exact unit required to achieve the desired level. The formula to obtain the amount requires is patient body weight in kilogram multiplied by desired level multiplied to 0.5. In case of children it should be transfused at the rate of 100 unit per minute. The half life of factor VIII is approximately 10 to 12 hours. Therefore, factor VIII should be given in continuous infusion to maintain steady plasma level. Factor IX is also given by calculating the dose through the formula where desired factor level is multiplied by the body weight (kg). The half life of factor IX is approximately 18 to 24 hours, therefore, it does not need to be given as often.

Replacement materials should be infused to achieve a level of 80 units/dL of factor IX and 100 units/dL of factor VIII; the levels should be maintained at greater than 50 to 60 units/dL for 7–10 days postoperatively. Lower doses to maintain levels at greater than 20–30 units/dL for an additional 1–2 weeks may then be used and continued till complete healing has occurred.

Prothrombin complex concentrate (PCC) can be an effective and alternative therapy in haemophilia. PCC is thrombogenic and risk of thrombosis increased in patient using high or repetitive doses, in patient with impaired fibrinolysis (liver disease or after the treatment with antifibrinolytic agents), and in patient with impaired ability to clear activated clotting factors (liver disease).[35] International Society of Thrombosis and Hemostasis has recommended adding of 100 units of heparin to each of 500 units of factor IX concentrate.

Sometimes acquired factor VIII or IX inhibitors coagulopathy are seen in patients with repeated transfusions. These patients have produced antibodies against these factors and become prone to increase blood loss during surgery in spite of factor transfusion. In these patients bypass agents recombinant factor VIIa or activated prothrombin complex concentrates transfusion is beneficial. About 10–15% of haemophilia A and 1–3% of haemophilia B patients may develop inhibitors against the factors and fail to respond routine replacement therapy. Most of the inhibitor develops as early as after 10–20 days of exposure in case of severe genetic disorder. Therefore, all known bleeding disorder should be screened for both factors as well as for inhibitors. The Bethesda assay has been used to know the inhibitor levels. On the basis of Bethesda titre, the patients are divided into two categories. High responder has Bethesda titre more than 10 and having high titre antibody which may become hundreds or thousands on repeated exposure. Low responder has Bethesda titre less than 10 and maintain at this even on repeated exposure. Very low titre cannot be detected and show low clinical recovery and short half life of clotting factor. Children should be screened every 3–12 months or 10–20 exposure days. Low responder can be treated with factor VIII concentrate infusion but high

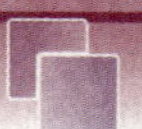

Table 9.9 Anaesthesia consideration in hemophilia

Preoperative
Hematologist consultation
Identify and treatment plan
Multiple surgery in one time
Preoperative DDAVP as it increases the factor VIII significantly
Discontinuation of anti-platelet drugs
Inhibitor level
Intraoperative
Judicious use of regional anaesthesia, intramuscular injections, nasogastric tube insertion, nasal intubation
Judicious use of potential bleeding medication
Coagulation profile for factors VIII and IX
Consider transfusion of factor concentrates if not responding check for inhibitor levels
Recombinant activated factor VII in severe bleeding
Postoperative
Maintain factor level for specified time period as advised by hematologist
Available blood products
Anticipate and treat bleeding episode

Source: Modified and adapted from Essential of Haematology, Ch-9 Charles J. Cote. A practice of anaesthesia for infants and children

responder needs aggressive treatment with porcine factor VIII concentrate, recombinant factor VIIa, or with PCC. Recombinant factor VIIa is administered as a bolus injection and a treatment consists of 90 µg/kg every two hours for three doses. The concurrent administration of tranexamic acid increases clot stability. An alternative therapy is an activated prothrombin complex concentrate. This is a plasma-derived product, and is given at a dose of 50–100 units/kg, maximum daily dose of 200 units/kg. The use of tranexamic acid should be avoided with PCC as it may increase the risk of thromboembolism.

Antifibrinolytic drugs such as tranexamic acid, epsilon amino caproic acid in case of mucosal bleed as an adjunct. These durgs should not be given with PCC as there is potential thrombotic complication may occur. Avoid antifibrinolytics in case of renal bleeding as unlysed clot behave like stones causes ureteric colic and obstructive nephropathy.

Avoid platelet inhibitory drugs such as acetylsalicycilic acid and non-steroidal anti-inflammatory drugs such as acetoaminophan paracetamol can be given safely.

Apart from these measures researchers are going on to treat haemophilia with genetic modifications. Gene therapy, cell therapy and tissue engineering have been recently developed modalities helpful in treating haemophilia. Induced pluripotent stem cells technology is also one of the recently developed techniques in treating haemophilia.

von Willebrand Disease

von Willebrand disease (vWD) is a most common hereditary bleeding disorder where von Willebrand factor (vWF) is defective or deficient. The vWF is essential plasma protein for the initial adherence of platelet to the injured endothelium and it also acts as carrier protein for the clotting factor VIII. The prevalence is 1 in 1000 to 3 in 100,000 of population.

vWF is produced from megakaryocytes and endothelial cells and stored in cellular granules known as Weible-Palade body in the endothelial cells and alpha granules in platelets.

vWD is broadly divided into three type. Type 1 and type 2 are autosomal dominant while 3 is ressecive type

Type 1: This is most common (75%) variant of vWD. It is characterized by decrease quantity of normal vWF. Patients show mild to moderate bleeding.

Type 2: This has qualitative defect in vWF and subdivided into 2A, 2B, 2M, 2N. Each subgroup has different genetic determinants but shows no clinical difference. They usually manifest moderate bleeding.

Type 3: Double heterozygous for vWF antigen is most severe but rare variant. This is characterized by absence of vWF as well as decrease vWD activity and factor VIII.

Clinical picture: Most common manifestation of this disease is mucocutaneous bleeding such as gum bleeding, epistaxis, skin bruise, menorrhagia and gastrointestinal bleeding. They experience excessive bleeding during trauma and surgery. Rare cases require blood transfusion.

Laboratory findings: Apart from routine investigations and cogulation profile, specific tests include vWF antigen assay, factor VIII asssay and ristocetin cofactor assay (it is a functional assay of platelet aggregation in presence of ristocetin). Bleeding time is prolonged. In mild case APTT is normal but in severe cases it is prolonged.

Anaesthetic Consideration

Both the disorders of clotting pathway can be presented with same complaints of repeated brusing and epistaxis but the large haematomas and haemathroses are associated mainly with haemophilia. History of recurrent epistaxis, bruising and postoperative bleeding after surgery especially tonsillectomy in either parents is also helpful in making diagnosis. A careful family history may identify the same symptoms in the parents or a sibling is suggestive of familial disorder. Patient should be optimised before surgery once diagnosis confirmed or in case of emergency surgery keep adequate blood and blood products ready. Patients who are more than 2 years of age, who have vWD and had not received vaccination, should be immunized against hepatitis A and B. Anaesthetic goal is cessation of bleeding or prophylaxis for surgical procedures. Avoid NSAIDs especially aspirin and other platelet inhibitory drugs. Avoid using blood components to control bleeding in the most of the cases of vWD. The DDAVP should be administered 90 minutes before the operation at a dose of 0.3 µg/kg which will increase the vWF and factor VIII to normal (>100 IU/mL). One thing is very important in using DDAVP that fluid restriction should be needed as younger children are prone to develop hyponatremia and seizures. In case of qualitative deficiency of vWF, vWF concentrates and factor VIII concentrates transfusions are required. In the post operative period the minor bleeding can be controlled with antifibrinolytic agent tranexamic acid.

Table 9.10 Anaesthesia consideration in vWD

Preoperative
Haematologist consultation
Determination of actual and desired factor
Discontinue platelet inhibitory drugs
Intraoperative
Judicious use of regional anaesthesia, intramuscular injections, nasogastric tube insertion, nasal intubation. Judicious use of potential bleeding medication
Coagulation profile
Consider transfusion of blood and factor concentrates
Consider use of antifibrinolytic drugs (e-aminocaproic acid, tranexamic acid)
Recombinant activated factor VII in severe bleeding
Postoperative
Factors levels VIII and vWF
Blood and blood products
Appropriate management of bleeding episodes
Watch for thromboembolic phenomenon

Source: Modified and adapted from Essential of Haematology, Ch-9 Charles J. Cote. A practice of anaesthesia for infants and children

DISORDER OF PLATELETS

Platelets are small cells of 1 to 4 mm diameter. The normal platelet count is 150,000–450,000/µL. The lifespan of a platelet is normally 7–10 days. Two-thirds of total platelets are present in the blood and approximately one-third are sequestrated in the spleen at any one time. Therefore, approximately 15,000 to 45,000/µL must be produced every day to maintain steady state. Platelets are important and essential component of hemostasis. Primary hemostasis is achieved by forming the platelet plug. Excessive bleeding may occur, if platelet count is low or platelet function is defective. The clinical manifestations of platelet type bleeding are of skin or mucous membrane bleed. Patechiae, eccymosis, epistaxis, menorrhagia, and gastrointestinal bleeding are common manifestation. Rarely hemarthrosis and deep muscle bleed. Platelet count is low may be because of reduced production or increase consumption.

Platelet membrane provides receptors for the formation of coagulation-complex. These receptors are integrin α/β heteroduplexes, the leucine rich receptor glycoprotein GPIb-IX complex, the G-protein-coupled-receptors (GPCRs) and immunoglobulin. Inherited platelet disorder occurs due to defect in these receptors. Children show early onset of skin and mucous membrane bleeding.

Glanzmann Thrombasthenia

Glanzmann thrombasthenia is the disorder of defective platelet integrin αIIb-β receptor. It is an autosomal recessive disorder characterized by failure of platelets to bind fibrinogen and aggregation. Clinical manifestations are repeated mucocutaneaous bleeding, gastrointestinal bleeding, joint bleeding and intracranial bleeding. Menorrhagia is a severe condition in teenage girls. Surgical procedure may bleed excessively. These patients require platelet transfusion therapy and in severe condition recombinant activated factor VII therapy as supplement to platelet transfusion.[35]

Bernard-Soulier Syndrome

Bernard-Soulier syndrome is also an inherited bleeding disorder of defective GPIb-IX complex platelet receptor. Syndrome is characterized by low platelet count along with deranged qualitative function of platelet and presence of macrothrombocytes. Clinical manifestations are same of skin and mucous membrane bleeding. Platelet transfusion, DDAVP and recombinant activated factor VII have been using as treatment modalities to optimise the patient.

Thrombocytopenia absent radii

Thrombocytopenia absent radii (TAR) is the congenital condition with decrease platelet count. Child is born with hypomegakaryocytic thrombocytopenia and bilateral absence of the radii. The platelet count is as low as 10^4/mL but soon improves with age and become normal after the age of one year. The child may have severe thrombocytopenia if expose to environmental stresses such as a viral infection. Child often has other skeletal abnormalities apart from obvious bilateral absence of and along with these approximately 30% may have associated cardiac anomalies such as tetralogy of fallots and atrial septal defect. Severe anaemia occurs owing to blood loss.

Fanconi Anaemia

It is primarily an autosomal genetic disorder and is characterized by pancytopenia resulting from complete bone marrow failure. There is macrocytosis/megaloblastic anaemia with unusual large red blood cells, neutropenia and thrombocytopenia, subsequently patient may develop acute myelogenous leukemia. The clinical manifestation arises by the age of 7 years with Fanconi anaemia, however, thrombocytopenia has been reported in neonates. Patient is short stature, abnormalities of skin, arm, head, kidney, ear and developmental disabilities. Bone marrow transplant is curative treatment in severe bone marrow failure.

May-Hegglin Anomaly

There is circulating giant platelets and Döhle bodies in white blood cells. Patient has thrombocytopenia with increase risk of bleeding.

Wiskott-Aldrich Syndrome

It is an X-linked disorder characterized by eczema, immunodeficiency and thrombocytopenia. Circulating platelets are small in size. Defect in B and T lymphocytes leads to immune dysregulation. Patient may die in early age from overwhelming infection owing to immune thrombocytopenia or haemolytic anaemia. Patient may die in second decade from lymphoma like illness.

Treatment includes steroid, intravenous immunoglobin or vincristine or plasmapheresis. Splenectomy helpful in thrombocytopenia and bleeding but it increases the risk of opportunistic infection. Bone marrow transplant is effective treatment.

Idiopathic thrombocytopenic purpura (ITP)

This condition is also known as autoimmune thrombocytopenia as it usually occurs after the viral infection or immunisation. It is unrelated to drug ingestion. The diagnosis is made by excluding of other causes of thrombocytopenia. The incidence in children is about 50 cases in 1,000,000. Peak prevalence occurs in children of 2–4 years and approximately 40% patients are below the age of ten years. This is the most common condition present in operative setting owing to acute onset of thrombocytopenia. It is generally self limiting and benign condition. Acute ITP resolves spontaneously within 6–8 weeks, while chronic purpura lasts more than 6 months without specific cause. The neonate born from affected mother need to be observed for a few days as they may be affected by the disease and the platelet count would be dropped as soon as splenic circulation established.

Clinical Manifestation

There are petechiae or purpura over the bony prominences. Bleeding from gum, nostril and menorrhagia are common manifestations. Severely low platelet patients may have intracranial, gastrointestinal and other major organ bleeding. However, the rate of platelet production is high in the bone marrow to balance the rate of destruction. Microangipathic haemolytic anaemia occurs as red blood cell enters microvascular circulation they become distorted due to thrombosis.

Investigation

Low platelet count on complete blood count and may be as low as $<2000/\mu L$. Presence of autoantibodies against the platelets is found on antibody titre. Bone marrow examination is needed in case of difficult diagnosis.

Treatment

Corticosteroid, intravenous immunoglobulin (IVIG), intravenous anti-D rhesus immunoglobulin (IVRhIG) and platelet transfusion are the available treatment modalities. Corticosteroid may be helpful in increasing platelet count. But the long term therapy associated with toxicity which limits its use. The American Society of Haematology (ASH) guideline for treating children is based on platelet count while British Society of Haematology (BSH) is more towards conservative 'wait and watch'.[36] Children who have developed chronic ITP or refractory ITP may put on immunosupresssent or chemotherapeutic agents. Splenectomy must be considered in case of old children and chronic ITP with very low platelet count.

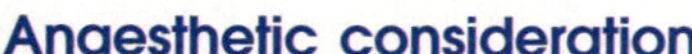

Anaesthetic consideration

Severe ITP with bleeding manifestations should be treated with high dose of parenteral corticosteroids, intravenous immunoglobulin and platelet transfusion. If children develop chronic ITP with very low platelet count (10,000 to 20,000 μ/L), splenectomy provides some protection. Approximately 50% of patients show permanent remission after splenectomy. These children should be vaccinated against capsular organism prior splenectomy and should be given antibiotic coverage postoperatively. In case of emergency surgery or intracranial bleed IVIG and platelet transfusion should be given first. Consider platelet transfusion if counts are below 50,000 μ/L with bleeding manifestations. Transfused platelet may improve ongoing process of hemostasis by participating in the process or there may be some posttransfusion increment and reasonable survival in the platelet. Child born with known ITP mother may have low platelet count but the known incidence is low. The platelet count may continue to fall 7 or more days following delivery, therefore, it is must checking the platelet count every 2 or 3 days until it shows rising trend. The platelet count may be improved in preparation for surgery using a course of intravenous immunoglobulins at a dose of 0.4 mg/kg daily for 5 days, a target platelet count of $80–100×10^9$/L being considered adequate to secure hemostasis at operation.[37] ASH guideline for managing platelet deficiency is given in Table 9.11 and for consideration of splenectomy is shown in Table 9.12.

Table 9.11 ASH guideline for managing platelet deficiency

ASH guideline	
Platelet count > 30,000 asymptomatic or minor purpura	No hospitalisation
Platelet count < 20,000 with significant bleeding	IVIG, anti-D IG or corticosteroid
Platelet count < 10,000 with minor purpura	Corticosteroid, IVIG
Platelet count < 10,000 with severe threatening bleeding	Parental high dose life corticosteroid, IVIG and platelet transfusion

Table 9.12 ASH guideline for considering platelet transfusion for elective splenectomy

Appropriate preoperative therapy	Inappropriate preoperative therapy
• Platelet count < 30,000 need to be given prophylactic IVIG • Platelet count < 10,000 need to be given prophylactic IVIG, parental glucocorticoids, anti-Rh (D)	• Platelet count > 50,000 IVIG, oral glucocorticoid, anti-Rh (D) • Platelet count > 30,000 parental glucocorticoid • Platelet count > 20,000 platelet transfusion

Splenectomy

For elective splenectomy patients ASH has given the guideline as appropriate and inappropriate preoperative therapy.

Disseminated intravascular coagulation (DIC)

Excessive consumption of clotting factor and platelets leads to DIC. It may occur due to gram negative sepsis, abruption placenta or amniotic fluid embolism (Table 9.14). The International Society on Thrombosis and Hemostasis (ISTH) has developed a consensus definition of DIC which is "...an acquired syndrome characterized by the intravascular activation of coagulation with loss of localisation arising from different cause. It can originate from and cause damage to the microvasculature, which if sufficiently severe, can produce organ dysfunction."

DIC is resulted due to hypofibrinogenemia as a process of exaggerated fibrinolysis. Owing to this there

Table 9.13 Anaesthesia consideration in ITP

Preoperative
Haemoglobin, platelet count
History of platelet transfusion
History of corticosteroid medication
History of infection
Presplenectomy antibiotic prophylaxis and immunisation
Haematologist consultation
Discontinuation of platelet inhibitory medications
Intraoperative
Antibiotic coverage
Stress corticosteroid coverage
Pharmacological therapy or platelet transfusion
Physiologic effects of laparoscopy on respiratory and circulatory function
Judicious use of regional anaesthesia, intramuscular injections, nasogastric tube insertion, nasal intubation
Judicious use of potential bleeding medication
Postoperative
Haemoglobin and platelet count
Infection
Steroid coverage
Postoperative analgesia

Source: Modified and adapted from Essential of Haematology, Ch-9 Charles J. Cote. A practice of anaesthesia for infants and children

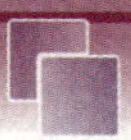

Table 9.14 Causes of DIC

Infection	Septicaemia, e.g. meningococcal Protozoa: malaria
Obstetric causes	Abruption placenta, placenta previa, pre-eclampsia, amniotic fluid embolism, placental laceration
Malignancy	Haematological malignancies
Shock	Trauma, burn
Extracorporeal circulation	Cardiopulmonary bypass
Intravascular haemolysis	ABO incompatible blood transfusion

are fibrin (ogen) degradation products and D-dimer increased in the blood. There is fibrin deposition in the microvasculature, consumption of clotting factors, and endogenous production of thrombin and plasmin. This damage to microvascular circulation leads to vasodilation, loosening of endothelial gap and capillary leak leading to shock. Furthermore, activation of coagulation cascade excessive thrombin formation occurs resulting into widespread microthrombus formation and ischeamic damage to multiple organs. This consumption of clotting factors and platelets has been led to disseminated bleeding.

Table 9.15 Anaesthesia consideration in DIC

Preoperative
Find out the primary cause and treat accordingly
CBC with platelets, coagulation profile including APTT and D-dimer
Preoperative transfusion of factors to achieve the required level
Platelets, FFPs, cryoprecipitate transfusion
Keep adequate blood and blood products ready
Intraoperative
Peripheral wide bore intravenous lines
Planned general anaesthesia with all resuscitative measures
Maintain good haemodynamics by infusing blood and blood products
Maintain adequate urine output, temperature
Inotropic supports if required. If septicaemia is the primary cause, then appropriate antibiotic coverage
Continue mechanical ventilation
Postoperative
Postoperative mechanical ventilation
CBC, platelet count and coagulation profile
Chest X-ray
Appropriate antibiotic

Clinical Manifestation

Child presents with shock, widespread purpura and petechiae.

Laboratory Investigation

Diagnosis is made with clinical picture of the sick child. Biochemical markers such as low platelet count on quantitative analysis of blood for platelets, there would be low level of clotting factors II, V and VIII. D-dimer is also increased (>2 µg/mL). PT and APTT are also prolonged. But no single investigation is reliably diagnoses DIC.

Treatment and Anaesthesia Consideration

As DIC is a secondary disease the primary underlying cause should be treated first. Child may not require replacement therapy. Appropriate and higher antibiotic coverage with transfusion of platelets and other clotting factors are considered for the treatment of DIC. FFP 10–15 mL/kg, cryoprecipitate 5 mL/kg (rich in fibrinogen), factors concentrate and platelets concentrate have been used to treat the ongoing bleeding. Cryoprecipitate 1 U/5 kg will raise the plasma fibrinogen level 50–100 mg/dL and it lasts for four to five days. Antithrombin III is useful to treat DIC in septicaemia. Also protein C concentrate is helpful in DIC in paediatric group but therapeutic support still needed. Prostacyclin may be used in case of known defective platelet activation pathology. Aprotinin may be advocated in case of fibrinolysis. But use of heparin is controversial, however, it has been proved its benefit in amniotic fluid embolism. Use of antifibrinolytics depends on coagulation profile though its use is complicated as it forms permanent fibrin clot, which is certainly not helpful in small renal vessels.

Paediatric Anaesthesia Pearl

More common form of bleeding is due to non-haematological cause and which is surgical bleeding which leads to cardiac arrest and must be anticipated and managed aggressively.

One Fact to Remember

One thing is very important in using DDAVP that fluid restriction should be needed as younger children are prone to develop hyponatremia and seizures.

Take Home Message

Avoid use of Platelet inhibitory drugs such as acetylsalicycilic acid and non-steroidal anti-inflammatory drugs for pain relief. Prefer paracetamol.

KEY POINTS

- Paediatric haematology differs in many aspects from adult haematology. Soon after birth transition of haematological components occurs from foetal to neonate and to infant.
- Foetal haemoglobin is present in highest concentration in the intrauterine life, however, level starts falling from third trimester.
- Soon after birth the rapid transition takes place and the concentration of foetal haemoglobin decreases while adult haemoglobin increases.

Table 9.16 Clinical pearls for all hematological disorders

Preoperative evaluation
History of familial bleeding disorder
History of transfusion
History of medication
History of recurrent infection
History of repeated bruising and epistaxis
Type and pattern of the disease
Clinical manifestation
Anaemia: Pallor, lethargy, weakness
Jaundice: Icterus, discoloration of urine
Splenomegaly: Abdominal pain and lump
Thrombocytopenia: Repeated bruising and epistaxis
Investigations
Routine
CBC, haemoglobin, reticulocyte count, platelet count
Liver function test, coagulation profile
Renal function test
Ultrasonography specific
Clotting factor assay
Echocardiography
Anaesthesia consideration
Preoperative optimisation with prophylactic pharmacological methods and transfusion
Available resources
Pre-splenectomy vaccination and antibiotic prophylaxis
Avoid triggering agents
Avoid hypoxia, hypercarbia, acidosis and shivering
Avoid intramuscular injections: In case of deranged coagulation profile avoid nasal intubation, nasogastric tube insertion, arterial cannulation
Avoid platelet inhibitory drugs: Aspirin, other NSAIDs
Monitoring includes haemodynamics, urine output, central venous pressure, temperature
Estimation of blood loss and appropriate transfusion
Postoperative haemoglobin level and coagulation profile

- After birth the larger part of total haemoglobin concentration is composed of HbA >95%, and lesser is of HbA2 <3.5% and HbF <2.5%
- Foetal haemoglobin has higher affinity towards oxygen, therefore, oxyhaemoglobin curve shifts to left. This property helps to extract oxygen from maternal haemoglobin.
- The haematological disorder manifests commonly early in life and requires early intervention.
- Red blood cell disorders lead to haemolytic anaemia, hyperbilirubinaemia, splenomegaly and cholelithiasis.
- Optimise the hematological indices preoperatively to reduce the risk of increase blood loss and also avoid triggering agents during intraoperative period leading to onset of hemolysis. Maintain near normal hemodynamics, temperature and adequate urine output.
- Red blood cell membrane disorders such as hereditary spherocytosis due to membrane protein deficiency.
- Enzymatic defect such as glucose-6-phosphate dehydrogenase deficiency makes the red blood cells vulnerable to oxidant injury.
- Haemoglobinopathies includes thalassemia and sickle cell anaemia.
- Coagulation cascade involves intrinsic or contact pathway, extrinsic or tissue pathway and common pathway. There are series of activation of clotting factors which coordinate process of haemostasis.
- Haemophilia occurs due to factor VIII or factor IX deficiency and requires factor transfusion to achieve normal level before surgery.
- von Willebrand disease occurs due to deficiency of von Willebrand factor which releases from endothelial cells and platelets.
- Platelet disorder leads to repeated bruising, petechiae, purpura and menorrhagia requires platelet transfusion.
- Disseminated intravascular coagulation is the secondary manifestation of primary aetiology and requires treatment of primary disease. It may require blood and blood components to improve outcome.

SUMMARY

Children with hematological disorders may present with anaemia, jaundice, thrombocytopenia and abdominal pain due to splenomegaly or cholelithiasis. They are vulnerable to bacterial and viral infection as their immunity has been compromised. They had history of repeated infections, multiple transfusions of blood and its components and also history suggestive of familial inheritance. Special care to be given to these patients and pre-anaesthetic check up requires proper evaluation to know the extent of various organs dysfunction due to haematological disorder. Preoperative optimisation of blood components should be done before the procedure. Intraoperative period includes proper planned anaesthetic management depending on the general condition of the patient. Postoperative care includes special attention towards the maintenance of asepsis and the optimisation of factors level required for wound healing.

FAQs with Answers

Q. What are the transfusion criteria for platelet transfusion in case of platelet disorder?

A. BCSH Guideline for platelet transfusion 2003.

The target platelet levels for different procedure and disease are given in Table 9.17.

Q. What is the sequence of preference for transfusion of blood products of different blood group in ABO blood group?

A. BCSH Guideline for ABO Transfusion is given in Table 9.18.

Group O FFP should only be given to patients of group O while group AB FFP can be given to patients of any ABO group.

Q. What do you mean by leucocyte depletion?

A. All components other than granulocytes should be leucocyte depleted that is not more than 5×10^6 leucocytes per unit at the time of preparation.

Q. How much volume can safely be transfused in children and neonates?

A. Consider Table 9.19.

Table 9.18 ABO blood group transfusion guideline

Blood group		RBC	Platelets	FFP
A	First choice	A	A	A/AB
	Second choice	O	O	—
B	First choice	B	B*	B/AB
	Second choice	O	A/O	—
O	First choice	O	O	O
	Second choice	—	A	A/B/AB
AB	First choice	AB	AB*	AB
	Second choice	A/B	A	A
	Third choice	O	—	—

*means group B and AB platelet concentrates may not be available.

Table 9.19 Safe volume transfusion in children and neonate

RBC	
1. Exchange transfusion:	
Term infant	80–100 mL/kg
Preterm infant	100–200 mL/kg
2. Top-up transfusion	10–20 mL/kg
Platelet concentrates	
Child <15 kg	10–20 mL/kg
Child >15 kg	Single apharesis unit/ standard pool
Crayoprecipitate	5–10 mL/kg
Children (15–30 kg)	5 units
Children (>30 kg)	10 units
FFP	10–20 mL/kg

Q. Should one do routinely haemoglobin level for children undergoing planned surgery and what is the haemoglobin level required?

A. One purpose of the routine preoperative measurement of Hb is to detect anaemia which is not clinically apparent. The conventional threshold

Table 9.17 Target platelets level in different procedure and disorder

Lumber puncture, epidural anaesthesia, gastroscopy and biopsy, laparotomy, transbronchial biopsy, liver biopsy	More than 50×10^9/L
Indwelling central venous cannulation, arterial line	More than 50×10^9/L
Brain and eye surgery	More than 100×10^9/L
Bone marrow aspiration and biopsy in severe thrombocytopenia	Can be done without platelet transfusion with adequate surface pressure
Trauma	Aim should be more than 50×10^9/L
DIC	Correct underline pathology and aim to maintain platelet level more than 50×10^9/L

for anaemia below which postponement of surgery or preoperative transfusion might be considered is an Hb level of 10 g/dL. Now, there is evidence to suggest that the risks of surgery do not rise significantly until the Hb level falls below 7 g/dL.

REFERENCES

1. Haberkern CM, Webel NE, Eisses MJ, et al. Essential of hematology. In Cote JC, Lerman J, Todres D (Eds). A practice of anaesthesia for infants and children. 4th edn. Saunders Elsevier, Philadelphia, 2009;177–194.
2. Mortan N, MacKinney A, Kosowe N, et al. Genetics of spherocytosis. American Journal of Human Genetics. 1962;14:170–184.
3. Jensson O, Jonasson JL, Magnusson S. Studies on hereditary spherocytosis in Iceland. Acta Medica Scandinavica 1977;201:187–195.
4. Grace RF, Lux SE. Disorders of The Red Cell Membrane. In Nathan DG, Orkin SH, Ginsburg D, Look AT, Fisher DE, Lux SE, (Eds). Haematology of infancy and childhood, 7th edn. Philadelphia, WB Saunders, Elsevier 2009;659–838.
5. Summerfield GP, Wyatt GP. Human parvovirus infection revealing hereditary spherocytosis. Lancet 1985;2:1070.
6. Bolton-Maggs PHB, Steven RF, Dodd NJ, et al. Guidelines for diagnosis and management of hereditary spherocytosis. British Journal of Hematology 2004;126:455–474.
7. Caprotti R, Franciosi C, Romano F, et al. Combined laparoscopy splenectomy and cholecystectomy for the treatment of hereditary spherocytosis: Is it safe and effective? Surgical Laparoscopy Endoscopy and Percutaneous Techniques. 1999;9:203–206.
8. Sandler A, Winkel G, Kimura K, et al. the role of prophylactic cholecystectomy during splenectomy in children with hereditary spherocytosis. Journal of Paediatric Surgery. 1999;34:1077–1078.
9. Das A, Bansal D, Ahluwalia J, et al. Risk factors for thromboembolism and pulmonary artery hypertension following splenectomy in children with hereditary spherocytosis. Pediatr Blood Cancer 2014 Jan;61(1):29–33.
10. Danielson PD, Shaul DB, Phillips JD, et al. Technical advances in pediatric splenectomy have had a beneficial impact on splenectomy. Journal of Paediatric Surgery 2000; 35:1578–81.
11. Curren TJ, Foley MI, Swanstrom LL, et al. Laparoscopy improves outcomes for pediatric splenectomy. Journal of Paediatric Surgery 1998;33:1498–1500.
12. Glader BE, Wintrobe's clinical hematology. 10th edn. Baltimore: Williams & Wilkins; Glucose-6-phosphate dehydrogenase deficiency and related disorders of hexose monophosphate shunt and glutathione metabolism; 2008; 1176–1190.
13. Luzzatto L, Mehta A, Vulliany T. Glucose-6-phosphate dehydrogenase deficiency. In: Scriver CR, Beaudet AL, Sly WS, et al. (Eds.). The Metabolic and Molecular Basis of Inherited Disease. 8th edn. Columbus: McGraw-Hill; 2001;4517–53.
14. Cappellini MD, Fiorelli G. Glucose-6-phosphate dehydrogenase deficiency. Lancet. 2008;371:64–74.
15. Habibi B, Basty R, Chodez S, Prunat A. Thiopentone related immune haemolytic anaemia and renal failure. Specific involvement of red cell antigen 1. N Engl J Med. 1985; 312:353–5.
16. Petz LD, Garratty G. Immune hemolytic anemias, 2nd edn. Philadelphia: Churchill Livingstone. 2004;261–317. Beutler E. The Molecular biology of enzymes of erythrocyte metabolism. In: Stamatoyannopoulos G, Nienhus AW, Majerus PW, et al. (Eds). The Molecular Basis of Blood Disease. Philadelphia: WB Saunders; 1993.
17. Altikat S, Ciftci M, Buyukokuroglu ME. In vitro effects of some anesthetic drugs on enzymatic activity of human red blood cell glucose-6-phosphate dehydrogenase. Polish J Pharmacol. 2002;54:67–71.
18. Hegedus F, Herb K. Benzocaine-induced methaemoglobinemia. Anesth Prog. 2005;52:136–139.
19. Srikanth MS, Kahlstrom R, Oh KH, et al. Topical benzocaine (hurricaine) induced methaemoglobinemia during endoscopic procedures in gastric bypass patients. Obes Surg. 2005;15:584–590.
20. Sarnaik SA. Thalassemia and related haemoglobinopathies. Indian J Pediatr. 2005 Apr; 72(4):319–24.
21. Sinha S, Black ML, Agarwal S, et al. Profiling β-thalassaemia mutations in India at state and regional levels: Implications for genetic education, screening and counselling programmes. Hugo J 2009 Dec;3(1–4):51–62.
22. Heeney M, Dover GJ. Sickle cell disease. In Nathan DG, Orkin SH, Ginsburg D, et al. (Eds). Hematology of infancy and childhood 7th ed. Philadelphia, WB Saunders, Elsevier. 2009;949–1014.
23. Akinsheye I, Alsultan A, Solovieff N, et al. Fetal haemoglobin in sickle cell anemia Blood. Jul 7, 2011;118(1):19–27.
24. Kotila TR, Fawole OI, Shokunbi WA. Haemoglobin F and clinical severity of sickle cell anemia among Nigerian adults. Afr J Med Sci. 2000 Sept–Dec;29(3–4):229–31.
25. Gumiero AP, Bellomo-Brandão MA, Costa-Pinto EA. Gallstones in children with sickle cell disease followed up at a Brazilian hematology center. Arq Gastroenterol. 2008; 45:313–8.
26. British Journal of Haematology 2004;124:433–53.
27. Bunn HF. Pathogenesis and treatment of sickle cell disease. N Engl J Med 1997;337:762–69.
28. Koshy M, Weiner SJ, Miller ST, et al. Surgery and anaesthesia in sickle cell disease: Cooperative Study of Sickle Cell Disease. Blood. 1995;86:3676-84.
29. Lusher JM. Clinical and laboratory approach to the patient with bleeding. In Nathan DG, Orkin SH, Ginsburg D, (Eds). Hematology of infancy and childhood, 6th edn. Philadelphia, WB Saunders, Elsevier. 2003;1515–26.

30. Ramgren O. A clinical and medico-social study of haemophilia in Sweden. Acta Med Scand 1962; 171:759.
31. Pollman H, Richter H, Ringkamp H, et al. When are children diagnosed as having severe haemophilia and when do they start to bleed? A 10 year single centre PUP study. Eur J Pediatr. 1999;158:S166–S170.
32. Schneider T. Circumcision and 'uncircumcision.' S Afr Med J. 1976;50:556–58.
33. Bray GL, Luban NL. Haemophilia presenting with intracranial hemorrhage. An approach to the infant with intracranial bleeding and coagulopathy. Am J Dis Child 1987; 141:1215–1217.
34. Royal children's hospital, Melbourne. www.rch.org. au.
35. Montgomery RR, Gill JC, Scott JP. Haemophilia and von Willebrand Disease. In Nathan DG, Orkin SH, Ginsburg D, et al. (Eds). Hematology of infancy and childhood, 6th edn. Philadelphia, WB Saunders, Elsevier, 2003;1547–76.
36. Shad AT, Gonzalez CE, Sandler SG. Treatment of immune thrombocytopenic purpura in children: current concepts. Paediatr Drugs. 2005;7(5):325–36.
37. Martlew VJ. Perioperative management of patients with coagulation disorders. Br J Anaesth 2000;84: 446–55.

Essentials of Pharmacology in Infants and Children

Sushama Raghunath Tandale

ABSTRACT

Maturation of anatomical and physiological system distinguishes Paediatric group as a specific population with major pharmacological differences from their older counterparts.

Larger body water content, immaturity of hepatic biotransformation pathway, increase organ blood flow, decrease protein binding and high metabolic rate are the essential findings in paediatric population. The following chapters discuss the ways in which this difference affects response to drug.

INTRODUCTION

When administering anaesthesia to paediatric population it is vital to understand developmental pharmacology in them. There are numerous reasons for altered pharmacokinetics and pharmacodynamics in neonates, infants and children.

Let us understand following terms:

Pharmacokinetics: Describes the absorption, distribution, metabolism and elimination of drugs. Another way of describing it is "the effects of the body on Drugs".[1]

- **Pharmacodynamics:** Describes the effects of drugs on the body.[1]
- **Phase I metabolism:** Biotransformation to render the drugs more polar (to prepare for elimination) by means of oxidation, reduction or hydrolysis.[1]
- **Phase II metabolism:** Biotransformation to render the drug more polar (to prepare for elimination) through conjugation reactions such as glucuronidation, sulfation and Acetylation.[1]
- **Volume of distribution (V_d)**: Volume of distribution denotes the volume of fluid and tissue into which drug appears to distribute with concentration equal to those in plasma.[2] Drugs with a less volume of distribution are mainly present in plasma or they are extensively bound by plasma proteins (e.g. heparin, warfarin). Drugs with a slightly higher volume of distribution are mainly present in extracellularfluid (e.g. muscle relaxants). Drugs with higher volume of distribution have extensive tissue distribution of drug.[1]
- **Half-life**: Half-life of drug is the time taken for half of the drug dose to get eliminated. Shorter the half-life, quicker it is eliminated. When drug concentration is around 5%, it is said to be negligible. Therefore, around 4 or 5 half-life must elapse until drug is eliminated, e.g. if half-life of drug is say 4 hrs and drug strength is 1000 mg, after 4 hrs, 500 mg is left, after 8 hrs 250 mg is left and after 12 hrs 125 mg is left and so on. A prolonged terminal half-life may reflect an increase volume of distribution or reduced clearance or both. Similarly shorter terminal half-life may represent decrease volume of distribution or increased clearance or both.[1]
- **Bioavailability:** Describes the extent and rate of uptake of an active drug into the body. It is expressed as a percentage when compared to intravenous administration of same drug.
- **Clearance**: It is the ability of body to eliminate drug.
  1. ***Hepatic clearance:*** It quantifies the loss of drug during its passage through liver which results due to hepatic metabolism and biliary excretion.

It is determined by following parameters:

a. *Hepatic blood flow:* Which reflects drug delivery to liver. It is decreased in congestive cardiac failure, volume depletion, hypocapnia, circulatory shock, patients on beta blocker, increased abdominal pressure.[3,4]
b. *Plasma protein binding:* Decrease protein binding results in increase free drug concentration which interacts with liver enzymes, thus augments hepatic clearance of drug, e.g. hypoalbunemia, drug displacement by other substance present in blood like bilirubin, free fatty acids, etc. increase protein binding of drug results in decrease hepatic clearance of it.[1]
c. *Intrinsic clearance:* It is the ability of hepatic enzyme to metabolise drug. Variation in liver enzyme activity affects clearance, e.g. liver failure.[1]

Liver is an important organ for drug elimination hence it is vital to know whether drug has high or low hepatic extraction ratio.

Drugs with high extraction ratio (lignocaine, propranolol, ketamine, fentanyl, sufentanyl, morphine, nitroglycerine, verapamil) and intermediate extraction ratio (methohexital, midazolam, alfentanyl) are almost completely removed from liver and their metabolism is limited by hepatic blood flow. A drug with low hepatic extraction ratio (bupivacaine, ropivacaine) elimination of drug depends upon hepatic enzyme activity and is independent of hepatic blood flow.[2]

2. ***Renal clearance:*** It is a function of glomerular filtration, secretion from peritubular capillaries to the nephron and reabsorption from nephron back to peritubular capillaries.

Clearance = glomerular filtration + tubular secretion – tubular reabsorption

Clearance is influenced by plasma concentration and reabsorption of drug by renal tubule. Reabsorption depends upon lipid solubility of drug and concentration gradient in tubular fluid. As water is absorbed from tubule, drug concentration in tubular fluid raises establishing concentration gradient and reabsorption of drug occurs. Drugs which are strong acids exist in urine in ionized form and are poorly absorbed. Drugs which are weak acids, e.g. barbital, which exist in non-ionized form in urine are almost all reabsorbed.[2]

PHARMACOKINETICS IN PAEDIATRIC POPULATION

Absorption

For a drug to exert its pharmacological effect it should bind to a receptor. Availability of drug to receptor site depends on concentration of drug in plasma. Absorption of drug into systemic circulation varies as per the route of administration.

Various routes of administration are as follows:

Oral

More acceptable route in children. The pH and volume of gastric fluid determines the absorption characteristics and hence the bioavailability of drug. Gastric pH reaches to adult value by 6 months to 3 years of age resulting in variable absorption of drug.[2,5] Small, lipid soluble, unionized molecules with favourable dissolution characteristics in gastric juice are better absorbed than larger ionized molecules.[1] An acidic drug such as penicillin, salicylate becomes less ionized as pH is reduced. Premedication with atropine and glycopyrrolate raises the pH of gastric contents.[2] Neonates have less gastric and bile acid secretion with variable gastric emptying. Gastric emptying is further slowed by increase in caloric density following neonatal formula feeds thus delaying the drug absorption.[2,5] Problems with oral route are emesis, degradation due to gastric juices, interference in absorption due to food or other drugs and first pass metabolism.[5]

Intramuscular and Subcutaneous

Absorption depends on lipophilicity of drug, local circulation and site of injection. Drug uptake is less in patients with shock, hypothermia and acidosis due to compromised local circulation.[2,5] Reduced skeletal muscle blood flow due to low arterial blood pressure and less muscular activity may reduce drug absorption in neonates.[5] Infants have dense capillary plexus in skeletal muscle which results in rapid drug uptake.[5] Drugs injected at upper extremity are rapidly absorbed than at lower extremity. Drugs with high pH like midazolam, phenobarbital is associated with tissue necrosis, pain and sterile abscess following intramuscular injection.[2]

Transdermal

Absorption is directly proportional to skin blood flow and indirectly proportional to thickness of stratum corneum.[2,5] Transdermal patch of NTG, clonidine, fentanyl and EMLA cream is available.[2] It provides sustained therapeutic plasma concentration as skin act as a reservoir for drug and also absorption continue for many hours after removal of patch.

Intravenous

Preferred route as it avoids problems with uptake. Onset is rapid and immediate.[1] Bioavailability is 100%. Problems with this route are adsorption of drug to plastic or glass tubing, hence with slow rate of infusion large amount of drug is adhered to tubing which gives incorrect conclusion regarding patients requirement.[2]

Rectal

Preferred route in emesis and upper gastrointestinal pathology. Small surface area of rectal mucosa results in slow and erratic absorption of drug.[2] Uptake depends upon formulation of drug and metabolism by gut wall and intestinal flora.[2,5] Drugs deposited below anorectal line escapes first pass metabolism and circulated to brain and heart before they reach liver results in increase bioavailability of drug.[2,5] Drugs use per rectally are diazepam, thiopentone, methohexitone, paracetamol, midazolam, ketamine and atropine.[2]

Transmucosal

Drugs administered via oral transmucosal or nasal mucosal route bypass the hepatic first pass metabolism.[5] Therefore, they have a higher bioavailability, e.g. bioavailability of nasal midazolam is 57%, whereas of oral midazolam it is 30%. Sublingual NTG, ketamine spray and fentanyl lollypops are the available preparations.

Distribution

Distribution of drug in body depends upon the following factors.

Body Composition

Ageing is associated with decrease in total body water content and increase in fat and muscle content which affects drug deposition in paediatric patient (Table 10.1).

Increase in total body water and extracellular fluid results in higher distribution of water soluble drug.

Table 10.1 Body composition in paediatric age group[3]

Body compartment	Premature infant 1.5 kg	Full term infant 3.5 kg	Adult 70 kg
TBW (% body weight)	83	73	60
ECF (% body weight)	62	44	20
Muscle mass (% body weight)	15	20	50
Fat (% body weight)	3	12	18

Hence neonates may require larger loading dose compared to older children to achieve same effects, e.g. succinyl choline and theophylline. Larger dose may increase the store of drug and prolongs drugs half-life.[2]

Less volume of muscle and fat accounts for less uptake and thus smaller reservoir for fat soluble drug.[3,6]

Plasma Protein Binding

Drugs with reduced plasma protein binding have increased volume of distribution, e.g. ampicillin, theophylline, barbiturate, bupivacaine, lignocaine and diazepam.[2] Free fraction of drug binds to receptor and responsible for pharmacological effect and clearance of drug. Protein bound drug is reservoir that helps in maintaining concentration of free drug in plasma and tissues. Acidic drugs (salicylate) mainly bind to albumin and basic drug (local anesthetics, opioid, and diazepam) binds to $\alpha_1$acid glycoprotein and to lesser extent to globulin and lipoprotein.[2,3,5] Renal disease, liver disease, CCF and malignancies decrease albumin production. Trauma (including surgery), infection, pain increases α_1 acid glycoprotein. Neonates have low serum albumin level (increase to adult level by 5 months of age), their albumin has low binding capacity as well as affinity for drugs and substance found in plasma of neonate like FFA, bilirubin, maternal steroid and sulphonamide decreases protein binding of drugs.[2] It is of particular importance in highly protein bound drugs such as phenytoin, diazepam, bupivacaine, barbiturates, antibiotics and theophylline. α_1 acid glycoprotein levels are low in both neonates and infants.[6]

Cardiac Output and Regional Blood Flow

On intravenous administration initial drug uptake occurs primarily in well perfused tissues like heart, brain, liver, kidney and later in less well perfused tissues like fat and muscle.[2] Therefore, concentration of drug in CNS rises quickly and remains high for long time as brain receives higher cardiac output compared to adult. Due to less fat and muscle drug that depends upon redistribution into them for termination of its action will have longer clinical effect like thiopentone and fentanyl.[2]

Tissue Membrane Permeability

Immature blood–brain barrier in neonate and infant coupled with incomplete myelination results in entry of drug in CNS and prolonged clinical effect with drugs like barbiturate and morphine.[2,3,5]

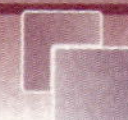

Blood Tissue Partition Coefficient

It depends upon binding of drug in blood and tissue and lipid solubility of drug.[2,3]

Metabolism

Liver is principal site of metabolism and is dependent on hepatic blood flow.[6] Hepatic blood flow is low at birth and increases during infancy.

Enzyme systems involved in drug metabolism matures at different rate. Enzymes of phase I metabolism matures by 6 months of age and some phase II reactions (sulfonation) are mature at birth and some (acetylation, glycination, glucuronidation) are not. All becomes mature by 1 year of age.[2] Both these reactions are decreased in neonates but can be induced by barbiturate.[2] Drugs undergoing phase I metabolism are metabolized by cytochrome p450 system, e.g. CYP3A4 is responsible for metabolism of midazolam, diazepam and paracetamol. Paracetamol is conjugated by both glucuronidation and sulfonation, hence elimination half life is similar in neonates and adult (3.5 hrs).

Excretion

Elimination of drug and its metabolite depends upon GFR, tubular secretion and tubular reabsorption.[3,6] All of them are decreased in neonate and infant. GFR mature to adult level by 1 month and tubular function by 12–18 months as the renal blood flow improves.[2,3,6] Therefore, drugs reliant on glomerular and tubular function for elimination are particularly affected and results in prolonged half life, hence may require reduction in initial dose and increase dosing interval between subsequent doses.

Neonate exhibits delayed excretion due to large volume of distribution, immature renal and hepatic function and altered protein binding. Older children have mature renal and hepatic function with normal adult values for protein, fat and muscle content and high cardiac output to liver and kidney, hence excretion is less affected.[7]

Table 10.2 Pathway for drug metabolism[4]

Reactions	Drug
Phase I reaction	
Oxidation	Thiopental
Aliphatic hydroxylation	Pentazocine, ketamine
Aromatic hydroxylation	Lignocaine, bupivacaine, fentanyl, propranolol
O-dealkylation	Pancuronium, vecuronium
N-dealkylation	Morphine, fentanyl, diazepam, ketamine, atropine
N-oxidation	Morphine
Oxidative deamination	Epinephrine
Desulfuration	Thiopentone
Dehalogenation	Halogenated anesthetics
Ester hydrolysis	Succinyl choline
Phase II reaction	
Glucuronide	Morphine, fentanyl, naloxone
Sulphate	Paracetamol, morphine
Glutathione	Paracetamol

PHARMACODYNAMICS OF INDIVIDUAL DRUGS

Intravenous Induction Agent

Propofol

It belongs to alkyl phenol group and available as emulsion containing soyabean oil, glycerol and egg lecithin,[4] high lipid solubility results in rapid onset of action. Dose required in young children (2.9 mg/kg) is high compared to older child (2.2 mg/kg) and adult (2 mg/kg) due to increase volume of distribution and clearance.[2,4,7] Pharmacokinetic study in children shows 50% greater central volume of distribution and 25% greater clearance than adult for maintenance.[6] It undergoes extensive hepatic and extrahepatic clearance. Side effects are reduction in MAP, SVR and cardiac index with variable change in heart rate.[3,6] Apnoea, suppression of airway reflex, involuntary movement and pain on IV injection.[6] Use of propofol infusion for long term sedation in critically ill child is associated with lactic acidosis, rhabdomyolysis, cardiac and renal failure.[2,4,7]

Thiopentone

It is a sodium salt of barbiturate with high alkalinity (pH of 2.5% solution is >10). High lipid solubility and non-ionized fraction is responsible for maximal uptake in brain in spite of high protein binding.[4] Dose requirement in infant (7 mg/kg) is higher than older children and adult (4–5 mg/kg) due to large volume of distribution.[3,4] In neonate drug requirement is less (3–4 mg/kg) due to decrease protein binding and impaired clearance.[4,7] Large dose increase store in body and cause delay awakening.[5] Termination of action is due to redistribution of drug in muscle and fat.[7] Side effects are decrease in BP, increase in heart rate, depression of ventilation, and decrease in intraocular and intracranial pressure.

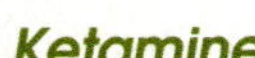

Ketamine

It is a cyclohexidine derivative. It produces dissociative anaesthesia by blocking the afferent impulses in diencephalon and associated pathway of cortex, sparing the reticular formation of brain stem[3] because of its analgesic property it is preferred for procedural sedation. High doses are required for induction in younger patient due to increase in volume of distribution (2–3 mg/kg).[2] Patient loses consciousness in 10 seconds and duration is 10–15 minutes[2] gag and cough reflex is maintained[2] clearance is reduced in neonates and infant due to reduced metabolism and excretion resulting in prolonged recovery.[2,5] It is used for sedation, induction and maintenance of anaesthesia. It is metabolized by liver; norketamine is principal metabolite which has 30% activity of parent compound. Problems are increase secretion, vomiting, dreaming, hallucination. Contraindications are URTI, raised ICT, open globe injury, psychiatric and seizure disorder; preservative free ketamine is used in epidural space because preservative causes neurotoxicity.[3,8]

Inhalational Anaesthetic Agent

Neonates, infants and young children have relatively higher alveolar ventilation and lower FRC compared with older children and adults. This higher minute ventilation to FRC ratio (5 : 1 in infant and 1.4 : 1 in adult) with relatively higher blood flow to VRG (Vessel rich group is 18% of body weight in infant compared to 8% in adult) and decrease in fat and muscle content results in rapid rise in alveolar anesthetic concentration and speeds inhalational induction. Blood gas coefficient is lower in neonates than adults thus allows faster induction. MAC is higher in infants than neonates and adult for halogenated agent except Sevoflurane which has same MAC in neonates and infants.[3,4,6,7] Cardiovascular system of neonates and infants is more sensitive to volatile agents because of not fully developed compensatory mechanism, e.g. vasoconstriction and tachycardia and immature myocardium is sensitive to myocardial depression.[2–4]

Table 10.3 Dose of ketamine[4]

Route of administration	Sedation dose (ml/kg)	Induction dose (ml/kg)
Per oral	6–10	—
Intravascular	0.5–1	2–3
Intramuscular	2–3	6–10
Per rectal	—	10

The MAC for almost all anesthetic agents is less in neonates than in infants. Typically MAC value peak at 1–6 months of age before decreasing to adult values.[3,8]

Sevoflurane

Pleasant smell and blood gas solubility coefficient 0.68 allows rapid induction and recovery, hence preferred in nonpremedicated children.[6] It is cardio stable (less tachycardia, myocardial depression and less sensitization of myocardium to catecholamine), causes dose dependent depression in tidal volume and respiratory rate with minimal airway irritation.[6] Breathholding, coughing, laryngospasm, desaturation during induction is infrequent, epileptiform and slowing of heart rate is reported.[3]

High incidence of excitement during emergence (33%) is noted.[7] It is not related to pain, inversely related to age, frequent in less than 5 years and low incidence with premedication.[7] Possible risk of exothermic reaction with dry dessicant and compound A formation if fresh gas flow is less than one liter.[7]

Isoflurane

It is not preferred for induction in paediatric patient due to irritation of airway and pungent smell. Wash in and wash out is slower due to high solubility in blood and tissue.[3,7] It causes less myocardial depression than halothane with a little change in heart rate. It causes

Table 10.4 Age related estimates of gas and tissue volume and blood flow[3]

Tissue volume	Gas and tissue volume (mL/kg)		Tissue blood flow % cardiac output	
	Adult	Infant	Adult	Infant
Tidal volume	7	7	—	—
FRC	40	20	—	—
Blood volume	70	90	—	—
Viscera	88	175	73	80
Muscle	425	180	11	10
Fat	150	100	6	5
Poorly perfused tissue	270	70	10	5

Table 10.5 MAC in paediatric patient[4]

MAC	Neonate	Infant	Child	Adult
Halothane	0.87	1.1–1.2	0.87	0.75
Sevoflurane	3.3	3.2	2.5	2
Isoflurane	1.6	1.8–1.9	1.3–1.6	1.2
Desflurane	8.9	9–10	7–8	6

greater reduction in $CMRO_2$ which is beneficial in anaesthesia for raised ICT patient.

Halothane

It causes potent myocardial depression. Sensitize the myocardium to catecholamine in presence of hypercapnia or inadequate depth.[3,7]

Desflurane

Its wash in and wash out is extremely fast but still induction is not recommended because triggering of upper airway reflex (50% breath holding and 40% laryngospasm).[3] Maintain cardiovascular homeostasis except for tachycardia.

Neuromuscular Blocking Agent

Immature neuromuscular junction and small reserve of acetylcholine makes neonate three times more sensitive to non-depolarizing muscle relaxant than adult. But this sensitivity is balanced by almost identical increase in volume of distribution so required dose is unaffected.[5,6] They also exhibits prolonged duration of action of neuromuscular blocking agent due to decreased hepatic and renal clearance, hence dose of additional relaxant should be reduced and given less frequently.[5,7]

Depolarizing Muscle Relaxant

Succinyl choline: It is available depolarizing muscle relaxant. It binds to acetyl choline receptor causing membrane ionic channel to open in the same fashion as acetylcholine. Molecule remains bound to receptor for extended period because they are not metabolized by acetyl cholinesterase and their concentration in synaptic cleft do not fall rapidly. This results in prolonged depolarization of muscle end plate.[3,4] With prolonged and repetitive exposure succinyl choline induced block begins to assume characteristics of nondepolarising block.[3] Dose required is high in neonates and infant (2–3 mg/kg IV) than in older children (1–2 mg/kg IV, 2–4 mg IM) and adult (1–1.5 mg/kg IV) [3] and duration is 3–10 minutes.[2,3] Difference in butyryl cholinesterase activity, receptor sensitivity and volume of distribution explains age related difference in succinyl choline requirement.[3] Patient should receive vagolytic doses of atropine prior to its administration. It has potential for rhabdomyolysis, hyperkalemia, masseter spasm and malignant hyperthermia.[4,7]

Non-depolarizing Muscle Relaxant

They act as a competitive antagonist. All non-depolarizing agents produce neuromuscular blockade by competition with acetylcholine for its binding sites on the α_1 subunits of the postsynaptic cholinergic receptor.[4]

Atracurium: It is a muscle relaxant of intermediate duration, metabolized by nonspecific ester and Hofmann degradation[3] onset of block and recovery time is same for all group but in neonate dose is influenced by time and temperature. Neonates less than 48 hours require less dose and duration is long in temperature less than 36°C.[2] Infants exhibits shorter duration of action due to large volume of distribution, rapid clearance and short half-life.[3]

Vecuronium: Sensitivity to Vecuronium is same in neonates, infants and children. Longer duration and prolonged recovery is seen in neonate due to large volume of distribution and delayed clearance.[2] Children recover rapidly than adults. Volume of distribution and mean residence time were greater in infants due to large volume of distribution and fixed clearance which results in prolongation of neuromuscular block.[3] Duration of effect (time from injection to 90% recovery) was longest in infant (73 min), children (35 min) and adult (53 min).[3] Infusion of 2.4 mcg/kg/min is required to maintain 95% of block in children during nitrous and narcotic anaesthesia which is higher than adults (0.9 mcg/kg/min)[3] in patients with renal and hepatic impairment duration is prolonged.[3]

Rocuronium: It is a muscle relaxant of intermediate duration with rapid onset (60–90 seconds). It is similar to Vecuronium but with one-tenth the potency[3] induction. Dose is 1 to 1.5 mg/kg.[2] With IV use of 0.6 mg/kg (increase heart rate by 15 beats), it produces complete neuromuscular block in infants and children at 50 and 80 seconds. In children if increase to 0.8 mg/kg neuromuscular block results in 30 seconds. Recovery is (0.6 mg/kg) twice longer in infant than children[3] thus infant exhibits potentiation of effect.

Opioid

Pharmacokinetics of opioid in younger children[4,8]

1. Increased free drug concentration due to decreased plasma protein binding (low levels of albumin and α_1 acid glycoprotein)
2. Easy entry of drug across brain due to immature blood–brain barrier.
3. Decrease metabolizing and excretory capacity due to immature hepatic and renal function.
4. Increased sensitivity to respiratory centre, hence susceptible to respiratory depression.

Table 10.6 Comparison of non-depolarizing neuromuscular blocking agents

Agent	Onset time (in sec)	Duration of action (in min)	Side effects	Clinical use	Refrigeration Storage
Atracurium	90	30 min or less	Hypotension, transiently, by release of histamine Toxic metabolite called laudanosine, greater accumulation in individuals with renal failure	Widely	Yes
Cisatracurium	90	60–80	Does not cause release of histamine	—	Yes
Vecuronium	60	30–40	Few, may cause prolonged paralysis and promote muscarinic block	Widely	No
Rocuronium	75	45–70	May promote muscarinic block	Widely	No
Pancuronium	90	180 or more	Tachycardia (slight) (no hypotension)	Widely	No

Morphine

It is 30–35% protein bound in adult and 18–22% in neonates. It has high hepatic extraction ratio, hence metabolism is improved with increase in hepatic blood flow.[3,4] It is metabolized by N-demethylation, glucuronidation and sulfonation. Patients with renal impairment are sensitive to its effect due to its decrease metabolism and delayed clearance.[3] Patients with hepatic impairment have prolonged half-life and delayed clearance.[3] Volume of distribution is large in children than adult and clearance increases with age.[6]

Hydromorphone

It is a synthetic derivative of morphine and five times more potent than morphine.[3,9] Pharmacokinetic profile is almost similar in adult and children with elimination half-life of 3–4 hours and duration of action 4–6 hours.[3,9]

Table 10.7 Dose of hydromorphone in infants and children[9]

Route	Dose
Oral	40–80 mcg/kg every 4 hourly
IV Bolus	10–20 mcg/kg every 3–4 hourly
IV Infusion	3–5 mcg/kg/hr
Epidural infusion	1–3 mcg/kg/hr

Codeine

It is a derivative of morphine. Analgesic action is due to morphine which is the metabolite product from demethylation in liver.[2,9] Bioavailability is 60% following oral route. Onset is 20 min and peak at 1–2 hours. Elimination half life is 2.5 to 3 hours. It is administered with paracetamol for moderate painful procedure.[9] Recommended dose is 15 mg/kg of paracetamol with 0.5 mg/kg of codeine.

Fentanyl

It has high hepatic extraction and pulmonary intake. Mean elimination half life, total body clearance, volume of distribution was larger in paediatric age group compared to adults. Clearance is markedly reduced in premature infants and half life was reported as 6–32 hours.[3] In infants and children fentanyl plasma concentration were less than those in adults after similarly administered IV dose.[3] Fentanyl pharmacokinetics after continous infusion for less than 24 hours in critically ill children have shown increase steady state volume of distribution, increase terminal elimination half life and normal clearance.[3] It can be administered by various route like oral, transmucosal, intravenous, intranasal, transdermal. With oral transmucosal route (10–15 mcg/kg), it shows peak plasma concentration at 5–20 minutes with 50% bioavailability. Side effects are PONV, respiratory depression, sedation and itching.[8] Following transdermal route, it takes 18–66 hours to reach peak plasma concentration.

Remifentanil

It has been used for maintenance of anaesthesia intraoperatively in infant and children. It is an ultra-short acting opioid with elimination half-life of 3.4 to 5.7 minutes.[3] Infant exhibits rapid clearance though elimination half life is same in all age group.[3] It gives stable conditions intraoperatively and associated with less incidence of PONV. Analgesic supplementation is required during extubation and recovery due to its

Table 10.8 Continuous IV infusion for infants <4 months (intense monitoring and nursing observation recommended) dose is in mg/kg.[8]

Drug	Bolus dose	Infusion dose
Morphine	0.02–0.05 mg/kg	0.02–0.05 mg/kg/hr
Fentanyl	1–2 mcg/kg	2–4 mcg/kg/hr

Table 10.9 Dose of fentanyl[4]

Route	Dose in mL/kg/hr
Intravenous (analgesia)	1–2 mcg/kg
Intranasal (analgesia)	2 mcg/kg
Intravenous (anaesthesia adjunct)	1–5 mcg/kg
Intravenous (induction)	50–100 mcg/kg
Intravenous (maintenance infusion)	2–4 mcg/kg/hr

ultra-short action.[3] It has been used in dose of 0.25 mcg/kg during general anaesthesia as IV infusion.[3]

NSAIDS

Non-opioid analgesic used to control mild to moderate pain of surgery. They act by blocking prostaglandin synthesis.

Diclofenac

It is recommended in children more than one year in dose of 1 mg/kg 8 hourly via oral route.[3] Single dose of 0.3 mg/kg for intravenous, 0.5 mg/kg for suppositories and 1 mg/kg for oral Diclofenac in children aged 1–12 years are recommended as they yield a similar AUC to 50 mg in adults.[10] It should be avoided in infants less than 6 months, hypovolemia, asthma, deranged renal function, patients with single kidney, peptic ulcer disease, etc.

Paracetamol

It is a weak inhibitor of prostaglandin synthesis. Analgesic action is probably due to activation of descending serotonergic pathway. Oral dose is 10–15 mg/kg 6 hourly.[2,8] Per rectal initial loading dose of 35–40 mg/kg followed by 20 mg/kg with dosing interval of 6 hours for first 24 hours.[2] Maximum dose does not exceed 100 mg/kg in children, 75 mg/kg in neonates and 40 mg/kg in premature infants less than 32 weeks.[2]

Ibuprofen

Dose is 5–10 mg/kg 6 to 8 hourly for 3 days.[2,8] Side effects are antiplatelet activity, gastritis, interstitial nephritis, hepatic toxicity.[8]

Ketorolac

Dose is 0.5 mg/kg 6 hourly IV/IM or 10 mg/kg 6 hourly PO for 3 days.

Local Anaesthetics

Pharmacokinetics of LA in children[2,8]

1. Decrease concentration of serum albumin and α_1 acid glycoprotein in neonate and infant less than 2 months leads to high concentration of free drug, hence prone to toxicity.
2. Infants less than 6 months of age have low levels of plasma cholinesterase.
3. Metabolism of amide group of local anesthetic is slow in newborn and adult value reaches by 3–6 months. Hence continuous infusion of local anaesthetic can lead to toxicity.
4. Infants in comparison with adults have slow elimination, less duration of block and require larger dose to achieve block, hence have a low therapeutic index.
5. Children have a low threshold for seizure.

They are of two types, Ester (tetracaine, chlorprocaine, procaine) and Amide (lignocaine, bupivacaine, ropivacaine).[3] They act by blocking voltage gated sodium channels. Ester compound is metabolized by plasma cholinesterase and amide compound is degraded in liver. Toxicity following local anesthetic administration is of two types. Local toxicity involves spinal cord or peripheral nerve and occurs at site of injection.[3] Systemic toxicity preferentially involves central nervous system and cardiovascular system. It depends upon the dose and rapidity of injection.[3]

Ropivacaine

It is a long acting amide with less cardiac and CNS side effects. It produces less motor blockade.[3] In comparative study of caudal ropivacaine vs bupivacaine quality and duration of post-operative pain relief, motor and sensory effect, time to first micturition were similar.[3] Pharmacokinetics of ropivacaine after caudal block is similar to bupivacaine with regards to onset, time, efficacy, duration and incidence of motor block[3] infants have shorter clearance than children with epidural use of ropivacaine (1.7 mg/kg).[3] It has low hepatic extraction ratio. Ropivacaine duration can be prolonged with neostigmine, clonidine and ketamine.[3]

In practical experience Ropivacaine and Levo bupivacaine used in caudal block is much more safer than bupivacaine.

Lignocaine

Neonates have longer elimination half life (3.2 hrs) compared to adult (1.8 hrs) via epidural route. Free drug concentration of lignocaine is 30–40%.[3] It has a high hepatic extraction ratio.[3] Lignocaine has longer elimination half life and larger volume of distribution in children than adult after caudal anaesthesia.[3] Maximum dose of plain lignocaine is 4 mg/kg and lignocaine

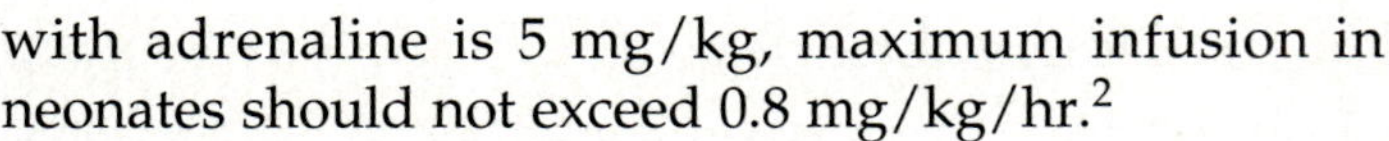

with adrenaline is 5 mg/kg, maximum infusion in neonates should not exceed 0.8 mg/kg/hr.[2]

Bupivacaine

It binds to α_1 acid glycoprotein which is low at birth and increases 3–5 times in first year of life, hence more free drug is found in plasma of neonate than older child.[6] In neonates clearance of bupivacaine is 10 mL/kg/min (adult—3 mL/kg/min), volume of distribution is 4.5 lit/kg (adult—1.2 lit/kg), elimination half life is 7 hours (adult—3 hrs) and also drug can easily cross brain due to immature blood–brain barrier (BBB). Hence they have more potential for toxicity than adult.[6] It has a low hepatic extraction ratio and it is highly protein bound. Free drug concentration for both ropivacaine and bupivacaine is 4–7%.[3] Drug clearance is low at birth but increases throughout life.[3] Infusion in neonates and infants less than 3 months should not exceed 0.2 mg/kg/hr and in infant more than 3 months and older children should not exceed 0.4 mg/kg/hr.[2]

> **Paediatric Anaesthesiology Pearl**
>
> The anaesthesiologist must recognize that there appears to be a plateau effect in dosing epidural local anesthetics. After some quantity of the local anesthetic has been injected, additional local anesthetic does not significantly increase block height.

Benzodiazepine

Diazepam

It is metabolized by hydroxylation and demethylation in liver and both these process are reduced in neonates (more marked in premature neonates), hence they have prolonged half-life.[2] Half-life of diazepam is 75 ± 38 hrs in preterm infants, whereas 18 ± 3 in children.[5] It produces good preoperative sedation with minimal cardiorespiratory side effects.[3,8] Dose is 0.1 to 0.3 mg/kg IV, IM or oral.[3,5,7] Onset is slow and at 30–90 minutes[7,8] t½ 80 hrs[5,7] IV injection is painful.

Midazolam

It is a short acting benzodiazepine. It exhibits pH-dependent ring phenomenon. At pH 4 diazepine rings open which makes drug more water soluble and at physiologic pH ring closes which makes drug more lipid soluble.[3] It has rapid onset of action.[2] It is preferred in paediatric age group due to mild cardiorespiratory depression, less pain on IV injection, short duration of action, decrease in separation anxiety and amnesia.[3] It is highly protein bound with 3–6% free drug concentration.[3] Metabolism is by hydroxylation in liver.[3] Some patients show postoperative problems like fearfulness, nightmare and food rejection seen after premedication with midazolam.[3] Problems with oral route are that it is bitter in taste, hence has to be mixed with flavor concentrate and bioavailability is 30 %, peak serum level is achieved after 45 minute and 85% shows peaceful separation[5] problems with nasal route is irritation of nasal mucosa, loss of volume, peak serum level in 10 minutes and animal study reveals neurotoxicity after topical application. Sublingual is 0.2–0.3 mg/kg as effective as 0.2 mg/kg intranasal (IN), rectal is 0.35 to 1 mg/kg, elimination half life is 2 hours.[7] If we used with narcotics it causes respiratory depression.[7] In neonate half-life is prolonged to 6–12 hrs.[7]

Fluid therapy in perioperative period

Fluid management is different in paediatric and adult patients because of the following reasons.[2,7,9]

I. Water requirement is more in young child due to high metabolic rate.
II. Greater evaporative loss due to high ratio of body surface area to body weight.
III. Thin stratum corneum allows greater evaporative loss especially in premature neonate.
IV. Insensible loss via respiration is greater as they have high minute ventilation.
V. Babies kept under overhead radiant heater often have increase loss of water and energy.
VI. Infants and child with renal insufficiency are not able to produce concentrated urine in presence of hypovolemia.

Fluid requirement is calculated based on the following methods[2,7,9]

1. **Calorie expenditure method:** Holliday Segar demonstrated that water requirement equals the

Table 10.10 Epidural infusion of bupivacaine in infants and children[2]

Age	Drug	Rate (mL/kg/hr)
>2–3 months	Bupivacaine 0.1% with fentanyl 2 mcg/cc	0.2–0.4
<2–3 months	Bupivacaine 0.1% with fentanyl 0.5 mcg/cc	0.1–0.2

Table 10.11 Dose of midazolam[3,4]

Intranasal	0.2–0.3 mg/kg	Onset–10 min
Per oral	0.5 mg/kg	15–30 min
Intramuscular	0.1 to 0.15 mg/kg	10 min
Per rectal	0.4 to 1 mg/kg	10 min
Oral transmucosal	0.2 mg/kg	10 min

total energy expenditure at rest in children. He has proposed the following formula to estimate the water requirement for maintenance. It does not include loss due to fluid deficit in preoperative period, third space loss, blood loss, increase requirement due to hyperthermia, etc.

2. **Body surface area:** This method requires weight and height of the child. It ignores the variations in metabolic rate and thus the fluid requirement and also prone to errors.[2,11]

Fluid requirement in neonates[7]

Newborn has high extracellular fluid volume. In initial few days of life they often excrete excess water hence has decrease fluid requirement for the first week. Volume required in neonate is shown in Table 10.13.

Perioperative fluid in paediatric patients should include replacement for preoperative deficit, ongoing maintenance requirement, surgical blood loss and postoperative requirement.

Preoperative deficit: It includes loss due to starvation in preoperative period, medical conditions like diarrhoea, fever, burns and surgical conditions like intestinal obstruction, intestinal perforation, trauma, etc. Starvation fluid is calculated by multiplying the hours of starvation with maintenance fluid requirement per hour. 50% of volume is replaced with isotonic fluid (isotonic saline or ringer lactate) in first hour and 25% each in the next two hours.[9]

Deficit due to starvation can be minimized by allowing clear liquid two hours prior to surgery. Intake of clear liquid has no effect on residual gastric volume and pH, it decreases the irritability due to thirst and hunger, decreases incidence of hypovolemia at induction and decreases the incidence of postoperative nausea and vomiting.[2,7] Patients with loss due to medical and surgical conditions should be assessed for severity of fluid deficit with the help of clinical parameters, urine output and acid–base status. Such patients needs aggressive resuscitation with crystalloid and if required colloid and blood depending upon the type of deficit in preoperative period.[2]

Table 10.12 Holliday-Segar formula[7]

Body weight	Requirement of maintenance fluid per hour
< 10 kg	4 mL/kg/hr
10–20 kg	40 mL + 2 mL/kg/hr for each kg for > 10 kg
> 20 kg	60 mL + 1 mL/kg/hr for each kg for > 20 kg

Table 10.13 Fluid requirement in neonate[7]

Day of life	Volume required per day
Day 1	70 mL/kg
Day 3	80 mL/kg
Day 5	90 mL/kg
Day 7	120 mL/kg

Intraoperative loss: It includes third space loss, fluid loss through RT aspirate, drains, ongoing maintenance requirement and surgical blood loss.[9]

Third space loss: Refers to transfer of relatively isotonic fluid from extracellular volume space to interstitial space. It should be replaced with isotonic (ringer lactate), non-glucose containing fluid.[9] Replacement of loss depends on severity of surgical trauma.[10]

Fluid loss with gastrointestinal secretions—ileostomy drain output is rich in K^+ and HCO_3, whereas pancreatic secretions are rich in Cl^-, hence replacing such loss with balance salt solution is preferred.[11]

Table 10.14 Estimation of fluid loss in neonates and infant[11]

Signs and symptoms	Mild	Moderate	Severe
Weight loss	3–5%	6–9%	>10%
General condition	Alert, restless	Thirsty, lethargic	Cold, sweaty, limp
Pulse	Normal rate, volume	Rapid, weak	Rapid, feeble
Respiration	Normal	Deep, rapid	Deep, rapid
Anterior fontanelle	Normal	Sunken	Very sunken
Systolic BP	Normal	Normal or low	Low or recordable
Skin turgor	Normal	Decreased	Markedly decreased
Eyes	Normal	Sunken, dry	Grossly sunken
Mucous membrane	Moist	Dry	Very dry
Urine output	Adequate	Less, dark colour	Oliguria, anuria
Capillary refill time	Normal	< 2 seconds	> 3 seconds
Estimated deficit	30–50 mL/kg	60–90 mL/kg	100 mL/kg

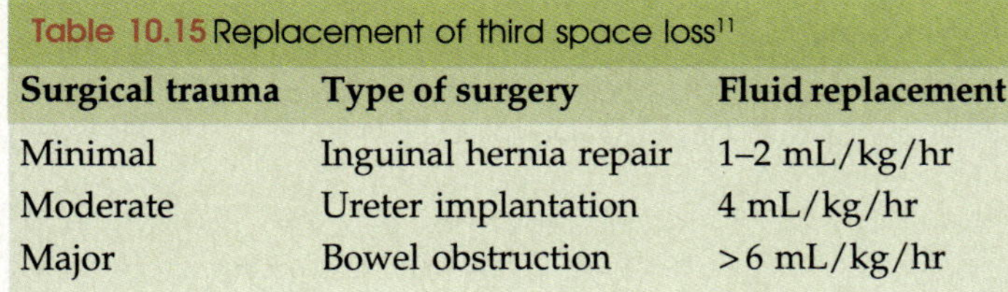

Table 10.15 Replacement of third space loss[11]

Surgical trauma	Type of surgery	Fluid replacement
Minimal	Inguinal hernia repair	1–2 mL/kg/hr
Moderate	Ureter implantation	4 mL/kg/hr
Major	Bowel obstruction	>6 mL/kg/hr

Maintenance requirement: It includes the loss due to evaporation, loss through skin and lungs and loss through stool and urine. Evaporative loss is dependent on gestational age, exposed surface area and ambient temperature and humidity.[11] Infants have greater fluid loss through respiration due to high minute ventilation. They can be minimized by providing humidified gases for ventilation. Skin wrap with plastic drape or cotton should be done to prevent evaporative loss.[2] Requirement of fluid is calculated by Holliday-Segar formula.[11]

Surgical blood loss: Maximal allowable blood loss (MABL) should be calculated for child undergoing surgery. It takes into consideration age, weight and starting haematocrit of child.[7] Target haematocrit is considered 40% in neonates and 30% in older children. It is calculated by following formula.[7]

$$\text{MABL} = \frac{\text{EBV} \times \left(\text{Pre-blood loss haematocrit} - \text{Target haematocrit}\right)}{\text{Pre-blood loss haematocrit}}$$

While replacing MABL, each mL of blood is replaced with 3 mL of crystalloid or 1 mL of colloid.[9,11] If blood loss is less than MABL there is no need for transfusion of PRBCs. If blood loss exceed MABL, Transfusion of blood is indicated.[7] Healthy children usually tolerate anaemia with adequate replacement of intravascular volume deficits. Preterm infants, term newborns, children with cyanotic congenital heart disease or those with respiratory failure in need of high oxygen-carrying capacity may not tolerate anaemia well and require early transfusion.[7] Incidence of apnoea is higher in neonates and preterm infants who have haematocrit values below 30%.

Table 10.16 Estimated blood volume (EBV) in Paediatric patients [7]

Age of child	Blood volume
Preterm neonate	100–120 mL/kg
Full term neonate	90 mL/kg
Infant	80 mL/kg
Child more than 1 year	70 mL/kg

Use of dextrose containing fluid in intraoperative period

Perioperative hypoglycemia is infrequent in healthy children even after prolonged fasting.[2,9,11]

1. Perioperative hyperglycemic stress response
2. Decrease glucose uptake by muscle
3. Ineffective utilization of glucose due to impaired effectiveness of insulin.

Problems with dextrose containing fluid are osmotic diuresis with rapid IV administration, impaired wound healing and increased susceptibility for damage to brain, heart and intestine during ischemic events.[2,9] Hence healthy children do not need glucose intraoperatively.[11] Children who receive clonidine in preoperative period and neuraxial block prior to surgery may not develop intraoperative hyperglycemic stress response, hence they require blood glucose monitoring at regular interval and if required dextrose containing fluid.[9] Use of 1–2% dextrose containing fluid may provide balance between risk of developing hypoglycemia or hyperglycemia during procedure.[11]

Children at risk for hypoglycemia are[2,9]

1. Premature neonate
2. Infant of diabetic mother
3. Sick children with chronic illness
4. Children on total parenteral nutrition
5. Children with inborn error of metabolism
6. Intolerance to oral feed

Such children have high requirement of intraoperative glucose (5–10%) and should be supplemented. It should be supplemented at maintenance rate with avoidance of bolus doses. Blood sugar monitoring should be done at regular interval.

Post-operative period: Tissues often retain excess water due to elevated ADH secondary to surgical trauma, pain, etc.[2] Hence replacement should be done with isotonic fluid and not hypotonic fluids as the latter cause hyponatremia and its clinical effects.

Colloid administration in paediatric patient

Replacement of fluid deficit should begin with crystalloid due to their low cost, lack of effect on coagulation, no risk of anaphylaxis and transmission of infection.[7,12] Bolus of 15–20 mL/kg of ringer lactate or isotonic saline over 15 to 20 minutes helps in maintaining cardiovascular stability.[12] Administration of colloid is indicated after 30–50 mL/kg of crystalloid infusion.[12]

Colloid in clinical use are albumin, hydroxy ethyl starch, gelatin and dextran.

Albumin: Albumin 5% is osmotically equivalent to plasma thus helps in expanding intravascular volume. It has been found harmful in children with traumatic brain injury and with increased intravascular permeability due to worsening of oedema.[12]

Hydroxyethyl starch: It is synthetic colloid derived from polysaccharide.[2,12] Dose should not exceed >20 mL/kg/day.[2] It is relatively safe in neonate and infant for plasma volume replacement.[12] Complications like coagulation abnormality (affects the activity of vWF, factor VIII, platelet), renal dysfunction (renal tubule cell swelling) and pruritus (accumulation in skin) are common with high molecular weight substance.[2,12] Newer generations are available with less side effects and prolonged volume expansion (4–6 hrs).

Gelatin: It is a polypeptide obtained from degradation of bovine collagen.[12] Effects are less on coagulation profile, allergic reaction and renal function following its administration.[2,12] Recent study has revealed risk of necrotizing enterocolitis in preterm infant and worsening of capillary leak in septic newborn with use of gelatin.[12]

Dextran: It is a glucose polymer synthesized by specific bacteria from sucrose.[2,12] Dose should not exceed 20 mL/kg/day.[12] It improves microvascular flow. Problems with use of dextran are interference with cross matching, platelet dysfunction, elevation of blood glucose and anaphylaxis.[2,12]

Take Home Message

1. There are many pharmacokinetic and pharmacodynamic changes occur as a child develops.
2. In general, caution is particularly needed in the premature and term neonate to avoid pharmacological errors.
3. The pharmacological variation amongst neonates and infants emphasize the need to titrate many drugs to effect.
4. Physiological and pathological factors can alter drug handling.
5. Enzyme systems in the developing child are variable and complex. This gives reduced predictability of how a drug will affect a young child.
6. The paediatric patient's ability to clear a drug changes rapidly in the first few months of life; often a child can clear drugs faster than an adult.
7. Anaphylaxis is rare in children. If it seems to be anaphylactic reaction, it probably is. Treat immediately starting with use of adrenaline.

Contd...

Take Home Message *(Contd...)*

8. Do not inject any pharmacological product that you did not draw up and label or have seen being done with your own eyes.
9. Perioperative fluid therapy should include preoperative fluid deficits, intraoperative loss due to surgery, third space loss, evaporative loss and postoperative requirement.
10. Majority of intraoperative loss is replaced with isotonic fluid (ringer lactate, isotonic normal saline).
11. Majority of healthy children do not require dextrose containing fluid in perioperative period. But children at risk of hypoglycemia should receive dextrose containing fluid.
12. Fluid therapy should be monitored by clinical parameters, input–output charting, acid–base status and serum electrolytes.

REFERENCES

1. Calvey TN, Williams NE, et al. (Eds). Principle and practice of pharmacology for anesthetist. 5th edn. USA: Blackwell publishing. 2008.
2. Gregory GA, et al. Pharmacology in Paediatric Anaesthesia. 2nd edn. New York: Churchill Livingstone. 1994.
3. Motoyama EK, Davis PJ, et al. (Eds). Smith's Anaesthesia for infants and children. 7th edn. Philadelphia; Mosby, an imprint of Elsevier. 2005.
4. Morgan GE, Mikhail MS, Murray MJ, et al. (Eds). Clinical Anaesthesiology. 4th edn. New York: McGraw-Hill, Medical Publishing Division; 2006.
5. Jacob R, Krishnan BS, Venkateshan T, et al. Pharmacokinetics and pharmacodynamics of anaesthetic drug in paediatrics. Indian Journal of Anaesthesia 2004;48(5): 340–346.
6. Webber SJ, Barker LN, et al, (Eds). Paediatric anaesthetic pharmacology. British Journal of Anaesthesia. 2003;3(2).
7. Miller RD, Eriksson LI, Fleisher LA, et al, (Eds). Miller's Anaesthesia 7th edn., Churchill Livingstone, an imprint of Elsevier. 2010.
8. Charlotte Bell et al, Zeev N Kain, et al. (Eds). Paediatric Anaesthesia Handbook 2nd edn, Yale university school of medicine, Mosby year book. 1997.
9. Ronald S Litman, Roberta L Hines, et al. (Eds). Pediatric Anesthesia Requisites in Anesthesiology. 1st edn. Elsevier Mosby. 2004.
10. Standing JF, Tibboel D, et al. Diclofenac-Pharmacokinetics, Meta-analysis and Dose recommendation for surgical pain in children aged 1–12 years. Paediatric Anaesthesia 2011. Mar; 21(3):316–24.
11. Suresh N, Rakhi B, et al. Perioperative fluid and electrolyte management in Paediatric patients. Indian Journal of Anaesthesia 2004;48(5):355–64.
12. Virendra AK, et al. Basics of fluid and blood transfusion therapy in Paediatric surgery patients. Indian Journal of Anaesthesia 2012;56(5):454–462.

CPCR in Paediatrics

Minal Harde and Rakesh Bhadade

ABSTRACT

Cardiopulmonary arrest is the most serious emergency in the medical practice and treatment must start without a second's delay. Cardiopulmonary cerebral resuscitation (CPCR) is an attempt to restart the heart and restore the brain functioning after cardiac arrest. Paediatric cardiopulmonary arrest is a unique from adult with respect to causes, pathophysiology and management.

American Heart Association (AHA) Guidelines for Cardiopulmonary Resuscitation (CPR) and Emergency Cardiovascular Care (ECC) completed 50 years of modern CPR in 2010.

This chapter describes essential elements of CPR based on most recent guidelines by AHA, key changes in CPCR guidelines in 2010 and the latest algorithms for paediatric and neonatal resuscitation.

Recognition of arrest and prompt action by the rescuer continue to be priorities for the 2010 AHA Guidelines for CPR and ECC. High quality CPR with monitoring is highly emphasized. Algorithms and the use and timing of drugs have been simplified.

Prevention of cardiac arrest situation is the most important step in paediatrics. Anticipation, extreme vigilance, early recognition, adequate preparation, prompt basic life support (BLS), and rapid paediatric advanced life support (PALS) are essential for survival and best quality of life.

INTRODUCTION

Cardiac arrest (CA) is cessation of cardiac mechanical activity. Paediatric cardiopulmonary arrest is a unique from adult CA as asphyxia is the commonest cause for CA.[1]

Approximately 16,000 children suffer a cardiac arrest each year in America.[2] Incidence in India is unknown. Overall outcome in-hospital resuscitation are better with survival of 27% as compared to an out-of-hospital arrest with survival of only 6%.[1,2] This can be improved by timely bystander CPR.[3,4] Children are more likely to survive in-hospital arrests than adults, and infants have a higher survival rate than children.[4,5]

The essential components of paediatric cardiopulmonary resuscitation (CPR) are:

- Prevention of cardiac arrest situation,
- Recognition of cardiac arrest and early CPR and basic life support (BLS),

Fig. 11.1 Paediatric chain of survival
Source: Part 13—Paediatric Basic Life Support 2010, American Heart Association Guidelines for Cardiopulmonary Resuscitation and Emergency Cardiovascular Care

- Prompt access to the emergency response system
- Paediatric advanced life support (PALS), followed by
- Integrated post-cardiac arrest care.

The above 5 links form the American Heart Association (AHA) Chain of Survival for paediatric patients, the first 3 links of which constitute paediatric BLS (Fig. 11.1).[1]

CAUSES OF PAEDIATRIC CARDIOPULMONARY ARRESTS

Neonates and children have very unique causes of cardiac arrest. Most paediatric cardiac arrests occur in children younger than one year of age and 90% are respiratory arrest. In infants, the leading causes of death are congenital malformations, complications of prematurity, and sudden infant death syndrome (SIDS). In children over 1 year of age, injury is the leading cause of death. In hospital and perioperative causes of CA are unique.

Causes of CA in children can be categorised as follows:[3, 7–11]

- **Respiratory**
  1. Foreign body obstruction
  2. Trauma
  3. Drowning
  4. Poisoning
  5. Bronchial Asthma exacerbation
  6. Infection
     - Supraglottitis
     - Bronchiolitis
     - Pneumonia
- **Circulatory disturbances leading to CA**
  1. Sepsis
  2. Metabolic disorders
  3. Electrolyte distubances
  4. Drug toxicity
  5. Haemorrhage

Sudden cardiac arrest syndrome

In cases of sudden collapse in older paediatric patients and patients with congenital heart disease, a primary cardiac cause should be considered. It can be structural/functional:

1. Cardiomyopathy (Hypertrophic/dilated/restrictive)
2. Coronary artery anomalies
3. Aortic rupture/Marfan syndrome
4. Myocarditis
5. Left ventricular outflow tract obstruction
6. Mitral valve prolapse
7. Coronary artery atherosclerotic disease
8. Arrhythmogenic right ventricular cardiomyopathy
9. Congenital heart disease
10. Primary pulmonary hypertension

Electrical

1. LQTS
2. Wolff-Parkinson-White syndrome
3. Brugada syndrome
4. Catecholaminergic polymorphic ventricular tachycardia
5. Short QT syndrome
6. Complete heart block

- **Perioperative causes of CA**
  1. Cardiovascular depression from the inhaled agents.
  2. Hypovolemia (often from hemorrhage)
  3. Complications of massive transfusion (usually hyperkalemia)
  4. ASA Physical Status 3–5
  5. Procedure related complications
  6. Local anaesthetic agent toxicity
  7. Respiratory events
     - difficult intubation, malpositioned endotracheal tube, inadvertent extubation
     - airway obstruction, laryngospasm, bronchospasm
     - equipment failure
     - cardiac tamponade
     - pneumothorax

Phases

There are four phases of CA: Pre-arrest, no-flow, low flow and post-resuscitation, with distinct pathology and management.[2,11–15]

The pre-arrest phase consists of events leading to CA and prevention is the goal.

- Reduced SIDS with "Back to sleep"
- Implementation of swimming safety norms to reduce drowning.
- Use of child passenger safety seats.

In the pre-hospital and hospital settings, this is achieved by the education of health care providers by early recognition of paediatric pathology leading to CA: respiratory and cardiovascular failure. Identifying patients at risk for cardiopulmonary arrest are as important as providing good CPR. This requires constant clinical evaluation and identification of risk factors. Critically ill patients are often at increased risk for cardiac arrest during airway manipulation, change in therapy, or manipulation of the patient or bed and when doctors and nurses change shifts.[15] Nearly 20% of anaesthesia-related paediatric cardiopulmonary arrests (CPAs) occur during emergence or recovery emphasizing the importance of extreme vigilance.[16]

The no-flow phase represents untreated CA prior to recognition by a lay bystander in the community or a medical provider in the hospital setting. The no-flow phase is longer in out-of hospital paediatric CA as compared to in-hospital CA.

The low-flow phase begins at the initiation of CPR. Chest compressions combined with ventilation provide coronary and cerebral perfusion. High-quality CPR with early ACLS will improve the chances of survival.[12]

The post-resuscitation phase begins with return of spontaneous circulation (ROSC). While ROSC is the initial therapeutic goal in CA and is a measure of the initial success, post-resuscitation care must be focused on reducing neuronal injury.

The Classification of Recommendations (COR) and Level of Evidence (LOE)

The American College of Cardiology Foundation (ACCF), the American Heart Association (AHA), International Liaison Committee on Resuscitation (ILCOR) and AHA Task Force on Practice Guidelines apply COR by developing, updating, and revising practice guidelines for cardiovascular diseases and procedures.[17,18] Writing committees assess the evidence with literature review; weigh the strength of evidence and update, or revise recommendations for clinical practice. Class and level of evidence is mentioned for tests, treatments, or procedures done during paediatric CPR. The Classification of Recommendations (COR) and Level of Evidence (LOE) is summarized in Table 11.1.

GUIDELINES IN PAEDIATRIC CARDIOPULMONARY RESUSCITATION (CPCR)

Cardiopulmonary resuscitation is a series of life-saving actions that improve the chance of survival following cardiac arrest. Recognition of arrest and prompt action by the rescuer continue to be priorities for the 2010 AHA Guidelines for CPR and ECC.

Recommended sequence of CPR has previously been known by the initials "ABC": Airway, Breathing/ventilation, and Chest compressions (or Circulation).

The 2010 AHA Guidelines for CPR and ECC recommend a "CAB" sequence (except for newly born) for the following reasons.

- During CPR, perfusing the heart and brain are the priorities and oxygen delivery is limited by blood flow rather than by arterial oxygen content, hence circulate the blood by starting ECC.
- Compressions can be initiated almost immediately, while positioning the head and attaining a seal for mouth-to-mouth or a bag-mask apparatus for rescue breathing take time and delays the initiation of chest compressions.
- AHA recommends CAB sequence for paediatric resuscitation in order to simplify training and more victims of sudden cardiac arrest will receive bystander CPR. It also offers the advantage of consistency in teaching rescuers, whether their patients are infants, children, or adults. However, for asphyxial cardiac arrest which is more common in infants and children, ventilations are also important in paediatric resuscitation. A recent large paediatric study shows that resuscitation results for asphyxial arrest are better with a combination of ventilations and chest compressions.[4]

Key Note:
The 2010 AHA Guidelines for CPR and ECC recommend a CAB sequence for paediatric resuscitation.

Table 11.1 Applying Classification of Recommendations (COR) and Level of Evidence (LOE)

Level of Evidence	Class I Benefit >>> Risk	Class IIa Benefit >> Risk	Class IIb Benefit ≥ Risk	Class III No Benefit, No Risk
A Data from multiple randomised controlled trials	Useful, effective, should be used	Useful, effective, reasonable to use	Useful, effective, may be considered	May not be useful, may be harmful
B Single or randomised controlled trials Non-randomised controlled trials	Useful, effective, should be used	Useful, effective, reasonable to use	Useful, effective, may be considered	Useful, effective, may be considered
C Only consensus opinion of experts, case studies	Useful, effective, should be used	Useful, effective, reasonable to use	Useful, effective, may be considered	Useful, effective, may be considered

Paediatrics BLS Algorithm (Fig. 11.2)

Activate (AHA) paediatric chain of survival. Safety of rescuer and victim is very important in field situations. If the infant or child is unresponsive and not breathing or only gasping (gasps do not count as breathing), health care providers may take up to 10 seconds to check for a pulse preferably brachial in an infant and carotid or femoral in a child (Class IIa, LOE C). CPR is not harmful but inaction, hence start CPR when in doubt about CA.

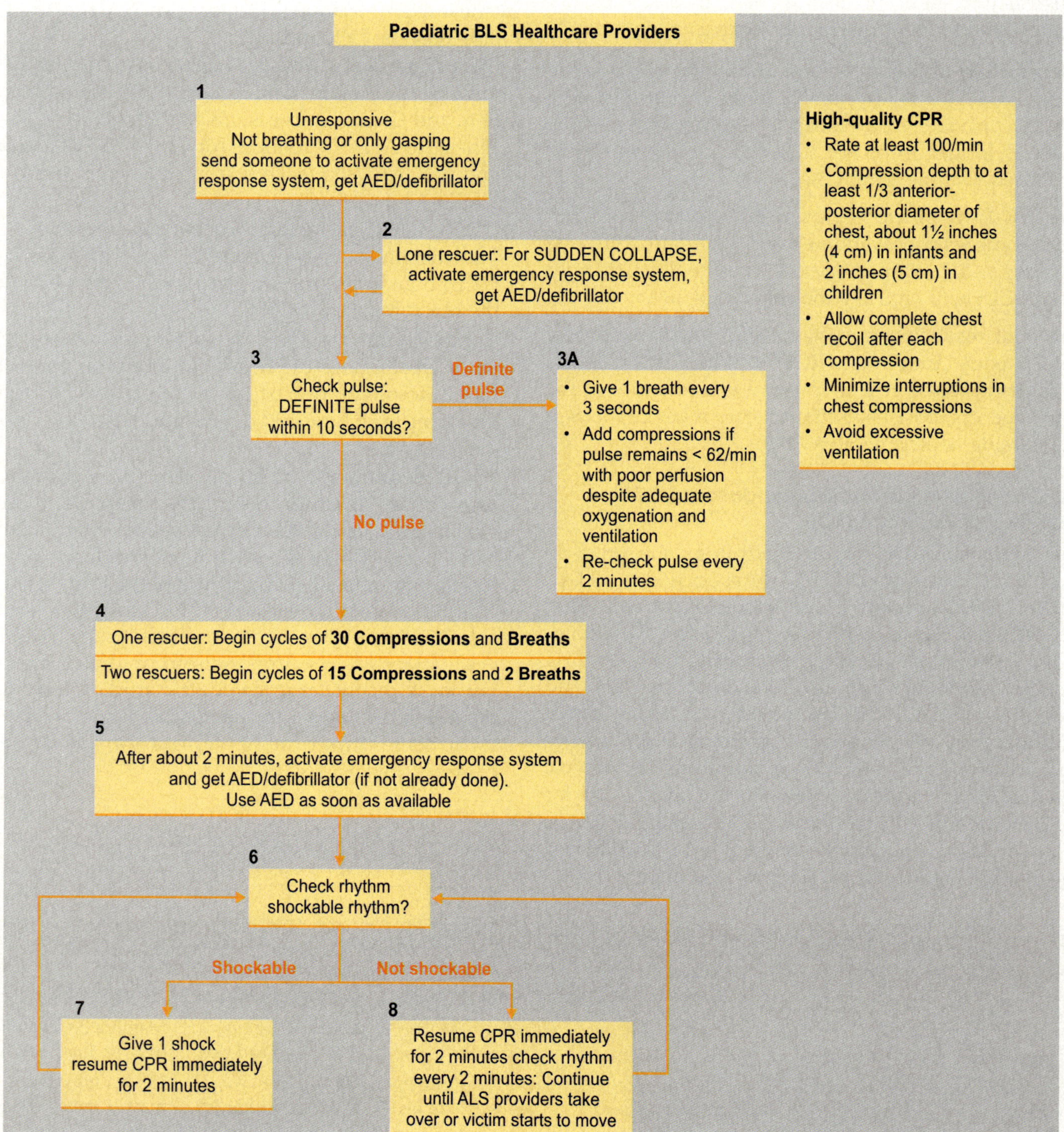

Fig. 11.2 Paediatric BLS Algorithm

Source: Part 13—Paediatric Basic Life Support 2010, American Heart Association Guidelines for Cardiopulmonary Resuscitation and Emergency Cardiovascular Care

Key Notes: Diagnosis of CA and need for CPR

1. Unresponsive
2. Not breathing/gasps
3. No pulse (only health care providers up to 10 seconds)

Chest Compressions

During cardiac arrest, high-quality chest compressions generate blood flow to vital organs and increase the chances of ROSC. Give 30 chest compressions on a firm surface.[1,19] For an infant, compressions can be given by 2 fingers placed just below the intermammary line or the 2-thumb–encircling hands technique (Figs 11.3 and 11.4).

The 2-thumb–encircling hands technique is preferred over the 2-finger technique because it produces higher coronary artery perfusion pressure, results more consistently in appropriate depth or force of compression, and may generate higher systolic and diastolic pressures.[19–21] For a child, compress the lower half of the sternum with the heel of 1 or 2 hands. Do not press on the xiphoid or the ribs.[1,22]

The characteristics of high-quality CPR and the reason for key changes in 2010 guidelines are as follows:

- ***"Push fast"****:* Push at a rate of at least 100 compressions per minute from up to 100/minute.

  "Push hard"*:* Push with sufficient force to depress at least one third the anterior-posterior (AP) diameter of the chest or approximately 1½ inches (4 cm) in infants and 2 inches (5 cm) in children (Class I, LOE C). Chest compressions of appropriate rate and depth are essential for effective CPR.

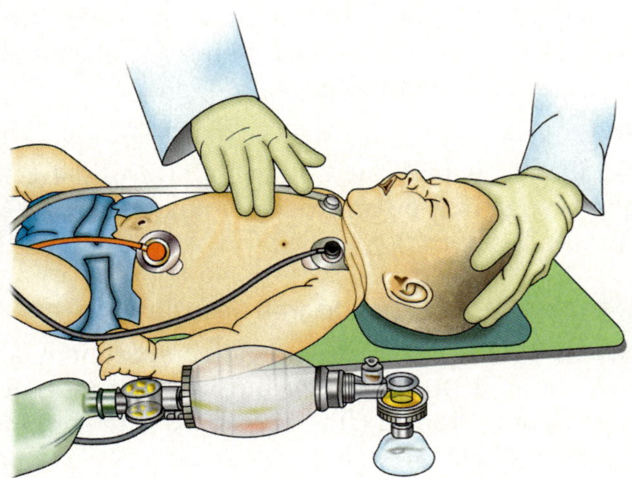

Fig. 11.3 Two finger technique ECM in infant
Source: Part 13—Paediatric Basic Life Support 2010, American Heart Association Guidelines for Cardiopulmonary Resuscitation and Emergency Cardiovascular Care

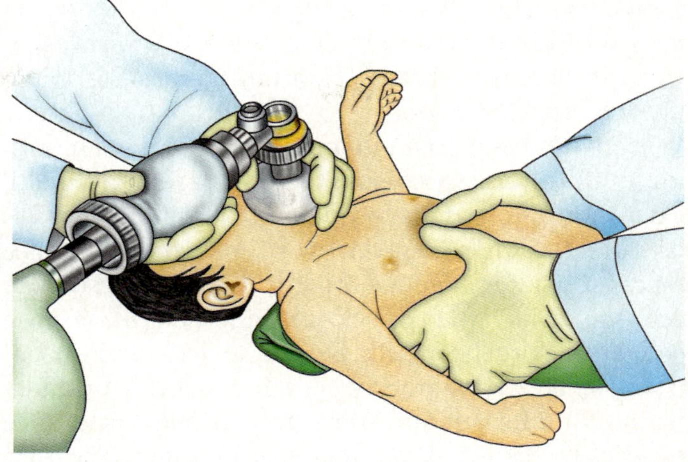

Fig. 11.4 Two thumb-encircling technique ECM in infants and newborns with bag and mask ventilation (2 rescuers)
Source: Part 13—Paediatric Basic Life Support 2010, American Heart Association Guidelines for Cardiopulmonary Resuscitation and Emergency Cardiovascular Care

- ***Maintain compression: Relaxation Ratio: 1:1*** and allow complete chest recoil after each compression to allow the heart to refill with blood, thereby improving blood flow to the vital organs during CPR (Class IIb, LOE B).
- ***Minimize interruptions of chest compressions*** as after interruption when chest compressions are resumed, several chest compressions are needed to restore coronary perfusion pressure. Thus, interruptions of chest compressions prolong the duration of low coronary perfusion pressure and flow.
- ***Avoid excessive ventilation*** as it increases intrathoracic pressure, which impedes venous return, thus reducing cardiac output and cerebral and coronary blood flow (Class III, LOE C).

Rescuers should rotate the compressor role approximately every 2 minutes to prevent compressor fatigue and deterioration in quality and rate of chest compressions.[23] Resuscitation outcomes in infants and children are best if chest compressions are combined with ventilations.

Airway and Breathing

Maintaining a patent airway and providing adequate ventilation is extremely important in paediatric CPR. After the initial set of 30 compressions, open the airway and give 2 breaths. In an unresponsive infant or child, the tongue may obstruct the airway and interfere with ventilations. Look, Listen and Feel for breathing is no longer recommended in 2010 AHA Guidelines for CPR, as precious time is lost in this process. Open the airway using a head tilt-chin lift manoeuvre and use only jaw thrust if there is evidence of trauma suggesting spinal injury (Class I, LOE B).[1]

To give breaths to an infant, use a mouth-to-mouth or mouth-to-nose technique; to give breaths to a child, use a mouth-to mouth technique (Class IIb, LOE C).[1] Each breath should be given over 1 second and observe the chest rise for effective breaths. In mouth-to-mouth technique, pinch the nose closed and in mouth-to-nose technique, close the mouth. Barrier devices can be used, however, they have not reduced the low risk of transmission of infection and some may increase resistance to airflow.[24] Bag-mask ventilation technique can be used by health care providers.

Coordination of Chest Compressions and Breathing is recommended with compression-to-ventilation ratio of 30 : 2 for single rescuers. Deliver ventilations with minimal interruptions in chest compressions (Class IIa, LOE C). Optimal CPR in infants and children includes both compressions and ventilations, but compressions alone are preferable to no CPR. If child returns to spontaneous circulation turn the child to one side (recovery position), which helps maintain a patent airway and decreases risk of aspiration. Optimal CPR in infants and children includes both compressions and ventilations, but compressions alone are preferable to no CPR (Class I LOE B).

High-quality CPR is very important because effective paediatric advanced life support (PALS) depends on good BLS.

Key Notes: High-quality CPR

1. Rate of chest compressions should be at least 100 compressions per minute.
2. "Push fast" and "Push hard"
3. Push at least 4 cm in infants and 5 cm in children.
4. Allow complete chest recoil after each compression.
5. Minimize interruptions in chest compressions.
6. Avoid excessive ventilation.
7. Maintain high-quality CPR.

ELECTRICAL INTERVENTIONS IN CARDIAC ARREST

Defibrillation

The 2010 AHA Guidelines for CPR and ECC recommend rapid defibrillation and Integrated Automated External Defibrillator (AED) in the Chain of Survival in BLS outside hospitals. The term defibrillation (shock success) is defined as termination of VF for at least 5 seconds following the shock.[25] Shock temporarily depolarizes or stuns an irregularly beating heart terminating fatal arrhythmia for at least 5 seconds and allows more coordinated contractile activity to resume. Children with sudden witnessed cardiac arrest are likely to have ventricular fibrillation (VF) or pulseless ventricular tachycardia (VT) and need immediate CPR and rapid defibrillation. VF and pulseless VT are referred to as "shockable rhythms" because they respond to defibrillation. (Class I, LOE B)

Defibrillators

Defibrillators are either manual or automated, with monophasic or biphasic waveforms. AEDs are sophisticated, computerized devices that guides for safe defibrillation by using voice and visual prompts. For infants a manual defibrillator is preferred but if not available AED with a paediatric dose attenuator can be used (Class IIa, LOE C).[26] If neither is available, an AED without a dose attenuator can be used.

Universal steps of AED operation:

- Step 1: Power ON the AED and attach electrode pads
- Step 2: 'Clear' the patient and ANALYSE the rhythm
- Step 3: PRESS the SHOCK button if shock is indicated

Manual defibrillators have adult (8–10 cm) and infant (4–5 cm) hand-held paddles or self-adhesive pads also can be used. Pads should be pressed firmly on the chest so that the gel on the pad completely touches the child's chest. Place manual paddles over the right infraclavicular area and the apex of the heart so the heart is between the two paddles (Figs 11.5A and B).

Energy dose: The recommended first energy dose for defibrillation is biphasic 2 J/kg followed by 4 J/kg, higher energy may be considered but not beyond 10 J/kg (Class IIb, LOE C).

Integration of Defibrillation with Resuscitation

Rescuers should coordinate chest compressions and shock delivery to minimize interruptions in chest compressions. Resume CPR, beginning with compressions, immediately after shock. No pulse check is recommended after defibrillation. Give 2 minutes of uninterrupted CPR and limit interruptions to < 10 seconds; interrupt only during intubation and when you are ready to deliver a shock.

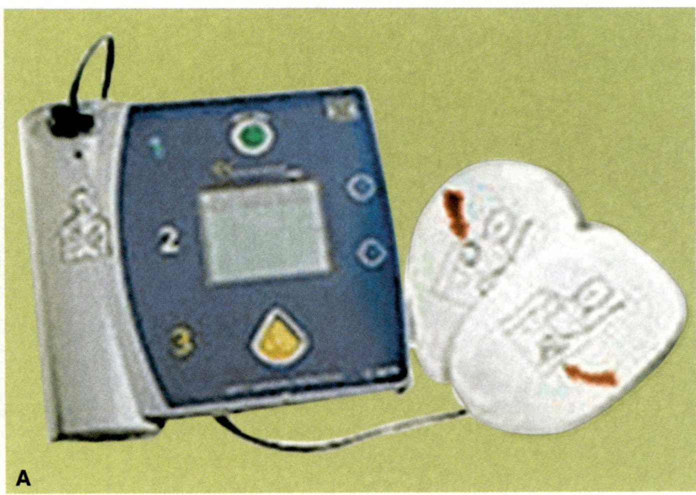

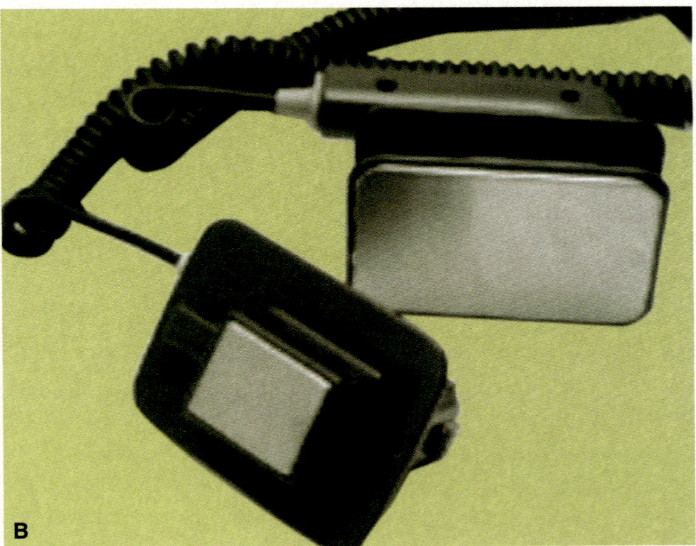

Fig 11.5A and B Defibrillator—(A) AED with adhesive pads (*From NET*) and (B) Pediatric paddles in conventional defibrillator

PAEDIATRIC ADVANCED LIFE SUPPORT

Paediatric advanced life support (PALS) is the organized response in an advanced healthcare environment where coordinated actions are performed simultaneously by a team. Organization of the rescuers into an efficient team for successful resuscitation is important.[27]

Chest compressions should be immediately started by one rescuer, while a second rescuer prepares to start ventilations with a bag and mask and other rescuers should obtain a monitor defibrillator, establish vascular access and calculate and prepare the anticipated medications. Ventilation is extremely important in paediatrics because of the large percentage of asphyxial arrests in which best results are obtained by a combination of chest compressions and ventilations.[4] Ventilations are sometimes delayed because equipment (bag, mask, oxygen and airway) must be mobilized. Therefore, start CPR with chest compressions immediately, while a second rescuer prepares to provide ventilations (Class I, LOE C). The effectiveness of PALS is dependent on high-quality CPR (Fig. 11.6).

Airway

After doing triple manoeuvre to open the airway, oropharyngeal and nasopharyngeal airways help maintain an open airway by displacing the tongue or soft palate from the pharyngeal air passages. Bag-mask ventilation should be done with a correct mask size, maintaining an open airway, providing a tight seal between mask and face (Class IIb, LOE C). Supraglottic devices like Laryngeal Mask Airway (LMA) can be used (Class IIa, LOE C).[28]

Use only the force and tidal volume needed to just make the chest rise visibly, avoid delivering excessive ventilation. Excessive ventilation during cardiac arrest increases intrathoracic pressure, which impedes venous return, thus reducing cardiac output and cerebral and coronary blood flow. It also increases the risk of stomach inflation, regurgitation and aspiration. Gastric inflation may interfere with effective ventilation and cause regurgitation, aspiration of stomach contents, and further ventilatory compromise.[29] These can be decreased by avoiding excessive peak inspiratory pressures, applying cricoid pressure or passing a nasogastric or orogastric tube to relieve gastric inflation (Class IIa, LOE B). Cricoid pressure is not routinely recommended as interferes with ventilation or the speed or ease of intubation.[29]

Endotracheal Intubation

Endotracheal intubation is the gold standard. Both cuffed and uncuffed endotracheal tubes (ETT) are acceptable for intubating infants and children but 2010 AHA Guidelines for CPR and ECC emphasize for use of appropriately sized cuffed ETT.[30] Verification of tube placement should be done by direct visualisation, clinical signs or the presence of water vapour in the tube and confirmed by End-Tidal CO_2 ($PETCO_2$) (Class I, LOE B).[31] During cardiac arrest, if exhaled CO_2 is not detected, confirm tube position with direct laryngoscopy because the absence of CO_2 may reflect very low pulmonary blood flow rather than tube misplacement.

After intubation, secure the tube and ventilate with an inspiratory time of approximately 1 second and at a

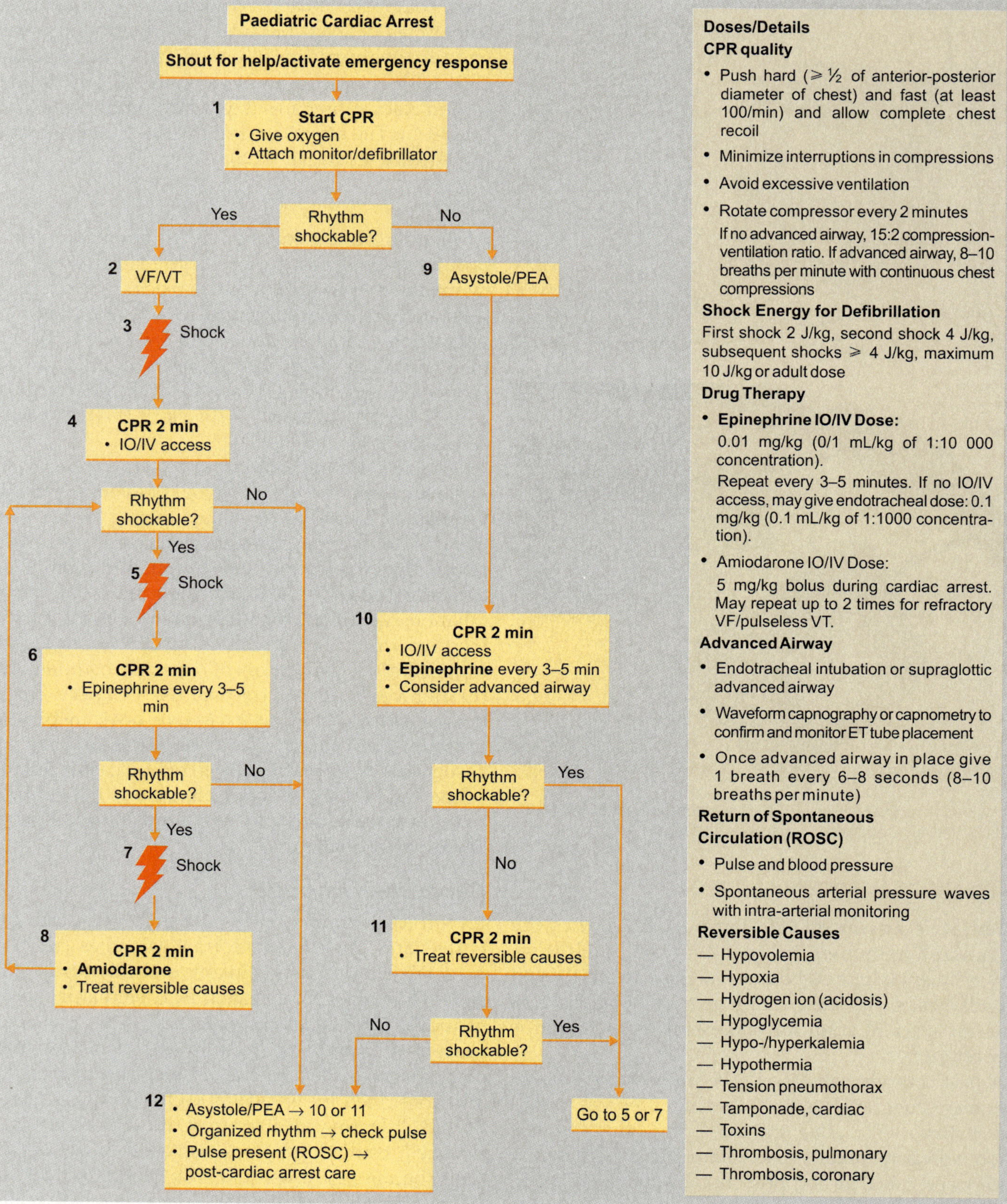

Fig. 11.6 Paediatric advanced life support (PALS) algorithm
Source: Part 14—Paediatric Advanced Life Support 2010, American Heart Association Guidelines for Cardiopulmonary Resuscitation and Emergency Cardiovascular Care

rate of about 8 to 10 per minute without interrupting chest compressions (Class I, LOE C).

Oxygen

Ventilate with 100% oxygen during CPR once ROSC is achieved; adjust the FiO_2 to the minimum concentration needed to achieve arterial oxyhemoglobin saturation at least 94%, with the goal of avoiding hyperoxia while ensuring adequate oxygen delivery (Class IIb, LOE C).[27]

VASCULAR ACCESS

Vascular access is essential for administering medications and fluids. Peripheral venous access is preferred but can be difficult in children during an emergency.

Venous Access: Peripheral IV access is acceptable and can be placed rapidly, but placement may be difficult in a critically ill child. A central venous catheter (CVC) placement is time consuming and requires training and experience. If both central and peripheral accesses are available, administering medications like sympathomimetics and antiarrythmics are preferred through CVC.[32]

Intraosseous (IO) access can be quickly established with minimal complications. IO access is a rapid, safe, effective, and acceptable route for vascular access in children (Class I, LOE C). Proximal tibia is the preferred site in children as it has a broad flat surface and the cortex, abundant marrow content and is easy to penetrate. Insertion site is the anteromedial surface of the tibia, 1–3 cms below the tibial tuberosity (Fig. 11.7).

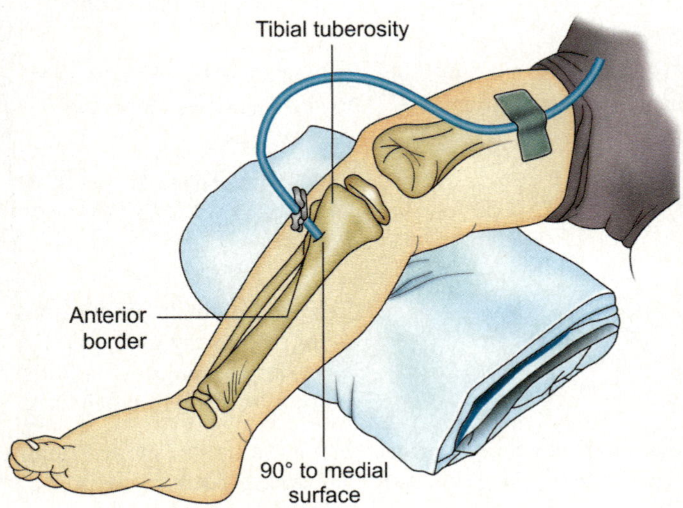

Fig. 11.7 Interosseous
Source: Critical Care Medicine Paediatric and Neonatal Intensive Care (Sec.-5;Ch-73-net)

All intravenous medications can be administered intraosseously and drug doses and fluid rates are the same as for intravenous route. Onset of action and drug levels for most drugs are comparable to venous administration.[32, 33] Each medication should be flushed with a saline bolus for prompt entry into the central circulation.

Endotracheal Drug Administration

The preferred method for drug delivery during CPR are IO or IV, but if it is not possible, lipid-soluble drugs, such as lidocaine, epinephrine, atropine, and naloxone can be administered via an endotracheal tube. After administering the drug through endotracheal tube flush 5 mL of normal saline and 5 consecutive positive-pressure ventilations. Exact endotracheal doses of medications are unknown. Recommended doses are double or triple the dose of lidocaine, atropine or naloxone. For epinephrine, a dose ten times the intravenous dose (0.1 mg/kg or 0.1 mL/kg of 1 : 1000 concentration) is recommended.

> **Key Note:**
> Drugs can be administered by endotracheal route are: **A**tropine, **l**idocaine, **o**xygen, **n**aloxone, and **e**pinephrine (mnemonic "ALONE").

PHARMACOLOGY OF RESUSCITATION (Table 11.2)

In the 2010 AHA Guidelines for CPR and ECC, the use and timing of drugs have been simplified and the following changes are made.

- Atropine is not recommended for routine use in the management of PEA/asystole.
- High-dose epinephrine is not routinely recommended.
- Adenosine is the drug of choice for supraventricular tachycardia and for management of stable undifferentiated regular monomorphic wide-complex tachycardia.
- Calcium, sodabicarbonate, magnesium are not indicated unless specific indications.

MONITORING

Electrocardiography

Continuous monitoring of cardiac rhythm is necessary for diagnosis of abnormal rhythm as well as to follow response to treatment and changes in clinical condition.[48]

Table 11.2 Pharmacology of CPR

Drug	Dose/Route	Action	Comments
Adenosine	0.1 mg/kg (maximum 6 mg) IV or IO followed by a rapid saline flush can be repeated as 0.2 mg/kg (maximum 12 mg). It should be preferably administered through the central line with continuous ECG monitoring.	Adenosine causes a temporary atrioventricular (AV) nodal conduction block and interrupts reentry circuits that involve the AV node. Pharmacologic cardioversion[34,35]	Adenosine is the drug of choice for supraventricular tachycardia. In 2010 AHA Guidelines recommended for management of stable undifferentiated regular monomorphic wide-complex tachycardia
Amiodarone[36, 37] (Class IIb, LOE C)	5 mg/kg IV/IO can be repeated twice up to 15 mg/kg with continuous monitoring of ECG and blood pressure. Maximum single dose 300 mg	Amiodarone slows AV conduction, prolongs the AV refractory period and QT interval, and slows ventricular conduction (widens the QRS).	It can be given IV push during cardiac arrest but slowly with perfusing rhythm. Caution when administering with other drugs that prolong QT
Atropine	0.02 mg/kg IV/IO, small doses of atropine <0.1 mg can produce paradoxical bradycardia because of its central effect. Maximum single dose is 0.5 mg	Parasympatholytic drug that accelerates sinus or atrial pacemakers and increases the speed of AV conduction	*In 2010 AHA guidelines* atropine not recommended for management of PEA/asystole. Indicated only in bradyarrythmia. Higher doses in organophosphate poisoning.[27]
Calcium chloride (Class III, LOE B)	Calcium chloride (10%) 20 mg/kg IV/IO Calcium gluconate 100 mg/kg over 5–10 minutes	Calcium chloride may be preferred because it results in a greater increase in ionized calcium but is more irritating to the vein	Indicated only in hypocalcemia, calcium channel blocker overdose, hypermagnesemia, or hyperkalemia.[38,39]
Epinephrine (Class I, LOE B)	0.01 mg/kg (0.1 ml/kg 1:10,000) IV/IO 0.1 mg/kg (0.1 mL/kg 1:1000) through endotrachael route and can be repeated every 3–5 minutes.	The α adrenergic-mediated vasoconstriction. Increases aortic diastolic pressure and coronary perfusion pressure. Redistribution of blood flow to vital organs.	High-dose epinephrine is recommended only for beta blocker overdose.[27,40,41] Do not administer catecholamines and sodium bicarbonate simultaneously
Glucose (Class I, LOE C)	(D25W) administered as 0.5–1 g/kg IV/IO (2–4 mL/kg)	Infants have a high glucose requirement and low glycogen stores, hence hypoglycaemia may develop when energy requirements increase.	Blood glucose concentration should be checked during the resuscitation and hypoglycemia to be treated promptly.[27,42]
Lidocaine	1 mg/kg IV/IO bolus, followed by infusion of 20–50 mcg/kg/minute.	Lidocaine decreases automatically and suppresses ventricular arrhythmias.[36,37]	It can be used in VF refractory to shocks and epinephrine
Magnesium sulfate	25–50 mg/kg IV/IO over 10–20 minutes can be administered rapidly in torsades de pointes and maximum single dose is 2 gm		Indicated in documented hypomagnesemia or for torsades de pointes.[43]
Naloxone	0.1 mg/kg		Indicated in the infant for reversal of respiratory depression, secondary to maternal opioids, given four hrs before delivery.
Procainamide	15 mg/kg IV/IO slowly with continuous monitoring of ECG and blood pressure.	Procainamide prolongs the refractory period of the atria and ventricles and depresses conduction velocity.	There is a limited clinical data on using procainamide in infants and children.[44]

Contd...

Table 11.2 Pharmacology of CPR *(Contd...)*

Drug	Dose/Route	Action	Comments
Sodium Bicarbonate (Class III, LOE B)	1 mEq/kg per dose IV/IO slowly after adequate ventilation.	To be administered with caution as may cause hypokalemia, hypocalcemia, hypernatremia, and hyper-osmolality; decrease the VF thresh-ld and impair cardiac function.	Indicated for treatment of hyperkalemic cardiac arrest, documented acidosis.[45]
Vasopressin	Vasopressin: 0.4 U/kg Terlipressin: 10–20 U/kg	Effective as a rescue therapy in refractory prolonged cardiac arrest when standard treatment fails.[46,47]	There is insufficient evidence for or against the routine use of vasopressin during paediatric CPR

Echocardiography may be considered to identify patients with potentially treatable causes of the arrest, particularly pericardial tamponade and inadequate ventricular filling (Class IIb, LOE C).[49,50] Minimize interruption of CPR while performing echocardiography.

End-Tidal CO_2 ($PETCO_2$)

The 2010 AHA Guidelines for CPR recommend monitoring quality CPR by continuous capnography for effectiveness of chest compressions. For high quality CPR maintain $PETCO_2$ consistently above 10–15 mmHg. (Class IIa,LOE C). There is a strong correlation between $PETCO_2$ and interventions that increase cardiac output during CPR or shock.[27,51] $PETCO_2$ must be interpreted with caution for 1 to 2 minutes after administration of epinephrine or other vasoconstrictive medications because these medications may decrease the end-tidal CO_2 level by reducing pulmonary blood flow. An abrupt and sustained rise in $PETCO_2$ is observed just prior to clinical identification of ROSC.[52]

Whenever feasible, monitoring of arterial pressure during the relaxation phase of chest compressions or central venous oxygen saturation ($ScvO_2$) are recommended.

ARREST RHYTHMS

The arrest pulse less rhythm is either "shockable" (e.g. VF or rapid VT) or "not shockable" (e.g. asystole or PEA). It may be necessary to momentarily interrupt chest compressions to determine the child's rhythm. Asystole and bradycardia with a wide QRS are most common in asphyxial arrest. VF is commomner in older children with sudden arrest.[1,27]

"Nonshockable Rhythm": Asystole/PEA

PEA is an organized electric activity slow, wide QRS complex without palpable pulse. This rhythm may be more reversible than asystole.

For asystole and PEA throughout resuscitation, emphasis should be on provision of high-quality CPR. During CPR administer epinephrine, 0.01 mg/kg (0.1 mL/kg of 1 : 10 000 solution) maximum of 1 mg (10 mL) repeated every 3 to 5 minutes. Check rhythm every 2 min with minimal interruptions in chest compressions.

If at any time the rhythm becomes "shockable," give a shock and resume chest compressions. If the rhythm is "nonshockable" continue with cycles of CPR and epinephrine administration until there is evidence of ROSC or termination of the effort. At this time treat the cause and not only the condition. Search for and treat reversible causes of CA which can be summerised as 6 Hs and 6 Ts (Table 11.3).

In case of bradycardia unresponsive to standard CPR and if associated with congenital or acquired heart disease, emergency transcutaneous pacing may be lifesaving (Class IIb, LOE C).[27]

"Shockable Rhythm" VF or Rapid Pulseless VT

Provide high quality CPR until the defibrillator is ready to deliver a shock; after shock delivery (2 J/kg), immediately resume CPR for 2 minutes, beginning with chest compressions. Minimize interruptions of chest compressions as defibrillation is successful after a period of effective chest compressions.[51] CPR may provide coronary perfusion, increasing the likelihood of defibrillation with a subsequent shock. If a "shockable" rhythm persists, give another shock (4 J/kg) and continue CPR, give epinephrine 0.01 mg/kg every 3 to 5 minutes.

Table 11.3 Differential diagnosis of cardiac arrest–6Hs and 6Ts

Hypoxia	Tablets (drug overdose)
Hypovolemia	Tamponade (cardiac)
Hydrogen ion (acidosis)	Tension pneumothorax
Hyperkalemia/Hypokalemia	Thrombosis-heart (AMI)
Hypothermia	Thrombosis-lungs (pulmonary embolus)
Hypoglycemia	Trauma

Check rhythm every 2 minutes with minimal interruptions in chest compressions. Outcome of shock delivery is best if the time between last compression and shock delivery is minimized.

During prolong VF, the myocardium is depleted of oxygen and other metabolic substrates. Chest compressions can deliver oxygen and energy substrates, increasing the chances of shock success and thus terminating VF and a perfusing rhythm may return.[53]

There is no upper limit to the number of shocks you can give as shockable rhythms have better prognosis and as long as the myocardium has energy to produce VF, it has energy to revert to normal sinus rhythm. However, high quality CPR to be maintained and rhythm appropriate medications as discussed in PALS to be administered. If the rhythm turns "nonshockable" continue with cycles of CPR and epinephrine administration until there is evidence of ROSC or termination of the efforts to declare death.

Extracorporeal Life Support (ECLS)

Extracorporeal life support (ECLS) is a modified form of cardiopulmonary bypass used to provide prolonged delivery of oxygen to tissues. ECLS should be considered for cardiac arrest occurring in ICU and which are refractory to standard resuscitation attempts, with a potentially reversible cause of arrest (Class IIa, LOE C). The expertise and equipment availability is limiting factor.[54]

With underlying cardiac disease, long-term survival when ECLS is initiated in a critical-care setting has been reported even after 50 minutes of standard CPR.

RECENT GUIDELINES IN NEONATAL RESUSCITATION (Fig. 11.8)

CPR recommendations are different for infants and for the newly born.[55–57] The aetiology of neonatal arrests is nearly always asphyxia, hence the A-B-C sequence has been retained for resuscitation. Resuscitation guidelines have been modified and C-A-B sequence is recommended for neonates with congenital heart disease, with single-ventricle anatomy, Fontan or hemi-Fontan/bidirectional Glenn physiology and pulmonary hypertension.[55]

Assessment of the foetus at birth using the Apgar score is a simple, useful guide to neonatal well-being and resuscitation. It is evaluated at 1 and 5 minutes[15,56] (Table 11.4) .

"The Golden Minute" The first minute is very important during which the following steps should be completed.

- Rapid evaluation
- Assessment of Apgar score
- The initial steps of resuscitation:
  1. To provide warmth by covering the baby in plastic wrapping (Class I, LOE A) or placing under a radiant heat source
  2. Positioning the head in a "sniffing" position to open the airway
  3. Clearing the airway, if necessary, however the role of peripartum suctioning has been deemphasized in active babies even in the presence of meconium
  4. Drying the baby and stimulating breathing

Oxygen saturations (SpO_2) monitoring is recommended when resuscitation is anticipated, with the probe attached to the right upper extremity. It guides for any need of supplementary oxygen, when cyanosis is persistent and when assisted ventilation is needed (Class I, LOE B).

For babies born at term, it is recommended to begin resuscitation with room air as hyperoxia can be toxic. If oxygen administered should be blended with air and SpO_2 monitored to guide titration of the blend delivered.[55]

Table 11.4 Relation of age, height, and weight to body surface area (BSA)

Sign	Score*		
	0	1	2
Heart rate	Absent	Less than 100/min	More than 100/min
Respiratory effort	Absent	Slow, irregular	Good, crying
Color	Blue, pale	Body pink, extremities blue (acrocyanosis)	Completely pink
Reflex irritability (response to insertion of a nasal catheter)	Absent	Grimace	Cough, sneeze
Muscle tone	Limp	Some flexion of extremities	Active motion

*Each variable is evaluated individually and scored from 0 to 2 in an infant at 1 and 5 minutes of age. The total score at each time is the sum of the scores of the individual variables. A total score of 10 is perfect.

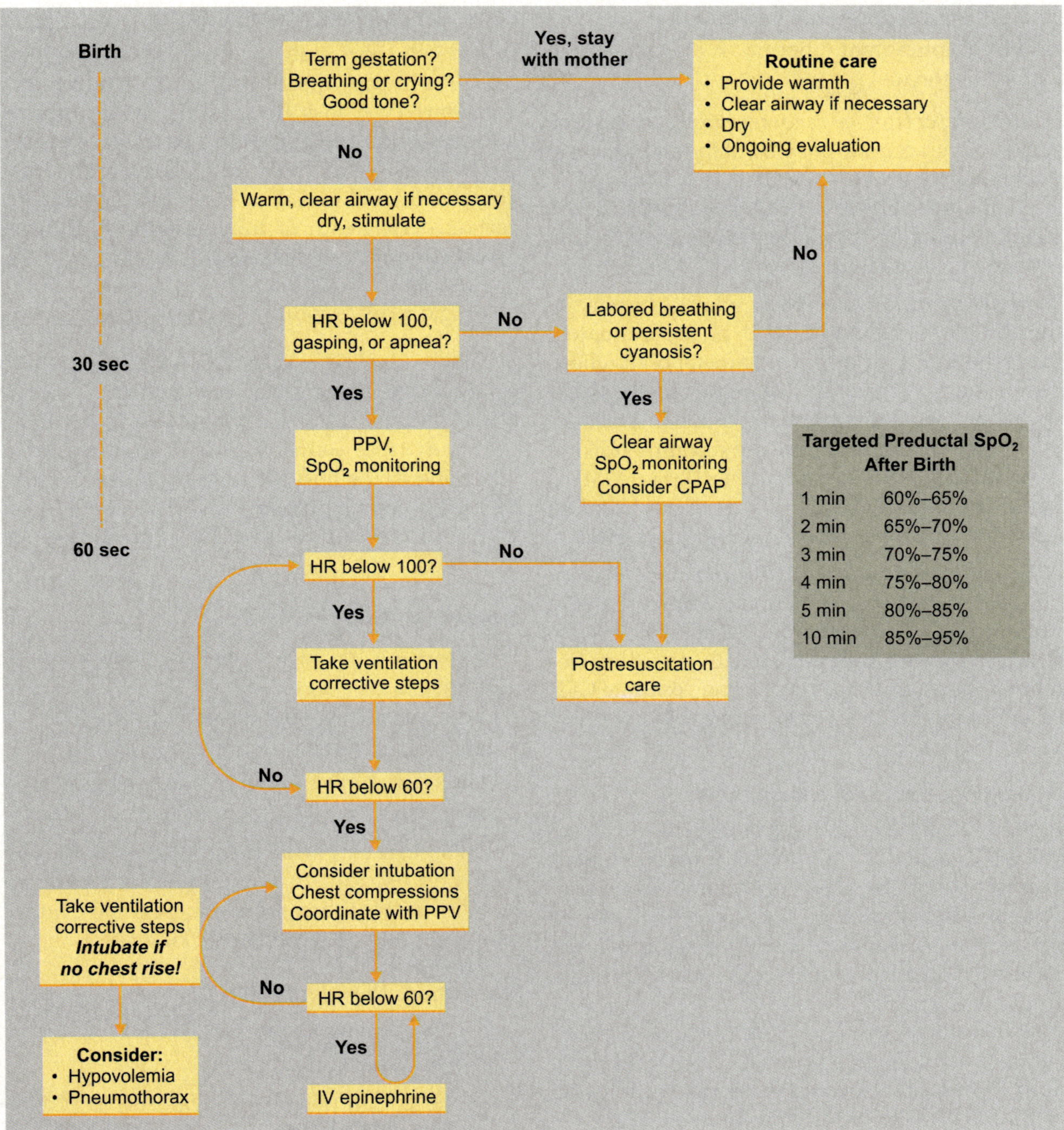

Fig. 11.8 Recent guidelines in neonatal resuscitation
Source: Part 14—Paediatric Advanced Life Support 2010, American Heart Association Guidelines for Cardiopulmonary Resuscitation and Emergency Cardiovascular Care

Spontaneously breathing preterm infants with respiratory distress may be supported with CPAP or with intubation and mechanical ventilation (Class IIb, LOE B).

Laryngeal mask airway (LMA) is effective for ventilating newborns weighing more than 2000 g (Class IIb, LOE B). LMA can be used during resuscitation if face-mask ventilation is unsuccessful and tracheal intubation is unsuccessful or not feasible.[55,57] (Class IIa, LOE B).

Indications of endotracheal intubation during neonatal resuscitation:

- Initial endotracheal suctioning revealing meconium
- Bag and mask ventilation is ineffective or prolonged

- When chest compressions are performed
- Congenital diaphragmatic hernia or extremely low birth weight neonate.

Exhaled CO_2 detection is recommended as a quick confirmation of the accurate position of the endotracheal tube in neonates (Class IIa, LOE B).

Ventilation is most effective in neonatal resuscitation and assisted ventilation should be delivered optimally before starting chest compressions.

Chest Compressions in new born should be on the lower third of the sternum to a depth of approximately one-third of the anterior-posterior diameter of the chest. The 2-thumb–encircling hands technique may generate higher peak systolic and coronary perfusion pressure than the 2-finger technique, hence are recommended in newly born infants[55, 58] (Class IIb, LOE C) (Fig. 11.4).

The chest should re-expand fully during relaxation, but the rescuer's thumbs should not leave the chest.

Ratio of 3:1 compressions to ventilations with 90 compressions and 30 breaths to achieve approximately 120 events per minute should be maintained. Assess heart rate, and oxygenation periodically avoiding frequent interruptions of compressions and continue CPR until the spontaneous heart rate is more than 60 per minute.

Pharmacology of neonatal resuscitation

The recommended IV dose of epinephrine is 0.01 to 0.03 mg/kg (Class IIb, LOE C). An isotonic crystalloid solution or blood can be used for volume expansion. The recommended dose is 10 mL/kg, which can be repeated. In premature infants, rapid infusions of large volumes may cause intraventricular haemorrhage. (Class IIb, LOE C).[55,57,59,60]

Glucose infusion should be given as soon as after resuscitation, to avoid hypoglycemia (Class IIb, LOE C).

Calcium, buffers or vasopressors are rarely indicated during CPR but may be useful after resuscitation.

Therapeutic hypothermia is recommended for babies born near term with evolving moderate to severe hypoxic-ischemic encephalopathy.

Key Points:

- Apnoea or gasping start ventilation at a rate of 40 to 60 breaths per minute.
- Heart rate is less than 60 per minute, then Start Chest compressions.
- The 2-thumb–encircling hands technique
- Ratio of 3:1 compressions to ventilations with 90 compressions and 30 breaths.

Discontinuing Resuscitative Efforts

In a newly born baby with no detectable heart rate for 10 minutes, discontinuing resuscitation can be considered[55] (Class IIb, LOEC). When extreme prematurity, birth weight < 400 g or congenital anomalies such as an encephaly, and major chromosomal abnormalities like trisomy 13 are associated with almost certain early death or unacceptably high morbidity, resuscitation is not indicated (Class IIb, LOE C).

FOREIGN-BODY AIRWAY OBSTRUCTION (CHOKING)

Foreign-body airway obstruction (FBAO) in children < 5 years of age is one of the commonest and potentially treatable cause of cardiac arrest. Sudden onset of respiratory distress with coughing, gagging, stridor, or wheezing in the absence of fever suggests FBAO.[1,61,62] Key to successful outcome is early recognition as signs are obvious but often fatal if undiagnosed and untreated.

Causes of FBAO

- Liquids are the most common cause of choking in infants
- Large, poorly chewed pieces of food
- Balloons, small toys
- Foods (e.g. round candies, nuts, and grapes)
- Loose teeth.

FBAO can be partial and presents with wheezing, cough and stridor or complete which presents with inability to speak, breathe or cough. Child Clutches neck and turns blue (Universal chocking sign).

Precautions to prevent FBAO

- Food cut into small pieces
- Slow and thorough chewing
- Avoiding laughing and talking during swallowing
- Safe toys for children

Management of FBAO (Figs 11.9A to C)

Chest Thrusts

- Used instead of Heimlich Maneuver in infants and children up to 8 years as abdominal thrusts may damage the infant's relatively large and unprotected liver.
- Give up to 5 upward chest thrusts with a fist of one hand positioned over the lower half of sternum.
- It should simulate artificial cough.

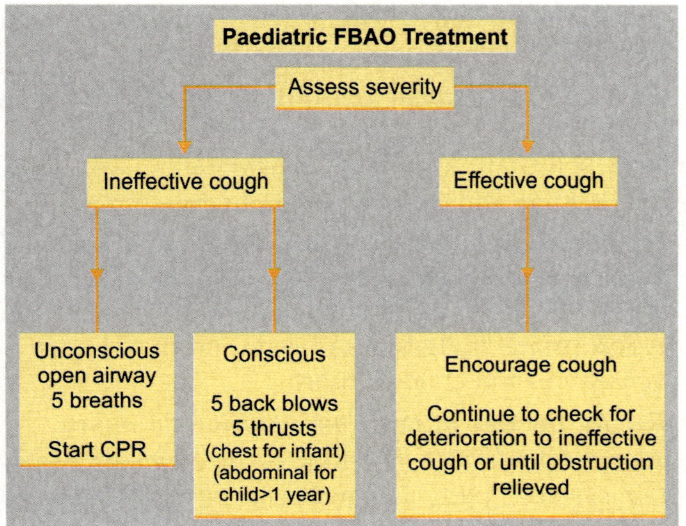

Fig. 11.9A Paediatric FBAO algorithm

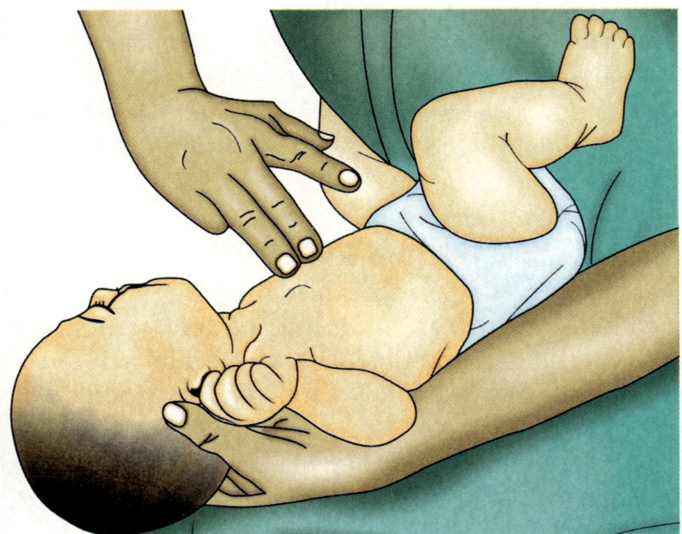

Fig. 11.9B Chest thrust in infant

Back Blows

- Infant: Prone, head low, supported between 2 forearms and on the thigh of rescuer.
- Deliver 5 back blows forcefully between shoulder blades with heel of hand ensuring an open mouth

If the child becomes unresponsive, start CPR with chest compressions. If foreign body is visible, remove it but do not perform blind finger sweeps. Attempt to give 2 breaths and continue with cycles of chest compressions and ventilations until the object is expelled.

Drowning

Drowning is one of the common causes of CA in children and preventon by implementation of swimming safety norms is must.[1,2] Outcome depends on the duration of submersion, the water temperature, and prompt and effective CPR.[63] Start resuscitation by safely removing the child from the water as rapidly as possible. Prompt initiation of rescue breathing is very essential and can be started in the water by trained person. Mouth-to-nose ventilation may be preferred. Chest compressions should be given outside the water. Routine stabilization of cervical spine in the absence of a spinal injury is not recommended. Do not attempt to remove water from lungs but remove visible foreign material from mouth. Hypothermia is suspected if submerged for long time, rewarm slowly.

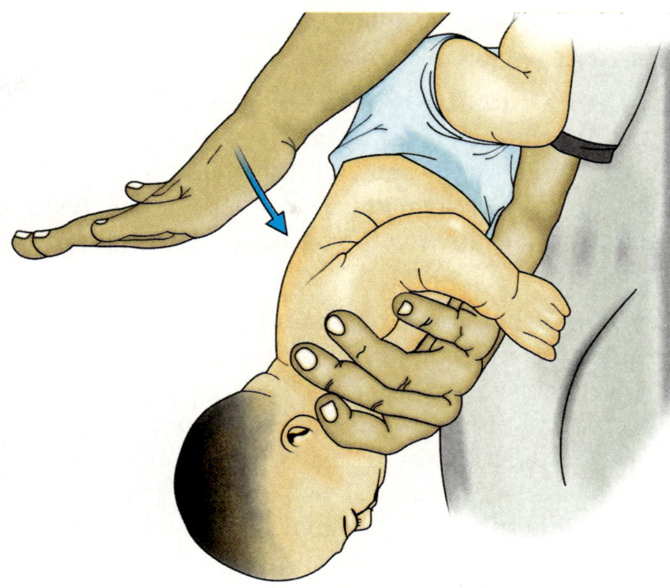

Fig. 11.9C Back blow in infants

Key Points:

- Do not attempt CPR in water.
- Begin rescue breathing as soon as possible
- Begin with 5 cycles (about 2 minutes) of CPR, then activate emergency response system

POST-CA SYNDROME

If ROSC is achieved quickly after the recognition of CA and initiation of treatment, a pathological post-resuscitation phase may not occur. Children have increased cerebral blood flow and higher metabolic needs as compared with adults, and undergo neuronal maturation and synaptogenesis at the time of the insult.[11]

Brain injury includes impaired cerebrovascular autoregulation, cerebral oedema and post-ischemic neurodegeneration. Clinically child may have seizures, cognitive dysfunction, myoclonus, signs of stroke, coma, persistent vegetative state and brain death.[64]

Myocardial dysfunction after paediatric CA is a reversible characterised by global myocardial hypokinesia, low cardiac output, with normal coronary blood flow. Clinically, it can manifest as hypotension, dysrhythmias and cardiovascular collapse which is usually normalized by 72 hours.

Systemic ischaemia/reperfusion response in CA is secondary to inadequate tissue oxygenation followed by reperfusion which may lead to increased coagulation, impaired vasoregulation, adrenal suppression and increased susceptibility to infection. Clinical manifestations include fever, hypotension, hyperglycemia and infection that may precipitate multiorgan failure.[64]

IATROGENIC COMPLICATIONS OF CPCR

Iatrogenic complications of CPCR are rare in infants and children. Clinically significant iatrogenic injuries occur in approximately 3% of cases.[65] Commonest complications are rib fractures, sternal fracture followed by pneumothorax, pneumoperitoneum, haemorrhage, retinal haemorrhages, etc.

Burns to the patients can occur due to poor contact between defibrillator paddles and patient's chest, hence proper use of conduction gel or self-adhesive pads are recommended. Fire in the oxygen rich environment can occur with sparking from defibrillator, hence resuscitation bag or ventilator should be left connected to endotracheal tube.

POST RESUSCITATION CARE

The 2010 AHA Guidelines for CPR and ECC emphasize increased importance of post-cardiac arrest care and bundled goal-oriented management.[27,66]

Objectives of post cardiac arrest care are:

- ***To optimize systemic perfusion***, restore metabolic homeostasis and support organ function.

  Monitor vital signs at frequent intervals and step up monitoring and secure central venous line and arterial line. Arterial lactate and central venous oxygen saturation to assess the adequacy of tissue oxygen delivery should be monitored.

  Vasoactive drugs administered to improve myocardial function and organ perfusion. Epinephrine or norepinephrine (0.1–0.5 mcg/kg/min) may be preferable to dopamine (5–10 mcg/kg/min) in infants with marked circulatory instability and decompensated shock. Dobutamine (5–10 mcg/kg/min) is preferred in children with poor myocardial function.
- ***Optimize mechanical ventilation to minimize lung injury***

  Goal is to reduce the risk of oxidative injury while maintaining adequate oxygen delivery.

  Keep lowest inspired oxygen concentration that will maintain the arterial oxyhemoglobin saturation around 94%. Monitor with blood gases and $PETCO_2$. Appropriate analgesia and sedation may improve ventilation and child comfort.
- ***Reduce the risk of renal and multiorgan injury***

  Avoid dehydration, nephrotoxic medications. Maintain systemic perfusion and urine output 0.5–1 mL/kg per hour in children.
- ***To preserve neurologic function, prevent secondary organ injury***

  A primary goal of resuscitation is to preserve brain function and avoid secondary damage.

  Interventions to reduce secondary brain injury, such as therapeutic hypothermia, can improve survival and neurological recovery.[66,67]

Targeted Temperature Management

Therapeutic hypothermia is recommended for neonate born near term with evolving moderate to severe hypoxic-ischemic encephalopathy and children who do not awaken after ROSC.[67] Not indicated in patients with major bleeding.

Cooling should be initiated in neonatal intensive care facilities and body temperature is reduced to 32–34°C immediately after ROSC. Commonly used methods are surface cooling and endovascular cooling. Favourable neurological outcome is documented by a few studies. Associated complications are shivering, bradycardia, hypotension, diueresis, hypokalemia, infections.[66,67]

TERMINATION OF RESUSCITATIVE EFFORTS AND ETHICAL ISSUES

There are no specific predictors of outcome to guide when to terminate resuscitative efforts in paediatrics.[27] In 2010 AHA Guidelines for CPR and ECC. The duration of resuscitation was reviewed. In a newly born baby with no detectable heart rate for 10 minutes, stopping resuscitation can be considered. When certain early death and an unacceptably high morbidity are known with gestation, birth weight, or congenital anomalies, resuscitation is not indicated.

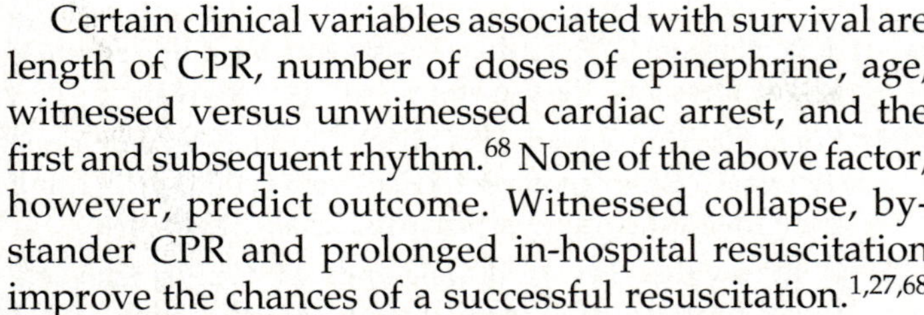

Certain clinical variables associated with survival are length of CPR, number of doses of epinephrine, age, witnessed versus unwitnessed cardiac arrest, and the first and subsequent rhythm.[68] None of the above factor, however, predict outcome. Witnessed collapse, by-stander CPR and prolonged in-hospital resuscitation improve the chances of a successful resuscitation.[1,27,68]

The death of the child is very devastating for the family. Family guilt is overwhelmed hence emotional support is essential. Whenever possible, provide family members with the option of being present during resuscitation of an infant or child.[69] (Class I, LOE B)

Prevention, anticipation, adequate preparation, extreme vigilance, accurate evaluation, and prompt initiation of CPR are critical for successful paediatric resuscitation.

Pearls
- Time is crucial
- Follow all steps of resuscitation well
- Treat the cause and not the condition
- Resuscitate the heart and restore the brain
- Emphasize importance of high quality CPR
- Follow simplified cardiac arrest algorithms
- Re-start the heart and keep it restarted

Take Home Message

CPR is not harmful; inaction is, hence start CPR when in doubt.

FAQs with Answers

Q. What constitutes Paediatric Chain of Survival?

A. Prevention of cardiac arrest, immediate recognition, early BLS, Prompt access to the emergency response system, PALS, Integrated post-cardiac arrest care.

Q. What are characteristics of High-quality CPR?

A. "Push fast" and "Push hard", complete chest recoil after each compression, minimize interruptions in chest compressions, avoid excessive ventilation, monitor quality CPR.

Q. What is the recommended energy dose for defibrillation in paediatrics?

A. The recommended first energy dose for defibrillation is biphasic 2 J/kg followed by 4 J/kg, higher energy may be considered but not beyond 10 J/kg

Q. What are different arrest rhythms?

A. The arrest pulse less rhythm is either "shockable" (e.g. VF or rapid VT) or "not shockable" (e.g. asystole or PEA).

Q. Which drugs can be administered by endotracheal route?

A. Atropine, lidocaine, oxygen, naloxone, epinephrine (ALONE) can be administered via endotracheal route

Q. What are signs of ROSC?

A. An abrupt and sustained rise in $PETCO_2$ occurs prior to clinical signs of ROSC like return of central pulsation.

Q. What are the key changes made in 2010 AHA Guidelines for CPR and ECC?

A. "CAB" sequence, high quality CPR with monitoring continuous capnography. BLS, PALS and neonatal algorithms and the use and timing of drugs have been simplified.

Q. What is the target temperature for therapeutic hypothermia?

A. For therapeutic hypothermia body temperature is reduced to 32–34°C immediately after ROSC.

Q. How do you monitor CPR quality?

A. For high quality CPR maintain $PETCO_2$ consistently above 10–15 mm Hg.

BLS

C - Closed Chest Compression ECM A- Open Airway (Jaw Thrust, Chin Lift and Head Tilt)
B - Positive Pressure Ventilation Expired Air/Resuscitation Bag
D - Defibrillation (Pulseless Patient with VT or VF)

ACLS

D - Defibrillation (Pulseless Patient with VT or VF)
A - Airway with ET Tube
B - Assess Adequacy of Ventilation
C - Closed Chest Compression ECM IV Access for Fluids and Drugs
D - Diagnosis: Treat and Reverse Cause of Arrest

REFERENCES

1. Berg MD, Schexnayder SM, Chameides L, et al. Part 13: pediatric basic life support: 2010 American Heart Association Guidelines for Cardiopulmonary Resuscitation and Emergency Cardiovascular Care. Circulation. 2010;122(suppl 3):S862–S875.1.
2. Topjian AA, Berg RA, Nadkarni VM. Pediatric cardiopulmonary resuscitation: Advances in science, techniques, and outcomes. Pediatrics. 2008 Nov;122(5):1086–98.
3. Atkins DL, Everson-Stewart S, Sears GK, et al. Epidemiology and outcomes from out-of-hospital cardiac arrest in children: the Resuscitation Outcomes Consortium Epistry-Cardiac Arrest. Circulation. 2009;119:1484–1491.

4. Kitamura T, Iwami T, Kawamura T. Conventional and chest-compression-only cardiopulmonary resuscitation bystanders for children who have out-of-hospital cardiac arrests: A prospective, nationwide, population-based cohort study. Lancet. 375 2010:1347–1354.

5. Nadkarni VM, Larkin GL, Peberdy MA, et al. First documented rhythm and clinical outcome from in-hospital cardiac arrest among children and adults. JAMA. 2006;295:50–57.

6. Meaney PA, Nadkarni VM, Cook EF, et al. Higher survival rates among younger patients after pediatric intensive care unit cardiac arrests. Pediatrics. 2006;118:2424–2433.

7. Winkel BG, Risgaard B, Sadjadieh G, et al. Sudden cardiac death in children (1–18 yrs): Symptoms and causes of death in a nationwide setting Eur Heart J 2014;35:13:868–875.

8. American Academy of Pediatrics. Pediatric sudden cardiac arrest. Pediatrics 2012;129:1094–1102.

9. Bhananker SM, Ramamoorthy C, Geiduschek JM, et al. Anesthesia-related cardiac arrest in children: Update from the Pediatric Perioperative Cardiac Arrest Registry. Anaesth Analg 2007;105: 344–50.

10. Morray JP, Bhananker SM. Recent Findings From the Pediatric Perioperative Cardiac Arrest (POCA) Registry. ASA Newsletter 2005;69(6):10–12.

11. Tress EE, Kochanek PM, Saladino RA, et al. Cardiac arrest in children. J Emerg Trauma Shock. 2010; 3(3):267–72.

12. Berg MD, Nadkarni VM, Zuercher M, et al. In-hospital pediatric cardiac arrest. Pediatr Clin North Am. 2008;55: 589–604.

13. Crewdson K, Lockey D, Davies G. Outcome from paediatric cardiac arrest associated with trauma. Resuscitation. 2007;75:29–34.

14. Moler FW, Meert K, Donaldson AE, et al. In-hospital versus out-of-hospital pediatric cardiac arrest: A multicenter cohort study. Crit Care Med. 2009;37:2259–67.

15. Zwass MS, Gregory GA. Pediatric and Neonatal Intensive Care ch. 84. Millers Anesthesia 7th edn. Ronald D Miller, Lars I Eriksson, Lee A Fleisher, Jeanine P Wiener-Kronish, and William L Young, Elsevierhealth. 2689–98.

16. Christensen R, Voepel-Lewis T, Lewis I, et al. Pediatric cardiopulmonary arrest in the postanesthesia care unit: analysis of data from the American Heart Association Get With The Guidelines-Resuscitation registry. Paediatr Anaesth. 2013;23(6):517–23.

17. Greenland P, Alpert JS, Beller GA, et al. 2010 ACCF/AHA guideline for assessment of cardiovascular risk in asymptomatic adults: a report of the American College of Cardiology Foundation/American Heart Association Task Force on Practice Guidelines. Circulation. 2010;122:e584–e636.

18. Field JM, Hazinski MF, Sayre MR, et al. Part 1: executive summary: 2010 American Heart Association Guidelines for Cardiopulmonary Resuscitation and Emergency Cardiovascular Care. Circulation. 2010;122(suppl 3):S640 –S656.

19. Nishisaki A, Nysaether J, Sutton R, et al. Effect of mattress deflection on CPR quality assessment for older children and adolescents. Resuscitation. 2009;80:540–545.

20. Braga MS, Dominguez TE, Pollock AN, et al. Estimation of optimal CPR chest compression depth in children by using computer tomography. Pediatrics. 2009;124:e69–e74.

21. Whitelaw CC, Slywka B, Goldsmith LJ. Comparison of a two-finger versus two-thumb method for chest compressions by healthcare providers in an infant mechanical model. Resuscitation. 2000; 43:213–216.

22. Aufderheide TP, Pirrallo RG, Yannopoulos D, et al. Incomplete chest wall decompression: a clinical evaluation of CPR performance by EMS personnel and assessment of alternative manual chest compression-decompression techniques. Resuscitation. 2005;64:353–362.

23. Ashton A, McCluskey A, Gwinnutt CL, et al. Effect of rescuer fatigue on performance of continuous external chest compressions over 3 min. Resuscitation. 2002;55:151–155.

24. Mejicano GC, Maki DG. Infections acquired during cardiopulmonary resuscitation: estimating the risk and defining strategies for prevention. Ann Intern Med. 1998;129:813–828.

25. Link MS, Atkins DL, Passman RS, et al. Part 6: electrical therapies: automated external defibrillators, defibrillation, cardioversion, and pacing: 2010 American Heart Association Guidelines for Cardiopulmonary Resuscitation and Emergency Cardiovascular Care. Circulation. 2010;122(suppl 3):S706–S719.

26. Atkins DL, Jorgenson DB. Attenuated pediatric electrode pads for automated external defibrillator use in children. Resuscitation. 2005;66:31–37.

27. Kleinman ME, Chameides L, Schexnayder SM, et al. Part 14: pediatric advanced life support: 2010 American Heart Association Guidelines for Cardiopulmonary Resuscitation and Emergency Cardiovascular Care. Circulation. 2010;122(suppl 3):S876–S908.

28. Park C, Bahk JH, Ahn WS, et al. The laryngeal mask airway in infants and children. Can J Anaesth. 2001;48:413–417.

29. Ellis DY, Harris T, Zideman D. Cricoid pressure in emergency department rapid sequence tracheal intubations: a risk-benefit analysis. Ann Emerg Med. 2007;50:653–665.

30. Newth CJ, Rachman B, Patel N, et al. The use of cuffed versus uncuffed endotracheal tubes in pediatric intensive care. J Pediatr. 2004;144:333–337.

31. Bhende MS, Karasic DG, Karasic RB. End-tidal carbon dioxide changes during cardiopulmonary resuscitation after experimental asphyxial cardiac arrest. Am J Emerg Med. 1996;14:349–350.

32. Horton MA, Beamer C. Powered intraosseous insertion provides safe and effective vascular access for pediatric emergency patients. Pediatr Emerg Care. 2008;24:347–350.

33. Guay J, Lortie L. An evaluation of pediatric in-hospital advanced life support interventions using the pediatric

Utstein guidelines: a review of 203 cardiorespiratory arrests. Can J Anaesth. 2004;51: 373–378.

34. Balaguer Gargallo M, Jordan Garcia I, Caritg Bosch J, et al. Supraventricular tachycardia in infants and children. An Pediatr (Barc). 2007;67:133–138.
35. Moghaddam M, Mohammad Dalili S, Emkanjoo Z. Efficacy of Adenosine for Acute Treatment of Supraventricular Tachycardia in Infants and Children. J Teh Univ Heart Ctr. 2008;3:157–162.
36. Somberg JC, Bailin SJ, Haffajee CI, et al. Intravenous lidocaine versus intravenous amiodarone (in a new aqueous formulation) for incessant ventricular tachycardia. Am J Cardiol. 2002;90:853– 859.
37. Dorian P, Cass D, Schwartz B, et al. Amiodarone as compared with lidocaine for shock-resistant ventricular fibrillation. N Engl J Med. 2002;346: 884–890.
38. Srinivasan V, Morris MC, Helfaer MA, et al. Calcium use during in-hospital pediatric cardiopulmonary resuscitation: a report from the National Registry of Cardiopulmonary Resuscitation. Pediatrics. 2008;121:e1144–1151.
39. Martin TJ, Kang Y, Robertson KM, et al. Ionization and hemodynamic effects of calcium chloride and calcium gluconate in the absence of hepatic function. Anesthesiology. 1990;73:62–65.
40. Battin M, Page B, Knight D. Is there still a place for endotracheal adrenaline in neonatal resuscitation? J Paediatr Child Health. 2007;43:504.
41. Rodriguez Nunez A, Garcia C, Lopez-Herce Cid J. Is high-dose epinephrine justified in cardiorespiratory arrest in children? An Pediatr (Barc). 2005;62:113–116.
42. Beiser DG, Carr GE, Edelson DP, et al. Derangements in blood glucose following initial resuscitation from in-hospital cardiac arrest: a report from the national registry of cardiopulmonary resuscitation. Resuscitation. 2009;80:624–630.
43. Hassan TB, Jagger C, Barnett DB. A randomised trial to investigate the efficacy of magnesium sulphate for refractory ventricular fibrillation. Emerg Med J. 2002;19:57–62.
44. Chang PM, Silka MJ, Moromisato DY, et al. Amiodarone versus procainamide for the acute treatment of recurrent supraventricular tachycardia in pediatric patients. Circ Arrhythm Electrophysiol. 2010;3:134 –140.
45. Lokesh L, Kumar P, Murki S, et al. A randomized controlled trial of sodium bicarbonate in neonatal resuscitation-effect on immediate outcome. Resuscitation. 2004;60:219–223.
46. Agrawal A, Singh VK, Varma A, et al. Therapeutic Applications of Vasopressin in Pediatric Patients. Indian Pediatr 2012;49:297–305.
47. Gil-Anton J, Lopez-Herce J, Morteruel E, et al. Pediatric cardiac arrest refractory to advanced life support: Is there a role for terlipressin? Pediatr Crit Care Med. 2010;11:139–141.
48. Li Y, Ristagno G, Bisera J, et al. Electrocardiogram waveforms for monitoring effectiveness of chest compression during cardiopulmonary resuscitation. Crit Care Med. 2008; 36:211–215.
49. Niendorff DF, Rassias AJ, Palac R, et al. Rapid cardiac ultrasound of in patients suffering PEA arrest performed by nonexpert sonographers. Resuscitation. 2005;67: 81–87.
50. Querellou E, Meyran D, Petitjean F, et al. Ventricular fibrillation diagnosed with trans-thoracic echocardiography. Resuscitation. 2009;80:1211–1213.
51. Ristagno G, Tang W, Chang YT, et al. The quality of chest compressions during cardiopulmonary resuscitation overrides importance of timing of defibrillation. Chest. 2007;132:70–75.
52. Pokorna M, Necas E, Kratochvil J, et al. A Sudden Increase in Partial Pressure End-tidal Carbon Dioxide [P(ET)CO2] at the Moment of Return of Spontaneous Circulation. J Emerg Med. 2009.
53. Eftestol T, Wik L, Sunde K, et al. Effects of cardiopulmonary resuscitation on predictors of ventricular fibrillation defibrillation success during out-of-hospital cardiac arrest. Circulation. 2004;110:10–15.
54. Huang SC, Wu ET, Chen YS, et al. Extracorporeal membrane oxygenation rescue for cardiopulmonary resuscitation in pediatric patients. Crit Care Med. 2008;36:1607–1613.
55. Kattwinkel J, Perlman JM, Aziz K, et al. Part 15: neonatal resuscitation: 2010 American Heart Association Guidelines for Cardiopulmonary Resuscitation and Emergency Cardiovascular Care. Circulation. 2010;122(suppl 3):S909–S919.
56. Forsbald K, Kallen K, Marsal K, et al. Apgar score predicts short-term outcome in infants born at 25 gestational weeks. Acta Paediatr 96:166, 2007.
57. Chadha IA. Neonatal resuscitation: Current issues. Indian J Anaesth. 2010 Sep–Oct;54(5):428–438.
58. Dorfsman ML, Menegazzi JJ, Wadas RJ, et al. Two-thumb vs two-finger chest compression in an infant model of prolonged cardiopulmonary resuscitation. Acad Emerg Med. 2000;7:1077–1082.
59. Wyckoff MH, Perlman JM, Laptook AR. Use of volume expansion during delivery room resuscitation in near-term and term infants. Pediatrics. 2005;115:950–955.
60. Salhab WA, Wyckoff MH, Laptook AR, et al. Initial hypoglycaemia and neonatal brain injury in term infants with severe fetal acidemia. Pediatrics. 2004;114:361–366.
61. Morley RE, Ludemann JP, Moxham JP, et al. Foreign body aspiration in infants and toddlers: recent trends in British Columbia. J Otolaryngol. 2004;33:37–41.
62. Prevention of choking among children. Pediatrics. 2010; 125:601–607.
63. Modell JH, Idris AH, Pineda JA, et al. Survival after prolonged submersion in freshwater in Florida. Chest. 2004;125:1948–1951.
64. Nolan JP, Neumar RW, Adrie C, et al. Post-cardiac arrest syndrome: epidemiology, pathophysiology, treatment, and prognostication: A Scientific Statement from the International Liaison Committee on Resuscitation; the

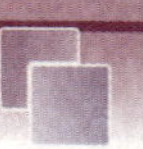

American Heart Association Emergency Cardiovascular Care Committee; the Council on Cardiovascular Surgery and Anesthesia; the Council on Cardiopulmonary, Perioperative, and Critical Care; the Council on Clinical Cardiology; the Council on Stroke. Resuscitation. 2008;79:350–79.

65. Bush CM, Jones JS, Cohle SD, et al. Pediatric injuries from cardiopulmonary resuscitation. Ann Emerg Med July 1996;28:40-44.
66. Peberdy MA, Callaway CW, Neumar RW, et al. Part 9: post-cardiac arrest care: 2010 American Heart Association Guidelines for Cardiopulmonary Resuscitation and Emergency Cardiovascular Care. Circulation. 2010;122(suppl 3):S768–S786.
67. Doherty DR, Parshuram CS, Gaboury I, et al. Hypothermia therapy after pediatric cardiac arrest. Circulation. 2009;119: 1492–1500.
68. Lopez-Herce J, Garcia C, Dominguez P, et al. Characteristics and outcome of cardiorespiratory arrest in children. Resuscitation. 2004;63:311–320.
69. Boyd R. Witnessed resuscitation by relatives. Resuscitation. 2000;43:171–176.

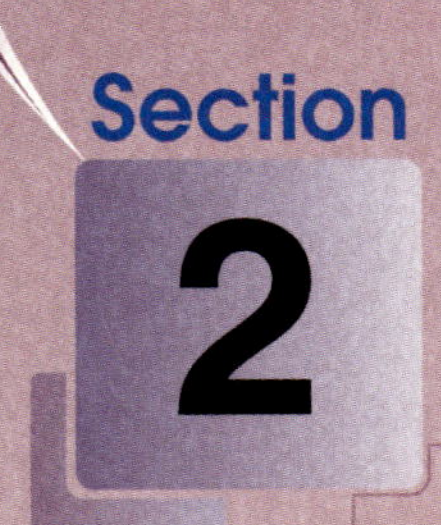

Scientific Basis for Practice of Paediatric Anaesthesia

12. Preoperative Evaluation, Preparation and Psychological Aspects of Paediatric Anaesthesia
13. Postanaesthesia Care Unit Management
14. Equipment
15. Blood Transfusion and Strategies for Blood Conservation in Infants and Children
16. Acute and Chronic Pain Management in Infants and Children
17. Regional Blocks in Paediatrics
18. Ultrasound in Paediatric Anaesthesia

12

Preoperative Evaluation, Preparation and Psychological Aspects of Paediatric Anaesthesia

Neerja Bhardwaj

INTRODUCTION

The perioperative period can be an extremely distressing period for a child who is undergoing a surgical procedure. An anaesthesiologist has to ensure that children undergoing surgery are evaluated not only for the presence of associated diseases but also to identify children who are anxious and would therefore need adequate psychological preparation. The stress of surgery and separation from parents may present in the form of anxiety which if not managed can lead to adverse postoperative outcomes and behavioral disturbances. Therefore, an understanding and management of anxiety is essential to avoid adverse psychological and physiological outcomes. Various methods both pharmacological and non-pharmacological have been extensively investigated for their efficacy in reducing or alleviating anxiety in children undergoing a surgical procedure. This chapter aims to discuss the various issues pertaining to the preoperative assessment and psychological preparation of children presenting for surgery as well as various pharmacological agents available for premedication.

PREOPERATIVE EVALUATION

Perioperative care begins with a comprehensive pre-anaesthetic evaluation of children. This preoperative evaluation enables the anaesthesiologist to assess the medical problems of the children which may influence anaesthetic management, as well as a chance to win the confidence of the patient and the parents. Generally children presenting for surgery have normal health but some of them may have complex medical problems which are predominantly congenital or developmental in origin. Therefore, the primary aim of the anaesthesiologist is to identify the presence and the severity of the disease condition so that a safe anaesthesia plan can be formulated.

At the pre-anaesthetic visit, focus should be on reviewing of the medical record, particularly focusing on any previous anaesthetic exposure, problems encountered during the postoperative period like post-operative nausea and vomiting, delirium, malignant hyperthermia and the techniques utilized for airway management.[1,2] A history of cardio-respiratory diseases or airway anomalies should be elicited. Children with syndromes have multisystem involvement and require more thorough preoperative assessment with a focus on cardiac and airway assessment. One should also take history of medical or environmental allergies, current drug therapy including herbal medications and the possibility of its interaction with the anaesthetics. Parents should be questioned for the presence of upper respiratory infection (URI) because many studies report that a child anaesthetized while having a URI is at increased risk for developing laryngospasm, broncho-spasm, coughing, breath holding and arterial oxygen desaturation.[3–5] Also upper respiratory tract infection is associated with an increased risk for these peri-operative respiratory adverse events only when symptoms are present at time of assessment or less than 2 weeks before the procedure.[3] The relevant obstetric and perinatal issues should be reviewed like gestational age at birth, problems of prematurity and requirement and duration of respiratory support if any. Relevant laboratory investigations should then be reviewed.

Baseline clinical examination should include height, weight, heart rate, blood pressure, respiratory rate, temperature and arterial oxygenation saturation if indicated. Airway examination should focus on identification of potential predictors of difficult intubation such as limited mouth opening, stridor, loose teeth, mandibular hypoplasia/retrognathia, macro-glossia, cleft or high arched palate and restricted cervical spine movement. This is because all these features may be a part of a syndromic child. Also the parameters and scoring systems used for predicting airway difficulty in adults have not been validated in children. Spinal anatomy should be examined if a neuraxial technique is being planned and the sites for intravenous cannulation should be identified. Children in the age group of 4–8 years should be examined for loose primary teeth.

PREOPERATIVE INVESTIGATIONS

The goal should be to perform a clinical examination which can then lead to selective and targeted investigations. Preoperative haemoglobin testing is not routinely indicated since mild to moderate anaemia produces minimal adverse effects in healthy children undergoing minor surgery. Severe anaemia reduces oxygen-carrying capacity and can impair tissue oxygen supply. It is definitely indicated in children where clinical assessment gives a suspicion of severe anaemia, children of <1 year, former preterm infants and as a baseline in surgeries expected to cause severe blood loss.[2] In surgeries where a large amount of blood loss is expected, blood for grouping and cross matching should be drawn. Routine testing for urea, creatinine, electrolytes and coagulation studies is not required but should be tested based on the clinical history of liver and kidney diseases, family history of bleeding disorders or easy bruising. Routine chest X-ray is not needed in paediatric population but can be considered in children with cardiac, respiratory and malignant disease like lymphoma where chest X-ray is done to exclude a mediastinal mass.

FASTING GUIDELINES

Children need to be fasted before surgery to reduce the risk of regurgitation and aspiration. The duration of fasting is important because prolonged fasting can lead to dehydration, hypoglycemia and patient discomfort.[6] The modern fasting guidelines are more liberal and are presented in Table 12.1.[7] Clear fluids if given until 2 h preoperatively do not increase the gastric volume, nor reduce pH and has been found to cause less dehydration and making children less thirsty and hungry and better behaved.[8] Breast milk is slow in clearance as compared to clear fluids but faster than formula preparations.[9] Fasting for formula milk in different hospitals ranges from 4–6 hours based on factors like osmolality, protein content, energy density and pH, all of which can alter rate of gastric emptying. Whey-predominant formula empties faster than casein-predominant formula.[10] Cow's milk is treated as solid food because of its high lipid content, requiring 6 hours fasting.

Table 12.1 American Society of Anesthesiologists fasting recommendations[7]

Ingested material	Minimum fasting period (hours)
Clear fluids	2
Breast milk	4
Infant formula	6
Non-human milk	6
Light meal	6

PSYCHOLOGICAL EFFECTS OF HOSPITALIZATION AND SURGERY

It is estimated that about 50–70% of children develop significant anxiety and fear before their surgery. The most stressful period during the perioperative period has been found to be the induction of anaesthesia.[11] Anxiety in children undergoing surgery is characterized by a subjective feeling of tension, apprehension, nervousness and worry that may be expressed in various forms like crying, screaming, protesting, attempting to escape the procedure and resisting face mask placement. An increased preoperative anxiety can lead to decreased parental satisfaction, impaired perioperative neuroendocrine response and problematic postoperative clinical and psychological recovery.[12] This may present as negative behavioral changes, increased postoperative pain and analgesic requirement and increased nausea and vomiting.[13,14] Postoperative maladaptive behaviours, such as new onset enuresis, feeding difficulties, apathy and withdrawal and sleep disturbances, may also result from anxiety before surgery. Several studies have shown that about 40–55% of children undergoing elective surgery exhibit new-onset maladaptive behavioral changes such as nightmares, separation anxiety, eating problems, and increased fear of doctors which may persist long after the hospital experience has passed.[11] This particularly occurs when children do not receive preoperative sedation or preparation and cry or thrash or scream at the time of induction. In the same study children showed increased incidence of emergence delirium, need for more medications, delayed discharge and also sleep was adversely affected. Kain et al reported negative behavioral responses in 54% of children 2 weeks after surgery; these persisted up to 6 months in 20% and up to 1 year in 7% of children.[11] The same authors also showed a relationship between preoperative anxiety, emergence delirium and postoperative maladaptive behavior.[15]

Preoperative anxiety also activates the human stress response, leading to increased serum cortisol, epinephrine and natural killer cell activity.[16] Stress activates the hypothalamic pituitary-adrenal axis, increases circulating glucocorticoids and is associated with alterations of immune function and susceptibility to infection. The surgical stress response may produce detrimental effects where neuroendocrine hormones (e.g. cortisol, catecholamines) and cytokines (e.g., interleukin-6) provoke a negative nitrogen balance and catabolism, delay wound healing and cause postoperative immunosuppression.[17] Children are particularly vulnerable to the global surgical stress response because of limited energy reserves, larger brain masses and obligatory glucose requirements.

> **Warning**
> 50–70% of children develop significant anxiety and fear before their surgery which is characterized by a subjective feeling of tension, apprehension, nervousness and worry that may be expressed in various forms like crying, screaming, protesting, attempting to escape the procedure and resisting face mask placement.

Risk Factors for the Development of Preoperative Anxiety

It is important to identify children at higher risk for developing preoperative anxiety and direct resources to those children. Children may feel anxious because of parental separation, fear of pain or discomfort, loss of control, uncertainty about "going to sleep" and masked operation room personnel. The various risk factors which have been identified to increase chances of separation anxiety include:

Age: A number of studies have shown that younger children between the ages of one and five years are more at risk for developing preoperative anxiety than older children.[11,18,19] In the first week of life, infants are able to discriminate among people but will accept care and comfort from adults other than their parents. By 3 months of age, however, infants begin to respond differently to familiar and unfamiliar people. Older infants smile more at familiar people and may even try to engage their attention. Separation anxiety usually begins at 7–8 months of age and peaks around 1 year of age.

Temperament and baseline anxiety: Children with high-trait (baseline) anxiety or those with a shy and inhibited temperament have higher levels of anxiety on the day of surgery.[11,20,21] Also, children with a passive coping style, e.g. children who use avoidance, withdrawal, and wishful thinking to deal with the stress of surgery are at higher risk of preoperative anxiety.[22]

Past medical encounters: Children who have had a previous bad medical experience and previous surgery tend to have higher anxiety.[11,18,21] However, some authors have not found previous surgery to be associated with more anxiety.[23] However, parents of children undergoing repeat surgery have less anxiety when compared to the first exposure.[23]

Parents' Level of Anxiety

The parental state (or contextual) anxiety, trait (or baseline) anxiety and monitoring and coping styles have all been linked to heightened children's anxiety.[11,21] Divorced parents and parents with lower educational levels have more anxiety preoperatively.[11,19]

Management of Preoperative Anxiety in Children

Several modalities are used currently to decrease preoperative anxiety in children like parental presence during the induction of anaesthesia, psychological preparation programs and sedative premedications. Various studies have been conducted to document the superiority of one method over the other.[24–28] However, there is a lot of discrepancy in the results of these studies. Yip et al reviewed 17 clinical trials including 1796 children, parents or both, subjected to parental presence, clown doctors, interactive cartoon computer packages, midazolam, handheld video games, hypnotherapy, decreasing sensory stimulation at induction, music therapy, and relaxational parental acupuncture. From their study it was inferred that parental presence does not reduce anxiety or improve cooperation of children.[24] Other interventions were, however, helpful in reducing the children's anxiety and improving cooperation.

PSYCHOLOGICAL PREPARATION PROGRAMS

The concept that children undergoing surgery need psychological preparation was introduced about 50 years back.[29] It started with provision of information to the child regarding the surgery and anaesthesia and enabled the building up of rapport between medical persons and the child.[30,31] This was followed in the 1970s by use of modelling preparation programs which included use of illustrated books, video programs and puppet shows.[31–33] In the 1990s children were taught coping skills by child-life specialists who facilitate perioperative adjustment of both children and parents by using play experiences.[34,35] These specialists also teach them relaxation skills. Although it is established that these preparation programs are effective in reducing anxiety of children in the holding area, it is not proven that they are as effective at time of induction. Also the psychological preparation programs should be individualised and targeted to the needs of each child and also should be timed in relation to the time of surgery.[19,32,36] This is because older children need adequate time to process new information and younger children <3 years are unable to separate fantasy from reality. Preparation programs for children who have been previously hospitalized are difficult and simple modelling and play programs are not beneficial.

Programs for parents are also essential since it is known that parents become very anxious at the prospect of surgery on their children.[19] This also becomes a significant risk factor for producing anxiety in children. Parents who undergo a preoperative preparation program or who view a preoperative videotape featuring factual information about anaesthesia, display reduced preoperative anxiety on the day of surgery.[19,37] However, this anxiolytic effect is temporary and does not remain during the anaesthetic induction, nor does it extend to the recovery room or at 2 weeks postoperatively.

Web-based age-specific information systems like www.narkoswebben.se are the future of psychological preparation programs. The computerized multimedia displays and interactive technology can provide specific interventions for children with a vast variety of medical problems and coping styles.[38]

Parental Presence During Induction of Anaesthesia

It has been observed that parents prefer to be present with their children during minor procedures as well as during emergency procedure, lumbar puncture, resuscitation and induction of anaesthesia. Various surveys have shown that parents prefer to be present at the time of induction of anaesthesia irrespective of the child's age and previous surgical experience.[39,40] Studies have shown that parents who were present during the induction of anaesthesia of their child were significantly more satisfied with the overall quality of care that was provided to their child as well as with the quality of separation from their child on entrance to the operating room.[27,41] A study was conducted by Kain et al to determine if it was safe to allow parents to be present in the operating room at the time of induction of anaesthesia. They found that the parents who were allowed to be present in the OT had higher pulse rate and skin conductance levels.[42] However, they could not demonstrate any ECG abnormalities or rhythm disturbances in this group of patients confirming its safety. Multiple studies based on this technique of allowing parental presence have shown contradictory results.[27,43] In evidence based review of parental presence on child anxiety Chundamala et al did not find any role of parental presence in alleviating child or parent anxiety.[44] However, Caldwell et al have criticized this technique quoting that the mere presence of parents is not an effective technique. Rather their preparation should be based on a mandatory preoperative visit by the parents approximately 3 days before surgery; a 30-minute preparation session with a researcher; watching a videotape developed by the research group at least twice at home; a home visit by a researcher on two separate evenings to answer any questions and remind the parents to watch the video; a short (10 min) preparation period on the day of surgery conducted by the researcher; the use of a specially selected group of toys on the day of surgery; and giving the child a "surprise box" for the induction of anaesthesia. The authors after this type of extensive preparation found the children in this intervention group to be less anxious than the nonprepared group.[45] However, parental presence is not routinely practised in our hospital owing to a large work load and lower educational level of parents.

The drawbacks of parental presence include concerns about disruption of the operating room routine, crowded operating rooms, and parents' possible adverse reactions. In addition, increased parental anxiety can result in increased child's anxiety, prolonged anaesthetic induction, and additional stress on the anaesthesiologist, especially if a complication develops.

Sedative Premedication

Despite the advantages of non-pharmacological methods in reducing anxiety, anaesthesiologist's still

Table 12.2 Routes and doses of premedicant drugs

	Oral/ Rectal	Mucosal	IN	IV
Midazolam (mg/kg)	0.5	0.2	0.2–0.5	0.5–5 y: 0.05–0.1 >5 y: 0.025–0.5
Clonidine (µg/kg)	3–4/5	—	4	0.5–1
Dexmedetomidine (µg/kg)	1–2	2–3	2	0.5
Ketamine (mg/kg)	2–6	4–5	1	1–2

IN: Intranasal, IV: Intravenous, IM: Intramuscular

prefer using sedatives for reducing anxiety of children. Multiple randomized controlled trials have found that midazolam is far superior to either preparation program or parental presence at time of induction in terms of preoperative anxiety and compliance during induction of anaesthesia.[27,44] Also sedative premedication with midazolam causes less anxiety and makes children more compliant. The most commonly used drugs for premedication include midazolam, a agonists like clonidine and dexmedetomidine and ketamine. The drugs and their doses by various routes are mentioned in Table 12.2.

Midazolam

Midazolam is a short-acting benzodiazepine that is very lipophilic in physiological pH, which contributes to its rapid onset of action. Midazolam has been shown to induce satisfactory sedation and anxiolysis within 20 min with a dose of 0.25–0.5 mg/kg administered orally producing easy separation from parents and acceptance of face mask placement. The advantages of midazolam include its rapid and reliable onset, anxiolysis with minimal sedative effects,[47] minimal delay in recovery room discharge,[48] administration via multiple routes (oral, intranasal, rectal, sublingual, intramuscular, intravenous)[49] and reduction in the incidence of emergence delirium.[50] The anxiolysis and amnesia that result from administration of midazolam are not only beneficial for reduction of preoperative anxiety but also improve the postoperative outcome. The drawbacks with midazolam are its bitter taste which has to be masked with additives and low bioavailability with oral route. Midazolam is metabolized by CYP3A4 mediation to produce the primary metabolite 1-hydroxymidazolam. Several fruit juices such as grapefruit, black mulberry, pomegranate and black raspberry have a potential inhibitory effect on CYP3A4-catalysed midazolam 1-hydroxylation.[51]

The nasal route produces an unpleasant burning of the nasal cavity but it produces a higher plasma concentration compared to oral route. Benzodiazepines produce anterograde amnesia and Stewart et al showed that midazolam impaired the explicit memory while leaving the implicit memories intact.[52] This makes the children remember stressful events immediately before surgery by preserving the implicit memory but the child will be unable to bring them to mind to process it sensibly because of poor explicit memory.

Key Point

Midazolam anxiolysis and amnesia are not only beneficial for reduction of preoperative anxiety but also improve the postoperative outcome.

Clonidine

Clonidine is an α_2-adrenergic agonist which when compared to benzodiazepines produces superior preoperative sedation and anxiolysis in children, acts as an analgesic, decreases volatile anaesthesia requirements, reduces emergence agitation[53] and improves perioperative hemodynamic stability.[54–58] It has advantages over midazolam in that it does not have any psychotropic effects, does not have amnestic effect and is not bitter to taste.[59] Clonidine can be administered orally (4 µg/kg) and intranasally (2 µg/kg). Nasal clonidine is not associated with nasal burning. One major drawback of clonidine as a premedicant is prolonged onset time, which requires it to be, administered at least 45–60 min before the induction. In contrast, because clonidine is associated with analgesia, its use is beneficial when postoperative analgesia is needed. In safety terms, clonidine has an excellent therapeutic index and is associated with minimal hemodynamic changes in healthy children.

One Fact to Remember

Clonidine has an excellent therapeutic index and is associated with minimal hemodynamic changes in healthy children.

Dexmedetomidine

Dexmedetomidine is a more selective α_2-adrenergic receptor agonist than clonidine with sedative, anxiolytic and analgesic effects with a shorter elimination half-life and is being used in children for premedication.[60] It is currently only approved by the US FDA for continuous infusion of up to 24 h in the adult intensive care unit and its use in children is 'off-label'. It can be used by oral, nasal, intravenous and buccal routes. The bioavailability of dexmedetomidine via oral route is 15% but when administered via the buccal mucosa, it is 80%.[61] Given intravenously in a bolus dose of 0.5–1 μg/kg followed by an infusion of 0.5–1 μg/kg/h, it produces effective sedation. It has a good systemic absorption when administered through the oral route with doses ranging between 3 and 4 μg/kg administered 30–50 min before induction of anaesthesia. Clinical investigations have demonstrated its sedative, analgesic, anxiolytic and sympatholytic effects without hemodynamic perturbations after intravenous, intranasal, buccal and oral administration in children.[62–64]

Ketamine

Ketamine is a phenylpiperidine derivative which produces "dissociative anaesthesia." It is a lipophilic drug which is poorly bound to the plasma proteins. It has a large volume of distribution and a short elimination half-life of 1–2 h. It can be administered by various routes intravenous, intramuscular, oral, sublingual, rectal and nasal. Orally it can be given alone in a dose of 3–8 mg/kg because oral dose has high hepatic first-pass effect.[65,66] Also high dose of ketamine can cause excessive secretions, dysphoria and hallucinations.[67] Ketamine (2–3 mg/kg)is usually combined with midazolam (0.5 mg/kg) to produce a synergistic effect in children who are difficult to sedate.[66,68–71] For the child who is combative, refuses to accept other routes of administration, and in whom the procedure cannot be delayed or rescheduled, intramuscular ketamine is indicated. When given in a dose of 2 mg/kg IM it is highly effective at producing a satisfactory state of mask acceptance in children and does not result in an increased length of stay in the recovery room.[72]

SUMMARY AND CONCLUSIONS

Children encounter anxiety before surgery which is related to separation from parents and the fear of unknown. This stress related anxiety in children if not addressed can lead to adverse postoperative behavioral outcomes in the form of nightmares, hallucinations, demand for more analgesics, bed wetting and feeding difficulties. The management of separation anxiety requires identification of children who are at risk so that resources are focused on them. Both behavioral and pharmacological interventions have been investigated for their role in prevention of separation anxiety. The choice of intervention for managing this anxiety in children depends on the hospital policy and availability of resources.

FAQ with Answer

Q. Which is more selective α_2-adrenergic receptor agonist than clonidine with sedative, anxiolytic and analgesic effects with a shorter elimination half-life?

A. Dexmedetomidine is more selective α_2-adrenergic receptor agonist which is sedative, analgesic, anxiolytic and sympatholytic effects without hemodynamic perturbations and can be used by intravenous, intranasal, buccal and oral route.

REFERENCES

1. Krane EJ, Davis PJ. Preoperative preparation for infants and children. In: Motoyama EK, Davis PJ, (Eds). Smith's Anaesthesia for Infants and Children. 7th edn. Philadelphia: Mosby Elsevier; 2006;p 255–71.
2. Davidson A, Howard K, Browne W, et al. Preoperative evaluation and preparation, anxiety, awareness and behaviour change. In: Gregory GA, Andropoulos DB, (Eds). Gregory's Paediatric Anaesthesia. 5th edn. West Sussex: Wiley-Blackwell; 2012;p 273–99.
3. von Ungern-Sternberg BS, Boda K, Chambers NA, et al. Risk assessment for respiratory complications in paediatric anaesthesia: A prospective cohort study. Lancet 2010;376: 773–83.
4. Parnis SJ, Barker DS, van der Walt JH. Clinical predictors of anaesthetic complications in children with respiratory tract infections. PaediatrAnaesth 2001;11:29–40.
5. Tait AR, Malviya S, Voepel–Lewis T, et al. Risk factors for perioperative adverse respiratory events in children with upper respiratory tract infections. Anesthesiology 2001;95:299–306.
6. Brady M, Kinn S, Ness V, et al. Preoperative fasting for preventing perioperative complications in children. Cochrane Database Syst Rev 2009 Oct 7;(4):CD005285.
7. Practice guidelines for preoperative fasting and the use of pharmacologic agents to reduce the risk of pulmonary aspiration: Application to healthy patients undergoing elective procedures: A report by the American Society of Anesthesiologists Task Force on preoperative fasting. Anesthesiology 2011;114:495–511.
8. Splinter WM, Schaefer JD. Unlimited clear fluid ingestion two hours before surgery in children does not affect volume or pH of stomach contents. Anaesth Intensive Care 1990;18:522–6.
9. van den Driessche M, Peeters K, Marien P, et al. Gastric emptying in formula-fed and breast-fed infants measured with the 13C-octanoic acid breath test. J Pediatr Gastroenterol Nutr 1999;29:46–51.
10. Billeaud C, Guillet J, Sandler B. Gastric emptying in infants with or without gastro-oesophageal reflux according to the type of milk. European J Clinical Nutrition 1990;44:577–83.

11. Kain ZN, Mayes LC, O'Connor TZ, et al. Preoperative anxiety in children: Predictors and outcome. Arch Pediatr Adolesc Med 1996;150:1238–45.
12. Kain ZN, Caldwell-Andrews AA, LODolce ME, et al. The perioperative behavioral stress response in children. Anesthesiology 2002;96:A1242.
13. Kain ZN. Postoperative maladaptive behavioral changes in children: Incidence, risk factors and interventions. Acta Anesthesiol Scand 2000;51:217–26.
14. Kain Z, Mayes L, Caramico L, et al. Distress during induction of anaesthesia and postoperative behavioral outcomes. Anesth Analg 1999;88:1042–7.
15. Kain ZN, Caldwell-Andrews AA, Maranets I, et al. Preoperative anxiety and emergence delirium and post-operative maladaptive behaviors. Anesth Analg 2004;99: 1648–54.
16. Kain Z, Sevarino F, Rinder C. The preoperative behavioral stress response: Does it exist? [abstract] Anesthesiology 1999;91:A742.
17. Chrousos G, Gold P. The concepts of stress and stress system disorders. JAMA 1992;267:1244–52.
18. Vetter T. The epidemiology and selective identification of children at risk for preoperative anxiety reactions. Anesth Analg 1993;77:96–9.
19. Kain ZN, Mayes LC, Caramico LA. Preoperative preparation in children: A cross-sectional study. J Clin Anesth 1996;8:508–14.
20. Melamed BG, Ridley-Johnson R. Psychological preparation of families for hospitalization. Dev Behav Pediatr 1988;9: 96–102.
21. Kain ZN, Mayes L, Caramico L, et al. Social adaptability and other personality characteristics as predictors for children's reaction to surgery. J Clin Anesth 2001;12: 549–54.
22. Thompson ML. Information seeking coping and anxiety in school-age children anticipating surgery. J Child Health Care. 1994;23:87–97.
23. Kain ZN, Caldwell-Andrews AA, Wang SM, et al. Parental intervention choices for children undergoing repeated surgeries. Anesth Analg. 2003;96: 970–5.
24. Yip P, Middleton P, Cyna AM, et al. Nonpharmacological interventions for assisting the induction of anaesthesia in children. Evid Based Child Health. 2011;6:71–134.
25. Vagnoli L, Caprilli S, Messeri A. Parental presence, clowns or sedative premedication to treat preoperative anxiety in children: What could be the most promising option? Paediatr Anaesth. 2010; 20:937–43.
26. Kain ZN, Mayes LC, Wang SM, et al. Parental presence during induction of anaesthesia versus sedative premedication: Which intervention is more effective? Anesthesiology 1998;89:1147–56.
27. Kain ZN, Mayes LC, Wang SM, et al. Parental presence and a sedative premedicant for children undergoing surgery: A hierarchical study. Anesthesiology. 2000;92: 939–46.
28. Martin SR, Chorney JM, Tan EW, et al. Changing healthcare providers'behavior during paediatric inductions with an empirically based intervention. Anesthesiology, 2011;115: 18–27.
29. Mellish RWP. Preparation of a child for hospitalization and surgery. Pediatr Clin North Am. 1969;16:543–53.
30. Melamed BG, Ridley-Johnson R. Psychological preparation of families for hospitalization. Dev Behav Pediatr. 1988;9: 96–102.
31. Melamed BG, Siegel LJ. Reduction of anxiety in children facing hospitalization and surgery by use of filmed modeling. J Consult Clin Psychol. 1975; 43:511–21.
32. Melamed B, Meyer R, Gee C, et al. The influence of time and type of preparation on children's adjustment to hospitalization. J Pediatr Psychol. 1976;1:31–7.
33. Melamed BG, Yurcheson R, Fleece EL, et al. Effects of film modeling on the reduction of anxiety-related behaviors in individuals varying in level of previous experience in the stress situation. J Consult Clin Psychol. 1978;46:1357–67.
34. Melamed BG. Putting the family back in the child. Behave Res Ther. 1993;31:239–47.
35. American Academy of Paediatrics Committee on Hospital Care: Child life programs. Paediatrics. 1993;91:671–3.
36. Robinson PJ, Kobayashi K. Development and evaluation of a presurgical preparation program. J Pediatr Psychol. 1991;16:193–212.
37. Cassady JF Jr, Wysocki TT, Miller KM, et al. Use of a pre-anesthetic video for facilitation of parental education and anxiolysis before paediatric ambulatory surgery. Anesth Analg. 1999;88:246–50.
38. Kain ZN. Psychological aspects of paediatric anaesthesia. In: Motoyama EK, Davis PJ (Eds). Smith's Anaesthesia for Infants and Children. 7th edn. Philadelphia: Mosby Elsevier. 2006;p 241–54.
39. Kain Z, Ferris C, Mayes L, et al. Parental presence during induction of anaesthesia: Practice differences between the US and Great Britain. Paediatr Anaesth. 1996;6:187–93.
40. Kain Z, Mayes LC, Bell C, et al. Premedication in the United States: A status report. Anesth Analg. 1997;84:427–32.
41. Hannallah RS, Rosales JK. Experience with parents' presence during anaesthesia induction in children. Can Anaesth Soc J. 1983;30:286–9.
42. Kain ZN, Caldwell-Andrews AA, Mayes LC, et al. Parental presence during induction of anaesthesia: physiological effects on parents. Anesthesiology 2003;98:58–64.
43. Schulman JL, Foley JM, Vernon DT, et al. A study of the effect of the mother's presence during anaesthesia induction. Paediatrics. 1967;39:111–4.
44. Chundamala J, Wright JG, Kemp SM. An evidence-based review of parental presence during anaesthesia induction and parental/child anxiety. Can J Anesth. 2009;56:57–70.
45. Caldwell-Andrews AA, Blount RL, Mayes LC, et al. Behavioral interactions in the perioperative environment: A new conceptual framework and the development of the

perioperative child–adult medical procedure interaction scale. Anesthesiology. 2005;103:1130–5.

46. Cote CJ, Cohen IT, Suresh S, et al. A comparison of three doses of a commercially prepared oral midazolam syrup in children. Anesth Analg. 2002; 94:1–3.
47. Cox RG, Nemish U, Ewen A, et al. Evidence-based clinical update: Does premedication with oral midazolam lead to improved behavioural outcomes in children? Can J Anaesth. 2006;53:1213–19.
48. McMillan CO, Spahr-Schopter IA, Sikich N, et al. Premedication of children with oral midazolam. Can J Anaesth. 1992;39:545–50.
49. Kogan A, Katz J, Efrat R, et al. Premedication with midazolam in young children: A comparison of four routes of administration. Pediatr Anaesth. 2002;12:685–9.
50. Ko YP, Huang CJ, Hung YC, et al. Premedication with low dose oral midazolam reduces the incidence and severity of emergence agitation in paediatric patients following sevoflurane anaesthesia. Acta Anaesthesiol Sin. 2001;39: 169–77.
51. Bozkurt P. Premedication of the paediatric patient—anaesthesia for the uncooperative child. Curr Opin Anaesthesiol. 2007;20:211–5.
52. Stewart SH, Buffett-Jerrott SE, Finley GA, et al. Effects of midazolam on explicit vs implicit memory in a paediatric surgery setting. Psycho pharmacology (Berl). 2006;188: 489–97.
53. Nishina K, Mikawa K, Uesugi T, et al. Oral clonidine premedication reduces minimum alveolar concentration of sevoflurane for laryngeal mask airway insertion in children. Pediatr Anesth. 2006;16:834–839.
54. Dahmani S, Brasher C, Stany I, et al. Premedication with clonidine is superior to benzodiazepines. A meta analysis of published studies. Acta Anaesthesiol Scand. 2010;54: 397–402.
55. Almenrader N, Passariello M, Coccetti B, et al. Premedication in children: A comparison of oral midazolam and oral ketamine. Paediatric Anesth. 2007;17:1143–9.
56. Jatti K, Batra YK, Bhardwaj N, et al. Comparison of psychomotor functions and sedation following premedication with oral diazepam and clonidine in children. Int J Clin Pharmacol Ther. 1998;36:336–9.
57. Ramesh VJ, Bhardwaj N, Batra YK. Comparative study of oral clonidine and diazepam as premedicants in children. Int J Clin Pharmacol Ther. 1997; 35:218–21.
58. Cao J, Shi X, Miao X, et al. Effects of premedication of midazolam or clonidine on perioperative anxiety and pain in children. Bio Science Trends. 2009;3:115–8.
59. Bergendahl H, Lonnqvist P, Eksborg S. Clonidine in paediatric anaesthesia: Review of the literature and comparison with benzodiazepines for premedication. Acta Anaesthesiol Scand. 2006;50:135–143.
60. Yuen VMY. Dexmedetomidine: perioperative applications in children. Pediatr Anesth. 2010;20: 256–64.
61. Anttila M, Penttila J, Helminen A, et al. Bioavailability of dexmedetomidine after extravascular doses in healthy subjects. Br J Clin Pharmacol. 2003; 56:691–3.
62. Yuen VM, Hui TW, Irwin MG, et al. A comparison of intranasal dexmedetomidine and oral midazolam for premedication in paediatric anaesthesia: A double-blinded randomized controlled trial. Anesth Analg. 2008;106: 1715–21.
63. Sakuri Y, Obata T, Odaka A, et al. Buccal administration of dexmedetomidine as a preanesthetic in children. J Anesth. 2010;24:49–53.
64. Schmidt AP, Valinetti EA, Bandeira D, et al. Effects of preanesthetic administration of midazolam, clonidine or dexmedetomidine on postoperative pain and anxiety in children. Pediatr Anesth. 2007; 17:667–74.
65. Alderson PJ, Lerman J. Oral premedication for paediatric ambulatory anaesthesia: a comparison of midazolam and ketamine. Can J Anaesth. 1994; 41:221–6.
66. Darlong V, Shende D, Subramanyam MS, et al. Oral ketamine or midazolam or low dose combination for premedication in children. Anesth Intens Care 2004;32:246–9.
67. Gingrich BK. Difficulties encountered in a comparative study of orally administered midazolam and ketamine. Anesthesiology. 1994;80:1414–5.
68. Funk W, Jakob W, Riedl T, et al. Oral preanesthetic medication for children: double-blind randomized study of a combination of midazolam and ketamine vs midazolam or ketamine alone. Brit J Anaesth. 2000;84:335–40.
69. Ghai B, Grandhe RP, Kumar A, et al. Comparative evaluation of midazolam and ketamine with midazolam alone as oral premedication. Pediatr Anesth. 2005;15:554–9.
70. Horiuchi T, Kawaguchi M, Kurehara K, et al. Evaluation of relatively low dose of oral transmucosal ketamine premedication in children: A comparison with oral midazolam. Pediatr Anesth. 2005;15:643–7.
71. Jia JE, Chen JY, Hu X, et al. A randomized study of intranasal dexmedetomidine and oral ketamine for premedication in children. Anaesthesia. 2013;68: 944–9.
72. Hannallah RS, Patel RL. Low-dose intramuscular ketamine for anaesthesia preinduction in young children undergoing brief outpatient procedures. Anesthesiology. 1989;70: 598–600.

Post-anaesthesia Care Unit Management

Arachana C Prabhu and Pallavi L Butiyani

BACKGROUND

Post-anaesthesia Care Unit (PACU), is a critical care area, where the paediatric patients are managed during the transition phase from anaesthesia to recovery. With advances in the anaesthesia techniques and newer short acting anaesthesia drugs, this phase has significantly reduced. Still PACU remains to be a challenge to anaesthesiologist. In PACU, every patient should get vigilant care, standard monitoring, adequate analgesia and timely management of any untoward complication. In this chapter we will discuss most common post-operative issues and their management.

EMERGENCE DELIRIUM (ED)

Introduction

Emergence delirium, also called emergence agitation or emergence excitement, is defined as a condition, in which emergence from general anaesthesia is accompanied by psychomotor agitation.

Presentation

ED is characterized by irritable, uncooperative, inconsolably crying, moaning, kicking or thrashing child.[1,2] ED is generally self-limiting and short lived, but in rare cases, it can be severe and lasts longer (as long as two days in one reported case). This behavior may result in harm to the child or to surgical site and also to the care giver.[3]

Risk Factors

Rapid emergence from anaesthesia,[4] use of newer volatile anaesthetics like sevoflurane, desflurane, 2–5 years old children,[5] patients undergoing Opthal and ENT surgeries,[6] preoperative anxiety are some of the risk factors.

Severity Scales

Various scales have been developed to measure the severity of ED, e.g. PAED scale (developed by Bajwa and colleagues), Watcha scale, Cravero scale, etc.

Watcha Scale

Behaviour	Score
Asleep	0
Calm	1
Crying but can be consoled	2
Crying but cannot be consoled	3
Agitated and thrashing around	4

Preventive Strategies and Treatment Options

1. **Counselling:** Adequate preoperative counselling of both child and parents with videos, pictures, etc. helps in reducing anxiety, which is a predisposing factor for ED.
2. **Sedation:** Intravenous sedation with midazolam, fentanyl, propofol.
3. **Parental reunion:** May help.

Take Home Messages

ED is a potentially dangerous, common postoperative issue in paediatric patients, especially associated with use of potent inhalational agents like sevoflurane and desflurane. Intravenous sedation with propofol, midazolam, and fentanyl is useful.

AIRWAY MANAGEMENT AND POSTOPERATIVE RESPIRATORY COMPLICATIONS IN PACU

Introduction

Post-anaesthesia recovery period is a time of significant risk for paediatric patients, especially neonates and infants. A large percentage of otherwise healthy infants and children develop oxygen desaturation during transport and on arrival in PACU. Therefore, the anaesthesiologist must be vigilant about the breathing pattern of child during transport, and child should get oxygen supplementation during transport.[7]

Ideal Airway Practice in PACU should be, on arrival in PACU, the anaesthesiologist should confirm the patency of airway, assess the adequacy of ventilation, and ensure adequate supply of humidified oxygen.

Common Airway Complications in PACU are: Airway obstruction, post-intubation croup, laryngospasm, pulmonary edema, respiratory insufficiency, etc.

Airway Obstruction

Diagnosed by observing paradoxical see-saw breathing pattern, intercostal in drawing, subcostal and/or sternal recession, tracheal tug,[8] and oxygen desaturation.[9] Most common causes of airway obstruction in immediate postoperative period are tongue fall, but secretions, blood and mucus in the airway and airway edema can also cause airway obstruction.

Management

Neck extension, mouth opening and jaw thrust alone or in combination are generally sufficient to relieve obstruction. Tongue fall can be prevented by positioning the patient in lateral position with neck extension. If these maneuvers fail to relieve the airway obstruction, insertion of nasopharyngeal or oropharyngeal airway can be considered. Nasopharyngeal airway is better tolerated. Video analysis of airway obstruction in children showed that, addition of CPAP of 10 cm of H_2O improves airway patency and significantly decreases the stridor score.[10] Following surgeries of the oral cavity, adenotonsillectomy, dental procedures, in addition to, secretions and blood clots, throat packs and airway edema can also result in airway obstruction. Throat inspection and pharyngeal suction under direct vision will prevent such obstruction.

Postintubation Croup

The reported incidence of post intubation croup is 1–6%.[11] The most common cause is tight fitting endotracheal tube, without leak at 25 to 40 cm of H_2O with IPPV. Other causes may include traumatic or repeated intubation, 'bucking' or coughing with endotracheal tube in place, changing head position, surgery lasting more than one hour, head and neck surgery.

Management

Cool and humidified oxygen administered after extubation may help in mild cases.

Racemic epinephrine, 0.25–0.5 mL of 2.25% solution, diluted in 3–5 mL normal saline nebulized with oxygen. It helps by producing mucosal vasoconstriction and shrinking the swollen airway mucosa. Child should be observed for at least four hours to manage 'Rebound effect". Dexamethasone is not very useful in immediate postoperative period, but a dose of 0.5 mg/kg used 6 hrly for first 24 hrs is useful to prevent rebound effect. Rarely a child might need reintubation with smaller size tube.

Laryngospasm

The incidence of perioperative laryngospasm is about 18/1000 in the age group of 0–9 yrs. Infants of 1–3 months age have highest incidence.[12] Many studies have shown that, active or recent upper respiratory infection is most commonly associated with perioperative laryngospasm. Other causes are airway surgery, airway irritation. There is controversy, as to, whether extubation should be at a deep or light plane of anaesthesia, in an attempt to prevent laryngospasm, but the available data is insufficient to prevent either view.

Management

Initial management is with chin lift, jaw thrust and application of CPAP with mask. Most of the time only this much is sufficient. Sometimes a small dose of propofol is required in addition. But rarely, severe laryngospasm fails to respond to above management and progresses to hypoxia and bradycardia. This needs muscle relaxation with succinyl choline.

Pulmonary Oedema

Pulmonary oedema developing shortly after the relief of airway obstruction is known as post-obstructive or negative pressure pulmonary edema. Presents with rales, wheezing, desaturation and copious production of pink frothy respiratory secretions.

Once airway obstruction is relieved, child should receive CPAP by mask (5–10 cm of H_2O), with high concentration of oxygen. Diuretics and fluid restriction is also helpful. If hypoxia persists, consider reintubation.

Respiratory Insufficiency

Residual effect of anaesthetics (especially opioids) or muscle relaxants, apnoea of prematurity and obstructive sleep apnoea are important causes.

Management

Opioid overdose: Diagnosed by hypoventilation, bradycardia, sedation and hypoxia.

Treatment is with Naloxone. A dose of 0.01 mg/kg repeated after every 2–3 min is recommended. Because of its shorter half-life, it requires repeated doses or continuous infusion. It has to be kept in mind that, naloxone reverses the analgesic effect of opioids. Rarely severe respiratory depression may need reintubation and ventilation.

Inadequate reversal of muscle relaxation: Diagnosed clinically simply by observing the child's breathing pattern, muscle weakness or with the help of peripheral nerve stimulator. Managed with additional dose of antagonist or reintubation and ventilation.

Apnoea of prematurity: Children born at less than 37 weeks of gestation are at risk for apnoea following general anaesthesia,[13] and can persist until 50 to 60 wks post-conceptual age.[14] Therefore, these infants should be in hospital overnight and observed after general anaesthesia.[15] Whenever possible, use of regional anaesthesia without sedation should be practiced. Caffeine in a dose of 10 mg/kg is found to be useful.[16]

Obstructive sleep apnoea: With increased incidence of childhood obesity, the incidence of OSA is also high. Most commonly done surgery in OSA is adenotonsillectomy. Commonly these patients can be treated on an outpatient basis, but severe OSA needs observation in post-operative period. These patients are sensitive to opioids, so should be used carefully. Use regional anaesthesia whenever possible.

Practical Key Points to Remember

Respiratory system management is the most vulnerable part in PACU. Respiratory reserve of child is significantly less, which makes the safety window small. Each paediatric patient should get supplemental oxygen and SpO_2 monitoring in PACU. High index of suspicion as well as early recognition and timely intervention is essential to prevent serious life threatening complications.

INTRAVENOUS FLUID THERAPY IN POSTOPERATIVE PERIOD

Introduction

Perioperative intravenous fluid therapy in paediatric patients is a topic for huge controversy since long. In 1957, Holliday and Segar described the maintenance fluid therapy concept, and the famous 4,2,1 formula was widely accepted.[17] But recent work has challenged this concept.

Fluid and Electrolyte Physiology in Children

Under normal conditions, 1 ml of water is required to metabolize 1 Kcal. So the energy and water consumption are equal.[18] Daily requirements of sodium and potassium are 3 mmol/kg and 2 mmol/kg respectively. Thus the daily requirement of fluid and electrolyte collectively results in hypotonic electrolyte solution. This explains the profound use of hypotonic solutions in paediatric practice. But this practice results in postoperative hyponatremia, which is the most frequent electrolyte disorder in paediatric patients. Severe hyponatremia (<120 mmol/L) can result in transient or permanent brain damage.[19]

Hypoglycemia is one of the most commonly feared risk in postoperative period in paediatric patients, especially very young population. So there is a trend towards using high concentration dextrose solutions both by anaesthesiologist and surgeons. In 1988, Lindahl found that energy expenditure in anaesthetized child was 50% lower than that calculated by Holliday and Segar.[20] Thus in practice it is found that use of high concentration dextrose solutions used in postoperative periods, causes significant hyperglycemia in patients.

Hyperglycemia induces osmotic diuresis and consequently dehydration and electrolyte disturbances.In various studies using different percentages of dextrose solutions and mixtures of dextrose and RL, it is found that , blood glucose and sodium values were maintained within acceptable limits with RL+1% Dextrose solution.[21–24]

By a series of clinical studies done in early 1990s the idea of developing a near ideal maintenance fluid for paediatric surgical patients leads to developing polyionique B66.[25] Composition of Polyionique B66 in mmol/L is, Sodium-120, Potassium-4, Calcium-2, Chloride-108, Lactate-20, and Dextrose-50.5. It is the fluid of choice in infants and young children (3 yrs).

For minor surgical procedures the intraoperative administration of large volumes of RL or Polyionique

B66 (10–20 mL/kg) is generally sufficient to replace preoperative fasting deficit as well as postoperative maintainance fluid replacement. This condition is called superhydration and is also found to reduce the incidence of postoperative nausea and vomiting in paediatric as well as adult patients.[26] In neonates the IV fluid of choice is dextrose 10% till first 3 days of life at a rate of 100–120 mL/kg/24 hrs.[27]

Recommendations for postoperative IV fluid therapy

1. Hypovolemia should be rapidly treated with isotonic fluid bolus of 10–20 mL/kg.
2. Preferred maintenance IV fluid for neonates is 10% dextrose, infants and children <3 years is RL with 1% dextrose or polyionique 66 and children >3 years is RL.
3. Adequacy of IV fluid therapy should be monitored time to time by clinical parameters like pulse rate, blood pressure, urine output, CRT, skin turgor.
4. Fluid used to dilute drugs should also be calculated. Preferably dilute in normal saline.

The Lindahl Formulae for calories, Fluid and Electrolyte requirement[28]

Caloric requirements = 1.5 × kg + 5 = Maintenance cal/hr (kcal/hr)

Fluid requirement = 2.5 × kg + 10 = Maintenance fluid/hr (mL/hr)

Sodium requirement = 0.045 × kg + 0.16 = Maintenance Na^+/hr (mEq/hr)

Potassium requirement = 0.03 × kg + 0.1 = Maintenance K^+/hr (mEq/hr)

POSTOPERATIVE PAIN MANAGEMENT

Introduction

Previously postoperative pain in children was of negligible consideration, because of the firm belief that small children might neither feel pain nor they have the memory of the incidence.[29]

Further, the negligence for effective postoperative pain relief is probably due to lack of knowledge and expertise, and fear of respiratory depression. Anand et al first described the effects of painful stimulus in neonates.[30]And now it is well accepted fact that even the fetus experiences pain and alleviation of pain is "Basic human right".[31]

Pain Assessment

In small babies it is very difficult to differentiate discomfort due to pain and that due to other causes like hunger, fear, etc. Most common scales[32–34] used to assess pain in newborns are: Premature infant pain profile (PIPP), CRIES postoperative pain scales. FLACC scale[35] is validated for assessment of postoperative pain in children between 2 months and 7 years. Around 3 to 4 years children may be able to report pain. Various self-report pain scales[36] are there for young children. For example, the Poker chip scale, Wong-Baker Faces scales, The Faces Pain scale-Revised (FPS-R), Oucher scale, etc. School children can generally use the same scales as adults without difficulty.

FLACC Behavioral Pain Assessment

FLACC behavioral pain assessment is given in Table 13.1.

Table 13.1 FLACC behavioral pain assessment

Categories	Scoring		
	0	1	2
Face	No particular expression or smile	Occasional grimace or frown, withdrawn, disinterested	Frequent to constant quivering chin, clenched jaw
Leg	Normal position or relaxed	Uneasy, restless, tense	Kicking or legs drawn up
Activity	Lying quietly, normal position, moves easily	Squirming, shifting back and forth, tense	Arched, rigid or jerking
Cry	No cry (awake or asleep)	Moans or whimpers, occasional complaints	Crying steadily, screams or sobs, frequent complaints
Consolability	Content, relaxed	Reassured by occasional touching, hugging, or being talked to, distractible	Difficult to console or comfort

ACUTE PAIN MANAGEMENT APPROACH

A. **Non-pharmacological:**[37]
- **Distraction** with games, toys, music, television.
- **Comforting** with parental contact, rocking, rubbing. Other therapies like hypnosis, acupuncture.

B. **Pharmacological:** Several drugs and routes are described for pain management in paediatric patients. Here we will discuss commonly used drugs and routes.

Drugs and Dosages

Non-opioid

- **Paracetamol**: Initial dose of up to 45 mg/kg[38,39] administered rectally before awakening from anaesthesia. Additional doses orally (10–15 mg/kg) or rectally (20 mg/kg) every 4–6 hrs. Total daily dose via any route should not exceed 100 mg/kg in children, 75 mg/kg for infants, 60 mg/kg for term and preterm neonates older than 32 wks, 40 mg/kg in preterm neonates less than 32 wks.[40,41]
- **Diclofenac:** More effective pain relief. 1 mg/kg every 8 hrly orally, rectally or intravenously.
- **Tramadol:** Can be used by oral, intravenously or rectal route in a dose of 1–2 mg/kg 8 hrly. Most troubling side effect is increased incidence of PONV. Other available drugs are ketorolac, ibuprofen.

Opioids

- **Fentanyl:** Short acting and potent in a dose of 1–2 µmg/kg. Side effects are sedation, respiratory depression, so needs close monitoring.
- **Codeine:** Especially if combined with paracetamol in a dose (0.5 mg/kg) is very useful.
- **Morphine:** 0.05–0.1 mg/kg.

Intravenous patient controlled analgesia: Can be used in older children. Morphine is the most commonly used drugs. The bolus dose and lock out period should be set according to individual patient.

Local anaesthetic: Can be used for local infiltration anaesthesia, ring blocks, e.g. penile block, nerve blocks and neuraxial blocks.

Caudal blocks: Very effective, and relatively safe. The volume and dose of drug is to be calculated according to dermatomes.

Armitage formula

0.5 mL/kg for a lumbosacral block
1 mL/kg for thoracolumbar block
1.25 mL/kg for mid-thoracic block

A mixture of 2% lignocaine and 0.25% bupivacaine, in equal parts gives faster onset and longer duration. Ropivacaine can also be used in caudal blocks.

Epidural: Can be used as single shot or continuous infusion. Insertion site depends on the site of incision. Bupivacaine: Initial loading dose is 2–2.5 mg/kg, infusion rate should not exceed 0.4–0.5 mg/kg/hr for neonates.[42]

Adjuvents: Opioids like fentanyl (1 µgm/kg), morphine, significantly increase duration of analgesia. Risk of respiratory depression is to be kept in mind. Others like Clonidine (1–2 µgm/kg), ketamine (1 mg/kg), tramadol (1–2 mg/kg), midazolam (50 µgm/kg) and neostigmine (20–50 µmg/kg) have also be found to be effective.

> **Paediatric Anaesthesia Pearls**
>
> Adequate pain relief is a Basic Human Right, and it has to be kept in mind in treating paediatric patients including neonates. Knowledge and skills in regional anaesthesia eases the job. Judicious use of Opioids and non-opioid analgesics helps in smooth recovery. Non-pharmacological methods like parental presence, distraction, comforting are very useful.

THERMOREGULATION IN CHILDREN

Introduction

Thermoregulation in human is a result of several feedback mechanisms with hypothalamus being the center. Thermoregulatory mechanisms are immature in neonates and young infants, they mature towards the end of first year of life.

Thermogenesis in Children

Normal thermogenesis in neonates and infants is by vasoconstriction and non-shivering thermogenesis[43] (Brown fat). In older children shivering also plays an important role.

Hypothermia: Defined as core body temperature less than 36° C.

Risk Factors for Hypothermia during Perioperative Period

Physiological factors[44] like large body surface area to body mass ratio, thin skin with less subcutaneous fat, large head size.

Environmental factors like cold operating room and PACU.

Anaesthesia and surgery related factors: General as well as neuraxial anaesthesia, use of cold anaesthetic gases, IV fluids and irrigation fluid, large surgical exposure and prolong surgeries.

Effects of hypothermia are increased oxygen consumption due to shivering[45] (40–100% but as high as 500%), increased perioperative blood loss due to platelet dysfunction and coagulopathy, longer post-anaesthetic recovery due to altered drug metabolism, wound infection and delayed wound healing.

Prevention and treatment of hypothermia:[46] Monitor core body temperature every 30 min., maintain ambient temperature around 24° C, cover patient adequately, active warming with forced air warmers, fan healers, warming blanket or overhead heater and supplement oxygen till the patient is normothermic.

Hyperthermia: Defined as core body temperature of 38°C and above.

Causes of hypothermia in PACU[47] are excessive warming, bacteremia, inflammatory stimulus of surgery, drug fever, rare causes, like malignant hyperthermia and neuroleptic malignant syndrome.

Treatment[48] consists of minimizing clothing and blankets, exposing the skin to air, increase air circulation, sponging with cold water, and consider antipyretic such as paracetamol.

MALIGNANT HYPERTHERMIA

Introduction

It is a hyper metabolic state, described by Denborough in 1960.[49] It has autosomal dominant inheritance, defect located on long arm of chromosome 19.

Causes and risk factors are exposure to certain drugs, most commonly inhalational anaesthetics, depolarizing muscle relaxants, catecholamines,[50] males are more commonly affected. Previously it was thought that muscular dystrophies (like duchenne, becker) have definite association with susceptibility for MH but now this association is being questioned.[51]

Signs and Symptoms

Most commonly occurs in anaesthetized patients in operating room but can occur in early postoperative period.[52] The signs and symptoms include, high body temperature (the rate of increase is very important. It can be as rapid as 1 °C every 5 min. Temperatures have been reported as high as 46 °C[53]), muscle rigidity, tachycardia, tachypnea, increased CO_2 production (can be >100 mmHg) and oxygen consumption, acidosis, hyperkalemia, rhabdomyolysis, myoglobin urea, etc.

Treatment: Dantrolene: Initial dose of 2.5 mg/kg repeated every 5 min until symptoms reverse or maximum dose of 10 mg/kg. Once patient is stabilized, maintenance dose of 1 mg/kg, every 4–8 hrly for 24–48 hrs. Cooling of the body by applying ice packs to exposed body, nasogastric lavage with iced solution. Treatment of associated electrolyte abnormalities, arrhythmias.

Must do a thing for paediatric patients under anaesthesia:

Thermoregulation in children is immature, making them more vulnerable to hypothermia. Preventing heat loss and active warming in intraoperative as well as postoperative period is essential.

SEIZURES IN PACU

Etiology: Hyponatremia (Na <120mEq/L), hypoglycemia, hyperthermia, hypoxia and hypercarbia. Patients with known seizure disorder can get seizures in PACU.

Management goals are to avoid injury to tongue, secure airway, supplement oxygen, control seizure, correction of underlying issue.

Objectives of Acute Management of Seizure

Maintenance of adequate airway, breathing and circulation (ABC): Open airway by manipulation or oropharyngeal airway. Clear the airway by suctioning secretions or mucous. Administer supplemental oxygen. Assist breathing, if required. May need endotracheal intubation and ventilation.

Terminate seizure with short acting benzodiazepines like midazolam, either IV or as nasal spray (0.2 mg/kg). Intravenous anaesthetic agents like propofol, thiopentone are also useful. In severe cases consider paralysis with muscle relaxants.

Find and treat the predisposing factor. Investigate for blood sugar, electrolyte and arterial blood gas abnormalities.

Anticonvulsants are generally not required and the seizures stop spontaneously. But in rare cases it may need further neurological investigations.[54]

PONV

Generally considered as a minor issue, but in fact it is a common cause of postoperative morbidity. School children have the highest incidence[55,56] of 34–50% while lowest in infants (5%). Middle ear surgery, tonsillectomy, strabismus repair, laparotomy and laparoscopy have increased risk.[57] Longer duration of surgery and gastric distention following inappropriate mask ventilation are also found to increase incidence of PONV. Severe PONV can lead to wound dehiscence, aspiration of gastric contents, bleeding, dehydration and electrolyte disturbances.

Most commonly used drugs to treat PONV are metoclopramide (0.25 mg/kg) or ondensetron (0.1–0.15 mg/kg). Droperidol (75 mcg/kg) is also useful but can cause sedation, lethargy, agitation, and extrapyramidal effects. Dexamethasone and propofol also have role in resistant cases.

SUMMARY AND CONCLUSION

Post-anaesthesia care unit (PACU), is a critical care area, where the paediatric patients are managed during the transition phase from anaesthesia to recovery. With advances in the anaesthesia techniques and newer short acting anaesthesia drugs, this phase has significantly reduced. A few critical areas discussed above are summarized as below:

a. ED is a potentially dangerous, common post-operative issue in paediatric patients.
b. Respiratory system management is the most vulnerable part in PACU. Respiratory reserve of child is significantly less, which makes the safety window small. Each paediatric patient should get supplemental oxygen and SpO_2monitoring in PACU.
c. Adequate pain relief is a Basic Human Right, and it has to be kept in mind in treating paediatric patients including neonates.
d. Thermoregulation in children is immature, making them more vulnerable to hypothermia. Preventing heat loss and active warming in intraoperative as well as postoperative period is essential.

REFERENCES

1. Linda J Mason. Pitfalls of paediatric anaesthesia, pedsanaesthesia.org 2004.
2. Vlajikovic GP, Sindjelic RP. Emergence delirium in children: many questions, few answers. Anesth analg 2007;104: 84–91.
3. Smessaert A, Schehr CA, Artusio JFJ. Observations in the immediate postanaesthesia period. II. Mode of recovery. Br J Anaesthesia 1960;32:181–185.
4. Laila Rodugue, Susan Vergese. Paediatric emergence delirium. Contin Educ. Anaesth Crit Care Pain 2012, doi 10.1093/bjaceaccp/mks051.
5. Aono J, Ueda W, Mamiya K, et al. Greater incidence of delirium during recovery from sevoflurane in preschool boys. Anesthesiology 1997;87:1298–1300.
6. Voepel-Lewis T, Malviya S, Tait AR. A prospective cohort study of emergence agitation in paediatric post-anaesthesia care unit. Anesth Analg 2003;96: 1625–1630.
7. Controversies in paediatric anaesthesia—CLSF News, Aug, 2001;10(5).
8. Dilip Pawar: Common postoperative complications in children, IJA Sep-Oct, 2012;56(5):496–501.
9. Paediatric anaesthesia, 4th edn, George Gregory, p. 242.
10. Meirer S, Geiduschek J, Paganoni R, et al. The effect of chin lift, jaw thrust and continuous positive airway pressure on the size of the glottis opening and on stridor score in anaesthetized spontaneously breathing children, Anaesth Analg 2002;94:494–499.
11. Understanding Paediatric Anaesthesia by Rebecca Jacob, p. 112.
12. Pankaj Kundra, Hari Krisnan S. Airway management in Children, IJA. 2005;49(4):300–307.
13. Gregory GA, Steward DJ: Life threatening perioperative apnea in 'Ex-Premie' Anaesthesiology. 1983;59:495.
14. Kurth CD, Spitzer AR, Broennle AM et al. Postoperative apnea in former preterm infants: prospective comparison of spinal and general anaesthesia. Anesthesiology 1987;66:483.
15. Paediatric Anaesthesia, 4th edn, George Gregory, p 243.
16. Henderson-Smart DJ, Steer P. Postoperative caffeine for preventing apnoea in preterm infants. Cochrane Database syst Rev. 2000;2:CD000048 PubMed.
17. Holliday M, Segar W. The maintenance need for water in parenteral fluid therapy. Paediatrics 1957; 19:823–832.
18. Isabella Murat, Marie-Claude Dubois. Perioperative fluid therapy in paediatric practice, Euroanaesthesia 2008.
19. Arieff AI. Postoperative hyponatraemia encephalopathy following elective surgery in children. Paediatric Anesth 1998;8:1–4.
20. Lindahl SG. Energy expenditure and fluid and electrolyte requirements in anaesthetized infants and children. Anaesthesiology 1988;69:377–382.
21. Aun CS, Panesar NS. Paediatric glucose homeostasis during anaesthesia, Br. J. Anaesth 1992;2:99–104.
22. Dubois M, Gouyet L, Murat I. Lactated Ringer with 1% Dextrose, an appropriate solution for perioperative fluid therapy in children. Paediatric anaesth 1992;2:99–104.
23. Hongnat J, Murat I, Saint Maurice C. Evaluation of current paediatric guidelines for fluid therapy using two different dextrose hydrating solutions Paediatric Anaesth 1991;1: 95–100.
24. Welborn LG, Hannallah RS, McGrill WA, et al. Glucose concentrations for routine intravenous infusions in paediatric outpatient surgery. Anaesthesiology 1987;67: 427–430.
25. Robert G. Hahn. Clinical fluid therapy in the perioperative setting.

26. Goodarzi M, Matar MM, Shafa M, et al. A prospective randomized blinded study of effect of intravenous fluid therapy on postoperative nausea and vomiting in children undergoing strabismus surgery. Paediatric Anesth. 2006;16:49–53.
27. Emma Dickson, Carolyn Smith. Infant 2006;2(5).
28. George Gregory. Paediatric Anaesthesia. 4th edn. p 8.
29. Aynsley, Green A, et al. Pain and stress in infancy and childhood-where to now? Paediatric Anaesth 1996;6: 167–172.
30. Anand KJS, Carr DB, Hickey PR. Randomized trial of high dose sufentanyl anaesthesia in neonates undergoing cardiac surgery; hormonal and hemodynamic stress responses. Anaesthesiology 1987;67:A502.
31. Frank HK. The society of Paediatric Anaesthesia, 15th Annual meeting, New Orleans, Louisiana oct 2001, Anesth Analg 2002;94:1661–1668.
32. Gurnau RV, Johnstan CC, Craig KD. Neonatal facial and cry responses to invasive and non-invasive procedures. Pain 1990;42:295–305.
33. Stevens B, Johnston C, Petryshen P, et al. Premature infant pain profile: development and initial validation. Clin J Pin 1996;12:13–22.
34. Lawrence J, Alcock D, McGrath P, et al. The development of a tool to assess neonatal pain. Neonatal netw. 1993;12:59–66.
35. Merkel S, Shayevitz JR, Voepel Lewis T, et al. The FLACC: A behavioral scale for scoring postoperative pain in young children. Paediatric Nurs. 1997;23:293–297.
36. American Medical Association, Module 6, Paediatric pain management updated 2013.
37. Travers Am, Diedericks J. Postoperative pain relief in children. Specialist medicine March 1994;12–9.
38. Susan T Verghese, Raafat S Hannallah. Acute pain management in children. J Pin Res. 2010;3:105–123.
39. Montogomery CJ, MC Cormack JP, Reichert CC, et al. Plasma concentrations after high dose (45 mg/kg) rectal acetaminophen in children. Can J Anaesth 1995;42:982–986.
40. Berde CB, Srthna NF. Analgesics for treatment of pain in children, N Engl J Med 2002;347:1094–1103.
41. Anderson BJ, Holford NH, Woollard GA et al. Perioperative pharmacodynamics of acetaminophen analgesia in children. Anesthesiology 1999; 90:411–421.
42. Berde CB. Convulsions associated with paediatric regional anaesthesia. Anesth Analog 1992;75:164–166.
43. Bajwa SJS, Swati. Perioperative hypothermia in Paediatric patients: Diagnosis, prevention and management, Anaesth pain and intensive care 2014;18(1):97–100.
44. Arndt K. In advert Hypothermia in OR.AORNJ. Aug, 1999; 70(2):204–6, 208–14.
45. Bay J, Nunn JF, Pry S, et al. Factors influencing arterial PO_2 during recovery from anaesthesia. Br J Anaesth. 1968;40(6):398–407.
46. AORN Recommended Practices committee: Recommended practices for the prevention of unplanned perioperative hypothermia. AORN J. May 2007;85(5):972–4, 976–84, 986–88.
47. George Gregory. Paediatric anaesthesia. 4th edn. p 76.
48. Great Ormond street hospital for children, guidelines for recovery care of the child/young person.
49. Denborough MA, Lovell RRH, et al. Anaesthetic deaths in a family. Lancet 1960;2:45.
50. Rosenber H, Daris M, James D, et al. Orphanet J of rare diseases 2007;2–21.
51. Maslow A, Lisbon A. Anaesthetic considerations in the patients with mitochondrial dysfunction Anaesth Analog 1993;76:884–886.
52. James W Chaplin: Malignant hyperthermia, Medscape Feb. 11, 2013.
53. Course study: 9076: Postoperative complications.
54. Robert Tasker. Arch dis child 1998:79;78–83, doi 1136/abc 79.1.78.
55. Watcha MF, White PF. Postoperative nausea and vomiting. Its etiology, treatment and prevention. Anesthesiology. 1992;77:162–84.
56. Cohen MM, Cameron CB, Duncan PG. Paediatric anaesthesia morbidity and mortality in perioperative period. Anesthe Analg. 199;70:160–167.
57. JB Rose, MF Watcha. Postoperative nausea and vomiting in paediatric patients. Br J Anaesthesia. 1999;83(1):104–117.

14

Equipment

RD Patel, Amit Padvi and Namrata Padvi

INTRODUCTION

Improvement in the paediatric anaesthetic care occurs with the innovation in equipment. Remarkable changes such as laryngeal mask airways, fibreoscopes, cuffed endotracheal tubes and double lumen tubes significantly alter our practical approach towards different paediatric surgeries and patients.

Medical equipment designs with innovative changes have dramatic impact on paediatric anaesthesia practice since past few years.

In this chapter we will discuss the commonly used paediatric anaesthesia equipments.

PAEDIATRIC FACE MASKS (Table 14.1)

I. It is frequently used airway equipment (Fig. 14.1)

II. Face masks provide an interface between the child and the breathing system.

III. An ideal face mask for paediatric use should:

a. Properly fit with adequate seal covering nasal bridge to just below lower lip without compressing the nasal passage (to prevent leaks during positive pressure ventilation and dilution of anaesthetic gases during spontaneous ventilation).

b. Minimal dead space

c. Have a soft rim to minimize pressure and prevent trauma.

d. Be of the correct size to avoid pressure on the eyes.

e. Transparent which allows the inspection of visible breathing (humidity), secretions (vomiting) and lip colour (cyanosis).

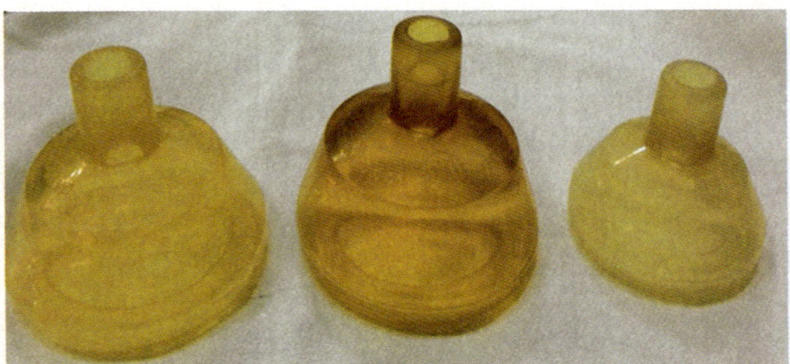

Fig. 14.1 Paediatric face masks

Table 14.1 Face mask sizing

Size	Age
00	Preterm
0	Neonate–3 months
1	3 months–Up to 1 year
2	1–5 years
3	More than 5 years
4	Adult

Indications

1. It is used for pre-oxygenation prior to induction.
2. Mask ventilation during inhalational induction, maintenance with spontaneous ventilation.
3. Positive pressure ventilation before intubation.

- Round, transparent, plastic face masks with an inflatable rim are used for neonates and infants (sizes 1 and 2). They have a larger dead space, they are easier to position.
- A teardrop shape is generally used for older children (sizes 3 and 4).

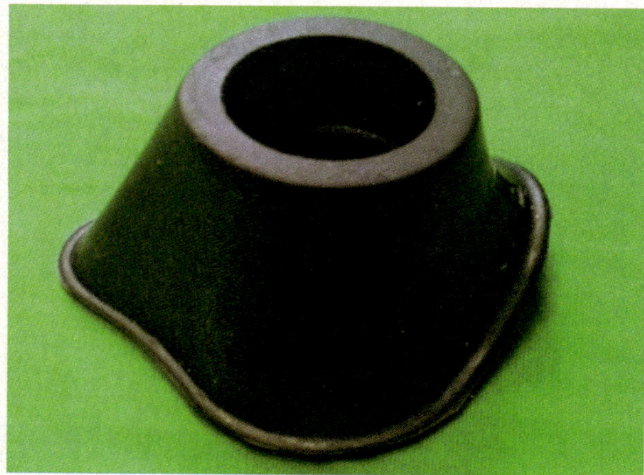

Fig. 14.2 Rendell-Baker face mask

- Acceptability to the child can be improved by the use of scented masks.
- The Rendell-Baker face mask, although originally devised to minimize dead space, does not have an inflatable cuff and is now rarely used (Fig. 14.2).

Face masks or angle pieces can be adapted for the passage of a fibreoptic bronchoscope called Patil Syracuse mask.

OROPHARYNGEAL AIRWAYS

- The oropharyngeal Guedel airways are widely used in paediatric patients (Fig. 14.3 and Table 14.2).

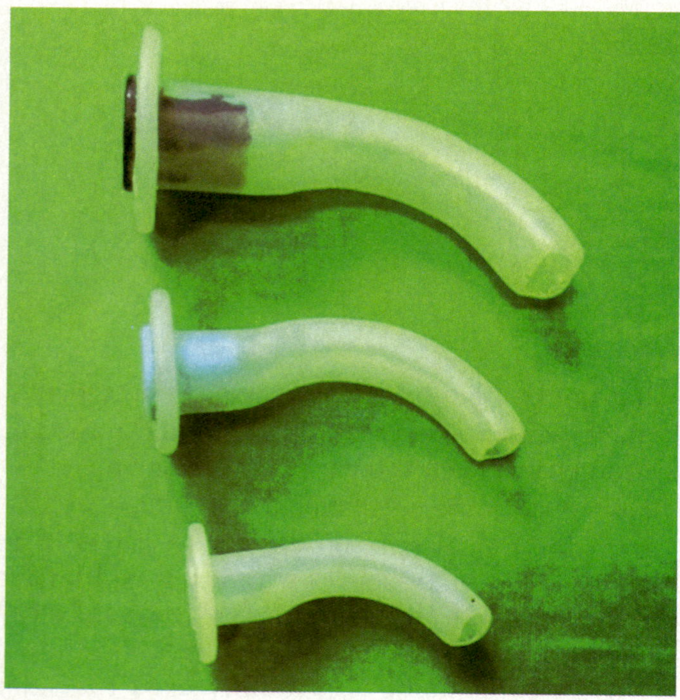

Fig. 14.3 Oropharyngeal Guedel airways

Table 14.2 Guedel oropharyngeal airways

Size	Age
00,000	Preterm
0	Neonate–3 months
1	3 months–Up to 1 year
2	1–5 years
3	More than 5 years
4	Adult

- It is used to prevent the tongue and epiglottis from occluding the upper airway.
- It can be used for the prevention of gastric distension during mask ventilation.
- It is very helpful for the airway management of children with micrognathia, a large tongue (e.g. Down's) or Pierre Robin, Hurler's, Hunter's, or Goldenhar syndromes, etc.
- The use of correct size airway is a necessity for its effective application. The correct length is determined by the distance between the centre of the incisors and the angle of the jaw. The distal end should lie just above the epiglottis. An incorrect choice of airway size can worsen airway obstruction and cause trauma and laryngospasm.

Clinical Pearls

1. The correct length of oropharyngeal airway is determined by the distance between the centre of the incisors and the angle of the jaw.
2. Insertion of airway during lighter planes of anaesthesia can trigger laryngospasm or vomiting if pharyngeal reflexes are not sufficiently depressed.

NASOPHARYNGEAL AIRWAY (NPA)

1. It helps to maintain the patency of nasal passage from nostril to nasopharynx (Fig. 14.4).
2. Can be of use in children with airway problems.
3. The distance from the tip of the nostril to the tragus of the ear gives the correct length of NPA so that the distal end should lie just above the epiglottis.[1]
4. Nasopharyngeal airways should be well lubricated before insertion.
5. Avoid the use if there is evidence of coagulopathy or nasal deformity.
6. It is contraindicated in children with basal skull fracture.
7. Nasopharyngeal airways may also be used for the provision of nasal CPAP in small infants.[2]

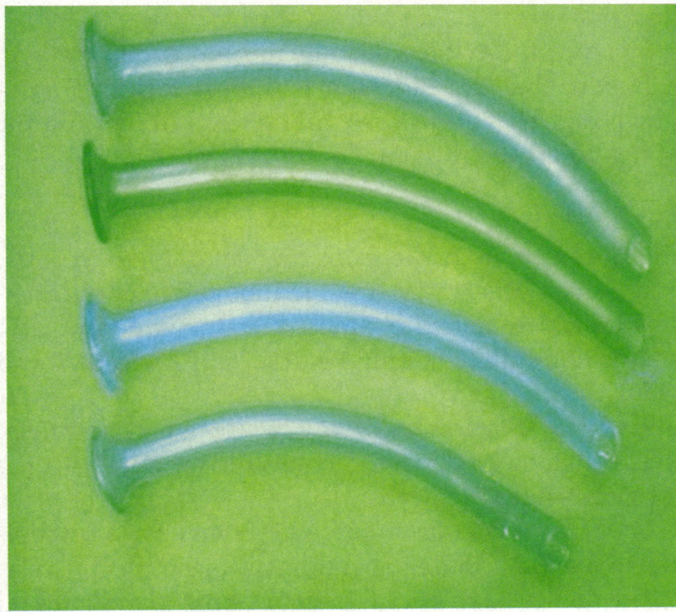

Fig. 14.4 Nasopharyngeal airway

LARYNGEAL MASK AIRWAY (LMA)

1. The laryngeal mask airway (LMA) is a supraglottic airway device.
2. LMA was developed by Dr Archie I. J Brain in 1983.
3. LMAs are classified according to design 1st and 2nd generations.
4. Relatively non-invasive as compared to endotracheal intubation.
5. LMA provides a low pressure seal over the glottis.
6. Easy to insert and remove as compared to endo-tracheal tube.
7. Minimal disturbances in the cardiovascular and respiratory system observed during the use of LMA compared to ETT.
8. Lesser risk of airway injury

Successful placement depends upon

1. Selection of optimal size of LMA
2. Pharyngeal tone, position of head and neck, shape of the palato-pharyngeal curve, and depth of anaesthesia.
3. Adequate inflation volume of LMA cuff to achieve airtight seal.

Techniques of insertion[3]

1. Using the thumb and index finger to guide the LMA against the hard palate.
2. Using a modified preconfigured styletted LMA.
3. Inserting a partially inflated LMA laterally 45° against side of tongue, advancing until resistance is met and then rotating back into midline.

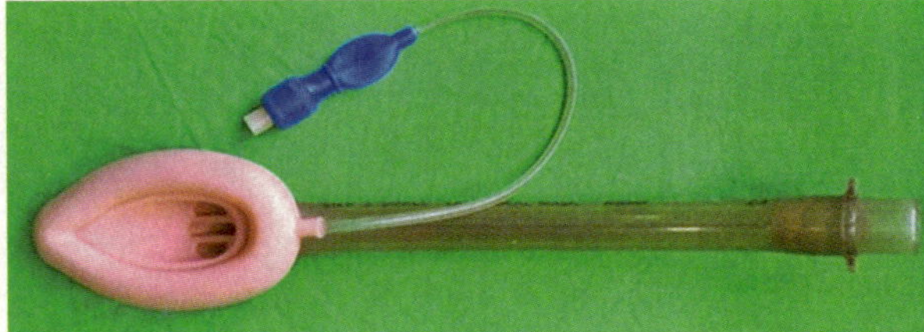

Fig. 14.5 LMA Classic™

4. Inserting the LMA with its cuff facing the palate and turned 180° as entering hypopharynx—similar to inserting an adult Guedel airway.

First Generation LMA

Classic™ LMA (cLMA)

1. The LMA Classic™ was first introduced in U.K. in 1988 as an alternative to the face mask (Fig. 14.5).
2. The soft silicone cuff reduces the likelihood of throat irritation and stimulation.
3. It has the widest range of sizes, from neonate to large adults.
4. The LMA Classic™ is ideally suited for elective, outpatient surgical procedures.
5. It is most often used in spontaneously breathing patients, but can also be used with assisted and controlled ventilation up to 20 cm H_2O.
6. It can be used successfully in emergency situations, including difficult airways and neonatal resuscitation.
7. Clinical advantages:
   a. More secure ventilation than a face mask.
   b. Allows single-handed ventilation.
   c. Rapid, blind insertion (without laryngoscopy).
   d. Part of the ASA difficult airway algorithm.

Clinical Pearl

The classic laryngeal mask airway (cLMA), in paediatric patients forms a less effective glottic seal in children than in adults.[4,5]

Second Generation LMA

A. Pro-Seal® laryngeal mask airway (PLMA)
B. i-gel® LMA

Advantages of second generation LMA[6]

1. Improved pharyngeal seal enabling controlled ventilation.
2. Increased oesophageal seal preventing the regurgitant fluid aspiration.
3. A drain tube which provides oesophageal seal.

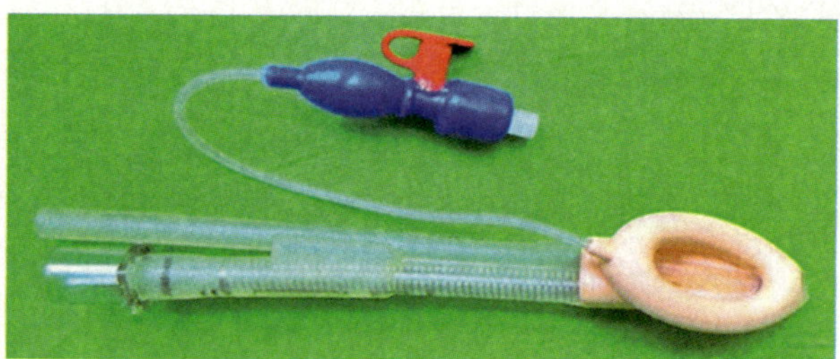

Fig. 14.6 Pro-Seal® laryngeal mask airway (PLMA)

It helps to:
a. Assist insertion.
b. Confirm correct device positioning.
c. Suction the stomach.
d. Minimizes chances of regurgitation in oropharynx.

Pro-Seal® Laryngeal Mask Airway (PLMA)

It is a supraglottic airway device with a gastric drain tube (Fig. 14.6 and Table 14.3)).

The LMA Pro-Seal® has four main components:

1. **Mask:** The mask has a main cuff that seals around the laryngeal opening and the larger sizes also have a dorsal cuff which helps to increase the seal.
2. **Inflation line with pilot balloon:** It is terminating in a pilot balloon and valve for mask inflation and deflation. A red plug is also fitted to the valve to aid effective steam sterilisation.
3. **Airway tube:** The airway tube is wire reinforced to prevent collapse and terminates with a standard 15 mm connector.
4. **Drain tube:** A drain tube passes lateral to the airway tube and traverses the floor of the mask opening at the mask tip opposite the upper oesophageal sphincter. It allows for blind insertion of standard oro-gastric tubes, in any patient position, without the need to use Magill's forceps.
5. **Introducer tool:** PLMA is provided with an introducer tool to aid into successful insertion.

Table 14.3 Inflation cuff volume for LMA Pro-Seal® according to weight

Size	Child's weight		Volume of cuff inflation	Oro-gastric tube
1	Infant	<5 kg	5 mL	8 fr
1½	Infant	5–10 kg	7 mL	10 fr
2	Child	10–20 kg	10 mL	10 fr
2½	Child	20–30 kg	14 mL	14 fr
3	Child	30–50 kg	20 mL	16 fr
4	Adult	50–70 kg	30 mL	16 fr
5	Adult	70–100 kg	40 mL	18 fr

Sterilisation

1. Steam autoclaving is the only recommended method.
2. Ensure that the red plug is opened prior to autoclaving. This allows any air or moisture within the cuff to escape thus preventing rupture.

i-gel® LMA

The i-gel gets its name from the soft gel-like material from which it is made. It is the innovative application of material that has enabled the development of a unique non-inflatable cuff (Fig. 14.7 and Tables 14.4 and 14.5).

1. The i-gel® is a unique airway device which is cuffless.
2. The shape, softness and contours accurately to the perilaryngeal anatomy.
3. The non-inflatable cuff of i-gel® is made of a soft gel-like medical grade thermoplastic elastomer.
4. The device has a buccal cavity stabilizer and integral bite block, epiglottic rest with a protective ridge which prevents down folding of the epiglottis during insertion.

ENDOTRACHEAL TUBE

"The endotracheal tube is the link between our most expensive and our most sophisticated object, our anaesthesia machine, and our most delicate and most precious subject, our paediatric patients."

Andreas C Gerber[7]

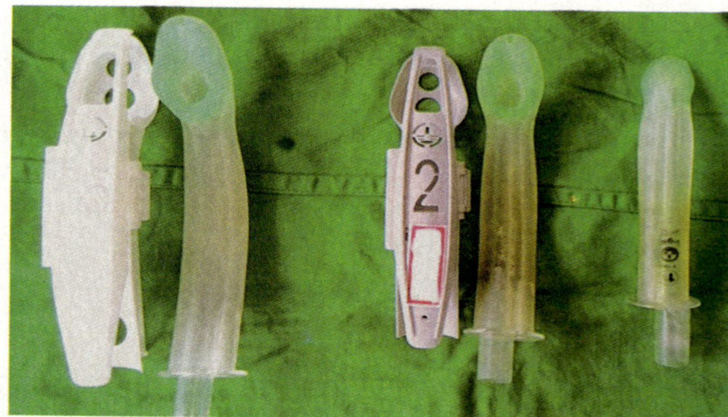

Fig. 14.7 i-gel® supraglottic airway is supplied in colour-coded poly-propylene 'cage pack'

Table 14.4 i-gel® supraglottic airway is supplied in colour-coded polypropylene 'cage pack'

i-gel® LMA	Sizes	Weight	Colour code
	1.0	2–5 kg	Pink
	1.5	5–12 kg	Blue
	2	10–25 kg	Grey
	2.5	25–35 kg	White

Table 14.5 Summary of supraglottic airway devices

Sl. No.	Supraglottic devices	Paediatric sizes; recommended weight range	Generation
1	cLMA	1.0: <5 kg 1.5: 5–10 kg 2.0: 10–20 kg 2.5: 20–30 kg	1st
2	PLMA	1.0: <5 kg 1.5: 5–10 kg 2.0: 10–20 kg 2.5: 20–30 kg	2nd
3	i-gel	1.0: 2–5 kg 1.5: 5–12 kg 2: 10–25 kg 2.5: 25–35 kg	2nd

2nd generation devices incorporate design features to reduce regurgitation risk.

1. Endotracheal tube is gold standard mean of establishing and maintaining a patent airway to ensure adequate exchange of oxygen and carbon dioxide (Fig. 14.8).
2. Originally made from red rubber, most modern tubes are now made from polyvinyl chloride, but tubes constructed of silicone rubber, latex rubber are available.
3. Types of endotracheal tube include oral or nasal, cuffed or uncuffed, preformed (e.g. RAE (Ring, Adair, and Elwyn) tube), reinforced tubes, and double-lumen endobronchial tubes (Fig. 14.9).
4. Finding the correct-sized tube is important, to avoid large leaks around the tube and to avoid airway trauma because of oversized ETT.

Clinical Pearl

Endotracheal tubes in small children are uncuffed, because of the anatomic differences of the larynx and cricoid ring being the narrowest portion.

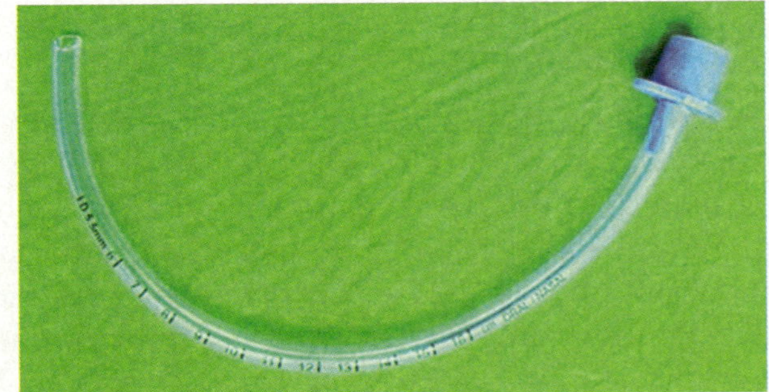

Fig. 14.8 Endotracheal tube

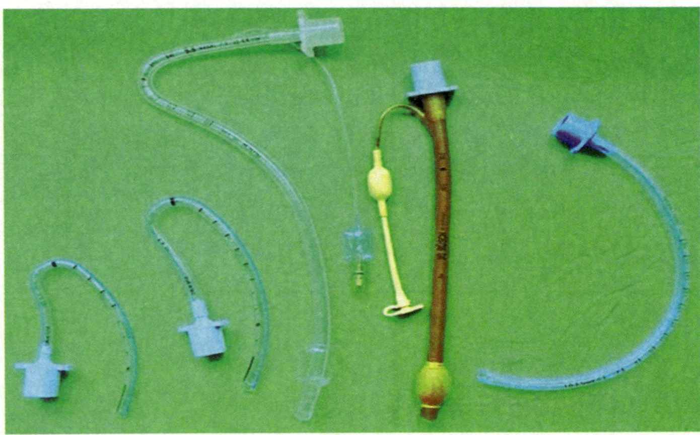

Fig. 14.9 Different types of endotracheal tube

Indications

1. To maintain the patency of airway to ensure adequate exchange of oxygen and carbon dioxide
2. To provide controlled ventilation in unconscious patient
3. To provide a secure airway for transport

Sizing

1. Uncuffed ETT size can be estimated by the equation: (Age in years/4) + 4 = size of endotracheal tube (ET) mm. This age-based formula has been shown to be more accurate than methods estimating ETT size based on width of the patient's fifth finger.[8]
2. Cuffed ETT size can be calculated from the Khine's equation: (Age in years/4) + 3 = size of endotracheal tube (ET) mm or one-half smaller size than the calculated cuffed ETT diameter.[9]
3. **Penlington's formula** (most common):
   - For age <6 years, (Age in years/3) + 3.5 = size of endotracheal tube (ET) mm
   - For age >6 years, (Age in years/4) + 4.5 = size of endotracheal tube (ET) mm
4. **For premature newborn:** Table 14.6.

Depth of ETT insertion: Distance at the lips

1. Visualise the tube passing through vocal cords avoiding endobronchial intubation.

Table 14.6 Endotracheal tube size and depth of insertion in newborns

Weight (kg)	Endotracheal size (mm internal diameter)	Depth of placement (cm)
Less than 1.5	2–2.5	6–7
1.5–2.5	2.5–3.0	7–8
>2.5	3–3.5	8

2. Black mark at the bottom of ET tube should be at cord level.
3. Multiply ET internal diameter by 3.
4. Newborns ('Tip to Lip' distance = 6 + Weight in kg)
   a. Weight 1 kg: Insert 7 cm depth
   b. Weight 2 kg: Insert 8 cm depth
   c. Weight 3 kg: Insert 9 cm depth
   d. Weight 4 kg: Insert 10 cm depth

   and

   a. Infant under 6 months: 10 cm
   b. Infant under 1 year: 11 cm
   c. Child under 2 years: 12 cm
   d. Child over 2 years: (Age in years)/2 + 12 cm

Clinical Pearl

For clinical use cuffed endotracheal tubes are available from size 5 mm ID.

Flexometallic or Armored Tube

1. The "armored" endotracheal tubes are cuffed, wire-reinforced, silicone rubber tubes which are quite flexible but yet difficult to compress or kink (Fig. 14.10).
2. It is useful if the neck is to remain flexed during surgery (head neck surgeries), airway surgeries, etc.
3. Difficult insertion: Stylet is required.
4. Spirals do not allow the tube to be cut to desired length.
5. Does not have a Murphy eye, hence may cause airway obstruction if the bevel abuts against tracheal wall.

Clinical Pearl

Armoured tubes are non-transparent and slippery, hence proper fixation is required.

Double-lumen Tube

1. Various types of double-lumen endotracheal tubes have been developed (Carlens, White, Robertshaw, etc.) for ventilating each lung independently—this is useful during thoracic operations. These allow single-lung ventilation, while the other lung is collapsed to make surgery easier (Fig. 14.11).
2. Double-lumen endotracheal tube is essentially two single lumen tubes of different length bound together and termed right or left sided depending on which mainstem bronchus the tube is designed to fit. The shorter tube terminates above the carina and the longer extends to the mainstem bronchus designed to fit.
3. The tube has two curves, namely an anterior curve to fit the oropharyngeal-laryngotracheal curvature and a bronchial curve to the right or left depending on the bronchus designed to fit.
4. The tube has two cuffs. One cuff seals the trachea and the other the bronchial stem which seals the main bronchus. Both cuffs have separate inflation tubes, pilot balloons and connectors which are colour coded.
5. Robertshaw (and others) developed double-lumen endobronchial tubes for thoracic surgery. The smallest available size is 26 Fr (for 8–10 years age).
6. Marraro tube is a bilumen tube for infants. It consists of two separate uncuffed tubes attached longitudinally at different lengths.

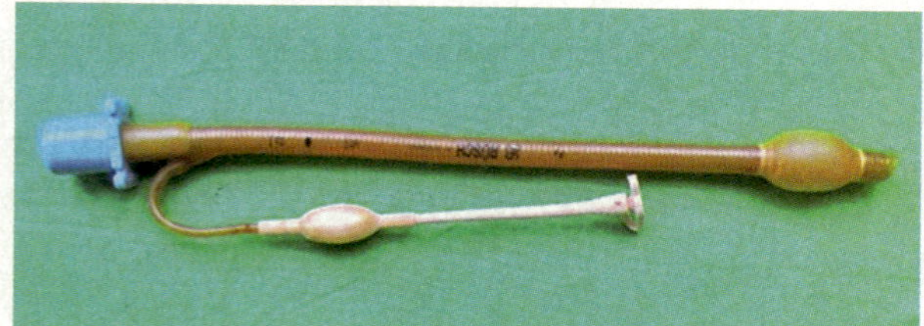

Fig. 14.10 Armored tube

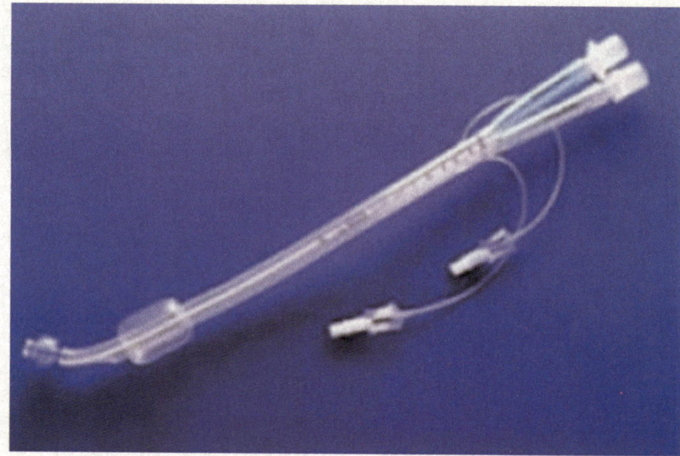

Fig. 14.11 Double-lumen tube

Preformed Tubes

Preformed tubes such as the oral and nasal RAE tubes are named after the inventors Ring, Adair and Elwyn. These may also be made of polyvinyl chloride or wire-reinforced silicone rubber. South pole tubes are used for cleft lip or palate repair and nasal surgeries. North pole tubes are used for facial, mandibular and intra-oral surgeries. Selection of a proper sized tube is essential as a smaller sized tube might not reach

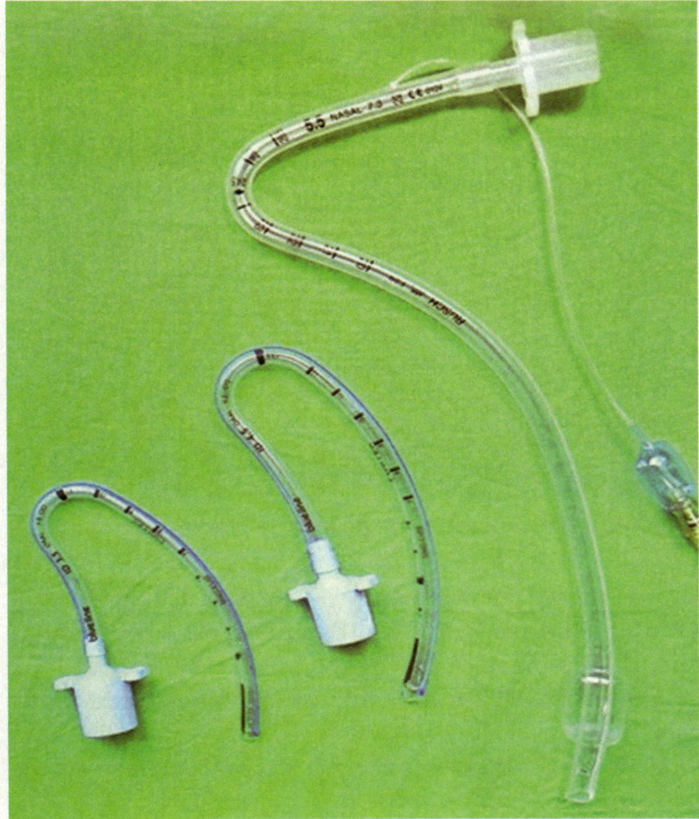

Fig. 14.12 Preformed tube

below the larynx. Child's height and weight is more important than age in selecting the correct size of tube (Fig. 14.12).

> **Clinical Pearls**
> 1. Prefixed shape tends to have endobronchial migration with change in position, therefore, accurate sized tube should be used.
> 2. Suctioning through preformed tube is technically difficult.
> 3. Prefixed tube offers more resistance to breathing than standard ETT.

MICROCUFF Paediatric Endotracheal Tube*

The Microcuff endotracheal tubes were invented in 2004 with ultra thin high volume low pressure polyurethane cuff (Fig. 14.13 and Table 14.7).

The improved features:

1. Polyurethane high volume low pressure cuff with improved sealing characteristics.
2. The cuff is placed more distally.
3. Cuff below the narrow cricoid ring and theoretically reduces the chance of main bronchus intubation.[10]

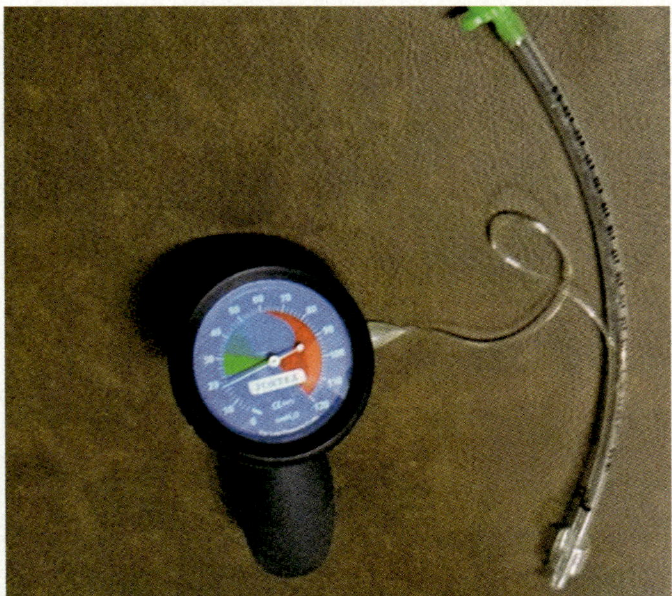

Fig. 14.13 Microcuff tube with cuff manometer

Table 14.7 Recommended size selection for Microcuff endotracheal tube

Age (years)/weight (kg)	Tube size I.D.
Term $\geq$ 3 kg to $<$8 months	3.0 mm
8 months to $<$2 years	3.5 mm
2 to $<$4 years	4.0 mm
4 to $<$6 years	4.5 mm

4. Adequate sealing:
   a. Preventing aspiration,
   b. Decreased tube exchange rate,[11]
   c. Decreased theatre pollution[12]
   d. Decreased cost of anaesthetic agents because there is no leak.
   e. More accurate capnography and gas analysis.[13]

> **Clinical Pearls**
> 1. Ensure black mark is placed at the level of vocal cords during intubation.
> 2. After intubation, audible air leak should be present at $\leq$ 20 cm H_2O airway pressure with the cuff fully deflated. If no air leak is detected, the tube may be too large; consider changing the tube.
> 3. Inflate the cuff to the effective sealing pressure but no higher than 20 cm H_2O cuff pressure.
> 4. Continuous monitoring of cuff pressure is a must to ensure pressure does not exceed 20 cm H_2O.
> 5. Avoid manual compression of the pilot balloon.

Disadvantages of Microcuff endotracheal tubes

1. Extra care is required for correct placement.
2. Trauma may occur if cuff is overinflated.
3. Cuff pressure must be monitored throughout the case.
4. More expensive
5. Cuff pressures vary due to temperature, gas exchange, cuff movement and anaesthetic depth.

> **Clinical Pearls**
>
> 1. The type of endotracheal tube that is chosen for a paediatric patient is at the discretion of the anaesthetist, but the utmost care should be taken to ensure that they are provided with the most suitable endotracheal tube and that no trauma is sustained on their developing airway and lungs.[14]
> 2. The microcuff paediatric tracheal tube with ultra thin high volume low pressure polyurethane cuff also available in preformed shape.[15]

Oxford Tube

1. It is L-shaped tube made of red rubber (Fig. 14.14).
2. It may cuffed or uncuffed used for upper face surgeries as it is non-kinkable.
3. Internal diameter is uniform throughout the tube but the thickness of wall varies.
4. Proximally it is thicker than the distal tip which prevents compression by mouth gag.
5. Bevel is situated at posteriorly at the tip and may abut against posterior wall if head is flexed.
6. Difficult to suction through and is non-transparent.

LARYNGOSCOPE

It is a viewing instrument for larynx (larynx + scopy) which facilitates tracheal intubation under direct vision. It was introduced by Kirstein in 1895 (Fig. 14.15).[16]

Laryngoscope is a left-handed instrument, with the operator's right hand being used to pass the tube.

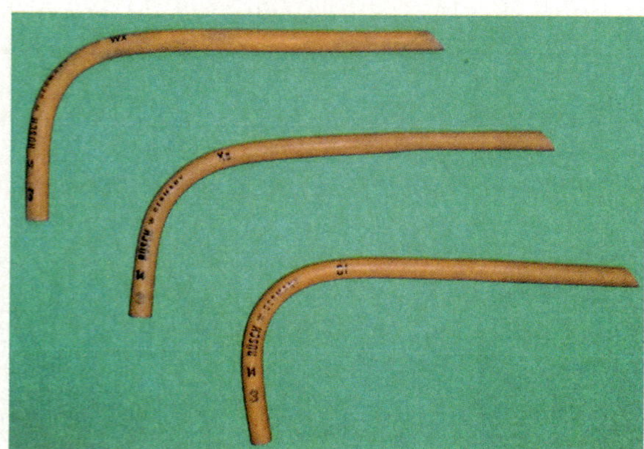

Fig. 14.14 Oxford tubes

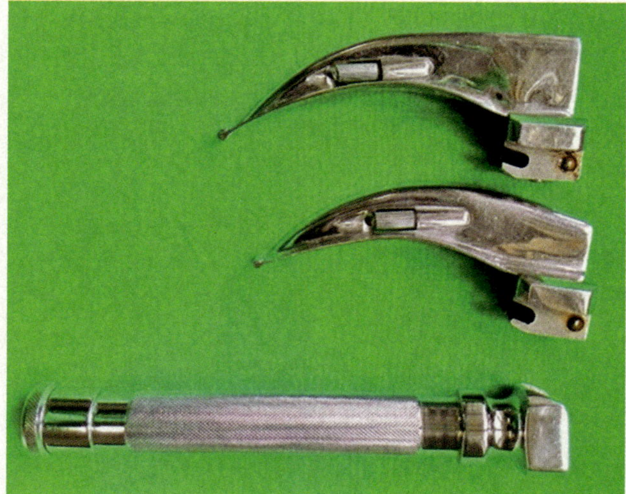

Fig. 14.15 Laryngoscope with Macintosh blades

Conventional laryngoscope consists of a handle containing batteries with a light source, and a set of interchangeable blades.

The principal components of a laryngoscope blade are:

1. Spatula—passes over the lingual surface of the tongue.
2. Flange—used to direct the tongue towards the left side of the mouth (passing over the patient's right buccal tongue surface).

> **Clinical Pearls**
>
> 1. Dental injury is a major concern during laryngoscopy.
> 2. The flange of the laryngoscope should never be leveraged backward against the teeth.
> 3. The curved blades need to reach the vallecula and apply pressure on the underlying hyoepiglottic ligament.

Two basic styles of laryngoscope blade (Fig. 14.16)

A. **Curved blade**

B. **Straight blade.**

A. Curved blade (Fig. 14.17)

1. Curved blades have a larger displacement volume (spatula and flange) and lift the epiglottis indirectly
2. Curved blades need to only reach the vallecula and apply pressure to the underlying hyoepiglottic ligament
3. The Macintosh blade is the most widely used of the curved laryngoscope blades.[17]
4. The Macintosh blade is positioned in the vallecula, anterior to the epiglottis, lifting it out of the visual pathway.

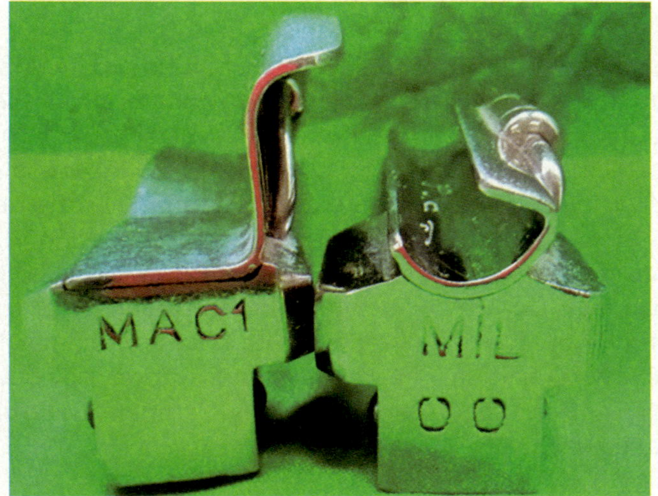

Fig. 14.16 Macintosh and Miller blades

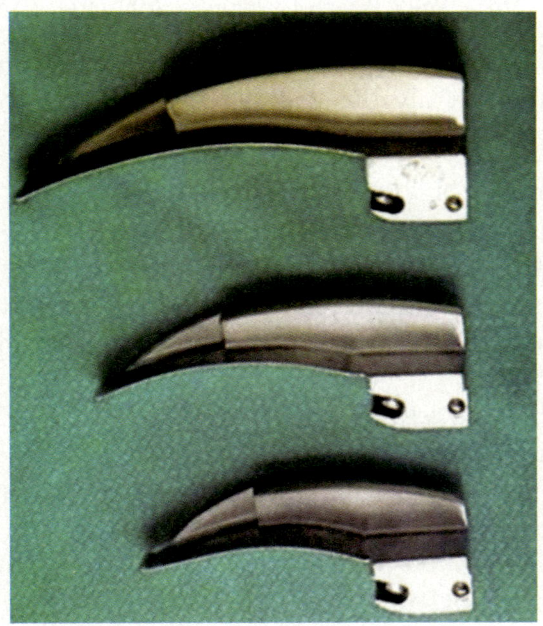

Fig. 14.17 Curved blade

B. Straight blade (Fig. 14.18)

1. Early laryngoscopes used a straight "Magill Blade", and this design is still the standard pattern veterinary laryngoscopes are based upon; however, the blade is difficult to control in adult humans and can cause pressure on the vagus nerve, which can cause unexpected cardiac arrhythmias. The Miller blade is the most popular style of straight blade.[18,19]
2. The Miller, Wisconsin, Wis-Hipple, and Robertshaw blades are commonly used for infants. It is easier to visualize the glottis using these blades than the Macintosh blade in infants, due to the larger size of the epiglottis relative to that of the glottis.

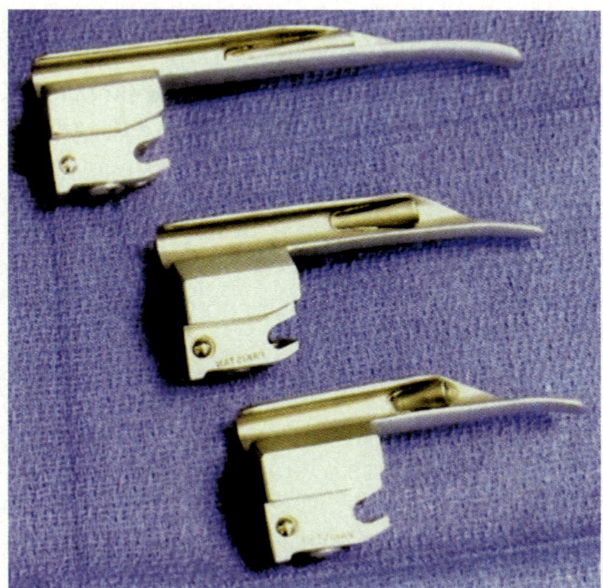

Fig. 14.18 Straight blade

3. Straight blade laryngoscopes lift the epiglottis directly.
4. Straight blades must be passed deeper, under the epiglottis.
5. Miller blade is positioned posterior to the epiglottis, trapping it while exposing the glottis and vocal folds.
6. Incorrect usage can cause trauma to the front incisors; the correct technique is to displace the chin upwards and forward at the same time, not to use

Table 14.8 Summary of different laryngoscope blades

Name of blade	Type of blade
Cranwall	Straight, no flange
Jackson	Straight
Janeway	Straight
Reduced Flange (RF Mac)	Curved reduced flange at heel
Macintosh	Curved
Magill	Straight
Miller	Straight
Parrott	Curved
Phillips	Straight
Robertshaw	Straight
Seward	Straight
Siker	Curved, with integrated mirror
Soper	Straight
Wis-Hipple	Straight
Wisconsin	Straight

the blade as a lever with the teeth serving as the fulcrum.

7. Both Miller and Macintosh laryngoscope blades are available in sizes 0 (neonatal) through 4 (large adult). Miller blade is available in size 00 also.
8. There are many other styles of curved and straight blades (e.g. Phillips, Robertshaw, Sykes, Wisconsin, Wis-Hipple, etc.) with accessories such as mirrors for enlarging the field of view and even ports for the administration of oxygen.

Clinical Pearl

The Miller, Wisconsin, Wis-Hipple, and Robertshaw blades are commonly used for infants. It is easier to visualize the glottis using these blades than the Macintosh blade in infants.

VENTILATING RIGID BRONCHOSCOPE

Components

1. A metal tube with a removable optical rod lens telescope (Fig. 14.19 and Table 14.9).
2. Vents in the wall allow ventilation of the contralateral lung when the distal end of the bronchoscope is positioned in a bronchus.
3. The side arm has a 15 mm attachment for an anaesthetic T-piece circuit.
4. Ventilation occurs between the lumen of the bronchoscope and the outer surface of the telescope.
5. With the telescope in place controlled ventilation can be done but the cross sectional area of lumen is reduced.
6. Using too large a bronchoscope leads to compression of tracheal mucosa and postoperative oedema with the risk of stridor.

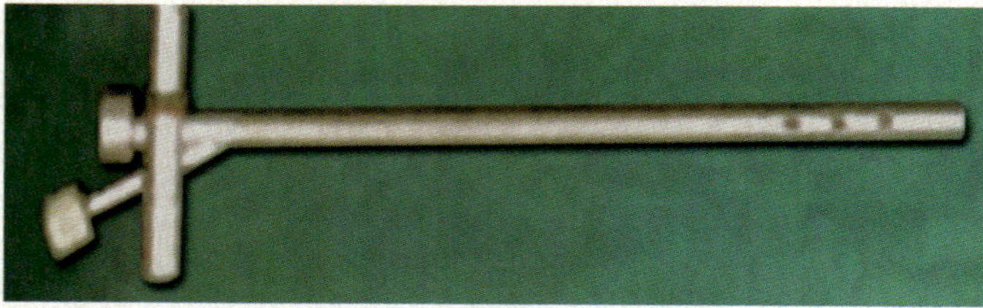

Fig. 14.19 Ventilating rigid bronchoscope

Table 14.9 Use of different sized ventilating rigid bronchoscope

Age	Cricoid airway diameter	Bronchoscope size ID (mm)	ED (mm)
1 year	5.5	3.5	5.7
2 years	6.5	3.5	5.7
3 years	7.0	4.0	6.7
5 years	7.5	5.0	7.8

FIBREOPTIC BRONCHOSCOPE

It consists of illumination fibreoptic bundle and imaging fibreoptics or a camera. There is channel for suction of secretions and blood, for the passage of topical medication and fluid for washing, and for the passage of various instruments for diagnostic retrieval of tissues or for therapeutic procedures. The eyepiece contains the lenses with adjustment ring, camera can be attached to eyepiece. Control lever for flexing the distal tip of the fibroscope. The rotator movement allows approximately 360° visualization. The small paediatric fibroscope does not facilitate the suction or biopsy channel due to its small size.

BREATHING SYSTEM

1. It delivers the intended inspired gaseous mixture from the anaesthetic machine to the alveoli.
2. The fresh gas flow (FGF) rate required to prevent re-breathing of alveolar gas is a measure of the efficiency of a breathing system.

Components of a Breathing System

There are several components which may be used in the construction of an anaesthetic breathing system:

1. A fresh gas entry port in the form of a delivery tube.
2. Carbon dioxide absorbent (only used in rebreathing system).
3. Adjustable Pressure Limiting (APL) valve.
4. Reservoir bag.

The tubing used is corrugated to prevent kinks and occlusion.

It also captures water vapour which is normally exhaled during expiration.

An Ideal Breathing System

1. Easy to use.
2. Possess safety features to prevent patient morbidity (e.g pressure limitation, no cross infection, etc.)
3. Should impose no additional inspiratory or expiratory resistance or compliance that adversely affects breathing.
4. Should impose no additional anatomical dead space in the form of apparatus dead space.
5. Should adaptable for various sizes and types of patients and can be used for both spontaneous and controlled ventilation.
6. Should minimize wastage of gases and permit satisfactory scavenging during spontaneous and controlled ventilation.

7. Should maintain temperature and humidity
8. Should permit easy use of monitoring.

Breathing System Commonly Used in Paediatric Anaesthesia

Jackson-Rees Circuit (JR Circuit) (Fig. 14.20)

It is most commonly used circuit for ages 5 years and below or less than 20 kg child. It is modification of Ayre's T piece.

The Ayre's T piece attached with a corrugated tube which acts as a reservoir and this modification termed Mapleson E circuit.

Jackson-Rees modified the Mapleson E circuit by adding a reservoir bag with open end which allows controlled ventilation and observation of spontaneous breathing and this is termed Mapleson F system.

Components

1. Fresh gas tubing (green) 8 mm diameter, 1 m long attached to T piece at right angle.
2. T piece 1 cm diameter
3. Corrugated tube with 0.5 L reservoir bag with open end or expiratory valve.

Advantages

1. Simple design, easy to use.
2. Light weight, minimal dead space, low resistance.
3. Easy to switchover from spontaneous to controlled ventilation.
4. Allows observation of spontaneous breathing, assessment of lung compliance, tidal volume.
5. Application of continuous positive pressure during spontaneous and positive end expiratory pressure (PEEP) is facilitated.

Clinical Pearl

Practical application of continuous positive pressure during spontaneous breathing at the time of extubation helps to expel the secretions once the tube is removed thus reducing the chances of post-extubation airway complications.

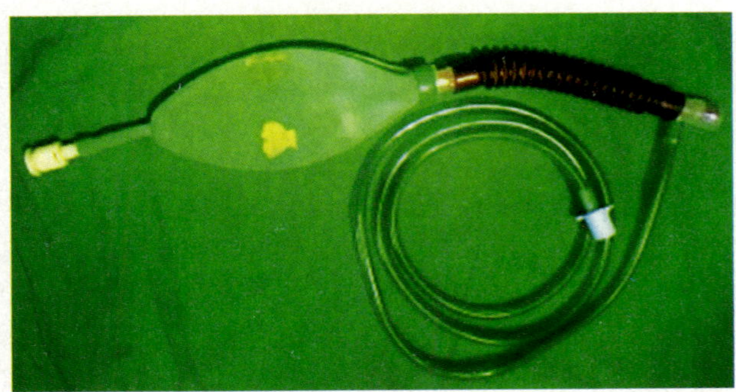

Fig. 14.20 Jackson-Rees circuit

Recommended Fresh Gas Flows (FGF) to Maintain Normocarbia

1. Spontaneous ventilation 200 mL to 300 mL/kg.
2. Controlled ventilation 70 mL/kg

Or

1. Spontaneous ventilation 2.5 times the minute ventilation.
2. Controlled ventilation 1000 mL + 200 mL/kg.

Bain's Circuit

1. Bain's breathing circuit is a modified Mapleson D circuit. It is co-axial type (tube within a tube) (Fig. 14.21).
2. It is called universal circuit as it can be used in children as well as in adult, for spontaneous as well as control ventilation.

Components

The green fresh gas tube with 7 mm internal diameter lies within larger corrugated tube with 22 mm internal diameter. The reservoir bag with APL valve placed away from the patient end facilitates its use during head, neck, face surgeries.

Advantages

1. It is a compact, easy to handle and portable circuit.
2. Warming of inspired gases occurs due to co-axial circuit.
3. Partial rebreathing improves humidification
4. APL controls system pressure
5. Low dead space, low resistance to breathing.
6. Facilitates scavenging of waste gases.

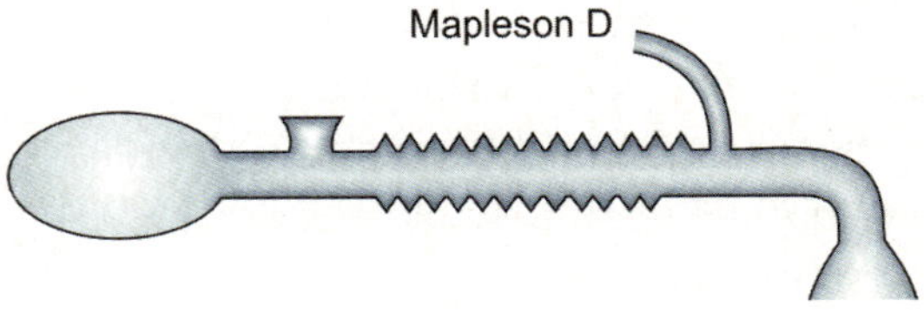

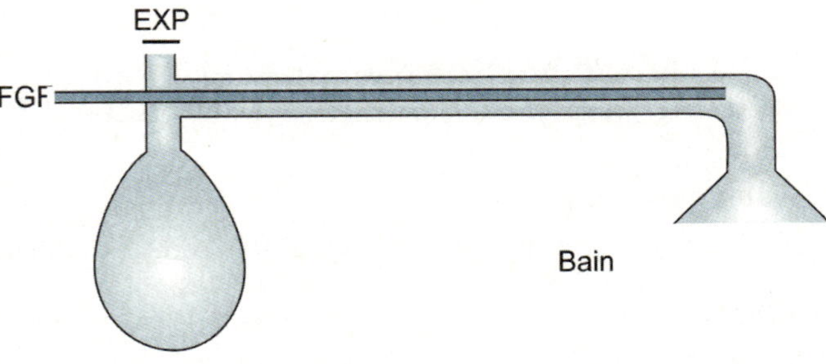

Fig. 14.21 Modification of Mapleson D circuit

Disadvantages

1. High fresh gas flow required.
2. High gas flow rates—for example, if the oxygen flush valve is used, it may cause lung barotrauma.
3. If the inner tube becomes disconnected or breaks, the entire breathing tube becomes dead space.

> **Clinical Pearls**
>
> Two tests are established to test the patency of inner tube.
>
> **1. Pethick's Test:**[20]
>
> It is tested by closing the APL valve and activating the oxygen quick-flush. If the inner tube is intact, the Venturi effect of the rapidly moving stream of gas leaving the inner tube will suck gas out of the bag and the bag will empty. If the inner tube is damaged, the stream of gas will be directed into the bag and it will fill.
>
> **2. Foëx and Crampton-Smith Test:**[21]
>
> It is known as the occlusion test. The inner tube is occluded (using, for example, the plunger from a 2 mL syringe) while gas flows into the breathing system and pressurisation of the backbar is observed by dipping of the rotameters.

Bain's System Flow Rates

1. Spontaneous ventilation: 200–300 mL/kg/min
2. Controlled ventilation: Infants and less than 10 kg—3–5 L/m, 10–50 kg—5–6 L/m or 2–3 times minute ventilation, whichever is greater.
3. Depends on fresh gas flow, to flush out CO_2
4. Spontaneous ventilation: 200–300 mL/kg/min
5. Controlled ventilation: 70 mL/kg/min

CIRCLE SYSTEM

1. It allows rebreathing of anaesthetic gases
2. It requires lower FGF rates
3. There is less pollution, CO_2 absorption
4. It conserves heat and humidity

   The circle system consists of seven components:
   a. Fresh gas inflow source
   b. Inspiratory and expiratory unidirectional valves
   c. Inspiratory and expiratory corrugated tubes
   d. A Y-piece connector
   e. Overflow or pop-off valve, referred to as the APL valve
   f. A reservoir bag
   g. A canister containing a carbon dioxide absorbent.

Absorbent

Three formulations

1. Soda lime
2. Baralyme
3. Calcium hydroxide lime (Amsorb)

Indicators

They indicate the exhaustion of absorbent. Most commonly used is ethyl violet.

1. **Soda lime** (most commonly used)

   80% calcium hydroxide, 15% water, 4% sodium hydroxide, and 1% potassium hydroxide (an activator) silica

   The equations:
   a. $CO_2 + H_2O \Leftrightarrow H_2CO_3$
   b. $H_2CO_3 + 2NaOH(KOH) \Leftrightarrow Na_2CO_3(K_2CO_3) + 2H_2O + \text{Heat}$
   c. $Na_2CO_3\ (K_2CO_3) + Ca(OH)_2 \Leftrightarrow CaCO_3 + 2NaOH(KOH)$
2. **Baralyme:** 20% barium hydroxide and 80% calcium hydroxide
3. **Calcium hydroxide lime:** Lack of sodium and potassium hydroxides

   It forms carbon monoxide and the nephrotoxic substance known as compound A.

Compound A formation:

Sevoflurane interaction with carbon dioxide absorbents and forms:

- Compound A [fluoromethyl-2,2-difluoro-1-(trifluoromethyl)vinyl ether].

Contributing Factors

1. Low-flow or closed-circuit
2. Concentrations of sevoflurane
3. Higher absorbent temperatures
4. **Humphrey A, D or E system:** It is a versatile hybrid system that can perform functionally as Mapleson A, D or E circuit.

SELF-INFLATING RESUSCITATION BAG

1. It is a manual resuscitator or "self-inflating bag", which is commonly used to provide positive pressure ventilation to patients who are not breathing or not breathing adequately (Fig. 14.22).
2. It is a required part of resuscitation as part of standard equipment on a crash cart, in emergency rooms or operation theatre and other critical care settings.
3. The full-form of AMBU is Artificial Manual Breathing Unit.

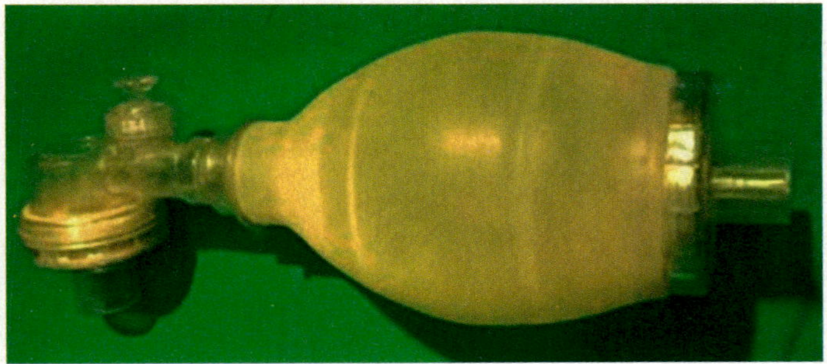

Fig. 14.22 Self-inflating resuscitation bag

Components

1. **Mask:** The mask provides seal over the patient's face.
2. **Valve:** There is a non-rebreathing valve to prevent backflow into the bag itself.
3. **Pressure relief valve:** This is additional feature available with paediatric size unit with pressure limit for 40 cm of H_2O.
4. **Self-inflating bags:** A soft bag which is squeezed to expel air to the patient. It is a flexible air chamber; it self-inflates from its other end, drawing in either ambient air or a low pressure oxygen flow supplied by a regulated cylinder, while also allows the patient's lungs to deflate. A separate reservoir bag which can be filled with pure oxygen which can increase the amount of oxygen delivered to the patient to nearly 100%.

SUMMARY

The innovation and revolution in the design of supraglottic airway devices has secured its place in airway management and is promising. They are playing significant role in the improvement of perioperative outcomes in the paediatric patient. But high end clinical trials with large sample size are required to give an edge to a revolution in paediatric anaesthetic practice.

Use of proper instrument sharpens the anaesthesia skill. Fine clinical judgement, the periodic checking of all equipment, ensuring the uninterrupted delivery of anaesthetic to patients via intact circuits and intravenous access and the use of familiar, appropriate techniques by competent anaesthesiologist enhances the surgical outcome of our small precious patients.

REFERENCES

1. Daniel L, Michael F. Emergency Care O'Keefe. Edward TD, (Ed.) 10th edn. Pearson, Prentice Hall. Upper Saddle River, New Jersey. 2005;147.
2. Aruna S. Equipments for Paediatric Anaesthesia Indian J Anaesth. 2004;48(5):365–371.
3. Bhavesh P, Robert B. Laryngeal mask airway and other supraglottic airway devices in paediatric practice. Contin Educ Anaesth Crit Care Pain. 2009;9(1):6–9.
4. Lopez-Gil M, Brimacombe J, Keller C. A comparison of four methods for assessing oropharyngeal leak pressure with the laryngeal mask airway in paediatric patients. Paediatr Anaesth. 2001;11:319–21.
5. Keller C, Brimacombe J, Keller K, et al. Comparison of four methods for assessing airway sealing pressure with the laryngeal mask airway in adult patients. Br J Anaesth. 1999;82:286–7.
6. 4th National Audit Project of the Royal College of Anaesthetists and the Difficult Airway Society: Major Complications of Airway Management in the United Kingdom. Dr Tim Cook, Dr Nick Woodall and Dr Chris Frerk (Eds). Report and findings: March 2011.
7. Gerber AC. New Advances in Paediatric Ventilation: Revolutionizing the Management of Paediatric Intubation with Cuffed Tubes. Kimberly-Clark, Adair Greene McCann. Microcuff paediatric tube: Now anaesthesiologists can use cuffed endotracheal tubes in children. 2008;10–15.
8. King BR, Baker MD, Braitman LE, et al. Endotracheal tube selection in children: A comparison of four methods. Ann Emerg Med. 1993;22:530–4.
9. Khine HH, Corddry DH, Kettrick RG, et al. Comparison of cuffed and uncuffed endotracheal tubes in young children during general anaesthesia. Anaesthesiology 1997;86:627–31.
10. Litman R, Maxwell L. Cuffed versus Uncuffed endotracheal tubes in Paediatric Anaesthesia: The debate should finally end. Retrieved 2013 August 1 from http://journals.www.com/anaesthesiology/Fulltext/2013/03000/Cuffed_versus_Uncuff ed_Endotracheal_Tubes_in.12.aspx (2012).
11. Fine GF, Fertal K, Motoyama EK. The effectiveness of controlled ventilation using cuffed versus uncuffed ETT in infants. Anaesthesiology 2000;93:1251.
12. Khine HH, Corddry DH, Kettrick RG, et al. Comparison of cuffed and uncuffed endotracheal tubes in young children during general anaesthesia. Anaesthesiology 1997;86:627–31.
13. Orliaguet GA, Renaud E, Lejay M, et al. Postal survey of cuffed or uncuffed tracheal tubes used for paediatric tracheal intubation. Pediatr Anesth. 2001;11:277–81.
14. Allman K, Wilson I. Oxford Handbook of Anaesthesia: 3rd edn. Oxford University Press: UK 2011.
15. Dullenkopf A, Schmitz A, Frei M, et al. Air leakage around tracheal tube cuffs. Eur J Anaesth 2004;21:448–53.
16. Hirsch NP, Smith GB, Hirsch PO. "Alfred Kirstein. Pioneer of direct laryngoscopy". Anaesthesia. January 1986;41(1):

42–5. doi:10.1111/j.1365-2044.1986.tb12702.x. PMID 3511764.

17. Scott J, Baker PA (2009). "How did the Macintosh laryngoscope become so popular?". Paediatric Anaesthesia 19 (Suppl 1):24–9. doi:10.1111/j.1460-9592.2009.03026.x. PMID 19572841.
18. Robert Reynolds Macintosh. "A new laryngoscope". The Lancet. 1943;1(6):205. doi:10.1016/S0140-6736(02)95524–8.
19. Magill IW. "An Improved Laryngoscope for Anaesthetists". The Lancet. 1926;207:(5349):500. doi:10.1016/S0140-6736(01)17109–6.
20. Pethick SL. Letter to the Editor. Canadian Anaesthetists Society Journal. 1975;22:115.
21. Foëx P, Crampton Smith A. A test for co-axial circuits. Anaesthesia 1977;32:294.

15

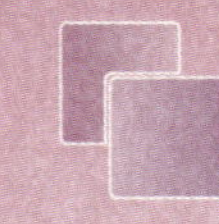

Blood Transfusion and Strategies for Blood Conservation in Infants and Children

Shruti Kamdi and Prashant Kamdi

ABSTRACT

Management of bleeding in paediatric population presents its own set of dilemmas and challenges. One of the primary problems is the lack of good scientific evidence regarding the best management strategies for children. There is increasing concern about the safety of homologous blood transfusion during paediatric surgery, and a conservative transfusion practice is associated with improved outcome. In every paediatric surgical unit, a strategy to decrease or avoid blood transfusion must be implemented. A multidisciplinary approach allows the optimal use of all available resources. A strategy to minimize transfusion requirement requires a combined effort involving the entire surgical team with pre-, peri-, and post-operative planning and management. Good teamwork, understanding, and communication between paediatric surgeons, anaesthesiologists and all associated specialities including transfusion medicine allow for a synergistic relationship to enhance patient care and give the best end result.

INTRODUCTION

Challenges unique to paediatrics

- Legal considerations
- Small blood volume
- PAD has limited utility (smaller patient blood volume)
- Evolution of pathology (e.g. sickle cell disease and CHD)
- Undiagnosed bleeding disorders
- One size does not fill all
- Many medications lack FDA paediatric approval

To minimize risks and costs, the transfusion of homologous blood should be kept to a minimum by a team approach to blood conservation.

TRANSFUSION GUIDELINES WITH LOWER PERIOPERATIVE HAEMOGLOBIN[1]

These guidelines are given in Tables 15.1–15.5.

Table 15.1 Blood components and dosing of small volumes in neonatal and paediatric patients[1]

Component	Dose	Expected increment
Red blood cells	10–15 mL/kg	Haemoglobin increases 2–3 g/dL
Fresh frozen plasma	10–15 mL/kg	15–20% rise in factor levels (assuming recovery)
Platelets whole-blood derived (WBD) or apheresis	5–10 mL/kg or 1 WBD unit/ 10 kg (patients ≥ 10 kg)	50,000/µL rise in platelet count (assuring recovery)
Cryoprecipitated AHF	1–2 units/10 kg	60–100 mg/dL rise in fibrinogen (assuring recovery)

Table 15.2 Transfusion guidelines for RBCs in infants less than 4 months of age

1. Haematocrit <20% with low reticulocyte count and symptomatic anaemia (tachycardia, tachypnea, poor feeding)
2. Haematocrit <30% and any of the following:
   a. On <35% oxygen hood.
   b. On oxygen by nasal cannula.
   c. On continuous positive airway pressure and/or intermittent mandatory ventilation on mechanical ventilation with mean airway pressure, 6 cm of water.

Contd...

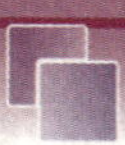

Table 15.2 Transfusion guidelines for RBCs in infants less than 4 months of age (*Contd...*)

d. With significant tachycardia or tachypnea (heart rate > 180 beats/minute for 24 hours, respiratory rate > 80 beats/minute for 24 hours).
e. With significant apnoea or bradycardia (> 6 episodes in 12 hours or 2 episodes in 24 hours requiring bag and mask ventilation while receiving therapeutic doses of methylxanthines).
f. With low weight gain (< 10 g/day observed over 4 days while receiving ≥ 100 kcal/kg/day).

3. Haematocrit < 35% and either of the following:
   a. On > 35% oxygen hood.
   b. On continuous positive airway pressure/intermittent mandatory ventilation with mean airway pressure ≥ 6–8 cm of water.
4. Haematocrit < 45% and either of the following:
   a. On extracorporeal membrane oxygenation.
   b. With congenital cyanotic heart disease.

Table 15.3 Transfusion guidelines for RBCs in patients > 4 months of age

1. Emergency surgical procedure in patient with significant postoperative anaemia.
2. Preoperative anaemia when other corrective therapy is not available.
3. Intraoperative blood loss >15% total blood volume.
4. Haematocrit < 24% and:
   a. In perioperative period, with signs and symptoms of anaemia.
   b. While on chemotherapy/radiotherapy.
   c. Chronic congenital or acquired symptomatic anaemia.
5. Acute blood loss with hypovolemia not responsive to other therapy.
6. Haematocrit <40% and:
   a. With severe pulmonary disease.
   b. On extracorporeal membrane oxygenation.
7. Sickle cell disease and:
   a. Cerebrovascular accident.
   b. Acute chest syndrome.
   c. Splenic sequestration
   d. Aplastic crisis
   e. Recurrent priapism
   f. Preoperatively when general anaesthesia is planned (target haemoglobin 10 mg/dl).
8. Chronic transfusion programs for disorders of red cell production (e.g. β thalassemia major and Diamond-Blackfan syndrome unresponsive to therapy).

Table 15.4 Transfusion guidelines for platelets in neonates and older children

With thrombocytopenia

1. Platelet count 5000–10000/µl with failure of platelet production.
2. Platelet count < 30,000/µl in neonate with failure of platelet production.
3. Platelet count < 50000/µl in stable premature infant:
   a. With active bleeding, or
   b. Before an invasive procedure, with failure of platelet production.
4. Platelet count < 100000/µl in sick premature infant:
   a. With active bleeding, or
   b. Before an invasive procedure in patients with DIC.

Without thrombocytopenia

1. Active bleeding in association with qualitative platelet defect.
2. Unexplained excessive bleeding in a patient undergoing cardiopulmonary bypass.
3. Patients undergoing ECMO with:
   a. A platelet count of < 100000/µl or
   b. Higher platelet counts and bleeding.

DIC=disseminated intravascular coagulation, ECMO=extra-corporeal membrane oxygenation

Table 15.5 Transfusion guidelines for plasma products in neonates and older children

Fresh frozen plasma (FFP)

1. Support during treatment of disseminated intravascular dissemination.
2. Replacement therapy:
   a. When specific factor concentrates are not available, including, but not limited to, antithrombin C or S deficiency, and factor II, factor V, factor X, and factor XI deficiencies.
   b. During therapeutic plasma exchange when FFP is indicated (cryo-poor plasma, plasma from which cryoprecipitate has been removed).
3. Reversal of warfarin in an emergency situation, such as before an invasive procedure with active bleeding.

Note: FFP is *not* indicated for volume expansion or enhancement of wound healing.

Cryoprecipitated AHF

1. Hypofibrinogenemia or dysfibrinogenemia with active bleeding.
2. Hypofibrinogenemia or dysfibrinogenemia while undergoing an invasive procedure.
3. Factor XIII deficiency with active bleeding or while undergoing an invasive procedure in the absence of factor XIII concentrate.

Contd...

Table 15.5 Transfusion guidelines for plasma products in neonates and older children (*Contd...*)

4. Limited directed-donor cryoprecipitate for bleeding episodes in small children with haemophilia recombinant and plasma-derived factor VIII products are not available.
5. In the preparation of fibrin sealant.
6. von Willebrand disease with active bleeding, but only when both of the following are true:
   a. DDAVP is contraindicated, not available, or does not elicit response.
   b. Virus-inactivated plasma-derived factor VIII concentrate (which contains von Willebrand factor) not available.

AIMING FOR REDUCED BLOOD LOSS[2]

Management of bleeding in paediatric population presents its own set of dilemmas and challenges. The key to success in the predicament is firstly to ensure that the anaesthetist has a clear understanding of the underlying normal physiology of the young child's haematologic status. Then by adding knowledge of the abnormal pathology that is being presented, the anaesthetist can at least understand what anomalies he or she is facing.

The New Paradigm
- **Anaemia** is common in ill children;
- **Transfusions** may not be safe nor as beneficial

Anaesthetic Techniques to Reduce Blood Use

General

There are some basic things that the anaesthetist and surgeon can do to reduce blood loss during surgery:
- positioning of the anaesthetized patient so as to minimize any venous congestion in the operating field
- the use of local vasoconstrictors

Specific

There are also some specific procedures that may help in reducing transfusion and these are discussed below.

- **Preventing Hypertension**

  Good anaesthetic management should involve preventing the patient becoming hypertensive (and provoking excessive bleeding), and in major surgery this needs to be supported by good postoperative analgesia (lest the patient bleeds excessively post-operatively). This is especially important in cases where there are suture lines in major vessels, e.g. cardiac or vascular cases.

- **Preventing Hypothermia**

  Unintentional hypothermia is to be avoided as this will contribute to postoperative shivering, acidosis and possibly even coagulopathy. Temperature monitoring and use of warming devices will help in preventing unintentional hypothermia.

- **Controlled Hypotension**
- **Aprotinin, DDAVP and Tranexamic acid**

  Aprotinin and Tranexamic acids were both proven to be effective, whereas routine use of DDAVP was not.

  Aprotinin is a non-specific protease inhibitor that has been shown to be effective in reducing blood loss in cardiac surgery. The routine use of these drugs in cardiac surgery will continue to be controversial. Their use in specific situations like redo valve surgery, and in patients with active endocarditis who require urgent surgery is proven and uncontroversial.

Fibrin Sealant

Fibrin sealants have been used in surgery for over 20 years. They generally contain fibrinogen (with or without factor XIII) and thrombin (plus calcium with or without antifibrinolytic drugs) which can be applied to a wound surface sequentially or simultaneous.

Transfusion-free **paediatric cardiac surgery** is unrealistic for the vast majority of procedures in neonates or small infants; however, considerable progress has been made by using techniques that decrease the need for homologous blood products or even allow bloodless surgery in older infants and children. These techniques involve a decrease in prime volume by downsizing the bypass circuit with the help of vacuum assisted venous drainage, microplegia, autologous blood predonation with or without infusion of recombinant (erythropoietin), cell salvaging, ultrafiltration and retrograde autologous priming. The three major techniques which are simple, safe, efficient, and cost-effective are: a prime volume as small as possible, cardioplegia with negligible hydric balance and circuit residual blood salvaged without any alteration. Furthermore, these three techniques can be used for all the patients, including emergencies and small babies.

Reduction in Prime Volume using a Reduced Bypass Circuit

Reduction in prime volume is a major factor in blood conservation. If we assume a blood volume of about 80 mL/kg for neonates, the blood volume of a 3 kg baby is 240 mL. For this category of patients the prime volume is often equivalent or even higher than their blood volume. Therefore asanguineous priming is unrealistic except for rare cases with a high haematocrit level prior to surgery. However, it is possible to downsize the bypass circuit and thus decrease the prime volume.

It is interesting to note the following observations: (1) the internal diameter of the arterial line may be decreased to 1/8 inch for patient weight up to 5 kg, or to 5/32 inch (which is about 4 mm) for patients up to 7 kg; (2) the arterial filter, usually known as a safety device, is no longer considered essential; and (3) the hemofilter is not a constant component of the bypass circuit (filling of the filter and its connective tubing increased prime volume, and thus hemodilution). Another positive side effect of the miniaturized circuit is reduced blood contact with the surface of the cardiopulmonary bypass circuit; this contact is thought to activate the systemic inflammatory response.

Vacuum-assisted Venous Return

Vacuum-assisted venous return is helpful to further decrease prime volume. Such assisted venous drainage allows us to decrease declivity of the membrane oxygenator, and thus, to significantly decrease the length of the venous, arterial and suction lines. This technique was first developed in adult surgery and was considered a powerful system to decrease hemodilution during cardiopulmonary bypass. Furthermore, vacuum-optimized venous return flow, and full support blood flow rates can be achieved through cannulae that demonstrate limited flow capacity under siphon drainage conditions. An increase in gaseous microemboli is a complication related to vacuum-assisted venous drainage. However, this drawback is avoidable by adhering to specific parameter. If the maximal value of the vacuum remains under –40 mmHg, the level of embolic activity is equivalent to that seen during gravity-siphon venous drainage. When using vacuum-assisted venous drainage, a pressure relief valve is an essential component of the circuit. The hypothesis of an increase in haemolysis during use of the vacuum was ruled out by several investigators. Vacuum-assisted venous return is a technique, without any obvious drawbacks, that is used by several paediatric centres with consistent ability to reduce homologous blood transfusion.

Microplegia or Miniplegia

The original composition of blood cardioplegia described by Buckberg was a mixture of 4 parts blood added to 1 part crystalloid; this has become the standard for cold blood cardioplegia. Alteration of this composition was proposed by several authors when warm, or at least tepid, and blood cardioplegia was adopted because the only rationale for dilution was to decrease high blood viscosity associated with hypothermia. Furthermore, at that time cardioplegia was retrograde and performed continuously through the coronary sinus. The risk of fluid overload and of clotting factor dilution was real with standard blood cardioplegia. Microplegia was then also used for intermittent warm blood cardioplegia.The technique for continuous or discontinuous microplegia injection is identical. Blood is diverted from the arterial line or from a specific built-in port of the oxygenator through an occlusive roller pump. Downstream of the roller pump, the arresting agent is added *via* a syringe pump.

The theoretical advantages of non-diluted cardioplegia are as follows:

1. A higher myocardial oxygen supply because of a higher haemoglobin level and a rightward shift of the oxyhaemoglobin dissociation curve;
2. A negligible fluid balance of the cardioplegia (the volume of blood diverted from the circuit is sucked from the coronary sinus to the cardiotomy reservoir so that the balance is limited to a few milliliters of crystalloid arresting agent);
3. A decreased tendency for tissue oedema with non-diluted *vs* diluted cardioplegia demonstrated in experimental data and
4. Cost-effectiveness when compared to the standard cardioplegia technique.

The benefit to hydric balance of microplegia *vs* standard cardioplegia is well documented. When using standard cardioplegia with a blood to crystalloid ratio of 4:1, cardioplegia is sucked into the cardiotomy reservoir, dilution of the circulating blood increases during each cardioplegia injection. The dilution is significant during complex procedures that require prolonged cross-clamp times. When standard cardioplegia is wasted, blood is also wasted; and crystalloid or colloid must be added to restore the level in the cardiotomy reservoir.

Cell-salvage Techniques

Cell salvage techniques scavenge blood loss. There are two main techniques of cell-salvage: the blood is either collected and reinjected without any treatment (non-wash technique), or the blood is treated and anticoagulated, washed and centrifuged in a cell-saver machine to obtain a concentrate of red blood cells. The washing technique is said to remove debris from shed blood thus reducing the risk of cerebral thromboembolism and improving neurological outcome. Washing also removes platelets, coagulation factors and other plasma proteins leading to coagulopathy, and an increased risk of organ failure and of systemic inflammatory response. However, the safety of the cell salvage technique has been shown in multiple studies. The benefits of cell salvage in reducing allogeneic blood transfusion is controversial. A meta-analysis failed to find any significant benefit from cell salvage in cardiac surgery, while other studies demonstrated a significant reduction in blood transfusion with washed salvaged blood. One of the major limitations of washing blood in paediatric surgery is that it is time-consuming during which the blood is unavailable to the patient. Recent progress has been made with the introduction of a small-volume centrifugal bowl dedicated to paediatric patients the results of the cell-saver technique are widely influenced by surgical haemostasis by the motivation for blood preservation. Another component influencing the results of cell salvage is the use of residual volume in the circuit after coming off cardiopulmonary bypass. Some centres add this residual blood to the cell-saver for washing while transfuse it directly into the patient. Some centres advocate collection of residual blood from the circuit without any further treatment. The quality of this blood is exactly the same as the quality of the patient's blood at the time of discontinuation of cardiopulmonary bypass. This blood is used during the post-bypass period when necessary. This blood contains coagulation factors that are otherwise removed during cell-saver treatment. It also contains heparin which can be removed by adding additional protamine as needed. This policy has proven to be safe, efficient, simple and less expensive than cell salvage.

PROACTIVE HYPOTENSION WITH PURPOSE

For a procedure to be used to reduce exposure to allogeneic blood, the procedure should itself have a safety level that is comparable with allogeneic blood. In the case of controlled hypotension, this is arguable. The technique has been associated with adverse events such as unexplained visual loss following spinal surgery it appears to be contra-indicated in surgery for subarachnoid haemorrhage and has been described by Jones as "a controversial technique and it may be argued that it is inappropriate in modern anaesthetic practice". The technique cannot be advocated for widespread use until it is supported by better safety data.

Due to the potential for the transmission of infectious diseases with the homologous transfusion of blood products, there has been an increased interest in measures to limit intraoperative blood loss and avoid the need for homologous transfusion during high-risk surgical procedures including spinal surgery. Controlled hypotension (also referred to as deliberate or induced hypotension), defined as a reduction of systolic blood pressure to 80 to 90 mmHg, a reduction of mean arterial pressure (MAP) to 50 to 65 mmHg or a 30% reduction of baseline MAP, is one technique that has been used to limit intraoperative blood loss. When considering the paediatric-aged patient, studies have reported the use of the inhalational agent sevoflurane, the alpha (2)-adrenoceptor agonist dexmedetomidine as well as various vasodilators including sodium nitroprusside, nitroglycerin, fenoldopam, and alprostadil for controlled hypotension. Sevoflurane offers the advantages of easy dosage titration, no need for an additional intravenous infusion as well as providing anaesthesia in addition to controlled hypotension. Disadvantages include a slightly higher cost than some of the intravenous agents and the inability to monitor evoked potentials with high sevoflurane concentrations. Whereas sodium nitroprusside, nicardipine and fenoldopam all provide the desired level of hypotension in paediatric-aged patients, nitroglycerin was not effective in this age group of patients in one study. When comparing nicardipine and sodium nitroprusside, nicardipine offers the potential advantages of fewer episodes of excessive hypotension, less rebound tachycardia and, in one study, less blood loss. Although fenoldopam has been shown to be effective, cost issues may limit widespread application for this technique. The pharmacologic profile of dexmedetomidine indicates that this drug has potential in controlled hypotension and clinical data are needed to define its role.

AUTOLOGOUS BLOOD TRANSFUSION[3]

Paediatric autologous donation is most successful when the likelihood of transfusion is high. For the adolescent and preteen patient, preoperative donation of autologous red cells and frozen plasma components may offer the best choice in many situations. Autologous donation is a recognized alternative in planned orthopedic procedures. One or more donations of whole blood may be adequate to provide the anticipated products.

Stable patients undergoing elective surgical procedures potentially requiring blood transfusion, such as orthopedics, are candidates for preoperative WB collection. Autologous donation can significantly reduce patient exposure to allogeneic red cell antigens and also infectious elements (Henry 2002). To safely donate autologous blood, a patient's haemoglobin should be at least 11 g/dL. Blood donation ≥ 4 weeks before the surgical procedure is recommended to allow time for adequate compensatory erythropoiesis. This time lag reduces the risk of anaemia at the time of surgery by allowing the patient to produce adequate volume recovery. Weekly collection is most common and dietary supplementation with iron is recommended before initiation of autologous blood collections. The WB product is stored at 4°C for up to 35 days, after which it must be frozen or discarded. If the product is not used, it cannot be crossed over for allogeneic use, because autologous donors do not meet the strict criteria required for the general blood donor population. Absolute contraindications to autologous donation are as follows: infection or risk of bacteremia, aortic stenosis, unstable angina, active seizure disorder, myocardial infarction or cerebrovascular accident during previous 6 months, high-grade left main coronary artery disease, cyanotic heart disease, uncontrolled hypertension, and significant pulmonary or cardiac disease.

Acute Normovolemic Haemodilution (ANH)

This technique involves WB collection from patients immediately prior to a procedure in which blood loss is anticipated. Rapid replacement of the removed blood volume with crystalloid or colloid solution is done prior to surgery. Re-infusion of the collected blood typically occurs toward the end of the procedure, or as soon as major bleeding has stopped. The reduction of RBC loss during surgery is the purpose of this technique and is sometimes preferred to the cell-saver WB collection, which ends up with lower haematocrits than ANH blood products.

Postoperative Blood Collection

This procedure involves recovery of blood from surgical drains and is usually filtered but not always washed before reinfusion. The salvaged product may be haemolysed and dilute. The product must be transfused within 6 hours or it must be discarded. The primary indications for postoperative blood collection are cardiac and orthopedic surgery cases (Table 15.6).

HAEMOGLOBIN-BASED OXYGEN CARRIERS, PERFLUOROCHEMICAL SOLUTIONS[4]

Properties of an ideal blood substitute:

- Adequate oxygen delivery to the tissues
- Long circulation time
- Non-toxic
- Rapidly excreted without causing harm
- Stable at room temperature
- Easily sterilized
- Cheap to manufacture
- Long shelf-life and easy to store
- Widely applicable without cross-matching
- Free of side effects

Haemoglobin-based Oxygen Carriers

1. Conjugated Hb (surface modified Hb)
2. Cross linked Hb
3. Polymerised Hb
4. Encapsulated Hb
5. Haemoglobin with antioxidant properties

Conjugated Haemoglobin

Combination of haemoglobin molecules with large molecules like, dextran, polyoxyethylene polyethylene glycol.

Table 15.6 Autologous donation

Advantages	Disadvantages
1. Prevents transfusion-transmitted disease	1. Risk of bacterial contamination or volume overload remains
2. Prevents red cell alloimmunisation	2. Does not eliminate risk of administrative error with ABO incompatibility
3. Supplements the blood supply	3. More costly than allogenic blood
4. Provides compatible blood for patients with alloantibodies	4. Wastage of blood not transfused
5. Prevents some adverse transfusion reactions	5. Causes perioperative anaemia and increased likelihood of transfusion

Conjugated Hb has increased intravascular half life, reduced antigenicity, high osmotic pressure and high viscosity.

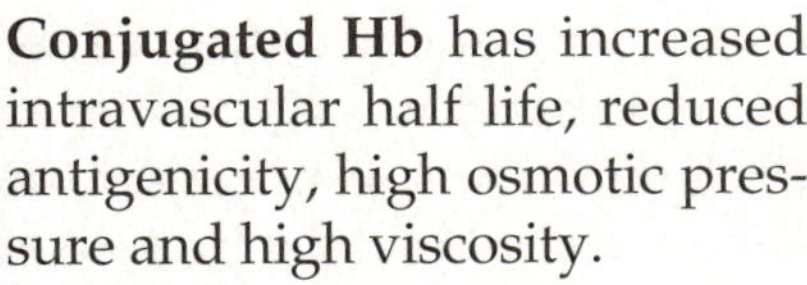

Cross-linked Haemoglobin

Cross-linked means a covalent bond between 2 globin chains through chemical modifications

Advantages of cross-linked Hb

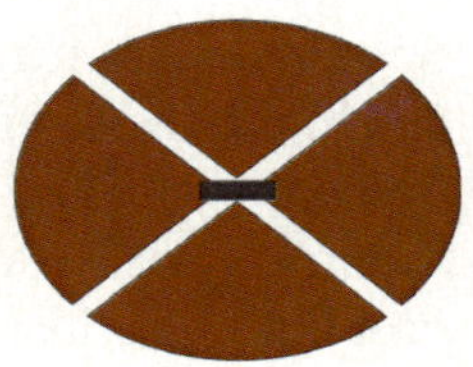

- Higher P50 than normal haemoglobin
- An increase in the plasma half-life of up to 30 hrs
- Eliminates nephrotoxicity

Polymerised Haemoglobin

- Problem of vasoconstriction was solved with polymerisation
- Polymerisation is done with various chemical agents like O-raffinose, Glutaraldehyde, Sebacyl chloride

Encapsulated Haemoglobin

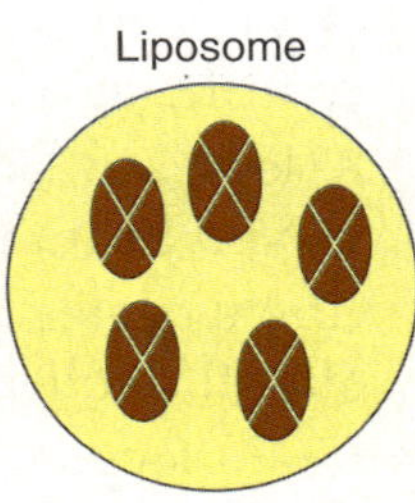

Natural Hb can be encapsulated in synthetic liposomes, made from natural lecithin or synthetic phospholipids. Liposome encapsulated haemoglobin (LEH) mimics natural red cells, and called *Neohemocytes*. LEH are taken by RE cells and their breakdown products cause lasting damage to the cells.

Complexes with Superoxide Dismutase and Catalase (polyhb-sod-cat)

Hb solutions with *antioxidant* properties significantly removes oxygen radicals and peroxides, stabilize the cross-linked Hb and decrease oxidative iron and heme release which in turn reduces ischaemia-reperfusion injury.

Perfluorocarbons (PFCs)

Greenhouse gases developed during aluminium production PFCs are about 1/100th the size of a red blood cell and capacity to dissolve up to 50 times more oxygen than plasma (Figs 15.1 and 15.2).

- Binding curve of PFC is a *linear* function
- Oxygen can be transported in relevant amount to the patients in PFC only when the inspirational oxygen fraction is high enough

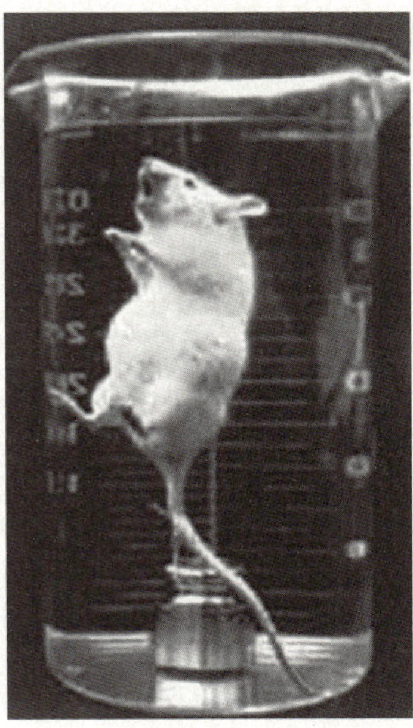

Fig. 15.1 The first real success in fluid breathing[5]

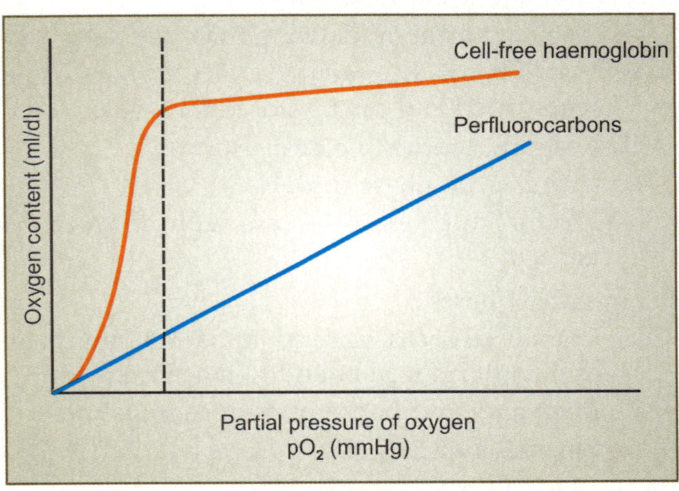

Fig. 15.2 Gas carriage by PFC emulsion

- So, patients on PFCs always need *oxygen supplementation.*
- PFCs are insoluble in water so they need to be emulsified.
- PFCs are chemically and physically inert.
- Relatively inexpensive to produce and contain no biological product (free from infectious disease).

Disadvantages of PFC Emulsion

1. Oxygen toxicity
2. Unstable emulsion, need to be stored in frozen stage
3. Retention in liver and spleen
4. 1st generation PFCs associated with complement activation and immunologic reaction

Table 15.7 Types of PFC

1st Generation	2nd Generation
Dissolved in Puronic F–68	Dissolved in lecithin solution
Associated with complement activation	No complement activation
Example: Flusol-DA	Example: Oxygent (Alliance)

5. PFCs may result in immunosuppression, fever, transient leucopenia, self-limiting transient thrombocytopenia.

Platelet Substitutes

Attempts were made to make synthetic platelet analogs to increase and extend the function of autologous platelets in circulation.

Three types of platelets substitutes are under development:

1. Infusible platelets membranes

- i. Prepared from outdated human platelets
- ii. Platelets are fragmented, virally inactivated, lyophilized and can be stored for 2 years
- iii. Resistant to immune destruction
- iv. Currently in phase II trials
- v. Product appears to be safe with no thrombogenecity

2. Thrombospheres

- i. Composed of cross-linked human albumins with human fibrinogen bound to the surface
- ii. It appears to enhance platelet aggregation
- iii. Entered clinical trial in Europe

3. Liposome based agents

- i. Plateletosomes
- ii. Factor Xa with phospholipids vesicles
- iii. Plateletosomes are lipid vesicles with platelet glycoproteins on their surface
- iv. Both are hemostatically effective in vitro but they have shown high toxicity in animal models.

BLOOD COMPONENT THERAPY, PLATELETS, WHITE CELLS AND PLASMA[6]

Blood components are usually requested and prepared based on the individual need of a patient. Several "special" product requirements that may be requested for the neonatal or older paediatric patient include: (1) "Fresh" red blood cells (RBCs) or wholeblood, (2) Cytomegalovirus (CMV) "safe" components, (3) Leukocyte-reduced blood components, (4) Irradiated cellular components, (5) Units that are negative for haemoglobin S, (6) Volume-reduced platelet products, and (7) Components that are packaged into small volume containers.

Granulocytes

The subgroups where the most success in reducing mortality has been demonstrated have been in neonates with severe neutropenia and sepsis because of the use of a higher dose of granulocytes per size of the recipient (neonate) and the use of repetitive transfusions over a minimum of 5 days. Granulocyte transfusions should probably be considered in:

- Severely neutropenic patients (ANC $<500 \times 10^9$) with bacterial sepsis or infection with yeast and fungi, in whom antimicrobials or antifungals have failed and in whom bone marrow recovery is expected to be delayed at least 3 weeks.

  Allogeneic granulocyte donors should be mobilized with G-CSF (5 mg/kg/day) and dexamethasone (8 mg po), 12 hours before the scheduled collection.
- Granulocytes should be collected by continuous flow centrifugation techniques.
- At least 2 to 3×10^{10} granulocytes (not less than 1×10^{10}) should be transfused daily for a minimum of 5 days.
- Granulocytes should be transfused as soon as possible after the collection.
- Granulocytes should be obtained from compatible donors if possible (by HLA match and/or leukocyte cross-matching).

REFERENCES

1. Cassandra D Josephson. Neonatal and Paediatric Transfusion Practice, Technical manual AABB, 17th edn. p 645–63.
2. World J Cardiol 2010 February 26;2(2):27–33. ISSN 1949–8462 (online).
3. Alternatives to Transfusion: Perioperative Blood Management Lynne Uhl, Rossi's principles of Transfusion Medicine, 4th edn. 566–72.
4. Bhat Sudha, Shivram C. Transfusion Medicine For Clinicians, 2011;197–208.
5. Clark LC Jr. and Gollan F. Survival of mammals breathing organic liquids equilibrated with oxygen at atmospheric pressure. Science 1996;152:155.
6. David C Burghardt. Component Preparation and Storage, Handbook of Paediatric Transfusion Medicine, 2001;9–17.

16

Acute and Chronic Pain Management in Infants and Children

Dinesh Kumar Sahu and Anjana Sahu

INTRODUCTION

Neonates and infants are more sensitive to painful stimuli than adults. In the past it was believed that preterm and term neonates did not have fully developed pain pathway, therefore, they did not feel pain but now it has been proven that they do feel pain and respond well to the analgesics.[1] Children also report stronger pain for stimuli that evoke moderate tissue damage in comparison to adults. The pain perceptions differ in children from those of adults because of developmental changes in their understanding and previous pain experiences. As children mature they experience a wider diversity of pains varying in location, intensity, and quality. The nociceptive system in children is plastic therefore they respond differently to the same amount of tissue damage. In children, perception of pain depend on complex neural interactions, impulses generated by tissue damage are modified both by ascending systems activated by a noxious stimulus (e.g. touch) and by descending pain suppressing systems activated by various situational factors, such as a child's expectations about what he or she will feel.

Type of pain: Pain is defined as *"an unpleasant sensory and emotional experience associated with actual or potential tissue damage, or described in terms of such damage"* by International Association for Study of Pain (IASP). It is classified into nociceptive and neuropathic pain based upon the underlying pathophysiology. Determining the type of pain helps in identifying the cause of pain, which may guide treatment of choices.

- **Nociceptive pain** is caused by stimulation of intact nociceptors as a result of tissue injury and inflammation. It is divided into somatic pain and visceral pain. Somatic pain is due to pathology in skin, soft tissue, skeletal muscle, and bone; and it is well localized and described as sharp, aching, squeezing, stabbing, or throbbing. Visceral pain is due to pathology with receptors in internal organs, such as the kidney and gastrointestinal tract; and it is typically poorly localized, and is often described as dull, cramp, achy, and diffuse to localize.
- **Neuropathic pain** is caused by stimulation or abnormal functioning of peripheral or central nervous system neurones. It can be caused by compression, transection, infiltration, ischaemia, or metabolic injury to the nerves. It is often described as burning, shooting, electric, or tingling.
- **Acute pain** is of sudden onset, is felt immediately following injury, is severe in intensity, but is usually short-lasting. It arises as a result of tissue injury stimulating nociceptors and generally disappears when the injury heals.
- **Chronic pain** is continuous or recurrent pain that persists beyond the expected normal time of healing. Chronic pain may begin as acute pain and persist for long periods or may recur due to persistence of noxious stimuli or repeated exacerbation of an injury. Chronic pain may also arise and persist in the absence of identifiable pathophysiology or medical illness (Table 16.1).

Key Points

- Infants have immature nervous systems but they do feel pain.
- Untreated acute pain in children does have long-term adverse effects.
- Children do not carry a higher risk of drug addiction when they receive opioids for pain control.

Contd...

Table 16.1 Common type of chronic pain occur in children

1. Neuropathic pain
   - Complex regional pain syndrome type I
   - Complex regional pain syndrome type II
     - peripheral nerve injuries
     - postamputation pain
     - deafferentation pain
2. Headache
3. Chest pain
4. Recurrent abdominal pain
5. Chronic illness
   - Sickle cell disease
   - Cystic fibrosis
   - Collagen vascular disease (e.g. juvenile rheumatoid arthritis, systemic lupus erythematosus)
   - Myofacial pain, fibromyalgia
6. Cancer pain

Key Points *(Contd...)*
- Pain can be measured in infants and children.
- Children do suffer from chronic pain.
- As many as 40% of otherwise healthy children experience recurrent pain problems such as headache, abdominal pain, and lower limb pain.

ASSESSMENT OF PAIN SEVERITY AND COGNITION

Several pain scales that can be used for children, including infants comprised of itemized lists of the various distress behaviors, have been designed to more specifically assess pain intensity. In children, assessment of the severity of pain is performed by the following two methods:

- Self-reporting
- Observational scales

Self-reporting

Self-reporting relies upon the cognitive ability of the child. In younger children, evaluation of paediatric pain typically uses age-based, pain rating scales.

- **Younger children (3 to 8 years of age):** Some children as young as three years of age are capable of quantifying their pain and being able to translate it to a visual representation. In this age group, pain is quantified by using visual analog pain scales based upon a series of faces showing an increase in distress or pain (Fig. 16.1).[2–4]
- **Older children (8 to 11 years of age):** Pain assessment in this age group is generally performed using visual analog tools that rate the intensity of pain on a horizontal or numeric scale (e.g. 0 to 10 scale).

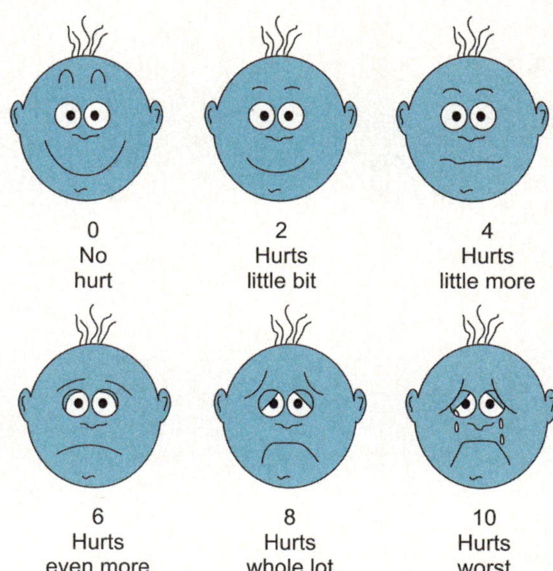

Fig. 16.1 Wong-Baker FACES® pain rating scale

- **Adolescents:** Adolescents can rate their pain using a numerical rating scale without the use of an accessory pain assessment tool. In this age group, a description of the following components of pain usually can be obtained from the history:
  - *Description:* Sharp, stabbing, dull, burning, or tingling
  - *Location and radiation:* Point the pain start and spread pattern
  - *Intensity:* On a scale of 1 to 10
  - *Duration and constancy:* Continuous or remission
  - Frequency.
  - Factors that aggravate or relieve pain
- **Pain-location tools:** Several graphic-based pain-location tools have been used to determine the location of pain in children and adolescents including the adolescent and paediatric pain tool and the paediatric pain questionnaire. These tools typically use a graphic outline of the body, and the patient is asked to "colour" in the areas where he/she is experiencing pain.

Observational Tools

The following observational tools are used to assess pain in infants and children who are unable to self-report. These pain scales are based upon scoring facial expressions, ability to be consolved, level of interaction, limb and trunk motor responses, and verbal responses.[5–7]

- Revised face, legs, activity, cry, consolability (r-FLACC) tool:[8,9] Nonverbal children (Table 16.2).
- Non-Communicating Children's Pain Checklist-Postoperative Version (NCCPC-PV):[10] Nonverbal children.

- Nursing Assessment of Pain Intensity (NAPI):[16] Newborn to 16 years of age.
- CRIES neonatal post-op pain measurement score (Table 16.3).

In a study that compared the r-FLACC, NCCPC-PV, and NAPI assessment tools, the r-FLACC received the highest clinical utility score followed by the NAPI. Based upon the limited data, no tool can be recommended over another. It is important that each center adopt guidelines of routine assessment for the detection of pain and provide staff training in the use of the selected pain assessment tool.

Nonverbal children with neurological impairment—Nonverbal children with neurological impairment (NI) present unique challenges in evaluating the presence and severity of pain as they cannot self-report their pain. For many such children, pain can remain a frequent, recurrent problem that often remains undertreated without appropriate evaluation.

History and behavior patterns should be obtained from parents or caregiver. Specific behaviors that are associated with pain in nonverbal children with NI include:

- Vocalizations (crying, moaning).
- Facial expression (grimacing).
- Inability to be consoled.
- Increased movement, tone and posture (arching, stiffening), and physiological responses.
- In addition, some children display atypical behaviors such as laughing, becoming withdrawn, and lack of facial expression.

The pain assessment for nonverbal children with NI should be done with observational tools.

MANAGEMENT

Pain treatment should always be started moment patient starts complaining of pain. The best way to start a pain medication is to record VAS of the patient. Many hospitals are now including VAS as 5th vital sign to be noted routinely. The management should be protocol based.

Protocol

Four simple concepts should be followed when administering analgesics to children:[11]

1. by the ladder,
2. by the mouth,
3. by the clock,
4. by the child

By the ladder

It means a three-step approach for selecting progressively stronger traditional analgesic drugs

Table 16.2 r-FLCC pain assessment scale

Criteria	Score 0	Score 1	Score 2
Face	No particular expression or smile	Occasional grimace or frown, withdrawn, uninterest	Frequent to constant quivering chin, clenched jaw
Legs	Normal position or relaxed	Uneasy, restless, tense	Kicking, or legs drawn up
Activity	Lying quietly, normal position, moves easily	Squirming, shifting, back and forth, tense	Arched, rigid or jerking
Cry	No cry (awake or asleep)	Moans or whimpers; occasional complaint	Crying steadily, screams or sobs, frequent complaints
Consolability	Content, relaxed	Reassured by occasional touching, hugging or being talked to, distractible	Difficult to console or comfort

The scores are added together to get a 0–10 pain score, 0 = No pain, 10 = Maximum pain.

Table 16.3 CRIES neonatal postoperative pain measurement score*

Score#	0	1	2
Crying	No	High pitched	Inconsolable
Requires O_2 for Sat >95%	No	<30%	>30%
Increased vital signs	HR and BP, = or < of preop	HR or BP increased <20% of preop	HR or BP increased >20% of preop
Expression	No expression or smile	Grimace	Grimace/Grunt
Sleepless	No	Wakes up at frequent intervals	Constantly awake

*Neonatal pain assessment tool developed at the University of Missouri-Columbia, by S Krechel, MD and J Bildner, RNC, CNS.
#Medication should be given to infant, if score is 4 or greater.

(acetaminophen, codeine, or morphine) according to a child's level of pain (mild, moderate, or strong). Even when children need opioid analgesics, they should continue to receive nonsteroidal antiinflammatory drugs as supplemental analgesics.

Recently, attention has focused on ''thinking beyond the ladder'' and using adjuvant analgesics as the first step for children whose pain has neuropathic origin. Adjuvant analgesics include a variety of drugs with analgesic properties that were initially developed to treat other health problems, such as convulsions and depression. These drugs more specifically target neuropathic mechanisms and are critical analgesics for certain types of pain (Table 16.4).

By the mouth

It means the oral route of drug administration. Medication should be administered to children by the simplest effective route, usually by mouth as far as possible. Because children are afraid of injections, they may deny that they have pain or may not request medication.

By the clock

It means timing for administering analgesic medications. Analgesics should be administered on a regular schedule, e.g. every 4 or 6 hours, based on the drug's duration of action and the severity of the child's pain, not on as-needed (SOS) basis, unless a child's episodes of pain are truly intermittent and unpredictable.

By the child

It means individualization of drug dose as per child's conditions. The goal is to select a dose that prevents children from experiencing pain before they receive the next dose. It is essential to monitor a child's pain regularly and adjust analgesic doses as necessary.

Table 16.4 Ladder approach

VAS	Grade of pain	Medication	WHO analgesic ladder steps
1–2	Mild	Preferably no medication, Reassurance	1
3–4	Mild	Preferably Paracetamol if not controlled, then NSAID	2
5–7	Moderate	Paracetamol ± Weak Narcotic	2
8–10	Severe	Paracetamol ± Strong Narcotic ± NSAID ± Interventional procedure	3

Pain Medications

- Nonopioid analgesics (Paracetamol, NSAIDs).
- Opioid analgesics (Codeine, Morphine, Fentanyl).
- Local anaesthetics.
- Co-analgesics (or adjuvant analgesics).
- Corticosteroids.

Non-pharmacological Treatments

- Psychological interventions (cognitive therapy, behavioural therapy).
- Transcutaneous electrical nerve stimulation.
- Physical therapies.

PAIN MEDICATIONS

Neonates and infants require the same analgesic drugs as older children. However, the difference in pharmacokinetics and pharmacodynamics among neonates, preterm infants, and full-term infants warrants special dosing considerations and close monitoring when they receive opioids. Paracetamol can be safely administered to neonates and infants without concern for hepatotoxicity when given for short courses at the recommended dose. The starting doses for opioid analgesics in infants under 6 months of age are one-quarter to one-half of the suggested doses. As for children, the dosage and mode of administration of opioids need to be titrated between the degree of analgesia required and a reasonable level of sedation. While prescribing analgesics one should keep in mind the possible side effects and adjuncts to minimize them, should also be prescribed.

NONOPIOIDS ANALGESICS

Aspirin, paracetamol, non-selective non-steroidal anti-inflammatory drugs (NSAIDs), cyclooxygenase-2 selective inhibitors (coxibs) are the commonly available nonopioid analgesics. NSAIDs commonly used in children are Ibuprofen and Diclofenac (Table 16.5). The combination of paracetamol and NSAID was clearly more effective than paracetamol alone. Paracetamol is also an effective adjunct to opioid analgesia. Opioid requirements are reduced by 20% to 30% when combined with a regular regimen of oral or rectal paracetamol.

OPIOID ANALGESICS

Opioid drugs available in India for pain management are buprenorphine, pentazocine, pethidine, codeine,

Table 16.5 Nonopioid analgesics

Drug	Dosage	Comment
Aspirin	10–15 mg/kg PO, every 4–6 h	Very useful in Juvenile rheumatoid arthritis and other rheumatological conditions. Contraindication in viral infection and platelet dysfunction.
Paracetamol	10–15 mg/kg PO, every 4–6 h 35–45 mg/kg Rectal, every 6–12 h	No GIT and haematological effect; lacks anti-inflammatory effects, hepatic failure with overdose. Avoid in glucose-6-phosphate dehydrogenase deficiency.
Ibuprofen	5–10 mg/kg PO, every 6–8 h	Anti-inflammatory activity. Risk of GIT bleeding, platelet dysfunction
Naproxen	10–20 mg/kg/day, PO, every 12 h Dose limit of 1 g/day	Avoid in patients with severe renal impairment
Diclofenac	1 mg/kg PO, every 8–12 h Dose limit of 50 mg/dose. 0.3 mg/kg IV, 0.5 mg/kg Rectal	Avoid in GI ulcer, bronchial asthma, renal and hepatic dysfunction.

PO—by mouth, IV—intravenous, GIT—gastrointestinal

dextropropoxyphene, fentanyl, sufentanil, morphine and atypical opioids are tramadol and tapentadol. Out of this fentanyl, sufentanil and morphine come under narcotic rules and regulations. Opioids are most commonly used analgesics for moderate to severe acute pain. Owing to immature development of hepatic and renal system opioids have longer elimination half life and slower elimination in neonates and infants. During initial 3–4 months of age these infants have decreased ventilatory drive to hypoxia and hypercarbia therefore continuous cardiorespiratory monitoring is recommended. opiods can be administered through oral, intravascular, intramuscular, rectal, subcutaneous, transdermal or transmucosal route (Table 16.6).

Table 16.6 Opioid dosing regimen[12]

Opioid	Routes/Age groups	Dosage
Morphine	PO, infants and children	0.3 mg/kg every 3–4 h
	IV bolus:	
	Pre-term neonate	10–25 μg/kg every 2–4 h
	Full-erm neonate	25–50 μg/kg every 3–4 h
	Infants and children	50–100 μg/kg every 2–4 h
	IV infusion:	
	Pre-term neonate	2–5 μg/kg/h
	Full-term neonate	5–10 μg/kg/h
	Infants and children	15–30 μg/kg/h
	Epidural bolus:	
	Infants and children	25–30 μg/kg
	Epidural infusion:	
	Infants and children	4–8 μg/kg/h
Fentanyl	Oral transmucosal	10–15 μg/kg
	Intranasal	1–2 μg/kg
	Transdermal	25, 50, 75, 100 μg/h
	IV bolus	0.5–1 μg/kg every 1–2 h
	IV infusion	0.5 μg/kg/h
	Epidural bolus	0.5–1 μg/kg
	Epidural infusion	0.2–1 μg/kg/h
Pethidine	**IV bolus:**	
	Infants and children	0.8–1 mg/kg every 3–4 h
Codeine	PO, infants and children	0.5–1 mg/kg every 4 h

Opioid-related Side Effects in Children

The most common side effects of opioids are nausea, vomiting, pruritus, constipation, and sedation. Children may not tell all side effects (i.e. constipation, dysphoria) voluntarily, therefore these problems should be asked individually. Some side effects may subside within first or second week of the treatment as the child develops tolerance to them (e.g. nausea, vomiting, and drowsiness). Children should be properly instructed about these problems and should be encouraged to be with the treatment. If side effects persist, then appropriate measurement should be taken in the form of slow titration of the dosage or shift to alternate opioid. if respiratory depression occurs, can be reversed with administration of μ receptor antagonist naloxone (0.1 mg/kg) in infants and children.

As opioids may induce physical dependence and tolerance, the dose should be adjusted according to the need of controlling pain. Physical dependence may develop after a week of treatment and similarly tolerance too. However, these two effects are different from addiction and there is no reported evidence of children addiction for opioid analgesics administering for pain management.

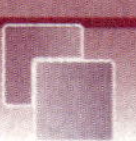

Clinical Pearls for Opioid used in Children

1. Choose an appropriate route, oral is preferred. Whenever continuous IV infusion is used, hourly SOS rescue doses with short-onset opioids should be available. A rescue dose is usually 50–200% of continuous hourly dose. If more than six rescues are necessary in a 24-hour period, increase the hourly infusion rate by the total amount of rescues for the previous 24 hours divided by 24. An alternative is to increase infusion rate by 50%.
2. Choose an appropriate drug and dose. If inadequate pain relief and no toxicity at peak onset of opioid action, increase dose in 50% increments.
3. To change opioids: Because of incomplete cross-tolerance, if changing between opioids with short duration of action, start the new opioid at 50% of the calculated equianalgesic dose. Titrate to effect. If changing between opioids from short to long duration of action (i.e. morphine to fentanyl), start at 25% of equianalgesic dose and titrate to effect.
4. When discontinuing drug or tapering opioids: For anyone receiving opioids for more than 1 week, the dose should be tapered to avoid withdrawal symptoms. Taper by 50% for 2 days, then decrease by 25% every 2 days. When dose is equianalgesic to an oral morphine dose of 0.6 mg/kg/day, it may be stopped. Some patients on opioids for prolonged periods may require much slower tapering.
5. Pethidine is not recommended for chronic use because norpethidine may accumulate,which is a toxic metabolite with a long serum half-life, can cause myoclonus, hyper reflexia, and seizures.

LOCAL ANAESTHETICS

Commonly used local anaesthetics are lignocaine, bupivacaine, levobupivacaine and ropivacaine. These medications should be used only in supervised atmosphere where resuscitation facilities are available. Adverse effects can occur with local anaesthetics and are usually dose-related. These include sensory and motor deficits when these agents are administered regionally or intraspinally. Neurologic or mental status change may signify systemic toxicity from increasing blood levels of medication. Dizziness, confusion, circum-oral numbness, metallic taste, and seizures are some of the signs that suggest neurotoxicity. Potential cardiovascular reactions include dysrhythmias, hypotension, and severe cardiovascular collapse. Allergic reactions to local anaesthetics can occur but are rare (Table 16.7).

COANALGESICS

Adjuvant therapy can be used with any child with pain regardless of intensity. It can enhance analgesic efficacy, treat concurrent symtoms, and/or independent analgesic activity for specific type of pain. Adjuvant therapy is particularly helpful for neuropathic pain and chronic pain, especially children with cancer. Adjuvant therapy in children include the following classes of drugs:

- Antidepressant for neuropathic pain (Tricyclic antidepressant—0.1–0.2 mg/kg titrated up to 1 mg/kg/day)
- Anticonvulsant for neuropathic pain (Gabapentine—2 mg/kg tds, Carbamazepine—10 mg/kg/day divided into 2–4 doses)
- Gucocorticoid for hepatic distention and cerebral oedema
- Salmon calcitonin and biphosphonite for bone pain
- Radiation therapy for bone pain due to tumor
- Complementary and alternative medicines—vitamins and minerals
- NMDA-receptor antagonists—ketamine as systemic analgesic
- Alpha-2 agonists—adjuvants to LA for nerve blocks (Clonidine and dexmedetomidine)
- Neurolytic agents—sympathetic blockades (alcohol, phenol)

CORTICOSTEROIDS (Anti-inflammatory Drugs)

Most commonly used drugs are dexamethasone, hydrocortisone, prednisolone, triamcenalone, methyl prednisolone. These are good adjuncts especially in inflammatory pain or terminally ill cancer pain patients. These should be used in short bursts and should be

Table 16.7 Local anaesthetics dosage

Local anaesthetics	Maximum dose	Comments
Lignocaine	5 mg/kg 7 mg/kg with adrenaline	Cardiac depressant at higher doses
Bupivacane	2.5 mg/kg	More cardiac depressant than lignocaine
Levobupivacaine	2.5 mg/kg	Less cardiotoxic than bupivacaine
Ropivacaine	2.5 mg/kg	Less cardiotoxic than bupivacaine and levobupivacaine

discontinued after giving it for a few weeks to prevent steroid related side effects. Oral dosage should be started if patient is managed in outpatient department. Intravenous loading dosage of prednisolone or Dexamethasone can be given if patient is inpatient.

Steroid	Dosage	Half life
Dexamethasone	0.2 mg/kg	36 to 72 hrs
Prednisolone	2 mg/kg	18 to 36 hrs
Hydrocortisone	10 mg/kg	8 to 12 hrs
Methyl prednisolone	2 mg/kg	18 to 36 hrs

Methods of Administration

a. Systemic administered analgesia
   - Oral route
   - Intravenous route
   - Intramuscular and subcutaneous routes
   - Rectal route
   - Transdermal route
   - Transmucosal routes

b. Regionally and local administered analgesia
   - Epidural analgesia
   - Intrathecal analgesia
   - Regional analgesia and peripheral nerve block
   - Other local analgesic techniques

c. Patient-controlled analgesia (PCA)
   - Epidural PCA analgesia (PCA IV)
   - Intravenous PCA analgesia (PCEA)

METHODS OF ADMINISTRATION

Systemic Administered Analgesia

One of the following methods can be used:

1. **Oral route:** Paracetamol, NSAIDs, COX-2 inhibitors, tramadol, codeine, morphine, etc.
2. **Intravenous route:** Most of the drugs can be given with this route either intermittent or continuous in acute conditions.
3. **Intramuscular and subcutaneous routes:** Inj diclofenac, inj tramadol, inj pentazocine or inj morphine. Morphine can also be used through SC route.
4. **Rectal route:** Paracetamol, diclofenac, tramadol are available for this route
5. **Transdermal route:** Diclofenac Sodium, Fentanyl, Buprenorphine are used with this route
6. **Transmucosal routes:** Fentanyl as lollypop preparation.

Regional and Local Administered Analgesia

1. **Epidural analgesia:**
   - Continuous epidural analgesia: Patient is connected to continuous infusion through epidural catheter with 'syringe pump'or 'automatic reservoir pump/elastomeric pump'.
   - Intermittent epidural analgesia: It can be given where infusion is to be avoided in certain patient, syringe pump is not available or those patient showing persistent side effects like nausea, vomiting, itching or hypotension.
2. **Intrathecal analgesia:** Opioids are added to local anaesthetics to prolonged analgesic effect. Clinical experience with morphine, fentanyl and sufentanil has shown no neurotoxicity or behavioural changes at normal intrathecal doses.
3. **Regional analgesia and peripheral nerve block:** Brachial plexus block, celiac plexus block, femoral nerve block, intercostals block are given to relief acute pain with dose adjusted for paediatric patient.
4. **Other local analgesic techniques:** Intra-articular injection, wound infiltration with local anaesthetics, etc.

Patient-controlled Analgesia

It is used in acute settings for usually indoor patients in hospitals. It has also been used for cancer patients at home. PCA pumps are microprocessor based portable devices, which run on battery or electricity. The electronic pump gives continuous background infusion superimposed on patient controlled boluses. It can be programmed to deliver a specific dose by patients themselves on an as-needed basis, the minimum interval between doses (lockout period) and maximum dose of drug that can be given in a given period. Patients can be ambulating and do exercise also by carrying electronic PCA pump with them. The pump is connected to epidural catheter, peripheral nerve block catheter or IV cannula (Tables 16.8 and 16.9).

Table 16.8 PCA IV dosage

Drug	Demand dose (µg/kg)	Lockout interval (min.)	Basal infusion (µg/kg/h)	1 hour max. limit (µg/kg)	SOS rescue dose (µg/kg)
Morphine	20	8–10	0–20	100	50
Fentanyl	0.5	6–8	0–0.5	2.5	0.5–1

Table 16.9 PCA IV dosage (lumbar epidural)

Drug	Demand dose (mL/kg)	Lockout interval (min.)	Basal infusion (mL/kg/h)	1 hour max. limit (mL/kg)	Adjuvants
Bupivacaine 0.0625–0.1%	0.05–0.1	20–30	0.1–0.2	0.2–0.4	Fentanyl 5 µg/mL or Morphine 0.5 mg/mL
Ropivacaine 0.1–0.2%	0.05–0.1	20–30	0.1–0.2	0.2–0.4	Fentanyl 5 µg/mL or Morphine 0.5 mg/mL

NON PHARMACOLOGICAL TREATMENTS

Nonpharmacologic therapies are as important as medications in relieving pain. They involve physical modalities, such as acupuncture, massage, positioning, deep breathing, and application of heat or cold, and psychosocial modalities, such as distraction, biofeedback, and imagery. TENS has also been used in acute pain conditions apart from chronic pain.

Cognitive	Behavioral	Physical
Information Choices and control Distraction and attention Guided imagery Hypnosis	Exercise Relaxation therapy Biofeedback Behavioral Psychotherapy	Massage Physiotherapy Thermal stimulation Sensory stimulation TENS Acupuncture

Cognitive Therapies in Paediatric Clinical Practice

Cognitive therapies are an essential component of pain control because treatment should be directed at all of the causes of children's pain and suffering. Cognitive therapies are directed at a child's beliefs, expectations, and coping abilities. They encompass a wide range of approaches from basic patient education to formal psychotherapy. Cognitive interventions are the most powerful and versatile nondrug pain therapies for children. A basic cognitive intervention comprises providing children with age-appropriate information about pain and teaching them how to use simple coping strategies. When children receive accurate information about what will happen to them and what they may feel, they can improve their understanding, increase their control, lessen their distress, and reduce their pain. Healthcare providers should emphasize the sensory aspects (i.e. tingling, cool, sharp) rather than the hurting aspect when they prepare children for invasive procedures.

Distraction and focused attention, as well as guided imagery, are practical tools that health professionals and parents can routinely use when children experience pain. Music, lights, colored objects, tactile toys, sweet tastes, and other children are effective attention-grabbing stimuli, particularly in young children. Conversation, games, computers, and interesting movies are effective distracters for older children and adolescents.

Behavioral Therapy in Pain Management for Children

Behavioral therapies are designed to change either children's own behavior or the behavior of the adults who interact with them. The therapeutic objective is to lessen behaviors that can increase children's pain, distress, and disability, while increasing behaviors that can reduce pain. Progressive muscle relaxation and simple repetitive physical exercise (depending on the patient's preference) are convenient methods for most children to use during painful medical treatments. During stressful treatments, many children seem naturally to tense their muscles and hold their breath. Some children can learn to relax by alternately tightening and loosening their fists, by rhythmically moving a leg, or by deep, paced breathing.

General exercise regimens are an important component of pain management for children experiencing recurrent or persistent pain, as well as for children requiring multiple and repeated painful treatments. The objective is to restore as many of a child's normal activities as possible to provide them with enjoyment, increase their participation in social events, increase their independent pain management, and help them reduce their stress.

CHRONIC PAIN

Assessment

Psychosocial assessment of the child and family focuses on an assessment of the child's emotional functioning, coping skills, and impact of pain on daily life including sleeping, eating, school, social and physical activities, and family and peer interactions. A complete physical and neurological examination that includes observation of the child's general appearance, posture, and gait should be performed with the focus on but not limited to the affected area. Basic vital signs and growth parameters should be obtained during at least the first evaluation. Judicious laboratory and radiological studies are useful if a specific disease is suspected.

Chronic Headache

The most common type of headaches that occur in children are tension headache, migraine and mixed tension migraine headache. Migraine headache are slightly more common in boys before age of puberty and in girls after menarche. There is strong family history of migraine. Many children with migraine may not describe the classic visual or auditory aura but may instead report fatigue, irritability, dizziness, or nausea prior to development of the headache. Children mostly have throbbing unilateral of frontal headaches that are frequently associated photophobia, nausea, and vomiting. More than 90% children get relief from sleep only. Tension headache are frequently described as squeezing pain that occurs bilaterally, and circumferentially, or in a occipital region. Tension headaches are without aura.

Drug therapy of migraine, includes abortive drugs and prophylactic drugs.

Abortive: NSAIDs are the first line drugs paracetamol 10–15 mg/kg orally, ibuprofen 6–10 mg/kg orally. Injectable diclofenac or ketorolac can be used in patient with vomiting. Sumitriptan is 5-HT serotonin antagonist can be used orally, nasally, or intramuscularly.

Prophylactic: B-Blocker, anticonvulsants, and antidepressants are drugs for prophylactic migraine therapy. propranolol 1–2 mg/kg daily, low dose TCA such as nortriptyline 0.2 mg/kg orally bedtimes (titrated up to 1 mg/kg/day).

Abdominal pain

About 10–20 percent of school-age children experience recurrent abdominal pain, out of these 10% of cases has organic cause.[12] A thorough history, physical examination, and review of systems is crucial in determining organic causes of abdominal pain. A psychological history is mandatory to understand, how the child and family cope with pain, and to explore any behaviour suggesting school avoidance and social isolation.

Common causes: Constipation, lactose intolerance, irritable bowel syndrome

Treatment strategies: Improve pain coping skill through behavioral approaches, diet modification, and to treat organic cause, if any. The routine use of pain medication should be avoided.

Chest Pain

It is a frequent complaint among children and adolescents. The most common aetiologies of chest pain include musculoskeletal conditions particularly costochondiritis. Other causes are idiopathic chest pain and psychogenic. In general, cardiac causes are usually suggested by history, physical exam, and family history. Abdominal and GIT diseases such as reflux esophagitis, eosophageal spasm or gastritis may present with chest pain.

NSAIDs are helpful for a musculoskeletal chest pain. Many children and adolescents get relief with nonpharmacological therapy like tens, heat therapy, exercise, and stress relaxation techniques.

Neuropathic Pain

IASP recommended that all neuropathic pain syndrome should be group together and called complex regional pain syndrome (CRPS). CRPS is divided into two different types: CRPS-I follows soft tissue injury, and CRPS-II follows a peripheral nerve injury.

CRPS-I

CRPS-I is characterised by persistent limb pain and allodynia, with cyanosis, mottling, coldness, increasing sweating, atrophy, or other sign of autonomic dysfunction including osteopenia. In children majority of patients are female and a lower limb involvement are common.

Treatment in adult, emphasis on early and aggressive use of sympathetic block, in contrast, children should be given noninvasive regimen first that emphasis active physical therapy and cognitive-behavioral interventions. Medication commonly tried includes TCA, anticonvulsants, and oral vasodilator with variable results. Sympathetic blocks are used in children who do not get relief with noninvasive therapy. To avoid multiple procedures, continuous catheter infusion technique is preferred.

CRPS-II

CRPS-II in children occur primarily as a result of extremity trauma, post-surgical nerve injury, nerve involvement of tumour, metabolic neuropathy, and congenital and traumatic paraplegia. It present as burning pain, pin-prick, or numbness sensations. Phantom limb sensation are described as a variety of sensory sensation like itching, tingling, and pain referred to the absent limb.

Treatments for neuropathic pain mainly include physical therapy including TENS, tricyclic antidepressants, anticonvulsants, cognitive-behavioral therapy and physical rehabilitation.

Chronic Illness

Other causes of chronic pain include cystic fibrosis, sickle cell disease, collagen vascular disease, etc.

Cyctic fibrosis: Children usually present with chest pain, headaches, back pain, compression fracture and arthritic pain. COX-2 inhibitors are preferred over NSAIDs due to less risk of exacerbating hemoptasis.

Sickle cell disease: It is characterise by both acute and chronic pain. Vaso-occlusive episodes produce severe ischaemia pain in abdomen and extremities.

Collagen vascular disease: Children with juvenile rheumatoid arthritis, systemic lupus erythematosus present with multiple joint pains.

Myofascial pain and fibromyalgia: Children frequently present with a spectrum of complaints related to myalgia, fatigue, dizziness, etc. Sedentary lifestyle and less outdoor activity are contributory factors. Children should be evaluated for nutritional deficiency.

Treatment for pain due to chronic illness should be "by ladder" approach along with non-pharmacological treatment.

Cancer Pain

Pain related to treatment

It is essential to provide children undergoing invasive procedures (e.g. bone marrow aspirations, catheter placements, lumbar punctures) with appropriate analgesic or anaesthetic treatments, such as topical anaesthetic creams before painful needle insertions and sedatives for aversive procedures. However, note that many children prefer not to be sedated, and wish to remain alert and aware. Children can use simple coping strategies to complement the analgesic regimen. Pain can be minimized when children have increased control, increased choice, and accurate information about what will happen. Imagery, distraction, and attention focusing are valuable tools for many children.

Pain related to tumour

Tumour may produce nociceptive pain as well as neuropathic pain. Treatment approach should follow WHO's "analgesic ladder". Pain in children with cancer should be viewed not as an isolated concern, but rather must be seen in the context of a condition that produces fear, anxiety, grief, loss, and suffering. Pharmacological treatment should always be accompanied by psychosocial support.

SUMMARY

Neonate, infant and smaller children unable to express their pain in words but they can show it by changing their behaviour. Nowadays various methods and modes are available to assess their pain and manage them effectively. Multimodal approach uses several modalities of pain management to provide a total pain free and stress-free state. Multimodal technique of pain management involves administration of two or more drugs or module that act by different mechanisms via a single route or different routes for providing superior analgesic efficacy with equivalent or reduced adverse effects. Pain management particularly chronic pain needs multidisciplinary approach in children with a psychologist, physiotherapist and a pain specialist.

REFERENCES

1. Anand KJS, Hickey PR. Pain and its effect in the human neonate and fetes. N Engl J Med. 1987;317:1321.
2. Wong DL, Hockenberry-Eaton M, Wilson D, et al. Wong's Essentials of Pediatric Nursing, Mosby, St Louis. 2001; Volume 6.
3. Wong DL, Baker CM. Pain in children: comparison of assessment scales. Pediatr Nurs. 1988;14:9.
4. Tomlinson D, von Baeyer CL, Stinson JN, et al. A systematic review of faces scales for the self-report of pain intensity in children. Pediatrics. 2010; 126:e1168.
5. Bush JP, Harkins SW, (Eds). Children in pain: Clinical and research issues from a developmental perspective, New York, 1991, Springer-Verlag.
6. McGrath PA. Chronic pain in children. In Crombie IK, (Ed). The epidemiology of chronic pain, Seattle, IASP Press. 1999;81–101.
7. McGrath P.A. Pain in the pediatric patient: Practical aspects of assessment. Pediatr Ann. 1995; 24:26–128.
8. Voepel Lewis T, Merkel S, Tait AR, et al. The reliability and validity of the Face, Legs, Activity, Cry, Consolability observational tool as a measure of pain in children with cognitive impairment. Anesth Analg. 2002;95:1224.
9. Malviya S, Voepel-Lewis T, Burke C, et al. The revised FLACC observational pain tool: Improved reliability and

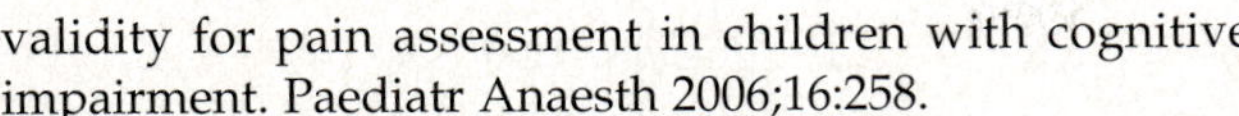

validity for pain assessment in children with cognitive impairment. Paediatr Anaesth 2006;16:258.

10. Breau LM, McGrath PJ, Camfield CS, et al. Psychometric properties of the non-communicating children's pain checklist-revised. Pain 2002;99:349.
11. Patric A McGrath, Stephen Brown. Pain in children. In: Argoff CE, McCleane G, (Eds). Pain management Secrets, 3rd edn. Philadelphia: Mosby Elsevier Publishers. 2009;221–234.
12. Jose B Rose. Pediatric Analgesia Pharmacology. In Ronald S Litman, (Ed). Pediatric Anaesthesia: The Requisites in Anesthesiology.Pennysylvania: Elsevier Mosby Press, 2004; p. 201.
13. Apley J, Naish N. Recurrent abdominal pain: a field survey of 1000 school children. Arch Dis Child 1958;33:165.0

Regional Blocks in Paediatrics

Pradnya Sawant

Application of regional anaesthesia techniques in infants and children is evolved around the turn of century when Bainbridge, in 1901, and Grey, in 1909, successfully employed spinal anaesthesia in infants and children. The role of regional blocks in paediatrics has revolutionized paediatric anaesthesia in the last two decades. In children regional is extensively used as sole anaesthetic method in conjunction with light general anaesthesia. Regional anaesthesia provides excellent intraoperative analgesia, which can be extended in the postoperative period. This results in a playful, pain-free and non-irritable child, thereby decreasing the morbidity. Regional anaesthesia also valuable role in diagnosis and management of cancer pain and certain chronic pain syndrome.

Advantages

- It provides complete block of sensory transmission, hence offering complete pain relief.
- It reduces the other anaesthetics requirement and has a sparing effect leading to faster and smoother recovery from anaesthesia.
- It can be extended to postoperative period for pain relief, especially after major surgeries.
- It has activation of the sympathetic stress response.
- It gives shorter hospital stay because of faster recovery, hence reduces cost.
- It gives prompt return to post-operation feeding schedule, hence chances of hypoglycaemia are less especially in small children.
- Non-irritable, playful and pain free child leading to better parental acceptance.

Disadvantages

1. Skilled or experienced personnel is required.
2. It has to be supplemented with sedation or general anaesthesia to minimize movement and crying of a child.

To practice safe and effective paediatric regional blocks, it is essential to know how children, especially neonates, are different from adult in various ways.

ANATOMICAL DIFFERENCES

In utero the cephalic end of the developing embryo and fetus differentiates first and grows more rapidly. The newborn has a large head compared to other parts of the body. During subsequent growth the pattern reverses leads to the adult configuration. Thus the anatomical relationship between the different structures change with increasing age and hence landmarks used in adults may not necessarily apply in children.

- In neonates and infants (under 1 year) the end of the spinal cord (L3), dural sac (S2–S4) are located more caudal than in adults. At approximately one year the spinal cord (L1) and the dural sac (S2) assumes the adult position.
- The intercristal line is found at L5 in children and L5–S1 interspace in premature babies and the neonates (adult level L4).
- The vertebral column forms a single shallow anteriorly concave curve extending from C1 to L5 at birth. The cervical curve appears when the head is held upright (at approximately 6 months) and the lumbar curve (at 1 year) develops with weight bearing.
- The spinous processes are thus more parallel and horizontal facilitating epidural puncture at all levels.

- In neonates the (L5–S1) interspace is the largest and most easily palpable.
- CSF volume is relatively high in infants weighing less than 1.5 kg, i.e. 4 mL/kg—body weight, in contrast to the adults and older children (2 mL/kg). CSF production is also increased (0.35 mL/min). Hence infants require proportionately more local anaesthetic dose for spinal block than older children and the incidence of the post spinal headache is extremely low in children.
- The spinal canal is triangular in shape and the spinal cord is ellipsoid in cross section.
- The ossification process of the sacral vertebrae is incomplete in children.
- Nerves are thinner with less myelination in neonates and young infants, allowing a lower concentration of local anaesthetic to be effective.

PHYSIOLOGICAL DIFFERENCES

There are important differences in the physiological effects of central blockade between children and adults.

Haemodynamically: Clinically significant hypotension is not a feature of central blockade in children, even without volume preloading. Children under five years show a little or no change in arterial pressure and heart rate after spinal blockade to levels of T_3–T_5. **I. Murat** found that following lumbar epidural, children older than eight years behaved like adults, whereas those younger than eight years showed no significant hypotension, irrespective of the level of blockade. According to **Bernard Dalenes**, pre-pubertal children do not develop significant hypotension. The explanation of this may be due to—

- Relative immaturity of the sympathetic nervous system in small children.
- The lower peripheral resistance so that sympathetic blockade is unlikely to decrease the blood pressure.
- Relative smaller volume of the lower extremities in proportion to the rest of the body. The volume below T10 in a 5-year old represents 30–40% of total body volume, whereas it represents up to 70% in an adult. Thus compensatory vasoconstriction in the vessels that remain unblocked in the upper body is large enough to maintain the blood pressure.

Indications

Indications depend on the general condition of the patient and type of surgery. It is essentially used for infra-umbilical extra-peritoneal procedures. Some of the special indications are stated below:

- **Low floppy infants:** Neuromuscular diseases with respiratory reserve be weakened pharyngeal or laryngeal reflexes.
- **Premature Babies:** Inguinal hernia with apnoeic spells
- History of malignant hyperthermia
- Children phobic of being made unconscious or the loss of self control under general anaesthesia.

Contraindications

Absolute

- Lack of parental consent
- Infection at the site of puncture
- Intracranial bleeding/increased ICT, meningitis

Relative

- Poorly controlled seizures
- Coagulopathy
- Anatomical anomalies—spina bifida
- Uncorrected hypovolemia
- Presence of CSF draining catheters

Advantages

- Safe
- Easy to perform
- Reliable
- Minimum physiological disturbances
- Allows prompt return to postoperative feeding schedules

Disadvantages

- Limited duration, e.g. spinal and if single shot block is used
- Supplementary sedation or general anaestheia is required, to minimize upper limb movements or crying
- Bloody or dry tap
- Level of analgesia is sometimes unpredictable

Regional blocks are divided into:

1. Central neural block (CNB)
2. Peripheral neural block (PNB)

CNB comprises

1. **Epidural:**
   - Caudal
   - Trans sacral
   - Lumbar
   - Thoracic
   - Cervical

2. **Subarachnoid block:** CNB can be given either as single shot or continuous by inserting catheter, using local anaesthetic with or without additives.

Caudal Epidural

Most commonly given in paediatric age group. Caudal is given through sacral hiatus which is a bony defect, triangular in shape in the form of inverted U or V with sacral cornu on each side covered by sacrococcygeal membrane. Two posterior superior iliac spines form the equilateral triangle and the apex being the hiatus (Figs 17.1 and 17.2).

Caudal is performed in lateral or prone positions using short beveled 22 gauge disposable needle. Local anaesthetic like 2% lignocaine with or without adrenaline or 0.5% bupivacaine with or without additives like narcotics, ketamine, midazolam, conidine and now dexmedetomidine, etc. can be used. Volume of the solution is determined by the level of analgesia required.

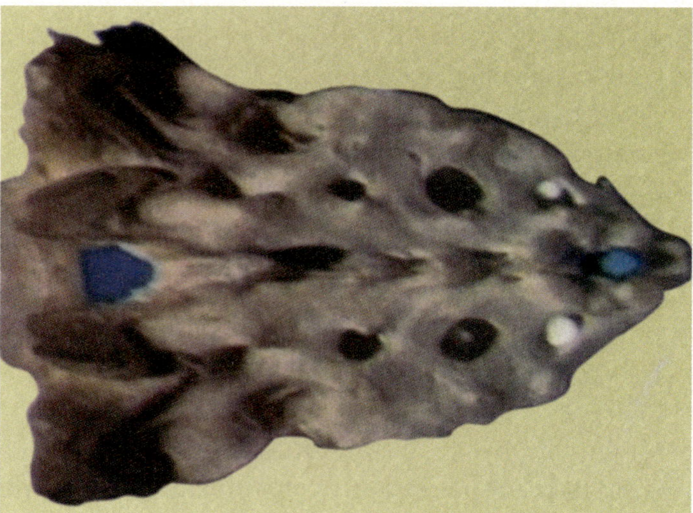

Fig. 17.1 Anatomy for candal anaesthesia

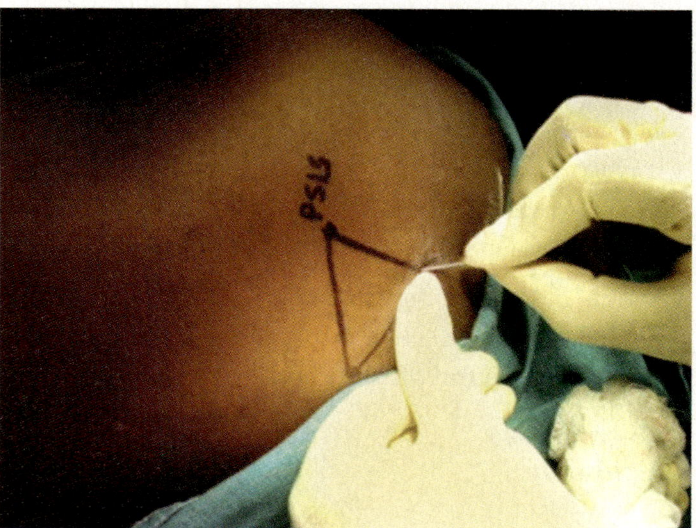

Fig. 17.2 Procedure for candal anaesthesia

Armitage formula seems most practical

Volume required = 0.5 mL/kg – lumbosacral
1.0 mL/kg – thoracolumbar
1.5 mL/kg – midthoracic
not to exceed 20 mL

Continuous caudal can be given by inserting catheter through caudal space. For infants and children less than 1 year ideally 19 gauge should be used. Since 19 gauge is very expensive, 18 gauge catheter can be passed through simple 18 gauge hypodermic needle. Epidural catheters are used for both intra and postoperative analgesia.

Trans sacral Block: It is similarly performed like caudal either 0.5 to 1 cm below or above the midline joining two posterior superior iliac spines.

Lumbar Epidural

A. **Lumbar approach:** Lumbar epidural block: The technique is same as that in an adult with the following differences:

1. **Depth of epidural space is small:** It is stated that rough estimate of the depth of the epidural space below the skin in children between 6 months and 10 years of age is approximately 1 mm/kg of body weight below the skin surface. Some of the formulae are mentioned below:
   - Depth of epidural space (cm) = 1 + 0.15 × age (years)
   - Depth (cm) = 0.8 + 0.05 × weight (kg)

   The mean depth of epidural space in neonates has been reported as 1 cm (SD 0.2, range 0.4–1.5 cm).
2. Ligaments are thinner; hence loss of resistance is sometimes difficult to feel.
3. Midline approach is preferred, as laminae are not well developed.

Technique:

- **Loss of resistance (LOR):** Saline should be used for LOR. Air should be avoided as it can give patchy block or cause air embolism.
- **Hanging drop technique:** A saline drop is placed on the hub of the needle after removing the stylet and as soon as the needle is in the epidural space, the drop is sucked in because of negative potential space.

Position:

1. Sitting—In cooperative adolescent group
2. Lateral

Methods:

1. Single shot
2. Catheter—Intermittent boluses
   Continuous infusion

Dose:

Volume—0.5 to 1 mL/kg

Drugs used:

Local anaesthetic agent	*Dose (mg/kg)*	*Conc. (%)*
Lignocaine	2–4	2
Lignocaine Tale	5–7	2
Bupivacaine	2–4	0.25–0.5
L-Bupivacaine		0.25
Ropivacaine	2–4	0.2 0.75

Additives:

Drug	*Recommended doses*	*Maximum dose*
Morphine	30 µg/kg	50 mcg/kg
Fentanyl	1–1.5 µg/kg	2.5 µg/kg
Sufentanil	0.25–0.5 µg/kg	0.75 µg/kg
Clonidine	1–1.5 µg/kg	1– 2 µg/kg
Ketamine	0.5 mg/kg	0.5–1 mg/kg

B. **Thoracic approach:** Technically difficult because of crowding of thoracic vertebrae and risk of spinal cord injury is high as cord is close to dura. In neonates thoracic approach is not preferred. Catheters are placed through caudal route. In older children 18 gauge is preparred.

Volume to be injected in epidural depends upon number of segments to be blocked.

Volume 0.5 mL/kg or
V (mL/neuromere) = 1/10 × age (in years) where V is volume

C. **Cervical epidural:** It is rarely given in children. Intra and postoperative continuous epidural can be given by bolus doses at certain time interval or by infusion using syringe or volumetric pumps.

Complications

- Complications of technical puncture—multiple punctures infections, injury to surrounding structures.
- Complications of epidural catheter—knotting, kinking, block, migration, etc.
- Complication of drugs—toxicity of local anaesthetics/narcotics/vasoconstrictors
- Haemodynamic alterations
- Failure of block—partial/complete

SUBARACHNOID BLOCK

Selection of Equipments

1. **Needles:** The ideal length of needle is 30 mm up to the age of 5 years and 45 mm between 5 and 10 years. Ideally needle should have a stylet to block CSF.
2. **Syringes:** Tuberculin or 2cc syringes
3. **Local anaesthetic agents** (Table 17.1)

Narcotics

Morphine is rarely used intrathecal in children because the risk of apnoea is very high.

Limitations of using narcotics are because of their side effects. Hence, for close observation experienced staff and narcotic antagonist should be readily available.

Technique

Position: Suitable positions for spinal anaesthesia (Figs 17.3A and B)

- Lateral position in a patient with poor physical condition (with extended head) (Fig. 17.4A)
- Sitting position in neonates and ex-premature infants less than 3 months old with support of head in both positions. It is mandatory to observe and maintain patency of the airway (Figs 17.4B and C).

Table 17.1 Dosages of the principle hyperbaric local anaesthetic agent used in children

Local anaesthetic	Concentration	Administered dose	Injected volume
Bupivacaine	0.5% + dextrose glucose 8%	<5 kg: 0.5 mg/kg 5–15 kg: 0.4 mg/kg >15 kg: 0.3 mg/kg	0.1 mL/kg 0.08 mL/kg 0.06 mL/kg

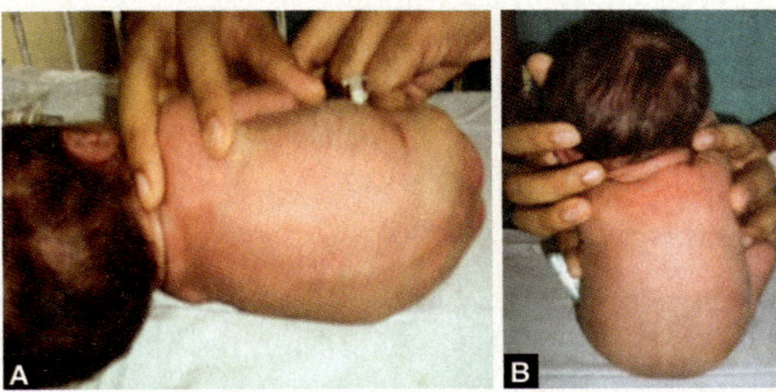

Fig. 17.3A and B Suitable positions for spinal anaesthesia

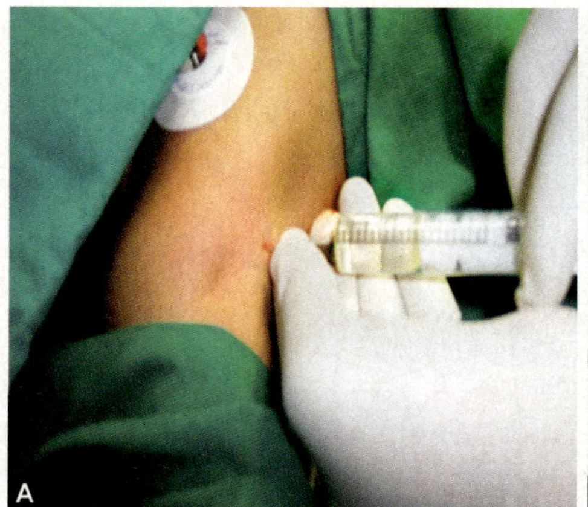
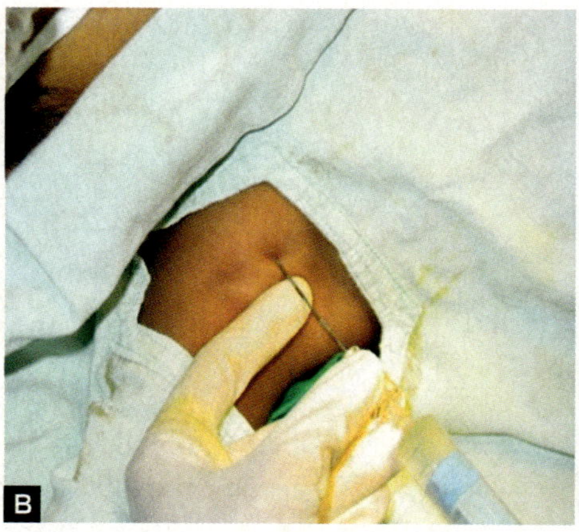
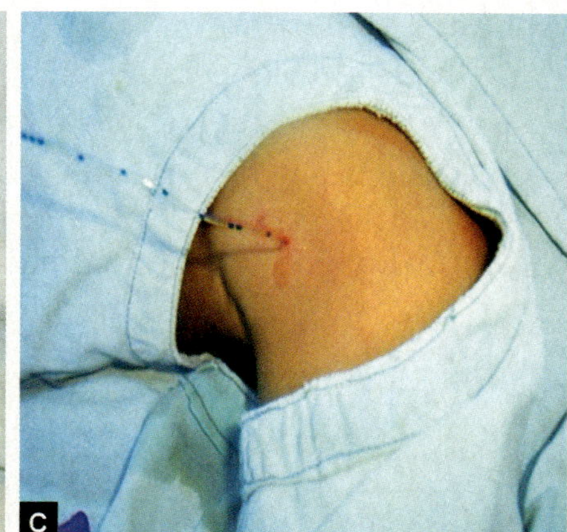

Figs. 17.4 (A) Lateral position, (B) and (C) Sitting position

Anatomical Landmark

The point of puncture should be between L4 and L5 or L5 and S1, as described by BUSONI. To avoid direct trauma to spinal cord.

Technique

The resistances of different tissues felt in a child are not the same as those in an adult. The depth of insertion is 12 mm in newborn, 15–25 mm in child up to 5 years level and 30–40 mm in 5 to 8 years level. In the presence of dry tap the space or the position of the patient should be changed.

Continuous spinal also can be given, as micro catheters are available but the risk associated with its use is unacceptable. It should be reserved for terminally ill oncological patients.

Spread of Anaesthesia

The spread of anaesthesia is to be detected in conscious child if bupivacaine is used as it results in motor paralysis. In children under general anaesthesia or when lignocaine is used, absence of response to surgical stimulus would indicate that analgesia is adequate. Child may require controlled ventilation if block extends above T5. Claude Saint Maurice ice cubes to skin is to determine the upper level of block and dose of local anaesthetic.

Complications and Sequelae

Specific to spinal

1. Meningitis	Septic and aseptic contamination of CSF leads to Meningitis.
2. Hypotension	When excessive doses are used.
3. Post spinal headache	It has a low incidence in children because of: • Inability to verbalize • No leakage of CSF, as CSF pressure is low • Highly elastic dura • Lack of ambulation

PERIPHERAL BLOCKS

Blocks can be performed

- In awake and cooperative older children.
- Under sedation.
- Under general anaesthesia.

Identification of nerve site can be done by the following methods.

- With the topographical landmarks.
- By eliciting paraesthesia caused by needles in contact with the nerve by electrical stimulations with nerve locator.
- By using Ultrasound Guided techniques.

Success of regional blocks depends upon various factors like:

1. Anatomical knowledge
2. Selection of equipment
   - **Needles:**
     - *Length:* Approx 30 mm because if it is too long chances of inadvertent damage to the surrounding structures are very high and if it is too short it may not reach the nerve site.
     - *Diameter:* Large enough to give rigidity to the needle. Short and blunt beveled needles are preferred so that there are fewer chances of injuring blood vessels and laceration of nerve fiber.
   - **Using nerve locator:** It helps in localization of a nerve more precisely.

Table 17.2 Local anaesthetic drug used most commonly in children and their recommended doses

Local anaesthetic agent	Dose (mg/kg)	Conc. (%)	Volume (mL/kg)	Latency (min)	Duration (hrs)	Toxic dose (mg/kg)
Lignocaine	5.0–7.0	0.5–2.0	0.1–0.5 Depending on size of nerve	5–10	0.75–2	More than 5–7
Bupivacaine	2.5–3.0	0.25–0.5	0.2–0.5	10–15	2–5	2.5–3

- **Local anaesthetic agents:** The local anaesthetic drug used most commonly in children and their recommended doses are shown in Table 17.2.

  Among the local anaesthetics Ropivacaine seems more promising and could replace Bupivacaine because it is equipotent and less cardio toxic.

3. **Addition of vasoconstrictor:** Addition of vasoconstrictor prolongs the duration of block; it decreases the peak plasma concentrations of LA drugs, hence reducing toxicity. Also it helps in detection of an inadvertent intravascular injection.
4. **Addition of narcotics:** Use of alone narcotic for block does not seem to be effective. Blocks can be given either single shot for short procedures and continuous by placing a catheter, either with intermittent boluses or continuous infusion of 0.075% to 0.125% of bupivacaine at a rate of 0.1–0.3 mL/kg/hr.

UPPER LIMB BLOCKS

Brachial plexus blocks can be given by various methods and at different like in Supraclavicular methods, Winnie's method of interscalene approach, Kulen Kamff's approach, Dalen's Parascalene approach, subclavian perivascular technique of Winnes and Collins. In infraclavicular method axilliary approach is used most commonly.

Supraclavicular approach (Dalen's parascalene method): The patient is placed in a supine position with role sheet under the shoulder and arm lying besides the body, the head turned away from the side to be blocked.

Anatomical Landmark

Mid-point of clavicle and sixth cervical tubercle (Chassaignac's tubercle) is projected on the skin at the intersection of the interscalene grove with the line passing through the cricoid cartilage. The needle is inserted perpendicular to the skin at a point junction of upper 2/3 and lower 1/3 on transection joining the mid point of clavicle to the sixth cervical tubercle. The plexus is situated at depth of 7–30 mm. from skin deep depending on age and weight of patient.

The spread of anaesthesia is limited to supraclavicular branches of brachial plexus. The block of the distal branches especially ulnar nerve is slower in onset and shorter in duration than that of proximal branches. Complications like damage to vertebral artery, epidural and intrathecal injections, damage to blood vessels in the neck, pneumothorax and undesirable nerve blocks are avoided by this approach.

Dose as per shown in Table 17.2.

Auxiliary approach: This is the safest approach to block brachial plexus.

Patient position: Supine with arm abducted at right angle to the body. Forearm flexion with supination with hand directed upwards lying close to the head.

Anatomical landmark: Axillary artery, the pectoralis major muscle and the coraco brachialis muscle.

Point of puncture: The typical "give way" is felt as needle enters the engulfing sheath and the pulsations of axillary artery are transmitted to the needle. For continuous axillary block epidural catheter no 19 Gz in smaller children and no18 Gz in older children are used.

The catheter can be introduced blindly by loss of resistance technique or through nerve locater needle. Like epidural catheter, it can be kept for 48 hrs to provide postoperative analgesia either by intermittent boluses or continuous infusion.

LOWER LIMB BLOCK

Most commonly used are sciatic, femoral, lateral cutaneous nerve of thigh and 3-in-1 block.

Sciatic nerve block: The sciatic nerve is the largest mixed nerve in the human body. The sciatic nerve can be blocked at three places, one at the site of its emergence from the sciatic foramen, one at the lower border of the gluteus maximus muscle and last in the mid thigh. The blocks are given by using loss of resistance technique like epidural. A continuous block can be given by placing a catheter near sciatic nerve. The mid-thigh approach is best suited for continuous block with a catheter as it stays undisturbed by patients' mobilization.

PENILE NERVE BLOCK (Fig. 17.5)

Indications: Circumcision, hypospadias repair, retraction of fore skin.

- Drug/dose: Bupivacaine 0.25%
- 2 mL for infants/10 mL for adolescent

Caution: Avoid epinephrine

Technique: Insert the needle 90° to the skin, just below the symphysis pubis into the shaft of penis "the pop" will be felt as the needle crosses Buck's fascia. Inject half the dose at 10 O'clock and half at 2 O'clock positions. The final 1 mL is given at the junction of scrotum and penis on the vertical side.

ILIOINGUINAL AND ILIOHYPOGASTRIC NERVE BLOCK

Anatomy: Ilioinguinal (L_1) and iliohypogastric (T_{12}–L_1) are the major branches of lumbar plexus.

Indications: Inguinal herniotomy, varicocele, orchidopexy.

Position: Supine

Puncture site: 0.5–1.0 cm medial and 1 cm inferior to anterior superior iliac spine above the inguinal ligament. A 22–23 gauge short beveled needle is directed at right angle to the skin advanced. The "pop off" is felt when aponeurosis is pierced. About 1–2 mL of 0.5% bupivacaine is injected. Then the needle with syringe is advanced while feeling the resistance to the needle tip a second pop off is felt as it pierces the internal oblique muscle. Additional 1–2 mL of bupivacaine is injected. Sometimes it is necessary to inject subcutaneously at a site of surgical incision.

INFRAORBITAL NERVE BLOCK (Fig. 17.7A and B)

The infraorbital nerve provides sensory innervation to the upper lip and lower eyelid.

Indication: Mainly cleft lip and lower eyelid surgery.

Technique: The block is given at the infraorbital foramen, which lies in the vertical line passing over

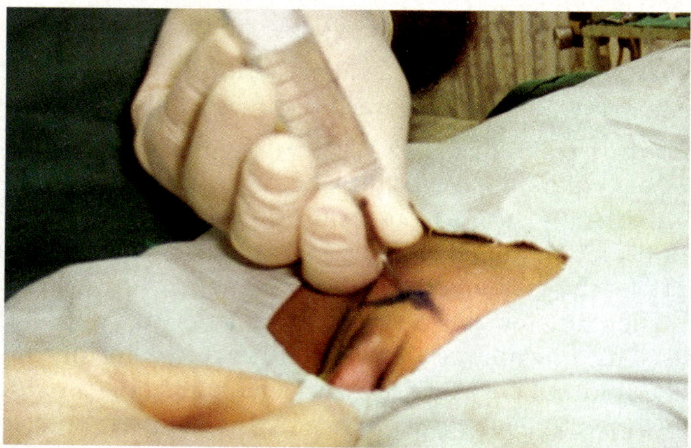

Fig. 17.5 Step 1 of Penile anaesthesia

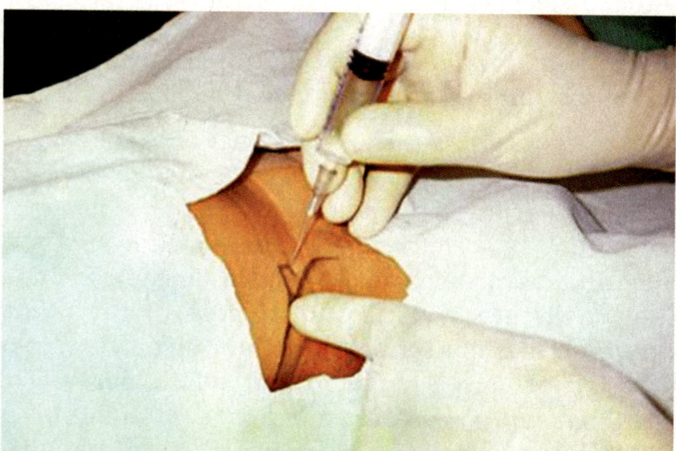

Fig. 17.6 Step 2 of Penile anaesthesia

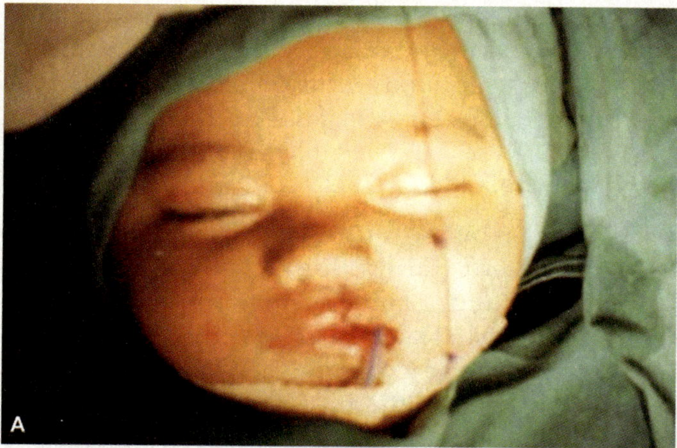

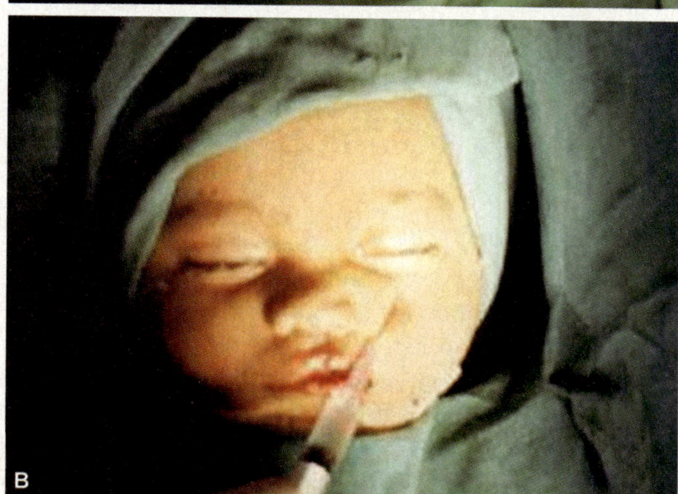

Fig. 17.7 (A) Anatomy and (B) Procedure of infraorbital nerve block

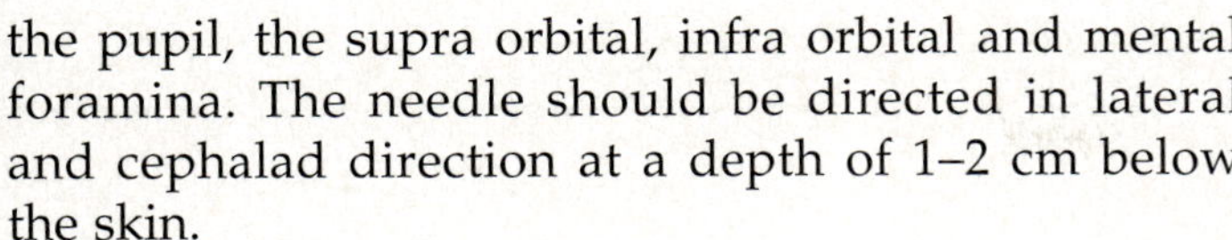

the pupil, the supra orbital, infra orbital and mental foramina. The needle should be directed in lateral and cephalad direction at a depth of 1–2 cm below the skin.

Dose: 1–2 mL of 0.2–0.5% bupivacaine.

SUMMARY OF RULES

1. General rule: Knowledge of surgical procedure and disease state is essential.
2. Preparation of patient:
   a. Proper valid consent
   b. Psychological management
   c. Premedication—better to give anxiolytics in older children.
3. Anatomical consideration:
   a. Bony landmarks are used as guide
   b. Do not elicit paraesthesia deliberately
   c. Knowledge of nerve physiology/segmental innervations
4. Anaesthetic aspects:
   a. Nerve blocking is a surgical procedure, hence aseptic precautions should be followed at patient's operative site by anaesthesiologist
   b. Facility of respiratory and cardiac resuscitation is a must
   c. Antagonist to narcotic drugs
5. Pharmacologic consideration:
   a. Least toxic drug is selected
   b. Period of latency is observed
6. Technical aspects:
   a. Avoid multiple insertions
   b. Withdraw and reinsert to change the direction
7. Aspiration test: Should be negative for blood.

REFERENCES

1. Brown TCK, Fisk GC. Regional and local anaesthesia chapter in Anaesthesia for Children, 2nd edn. Blackwell Scientific publications, London, Edinburgh, Boston, Melbourne.
2. Bernard Dalens. Regional anaesthesia in infant's children and adolescent, 1st edn. Williams and Wilkins. Baltimore, Maryland, 1995.
3. Charles B Berde. Paediatric regional anaesthesia. George Gregory (Ed). 3rd edn. Churchill Livingstone. New York, London, Edinburgh, Boston, Melbourne, Tokyo.
4. Regional Anaesthesia in Children; Beyond the Caudal Block.
5. Abajian JC, Melish PWI, Browne AE, et al. Spinal anaesthesia for high risk infants. Anaesthesia Analgesia. 1984;63:359.
6. Gray HT. A study of spinal anaesthesia in children and infants. Lancet Sept. 1909;25:913.
7. Harnik EV, Hoy GR, Potolicchio S, et al. Spinal anaesthesia in premature infants recovering from respiratory distress syndrome., Anaesthesiology. 1986;64–95.
8. Welborn LG, Rice LJ, Hannallah R, et al. Postoperative apnoea in former preterm infants: Prospective comparison of spinal and neural anaesthesia. Anaesthesiology. 1990; 72: 838.
9. Bernand DJ. Regional anaesthesia in children. In: Miller RD, (Ed). Miller's Anaesthesia. 7th ed. Philadelphia: Churchill Livingstone. 2010.
10. Davis PJ, Cladis FP, et al. Smith's anaesthesia for infants and children. 8th edn. 2012.

18

Ultrasound in Paediatric Anaesthesia

Rakesh Garg and Naveen Yadav

ABSTRACT

The paediatric anaesthesia is always very challenging. The application of regional blocks requires a good understanding of the anatomy for successful block. The use of ultrasound in clinical practice of anaesthesiology has improved the success of many interventions. Similarly ultrasound guided regional nerve blocks are being increasingly used not only in adults but also in children. The ultrasound guided nerve blocks not only provide more success but also reduces the complications rates. The ultrasound guided nerve blocks in adults have been amply described in the literature. However, description of ultrasound guided blocks in paediatric patients are not well described. The literature and the experts express the utility of the use of ultrasound for the nerve blocks in the children as well. We discuss some of the important aspects of ultrasound guided nerve blocks and describe the technique as reported in the literature. With the advancement and further reporting of the experience in ultrasound guided regional blocks in children, this knowledge needs an updating. Readers are advised to keep themselves with these updates related to ultrasound guided regional nerve blocks.

INTRODUCTION

Ultrasound has emerged as an important tool in the clinical practice of anaesthesiologists. Ultrasound is a simple, repeatable, real time, radiation free and non-invasive technique. It is being used for diagnostic and interventional procedures with acceptable accuracy for localization of the area of interest.[1,2] The interventional procedures may be vascular related interventions or related to nerve blocks. Either of the interventions may be real time or may be used for locating and marking the structure and then performing desired intervention.[3] Though, surgical pain may be managed with intravenous analgesics like opioids, but the associated side effects like respiratory depression remains a concern. Regional blocks are routinely used in children for selected procedures. Ultrasound has emerged as useful adjunct to regional blocks in children.[1–10] However, these remains challenging in view of small body size of children with variable depth and position of the nerves at varying age.[6] This fact may be further challenged by presence of critical structures in vicinity of nerves and thus decreasing the safety margin.[7] The use of ultrasound has been found to improve the success of the intervention in shorter time along with lesser complications rates. Ultrasound allows better visualization of the target including nerve, fascial plane or anatomical space for regional nerve block.[6] Ultrasound guided blocks improves sensory and motor block, have faster onset of block, and longer duration of sensory blockade as compared to conventional blocks.[8] Also, the volume of drug is reduced for a nerve block when administered under guidance of ultrasound and hence the risk of toxicity.[7] This is because ultrasound allows the deposition of drug in close vicinity to nerves and drug spread can be visualized real time.[3,9] In view of such advantages, use of ultrasound for peripheral nerve blocks in infants and children has been recommended.[10] It has been emphasized that the use of ultrasonography will improve the safety in regional anaesthesia for children.[11] The evidence for ultrasound guided regional nerve blocks is increasingly being reported in adults. However, similar extent is not being reported in children. We present the reported literature with regard to ultrasound guided procedures in children. It is important to understand the anatomy, the sonoanatomy and finally hand-eye coordination with regard to ultrasound probe and imaging for successful nerve block.[12]

INTRODUCTION TO THE MACHINE

Understanding of the machine is important prior to initiating an interventional procedure. Ultrasound waves are high-frequency sound waves generated in specific frequency ranges and sent through tissues.[1] Range of frequency decides how far the ultrasound wave will penetrate the tissues. Lower frequencies penetrate deeper than the high frequencies. As the sound passes through the tissues, it is absorbed, reflected or allowed to pass through, depending on the echo-density of the tissues. The propagation of reflected or transmitted waves is based on difference in acoustic impedance between the tissues forming the interface.[1] Substances with high water content (e.g. blood, cerebrospinal fluid) conduct sound very well and reflect very poorly. Since they reflect very little of the sound, they appear as dark area. Substances low in water content and high in material are poor conductors (like air, bone) and reflect almost all the light and appear very bright.

Ultrasound Transducers

Ultrasound assembly comprises a transmitter which generate precisely timed, high-amplitude voltage to energize the transducer.[1,4] Ultrasound transducers consist of arrays of piezoelectric crystals that produce high frequency sound waves in response to an electrical signal. These crystals interconvert both electrical and mechanical energies, allowing for both transmission and reception of sound waves. The receiver in the transducer and the processor detect the reflected waves and amplify them for the final display of the reflected signals. Linear array typically produces a rectangular image format. The piezoelectric crystals are arranged in a straight line. Curvilinear arrays produce images in a sector format. The choice of frequency of transducer is based on the area of interest required for nerve block and primarily based on depth of penetration and the resolution. The high-frequency (10–14 MHz) transducers produce higher resolution images with low tissue penetration and thus required for superficial structures.[1,12] The low-frequency (4–7 MHz) sound waves have higher penetration in tissues but with poor resolution and suitable for deeper structures. The area of interest should be within the focal area of the ultrasound beam to create an optimal image on the screen.

Imaging

The structures can be imaged either in short axis or long axis depending upon the area of interest and approach for nerve block.[13] If the probe is turned by 90 degrees in either direction, the short-axis view becomes a long-axis view.[1] Doppler mode helps to delineate the neural structures from vascular structures during regional block.[1] The B-mode ultrasound is most frequently used and allows transverse and longitudinal sections.[1,13] The needle for nerve block is better visualized in longitudinal section. The relationship to structures, however, are better seen in transverse section. So a combination of transverse and longitudinal scan appears to be an optimal option for successful block. Nerves are better identified by scanning its course and short axis (transverse) scanning along the course of the nerve is preferable. Also, imaging in short axis allows dynamic assessment of the local anaesthetic agent. For these reasons most practitioners prefer short axis view for ultrasound guided peripheral nerve blocks. The needle movements produce tissue distortion provides a clue for needle position and direction in addition to acoustic shadows.[1] Depth and gain settings need to be managed depending on the area of interest for nerve block and better visualization of structures and needle.

Transducer Manipulation

To optimally display the anatomy for image presentation, the transducer may be manipulated. Transducer movement involves sliding, tilting, rotating and compressing. The principle behind such movements is to locate and identify the nerve more precisely.

Approach Technique

There are two basic approaches to ultrasound guidance.[13] With the 'out of plane' technique, the needle tip crosses the plane of imaging as an echogenic dot. With the 'in plane' approach, the entire tip up to the shaft of that advancing needle can be visualised. Both the techniques have been used by the practitioners of ultrasound guided regional nerve blocks or vascular interventions.

Out of Plane approach: For this approach, the target is cantered in the field and depth is noted. The needle is inserted to this particular depth and a 'test dose' (small volume of drug) is injected to observe the spread around the target nerve.[13] There are certain advantages of out of-plane approach. It is most similar to other approaches of regional block. The path taken by the needle is shorter than the in plane approach. Since the out of plane approach is along the nerve path, it is most suitable with catheter placement. The disadvantages of out of plane approach are unimagined needle path and needle crossing the plane of image without recognition.

In-plane approach: The in-plane approach has most direct visualisation. Here, the target is imaged at one side of the field away from the needle insertion site. It requires some movements of the transducer to visualize the needle. The disadvantages include partial line ups which create false sense of security when needle tip is not correctly identified. The in-plane approach has longer path therefore more structures to cross with the block needle.

SONOANATOMY AND SCANNING

Sonoanatomy

The ability to recognise and localize the structures in an ultrasound scan is arguably the most important part of ultrasound guided regional anaesthesia. The knowledge of surface anatomy is another useful tool. It helps in determining initial transducer placement. Most regional anaesthetic techniques have at least one anatomically significant structure for localizing the target structure, e.g. the subclavian artery for the supraclavicular nerve block or femoral artery for femoral nerve block. Once this structure has been identified, the target structure, e.g. the cords of the brachial plexus around the subclavian artery, can be located on-screen. Centralizing the target structure on the screen ensures the shortest needle pathway required. The knowledge of the relevant sonoanatomy becomes even more important when a deep structure or a nerve not accompanied closely by a vessel is the relevant structure, e.g. the obturator nerve in the medial compartment of the thigh. The ultrasound image of nerves varies from round, oval or triangular.[13] It is interesting to know the same nerve may have different shapes at different sites and it varies with the angulations of the probe with regards to nerve location.

The ultrasound image of nerves depends on the plane, angle and frequency of the ultrasound beam. The nerves may differ in echogenicity at different parts of the body and size of the nerve. Also the actual echogenicity of a nerve appears only if ultrasound beam is focused perpendicularly to the nerve axis.[10] The peripheral nerves may appear hypoechoic (dark structures) or hyperechoic (bright structures).[10,13] The nerves appear as honeycomb structures with round or oval shapes in the transverse plane or short axis.[13] These appear as hypoechoic fascicles surrounded by hyperechoic tissues (epineurium).[1] While in the longitudinal plane, hypoechoic parallel bands are bordered by hyperechoic striations of the nerve fascicles.[1] At times, nerve may appear like tendon. Nerve may be identified by its 'fascicular pattern' while tendon shows 'fibrillar pattern', i.e. multiple hyperechoic continuous lines.[10,13] Also, nerve path may be traced fully while tendon will end in the muscle.[13]

Needle guidance: The visibility of the needle depends on size (gauge) of needle, type of needle and insertion angle.[13] The needle tip visibility is reduced with steep angles.[13] Larger gauge needles are better visualized. Also sono-friendly needles with improved echogenicity are commercially available and better visualized. The acoustic background also affects the needle visualization.[13] The needle tip is better localized in an anechoic background like fluid or blood.[12] The machine setting with lower gain mimics anechoic background and thus helps in locating the tip of the needle. The needle can be better visualized by certain maneuvers like hydrolocalisation (injecting small volume of liquid like drugs itself), rotating the needle (more ultrasound reflection from beveled end), to and from movement of the needle (jiggling).[13] The test volume of liquid allows repositioning of the needle if the liquid does not appear to spread around the target area. At times, some air in the needle makes needle tip better visualized. However, presence of air makes further tissue evaluation difficult and thus de-airing is preferable.

Drug injection: Administration of the local anaesthetic agent (unagitated drug) provides a good contrast making the visualization of the target nerve better.[13] Optimally placed drug volume, i.e. when it surrounds the target nerve makes nerve floating in the liquid and is better visualized. The removal of air is important during the drug injection as air in the tissue makes ultrasound evaluation difficult. Though the use of sodium bicarbonate to alkalinize the solution has been reported to hasten the onset, but during ultrasound guided block, the bicarbonate solutions hampers visualization as it releases carbon dioxide and thus sonographic capture deteriorates. Also the understanding of the fascial planes is important as drugs are required to be deposited in these planes so as to bathe the target nerves. After administration of the drug, sonographic evaluation should be done to assess the distribution of the nerve along the path of the nerve and in short axis.[13]

ERGONOMICS

Body Ergonomics

Ergonomics (or human factors) is the scientific discipline concerned with the understanding of interactions among humans and other elements of a system in order to optimize human well-being and overall system performance. The system in ultrasound guided regional anaesthesia includes the patient, the anaesthesiologist, the ultrasound machine, the anaesthesia machine and other operating room equipment. Ensuring good ergonomics among these components minimises operator and improves the operator's ability to control and coordinate the manipulation of both the transducer and the needle. The patient should be positioned such that the area of interest is at a level that does not require the operator to bend. The ultrasound screen should be placed in the direct line-of-sight of the operator. This has an impact on the accuracy of needle-to-target guidance. The operator's hands should be braced upon the patient for support and to steady the transducer.

The acronym, SCANNING, can be used for preparing to scan in an ergonomically optimal manner:

S: Supplies—arrange all supplies including the ultrasound machine, the block tray, and the nerve stimulator as required.

C: Comfortable positioning of the patient and the operator.

A: Ambiance

N: Name and procedure

N: Nominate transducer

I: Infection control

N: Note lateral/medial side on screen

G: Gain depth

Good ergonomics contributes to good needle-beam alignment and visibility in two ways. Firstly, it minimises operator fatigue, which has been shown to be a common shortcoming amongst novices. Secondly, it improves the operator's ability to control and coordinate the manipulation of both the transducer and needle while simultaneously looking away at the ultrasound screen. The patient should be elevated to a height that does not require the operator to bend over. The operator's hands should be braced on the patient for support; this also steadies the transducer, which might otherwise slip in the gel on the patient's skin. Proper hand and arm positions; both hands and arms are comfortably supported. The ultrasound screen should also be placed in a location where it is visible without the operator having to turn their head or torso away from the patient, i.e. direct line-of-sight.

ULTRASOUND GUIDED PERIPHERAL NERVE BLOCK

Upper Extremity Nerve Blocks

The regional blocks for upper limb surgery provide optimal analgesia perioperatively. Though interscalene block is not so popular in children, but other brachial plexus blocks (supraclavicular, infraclavicular and axillary block) are reported in the literature.[4]

Interscalene Nerve Block

Indications: The interscalene nerve block is helpful for shoulder and upper arm surgery.

Initial settings: Depth 3 cm, frequency 8–14 MHz, a short (50 mm), broad (21 gauge) echogenic needle, nerve stimulator @0.5 mA, linear transducer preferably a small footprint hockey stick probe.

Patient position: Supine or semi lateral with head turned away from side to be blocked. In paediatric patient the positioning can be optimised by using a head ring and a small roll between the scapulae.

Transducer position: Transverse orientation on neck over the pulse of carotid artery, approximately 3–4 cm over the clavicle. The transducer is slid laterally to the edge of sternocleidomastoid muscle (SCM). The anterior and middle scalene muscles (SA and SM respectively) are identified. In between the two muscles the hypoechoic trunks of the brachial plexus (IS) are sandwiched (Fig. 18.1).

Needle approach: A medial to lateral in plane approach is preferred. This approach help needle path away from the pleura. Nerve stimulation may be used to identify the localized nerve roots and thus improves the success of the block (twitching of the biceps, triceps).

Local anaesthetic dose: The minimum amount of local anaesthetic to fully surround the nerve roots should be used, which is estimated to be 0.15–1.25 mL/kg.

Complications: Phrenic nerve palsy, vascular puncture.

Key Pearls

- Repeated aspirations to avoid intravascular injection.
- Slight redirection of the needle during injection to ensure the spread of the drug around the plexus.

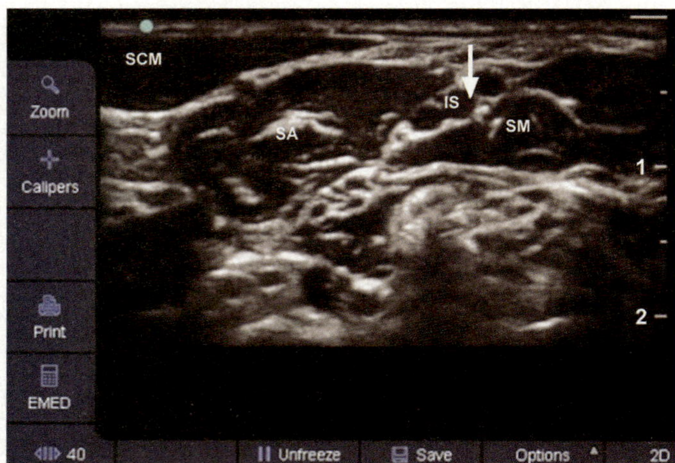

Fig. 18.1 Interscalene brachial plexus block (SCM-sternocleidomastoid muscle, SM-scalene muscle, IS-brachial plexus)

Supraclavicular Nerve Block

Indications: The supraclavicular block is indicated for arm, elbow, forearm and hand surgery.

Initial settings: Depth 3 cm, frequency 8–14 MHz, short (50 mm), broad (21 gauge) echogenic needle, nerve stimulator @0.5 mA.

Patient position: Supine or semi-lateral with head turned away from side to be blocked. Operator stands at the head of the patient with ultrasound machine facing them.

Transducer position: Transverse orientation, immediately superior and parallel to clavicle. Goal is to visualise pulsating subclavian artery (SCA). The brachial plexus can be seen as a bundle of hypoechoic round nodules (e.g. grapes) just lateral and superficial to the artery. Rib may be seen as hyperechoic line with dorsal shadowing at the medial and posterior of the artery (Figs 18.2 and 18.3).

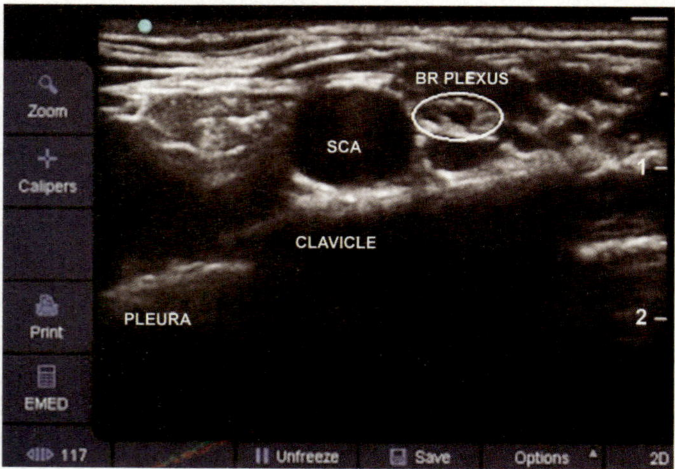

Fig. 18.2 Supraclavicular nerve block (SCA-subclavian artery, BR-brachial plexus)

Needle approach: The block needle is inserted in-plane toward the brachial plexus, in a lateral to medial direction.

Local anaesthetic dose: The initial injection of saline (in case of infants) or local anaesthetic should be made to ensure a good tip position before injection of 0.2–0.5 mL/kg local anaesthetic.

Complications: vascular puncture, pneumothorax.

Key Pearls

- In children apex of the lung lies in vicinity, so avoid any blind movement of the needle.
- Identify the structures lateral to carotid artery before negotiating the needle for the block.

Infraclavicular Nerve Block

Indications: Infraclavicular nerve block is indicated for the arm, elbow, forearm and hand surgery.[6]

Initial settings: Depth 3–5 cm, frequency 8–14 MHz, a short (50 mm), broad (21 gauge) echogenic needle, nerve stimulator @ 1 mA.

Patient position: The block is performed with the patient in supine position with the arm by the side.[14] By abducting the arm the plexus is brought more superficial. Positioning is optimised in paediatric patients by placing head in head ring and a small roll behind the scapulae. The orientation of the operator to

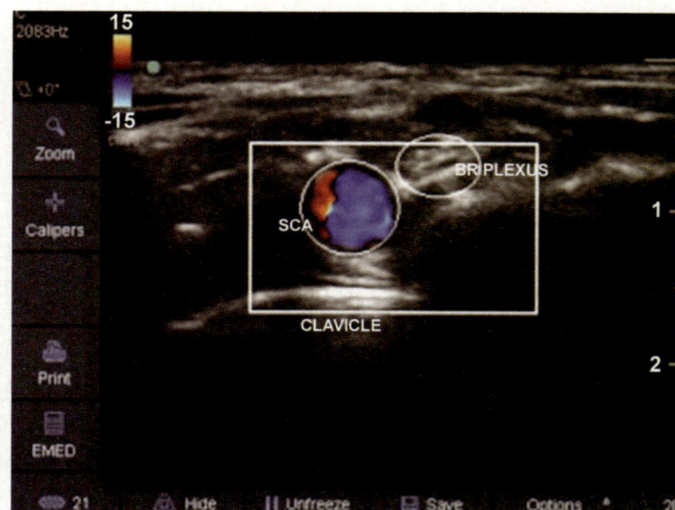

Fig. 18.3 Supraclavicular nerve block with Doppler mode 'on' (SCA-subclavian artery, BR-brachial plexus)

ultrasound machine is reversed compared to supra-clavicular block.

Transducer position: The linear probe is placed beneath the coracoid process in a parasagittal plane. The pectoral muscles are located initially followed by subclavian artery and vein. Proximally, the plexus lies cephalad and lateral to the artery, and more distally the cords take up their position around the artery—medial, lateral and posterior (Fig. 18.4).

Needle approach: The needle insertion site is chosen where the best view of cord, vessels and pleura is located. The needle is inserted in-plane from the cephalad aspect, with the insertion point just inferior to the clavicle. The needle is aimed toward the posterior aspect of artery and pass through the pectoral major and minor muscles.

Local anaesthetic dose: A test injection of saline or local anaesthetic is used to ensure the needle has passed through the fascia; following this 0.5 mL/kg of local anaesthetic is injected [r].

Complications: The infraclavicular block carries a significant risk of pneumothorax. Arterial puncture is most common complication in infraclavicular block.

Key Pearls

- Though lower frequency probe required for adults but in children high frequency probe provides better visualization.
- Be cautious anatomical variation of the nerves around the artery.
- Cervical pleura lies close to the medial location of the Infraclavicular fossa and thus avoid any blind needling.

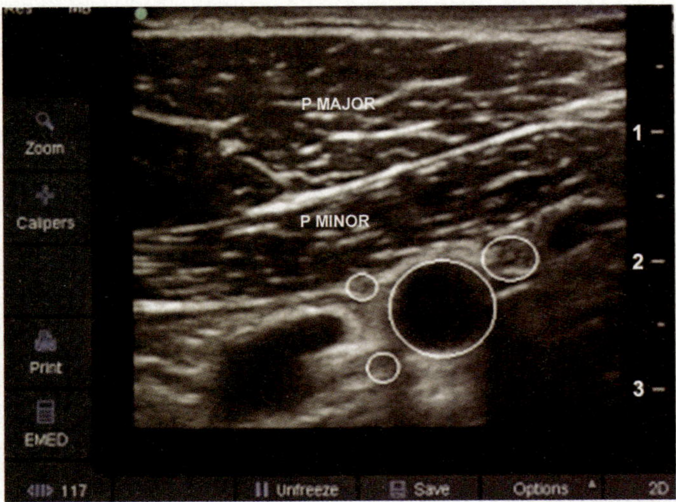

Fig. 18.4 Infraclavicular nerve block
(P Major-pectoralis major, P Minor-pectoralis minor, small circles represents brachial plexus and large circle represents subclavian artery)

Axillary Block

Indications: Axillary block is suitable for forearm and hand surgery.

Initial settings: Depth 3–5 cm, frequency 8–12 MHz, short (50 mm), broad (21 gauge) echogenic needle, nerve stimulator @1 mA, a hockey stick or small foot print probe.

Patient position: Supine with head turned away from the side to be blocked. Arm abducted and elbow flexed at 90°. The operator should stand at the head of the bed to view the ultrasound display across the patients arm.

Transducer position: Transverse, at the insertion point of pectoralis major muscle in humerus. Goal is to visualise the axillary artery in short axis. The biceps brachii appears medially. The triceps brachii appears medial and deep to biceps brachii. The anechoic axillary artery is in the centre with biceps brachii and coraco-brachialis on the sides. Initially the vessels should be identified then individual nerve to be seen and their identity confirmed by their course distally. The median nerve remains close to the artery throughout its course in the upper arm. The ulnar nerve begins medial to the artery and gradually moves away and more superficial as it travels to the ulnar groove. The radial nerve is usually located posterior to the artery and spirals posterior to the humerus (Fig. 18.5).

Needle approach: An in-plane approach from the lateral aspect of the arm is used for needle insertion. Slight reverse trendelenburg position will make the needle path more natural for the operator. Usually the three

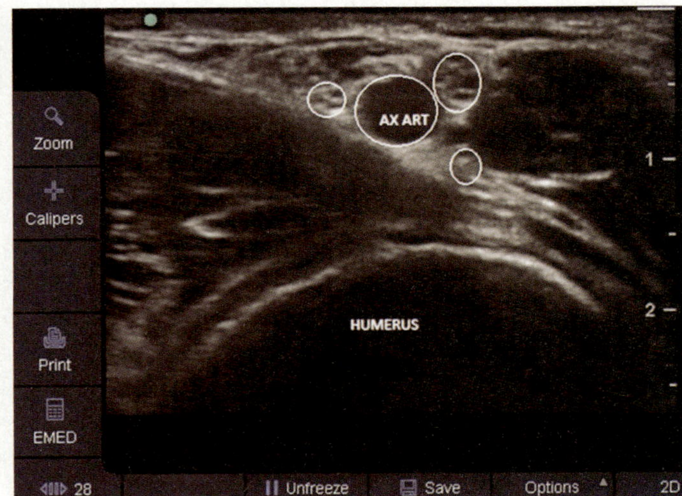

Fig. 18.5 Axillary nerve block
(AX ART–axillary artery, small circle represents medial ulnar and radial nerve)

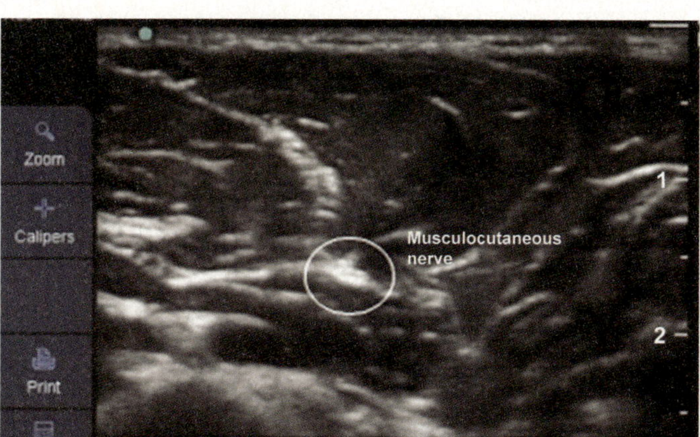

Fig. 18.6 Musculocutaneous nerve block

main nerves can be blocked individually by a single insertion site. But to block musculocutaneous nerve, it may be necessary to use a second needle insertion site (Fig. 18.6).

Local anaesthetic dose: A test injection of saline or local anaesthetic is used to ensure the needle has passed through the fascia, following this 0.5 ml/kg of local anaesthetic is injected.

Complications: A high risk of intravascular injection and high failure rate due to the musculocutaneous nerve exiting the sheath at the level of coracoids processes are main complications.

> **Key Pearls**
> - Scan distally to identify and localize the nerve for axillary block.
> - Use colour Doppler to identify vascular structures as these lies in close vicinity.

Lower Limb Blocks

The analgesia and anaesthesia for lower limb is usually provided with caudal block and to some extent with subarachnoid block.[6,8] The peripheral lower limb nerve blocks are not so common, probably because of lesser failure rate with caudal block and more expertise with the caudal block. However, the peripheral nerve block probably will have lesser complications with lesser requirement of local anaesthetics.[5,8]

Sciatic Nerve Block

Sciatic nerve blocks are performed either in the subgluteal or in the popliteal area depending on surgical intervention.[2,8]

Indications: Sciatic nerve block is suitable for foot and ankle surgery.[8]

Initial settings: Depth 6–8 cm, frequency 2–8 MHz, curved transducer or linear hockey stick, needle size 100–150 mm, 21 G short bevel insulated stimulating needle.

Patient position: For subgluteal block, the patient is positioned lateral with the non-operative leg lowermost and flexed and the operative leg uppermost and extended. This allows the probe to move up and down the thigh, mapping the course of the nerve down to its bifurcation into tibial and peroneal nerve (Fig. 18.7).

Transducer position: The probe is positioned in transverse plane and the block performed below the subgluteal crease where the nerve is best visualised. The nerve is located between gluteus maximus and quadratus femoris, appearing elliptical or flattened.

Needle approach: In most patients, an in-plane needle insertion technique from lateral to medial is preferred. Using a shallow needle trajectory will maximise needle visibility, but at the expense of the longer needle track. This may not be feasible where the nerve lies very deep as in case of obese teenagers. Here, an out-of-plane approach is preferred.

Local anaesthetic dose: The local anaesthetic needs to be seen spread circumferentially around the nerve, if this does not occur a second injection may be required.

> **Key Pearl**
> Choice of probe depends on the size of the child.

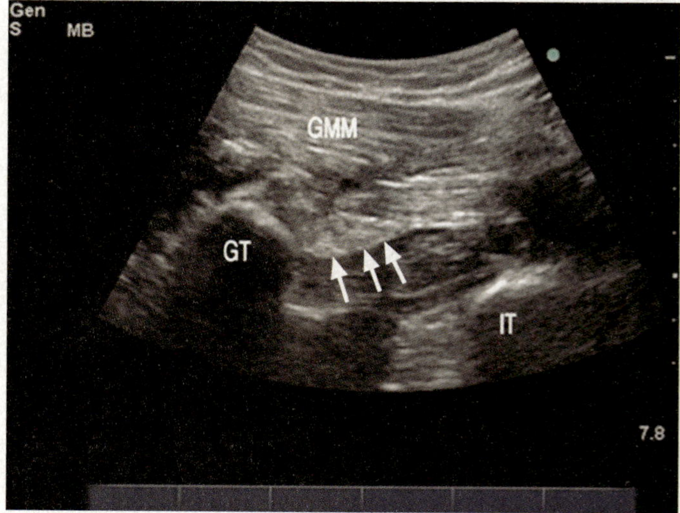

Fig. 18.7 Sciatic nerve block at subgluteal region (GT-greater trochanter, GMM-gluteus maximus, arrows represents sciatic nerve)

Complications

Femoral Nerve Block

Indications: Femoral nerve block provides anaesthesia and analgesia for anterior thigh, femur and knee surgery.[2] Together with the sciatic block, it is useful for surgery on or below the knee.

Initial settings: Depth 2–4 cm, frequency 8–14 MHz, Linear transducer preferably hockey stick probe, needle size 30–50 mm, 21 G short bevel insulated stimulating needle.

Patient position: Supine

Transducer position: The probe is positioned in transverse direction, initially over femoral artery, at or immediately inferior and parallel to inguinal crease. Goal is to visualize femoral artery. The nerve is visualized in short axis and is lateral to the anechoic large circular image (femoral artery). Doppler would help in identifying the vascular structure. The nerve is usually triangular shaped.[2] The superficial structures include fascia lata and iliaca and appear bright echogenic structures (Fig. 18.8).[2]

Needle approach: It can be performed both out-of-plane and in plane with the former being more useful for catheter insertion. The in-plane approach allows visualization of the needle tip when it enters fascia iliaca.[2]

Local anaesthetic dose: The volume sufficient to bathe the nerve appears to be optimal.

Complications: Femoral vessels puncture, intramural injection.

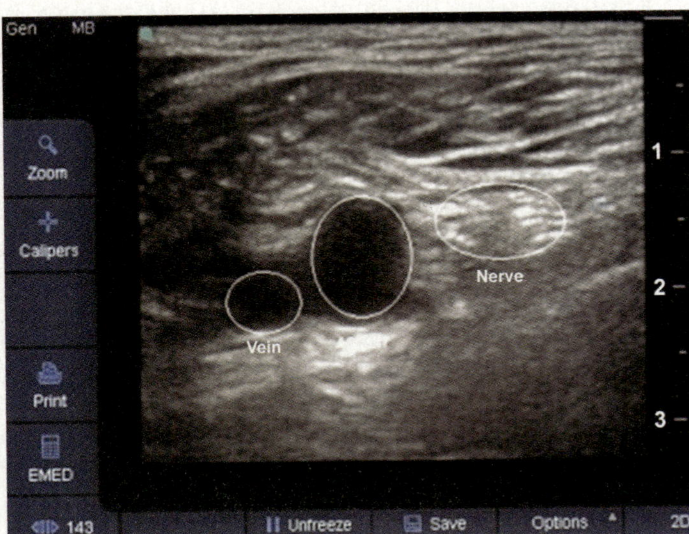

Fig. 18.8 Femoral nerve block

> **Key Pearls**
> - Observe for the local anaesthetic volume to surround the femoral nerve.
> - The needle placement is within fascia iliaca compartment for a successful block.

Popliteal Sciatic Block

Indications: The sciatic nerve block at popliteal region is useful for foot and ankle surgery.

Initial settings: Depth 3–5 cm, frequency 8–12 MHz, linear transducer, needle size 100–150 mm, 21 G short bevel insulated stimulating needle.

Patient position: It may be done in prone, supine and oblique position.

Transducer position: Transducer between tendon of hamstring muscle approx. 2–4 cm above the popliteal fossa crease. The goal is to visualise hyperechoic sciatic nerve superficial and lateral to popliteal artery and vein. The nerves can be identified by passive dorsiflexion and plantar flexion of the foot at the ankle, which will produce see-saw sign whereby the two nerves are seen to roll over each other within their common sheath as they are stretched.

Needle approach: Both in-plane and out-of-plane techniques have been described and are useful.

Local anaesthetic dose: Ultrasound image to observe the nerve bathed in local anaesthetic agent, usually around 5 mL.

Complications: Vascular puncture

> **Key Pearl**
> Popliteal vessels identification is a useful landmark.

Truncal Blocks

Truncal blocks are emerging useful blocks in children for providing analgesia for abdominal and umbilical procedures. The visualization of the muscles and associated fascial planes by ultrasound and also the spread of local anaesthetic agents in these planes ensure good success of the nerve blocks.

Ilioinguinal and Iliohypogastric Nerve Block

The ilioinguinal/iliohypogastric nerve block provides analgesia for surgical procedures in the sensory area of the ilioinguinal and iliohypogastric nerves.[6,15] However, this nerve block does not provide relief for visceral pain or due to peritoneal stretching as may happen during orchidopexy.[6]

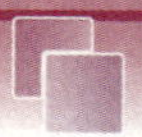

Indications: Inguinal surgeries (inguinal hernia, orchidopexy, varicocele)

Initial settings: Depth 3–6 cm, frequency 6–18 MHz, linear transducer preferably hockey stick probe, needle size 40 mm, 21 G short bevel insulated stimulating needle.

Patient position: Supine position, palpation of ASIS provides the initial landmark for transducer placement.

Transducer position:The probe is placed in a transverse position with one end of probe resting on anterior superior iliac spine, the other pointing towards the umbilicus. The ilioinguinal nerve is seen in short axis as hypoechoic ellipse between internal oblique and transverse abdominis muscle. The iliohypogastric nerve passes ventrally between external and internal oblique muscles and may not be seen.[2]

Needle approach: An in-plane approach directing the needle towards the anterior superior iliac spine is recommended to reduce the risk of breaching the peritoneum (which can be as close as 1.3 mm to the peritoneum)

Local anaesthetic dose: Volumes as low as 0.075 mL/kg have been shown to be affective.

Complications: Complications like bowel perforation, pelvic hematoma and unwanted femoral nerve have decreased drastically with the use of ultrasound but occasional complications are seen.

> **Key Pearls**
> - Both the nerves appear as hypoechoic structures.
> - Small volume of drug may be used to create the plane and confirm the spread of the drug between the muscles and close to the nerves.

Rectus Sheath Block

Rectus sheath blocks terminal branches of 9th, 10th and 11th intercostal nerve within the rectus sheath. Ultrasound guided block allows deposition of drug bilaterally within the space between the rectus abdominis muscle and the posterior sheath using real-time imaging.[16]

Indications: Useful for minor abdominal surgery via umbilical or a midline incision, e.g.umbilical and epigastric hernia repair, laparoscopic surgery and pyloromyotomy.[6,16]

Initial settings: Depth 3–6 cm, frequency 6–18 MHz, linear transducer, preferably hockey stick probe, needle size 50–100 mm, 21 G short bevel insulated stimulating needle.

Patient position: This block is performed in supine position.

Transducer position: The probe is placed just below the umbilicus (linea semilunaris) in the transverse plane. The lateral edge of rectus muscle is on the side of the screen.[2] The rectus sheath with its anterior and posterior layers along with enclosed rectus sheath is imaged. The sheath is hypoechoic on imaging. The peritoneum below appears hyperechoic (Fig. 18.9).

Needle approach: The needle is inserted at the semilunaris, and advanced in-plane from lateral to medial until the needle tip lies between the rectus muscle and posterior layer of the sheath. Prior to needle insertion, colour Doppler should be used to identify the inferior epigastric vessels as they travel within the rectus muscle. Usually two separate punctures are required to block the left and right sides. Ultrasound allows observing the spread of local anaesthetic within the posterior part of the rectus sheath.

Local anaesthetic dose: A volume of 0.1–0.2 mL/kg local anaesthetic has been shown to be effective.[6,16]

Complications: The vascular puncture and peritoneal perforation are the potential risks.

> **Key Pearl**
> The hydrodissection with small aliquots of drug volume helps to identify the plane for drug placement.

Transversus Abdominis Plane (TAP) Block

The transversus abdominis plane block has been reported for perioperative analgesia in abdominal procedures.[17] The ultrasound guided TAP block is technically feasible and avoids large volume of local anaesthetics required for local infiltration for abdominal

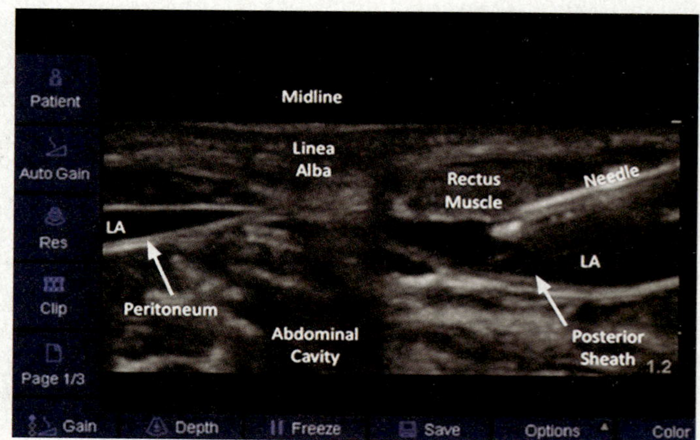

Fig. 18.9 Rectus sheath block

surgeries. The local anaesthetic in TAP block is deposited between the transversus abdominis and the internal oblique muscle.[6]

Indications: TAP block is useful in appendecitomy, inguinal hernia repair and abdominal surgery.

Initial settings: Depth 3–6 cm, frequency 6–18 MHz, linear transducer, needle size 50–100 mm, 21 G short bevel insulated stimulating needle.

Patient position: The block is performed in supine position.

Transducer position: The transverse abdominis plane (TAP) block is performed with the patient supine; the probe is positioned in sagittal plane between the 12th rib and the iliac crest over the mid axillary line. The three muscles (external oblique, internal oblique and transverse abdominis) can be easily identified due to muscle fibres running in different directions (Fig. 18.10).

Needle approach: The needle is inserted in-plane until the tip lies between internal oblique and transverse abdominis; the tip should be posterior to the mid axillary line to ensure that the lateral nerve branches are blocked.

Local anaesthetic dose: A volume of 0.5 mL/kg of local anaesthetic is generally recommended.

Complications: The peritoneal breach may occur.

> **Key Pearls**
> - The posterior movement of transversus abdominis muscle occurs with administration of the drug in correct plane.
> - Hydrodissection helps in identifying the correct plane.

Dorsal Nerve Block

The ultrasound guided dorsal nerve block has been reported to provide better and longer analgesia as compared to conventional dorsal nerve block (anatomical landmark based) and caudal epidural analgesia.[18,19]

Indications: Dorsal nerve block is indicated for perioperative analgesia for circumcision, penile procedures.

Initial settings: Depth 3–6 cm, frequency 6–18 MHz, linear transducer, needle size 40 mm, 21 G short bevel needle.

Patient position: Prone.

Transducer position: In this block, the drug is deposited under ultrasound guided into the sub-pubic space, deep to Scarpa's fascia on either side of the midline fundiform ligament.[20] In this technique, probe is placed vertically in sagittal plane along the shaft of the penis and the penile shaft structures and pubic symphysis are identified.[2]

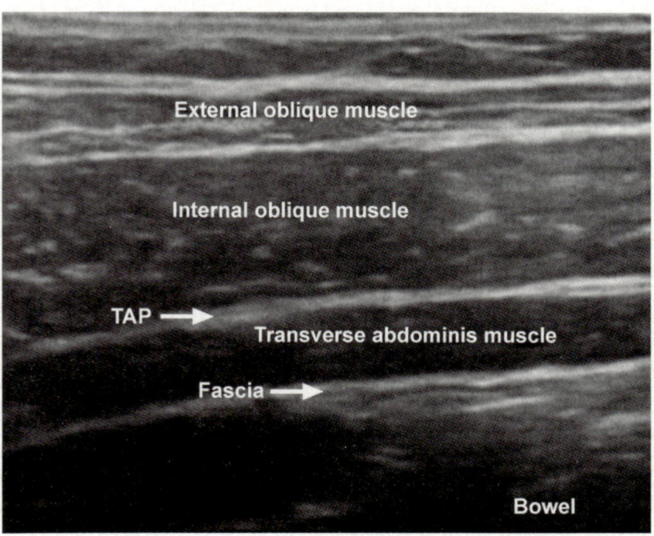

Fig. 18.10 Transversus abdominis plane (TAP) block

Needle approach: The needle is advanced into the subpubic space deep to Scarpa's fascia from either side of the ultrasound probe. After visualization of the paired neurovascular structures which lies deep to the deep fascia of the penis and on either side of the midline, local anaesthetic is injected on each side of the midline.

Local anaesthetic dose: The volume up to 3 years of age is 1–2 mL with an extra mL for every increment in three years with a maximum ceiling volume of 5–6 mL.[21]

> **Key Pearl**
> Spread of drug deep to scarpa's fascia needs to be imaged.

Central Neuraxial Blockade

Central neuraxial blockade is a valuable tool for perioperative pain management in children. While the use of ultrasound in neuraxial anaesthesia in adults is somewhat limited because of poor beam penetration through the ossified bony vertebral column, it could be much greater value in paediatric patients. In contrast to adults, children have limited ossification, thus allowing good visual resolution of the anatomy and block related equipment or solutions. The ultrasound guided neuraxial block specially real time visualization improves the success rate and safety of the block in experts hand.[22–25]

Epidural Block

Ultrasound allows visualization of ligamentum flavum, the dura mater, and the termination of the spinal cord.[22]

Also, depth of ligamentum flavum assessed by ultrasound has been found to correlate with depth of the ligamentum flavum evaluated clinically. Thus, ultrasound allows real-time identification of the tip of the needle within the epidural space. Ultrasound also allows visualization of the spread of the drug in the targeted space. Ultrasound imaging for epidural analgesia may be beneficial either preprocedurally (before puncture) or during (in real time)block performance to assess the depth to the epidural space as well as spread of local anaesthetic. The benefits of pre-procedural ultrasound may be more useful in obese children in whom the landmarks are more difficult to palpate. Ultrasound has also proven of help for epidural catheter placement in children.[23]

Indications: Caudal epidural anaesthesia is indicated for lower abdominal, urological, and orthopaedic procedures. The lumbar and thoracic blocks provide analgesia for chest and upper abdominal surgeries.

Initial settings: Depth 3–6 cm, frequency 6–18 MHz, linear transducer, needle size 50–100 mm, 21 G short bevel insulated stimulating needle.

Patient position: The patient should be positioned in lateral position with knee flexed.

Transducer position: To capture an overview of neuraxial structures, the probe should be placed both in transverse and longitudinal planes. In transverse view, the central vertebral body as appears as hyperechoic "V" in contrast to the more hypoechoic paravertebral muscles.[12] Bony structures such as the spinous processes are useful in identifying the midline. The ligamentum flavum and dura mater may be visualised as hyperechoic lines in the transverse view, although the dura mater becomes more difficult to see in children older than six months. Using a paramedian longitudinal view, the spinous process and laminae are easy to identify as slanted hyperechoic lines. Deep to the liganteum flavum and dura mater, the spinal cord appears as hypoechoic structure with two distinguishing features: a central line of hyperechogenicity representing the median sulcus, and a bright outer covering the pia mater.

Needle approach: For ultrasound assessed depth and location, the needle is placed in conventional manner keeping track the direction and depth of the space (i.e. skin to ligamentum flavum) as assessed with ultrasound. For real time, probe in paramedian longitudinal plane, needle is advanced, ventral displacement of the dura and widening of the space with loss of resistance ensures correct tip placement of the epidural needle.

Local anaesthetic dose: The dose remains as for conventional procedures of epidural anaesthesia and analgesia.

Complications: The epidural vessel rupture or inadvertently dural puncture as for conventional technique but with reduced risk.

Caudal Anaesthesia

Indications: Caudal blocks are for lower extremity and perineal perioperative analgesia are the most commonly practiced anaesthesia techniques in children.

Initial settings: Depth 3–6 cm, frequency 6–18 MHz, linear transducer, needle size 50–100 mm, 21 G short bevel insulated stimulating needle.

Patient position: The patient should be positioned in lateral position with knee flexed.

Transducer position: Preprocedural imaging in both transverse and longitudinal planes is important to identify the sacrococcygeal ligament, dural sac, and caudaequina. With the probe placed in the transverse plane at the level of coccyx, the sacral hiatus is visible between two hyperechoic reversed U-shaped structures which are bony prominence of sacral cornua.[24] Between the cornua, the two hyperechoic lines are imaged. The superior line represents the sacrococcygeal ligament while the inferior represents the dorsum of the pelvic surface of the sacrum. When the probe is placed in longitudinal plane between the sacral cornua, the dorsal surface of the sacrum, dorsal aspect of the pelvis surface of the sacrum, as well as the sacrococcygeal ligament are viewed. The ligament can be identified as a thick, linear, hyperechoic band that slopes caudally.

Needle approach: It may be beneficial to use both transverse and longitudinal planes. The sacrococcygeal membrane is punctured under ultrasound imaging in longitudinal plane and drug is injected. The drug deposition and its spread may be visualized using ultrasound in a longitudinal paramedian position.

Local anaesthetic dose: The dose remains as for conventional procedures of caudal epidural anaesthesia and analgesia.

Complications: The risk of subarachnoid administration or subperiosteal deposition is reduced as compared to conventional blocks.

CONCLUSION

The ultrasound has a very promising role for ultrasound guided regional nerve block in children. Further studies are required to study its outcome with regards to success and its feasibility in different peripheral nerve block. Ultrasound enables optimal placement of drug in lower doses with improved successful sensory and motor block. However, a formal training and practice needs to emphasized for a successful ultrasound guided nerve block.

REFERENCES

1. Gupta PK, Gupta K, Dwivedi AD, et al. Potential role of ultrasound in anaesthesia and intensive care. Anesth Essays Res. 2011;5:11–9.
2. Marhofer P, Sitzwohl C, Greher M, et al. Ultrasound guidance for infraclavicular brachial plexus anaesthesia in children. Anaesthesia. 2004;59:642–646.
3. Marhofer P, Greher M, Kapral S. Ultrasound guidance in regional anaesthesia. Br J Anaesth. 2005;94:7–17.
4. Robert S, Neary H. Paediatric ultrasound guided regional anaesthesia: Peripheral techniques. International Journal of Ultrasound and applied technologies in perioperative care. 2010;1:101–107.
5. Ganesh A, Gurnaney HG. Ultrasound Guidance for Pediatric Peripheral Nerve Blockade. Anaesthesiology Clin 2009;27:197–212.
6. Willschke H, Marhofer P, Machata AM, Lonnqvist PA. Current trends in paediatric regional anaesthesia. Anaesthesia. 2010;65:97–104.
7. Tsui BCH, Suresh S. Ultrasound imaging for regional anaesthesia in infants, children and adolescents. Anaesthesiology. 2010;112:473–92.
8. Oberndorfer U, Marhofer P, Bosenberg A, et al. Ultrasonographic guidance for sciatic and femoral nerve blocks in children. Br J Anaesth. 2007;98:797–801.
9. Brenner L, Marhofer P, Kettner SC, et al. Ultrasound assessment of cranial spread caudal blockade in children: The effect of different volumes of local anaesthetics. Br J Anaesth 2011;107:229–235.
10. Per-Arne L. Is ultrasound guidance mandatory when performing paediatric regional anaesthesia? Current Opinion in Anaesthesiology 2010;23:337–341.
11. Frederic L. Epidemiology and morbidity of regional anaesthesia in children. Current Opinion in Anaesthesiology. 2008;21:345–349.
12. Griffin J, Nicholls B. Ultrasound in regional anaesthesia. Anaesthesia. 2010;65:1–12.
13. Gray AT. Ultrasound-guided regional anaesthesia. Current state of art. Anaesthesiology. 2006;104:368–373.
14. Marhofer P, Sitzwohl C, Greher M, et al. Ultrasound guidance for infraclavicular brachial plexus anaesthesia in children. Anaesthesia. 2004;59:642–646.
15. Willschke H, Marhofer P, Bosenberg A, et al. Ultrasonography for ilioinguinal/iliohypogastric nerve blocks in children. Br J Anaesth. 2005; 95: 226–30.
16. Wilschke H, Bosenberg A, Marhofer P, et al. Ultrasonography guided rectus sheath block in paediatric anaesthesia—a new approach to an old technique. Br J Anaesth. 2006;97: 244–9.
17. Fredrickson MJ, Seal P. Ultrasound-guided transversus abdominis plane block for neonatal abdominal surgery. Anaesthesia and Intensive Care. 2009;39:469–472.
18. Sandeman DJ, Reiner D, Dilley AV, et al. A retrospective audit of three different regional anaesthetic techniques for circumcision in children. Anaesth Intensive Care. 2010;38:519–524.
19. Faraoni D, Gilbeau A, Lingier P, et al. Does ultrasound guidance improve the efficacy of dorsal nerve block in children? PediatricAnesthesia 2010;20:931–936.
20. Sandeman DJ, Dilley AV. Ultrasound guided dorsal nerve block in children. Anaesth intensive care. 2007;35:266–9.
21. Brown TCK, Weidner NJ, Bouwmeester J. Dorsal nerve of the penis block-anatomical and radiological studies. Anaesth Intensive Care. 1989;17:34–38.
22. Willschke H, Bosenberg A, Marhofer P, et al. Epidural catheter placement in neonates: Sonoanatomy and feasibility of ultrasonographic guidance in term and preterm neonates. Reg Anesth Pain Med. 2007;32:34–40.
23. Willschke H, Marhofer P, Bosenberg A, et al. Epidural catheter placement in children: comparing a novel approach using ultrasound guidance and a standard loss of resistance technique. Br J Anaesth. 2006;97:200–7.
24. Chen CPC, Tang SFT, Hsu TC, et al. Ultrasound guidance in caudal epidural needle placement. Anaesthesiology. 2004;101:181–4.
25. Sawardekar A, Szczodry D, Suresh S. Neuraxial anaesthesia in paediatrics. Anaesthesia and intensive care medicine. 2013;14:251–254.

Section

3

Anaesthesia for Special Surgical Procedure

Anaesthesia for Foetal Intervention and Surgery

Swati R Daftary and Rajen Y Daftary

ABSTRACT

In foetal intervention and surgery, the mother is a bystander while the foetus or foetuses are active recipients of foetal therapy. Anaesthesiologists dealing with these patients must consider the anaesthetic requirements of the mother and foetus, and hence should be aware of physiology of pregnancy and foeto-placental unit. As foetal surgery is increasingly becoming a beneficial intervention for many foetal anomalies diagnosed in utero, and with surgical approach varying from open surgery to minimally invasive surgery, a multidisciplinary approach becomes essential.

INTRODUCTION

Foetal surgery is the surgical treatment of a foetus in utero with certain life-threatening congenital anomalies. Its purpose is to correct problems that would be too advanced to correct after birth or would jeopardize the survival of the foetus till full term. The first successful therapeutic foetal procedure was done by Sir William Liley in 1963, where he gave intraperitoneal blood transfusion in a case of Erythroblastosis foetalis. The first successful foetal surgery was done by Michael Harrison in 1981 in a case of obstructive uropathy at UCSF Children's Hospital. Today there are number of centres all over the world doing foetal surgeries.[1] The ethical dilemma of foetal surgery, which is associated with high incidence of prematurity, foetal demise, maternal morbidity and huge costs is still debated. A few centres in India are successfully doing minimally invasive foetal surgeries today.[2,3]

Foetal Malformations and Management[4,5]

Management of foetal malformations depends on the type and whether they are compatible with postnatal life. Malformations not correctable and incompatible with postnatal life like acardiac/anencephalic twin or renal agenesis, the mother should undergo early termination of pregnancy. Malformations best corrected after birth are omphalocoele, gastroschisis, hydrocephalus, conjoined twins. Mother should undergo normal delivery/C-section in a tertiary care centre with facilities for immediate postnatal management of the neonate. Certain malformations if allowed till term, will result either in foetal demise or in a poor outcome, but are potentially correctable in utero like congenital diaphragmatic hernia (CDH), congenital cystic adenomatoid malformation (CCAM), sacrococcygeal teratoma (SCT), twin-twin transfusion syndrome (TTTS), twin reverse arterial perfusion (TRAP) sequence and meningomyelocele (MMC) which may benefit from foetal surgery.

Diagnosis of Foetal Malformations[6]

Advanced noninvasive and invasive antenatal diagnostic techniques like ultrasonography, foetal echocardiography, foetal magnetic resonance imaging, amniocentesis, umbilical blood sampling and chorionic villus sampling have improved our diagnosing these foetal malformations.

FOETAL ACCESS FOR SURGERY[7]

Depending on the pathology, different approaches for foetal interventions are described with different levels of invasiveness.

Table 19.1 Foetal surgical approaches

Type of intervention	Description	Examples
Open surgery	**Hysterotomy**· **Mid gestation:** 18–26 weeks· **At/near term:** Ex-utero intra-partum treatment (**EXIT**)	• CCAM–lobectomy • SCT–resection • MMC–repair • Cervical teratoma–resection • EXIT–Tracheal occlusion, Neck tumors, CDH (to ECMO), CCAM (to lobectomy)
Foetal endoscopic surgery • Developed in 1990s	Minimizes preterm labour Manipulation by visualizing the foetus in real time using both endoscopy and sonography	• Tracheal occlusion (CDH) • Laser ablation of vessels (TTTS) • Cord ligation/division • Cystoscopic ablation of PU valves· • Amniotic band division
Foetal image guided surgery • Least invasive· • Can be done under LA/RA (SA/EA)	Manipulation done entirely by sonography	• Amnioreduction/Infusion • Foetal blood sampling • RFA anomalous twins • Vesico/Pleuro amniotic shunts • Cord monopolar cautery • Balloon dilatation of aortic stenosis • In-utero pacing for 3° heart block

Basically there are three types of surgical approaches (Table 19.1). Open surgery which is either done between 18 and 26 weeks of gestation or done at or near term, also known as Ex-utero intrapartum treatment (EXIT). The other two approaches are minimally invasive and are becoming more popular due to complications associated with open surgery. Foetal endoscopic surgery minimizes preterm labour. Foetal image guided surgery is the least invasive type of foetal surgery. Providing anaesthesia for procedures ranging from complex open surgery to minimally invasive ultrasound-guided procedures can be challenging.

Anaesthetic Management

Foetal intervention involves the mother and foetus or foetuses. The mother is not a direct beneficiary from the intervention and may be at increased risk due to the procedure. These interventions involve a direct noxious stimulus to the foetus. Anaesthesiologists dealing with these patients should be well versed with maternal changes of pregnancy, physiology of uteroplacental circulation and foetoplacental unit. Anaesthesia for foetal surgery is a combination of obstetric anaesthesia and paediatric anaesthesia. Because of the high risk of these procedures, patient selection is an important consideration. The mothers must be at a sufficiently low anaesthesia risk and motivated to comply with frequent follow-ups and activity restrictions.[6,7]

MATERNAL, PLACENTAL AND FOETAL PHYSIOLOGY

Physiological Changes of Pregnancy

Marked anatomical and physiological changes occur in women during pregnancy. All the systems including circulatory, respiratory, haematological, gastrointestinal, liver, gall bladder, kidneys, endocrine, musculo-skeletal and nervous system undergo changes so as to adapt to the developing foetus and provide for its increased metabolic demands. It is beyond the capacity of this chapter to discuss these changes and hence the reader is referred to a standard textbook of obstetric anaesthesia.[8] What we will discuss is the anaesthetic implications of relevant maternal changes of pregnancy and appropriate adaptation of anaesthetic techniques for pregnant mothers undergoing foetal surgery.

Anaesthetic Implications[8]

Positioning: Preventing aorto-caval compression and impairment of uteroplacental blood flow by the gravid uterus is vital after twenty weeks of gestation. The uterus should be tilted to the left, through placement of a wedge underneath the right hip during surgery.

Changes in General Anaesthesia during Pregnancy

1. **Endotracheal intubation:** Vascular engorgement along with tissue oedema causes narrower and friable airway. These patients require smaller endotracheal tubes, have increased risk of failed intubation and bleeding with nasal instrumentation. Decreased lung capacities and increased oxygen demand makes them prone to hypoxia during apnoea.
2. Treat them as full stomach and premedicate with antacid and prokinetic agents. Good preoxygenation and rapid sequence induction and intubation with cricoid pressure is important.
3. **Inhalation and intravenous anaesthetics:** Induction dose of thiopentone sodium is decreased, whereas elimination half-life is prolonged. With propofol, both induction dose and elimination half-life remain unaltered. Inhalation anaesthetic agent's minimum alveolar concentration (MAC) is decreased and rate of uptake is increased.
4. **Muscle relaxants:** Succinylcholine's duration of blockade is unaltered or decreased, but pregnant women show increased sensitivity to rocuronium.
5. **Chronotropic agents and vasopressors:** Pregnancy reduces the chronotropic and pressor response to isoproterenol and adrenaline owing to the down-regulation of adrenergic receptors.

Changes in Neuraxial Analgesia and Anaesthesia

1. Technically becomes more difficult due to enhanced lumbar lordosis.
2. Widening of the pelvis results in a head-down tilt when a pregnant woman is in the lateral position. This tilt may increase the rostral spread of subarachnoid local anaesthetic.
3. Pregnant women exhibit a more rapid onset and a longer duration of spinal anaesthesia due to increased neural sensitivity to local anaesthetics.
4. Engorged epidural Batsons plexus causes narrowing of both subarachnoid and epidural space. Thus reducing the dosage/volume of the drug injected is important.
5. To treat hypotension, larger doses of vasopressors are required in pregnant patients.

Uteroplacental Physiology

Uteroplacental blood flow is the major determinant of oxygen and nutrient delivery and hence well-being of the foetus. Uterine blood flow is related to perfusion pressure (the difference between uterine arterial pressure and uterine venous pressure) and vascular resistance. The uteroplacental circulation is a widely dilated, low-resistance vascular bed with almost no ability for autoregulation.

The factors which reduce utero-placental blood flow are supine position (aortocaval compression), hypotension (sympathetic blockade, haemorrhage, drug induced), uterine contractions (oxytocin, hypertonus) and presence of endogenous and exogenous vasoconstrictors. Mechanical factors like kinking or compression of the umbilical cord and premature separation of the placenta from the uterus can also result in catastrophic reduction in foetal perfusion.[9] Mechanical hyperventilation during general anaesthesia leads to hypocapnoea and is associated with reduced uterine blood flow and foetal hypoxia and acidosis.[10] Maintenance of normal pCO_2, pO_2 can prevent foetal asphyxia. Neuraxial anaesthesia can increase uterine blood flow by reducing pain, stress and hyperventilation.

Drugs that cross placenta are atropine, scopolamine, β blockers, nitroglycerine, nitroprusside, diazepam, midazolam, thiopentone sodium, propofol, inhalational agents, local anaesthetics, opioids, ephedrine and drugs that do not cross placenta are glycopyrrolate, heparin, succinylcholine, nondepolarizing muscle relaxants.[11]

Foetal Physiology[7,12]

1. The human foetus responds to noise, pressure, pain and cold by mounting an autonomic response and a rise in stress hormones as early as 16 weeks. Foetal stress response can occur during foetal surgery and may act as a contributor to preterm labour.[13,14]
2. Altered coagulation factor predisposes foetus to increased bleeding. Associated low blood volume (110–160 mL/kg) can lead to hypovolemia.
3. Foetus is more sensitive to opioids, muscle relaxants and inhalational agents.
4. Foetus removed from the uterus during open surgery needs increased heat production. But this cannot be achieved because of absence of shivering and

nonshivering thermogenesis, immature skin barriers, and increased evaporative losses.

Foetal Surgery and Anaesthesia

In obstetric patients, regional anaesthesia is the technique of choice, but in open foetal surgery or EXIT, high concentration of potent inhalational agents are used to provide uterine relaxation and hence general anaesthesia is the technique of choice. Most of the endoscopic surgery on foetus, placenta and cord can be done under regional anaesthesia (spinal, epidural, combined spinal epidural). Image guided procedures can be done using local anaesthesia of the maternal abdominal wall alone.

The problem with general anaesthesia is that sometimes the surgeon feels the uterus is too relaxed, making the foetus unstable in position and causing difficulty with a percutaneous approach. Also, general anaesthesia with high concentration of potent inhalational agents could cause foetal cardiac depression.[15] Studies have shown that use of supplemental IV anaesthesia (SIVA) with remifentanil along with inhalational anaesthetics like desflurane, allows for decreased use of inhalational anaesthetics, resulting in better preservation of foetal cardiac function.[16,17]

Echocardiographic monitoring of the heart during foetal surgery demonstrates that acute cardiovascular changes take place during foetal surgery, which may be due to the physiology of the anomaly and the general effects of surgical stress, tocolytic agents, and anaesthesia.[15]

Hence for all foetal surgery, some basic anaesthetic objectives apply:

1. Maternal safety
2. Avoidance of teratogenic agents—avoid surgery in first trimester
3. Avoidance of foetal asphyxia
4. Adequate foetal anaesthesia and monitoring
5. Uterine relaxation
6. Prevention of preterm labor

Maternal safety: Anaesthesia for foetal surgery is an extension of obstetric anaesthesia and hence basic principles of obstetric anaesthesia must be followed. The only difference from regular obstetric patient is that preloading and fluid boluses to maintain normal BP or treat hypotension should be avoided in foetal surgery patients, as mother is at increased risk of pulmonary oedema due to aggressive tocolytic therapy.

Maternal Safety Key Points

- Thorough preoxygenation and anticipate airway difficulty
- Uterine displacement to left to avoid supine hypotensive syndrome
- Premedication with antacid and prokinetic agents, rapid sequence induction and intubation with cricoid pressure
- Avoid foetal asphyxia; maintain normal maternal pCO_2, pO_2 and BP
- Restrict maternal fluids to 500 mL
- Increased sensitivity to LA agents and reduced quantity of LA requirement in regional anaesthesia

Foetal Anaesthesia and Monitoring[18]

1. Whenever direct stimulation of the foetus is planned, an IM injection of fentanyl 20 µg/kg (to abolish stress response) and pancuronium/vecuronium 0.2 mg/kg (foetal immobility) is delivered to the foetus under direct vision or ultrasonographic guidance. Pancuronium is preferred for its vagolytic effect.
2. Foetal cutaneous and evaporative heat losses are reduced by warm ambient temperature, limiting surgical time and irrigation of warm fluids.
3. Fresh, warm O –ve, irradiated blood cross matched against the mother should be kept ready for foetal transfusion.
4. **Foetal monitoring** in the form of temperature, pulse oximetry, ultrasonography, echocardiography and blood sampling is carried out where indicated. Pulse oximetry (N = 60–70%) values >40% are suggestive of adequate foetal oxygenation. Sterile intraoperative echocardiography is also used to monitor FHR and stroke volume. It helps in detecting acute cardiovascular changes that take place during foetal surgery.[15]

Foetal Safety Key Points

- Avoid foetal asphyxia
- Carry out optimum foetal monitoring
- Take care of foetal hypothermia, anaemia, hypovolemia, stress

Uterine Relaxation and Prevention of Preterm Labour

Control of uterine tone by general inhalation anaesthesia is necessary for open and endoscopic foetal surgery requiring significant manipulation, so as to provide optimal operative exposure. This can be achieved by high concentration of potent inhalation agent (2–3 MAC) in 100% O_2 so as to have optimum uterine relaxation without maternal hypotension. Additional tocolysis can be achieved by preoperative insertion of indomethacin (50 mg) suppository and small doses of

IV nitroglycerine (50–100 mg). Epidural anaesthesia helps as adequate postoperative pain control is associated with lower maternal concentrations of oxytocin, reducing the risks of uterine contractions and preterm labor.

Magnesium sulphate, terbutaline, nifedipine are other tocolytic agents used alone or in combination in the postoperative period to prevent preterm labour.[13] While magnesium sulphate is associated with more maternal toxicity, indomethacin is associated with more foetal and neonatal toxicity. In February 2011, the US Food and Drug Administration (FDA) added a new Black Box Warning and contraindication to the use of terbutaline in preterm labour due to reports of death and serious adverse reactions.[19]

In EXIT procedure, tocolysis is terminated as soon as the cord is clamped followed by administration of oxytocin. In minimal access surgery which can be done under LA or RA, parental tocolytic agents are used.

Foetal Surgery—Prerequisites

For foetal surgery, a multidisciplinary team consisting of paediatric surgeon, anaesthesiologist, obstetrician, ultrasonologist, geneticist, social worker and nursing personnel are required to discuss the plan and obtain the consent. Mother must undergo extensive medical and psychosocial screening. She must be able to comply with the intensive demands postoperatively including bed rest and compliance with medications. The patient is an obligate c-section for both this and all subsequent deliveries if she is for open foetal surgery. The foetus should have a disease that merits intervention and the mother have low maternal risk for anaesthesia and surgery.[20]

OPEN FOETAL SURGERY

Mid-gestation Hysterotomy

Surgical considerations: It is performed between 18 and 26 weeks for defects like MMC, CCAM or SCT through a low transverse abdominal incision. The uterus is exteriorized and a wide hysterotomy is done after confirming the placental location by ultrasonography. Use of absorbable stapler allows performance of "bloodless hysterotomy". After hysterotomy, the foetal part is exteriorized for surgery. Once the defect has been repaired and returned inside the uterus, a watertight two-layer uterine closure is done. Warm saline or ringer lactate with antibiotic is infused into the amniotic sac to maintain uterine volume and decrease postoperative contractions. The skin is then closed and the maternal operation is completed.[18]

Anaesthesia Considerations:[20] Preparations

1. Type specific packed RBCs for the mother and O –ve packed RBCs for the foetus
2. Monitors: Two pulse oximeters (maternal and foetal), foetal echocardiography and arterial pressure transducer in addition to routine monitors
3. Epinephrine 10 μg/kg, atropine 20 μg/kg, fentanyl 20 μg/kg, and muscle relaxant prepared in a sterile manner in 1 mL syringes for possible foetal IM administration
4. Confirmation of maternal NPO status, large bore IV line
5. Lumbar epidural catheter inserted and test dosed for postoperative pain relief
6. Indomethacin suppository for postoperative tocolysis
7. Left uterine displacement maintained at all times

Intraoperative Management

1. Rapid sequence induction and intubation with IV thiopentone sodium or propofol and succinylcholine
2. Maintenance of GA with 0.5 MAC isoflurane or desflurane in 50% N_2O and O_2
3. Second IV line, radial artery cannulation, nasogastric tube, foley catheter insertion
4. IV fluid restricted to total of 500 mL to reduce the risk of postoperative pulmonary oedema
5. Before maternal skin incision, inhalation agent increased to 2–3 MAC to provide uterine relaxation and foetal anaesthesia. Foetal analgesia is provided with foetal IM fentanyl 20 μg/kg.
6. Maternal systolic BP maintained within 10% of baseline with the help of either ephedrine 5–10 mg IV or phenylephrine 1–2 μg/kg. Use of ephedrine is associated with higher incidence of foetal acidosis (pH <7.2).[21] Ephedrine is a logical choice if the maternal heart rate is slow, while phenylephrine should be used if the maternal heart rate is high.
7. Foetal monitoring
8. After closure of the uterus, the anaesthetic is converted to a regional technique. MAC is reduced to 0.5 and epidural catheter is dosed with LA and opioid. Tocolysis is instituted with a loading dose of magnesium sulphate 6 gm IV followed by IV infusion at 2–3 gm/hour.
9. Coughing or straining during emergence should be avoided to prevent disruption of the uterine closure.

10. Magnesium sulphate, well-functioning epidural analgesia and indomethacin are continued for 48 hours. After this the first line tocolysis is by oral nifedipine. If this fails then terbutaline is administered subcutaneously. Bed rest is recommended for remainder of the pregnancy.

Meningomyelocele (MMC): Combination of chronic chemical (amniotic fluid) and traumatic exposure of exposed spinal cord leads to progressive and irreversible damage. This results in absent lower extremity function (>20 weeks) and increased incidence of hindbrain herniation leading to shunt dependent hydrocephalus. In-utero treatment of hydrocephalus with ventriculoamniotic shunt was one of the earlier modalities, which is now no longer recommended.[22]

A randomized multicentric trial of prenatal (Intrauterine repair of MMC before 26 weeks of gestation) versus postnatal repair of myelomeningocele published in 2011, (MOMS) was conducted at three maternal–foetal surgery centres in the United States. The trial compared outcome in infants at 12 and 30 months and concluded that prenatal surgery for myelomeningocele reduced the need for shunting and improved motor outcomes at 30 months but was associated with maternal and foetal risks.[23]

Congenital cystic adenomatoid malformation (CCAM) and sacrococcygeal teratoma (SCT) are associated with high incidence of hydrops foetalis and foetal death. Large CCAM leads to cardiac and great vessel compression which is responsible for the pathology. Treatment includes foetal lobectomy, shunting or excision at EXIT.[18]

Presence of SCT is responsible for "vascular steal" phenomena, which leads to hydrops foetalis and foetal death. SCT can also lead to 'the maternal mirror syndrome' a state of maternal oedema that mirrors that of the foetus. Mother shows symptoms suggestive of preeclampsia and pulmonary oedema as a result of placentomegaly. This can be prevented by foetal surgery like open resection, radio frequency/LASER ablation of causative blood vessels or foetoscopic resection.[18]

Ex-utero Intrapartum Therapy (EXIT)

The EXIT procedure is used to achieve a patent foetal airway and to ensure adequate foetal oxygenation. EXIT procedure ends with the delivery of the foetus. An epidural or spinal anaesthesia has been used for short procedures but GA is preferred in longer procedures, keeping in mind maternal anxiety. Foetal anaesthesia is necessary when invasive procedures are planned and foetal pulse oximetry, foetal echocardiography and IV access become essential in prolonged invasive procedures. Surgical lesions eligible for EXIT procedure are cystic hygroma, cervical teratoma, obstructive upper airways (congenital or acquired), congenital hydrothorax and pleural effusion. It can also be used to put neonate on ECMO.[24]

Anaesthetic preparations are the same as those of mid-gestation open foetal surgery except that in EXIT procedure

1. Tocolytics are not used postoperatively and hence pulmonary oedema is less likely, and fluid management can be more generous.
2. Resuscitation equipment, neonatologist and additional operating room with anaesthesiologist may be required for direct post-delivery care and possible surgery of the newborn.

Intraoperatively during hysterotomy, the foetus is only partially exposed and maximum uterine relaxation and uterine volume is maintained so that placental perfusion is maintained and premature separation of placenta is avoided. For thoracic intervention when the foetus is fully delivered, care has to be taken to avoid stretching or compression of the umbilical cord.[18,20]

Once the airway is secured (direct laryngoscopy/fiberoptic bronchoscopy and intubation or tracheotomy) or lesion is resected, the lungs are ventilated.[25] Increases in oxygen saturation, the presence of end-tidal CO_2, and good chest movement are indicators of successful intubation. The umbilical cord is clamped and the foetus is delivered. Volatile agents are reduced after cord clamping and epidural catheter is dosed with LA and opioid analgesic. Oxytocin is administered immediately after clamping of the umbilical cord. Additional uterotonics such as methergine and prostaglandin may be used, if necessary. In spite of this, uterine atony and significant blood loss are known risks. Maternal trachea is extubated after surgical closure. It is important in the EXIT that no ventilation of the lungs occurs until the umbilical cord is to be clamped. Ventilation of the lungs will initiate the cascade of events leading to a transitional/neonatal circulation, and the benefits of operating on "placental support" are lost.[18]

EXIT is also used for reversal of tracheal occlusion in CDH and for placement on extracorporeal membranous oxygenation (ECMO) in cases of severe CDH, hypoplastic left heart syndrome and aortic stenosis with intact/restrictive atrial septum.

In short EXIT procedures, where regional anaesthesia is given to the mother,[26] intraoperative tocolysis is achieved by nitroglycerine 100–500 mg IV followed by continuous infusion at 1–20 mg/kg/min if required.

Foetal Endoscopic Surgery

Developed in 1990s, foetoscopic surgical procedures are the most common foetal interventions as they are less invasive than open foetal surgery and minimize preterm labor. These procedures involve the percutaneous placement of small trocars and foetoscopes into the uterus and visualizing the foetus in real time using both, an endoscope and sonograph.

Initially, these procedures were performed with general or neuraxial anaesthesia techniques, but these procedures are now done with sedation. Multiple regimens for sedation have been used successfully, including combinations of opioids and other sedatives such as benzodiazepines or propofol.[18,20]

Umbilical cord ligation and selective ablation of foetal connecting vessels are done for twin pregnancies complicated by twin reversed arterial perfusion sequence (TRAP) or twin-twin transfusion syndrome (TTTS), where the death of one or both twins is imminent.

Congenital Diaphragmatic Hernia (CDH)

In the late 1980s and early1990s, in utero anatomical diaphragmatic repair was carried out in the USA and Paris, but because of its associated complications, it fell in disrepute.

Today, midgestation tracheal occlusion in cases of severe CDH is an attempt to promote lung expansion. Study of foetuses with congenital high airway obstruction syndrome (CHAOS) showed that in foetuses with upper airway obstruction, lung fluid movement out of the airway is prevented, resulting in lung expansion. Hence the concept of PLUG ('Plug the lung until it grows') was applied to improve the outcome in CDH.[27] Foetoscopically placed titanium clips through the anterior neck dissection and foetoscopically placed detachable tracheal balloon, called percutaneous foetoscopic endoluminal tracheal occlusion (FETO) have been tried. These are removed in an EXIT procedure or reversed in utero around 34 weeks.[28] In a randomized, controlled study conducted by the Foetal Treatment Centre at UCSF from April 1999 through July 2001, foetal endoscopic surgery to occlude the trachea proved no better than planned delivery and high-level neonatal care at a tertiary care centre in improving the outcome for foetuses with severe congenital diaphragmatic hernia.[29]

Bladder outlet obstruction or lower urinary tract obstruction (LUTO) in a foetus can lead to oligohydramnios and result in renal failure from renal dysplasia and secondary pulmonary hypoplasia. Initially open foetal surgery to place a vesicoamniotic shunt or percutaneous vesicoamniotic shunt under USG was performed. Nowadays in-utero percutaneous cystoscopic LASER ablation of the PU valves is done.

Anaesthesia management of foetoscopic surgery remains same as open foetal surgery except that epidural catheters are removed after the surgery. Magnesium sulphate and indomethacin, followed by nifedipine is the mainstay of tocolytic management.[18,20]

Foetal Image Guided Surgery

FIGS is the latest addition to foetal surgery which is least invasive as manipulation is done entirely by ultrasonography. It can be done under local anaesthesia or regional anaesthesia. Examples are amniocentesis, foetal blood sampling, placement of catheter shunts in urinary bladder, abdomen or chest, radio frequency ablation of SCT blood vessels and cardiac manipulations like balloon dilatation of congenital aortic stenosis and percutaneous ultrasound guided transthoracic foetal heart pacing for foetal heart block.

Anaesthesia for balloon dilation of foetal aortic stenosis involves maternal general endotracheal anaesthesia and intramuscular administration of fentanyl, vecuronium, and atropine to the foetus as there is a need for a completely immobile mother and foetus, along with the potential need for foetal analgesia as the catheters and needles are advanced through the foetal chest wall and heart.[18]

SUMMARY

Foetal surgery treats the developing foetus as a patient. Providing anaesthesia for foetal surgery is challenging for many reasons. It requires integration of both obstetric and paediatric anaesthesia practice. Two patients must be anaesthetised for the benefit of one, and there is a little margin for error. Work is needed to study possible neurotoxicity caused by exposure of the developing brain to anaesthetic agents.

Foetal centres in the USA are moving away from open methods to minimally invasive techniques. Also, there is a movement away from total in utero repair towards only manipulating foetal pathophysiology in order to reverse life-threatening events, reduce operative time and lessen morbidity. With surgery, anaesthesia for foetal surgery continues to evolve. It is essential to have good communication and cooperation between surgeons, anaesthesiologists and perinatal physicians all through the perioperative period for safe management of the foetal surgery patient.

Take Home Messages

- In foetal surgery, maternal safety is most important
- The anaesthetic plan should be based on understanding of maternal and foetal physiology, requirements of surgery and the needs of the mother and foetus

REFERENCES

1. Jan A Deprest, Alan W Flake, Eduard Gratacos, et al. The making of fetal surgery—review of current practice. Prenat Diagn 2010;30:653–667.
2. Menon Prema, Rao KLN. Current Status of Fetal Surgery. Indian Journal of Paediatrics, 2005;72:433–436.
3. Saxena N Kirti. Anaesthesia for Fetal Surgeries. Indián J Anaesth. Oct 2009;53(5):554–559.
4. Charles B Cauldwell. Anaesthesia for fetal Surgery. Anesthesiology Clinics of North America 2002;20:1:211–226.
5. Laura B Myers, David Cohen, Jeffrey Galinkin, et al. Anaesthesia for fetal surgery. Paediatric Anaesthesia 2002;12:569–578.
6. Mark A Rosen. Anaesthesia for Fetal Surgery and Other Intrauterine Procedures. In: David H Chestnut, Linda S Polley, Lawrence C Tsen, Cynthia A Wong, (Eds). Chestnut's obstetric anaesthesia: Principles and practice 4th edn. Mosby Elsevior, Philadelphia, 2009;123–140.
7. Kha Tran, David E Cohen. Anaesthesia for Fetal Surgery. In: Peter J Davis, Franklyn P Cladis, Etsuro K Motoyama, (Eds). Smith's Anaesthesia for Infants and Children, 8th edn. Elsevior Mosby Inc., Philadelphia. 2011;589–604.
8. Robert Gaiser. Physiologic Changes of Pregnancy. In: David H Chestnut, Linda S Polley, Lawrence C Tsen, Cynthia A Wong, (Eds). Chestnut's obstetric anaesthesia: principles and practice, 4th edn. Mosby Elsevior, Philadelphia, 2009;15–36.
9. Warwick D NganKee. Uteroplacental Blood Flow. In: David H Chestnut, Linda S Polley, Lawrence C Tsen, Cynthia A Wong, (Eds). Chestnut's obstetric anaesthesia: Principles and practice, 4th edn. Mosby Elsevior, Philadelphia, 2009;37–55.
10. Gershon Levinson, Sol M Shnider, Alfred A deLorimier, et al. Effects of maternal hyperventilation on uterine blood flow and fetal oxygenation and acid-base status. Anaesthesiology, April 1974;40(4):340–347.
11. Mark I Zakowski, Norman L Herman. The Placenta: Anatomy, Physiology, and Transfer of Drugs. In: David H Chestnut, Linda S Polley, Lawrence C Tsen, Cynthia A Wong, (Eds). Chestnut's obstetric anaesthesia: principles and practice, 4th edn. Mosby Elsevior, Philadelphia, 2009;56–72.
12. Kenneth E Nelson, Andrew P Harris. Fetal Physiology. In: David H Chestnut, Linda S Polley, Lawrence C Tsen, Cynthia A Wong, (Eds). Chestnut's obstetric anaesthesia: principles and practice, 4th edn. Mosby Elsevior, Philadelphia, 2009;73–86.
13. Ritu Gupta, Mark Kilby, Griselda Cooper. Fetal surgery and anaesthetic implications. Continuing Education in Anaesthesia, Critical Care and Pain: 2008;8(2):71–75. *(TTTS, tocolyis, fetal stress response/analgesia).*
14. Marc Van de Velde, Frederik De Buck. Fetal and Maternal Analgesia/Anaesthesia for Fetal Procedures. Fetal Diagn Ther 2012;31:201–209 *(Fetal stress response).*
15. Jack Rychik, Zhiyun Tian, Meryl S, et al: Acute Cardiovascular Effects of Fetal Surgery in the Human Circulation. 2004;110:1549–1556.
16. Boat A, Mahmoud M, Michelfelder EC, et al. Supplementing desflurane with intravenous anaesthesia reduces fetal cardiac dysfunction during open fetal surgery. Paediatr Anaesth 2010; 20:748–56.
17. Pornswan Ngamprasertwong, Erik C Michelfelder, Shahriar Arbabi, et al. Anaesthetic Techniques for Foetal Surgery Effects of Maternal Anaesthesia on Intraoperative Foetal Outcomes in a Sheep Model. Anaesthesiology 2013;118:796–808.
18. Elaina E Lin, Kha M Tran. Anaesthesia for foetal surgery. Seminars in Paediatric Surgery 22 (2013); 50–55.
19. Michael G Ross: Preterm Labor Updated: Dec 5, 2011 http:/reference.medscape.com/Tocolytic Agents.
20. Hans P Sviggum, Bhavani Shankar Kodali. Maternal Anaesthesia for Foetal Surgery. Clin Perinatol 2013;40: 413–427.
21. NganKee WD, Lee A, Khaw KS, et al. A randomized double-blinded comparison of phenylephrine and ephedrine infusion combinations to maintain blood pressure during spinal anaesthesia for cesarean delivery: The effects on foetal acid-base status and hemodynamic control. Anesth Analg 2008;107:1295–302.
22. Manning FA, Harrison MR, Rodeck C. Catheter shunts for fetal hydronephrosis and hydrocephalus. Report of the International Foetal Surgery Registry. N Engl J Med. 1986;315:336.
23. Scott N Adzick, Elizabeth A Thom, Catherine Y Spong, et al. A Randomized Trial of Prenatal versus Postnatal Repair of Myelomeningocele. N Engl J Med 2011;364:993–1004.
24. Vinod Chinnappa, Stephen H Halpern. The ex uterointrapartum treatment (EXIT) procedure: maternal and fetal considerations, editorial. Can J Anesth, 2007;54(3):171–175.
25. Reza Rahbar, Adam Vogel, Laura B Myers et al. Foetal Surgery in Otolaryngology. Arch oto laryngol head neck surg. 2005;131:393–398.

26. Ronald B George, Abigail H Melnick, Erin C Rose, et al: Case series: Combined spinal epidural anaesthesia for Cesarean delivery and ex utero intrapartum treatment procedure. Can J Anesth. 2007;54(3):218–222.
27. Jan A Deprest, Kypros Nicolaides, Eduard Gratacos. Foetal Surgery for Congenital Diaphragmatic Hernia Is Back from Never Gone. Fetal Diagn Ther. 2011;29:6–17.
28. Deprest J, Jani J, Gratacos E, et al. Foetal intervention for congenital diaphragmatic hernia: The European experience. Semin Perinatol. 2005;29:94.
29. Michael R Harrison, Roberta L Keller, Samuel B Hawgood, et al. A Randomized Trial of Foetal Endoscopic Tracheal Occlusion for Severe Foetal Congenital Diaphragmatic Hernia. N Engl J Med. 2003;349:1916–24.

20

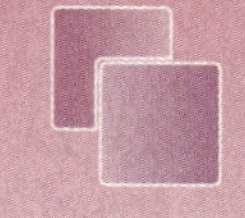

Premature Infants and Micropremies

Vidhya N Deshmukh

GENERAL CONSIDERATIONS

Prematurity is defined as birth before 37 weeks from the first day of the last menstrual period as per World Health Organization.[1] Preterm birth is associated with a high prevalence of clinical problems such as functional immaturities of a wide variety of organ systems, acquired problems, and problems associated with inadequate monitoring and/or follow-up plans. A better understanding of these issues will help guide an optimal treatment strategy.

Premature Infant Subgroups Depending on Gestational Age[2]

Late preterm	35–37 weeks	LBW <2500 g
Moderate preterm	30–34 weeks	Very LBW < 1500 g
Severe preterm	27–29 weeks	ELBW<1000 g
Ex preterm/ micropremie	<26 weeks	ELBW <1000 g

The etiology of preterm birth is multifactorial and involves a complex interaction between foetal, placental, uterine and maternal factors.

Identifiable Causes of Preterm Birth[1]

1. Foetal

a. Multiple gestations (twin pregnancy)
b. Foetal distress
c. Erythroblastosis foetalis
d. Nonimmune hydrops

2. Uterine

a. Bicornuate uterus
b. Premature cervical dilatation (incompetent cervix)

3. Placental

a. Placental dysfunction
b. Haemorrhagic disorder of pregnancy (placenta previa, Abruptio placenta)

4. Maternal

a. Hypertensive disorders of pregnancy (pre-eclampsia, eclampsia)
b. Chronic medical illness (renal disease, cyanotic heart disease)
c. Infection (*Listeria monocytogenes*, group B streptococcus, urinary tract infection, bacterial vaginosis, chorio-amnionitis)
d. Drug abuse (cocaine)

5. Others

a. Polyhydramnios
b. PROM (premature rupture of membranes)
c. Trauma
d. Iatrogenic

NEONATAL PROBLEMS ASSOCIATED WITH PREMATURE INFANTS[1]

The wide range of problems involving various organ systems is as follows:

1. Respiratory

a. Apnoea of prematurity
b. Respiratory distress syndrome (hyaline membrane disease)

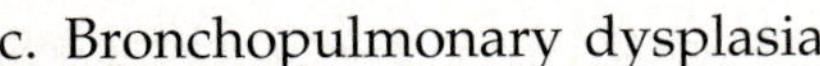

c. Bronchopulmonary dysplasia
d. Pneumothorax, pneumomediastinum, interstitial emphysema
e. Congenital pneumonia

2. Cardiovascular
a. Patent ductus arteriosus
b. Patent foramen ovale
c. Hypotension
d. Bradycardia (with apnoea)

3. Haematologic
a. Anaemia (early or late onset)
b. Thrombocytopenia

4. Gastrointestinal
a. Necrotizing enterocolitis
b. Poor gastrointestinal function—poor motility
c. Hyperbilirubinemia—direct or indirect
d. Spontaneous gastrointestinal isolated perforation
e. Spontaneous liver haemorrhage

5. Metabolic endocrine
a. Hypocalcemia
b. Hypoglycemia
c. Hyperglycemia
d. Hyperkalemia
e. Late metabolic acidosis
f. Hypothermia
g. Euthyroid but low thyroxine status

6. Central nervous system
a. Germinal matrix intraventricular haemorrhage (GMH-IVH)
b. Periventricular leukomalacia (PVL)
c. Encephalopathy of prematurity
d. Seizures
e. Retinopathy of prematurity
f. Deafness
g. Hypotonia
h. Perinatal stroke
i. Feeding difficulties

7. Renal
a. Hyponatremia
b. Hypernatremia
c. Hyperkalemia
d. Renal tubular acidosis
e. Renal glycosuria
f. Oedema

8. Others
Infections (congenital, perinatal, nosocomial: Bacterial, viral, fungal, parasitic).

Thermoregulation

Neonates loose heat by radiation, conduction, convection and evaporation. Extremely premature infants can lose 15 times more heat through transdermal water loss as compared with the term neonates.

Mechanism of Heat Loss for a Neonate in a Thermo-neutral Environment

- Radiation 39%
- Evaporation 24%
- Convection 34%
- Conduction 3%

Factors responsible for heat loss

- Cold environment (delivery rooms, operation theatre, NICU)
- High ratio of surface area to body weight
- Reduced subcutaneous fat and non-keratinized thin skin
- Less ability to maintain flexion of extremities
- Underdeveloped response of the temperature sensors in posterior hypothalamus to release thermogenic hormones such as norepinephrine and thyroxine.
- Underdeveloped ability to shiver in response to cold (reduced muscle mass).
- Insufficient stores of brown fat.

To compensate for increased heat loss constricts cutaneous blood vessels. Oxygen consumption and cell metabolism increases 2–3 folds.The major compensatory mechanism for cold in neonates is non-shivering thermogenesis. It occurs in brown fat which is stored in between the scapulae and around the abdominal organs.

Brown Fat Distribution

Brown fat distribution is shown in Fig. 20.1. Non-shivering thermogenesis is the result of stimulation triglyceride and fatty acid metabolism by norepinephrine and thyroid hormone. Prematurity, hypoglycemia and general anaesthesia exaggerate the poor metabolic response to hypothermia. Maintenance of normal body temperature is crucial as hypothermia increases pulmonary vascular resistance, decreases pulmonary blood flow, increases right to left shunting across foramen ovale and PDA. As compared with the

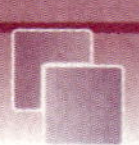

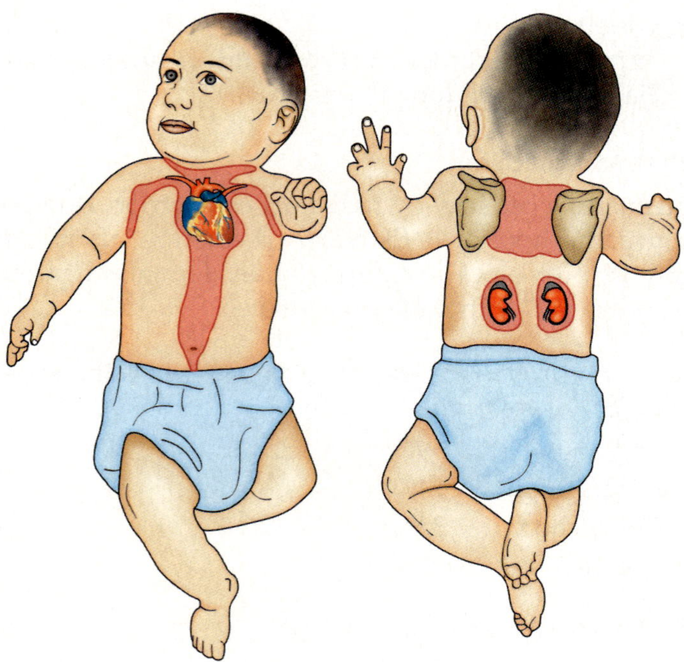

Fig. 20.1 Brown fat distribution

incubators, overhead warmers increase insensible water loss. There are several methods prevent heat loss mentioned below.

Protection against heat loss

- Transport the baby in a heated isolette
- Warm the operating room to more than 27° C (80° F)
- Use a warming mattress (water temperature of 40° C)
- Hot air mattress
- Heat and humidify gases to 36° C (at the trachea)
- Use a radiant heat warmer with servo controlled mechanism
- Wrap non-involved areas with plastic
- Cover head with hat/stockinet
- Warm intravenous fluids and blood
- Warm scrubbing and irrigation solutions
- Monitor the temperature in operating room.

> **Paediatric Anaesthesia Pearls**
>
> The anaesthesiologist must remember that patients cared for in overhead warmer may be hypovolemic and require correction of their intravascular volume preoperatively.

Respiratory System

Lung development is divided into five stages:[3]

1. The embryonic stage (4–6 weeks of gestation)—early upper airways appear.
2. The glandular stage (7–16 weeks)—the lower conducting airways form.
3. The canalicular stage (17–28 weeks)—the acini develop.
4. The terminal sac period (28–36 weeks)—the first respiratory unit for gas exchange (terminal air sacs and surrounding capillaries) make their first appearance.
5. The alveolar stage (36 weeks to 18 months of age)—alveoli develop.
   - Most alveoli develop after birth increasing from 20 million terminal air sacs at term to 300 to 400 million alveoli at 18 months of age.
   - The full term infant's diaphragm has 25% fatigue resistant, slow twitch, highly oxidative type-I fibers, and the preterm infant has only 10% (adult 55%).
   - The surface active material (surfactant) appears in foetal lungs by 20 weeks. By 35–36 weeks the surfactant amount increases and is secreted into the alveoli.
   - Pulmonary disorders such as respiratory distress syndrome (RDS), transient tachypnea of the newborn (TTN), pneumonia, and apnoea of prematurity are common and pose a greater risk of respiratory failure.
   - Tracheomalacia and bronchomalacia is common in premature infants. CPAP and PEEP increase FRC and decrease closing volume and helps to stent open the airway.
   - **RDS (Respiratory distress syndrome):** Surfactant is composed of phospholipids such as phosphatidylcholine (80%) and phosphatidylglycerol (5–10%). RDS results from qualitative and quantitative deficiency of pulmonary surfactant superimposed on cardiorespiratory immaturity. Around 35 weeks, there is a surge in surfactant release. Preterm infants lack phosphatidyl glycerol, thus predisposes them to RDS.
   - **TTN (Transient tachypnea of the newborn):** It results from timely clearance of pulmonary fluid from alveolar airspaces. Although Starling's forces and squeeze during vaginal delivery may play some role in clearing of lung fluid, amiloride sensitive sodium transport by lung epithelial cells through epithelial sodium channels (ENaCs) has emerged as the principal event in facilitating trans-epithelial alveolar fluid movement. Lower expression of these channels in preterm infants reduces their ability to clear lung fluid after birth.[4]

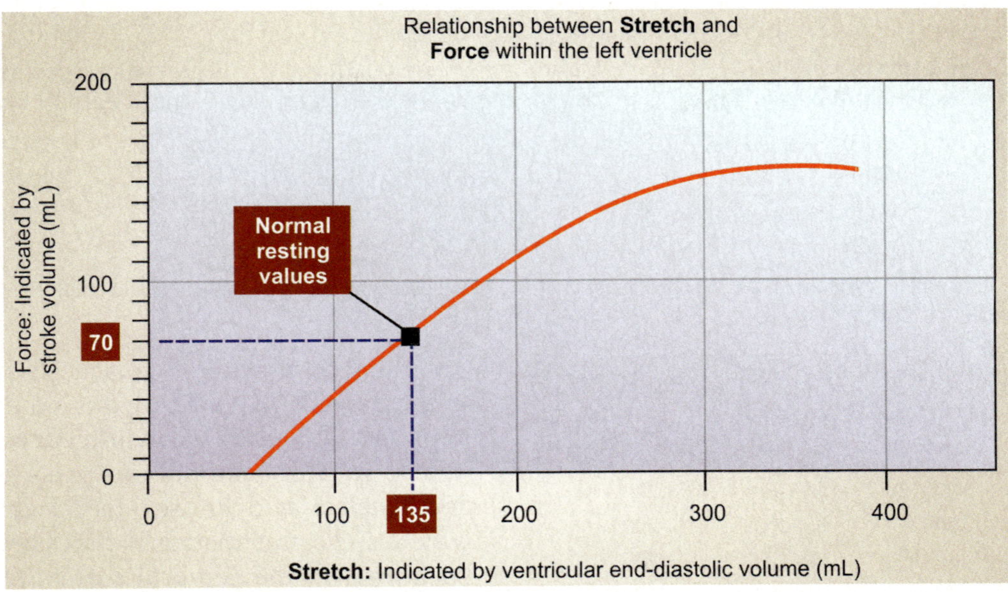

Fig. 20.2 Frank-Starling diagram

- **Hypoxic respiratory failure:** Some preterm infants develop severe hypoxic respiratory failure or persistent pulmonary hypertension of the newborn requiring additional therapies such as high frequency ventilation, inhaled nitric oxide, and extracorporeal membrane oxygenation.

Cardiovascular system

- The newborn's cardiac output per unit weight is the highest of any age group (approximately 200 mL/kg/min).
- The baseline state of the newborn myocardium is at the higher level of β adrenergic tone.
- The high resting cardiac output (CO) of the newborn limits its ability to increase CO in response to increased demand or changes in preload or afterload.

Frank-Starling (Fig. 20.2)

- The impaired ventricular function of the preterm and newborn is the result of the following factors:
  1. Fewer myofibrils,
  2. Decreased sympathetic innervation,
  3. Decreased β-adrenoreceptor concentration,
  4. Immaturity of the structure and function of the sarcoplasmic reticulum,
  5. Maturation specific mechanisms for calcium uptake, release, and storage
  6. Expression of various isoforms of contractile and non-contractile proteins, channels, exchangers and enzymes.
- The various ranges of systemic arterial blood pressures and heart rates in preterm infants are mentioned in Tables 20.1 to 20.3.

Table 20.1 Blood pressure ranges in healthy premature infants (501–2000 g)

	Systolic blood pressure (mmHg) Mean ± standard deviation		Diastolic blood pressure (mmHg) Mean ± standard deviation	
Age (days)	Minimum	Maximum	Minimum	Maximum
1	48 ± 9	63 ± 12	25 ± 7	35 ± 10
2	54 ± 10	63 ± 10	30 ± 0	39 ± 8
3	53 ± 9	67 ± 10	31 ± 8	43 ± 8
4	57 ± 10	71 ± 11	32 ± 8	45 ± 10
5	56 ± 9	72 ± 14	33 ± 9	47 ± 12
6	57 ± 9	71 ± 11	32 ± 7	47 ± 10

Source: Modified from Hegyi T, Anwar M, Carbone MT, et al. Blood pressure ranges in premature infants: II. The first week of life, Paediatrics 1996;97:336.

Table 20.2 Systemic arterial pressure in infants with birth weight 610–4220 grams

Birth weight	Systolic pressure (±95% confidence limits) (mmHg)	Diastolic pressure (±95% confidence limits) (mmHg)	Mean pressure (±95% confidence limits) (mmHg)
1	47(9)	27(10)	35(7)
2	54(9)	32(10)	40(7)
3	62(9)	37(10)	45(7)
4	69(9)	42(10)	50(7)

Source: Adapted from Versmold HT, Kitterman JA, Phibbs RH, et al. Aortic blood pressure during the first 12 hours of life in infants with birth weight 610–4220 grams, Paediatrics 1981;67:607.

Table 20.3 Acceptable heart rates in children

	Heart rates (beats/min)		
Age	Awake	Asleep	Exercise/fever
Newborn	100–180	80–160	<220
1 week–3 months	100–200	80–200	<220
3 months–2 years	80–150	70–120	<200
2–10 years	70–110	60–90	<200
>10 years	55–90	50–90	<200

Source: Data from Adams FH, Emmanouiides GC, (Eds): Moss's heart disease in infants, children, and adolescents, 3rd edn. Baltimore, 1983, Williams and Wilkins.[5]

The central nervous system

The brain goes through various developmental stages as follows:

- At mid gestation the brain is practically smooth except for the Sylvian fissure. By term all primary secondary and tertiary sulci are present with different gyri differentiating over the second half of gestation.
- The brain volume increases at a rate of 15 ml per week between 29 and 41 weeks.
- At 28 weeks brain volume is 13% of that observed at term.
- By about 34 weeks of gestation brain weighs 65% of that of term infant's brain.
- The white matter increases greatly as the term approaches with 5 fold increase during 35 to 41 weeks.
- Myelination begins at different times in different regions of the brain.
- The important structural changes are increases in neuronal connectivity, dendritic arborization, and connectivity, increasing synaptic junctions, maturation of neurochemical and enzymatic processes augmenting growth and maturation of the brain.
- **Encephalopathy of prematurity** is characterized by multifaceted gray and white matter lesions in preterm caused by multifactorial etiology such as acquired insults (cerebral hypoxia, ischaemia and systemic infection/inflammation that results in glutamate, free radical and/or cytokine toxicity to pre-oligodendrocytes, axons and neurons), altered development and reparative phenomena in different combinations. The white matter lesions comprise periventricular leukomalacia and diffuse cerebral white matter gliosis, whereas the gray matter includes neuronal loss and/or gliosis in the cerebral cortex, thalamus, hippocampus, basal ganglia, cerebellum and/or brainstem.[6]
- **Periventricular leukomalacia (PVL)** is the most common neurologic abnormality that occurs in infants born prematurely. It is defined as focal periventricular necrosis associated with diffuse reactive gliosis and microglial activation in the surrounding cerebral white matter. In various studies, it was found that PVL is more commonly seen in late preterm infants than in early preterm ones. At autopsy, the necrotic foci seen on histopathology were of two types acute and organizing, indicating the timing of injury. The two major inflammatory components of cerebral white matter injury are reactive gliosis and activated microglia. The clinical significance of peak in reactive gliosis and its relationship with the clinically mild neurological phenotype in late preterm infants is unknown. The neuronal loss in gray matter sites was always found in association with PVL with increasing incidence and severity in thalamus, globus pallidus and cerebellar dentate nucleus. It must be remembered that these various neuropathologic findings cannot be detected by the routine neuroimaging, under-appreciating its role in defining adverse neurological outcome in the late preterm infants.[6]
- **Intraventricular haemorrhage (IVH)** is also common in premature infants especially in micropremie. The incidence of germinal intraventricular haemorrhage (GMH-IVH) increases with decreasing gestational age. Based on various studies, GMH-IVH occurs infrequently in moderately preterm and late preterm infants. Routine cranial ultrasonography screening is recommended for infants less than 30 weeks of gestation once between 7 and 14 days, to be repeated

between 36 and 40 weeks of post-menstrual age. These recommendations are based on the higher incidence of IVH, which could affect the clinical management. The severity of IVH is graded as follows:[7]

Grade 1	Haemorrhage limited to germinal matrix
Grade 2	Haemorrhage extending into ventricular system
Grade 3	Haemorrhage into the ventricular system and ventricular dilatation
Grade 4	Haemorrhage extending into brain parenchyma

- **Maturation of feeding ability:** The most common clinical problem in moderate and late preterm infants is feeding difficulties. Feeding is a combination of complex events that requires efficient coordination between sucking, swallowing and breathing. Immaturity in these mechanisms presents as slow feeding, choking episodes, desaturation events, bradycardia, apnoea and prolonged hospital stay. The complex process of feeding depends on maturation of the central nervous system to provide coordination and synchronization of these functions. Interventions are available whereby patterned oro-cutaneous stimulation delivered through a pneumatic silicone pacifier can entrain preterm infants and facilitate suck development.
- **Hypoxic–ischaemic encephalopathy** affects foetuses and infants of all gestational age. It is final common pathways to multiple insults in perinatal period such as uteroplacental dysfunction, cord/placenta accidents, acute blood loss, infection and maternal hemodynamic compromise. Induced hypothermia is the only intervention proposed to ameliorate the brain injury in these patients. The whole body cooling with core temperature of 33–34°C or head and body cooling with core temperature of 34–35°C has shown to offer significant benefit in neonates at or beyond 36 weeks gestation. The therapeutic hypothermia is associated with various adverse effects such as disseminated intravascular coagulopathy, thrombocytopenia, arrhythmias, persistent pulmonary hypertension and subcutaneous fat necrosis.
- **Perinatal stroke**, though uncommon, do occur in preterm infants. It may remain clinically silent till developmental deficits become apparent later in childhood. It may be caused by the embolic event originating from placenta and passing through patent foramen ovale.

Renal function

- Permanent kidneys appear during fifth week of gestation.
- Nephrons appear by 8th week, initially in the juxtamedullary and cortical region.
- By 20 weeks 1/3rd of the final number of nephrons are present.
- By 35–36 weeks, the adult number of nephrons is present.
- Infants born prematurely develop new nephrons until about 34–35 weeks post-conceptual age.
- Premature neonates are less able to reabsorb and excrete Na. Hypoxia, respiratory distress, and hyperbilirubinemia further increases fractional Na excretion.
- Newborns, especially premature infants, have limited ability to concentrate their urine.
- The loss of bicarbonates increases pH. The premature newborns have low serum HCO_3^- concentration than term infants.

Age (gestational)	Serum bicarbonate level (mEq/l)
< 30 weeks	12–16
30–35 weeks	18–20
Term infants	20–22
Adults	25–28

- Glycosuria occurs in preterm infants at serum glucose concentrations below 100 mg/dL.
- High Na losses in proximal tubules increase Ca loss. Preterm neonates require supplemental intravenous Ca.
- Nonoliguric hyperkalemia (>5.0 mmol/L) characterized by rapid increase of serum K^+ during first 3 days of life, occurs in ELBW infants and preterm neonates with mild metabolic acidosis, because of rapid shifts of K^+ from intracellular to extracellular compartments.
- The total body water decreases with increasing gestational age (16 weeks – 94%, 32 weeks – 82%, term – 75%). Most of the extracellular water is in interstitial space especially more so in ELBW infants. During first 3–7 days of life, a healthy term infant loses around 5–10% of their body weight, whereas preterm loses more than 15% of their body weight.
- Maturation or renal function with age[8] is shown in Table 20.4.

Table 20.4 Maturation of renal function with age[8]

Measurement	Premature newborn	Full-term newborn	1–2 weeks	6 months to 1 year	1 to 3 years
GFR (ml/min/1.73 m^2)	14 ± 3	40.6 ± 14.8	65.8 ± 24.8	77 ± 14	96 ± 22
RBF (ml/min/1.73 m^2)	40 ± 6	88 ± 4	220 ± 40	352 ± 73	540 ± 118
Maximal concentration ability (mOsm/kg)	480	700	900	1200	1400
Serum creatinine (mg/dL)	1.3	1.1	0.4	0.2	0.4
Fractional excretion of sodium (%)	2–6%	<1	<1	<1	<1

Liver

1. Jaundice and hyperbilirubinemia are common in premature infants because of feeding difficulties and developmental immaturity of liver.
2. Preterm infants have higher rates of bilirubin production, shortened red cell life span, decreased hepatic uptake and conjugation, and an increased enterohepatic circulation as compared to term infants.
3. High concentration of unconjugated bilirubin can cause permanent neurologic damage known as kernicterus/chronic bilirubin encephalopathy.
4. Hyperbilirubinemia leads to injury in the basal ganglia (globus pallidus), central/peripheral auditory pathways, hippocampus, diencephalon, and subthalamic nuclei/midbrain.
5. On crossing the blood–brain barrier, bilirubin may damage neurons by interfering with energy metabolism in sub-cellular organelles, binding to/inhibiting function of specific organelles or cytoplasmic proteins, and/or directly damaging DNA.[9]
6. Acute kernicterus/acute bilirubin encephalopathy (ABE) results from unmonitored or insufficiently treated progressive hyperbilirubinemia.
7. Effective phototherapy and exchange transfusions are used as treat hyperbilirubinemia/ABE depending on the total serum bilirubin concentration.

Use of phototherapy and exchange transfusion in preterm infants

Gestational age (week)	Total serum bilirubin (mg/dL)	
	Phototherapy	Exchange transfusion
<28	5–6	11–14
28–29	6–8	12–14
30–31	8–10	13–16
32–33	10–12	15–18
34–35	12–14	17–19

Infants at increased risk of bilirubin toxicity are as follows:

1. Lower gestational age
2. Serum albumin levels <2.5 g/dL
3. Haemolytic disease (rapidly rising total serum bilirubin levels)
4. Clinically unstable infants (pH <7.15, sepsis with positive blood culture in first 24 hours, bradycardia and apnoea requiring bag-mask ventilation and intubation, hypotension requiring ionotropic support in first 24 hours, and mechanical ventilation).

Glucose homeostasis

- During foetal life, 80% of energy needs are met by glucose, which is transported across placenta by facilitative diffusion.
- The major storage of glucose is glycogen, which peaks in muscle and liver at term gestation.
- During the transition to postnatal life, glucose concentrations decrease accompanied by a surge in regulatory hormones (such as epinephrine, nor-epinephrine and glucagon) and decrease in insulin concentrations which increases mobilization of glycogen and fatty acids.
- The glucose production is achieved by glycogenolysis and gluconeogenesis. Premature infants are at increased risk of hypoglycemia because of reduced glycogen stores and low activity of gluconeogenic and glycolytic pathway.
- The incidence of hypoglycemia is increased during increased demands (sepsis, hypoxia, and cold stress) and when enteral intake is inadequate (abnormal suck and swallow or feeding intolerance).
- Symptomatic hypoglycemia must always be treated with intravenous glucose to avoid risk of neurologic injury. Symptoms of hypoglycemia include irritability, tremors, jitteriness, exaggerated Moro reflex, high-pitched cry, lethargy, floppiness, cyanosis, apnoea,

poor feeding, seizures. The trigger for treating symptomatic hypoglycemia infants is 40 mg/dL. Intravenous glucose dose is 200 mg/kg (10% dextrose at 2 mL/kg) and/or intravenous infusion at 5–8 mg/kg/min (80–100 mL/kg/day).

> **Paediatric Anaesthesia Pearls**
>
> Hypoglycemia is defined as blood sugar levels less than 40 mg/dL. It is treated with intravenous glucose bolus dose 200 mg/kg (10% dextrose at 2 mL/kg) and/or intravenous infusion at 5–8 mg/kg/min (80–100 mL/kg/day).

EXPREMATURE INFANTS/MICROPREMIES

These are a special category in premature infants who has specific systems affected more as compared to the other premature infants. The most common systems affected are respiratory system and central nervous system.

Respiratory System

Micropremies possess a biphasic ventilatory response to hypoxia. Initially ventilation increases during hypoxia followed after several minutes by hypoventilation and apnoea. The ventilatory response to CO_2 is decreased in micropremies and hypoxia further blunts this response. The combination of anaesthetic drugs and immature respiratory control system increases the risk of hypoxia, hypercapnia and apnoea in postoperative period.

The apnoea of prematurity is defined as episodes of apnoea lasting >20 seconds or <20 seconds associated with bradycardia or cyanosis. These episodes are common in micropremies and are inversely proportional to the advancing postconceptual age.

Apnoea in premature infants is exacerbated by following conditions:

1. Hypoxia,
2. Sepsis,
3. Intracranial haemorrhage
4. Metabolic abnormalities
5. Hypo/hypernatremia
6. Upper airway obstruction
7. Heart failure
8. Anaemia (haematocrit <30%),
9. Vasovagal reflexes and
10. Drugs including prostaglandins and anaesthetic agents.

The various treatments for apnoea of prematurity are as follows:

1. Stimulation
2. Bag and mask ventilation
3. Treatment of the underlying cause
4. Respiratory stimulants such as caffeine and theophylline
5. Neonatal continuous positive airway pressure (CPAP)
6. Ventilator support.

Broncho-pulmonary dysplasia is common in ex-premature/extreme low birth weight infants, occurring in approximately 60–90% of infants born at 23 weeks' gestation and approximately 50–70% of infants at 25 weeks' gestation. The arrest of lung growth is the most common cause of lung injury in the ELBW infants. Chronic lung disease (CLD) commonly co-exists with poor feeding and growth.

Cardiovascular System

The micropremie remains at greater risk of cardiovascular collapse during surgery and anaesthesia than a full term infant. The foetal heart has more connective tissue, less organized contractile elements, and increased dependence on extra-cellular calcium concentration than that of the infant. The less compliant foetal heart has a flatter Frank-Starling curve and is less sensitive to catecholamines because of near-maximal baseline β-adrenergic stimulation. The combination of limited ventricular stroke volume reserve, high heart rate, low blood volume, and little autoregulation predispose the micropremie to cardiovascular collapse during major surgery.

A patent ductus arteriosus (PDA) promotes pulmonary hypertension and congestive heart failure. Changes in systemic or pulmonary vascular resistance alter the direction of the flow through PDA. Hypoxia, hypercarbia, acidosis and hyperthermia increase the pulmonary vascular resistance predisposing to right to left shunt. Diuretic therapy and fluid restriction often used to treat heart failure increase the risk of hypotension during surgery.

Central Nervous System

The regions of central nervous system develop at different times during gestation.The impact of premature birth on the central nervous system depends on gestational age at birth and severity of cardiovascular, respiratory and other postnatal stressors. The most susceptible area of brain to injury is the periventricular white matter. The periventricular area is "watershed region" and is susceptible to poor perfusion and hypoxic-ischaemic injury during conditions of hypotension, low cardiac output, hypoxemia and hypocarbia.

The long term neurologic and developmental disabilities remain common in the micropremie and include cerebral palsy, cognitive deficits, behavioural abnormalities, visual and auditory impairment. Intraventricular haemorrhage (IVH) occurs in as many as one third of micropremature infants. The risk factors for development of early onset IVH (first day of life) include foetal distress, vaginal delivery, low Apgar score, metabolic acidosis, hypercapnia, and the need for mechanical ventilation. The risk factors for development of late onset IVH (days to weeks after birth) include respiratory distress syndrome, seizures, pneumothorax, hypoxemia, acidosis, severe hypocarbia, and use of vasopressor infusions. The multiple factors that decrease the incidence and severity of IVH include administration of sedation with opioids, antenatal glucocorticoids, or indomethacin.

Renal Function

In the micropremie, kidney function is decreased as a result of fewer nephrons and smaller glomerular size. The total body water (75–85% of body weight) in micropremie is higher than term infant. The ability to retain Na is not developed till 32 weeks of gestational age. The distal tubular response to aldosterone is low until 35 weeks of gestation and antidiuretic hormone increase eventually leads to hyponatremia. The elevation in potassium levels is seen in preterm infants during first few days of life as a result of shift from intracellular to extracellular space.

Retinopathy of Prematurity

Retinopathy of prematurity occurs in approximately 50% of extremely premature infants, with the incidence inversely proportional to the birth weight and gestational age. Its pathogenesis is discussed elsewhere in the chapter. Anaesthetic goals include minimizing inspired oxygen concentration and peak inspiratory pressures while maintaining oxygenation and ventilation.

Temperature Regulation

The micropremie is more susceptible to hypothermia than term infant. The thin less keratinized skin promotes evaporative heat loss and fluid loss in addition to increased susceptibility to damage from the most trivial trauma to skin. Non-shivering thermogenesis (NST) depends on the brown fat stores. NST is decreased in micropremie and regulation of skin flow is less efficient. Because of less fat for insulation and a large body surface area to mass ratio, the conductive and convective heat loss is increased. Amongst all other measures used, hot air mattress is the most effective means of warming.

Glucose Regulation

The micropremie is at risk of hypo/hyperglycemia. Decreased glycogen and fat stores predispose to hypoglycemia, whereas decreased insulin production with dextrose infusions, use of total parenteral nutrition and glucocorticoids lead to hyperglycemia. Hyperglycemia in neonates appears to protect the brain from ischaemic damage. The administration of dextrose containing fluids with an infusion pump so as to minimize wide fluctuations in glucose values and close monitoring of blood glucose levels is important during anaesthesia.

Hepatic and Haematologic Function

Immature hepatic function leads to reduction in many hepatic proteins necessary for drug metabolism. Reduced albumin synthesis decreases albumin levels as compared to term infants leading to increased free concentration of highly bound anaesthetic agents such as thiopental. The micropremie is at risk of developing spontaneous liver haemorrhage.

The haemoglobin level (13–15 g/dL) in micropremie is lower as compared to their term counterpart. The total blood volume is approximately 100–110 mL/kg. They are deficient in vitamin K and vitamin K dependent coagulation factors.[10] Thrombocytopenia (< 150000/mm^3) is commonly seen in approximately 70% of micropremature infants probably as a result of sepsis, disseminated intravascular coagulation and NEC.

Circulating blood volume in premature infants:[11]

	Blood volume (mL/kg)
Micropremie	110
Premie	100
Full-term neonate	90

ANAESTHETIC CONSIDERATIONS

Guidelines for admission and discharge of premature infants having surgery.[12]

1. Healthy term infants undergoing minor surgical procedure for short duration must be at least

44 weeks postmenstrual to be discharged on the same day. These include procedures performed under local anaesthesia with sedation.

2. Other full-term infants with a major medical problem having a minor procedure of short duration must be screened on an individual basis by the anaesthesiology department to be eligible for discharge on the same day.
3. Premature infants with minimal lung disease and no history of apnoea or bradycardia who present for a minor procedure of short duration must be at least 44 weeks postmenstrual to be discharged on the same day of surgery. This guideline includes infants who receive a regional anaesthetic or local anaesthesia with sedation.*
4. Premature infants (regardless of the gestational age with a history of apnoea and bradycardia), who may or may not have bronchopulmonary dysplasia and who have history of mechanical ventilation during the neonatal period must have: (1) a room air oxygen saturation of 96% or greater, (2) a normal Hb value (no anaemia or polycythemia) for their age, (3) no current requirement for home cardiorespiratory monitoring, (4) have uneventful course of surgery and anaesthesia, and (5) be cleared by anaesthesiologists to be discharged on the same day of surgery.*

Preoperative starvation

The guidelines for preoperative nil per os (NPO) are as follows:

Clear fluids	2 hours
Breast milk	4 hours
Formula feed	6 hours

Monitoring in Operating Room

General observation

- Colour (cyanosis, pallor)
- Chest mobility (bilateral expansion, respiratory pattern, and chest compliance)
- Palpation (temperature, pulses, and peripheral perfusion/capillary refill time)

Routine

- Precordial/oesophageal stethoscope (heart sounds, rate, rhythm, and breath sounds)
- Pulse oximeter
- Electrocardiogram
- Blood pressure
  - Noninvasive
  - Arterial line-umbilical artery catheter, radial, femoral (right radial artery in coarctation of aorta and left radial artery in presence of right Blalock-Tausig shunt)[13]
- Temperature
  - Core-rectal, oesophageal, nasopharyngeal
  - Skin
- End-tidal CO_2
- Peak inspiratory pressure, tidal volume, positive end expiratory pressure
- Fraction of inspired oxygen (FiO_2)
- Neuromuscular monitoring (peripheral nerve stimulator)
- Blood glucose

Optional

- Central venous pressure
- Blood gases—pH, pCO_2, pO_2
- Urine output
- Electrolytes

Common Intravenous Fluid and Electrolyte Requirements in the Newborn

Glucose

- Term newborn: 2–4 mg/kg/min
- SGA and LGA: >15 mg/kg/min on D1–D3

Sodium

- No sodium for first 24 hours (Na supplementation is not recommended during first few days of life because a transient negative Na balance may be necessary for the physiological reduction of extracellular fluid volume).[14]
- Day 2 onwards: 2–4 mEq/kg/day
- Requirement may change in response to gastrointestinal, genitourinary, transcutaneous, losses, drug or metabolic effects.
- The ELBW infants usually have huge transcutaneous fluid losses requiring replacement.

Potassium

- Minimum requirements in first 24 to 48 hours of life.
- Maintain with potassium 1–3 mEq/kg/day, in presence of normal urine output.

*These guidelines assume that these infants do not have other medical or surgical problems (e.g. hydrocephalus, ventriculo-peritoneal shunt) that would preclude same day discharge.

- Replace gastrointestinal, genitourinary, iatrogenic losses.

Calcium

- Daily requirements 200–400 mg/kg/day
- It varies with gestational age, history of asphyxia, and growth disturbance.

Blood loss replacement

Allowable blood loss = EBV (Hi – Hp)/Hav

EBV: Estimated blood volume, Hi: Initial haematocrit, Hp: Lowest allowable haematocrit, Hav: Average of these two haematocrits.

Maintainence of haematocrit to >35% (13 g/dL) in neonates with severe respiratory disease.

In infants with uncorrected cyanotic heart disease, the target Hb should be 13–18 g/dL.

Paediatric Anaesthesia Pearls

Sodium supplementation is not recommended, during first few days of life because transient negative sodium balance may be necessary for physiologic reduction of extracellular fluid volume that appears to be necessary for extra-uterine adaptation.[7]

Average fluid needs of low birth weight infants (mL/kg/d) during the first week of life (Table 20.5).

EQUIPMENT

Laryngoscope Blade Types and Sizes

Age	Miller	Macintosh
Premature neonate	0	0
Term neonate	0 to 1	1
1–12 months	1	1
1–2 years	1	2
2–6 years	2	2
6–12 years	2	3

Airway Device Details:[15]

Age	Pre-term	Full-term birth	6 months	1 year
Average weight (kg)		3.5	7	10
Approx. BSA (m^2)		0.25	0.38	0.49
ETT size (age +16)/4	2.5–3	3–3.5	3.5–4	4
Lip to mid-trachea (cm)	7–8	9	11	12
Nostril to mid-trachea (cm)	8–9	10	12	14

Table 20.5 Average fluid needs of low birth weight infants (mL/kg/d) during first week of life*

Age (days)	Component	Body weight (g) 751–1000	1001–1250	1251–1500	1501–2000
1	IWL†	65	55	40	30
	Urine‡	20	20	30	30
	Stool	0	0	0	0
	Total	**85**	**75**	**70**	**60**
2 – 3	IWL	65	55	40	30
	Urine	40	40	40	40
	Stool	0	0	0	5
	Total	**105**	**95**	**80**	**75**
4 – 7	IWL	65	55	40	30
	Urine	60	60	60	60
	Stool	5	5	5	5
	Total	**130**	**120**	**105**	**95**

Source: From Oh W: Fluid and electrolyte therapy in low birth weight infants, Pediatr Rev 1980;1:313.

*Allowance for increased metabolic rate (cold stress, increased activity) are not included; these infants are in incubator and naked.

†IWL-insensible water loss

‡Volumes required to achieve a urine osmolarity of 250 mOsm/kg of renal solute load during the first day (no sodium and protein added), 10 mOsm/kg/day on 2nd and 3rd days, and 15 mOsm/kg/day on 4th to 7th days.

The diameter of 5th finger roughly corresponds to the internal diameter of the ETT that can be inserted.

Calculations for estimating the length required for an endotracheal tube:

Height (in cm)/10 + 5
Weight (in kg)/5 + 12

Advance the endotracheal tube:
3 times the ID from the alveolar ridge
(Age in years/2) + 12

The tracheal length in preterm infants is 4 cm. In preterm infants weighing 1, 2, 3, 4 kgs should have ETT at gum margin at 7, 8, 9, 10 cm respectively.

Insert the endotracheal tube to the first or second black line marked on the tube.

Advance the endotracheal tube into a bronchus, withdraw it by 2 cm.

ETT, when inserted should allow a small leak during positive pressure ventilation at 20–25 cm of H_2O.

Supraglottic airway device details

Weight (kg)	LMA size	Laryngeal tube size	Cobra peri-laryngeal airway
0–5	1	0	0.5
5–10	2	1	1

Recommended ETT length to the nearest 0.5 cm by corrected gestation age (gestation age at birth + postnatal age) and weight at the time of intubation.

Corrected gestational age	Actual weight	ETT mark at lip (cm)
23–24	0.5–0.6	5.5
25–26	0.7–0.8	6.0
27–29	0.9–1.0	6.5
30–32	1.1–1.4	7.0
33–34	1.5–1.8	7.5
35–37	1.9–2.4	8.0
38–40	2.5–3.1	8.5
41–43	3.2–4.2	9.0

ANAESTHETIC AGENTS

Inhalational Agents

The very high partial pressures of inhalational agents develop rapidly in neonates than older children. The ratio of alveolar ventilation to FRC in neonates is 5:1 compared with 1.5:1 in adults. A greater fraction of cardiac output is distributed to the vessel rich group and brain. The solubility of inhalational agents is less in neonates. The brain tissue equilibrates swiftly to the alveolar concentration of anaesthetic and increases the risk of overdose. The minimum alveolar concentration (MAC) is related to post-conceptual age and is lowest in very premature infants. Sevoflurane is very popular agent for mask induction in paediatrics. It has been associated with prolongation of Q–T interval. The neonates usually have increased requirement of inhalational agents but it is decreased exponentially in very sick and expremature infants.

Intravenous Agent

Premature infants are more sensitive to thiopentone Na possibly because of decreased serum protein binding. Propofol has less negative ionotropic action compared to thiopental but is a powerful vasodilator and causes hypotension.[16] There is a little experience with the drug in premature infants. Ketamine stimulates the sympathetic nervous system. Increased blood pressure and intracranial pressure may be detrimental in infants with hydrocephalus or infants at risk of intracranial Haemorrhage. The duration of action of benzodiazepines such as midazolam is prolonged in by immature hepatic function in preterm neonate. Fentanyl is widely used in neonatal anaesthesia, especially in sick, premature infants. It has a wide margin of safety and has beneficial effects on hemodynamic stability. It can block pulmonary hypertensive crises. The doses used for induction are higher 30–50 μg/kg. Its clearance is lowest in premature infants (6–30 hrs) and increases with increasing gestational and postconceptual age. Remifentanil, a newer opioid gets metabolized by hydrolysis by tissue esterases therefore does not get accumulated and has lowered context sensitive half time (≈ 4 minutes).[17] The shorter context sensitive half time allows swift recovery expected in premature infants especially micropremies. There is a little experience with remifentanil in premature infants. Muscle relaxants are commonly used in neonatal anaesthesia. Succinyl choline, a depolarizing muscle relaxant is used sparingly as it causes bradycardia, hyperkalemia, muscle necrosis, and cardiac arrest in infants with myopathies. The ED_{95} in neonates is twice that of adults. The various non-depolarizing muscle relaxants used are cisatracurium, atracurium, vecuronium, and rocuronium. Most relaxants have prolonged duration of action in premature infants and frequency of dosing should be nerve stimulator guided.

Recovery from Anaesthesia

Immaturity of drug clearance systems prolongs recovery from anaesthetic agents in small, sick premature infants. Active warming is required to correct hypothermia before extubation. The neuromuscular block should be reversed. The infant should be hemodynamically stable and Hb should be near normal before reversal. The infant should resume regular rhythmic respiration with hip flexion and contraction of abdominal muscles. Laryngospasm may occur on extubation and anaesthesia personnel should be ready to re-intubate if necessary. Support of respiration can be achieved by short periods of CPAP post-extubation to prevent atelectasis. The risk of post-operative apnoea is high in premature infants and is inversely proportional to the gestational and post-conceptual age.

Regional Anaesthesia

Regional anaesthesia has been rarely used alone in neonates. It is usually combined with general anaesthesia or light sedation for decreasing the anaesthetic requirement intraoperatively and providing postoperative analgesia. Spinal and caudal anaesthesia are commonly used in the dosages mentioned above. Local infiltrations, dorsal penile nerve block, penile ring block are also effective. A regional anaesthesia without general anaesthesia is used in high risk neonates especially with bronchopulmonary dysplasia and infants at risk of postoperative apnoeas. Supplemental sedation during spinal anaesthesia increases the incidence of apnoeas. Ultrasound has made it easier and safer to give transversus abdominis plane (TAP) and rectus sheath block in neonates for umbilical hernia.

NECROTIZING ENTEROCOLITIS

Necrotizing enterocolitis is a multifactorial disorder that usually affects the premature infants with gestational age less than 36 weeks (usually fewer than 32 weeks). It is less commonly seen in term and late preterm infants. It is the leading cause of neonatal morbidity and mortality (10–30%). NEC is an acute ischaemic necrotizing disease of the gastrointestinal tract requiring emergency surgery. There is an inverse relationship between postmenstrual age and risk of NEC.

Signs and Symptoms

Early signs are nonspecific. Feeding intolerance increased pre-feeding gastric residues, emesis, abdominal distension, hematochezia (bloody stools).

Advanced signs are fulminant gastrointestinal signs, multiple organs dysfunction, and shock.

Abdomen appears shiny, distended and erythematous. The infant assumes the position of comfort, the frog leg position and is hypo-responsive. The abdomen feels firm, tender, tense and a tender mass may be palpable. The abdomen may have bluish discolouration. Erythema and bluish discolouration of scrotum is seen in male infants when peritoneal fluid from perforated bowel herniates into the scrotum.

Systemic signs include lethargy, hypotension, poor perfusion, pallor, increased episodes of apnoea and bradycardia, worsening respiratory function, temperature instability, tachycardia, hypoglycemia or hyperglycemia.

Laboratory Tests

Anaemia, left shift of neutrophils, neutropenia, thrombocytopenia, metabolic acidosis, and hyponatremia

Radiographic Findings

Abdominal plain or left lateral decubitus X-rays show following signs:

- Pneumatosis (intramural gas)
- Portal venous gas, thickened bowel wall
- Dilated bowel loops, a paucity of bowel gas
- Fixed dilated bowel loop (necrotic bowel loop)
- Dilated gas filled loops in centre of abdomen (ascites/free peritoneal fluid)
- Pnemoperitoneum (perforated viscus)
- Football sign (outlining of falciform ligament by air giving appearance of sutures in football).[18]

Ultrasound

- Free gas
- Abdominal fluid
- Ascites
- Qualitative assessment of peristalsis
- Arterial perfusion of bowel wall
- Portal venous gas.

Newer Monitoring Techniques:[19]

- Gastric tonometry
- Regional saturation of O_2 (rSO_2): Regional tissue O_2 level is dependent on balance of and O_2 utilized by tissue and amount of O_2 delivered by haemoglobin.
- Near infra-red spectroscopy (NIRS): It detects decrease in intestinal tissue oxygen in real time and measures the intestinal tissue oxygenation.
- Cerebro-splanchnic O_2 ratio (CSOR): It compares splanchnic O_2 levels with that in brain and is a way

Table 20.6 Modified Bell's staging for NEC[20]

Review of Bell's stages	Clinical findings	Radiographic findings	Gastrointestinal findings
Stage I	Apnoea, bradycardia, temperature instability	Normal gas pattern or mild ileus	Gastric residues, occult blood in stool, mild abdominal distention
Stage II A	Apnoea, bradycardia, temperature instability	Ileus gas pattern with one or more dilated loops and focal pneumatosis	Grossly bloody stools, prominent abdominal distension, absent bowel sounds
Stage II B	Thrombocytopenia, mild metabolic acidosis	Widespread pneumatosis, ascites, portal-venous gas	Abdominal wall oedema with palpable loops and tenderness
Stage III A	Mixed acidosis, oliguria, hypotension, coagulopathy	Prominent bowel loops, worsening ascites, no free air	Worsening wall oedema, erythema and induration
Stage III B	Shock, deterioration in laboratory values and vital signs	Pneumoperitoneum	Perforated bowel

to increase sensitivity for detecting intestinal ischaemia. Table 20.6 demonstrates modified Bell's staging for NEC.[20]

Pathogenesis of NEC

NEC is one of the devastating diseases seen in premature infants. The pathogenesis of NEC remains to be poorly understood. There are many factors implicated in the etiology of NEC mentioned below:

- Lack of adequate substrate and O_2 delivery to intestinal epithelial cells because of an incomplete microvasculature development or to an immature internal vascular tone.
- An inadequate intestinal barrier.
- An inflammatory response triggered by abnormal intestinal colonization.
- An immature immune response leading to inefficient killing of microbes leading to translocation through epithelium.
- Excessive production of inflammatory mediators, recruitment of neutrophils and subsequent necrosis. Figure 20.3 shows the pathophysiology of NEC.

The various inflammatory mediators found raised are as follows:

- Bacterial lipopolysaccharides
- Cytokines [nF-kB, toll-like receptors (TLR)/microbial associated molecular patterns (MAMP), interferon gamma, interleukin-6, interleukin-8, interleukin-10,

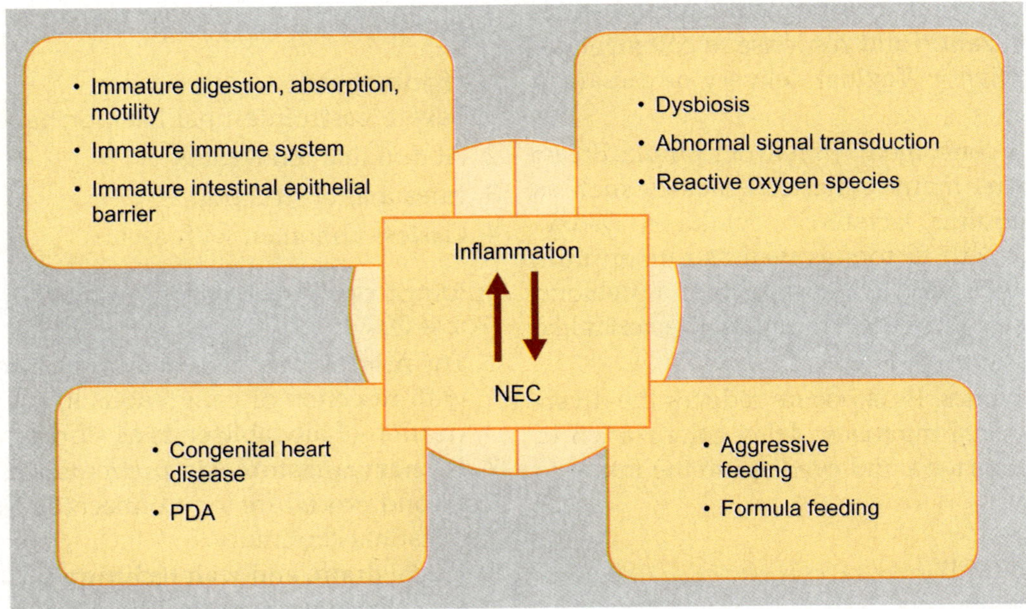

Fig. 20.3 Pathophysiology of NEC

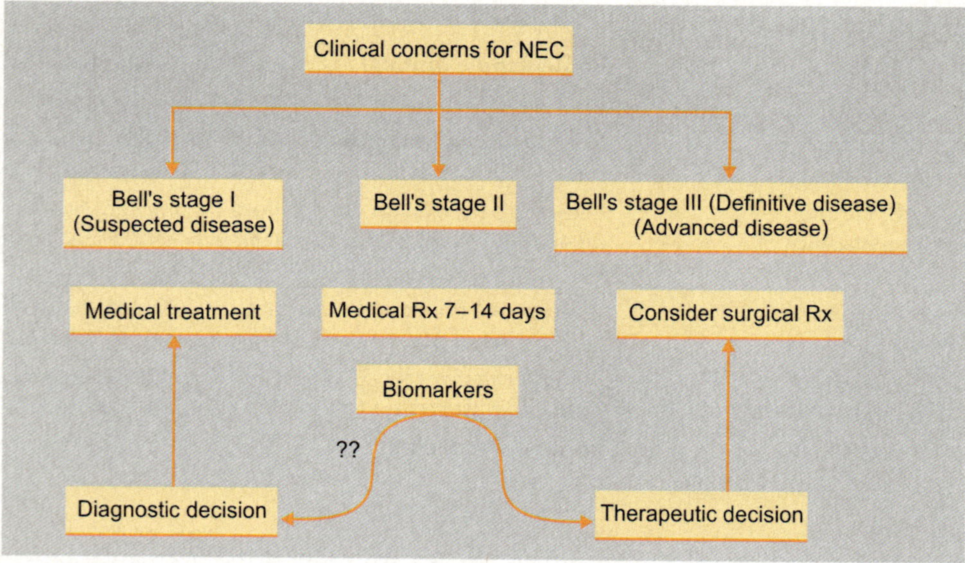

Fig. 20.4 Clinical concerns for NEC

interleukin-12, interleukin-18, tumor necrosis factor alpha (TNF-α), platelet activating factor (PAF), nitric oxide (NO), reactive oxygen species (ROS)]
- Neutrophils and macrophages.

ROLE OF PREBIOTICS, PROBIOTICS AND POSTBIOTICS[21]

Factors affecting the intestinal microbiota
1. **Prenatal**: Foetus swallows a large quantity of amniotic fluid during the last trimester of gestation thus getting exposed to the diverse microbes in amniotic fluid.
2. **Postnatal**: Following factors influence intestinal bacterial colonization and response to colonization.
   - Mode of delivery: Vaginal delivery or caesarean section
   - Type of milk consumed: Human or formula. Breast milk contains many beneficial factors such as immunoglobulins, lactoferrin, cytokines, lysozymes and growth factors as well as human milk oligosaccharides (HMO). HMO acts as a prebiotic stimulating the growth of commensal bacterias like Bifidobacterium species.
   - Use of antibiotics: Its exposure reduces the diversity of intestinal microbes, delay colonization of commensal bacteria and predispose the infant to NEC.

Indications for Surgery

Absolute indications
1. Pneumoperitoneum
2. Intestinal gangrene (positive paracentesis)
3. Intestinal perforation

Relative indications
1. Clinical deterioration
   a. Metabolic acidosis
   b. Ventilator failure
   c. Oliguria, hypovolemia
   d. Thrombocytopenia, leukopenia, leukocytosis
2. Portal venous gas
3. Erythema of abdominal wall
4. Fixed abdominal mass
5. Persistently dilated loop

Nonindications
1. Severe gastrointestinal haemorrhage
2. Abdominal tenderness
3. Intestinal obstruction
4. Gasless abdomen with ascites.

Surgical approaches for necrotizing enterocolitis
(Table 20.7)
1. The most widely accepted procedure is **laparotomy** with resection of gangrenous intestine and exteriorization of allviable ends as stomas.
2. **Primary anastomosis** prevents the necessity of a second procedure to reconnect the gut and establish intestinal continuity.
3. **Patch, drain, and wait technique:** The infant undergoes alaparotomy, and the major perforations are patched without resection.

Table 20.7 Surgical approaches for necrotizing enterocolitis

Approach	Relevant evidence	Current use
Bowel resection with enterostomy	**For:** Randomized controlled trials showing short-term outcomes equivalent to peritoneal drainage Preliminary studies suggesting improved neuro-developmental outcomes compared with primary peritoneal drainage **Against:** High peristomal complication rates	Standard of care when primary anastomosis is infeasible
Bowel resection with primary anastomosis	**For:** Avoidance of peristomal complications Improved survival in retrospective studies **Against:** Prospective studies, controlling for selection bias needed before use in non-ideal settings	Use in the settings of 1. Focal disease 2. Viable remaining intestine, and 3. Stable overall physiology
High jejunostomy	**For:** Case reports/series describing success in multi-segmental or pan-intestinal NEC **Against:** Prolonged dependence on total parental nutrition High peristomal complication rates	Used sparingly in multisegmental or pan-intestinal disease when initial resection would result in short bowel syndrome.
Clip and drop back	**For:** Case series describing utility in infants with extensive NEC **Against:** Lack of prospective evidence comparing this technique to laparotomy with enterostomy formation	
Patch, drain and wait	**For:** Case series describing utility in infants with extensive NEC **Against:** Lack of prospective evidence comparing this technique to laparotomy with enterostomy formation	Used sparingly
Primary peritoneal drainage	**For:** Randomized controlled trials showing short term outcomes equivalent to laparotomy Decreased invasiveness **Against:** Preliminary studies suggesting poorer neurodevelopmental outcomes when compared with laparotomy. As few as 11% of patients undergoing primary peritoneal drainage are managed successfully without requiring future laparotomy.	Ongoing debate regarding utility and long term outcomes. Used when infant too unstable to undergo laparotomy.

4. **Clip and drop back technique** can be used if there is extensive intestinal necrosis. Areas of obvious necrosis with perforation are resected, and the ends of the bowel are clipped or stapled closed.
5. **Peritoneal drains at the bedside:** Developed as a palliative procedure to decrease surgical morbidity and mortality in infants weighing <1,000 g. The purpose of peritoneal drainsis to decompress the peritoneal cavity of gas, necrotic debris and stool.

Management

Medical/Preoperative management

1. Prompt decompression of stomach using double lumen gastric tube (large lumen for aspiration and small lumen for irrigation and venting) with low constant suction, replacement of aspirated volume with Ringer lactate solution with extra potassium chloride lost in gastric aspirate.
2. Endotracheal intubation and ventilator support in infants with ventilator failure.
3. Frequent assessment of intravascular volume using serum electrolytes, haematocrit, and urine output. Parenteral nutrition with adequate protein (3.5–4 g/kg/d) to maintain positive nitrogen balance and allow repair of injured tissues.
4. Culture of blood and urine and prompt initiation of broad spectrum antibiotics.
5. Packed red cells to replace occult intestinal haemorrhage, judicious correction of thrombocytopenia, coagulopathy, and metabolic acidosis.

Intraoperative management

Arterial and central venous cannula is inserted for continuous monitoring, blood gas, and metabolic analysis. Red blood cells, fresh frozen plasma, and platelets are given to correct the coagulopathy. Inspired oxygen concentration is adjusted to 85–90% of arterial oxygen saturation. Nitrous oxide is avoided in presence of free air in gastrointestinal system and portal venous system.

High dose narcotic (fentanyl 50 mcg/kg) is delivered slowly as tolerated haemodynamically. Potent inhalational anaesthetics are poorly tolerated especially in presence of haemodynamic instability. Lower concentrations are used to supplement narcotics. Short acting neuromuscular blocking agents such as atracurium are given in presence of multiorgan dysfunction. Ionotropic agents are given to support cardiovascular system. Glucose intolerance is common in septic infants. High glucose content in red blood cell product provides additional glucose. Therefore, non-glucose containing intravenous fluids administered for resuscitation. Frequent glucose measurements are done to guide glucose control.

Postoperative management

1. Mechanical ventilation
2. Inotropic support
3. Parenteral nutrition.

Complications

- Intestinal stricture
- Short bowel syndrome: A rule of thumb is that greater than 30 cm of bowel with ileocecal valve or greater than 50 cm of bowel without the ileocecal valve is necessary for an infant to survive on enteral nutrition.
- Recurrent necrotizing enterocolitis
- Cholestatic liver disease: It occurs in infants on prolonged total parenteral nutrition. It is characterized by direct hyperbilirubinemia, elevated transaminases and hepatomegaly. It is treated with limited TPN and trophic enteral feeding.
- Anastomotic (marginal) ulcer.
- Neurodevelopmental impairment.

RETINOPATHY OF PREMATURITY

Retinopathy of prematurity is still a common cause of childhood blindness in high income countries, although it no longer occurs in epidemic proportions.

Risk factors for the development of retinopathy of prematurity:[22]

1. **Prenatal factors:** These factors reflect the degree of immaturity of retina at birth indicating its susceptibility to harm.
   - Gestational age
   - Birth weight
2. **Postnatal factors:** Factors that differ after preterm birth that do not match the intra-uterine environment of third trimester therefore prevent normal resumption of normal retinal neurovascular growth after birth.
   a. Exposure to oxygen, which is higher and more variable than in-utero and that, alters the oxygen regulated growth factors.
   b. Loss of the maternal and foetal interaction resulting in:
      - Increased metabolic demands in presence of loss of nutrition (essential fatty acids)
      - Decreased insulin like growth factor (IGF-1) and other factors resulting in poor postnatal growth and weight gain.

Classification of retinopathy of prematurity stages

Stage 1: Fine demarcation line is visible between vascular and avascular regions.

Stage 2: Broad ridge divides the vascular and avascular regions.

Stage 3: Neovascularization is note at the ridge, on the posterior surface and anteriorly towards the vitreous cavity.

Stage 4: Subtotal retinal detachment has occurred.

Stage 5: Total retinal detachment in an open or closed funnel configuration has occurred.

Pathogenesis of ROP

Normal retinal development

In the human, retinal vascular development occurs predominantly in second and third trimester in utero and reaches maturity at 36–40 weeks of post menstrual age through vasculogenesis and angiogenesis. Angiogenesis commences at 17 weeks and is complete just prior to the full term birth.

Phase I: Retinal vasculature formation occurs in utero in "physiologic hypoxia" with developmental progression. The oxygen saturation of the foetus in-utero is approximately 60–70%. Thus preterm birth into room air is often associated with increase in oxygen saturation, which is exacerbated by supplemental oxygen.

Hyperoxia causes down regulation of hypoxia inducible growth factors leading to disruption of normal vascular development. The losses of factors from maternal foetal interface (nutrition and other mediators of postnatal growth) also contribute to low serum IGF-1 and disruption in vessel growth, leading to phase-1 ROP.

Phase II: A proliferative phase follows the vessel loss of phase-1. It occurs when normal angiogenesis is taken over by pathologic angiogenesis. It begins to develop after 32 postmenstrual weeks. The transition to phase II occurs when the attenuated vasculature cannot supply enough oxygen and other nutrients to the developing retina, leading to increased expression of hypoxia induced factors. These factors (vascular endothelial growth factor/VEGF, insulin like growth factor-1/IGF-1) stimulate aberrant vessel formation at the junction between vascular and avascular retina. It has been postulated that increased oxygen supplementation may be beneficial during phase II ROP development. Increased tissue oxygen may reduce VEGF levels and arrest progression to severe ROP.[23] Neovascular proliferation may cause retinal folds, macular dragging and cicatricial changes ultimately causing retinal detachment and blindness.

Treatment of ROP based on understanding its pathogenesis (Fig. 20.5):

A. In utero
B. Phase I
C. Phase II
D. Resolution

Treatment of ROP

1. Laser photocoagulation: Hypoxic retina anterior to neovascularization in phase II of ROP, which produces VEGF and EPO, is destroyed to decrease pathologic blood vessel formation (promoting C to D).
2. Anti-VEGF therapy: Direct suppression of neovascularization with suppression of VEGF (promoting C to D).
3. Increasing IGF-1TO in utero levels after birth: Prevents vessel loss (phase-I) (preventing A–B) to prevent phase II (C).
4. Control of O_2 after preterm birth: Prevents hyperoxia induced suppression of hypoxia inducible factor, regulated factors VEGF and EPO that are necessary for normal retinal vascular development thus preventing vessel loss (preventing A–B).

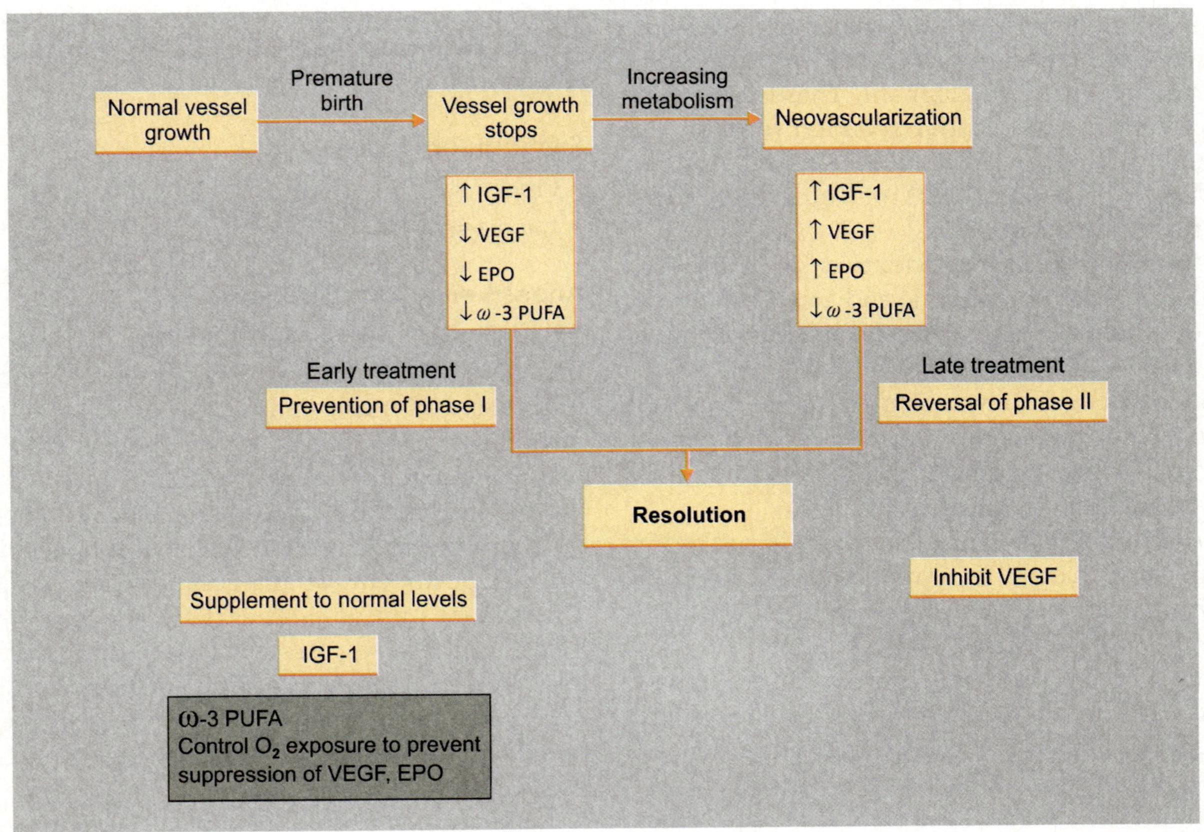

Fig. 20.5 Treatment of ROP

5. Maintaining adequate intake of the essential fatty acid DHA after preterm birth: Promotes normal vascularization and directly inhibits neovascularization (promote B to D and C to D).
6. Monitoring postnatal growth, this is based on rate of increase of postnatal IGF-1 levels: Predicts the future development of neovascular ROP(C).

Treatment

Prevention

1. Improved oxygen control with avoidance of fluctuations
2. Provision of sufficient nutrition as early as possible
3. IGF-1 replacement
4. DHA (docosahexanoic acid) supplementation
5. Suppression of VEGF
6. Vitamin E membrane stabilizing and antioxidant actions.

Anaesthetic considerations in infants undergoing premature infants with ROP:

1. **Anti-VEGF compounds:** The full anti-VEGF antibody, Avastin, is used in treatment. Intravitreal Avastin injection suppresses serum VEGF for weeks in preterm infants.
2. **Cryotherapy:** It involves placement of a probe chilled with nitrous oxide on the outer surface of the globe. Cryonecrosis of underlying retinal tissue decreases incidence of retinal detachment. These procedures are performed either under sedation (opioids and ketamine) with atropine and local anaesthesia that includes Sub-Tenon's block or complete general endotracheal anaesthesia.
3. **Laser photocoagulation:** Sedation with atropine, opioid analgesics or ketamine and local anaesthesia. Some ophthalmologists prefer the benefits of general anaesthesia.
4. **Scleral buckling or vitrectomy:** Once the ROP progresses to stage 4–5, it is performed to prevent blindness. These surgeries are always performed with general endotracheal anaesthesia.
5. **Examination under anaesthesia:** This procedure takes no more than 5–10 minutes. Premedication and anxiolysis are beneficial to the children requiring repeated examinations. Mask induction and maintenance of spontaneous respiration provide adequate conditions. Maintaining adequate depth of anaesthesia with swift and smooth emergence is necessary. Remifentanil along with propofol or sevoflurane are the ideal agents available at present because of their pharmacokinetic profile. More lengthy examinations require insertion of laryngeal mask airway with propofol or inhalational anaesthetic agents.

HERNIOTOMY

Embryology

Testicles descend from abdomen into scrotum through inguinal canal during seventh month. A peritoneal covering, processus vaginalis, encloses the tesicles during its descent. Processus vaginalis usually closes at term, but it remains patent in 15–38% of children. In premature infants, the incidence of closure is high, depending on the gestational age at birth. The continued patency of the processus vaginalis is responsible for the development of congenital hernias. Males are more affected than females. It is more common in first year of life. Right sided hernias are more common than left. Risk factors for inguinal hernia are prematurity, chronic respiratory illness and excessive intraperitoneal fluid (intraperitoneal shunts, ascites, and peritoneal dialysis). Complications related to inguinal hernias and their surgical repairs are common and include incarcerated bowel, intestinal obstruction, gonadal infarction, infection, hematoma, and recurrent hernias. Because of the risk of incarceration and bowel infarction, the hernia should be repaired as soon as the infant is medically ready.

Surgical Techniques

- Open
- Laparoscopic

Anaesthetic Considerations

Anaesthetic induction can be intravenous or inhalational technique. If airway cannot be maintained with bag and mask without distending the stomach, insertion of LMA or endotracheal tube is considered in infants younger than 1 year of age. Caudal epidural or ilio-inguinal and ilio-hypogastric block can be given to decrease the requirement of general anaesthetic and provide postoperative analgesia. Inadequate planes of anaesthesia and analgesia at the stage of spermatic handling can lead to laryngospasm and bradycardia. Premature infants have high incidence of inguinal hernia. Complications of general anaesthesia can be avoided in premature infants by using spinal or caudal epidural anaesthesia.

Laparoscopic herniorrhaphy requires endotracheal intubation. In patients with incarcerated or obstructed hernia require rapid sequence induction with cricoid pressure. Some anaesthesiologists prefer to intubate these infants awake to reduce the risk of aspiration. The microcuff endotracheal tubes made from polyurethane are available from 3.0 onwards which are used in moderate to late preterm infants. These tubes are known to provide a good seal to prevent aspiration and operation theatre pollution without causing pressure necrosis of tracheal mucosa.

Maintenance of anaesthesia is achieved using inhalational agents and nitrous oxide or air. Mechanical ventilation should be adjusted to minimize peak airway pressure (< 20 cm of H_2O) and maintain arterial oxygen saturation between 92 and 96%. If extubation is planned after the surgery, caffeine (10 mg/kg) is administered intravenously to prevent postoperative apnoea.

The micropremie with bronchopulmonary dysplasia requiring supplemental oxygen is an excellent candidate for regional anaesthesia. Regional anaesthesia circumvents the need to intubate the trachea, which may exacerbate BPD and make extubation after surgery difficult to achieve. For spinal anaesthesia, an intrathecal injection of a hyperbaric solution of tetracaine (1 mg/kg) or bupivacaine (0.1 mg/kg) provides 1–2 hours of surgical anaesthesia. For epidural anaesthesia 0.75 mL/kg of 0.25% bupivacaine with epinephrine is injected in the epidural space through sacral hiatus or lumbar epidural space. Preterm infants are more sensitive to local anaesthetic blockade than children and adults.

INTRATHECAL DRUG DOSE FOR BUPIVACAINE

Body weight (kg)	Bupivacaine (mg/kg)	Bupivacaine (ml/kg)
0–5	0.5	0.1
5–15	0.4	0.08
> 15	0.3	0.06

CRYPTORCHIDISM

Cryptorchidism or undescended testes affects 0.8% of 1 year old boys. The testicles may lie within the external ring just proximal to scrotum, inguinal canal or abdomen. The chance of developing malignancy in undescended testes is 10 fold higher than the normally descended ones.

The aim of repair is to alter the course of the spermatic artery from the renal pedicle to the internal ring to the external ring and to create a direct line from renal pedicle to scrotum. Inguinal exploration is needed for patients with non-palpable testes.It is either removed or placed in the scrotum by doing staged orchiopexy, auto-transplantation of testes or Fowler Stephens procedure. The Fowler Stephens procedure involves two stages. The first stage involves clipping of the spermatic vessels, whereas the second stage involves orchiopexy, several months later.

Anaesthetic Considerations

Anaesthesia can be induced by IV or inhalational technique. It can be maintained by bag and mask without insufflation of stomach. LMA can be inserted in infants below 1 year of age. Because of the traction and manipulation of testes and spermatic cord, incidence of intraoperative bradycardia and laryngospasm is increased. Its incidence can be reduced by caudal epidural or illio-inguinal and illio-hypogastric blocks. Endotracheal intubation is necessary in intra-abdominal exploration or laparoscopic orchiopexy. There is high incidence of postoperative pain and nausea, vomiting. Prophylactic antiemetic, such as Ondensetron (0.1 mcg/kg) are given in these cases. Spinal anaesthesia or caudal epidural anaesthesia is considered in ex-premature babies to avoid the complications associated with general anaesthesia. The anaesthetic considerations are same as mentioned for herniotomy.

PATENT DUCTUS ARTERIOSUS

Patent ductus arteriosus (PDA) is seen in approximately 10% of the patients with congenital heart disease. The male to female ratio is 1:2. In foetal life pulmonary blood is shunted from right to left through PDA to descending aorta bypassing the lung. Functional closure is seen immediately after birth. Anatomic closure is complete usually by 2–3 months of age. If the ductus is large, it does not close spontaneously shunting the blood from right to left side. The aortic end of the ductus is just distal to the origin of left subclavian artery, whereas the pulmonary end is located at the bifurcation of pulmonary artery.[24]

PDA is seen more commonly in infants with maternal rubella infection. It is a common occurrence in premature infants as the smooth muscle wall in premature is less responsive to high PO_2 and therefore less likely constrict after birth. In term infants, the wall of ductus lacks both the mucoid epithelial and muscular media layer, whereas in ductus in premature has normal structure. It undergoes spontaneous closure in many premature infants.

Pathophysiology

After birth increase in aortic pressure causes the blood to flow from left to right. In hemodynamically significant ductus, excessive blood flow to lung, left atrium, left ventricle results in enlargement of these structures and consequently congestive heart failure.[25] Elevation of pressure in left atrium leads to enlargement of foramen ovale with additional left to right shunt. The extent of shunt depends on the size of ductus and the ratio of pulmonary vascular resistance to systemic vascular resistance. Premature infants with respiratory distress and hypoxia continue the patency of the ductus needing aggressive ventilation. If the PDA is large, pulmonary artery pressure might increase to or beyond systolic blood pressure leading to reversal of the shunt if it is not corrected early.

Clinical Manifestations

If the ductus is small, it is usually asymptomatic. Large PDA leads to heart failure, growth retardation. The signs and symptoms include bounding arterial pulses with wide pulse pressure, cardiomegaly with prominent and heaving apical impulse, palpable thrill in left 2nd intercostal space radiating to left clavicle, left sternal border or towards apex. On auscultation a continuous machinery murmur is heard after onset of first heart sound localized in left 2nd intercostal space radiating to left clavicle and down to left sternal border.

Diagnosis

On chest radiography the following features are noted:

1. Prominent pulmonary artery
2. Prominent pulmonary vasculature marking along the ribs
3. Cardiomegaly

On 2-D Echo, large shunt, increased LA and LV dimensions are seen. Coloured and pulsed Doppler shows retrograde turbulent flow in pulmonary artery.

Cardiac catheterization shows normal or increased pressures in RV and PA and differing saturations of blood in various chambers of heart. Presence of oxygenated blood in pulmonary artery confirms the diagnosis of PDA.

Prognosis and complications

Spontaneous closure of PDA is rare.

Complications

- Infective endocarditis
- Pulmonary and systemic emboli
- Eisenmenger's syndrome
- Necrotizing enterocolitis
- Intracerebral and intraventricular haemorrhage

Treatment

Medical management is done with indomethacin or ibuprofen (10 mg/kg). Small PDA usually requires only prevention of infective endocarditis. Small PDA can be closed using catheter embolization with intravascular coils, whereas moderate to large sized can be closed using umbrella-shaped PDA closure devices under transesophageal echo guidance. Surgical correction is done either with classic left posterolateral thoracotomy or video-assisted thoracoscopic guidance (VATS).[24]

Indications for catheter embolization/surgical closure:

1. Contraindication to pharmacotherapy such as thrombocytopenia or renal failure.
2. Failure of pharmacotherapy
3. Signs and symptoms of congestive heart failure
4. Prevention of risk of infective endocarditis/ pulmonary complications
5. Before 1 year of age to prevent further complications
6. Failure of catheter embolization
7. Preterm or term PDA complications and too small for catheter based procedures.

Anaesthetic Management

Anaesthetic management depends on the patient age and clinical condition. Many patients are premature, sick, ventilator and ionotrope dependent with respiratory distress syndrome and heart failure. The physiologic goals are similar with other left-to-right shunts. The maneuvers that decrease PVR, SVR and myocardial contractility should be avoided. Invasive arterial pressure monitoring is necessary in sicker infants. Anaesthesia induction comprises fentanyl (30–50 mcg/kg) and muscle relaxant. Surgical dissection, lung retraction and creation of pneumothorax during open and VATS technique is known to cause hypoxemia, hypercarbia, and hypotension. Blood pressure and pulse oximeter should be applied in both upper (right arm preferable as clamping of aorta may be required if control of ductus is lost during dissection or ligation) and lower extremities. After ligation of the ductus there will be increase in the diastolic blood pressure and left ventricular afterload. At this stage ionotropes may be needed in the failing left ventricle. Patients are usually extubated at the end of the surgery.

Complications

- Blockage of endotracheal tube
- Profound haemorrhage from disruption or tearing of the ductus
- Inadvertent ligation of the major vessels such as left pulmonary artery or descending aorta
- Recurrent laryngeal nerve damage (can be reduced by intraoperative direct stimulation of the nerve or evoked electro-myographic monitoring)[25]
- Accidental extubation

Paediatric Anaesthesia Pearls

In neonates undergoing PDA correction, arterial blood pressure and pulse oximeter probes are placed on both right upper and lower extremities. Right arm is preferred as clamping of aorta might be required if the control of ductus is lost intraoperatively.

SUMMARY

Anaesthetizing preterm and expreterm neonates requires constant micro vigilance, rapid recognition of adverse events and trends, and swift intervention.

The anaesthetic considerations in the preterm neonate are based on the physiological immaturity of the various organ systems, associated congenital disorders, dramatic responses to various anaesthesia drugs, and cautious use of high concentrations of oxygen.

The benefit of providing adequate anaesthesia and analgesia must be carefully balanced with the significant cardiorespiratory depression in this fragile population. There can be exaggerated, unpredictable and dramatic responses to the multiple intravenous and inhalational anaesthetic agents.

Recently regional anaesthesia has been shown to be more safe and beneficial in the preterm infants and micropremies.

FAQ with Answer

Q. How to detect hypovolemia/hypotension in premature infants?

A. There are several ways to determine adequacy of fluid and blood replacement in preterm infants as follows:[26]

1. Mean arterial pressure is a better indicator of the intravascular volume status than systolic blood pressure.
2. A pressure more than two standard deviations below normal for that age group suggests hypovolemia.
3. Central venous pressure below 3 cm of H_2O indicates hypovolemia.
4. Adequate urine output is a good indicator of intravascular volume status.
5. Urine specific gravity of more than 1.009 indicates hypovolemia.
6. A fontanel below the inner table of the skull indicates volume depletion.
7. Delayed capillary refill time suggests hypovolemia.

REFERENCES

1. Waldemar A Carlo. Prematurity and Intrauterine growth restriction, Nelson's textbook of paediatrics, 19th edn. The high risk infant, 555–564.
2. George Gregory, Claire Brett. Neonatology for anesthesiologists, Smith's anesthesia for infants and children, 8th edn. 512–553.
3. Jay M Wilson, John W Difiore. Respiratory physiology and care, Pediatric anesthesia, Benson's Pediatric surgery, 5th edn. volume one. 71–88.
4. Rakesh Sahni, Richard A Pollin. Physiologic underpinnings for clinical problems in moderately preterm and late preterm infants, clinics in perinatology 40:645–663.
5. Maureen A Strafford. Cardiovascular Physiology and care, pediatric anaesthesia, Benson's Pediatric surgery, 5th edn. volume one. 103–133.
6. Robin Haynes, Lynn Sleeper, Joseph Volpe, et al. Neurologic studies of the encephalopathy of prematurity in late preterm infant, clinics in perinatology. 40:707–722.
7. Abbot R Laptook. Neurologic and metabolic issues in moderately preterm, late preterm and early term infants: Clinics of perinatology. 2013;40:723–738.
8. Demetrius Ellis. Regulation of fluids and electrolytes, Smith's Anaesthesia for infants and children, 8th edn. 116–156.
9. Matthew Wallenstein, Vinod Bhutani. Jaundice and kernicterus in the moderately preterm infant, clinic in perinatology 2013;40:679–668.
10. William Mauermann, Dawit Haile, Randall Flick, blood conservation, Smith's anaesthesia for infants and children, 8th edn. 395–417.
11. James P Spaeth, C Dean Kurth. The extremely premature infant (micropremie), 5th edn. Pediatric anesthesia by Charles and Cote. 735–746.
12. Ira Landsman, D Ryan Cook. Pediatric anesthesia, Benson's Pediatric surgery, 5th edn. volume one. 197–228.
13. John E Stork. Anaesthesia in the neonate, Neonatal and perinatal medicine by Martin Fararoff Walsch, 9th edn. 597–614.
14. Marc Rowe. The newborn as a surgical patient, Benson's Pediatric surgery, 5th edn. volume one. 43–70.

15. Robert Holzman. Airway management, Smith's anaesthesia for infants and children, 8th edn. 344–394.
16. Welzing L, Krips A, Eifinger F, et al. Propofol as an induction agent for endotracheal intubation can cause significant arterial hypotension in preterm neonates, Paediatric anaesthesia July 2010;20(7):605–11.
17. Carmen G, Maria S, Elisabetta V, et al. Remifentanil analgosedation in preterm newborns during mechanical ventilation, Acta Pediatrica, July 2009;98(7):1111–1115.
18. Barry D Kussman, Francis X McGowan (Jr). Congenital cardiac anaesthesia: Non-Bypass procedures, Smith's anesthesia for infants and children, 8th edn. 696–697.
19. James E Moore. Newer monitoring techniques to determine the risk of necrotizing eneterocolitis, clinics in perinatology, Necrotisingenterocolitis: March 2013;125–132.
20. Clair90e Brett, Peter J Davis. Anaesthesia for general surgery in the neonate, Smith's anesthesia for infants and children, 8th edn. 554–588.
21. Renu Sharma, Mark Lawrence Hudak. A clinical perspective of necrotizing enterocolitis past, present and future, Clinics in perinatology, Necrotising enterocolitis: March 2013;27–52.
22. Lois E Smith, Anna-Lena Hard, Ann Hellstrom. The biology of Retinopathy of Prematurity, Clinics in perinatology. June 2013;(40):201–214.
23. Brian W Fleck, Ben J Stenson. Retinopathy of prematurity and the oxygen conundrum, Clinics of perinatology 2013;40:229–240.
24. Daniel Bernstein, congenital heart diseases, Nelson's textbook of pediatrics, 19th edn. 555–559.
25. Barry D Kussman, Francis X McGowan (Jr). Congenital cardiac anesthesia: Non-Bypass procedures, Smith's anesthesia for infants and children. 8th edn. 696–697.
26. George Gregory. Anesthesia for premature infants: 3rd edn. Pediatric anesthesia. 351–373.

Anaesthesia for the Full-term Neonate

Ekta Rai

INTRODUCTION

With the advancement in the perinatal care, anaesthetists are involved in care of critically ill term, extremely preterm and low birth weight newborns for various surgical procedures which demands a good understanding of the physiology of their systems, pharmacokinetics and pharmacodynamics. This is an attempt for you to understand the basics and implement it in your clinical practice (Table 21.1).

DEFINITIONS

Gestational age: Time elapsed between the first day of the last normal menstrual period and the day of delivery.

Postnatal age/ Chronological age: Time elapsed after birth.

Postmenstrual age: Time elapsed between the first day of the last menstrual period and birth (gestational age) plus the time elapsed after birth (chronological age).

Corrected age: Corrected age is calculated by subtracting the number of weeks born before 40 weeks of gestation from the chronological age.

Table 21.1 Definitions

Terms	Definition
Preterm	<37 weeks of gestation at birth
Term	37–40 weeks of gestation at birth
Post term	>42 weeks of gestation at birth
Very low birth weight	<1500 g at birth
Extremely low birth weight	<1000 gm at birth
Small for gestational age	<5th percentile for gestational age

Conceptional age: Time elapsed between the day of conception and the day of delivery. Gestational age is 2 weeks longer than conceptional age.

> **Pearls**
>
> Corrected Gestational Age (CGA) influences the morbidity and mortality associated to preterm infants.

In preterm babies, the corrected gestation age (CGA) is important to describe as the morbidity and mortality is influenced by the CGA and PMA. For example, preterm baby born at 28 weeks is now 28 days will have PMA of 32 weeks only, whereas neonate (28 days) born at 40 weeks will have PMA of 44 weeks. Survival of neonatal surgery is inversely related to neonatal PMA, age at birth, weight at birth and at the time of surgery whereas it is directly related to expertise of the medical staff taking care of them.

Neonates who are large for gestation are mainly born to diabetic mothers and are liable to have low glucose level, birth injuries and polycythemia. The other causes for the large gestation are transposition of the great vessels, Beckwith-Wiedemann syndrome and postterm babies.

Physiology of The Systems

CNS

The central nervous system is not completely matured at birth in term babies. Intraventricular haemorrhage can result due to rapid fluctuation in the blood flow, volume, and cerebral venous pressure. Thus, the two important factors which are related to intraventricular haemorrhage are inefficient cerebral auto-regulation and the fragile cerebral vessels. There has been no casual relation has been proved between the two.

> **Fact to Remember**
>
> Intraventricular haemorrhage is associated with inefficient cerebral auto-regulation and fragile cerebral vessels.

IVH Grading

Intraventricular Haemorrhage Grading

IVH grading is based on head ultrasonography

Grade 1: Haemorrhage limiting to germinal matrix

Grade 2: Haemorrhage extending to ventricular system

Grade 3: Haemorrhage extending to ventricular system along with ventricular dilatation

Grade 4: Haemorrhage extending to brain parenchyma

> **Facts to Remember**
>
> - Severity of IVH determines the neurocognitive outcome of the preterm/term neonate
> - Pain management should be adequate as pain pathways are well developed.

In neonatal period, the pain excitatory pathways are well developed but the descending inhibitory pathways are not, thus the pain perceived are stronger with no negative feedback.[2–4] A beta myelinated fibre (light touch) is restricted to Lamina III and IV in adults, whereas in neonates it spreads to Lamina I and II also along with overlapping A delta and C unmyelinated fibre. It leads to more generalized response and lower threshold to pain.[4]

In neonates, the spinal cord extends to L2–3 and dural sac extends to S3–4 in contrast to adults (L1 and S2 respectively). Thus the spinal block should be attempted below L3 and there is higher incidence of the dural puncture in neonates than bigger children (the dura extends lower down). The spinal surface area and CSF volume are more and thus the volume of intrathecal drug requirement (mg/kg) is more in neonates. The myelination is slower thus the effective concentration of drug is lower.[1]

MCQ

Extension of spinal cord and dural sac at birth?

- Spinal cord at birth—L2–3 and in adults is L1.
- Dural sac at birth is S3–4 and in adults is S2.

Retinopathy of Prematurity (ROP)

ROP is also reported in term babies who got exposed to high concentration of oxygen. Hyperoxia is associated to ROP. ROP starts as the vascular narrowing and period to reduced blood flow which is followed by increased flow of blood leading to neo vascularisation and haemorrhage and the extremes results in retinal detachments.

CBF

Arterial CO_2 tension and hypoxia have pronounced effect on CBF. Hypocarbia causes vasoconstriction and can result in periventricular leukomalacia in preterm babies.[41] Hypoxia has vasodilatory effect. Sick neonates have almost nil cerebral autoregulation mechanism so are liable for intraventricular haemorrhage.[5]

CVS

Neonate heart is inefficient as filling chambers and contratile units.[6] It exhibits a flat Starling curve which means it has poor responsiveness to preload. Overfilling can lead to heart failure.[7] The myocardium of neonate is collection of disorganized myocardial cells, more non contractile tissues and water between the contractile tissues due to more ECF and TBW.[8,9]

Carbohydrate and short chain fatty acids are the energy source for neonatal heart. Diastolic relaxation improves in first month of life.[10] Neonatal heart has reduced L type channels and entry of ionized calcium occurs through T type channels, proteins and reverse Na/Ca exchange mechanism which is associated with calcium removal from cells.[11,12] Propogation of calcium is poor since the t tubular system is poor and limited ryanodine receptors at SR results into limited calcium release on trigger. Relaxation is inefficient as the uptake of the calcium in SR is inadequate. Thus cardiac contraction is extracellular calcium dependent.[13,14] This immature L type calcium channels, t tubule and SR matures by the end of month of life.[15]

Latest researches have supported the regenerative abilities of neaonatal heart due to presence of greater number of the stem cells and their ability to differentiate.[16]

> **Facts to Remember**
>
> - Neonate heart exhibits flat Starling curve response.
> - Haemodynamaic fluctuations are seen in neonates due to immature autonomic innervations.

Neonatal Heart and Response to Inotrope

Given to flat starling curve, the beta agonist are often used to improve the CO, but these drugs have intrinsic effect on the immature neonatal myocardium. In sick neonates, down regulation of beta receptors are found.[17] The current interest is in low dose vasopressin in PICU to overcome the resistance of inotropes.[18]

Autonomic innervations are present but immature in neonates thus they are prone for haemodynamic fluctuations. At birth, the sympathetic component is more dominant but in infancy it reverses and parasympathetic system becomes more prominent.[19–21] This reduced autonomic response results in reduced baroreceptor sensitivity.[22]

> **Fact to Remember**
>
> At birth, the sympathetic component is more dominant but in infancy it reverses and parasympathetic system becomes more prominent.

Respiratory System

Most of the complications and perioperative arrests in neonates are respiratory in origin. The rate of complications are inversely related to the age of the children.[23,24]

Respiratory Control

Complete maturation of the respiratory centre takes a few weeks to months after term birth.[25] The ventilator response to hypercapnia and hypoxia is impaired in neonates. The response to hypercapnia is present in term healthy babies, whereas it is attenuated in preterm neonates.[26,27] Breathing pattern is irregular in preterm and even term babies leading to life threatening apnoeas if not monitored adequately.[28] Excessive inflation of the the lung can lead to apnoeas in neonates and this reflex is Hering-Breuer inflation reflex. It is pronounced in preterm and term neonates[29] compared with older children. Anaesthetic drugs blunt the respiratory control to both hypoxia and hypercapnia.[30]

Apnoea of Prematurity (AOP)

Absence of air flow for more than 20 sec or apnoeic episode leading to desaturation is known as significant apnoea. It can be central, obstructive or mixed.[31,32]

Central Apnoea

Immaturity of respiratory control centre results in central apnoea. Methylxanthene is used in treatment of central apnoea.

Obstructive Apnoea

Obstruction of airway results in obstructive apnoea, mostly is seen in active sleep (REM phase) and the reduced tone of pharyngeal muscle causes the obstructive airway. CPAP or intubation relieves the obstruction.

Airway

Fact 1: Anatomic dead space is larger than older children
Reason: Large head

Fact 2: Neonate prefer to breathe through nose
Reason: Epiglottis is large and high in pharynx so the airway resistance is lower in nasal passage.

Fact 3: Airway collapse on deep inspiration.
Reason: Compliant airway

Fact 4: Higher airway resistance
Reason: Narrow airway

Fact 5: Greater WOB
Reason: Narrowing of airway, secretions, ETT, Laryngomalacia, tracheomalacia (more common in neonates) increases the WOB

Fact 6: PEEP is required essentially
Reason: For opening up the airway

Fact 7: Increased risk of atelectasis in neonates
Reason: Collateral connections between alveoli (pores of Kohn and bronchoalveolar canals of Lambert) are not present.[33] The absence of accessory interalveolar communications in neonates increases the risk of atelectasis

Hepatic

Gut function is not matured completely at birth. Risk of reflux of the stomach content is higher in neonates than adults due to slow emptying of the stomach and incompetent lower esophageal sphincter. Early feeding of neonate is always a critical issue as hypocaloric or trophic feeds is associated with food intolerance, indirect hyperbilirubenemia and cholestatic jaundice,[1] whereas the hypertonic feeds can result in necrotizing enterocolitis.[1]

Renal

Total body water is more for neonate and infants than adult. At full term, the GFR is only around 20–30% of the adult value. The GFR reaches adult value by one year of age. The tubular function and thus sodium retaining ability develops by 32 weeks of gestation.[1] The immaturity of kidneys also effect the metabolism and thus the duration of various drugs are prolonged.

Thus the water soluble drugs are required in larger quantities in relation to weight as first bolus but since the renal and hepatic functions is immature hence the further dosing is reduced.

Calcium Homeostasis

Hypocalcemia is been observed in nearly 40% of the sick neonates.[1] Neonatal hypocalcaemia is defined as the serum ionized calcium level less than 1 mmol/L in term neonate or 0.75 mmol/L or less in preterm.

Altered calcium metabolism because of blood transfusion, bicarbonate infusion and diuretics are important factors for the intra-operative hypocalcaemia. Hypocalcaemia can be asymptomatic or symptomatic (seizures, tremors).

Diagnosis rests on the serum level of ionized calcium with ion specific electrode.[1]

Treatment of hypocalcaemia is effective only once the hypomagnesemia is corrected along with the cause of the development of hypocalcaemia. Symptomatic hypocalcaemia is treated with 100 mg/kg of calcium gluconate (10%) by slow IV (over a period of 5 min).

Temperature Regulation

Heat Loss Mechanism

Convection: Less fat and more surface area leads to increased convective and conductive loss

Conduction

Radiation

Evaporation: Neonates especially the preterms have more evaporative loss due to lack of keratin in epidermis

Neonates have tendency to lose body heat as their head surface area is larger in relation to body which increases the heat loss. The source of body heat is mainly brown fat metabolism. Differentiation of brown fat cells is around 30 weeks of gestation hence is not present in extremely preterm neonates.[1] Warming of operation theatre (78–80 °F), underbody warming, and fluids will help in maintenance of the temperature in range for neonates.[1]

Most Effective Means of Warming in Neonates is Warming Mattress

Pharmacology

The pharmacokinetics (PK) is 'what the body does to drug' and Pharmacodynamics(PD) is 'what the drug does to body'. PK in paediatric population is affected by development of organ in terms of size and function along with the body composition, cellular function and metabolic activity.[34–38]

Sensitivity of receptors to drugs may be more in early age which will affect population specific PD.[34–38]

It is essential to understand that neonates are not small adults and to extrapolate the pharmacokinetics and dynamics to them can result into unpredictable results. Neonates, like adults, do have rapid uptake (alpha phase) and slower elimination phase (beta phase) but duration of these phase varies due to difference in body composition, protein binding, and maturation of organ function.[39]

PK deals with ADME (Absorption, Distribution, Metabolism and Elimination). Neonates have highest TBW (total body water) and maturation of organs like kidney and hepatobiliary are slow which results in slow clearance of the drug. Primary elimination clearance is by kidneys, whereas the metabolic clearance is by liver. It implies that water soluble drugs like cefazoline, suxmethonium, thiopentone, etc necessitating higher loading doses and prolong dosing intervals.[40–42]

FACT 1: TBW = 85–90%

Clinical Implication: Higher loading dose of water soluble drugs.

FACT 2: Total muscle weight = 30%

Clinical Implication: Lesser loading and long interval of muscle relaxants

FACT 3: Total fat = 15%

Clinical Implication: More sedation with Thiopentone as the effect diminishes due to redistribution rather metabolism.

FACT 4: Maturation of hepatic function is present for almost all the drugs but rate of conjugation is slow.

Clinical Implication: Duration of action of drugs are longer.

FACT 5: Most effected organ in neonate is kidneys

Clinical Implication: Slow elimination and thus frequency of administration is less

Preoperative Assessment

1. Corrected gestation age and weight of neonate: It is of utmost importance to find out the corrected gestation age of the babies as it directly effects the anaesthesia and postoperative care.
2. Associated congenital abnormalities:
3. Premedications: Sedation is not required as neonates do not have separation anxiety. Atropine can be used

for vagolysis and for reduction of secretions on routine basis or as per requirement. Ametop can be used for cannulation, EMLA is avoided in infants for the risk of methaemoglobinemia.

4. Parental anxiety: It is important to communicate with the parents and answer all the possible queries they have which will help to come down the anxiety of parents. Parental anxiety is inversely related to the age of the child which means the smaller the child more is the parental anxiety which is supported by the surgical mortality rates.[43] The rate of paediatric deaths attributable to anaesthesia has been reported to be 0.65–0.98/10,000 cases in both Australia (2008) and the USA (2011), which represents a two-third reduction in mortality since 1960.
5. Investigation:
   - **Hb:** Anaemia is related to apnoea in preterm babies and sometimes even in term neonates.

Normal Hb value		
	Birth Mean (range)	**1 month of age Mean (range)**
Hb	18 (14.5–21) g/dL	14 (10–16) g/dL
Reticulocyte	3–7%	0–1%

   - **Sickle cell disease testing:** Majority of the Hb present at birth is HbF which is replaced by HbA at around 3 month of age and in Sickle Cell Disease (SCD) by HbS. The Sickle dex screening may provide false negatives in neonates because of high HbF but electrophoresiscan still identify all Hb types at any age. At risk babies should be screened for SCD via cord blood.
   - **Bilirubin**
   - **Clotting studies**

Neonates are at risk of coagulation deficiencies due to the following reasons:

- immaturity of the coagulation system
- presence of sepsis, frequently associated with thrombocytopenia and coagulopathy
- jaundice
- vitamin K deficiency: Vitamin K is required for production of hepatic coagulation factors II, VII, IX and X. Vitamin K can be given through IM (single dose) or oral route (three doses). Vitamin K should be given routinely to all neonates preoperatively.

Fasting Orders

According to ASA fasting guidelines

- Clear fluids—glucose water; coconut water: Until 2 hours preoperative.
- Breast milk: Until 4th preoperatively.
- Formula milk feeds: Until 6 hrs preoperatively.
- Continuous feed via jejunal catheters: Until 4 hrs preoperatively.
- In case of delay in surgery: Consider rescheduling the fasting order or start IV fluids.

Preparation of OT

Preparation is key to success and thus the operation theatre preparation saves many difficult situations. Checked machine, circuit, equipment, drugs in appropriate dilutions, fluids connected to burette set with appropriate amount of fluid loaded, warming devices are kept ready before taking the neonate in the operation theatre.

Induction and Maintenance

A gaseous induction is not generally recommended, since all inhalation agents depress the heart long before they adequately depress airway reflexes, and because of the effects of inhalation agents on the airway: increased respiratory rate, decreased tidal volume, loss of intercostal muscle function (decreased functional residual capacity), and collapse of upper airway structures leading to upper airway obstruction (often relieved with 5–10 cm PEEP). If the infant has apparent normal airway anatomy, then a standard intravenous induction with muscle relaxant to facilitate intubation is indicated. Thiopentone is preferred induction agent in neonates as propofol is not licensed. Atracurium is the commonly used muscle relaxant as the enzymes are immature.

They are intubated and ventilated for most of the procedures as FRC is reduced so closing volume approaches tidal volume LMAs are prone to get dislodged on small movements or under light plane of anaesthesia. Intraoperative inspired O_2 should be minimal to maintain $SpO_2 > 95\%$. Regional blocks should be performed as and when possible as they help in reducing the systemic requirements of opiods and thus their side effects.

- **Euglycemia and Euthermia** should always be maintained.
- **Monitoring**: HR, ECG, SpO_2,[2] NIBP, $EtCO_2$ temperature, GRBS, airway pressures. Invasive monitors, if required.

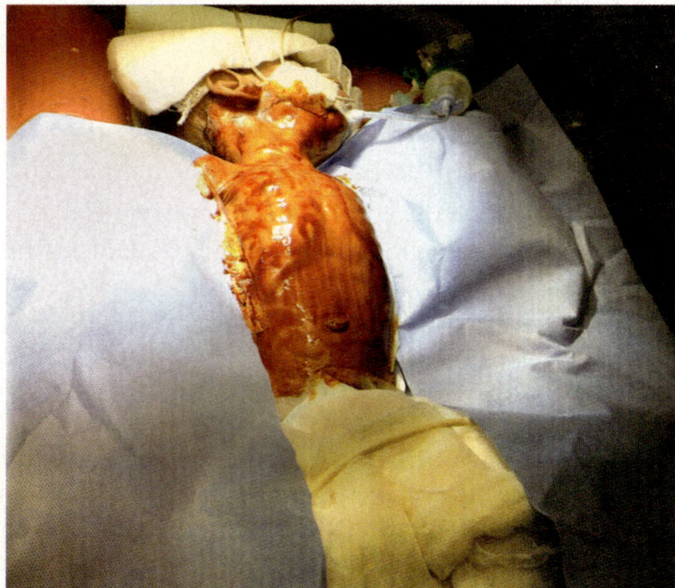

Fig. 21.1 Neonate undergoing surgery
Source: Department of paediatric surgery, Christian Medical College, Vellore

Analgesia:

Challenges in effective analgesia in neonates:

1. **Understanding of the pain pathway development:** The excitatory pathway are well developed in neonates but the inhibitory descending pathways are not developed thus the pain response is more than normal.
2. **Tendency to under treat the pain:**
   - Neonates cannot complaint verbally.
   - Opiods cause respiratory depression.
3. **Regional blocks:**
   - It is technically difficult to secure epidurals, nerve blocks, so expertise is required.
   - They are prone to local anaesthetics toxicity

CONGENITAL DIAPHRAGMATIC HERNIA

Compressive effect on the pulmonary structure and its cardiopulmonary sequelae is the hallmark of CDH.[1]

Incidence

Incidence of CDH is 1 : 2000–1 : 5000 of the live birth with male predominance.[1]

Embryology

Diaphragm completely develops by 7–10 weeks of gestation. The defect will thus allow the abdominal contents to enter the thoracic cavity at the time of elongation of the midgut (12 weeks).

Bochdalek type hernia (postero lateral) is most common CDH (90%). Neonates with Bochdalek type of hernia are more likely to be associated with congenital heart diseases and chromosomal abnormalities.[44]

Morgagni type hernia (9%) are anterior type and bilateral (1%) are very rare and often fatal.

CDH seems to be associated with genitourinary and gastrointestinal malformation and also with chromosomal abnormalities like trisomy 13, 18, tetrasomy and 12 p mosaicism.

Pathophysiology

Lung growth is severely effected during pseudoglandular phase wherein the proximal airway multiplies and pulmonary arterial vasculature is developing. Thus the CDH lung will have a few alveoli (lower surface area for effective gas exchange), decreased alveolar type II cells (reduced surfactant and hence atelectesis and intrapulmonary shunting). Unilateral hernia can effect both the lungs depending on the extent of the mass effect. The mass effect reduces the cross sectional area of the pulmonary vasculature and thus results in pulmonary hypertension. Right to left shunting via PFO, PDA causes severe hypoxemia and thus be life threatening.

Antenatal diagnosis: Antenatal diagnosis helps in preparing the parents and the doctors for the appropriate tertiary hospital with all the facilities and option of foetal (temporary tracheal plugging to stop the overflow of the surfactant rich fluid out of the lung and unplugging it at EXIT procedure and neonatal surgeries).[1] It also helps in risk stratification of foetus.

USG: Level 2 ultrasonography[1,44] helps in diagnosis of the condition and thus helps not only in the further management of the foetus but also in councelling the parents.

Findings suggestive of CDH are polyhydroamnios, intrathoracic gastric bubble and mediastinal shift away from the site of hernia.

Amniocentesis and Karyotyping: Karyotyping and amniocentesis will help in excluding any chromosomal abnormalities. Extremely low levels of maternal alphafeto protein are related to CDH.

Risk Stratification

High mortality can be predicted if:

- Presence of liver along with other abdominal content.
- Low lung to head ratio.

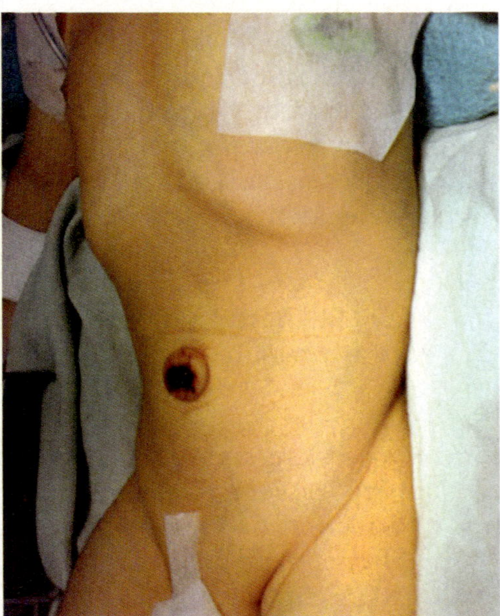

Fig. 21.2 Scaphoid abdomen—CDH
Source: Department of paediatric surgery, Christian Medical College, Vellore

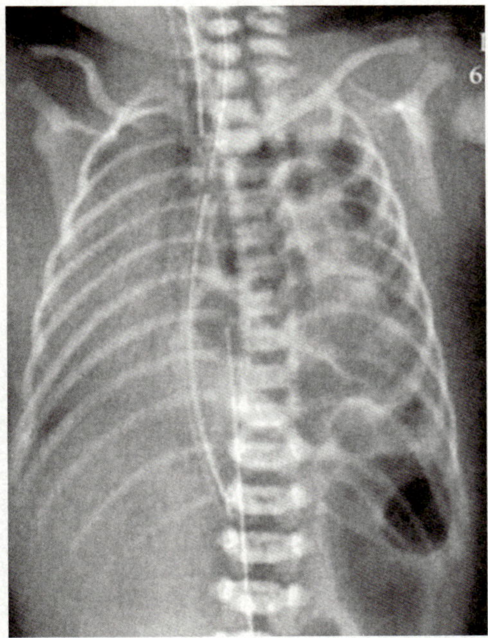

Fig. 21.3 Congenital diaphragmic hernia
Source: Department of paediatric surgery, Christian Medical College, Vellore

Diagnosis at Birth

- Tachycardia, tachypnoea, cyanosis are observed in neonate.
- The abdomen is classically described as "scaphoid abdomen".
- The mediastinum can be shifted depending on the mass effect.

Preoperative Optimization

Initial aim is to manage the respiratory failure by improving the oxygenation and ventilation. Definitive airway control is priority. Mask ventilation is avoided to limit the gas insufflations of stomach. Thus reducing the mediastinal shift or the mass effect in the cavity. Once airway is secured, nasogastric tube is secured to decompress the stomach. Ventilation is instituted in a sedated neonate in order to minimize the catecholamine release and thus reduce the pulmonary vascular resistance. Optimisation is guided by ABGs and CXR. Alveolar arterial gradient and PCO_2 level determines the survival.[1]

Preoperative Echo determines the cardiac functioning (especially the right side) and abnormalities. Cranial USG detects the intraventricular bleeding based on which the ECMO is initiated.

Various ventilation strategies have been targeted to minimize the barotraumas and pulmonary vascular resistance (hypoxemia, hypercarbia, acidosis, hypotension).[1] Thus low tidal volumes and limited peak inspiratory pressure will minimize the barotraumas and incidence of pneumothorax. Acidotic neonates will be treated with bicarbonate infusion as deliberate alkalosis will increase the pulmonary blood flow and thus reduce the ventilation–perfusion mismatch.

Refractory pulmonary hypertension is treated with inhaled NO as NO is short acting specific pulmonary vasodilator. It does not cause systemic hypotension.

ECMO has been tried in neonates where conventional treatment fails. It temporarily rests the lung till the maturation complete.[1] ECMO has also been used in post-operative patients who decompensate after the surgical correction (rebound hypertension). In neonates, veno arterial ECMO is utilized for oxygenation and hemodynamic stabilization. This invasive technique is associated with complications of anticoagulation, emboli, infection, circuit failure, etc.

Surgery

Surgery is planned once the target optimization is achieved.

Open repair is common as compared to laparoscopic technique[45,46]

Approaches: Abdominal, transthoracic or thoraco abdominal

Large defects may require patch placement.

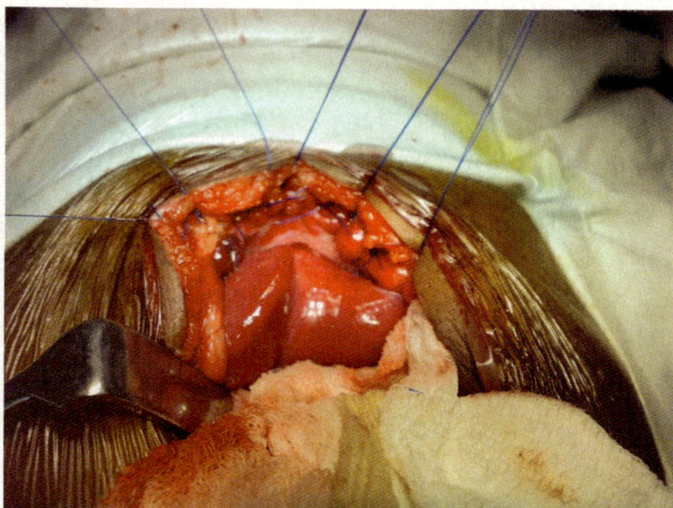

Fig. 21.4 Congenital diaphragmic hernia (CDH)
Source: Department of paediatric surgery, Christian Medical College, Vellore

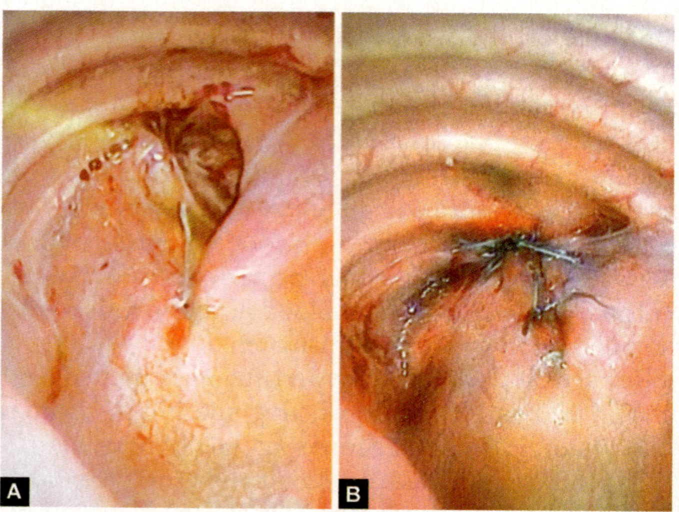

Fig. 21.5 Congenital diaphragmic hernia (CDH)
Source: Department of paediatric surgery, Christian Medical College, Vellore

CDH: Do's

Secure IV access in upper limb to avoid the effect of IVC compression after the reduction of hernia.

Anaesthesia

Anaesthetic care aims to support the perioperative and intraoperative care.

Transportation of the neonate is critical and should be done in incubator gently with continuing the same ventilation strategy as in NICU. Transportation of neonate on ECMO/HFOV/iNO is a challenge for anaesthetist.

INDUCTION AND MAINTENANCE

Unintubated neonates should undergo rapid sequence induction after decompression of the nasogastric tube in different positions to decompress the stomach. High dose opioids are used to reduced catecholamine levels. N_2O is not recommended.

Monitoring

HR, SpO_2,[2] $ETCO_2$, ECG, ABP, CVP, precordial stethoscope, ABG, Airway pressure.

Outcome

CDH survivors need long-term follow up in terms of respiratory support. The survivors who required ECMO or patch for correction had significant pulmonary disease.[47] Apart from pulmonary complication, growth retardation, GERD, neurocognitive delay,[48] behavioral disorder. Motor and language problem are as high as 70%.

OESOPHAGEAL ATRESIA AND TRACHEOESOPHAGEAL FISTULA

TEF

Oesophageal atresia is associated with TEF in 90% of the neonates but rarely it exists as isolated entity. TEF is linked to VACTERL anomalies in 25% of the neonates (vertebral abnormalities, imperforate anus, congenital heart disease, TEF, Radial aplasia, Renal abnormalities and Limb abnormalities.[49] As many as 20% to 25% of

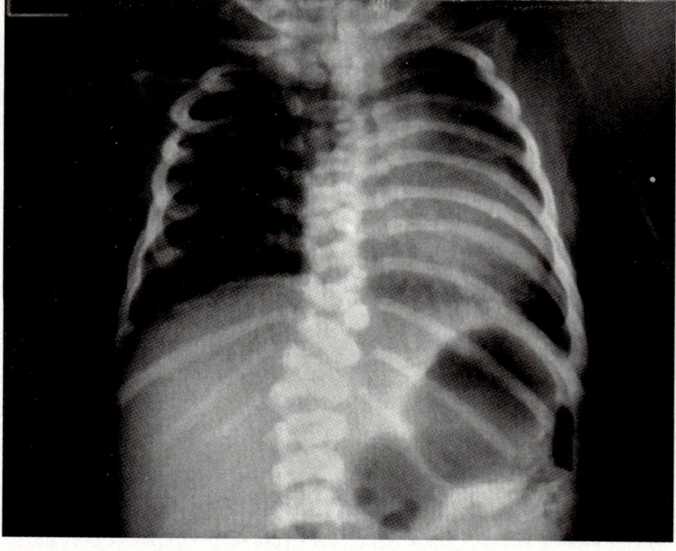

Fig. 21.6 Tracheoesophageal fistula (TEF)
Source: Department of paediatric surgery, Christian Medical College, Vellore

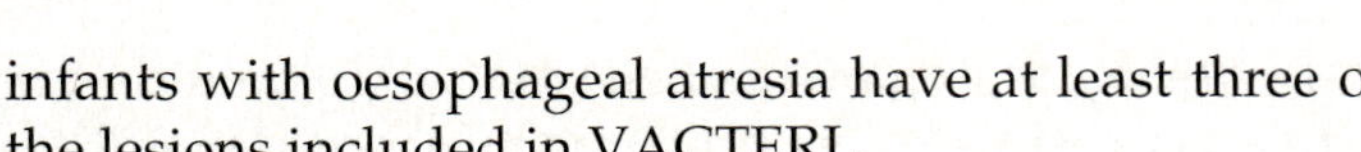

infants with oesophageal atresia have at least three of the lesions included in VACTERL.

Fact to Remember

TEF repair—urgent surgery but not emergent.

Spitz linked the higher mortality to **severity of heart disease** and **birth weight.**[50]

	Survival(%)
Group 1: Birth weight >1500 g No major cardiac anomaly	97%
Group 2: Birth weight <1500 g Major cardiac anomaly	59%
Group 3: Birth weight <1500 g Major cardiac anomaly	22%
Lopez et al. 2006 showed improved survival for the various categories: Category 1(98%); Category 2(82%) and Category 3(50%)	

Incidence

1:3000–1:4000 births[51]

Embryology

The embryology of TEF/EA is incompletely understood till date. Out of the many theories, a few are:

1. Trachea and esophagus originates from foregut during first 4–5 weeks
2. Ioannides et al postulated that foregut seperates into trachea and esophagus and abnormality in the differentiation of the separation can lead to TEF/EA.

Prenatal Diagnosis

Prenatal detection of the TEF/EA is as low as 40–50%.[52]

USG

- **Polyhydramnios**: Usually diagnosed around 24 weeks of gestation. (Pretorius et al. 1987).
- **Small or absent foetal gastric bubble**
- **Upper pouch sign (dilated blind ending pouch):** should raise the suspicion but is not diagnostic.[52]

Karyotyping: TEF has high incidence of co-existing chromosomal abnormalities.

Presentation

With the intake of the feed, the signs and symptoms are shown in most of the neonates with TEF.

- Excessive oral secretions,
- regurgitation of feeds,
- respiratory distress after the feeds,
- recurrent pneumonia (H type TEF)

H type fistula usually miss the early diagnosis and presents late in life (childhood).

Diagnosis

1. Inability to pass orogastric tube 9–10 cm into stomach
2. Radiographic studies with air contrast or dye demonstrating the blind esophageal pouch and bowel gas. In EA, presence of gas below diaphragm points out the presence of TEF
3. Abdominal distension.[53,54]

Preoperative evaluation

- **Pulmonary status** to decide for one lung ventilation and preprocedure Bronchoscopy
- Haemodynamic status
- Associated **congenital abnormalities**

Preoperative Optimization

1. Stop oral feeds. If nursing is allowed, it is done in prone or lateral position with 30 degree head up.
2. Position the neonate in reverse Trendelenberg and sump suction catheter placement in blind pouch to limit the pulmonary aspiration of secretions.
3. Central venous catheter is secured in sedation for parentral nutrition to encourage the growth.

Induction

Securing the airway is critical and is performed under sedation (fentanyl 0.2–0.5 mcg/kg or morphine 0.02–0.05 mcg/kg) in medically stable neonates. ETT is placed beyond the fistula in the trachea to minimize the gastric insufflations. To achieve this, the ETT is positioned endobronchial and then withdrawn just enough to have air entry equal bilaterally. There should be minimal gastric insufflations with final positioning of the ETT. Rigid/flexible bronchoscopy is integral part pre-operative evaluation of airway anatomy and to help in identifying the site, number of fistula and distance of the fistula from the carina which can guide the anaesthetist in securing the ETT.[55–57] Even after the exact evaluation, it may not be beneficial as the fistulas are most of the time close to carina and even the neck movement or positioning of neonate will result in the movement of the ETT within the trachea and the benefits of details found on bronchoscopy may be lost. Position of ETT distal to fistula and bevel facing anteriorly will occlude the fistula has been suggested.[58]

Monitoring

1. **Precordial Stethoscope**: Stethoscope on the left side of chest (left axilla) is vital in monitoring the position of the ETT through out the surgery.
2. **Routine Monitors**: HR, ECG, $ETCO_2$, SPO_2 (2 in number in patients with right to left shunting and pulmonary hypertension)
3. **ABP**: Regular blood sampling and beat to beat BP monitoring.
4. If gastrostomy is present at the time of intubation, it should be placed in water filled container so that the bubbling of the air entering the stomach can be seen and the ETT should be placed appropriately.

Surgery

Surgical approach:

1. Thoracoscopic[59]
2. Traditional Open Right thoracotomy (Left thoracotomy only if the aortic arch is right sided)

TEF neonates can get posted for primary repair (one staged or multi-staged) or rarely in unstable neonates palliative procedure (gastrostomy). Unstable neonates are stabilized (evaluation of other anomalies, mechanical ventilation and haemodynamic stabilization) usually within 48–72 hrs and definitive surgery is then planned. Gastrostomy not only helps in decompressing the stomach but also used for entral feeding if the surgery is delayed for some reason. Gastrostomy may lead to ventilator insuffiency by creating bronchocutaneous fistula resulting in inadequate ventilation.[55,60]

> Gap between the proximal and distal oesophagus determines the surgical procedure

If gap is

- **< 2 vertebral bodies**: Primary repair
- **Between 2 and 6 vertebral bodies**: Delayed anastomosis should be planned
- **> 6 vertebral bodies**: Primary repair not possible or
- Foker et al. described a long gap as a GAP > 2.5 cm

Maintenance

Spontaneous ventilation is preferred till the fistula is ligated but in preterm neonates with decreased lung compliance IPPV may be warranted. IPPV can lead to air leak, compromised ventilation and gastric insufflations causing the splinting of diaphragm and further compromising the ventilation.

To overcome, fogarty catheter is used to occlude the fistula via gastrostomy or by bronchoscopy depending on the condition of the neonate.[55,57]

After repair of the defect, transiently higher inspiratory time is required to overcome the absorption atelectesis.[61] Early extubation helps by reducing the pressure on the suture line.

> **Intraoperative Desaturation**
> - ETT displacement: Repositioning
> - Lung retraction especially in congenital heart disease neonate or the neonates with limited lung reserve.
> - Blockage of ETT: Mucous, blood, secretion
> - Surgical manipulation can obstruct the airway (kink)
> - Hypotension

Postoperative Issues[62]

Short Term	Long Term
Ventilation 2–3 days	GERD
Pain control	Recurrent chest infection
	Tracheomalacia
	Scoliosis

Ventilation

Postoperative ventilation usually is required for 24–48 hours to avoid collapse of alveoli due to tracheomalacia or surgical procedure. Pain is controlled during this period with either opioid infusion or regional analgesia.

Infants with long gap requires 5–7 days of elective ventilation with neuromuscular blocker and deep sedation to reduce the stress on the suture line.

Gastroesophageal Reflux

GER is the most common postoperative problem after TEF repair (35–50%). Dysmotility and abnormal esophageal function are found in around 75% of the patients and 100% of the delayed repair neonates. Dysmotility leads to dysphagia chocking which can result into cyanosis. Survivors need stringent follow up by multidisciplinary team to minimize the after effect of GER.

Recurrent Respiratory Infection

During first 3–4 years, respiratory chest infection is common. The contributing factors are GER, and abnormal tracheal epithelium at the site of TEF has no goblet cells and cilia resulting in impaired mucociliary clearance (Goyal et al. 2006).

Tracheomalacia

Tracheomalacia presents as brassy cough commonly known as TEF cough or stridor.

Tracheomalacia is seen in lower third of trachea close to the site of TEF. It is seen in 10% of the patients[63] and improves as the infant grows. Treatment is required in severe signs and symptoms. Treatment includes stenting[64] or aortopexy (posterior part of aorta is attached to trachea and suturing the aorta to sternum brings trachea forward).

Scoliosis

Postero lateral thoracotomies and vertebral anomalies may contribute to winged scapula and scoliosis. Scoliosis will further aggravate the pulmonary reserve compromise.

Risk factors for TEF neonates:[65]

- Congenital heart disease
- <2 kg neonate
- Poor lung reservoir
- Pericarinal fistula
- Thoracoscopic surgery

ABDOMINAL WALL DEFECTS: GASTROSCHISIS AND OMPHALOCELE

Gastroschisis

Gastroschisis (greek word) means "belly cleft".[66]

Gastroschisis and Omphalocoel are the most common abdominal defects with incidence of 1:10,000.[51] Pregnancies with elevated alpha fetoprotein (Anterior wall defects are related to high AFP) are evaluated with antenatal ultrasound scan. Antenatal ultrasounds are sensitive (95%) in the diagnosis of these wall defects after first trimester of pregnancy. This diagnosis is boon for the planning of such a delievery in well equipped tertiary medical centre. Vaginal delivery can be planned except for foetus with herniation of liver as the injury to liver can be lethal.

An omphalocoel is a central defect (>4 cms) of the umbilical ring through which the abdominal content (stomach, loops of intestine, rarely liver) herniated into the intact umbilical sac which has internal peritoneal membrane and external amniotic membrane.

A gatroschisis is a defect in abdominal wall (2–5 cm diameter) which usually occurs on the right side of umbilical cord through which the abdominal content (small and large intestine mostly) eviscerates. The contents are exposed to environment with no sac and thus is covered with exudative peel. The origin of this exudative peel is not so clear.

Abdominal Defects

Omphalocoel

- 1:5000
- Maternal age >40 years
- Central defect
- >4 cm
- Intact umbilical sac with internal peritoneal membrane and external amniotic membrane
- Embryology: Failure of fusion of the cephalic, caudal and lateral folds

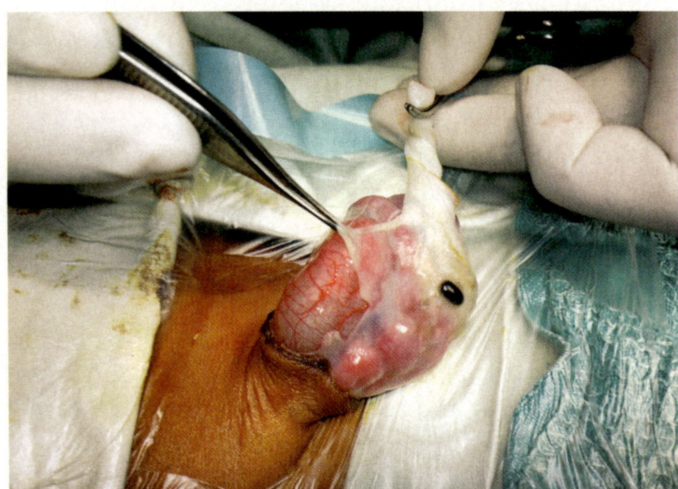

Fig. 21.7 Omphalocoel
Source: Department of paediatric surgery, Christian Medical College, Vellore

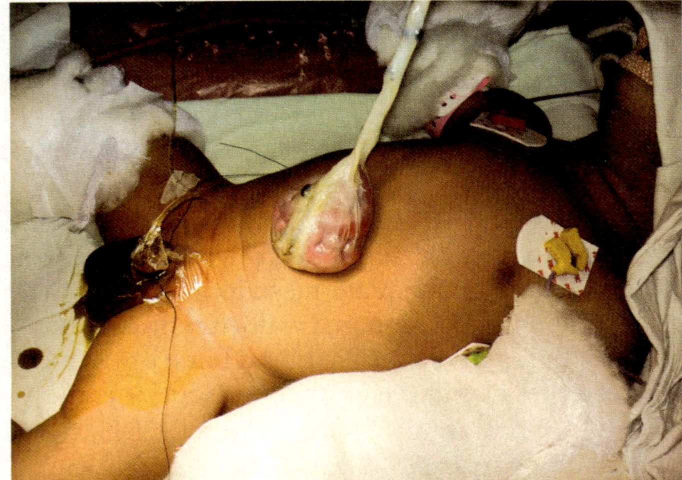

Fig. 21.8 Omphalocoel
Source: Department of paediatric surgery, Christian Medical College, Vellore

- Other anomalies: Cardiac defect (40%), genitourinary abnormalities, Chromosomal abnormalities (trisomy 13, 18 or 21), Beckwith-Wiedeman syndrome (10%), 10% premature
- Malrotation uncommon
- Surgery is semi-urgent as the sac is intact

Gastroschisis

- 1:3000
- Maternal age <20 years
- Peri umbilical defect (usually the right sided)
- 2–5 cm
- No umbilical sac present
- Embryology: Abnormal development of the right omphalo-mesentric artery or the right umbilical vein results in ischaemia of the right side of the umbilicus.
- Other anomolies are rare but LBW
- Malrotation is common
- Surgery is urgent and the abdominal content needs to be covered by cellophane

Embryology

Omphalocoel is described as failure of fusion of cephalic, lateral and caudal folds along with the abnormal differentiation of the myotomes to form abdominal musculature (7–12 weeks). During the midgut elongation, bowel herniates into umbilical cord. After 12 weeks, abdominal cavity enlarges and the midgut leaves the cords and enter into the abdominal cavity. Some postulates that the failure of content to return to abdominal cavity results in omphalocoel and small abdominal cavity.

Abnormal development of the right omphalo-mesentric artery or the right umbilical vein results in ischaemia of the right side of the umbilicus resulting in gastroschisis (Ruptured omphalocoel with intact umbilical cord).

Some postulates that imbalance between cell proliferation and cell death during the embryonic folding phase.[67] Inadequate mesoderm development results in abnormal abdominal wall growth, commonly found on the right of umbilicus and burst open due to increased pressure of the growing midgut.

Pentology of Cantrell[68] (Omphalocoel, CDH, sterna abnormalities, ectopic heart, gene Xq25 to Xq26.1 abnormalities) and OEIS (Omphalocoel, Extrophy bladder or cloacal, imperforate anus and sacrovertebral anomalies—meningomyelocoel) and Beckwith-Wiedemann syndrome are a few syndromes associated with Omphalocoel.

Preoperative Optimization

It is critical to obtain the haemodynamic stability along with the normothermia prior to operation.

Vigorous intravenous fluid therapy (150–300 mL/kg/day) aims to provide adequate hydration to compensate for the significant third space loss, peritonitis, and ischaemia. The target is urine output of 1–2 mL/kg/hr to resuscitate neonate from hypovolemia, hemoconcentration and metabolic acidosis.

Abdominal wall Defect

Preoperative optimisation includes

- Fluid and electrolyte optimisation
- Temperature regulation
- Avoid trauma to organs
- Treat infection

> Preoperative optimisation determines the outcome of neonate.

Intraoperative Management

Surgically, primary repair or staged repair with the help of" silo" is performed.[69] Silo" is made up of Teflon mesh that is sutured to the fascia of the defect. The organs are slowly reduced to peritoneal cavity over 3–10 days. Outcomes are better in slower reduction of abdominal organs. Forced closing of abdominal wall after forceful reduction of the content can lead to abdominal compartment syndrome (ACS). It not only impairs the respiratory function by restricting the diaphragm excursion but also diminishes the visceral blood flow, venous return.[70]

Monitoring

HR, ECG, $ETCO_2$, SpO_2 (2 in number—upper limb and lower limb to rule out the impaired perfusion) ABP, temperature monitoring, airway pressure, intragastric pressure (>20 mmHg is associated with ACS) and CVP (>4 mm of Hg associated with ACS),[70] regular GRBS monitoring.

Pre-oxygenation helps in building up the oxygen content in neonates prior to surgery. IV induction or inhalational induction after decompression of stomach can be preformed. N_2O should be avoided during the induction and maintenance and instead compressed air should be used. Neuromuscular agents relaxes the abdomen and thus facilitates the reduction of the contents. Reliable IV access is required not only intraoperative but also postoperative for nutritional support as the bowel motility is delayed after procedure.

Postoperative Care

Neonate with very small defect can be extubated on table.

Postoperatively, after an uncomplicated primary closure of an abdominal wall defect, mechanical ventilation is usually required for 24 to 48 hours or longer; thereafter, respiratory compliance usually improves dramatically.[67] Clearly, infants undergoing a gradual reduction after placement of a silo or similar device should be mechanically ventilated during this process. Inferior vena caval compression (evident by blueish lower limbs) or bowel ischaemia (necrotizing enterocolitis) can occur as a result of increased abdominal pressure and may require surgical decompression. Bowel hypomotility is most common in infants with gastroschisis. Survival improves drastically after successful reduction of abdominal contents back in the cavity.

The long-term outcome of infants with isolated abdominal wall defects is good.[68,71–73] The mortality rate is reported to be 61% for cases with associated anomalies, and only 15.5 to 20% without.[71–74]

Definition Abdominal Wall Defect

"Giant omphalocele"—The liver and biliary structures are part of omphalocele.

REFERENCES

1. Practice of Anesthesia for Infants and Children, 4th edn. Philadelphia, PA: Saunders Elsevier. 2009.
2. Baccei ML. Modulation of developing dorsal horn synapses by tissue injury. Ann N Y Acad Sci. 2010;1198: 159–167.
3. 11 Koch SC, Tochiki KK, Hirschberg S, et al. C-fiber activity-dependent maturation of glycinergic inhibition in the spinal dorsal horn of the postnatal rat. Proc Natl Acad Sci USA. 2012;109:12201–12206.
4. Fitzgerald M. The development of nociceptive circuits. Nat Rev Neurosci. 2005;6:507–520.
5. Greisen G. Autoregulation of cerebral blood flow in newborn babies. Early Hum Dev. 2005;81:423–428.
6. Andrew R. Wolf1, 2 and Adrian T Humphry. Limitations and vulnerabilities of the neonatal cardiovascular system: Considerations for anesthetic management. Pediatric Anesthesia. 2014;24:5–9.
7. Romero T, Covell J, Friedman WF. A comparison of pressure-volume relations of the fetal, newborn, and adult heart. Am J Physiol. 1972;222:1285–1290.
8. Marijianowski MM, van der Loos CM, Mohrschladt MF, et al. The neonatal heart has a relatively high content of total collagen and type I collagen, a condition that may explain the less compliant state. J Am Coll Cardiol 1994;23: 1204–1208.
9. Pelouch V, Kolar F, Milerova M et al. Effect of the preweaning nutritional state on the cardiac protein profile and functional performance of the rat heart. Mol Cell Biochem 1997;177: 221–228.
10. Kozak-Barany A, Jokinen E, Rantonen T, et al. Efficiency of left ventricular diastolic function increases in healthy full-term infants during the first month of life: A prospective follow-up study. Early Hum Dev. 2000;57:49–59.
11. Qu Y, Boutjdir M. Gene expression of SERCA2a and L- and T-type Ca channels during human heart development. Pediatr Res. 2001;50:569–574.
12. Qu Y, Ghatpande A, El-Sherif N, et al. Gene expression of Na^+/Ca^{2+} exchanger during development in human heart. Cardiovasc Res. 2000;45:866–873.
13. Schroder EA, Wei Y, Satin J. The developing cardiac myocyte: Maturation of excitability and excitation-contraction coupling. Ann N Y Acad Sci. 2006;1080:63–75.
14. Poindexter BJ, Smith JR, Buja LM, et al. Calcium signaling mechanisms in dedifferentiated cardiac myocytes: Comparison with neonatal and adult cardiomyocytes. Cell Calcium. 2001;30:373–382.
15. Wiegerinck RF, Cojoc A, Zeidenweber CM, et al. Force frequency relationship of the human ventricle increases during early postnatal development. Pediatr Res. 2009; 65:414–419.
16. Simpson DL, Mishra R, Sharma S, et al. A strong regenerative ability of stem cells derived from neonatal hearts. Circulation. 2012;126(Suppl 1):S46–S53.
17. Schranz D, Droege A, Broede A, et al. Uncoupling of human cardiac beta-adrenoceptors during cardiopulmonary bypass with cardioplegic cardiac arrest. Circulation. 1993;87:422–426.
18. Holmes C, Landry D, Granton J. Science review: Vasopressin and the cardiovascular system part 2–clinical physiology. Crit Care. 2004;8: 15–23.
19. Yiallourou SR, Sands SA, Walker AM, et al. Maturation of heart rate and blood pressure variability during sleep in term-born infants. Sleep. 2012;35:177–186.
20. Patural H, Pichot V, Jaziri F, et al. Automatic control of very preterm newborns: a prolonged dysfunction. Early Human Dev. 2008;84:681–687.
21. De Rogalski Landrot I, Roche F, Pichot V, et al. Autonomic nervous system activity in premature and full-term infants from theoretical term to 7 years. Auton Neurosci. 2007;136: 105–109.
22. Gournay V, Drouin E, Roze J. Development of baroreflex control of heart rate in preterm and full term infants. Arch Dis Child Fetal Neonatal Ed. 2002;86:F151–F154
23. Tay CL, Tan GM, Ng SB. Critical incidents in paediatric anaesthesia: An audit of 10000 anaesthetics in Singapore. Paediatr Anaesth. 2001;11:711–718.

24. Bhananker SM, Ramamoorthy C, Geiduschek JM et al. Anesthesia-related cardiac arrest in children: update from the pediatric perioperative cardiac arrest registry. Anesth Analg. 2007;105:344–350.
25. Carroll JL, Agarwal A. Development of ventilatory control in infants. Paediatr Respir Rev. 2010;11:199–207.
26. Gerhardt T, Bancalari E. Apnea of prematurity: I. Lung function and regulation of breathing. Pediatrics. 1984;74: 58–62.
27. Martin RJ, DiFiore JM, Korenke CB, et al. Vulnerability of respiratory control in healthy preterm infants placed supine. J Pediatr. 1995;127:609–614.
28. Mathew OP. Apnea of prematurity: pathogenesis and management strategies. J Perinatol. 2011;31:302–310.
29. Stocks J, Dezateux C, Hoo AF. et al. Delayed maturation of Hering-Breuer inflation reflex activity in preterm infants. Am J Respir Crit Care Med. 1996;154:1411–1417.
30. Kurth CD, Spitzer AR, Broennle AM. et al. Postoperative apnea in preterm infants. Anesthesiology 1987;66:483–488.
31. Mathew OP, Roberts JL, Thach BT. Pharyngeal airway obstruction in preterm infants during mixed and obstructive apnea. J Pediatr. 1982;100:964–968.
32. Dransfield DA, Spitzer AR, Fox WW. Episodic airway obstruction in premature infants. Arch Pediatr Adolesc Med. 1983;137:441–443.
33. Hislop A, Reid L. Development of the acinus in the human lung. Thorax. 1974;29:90–94.
34. Anderson BJ, Holford NH. Mechanistic basis of using body size and maturation to predict clearance in humans. Drug Metab Pharmacokinet 2009;24:25–36.
35. van den Anker JN. Developmental pharmacology. Dev Disabil Res Rev. 2010;16: 233–238.
36. de Wildt SN. Profound changes in drug metabolism enzymes and possible effects on drug therapy in neonates and children. Expert Opin Drug Metab Toxicol. 2011;7: 935–948.
37. Coté CJ, Ward RM, Lugo RA, et al. (section II, chapter 6). In: Coté CJ, Lerman J, Todres ID, (Eds). Pharmacokinetics and pharmacology of drugs used in children.
38. Hines RN. Developmental expression of drug metabolizing enzymes: Impact on disposition in neonates and young children. Int J Pharmdoi doi: 10.1016/j.ijpharm.2012.05.079.
39. Coté CJ, MD. Neonatal Anaesthesia. S Afr J Anaesthesiol Analg. 2010;16.
40. Shinwell ES, Eventov-Friedman S. Impact of perinatal corticosteroids on neuromotor development and outcome: Review of the literature and new meta-analysis. Semin Fetal Neonatal Med 2009;14:164–170.
41. Smits A, Kulo A, Verbesselt R, et al. Cefazolin plasma protein binding and its covariates in neonates. Eur J Clin Microbiol Infect Dis 2012;31:3359–3365.
42. Calder A, Bell GT, Andersson M, et al. Pharmacokinetic profiles of epidural bupivacaine and ropivacaine following single-shot and continuous epidural use in young infants. Pediatr Anesth. 2012;22:430–437.
43. Litman RS, Berger AA, Chhibber A. An evaluation of preoperative anxiety in a population of parents of infants and children undergoing ambulatory surgery. Paediatr Anaesth. 1996;6:443–447.
44. Wells LJ. Development of the human diaphragm and pleural sacs. In Contributions in Embryology, Washington DC. Carnegie Institution of Washington, 1954;35:109–159.
45. Camboulives J, Unal D. Anesthesia for congenital diaphragmatic hernia. Ann Anesthesiol Fr. 1980;2:135–141.
46. Guner YS, Khemani RG, Qureshi FG, et al. Outcome analysis of neonates with congenital diaphragmatic hernia treated with venovenous vs venoarterial extracorporeal membrane oxygenation. J Pediatr Surg. 2009;44(9):1691–1701.
47. Muratore CS, Utter S, Jaksic T, et al. Nutritional morbidity in survivors of congenital diaphragmatic hernia. J Pediatr Surg, 2001;36(8):1171–1176.
48. Bernbaum J, Schwartz IP, Gerdes M, et al. Survivors of extracorporeal membrane oxygenation at 1 year of age: the relationship of primary diagnosis with health and neuro-developmental sequelae. Pediatrics, 1995;96(5 Pt 1):907–913.
49. Diaz LK, Akpek EA, Dinavahi R, et al. Tracheoesophageal fistula and associated congenital heart disease: Implications for anesthetic management and survival. Pediatr Anesth. 2005;15:862–869.
50. Spitz L, Kiely EM, Morecroft JA, et al. Oesophageal atresia: At-risk groups for the 1990s. J Pediatr Surg, 1994;29:723–725.
51. Smith's anaesthesia for infants and children, 8th edn.
52. Houben CH, Curry JI. Current status of prenatal diagnosis, operative management and outcome of esophageal atresia/ tracheo-esophageal fistula. Prenat Diagn, 2008;28:667–675.
53. Crabbe DC. Isolated tracheo-oesophageal fistula.Paediatr Respir Rev. 2003;4:74–78.
54. Harjai MM, Holla RG, Kale R, et al. H-type tracheo-oesophageal fistula. Arch Dis Child Fetal Neonatal Ed. 2007.
55. Andropoulos DB, Rowe RW, Betts JM. Anaesthetic and surgical airway management during tracheo-oesophageal fistula repair. Pediatr Anesth. 1998;8:313–319.
56. Filston HC, Chitwood WR Jr, Schkolne B, et al. The Fogarty balloon catheter as an aid to management of the infant with esophageal atresia and tracheoesophageal fistula complicated by severe RDS or pneumonia. J Pediatr Surg. 1982;17: 149–151.
57. Reeves ST, Burt N, Smith CD. Is it time to reevaluate the airway management of tra-cheoesophageal fistula? Anesth Analg. 1995;81:866–869.
58. Salem MR, Wong AY, Lin YH, et al. Prevention of gastric distention during anesthesia for newborns with tracheoesophageal Fistulas. Anesthesiology 1973;38: 82–83.
59. Tokhais TA, Zamakhshary M, Aldekhayel S, et al. Thoracoscopic repair of tracheoesophageal fistulas: A case control matched study. Journal of Pediatric Surgery 2008;43: 805–809.

60. Richenbacher WE, Ballantine TV. Esopha–geal atresia, distal tracheoesophageal fistula, and an air shunt that compromised mechanical ventilation. J Pediatr Surg. 1990;25:1216–1218.

61. Cote, Lerman, Todres. Practice of Anaesthesia in infants and children. 4th edn.

62. Kovesi T, Rubin S. Long-term complications of congenital esophageal atresia and/or tracheoesophageal fistula. Chest. 2004;126:915–925.

63. Spitz L. Oesophageal atresia. Orphanet J Rare Dis. 2007; 2: 24.

64. Kovesi T, Rubin S. Long-term complications of congenital esophageal atresia and/or tracheoesophageal fistula. Chest 2004;126:915–925.

65. Anesthetic management of congenital tracheoesophageal fistula. Natasha Broemling and Fiona Campbell. Pediatric Anesthesia 2011;211092–1099.

66. Saxena AK, Hülskamp G, Schleef J, et al. Gastroschisis: 15 year, single-centre experience. Pediatr Surg Int. 2002;18:420–24.

67. Robinson JN, Abuhamad AZ. Abdominal wall and umbilical cord anomalies. Clin Perinatol. 2000;27:947–78.

68. Arnaoutoglou C, Pasqiuni L, Abel R, et al. Outcome of antenatally diagnosed fetal anterior abdominal wall defects from a single tertiary centre. Fetal Diagn Ther. 2008;24: 416–19.

69. Schuster SR. A new method for the staged repair of large omphaloceles. Surg Gynaec Obstet. 1967;125:837.

70. Greenwood RD, Rosenthal A, Nadal AS, et al. Cardiovascular malformations associated with omphalocoel. J Paediatr. 1974;85;818–821.

71. Wilson RD, Johnson MP. Congenital abdominal wall defects: An update. Fetal Diagn Ther. 2004;19:385–98.

72. Henrich K, Huemmer HP, Reingruber B, et al. Gastroschisis and omphalocele: Treatments and long-term outcomes. Pediatr Surg Int. 2008;24:167–73.

73. Yaster M, Buck JR, Dudgeon DL, et al. Hemodynamic effects of primary closure of omphalocele/gastroschisis in human newborns. Anesthesia. 1988;69:84–88.

74. Islam S. Clinical care outcomes in abdominal wall defects. Curr Opin Pediatr. 2008;20:305–10.

22

Anaesthesia for Paediatric Cardiovascular Surgery

Prasanna Salvi

INTRODUCTION

In the last three decades, tremendous improvements have been seen in the field of paediatric cardiac surgery, cardiology, anaesthesia, perfusion technology, intensive care as well as support systems like nursing and physiotherapy. Surgeries are now being performed in sicker as well as very small kids (premature) weighing as low as 550 gm. Any anaesthesiologist giving anaesthesia should be well versed with the pathophysiology of the lesion. A good TEAM is the key for the success of a paediatric cardiac surgical program (Fig. 22.1).

1. **Incidence:** The incidence of Congenital Heart Disease (CHD) is around 1% of all live births. Foetal echocardiography has made it possible to make an accurate diagnosis of CHD as early as 16 weeks of gestation. There are some lesions that are incompatible with life, while there are some (ASD, PDA, Bicuspid Aortic Valve) which may present later in life. CHD is more common in babies who are premature and SGA (small for gestational age), diabetic mothers, elderly mothers, consanguineous marriage, catch-22 spectrum and babies with trisomy-21 (Down's).[1]
2. **Prognosis:** The overall prognosis of these children has improved considerably. More emphasis is now laid on final corrective repair than on palliative procedures. Palliative procedures do still play a role in the optimisation of these sick kids, more so in the developing countries. With the knowledge of Extra Corporeal Membrane Oxygenation (ECMO) and cardiac transplantation, along with TEAM effort, more and more sicker and smaller babies are now being operated with favourable results.
3. **Spectrum of cases** (Fig. 22.2A to E):
   - Premature
   - Neonates
   - Infants
   - Adolescents
   - Adults (GUCH: Grown Up CHD)

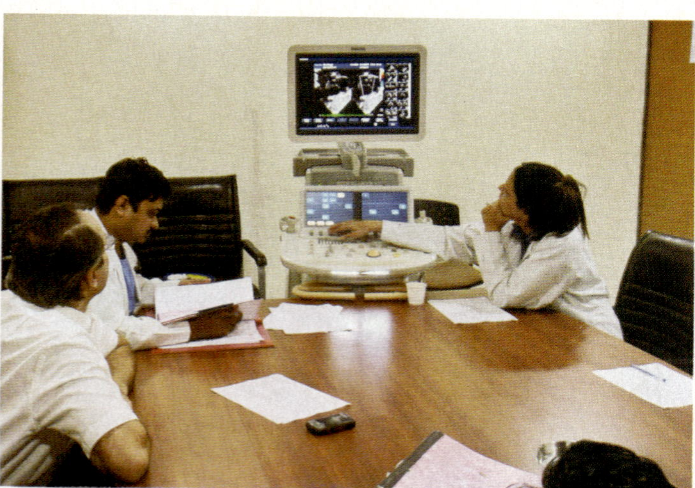

Fig. 22.1 Team work

FOETAL CIRCULATION

One needs to understand foetal circulation in order to understand the physiology of CHD. There is Ductus Venosus, Foramen Ovale and Ductus Arteriosus.

- **Ductus Venosus** carries oxygenated blood from the placenta through the umbilical vein to the liver and then to the inferior vena cava (IVC) into the right atrium.
- **Foramen Ovale:** Majority of the blood entering the right atrium from the IVC gets shunted to the left atrium through the foramen ovale.

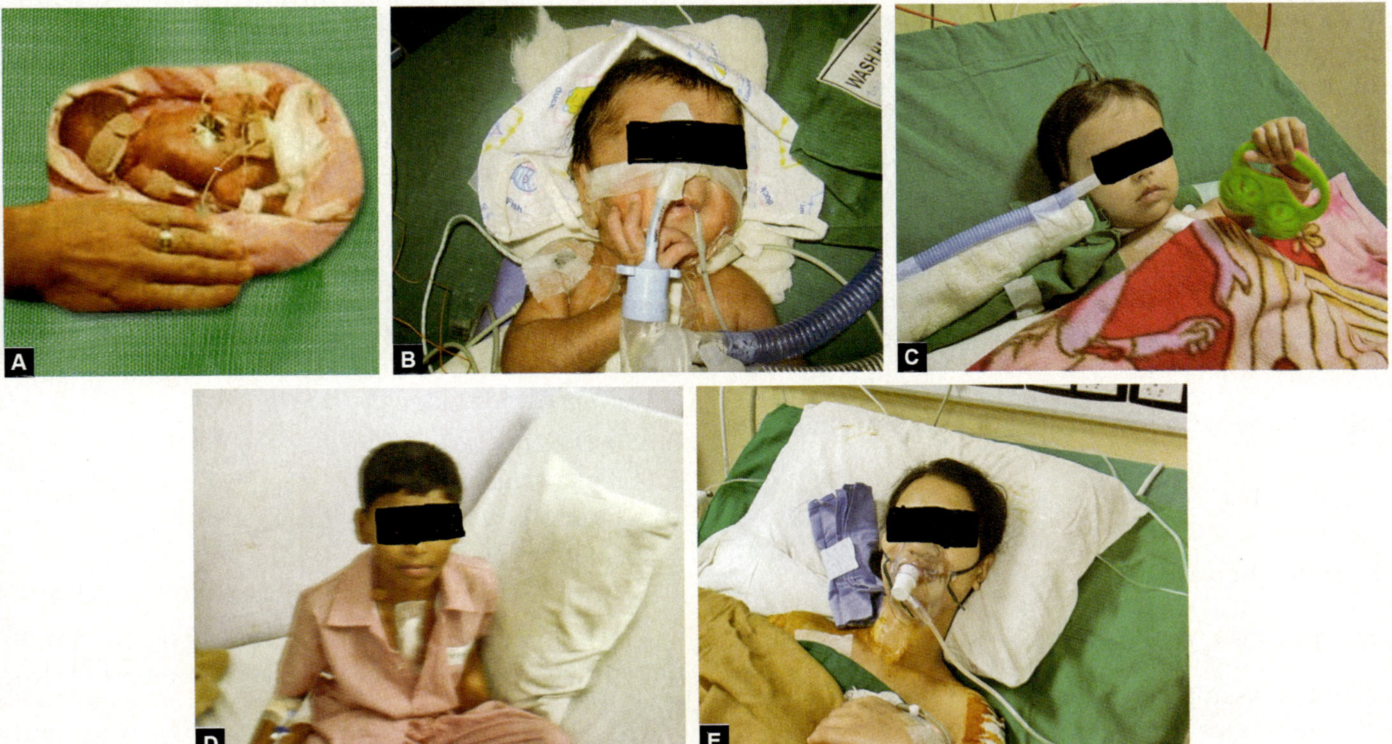

Fig. 22.2 (A) Premature, (B) Neonate, (C) Infant, (D) Adolescent and (E) Adult

Deoxygenated blood from the upper half of the body entering the right atrium via the superior vena cava enters predominantly into the right ventricle with only a small fraction crossing the left side through foramen ovale.

- **Ductus Arteriosus:** The RV blood then traverses via the ductus arteriosus into the descending aorta to supply the lower half of the body. The RV blood does not enter the pulmonary circulation as the pulmonary vascular resistance (PVR) is very high.

Take Home Message

1. High oxygen and glucose enriched blood entering the left atrium via foramen ovale perfuses the brain and the heart (coronaries)
2. In foetus, the circulation is parallel while in adult it is in series.

TRANSITIONAL CIRCULATION

At birth as the child cries, several modifications occur in the circulation so that the baby can adapt itself to the extrauterine life.

- Functional closure of the ductus arteriosus occurs within a few hours after birth. Anatomical closure may take several weeks.

High oxygen concentration causes the duct to constrict while a very low FiO_2 (fractional inspired oxygen concentration) causes the ductus to remain open. Hence in conditions where the patency of the ductus is obligatory for the survival of the child, the baby should preferably be ventilated with a very low FiO_2. Prostaglandin E_1 infusion (PGE_1) is started as it relaxes the ductal musculature. High doses of PGE_1 can cause apnoea and the baby may be needed to be supported by mechanical ventilation. Other side effects include seizures, systemic hypotension, inhibition of platelet aggregation, peripheral edema and unexplained fever.

- Functional closure of the ductus venosus and foramen ovale usually occur a few hours after birth. As the PVR falls, the pulmonary artery pressure also falls. It then becomes lower than the systemic pressure. The ductus shunts predominantly left to right. As a result, the left atrial pressure becomes more than the right atrial pressure and functionally closes the foramen ovale. Anatomical closure may not occur for months and about 25% of the adults still show probe patent foramen ovale.

In some defects like Tricuspid Atresia Type I, Pulmonary Atresia, Transposition of Great Arteries with intact septum, the foramen ovale and ductus may be necessary for the survival of the child. Hence an Emergency Balloon Atrial Septostomy (BAS) may be performed bedside under echo guidance and PGE_1 infusion is started to keep the duct open.

- The PVR which is very high in utero falls immediately after birth. It continues to fall down gradually till around 1–2 years of age.

If there are any intracardiac shunts like ASD, VSD, this decrease in PVR may cause increased pulmonary blood flow.

Factors which may prolong the transitional circulation

- Hypoxia
- Hypercarbia
- Acidosis
- Hypothermia
- Sepsis
- Prematurity
- CHD

ANATOMY OF CHILD'S HEART

1. The two ventricles are initially of the same size. As the pulmonary vascular resistance (PVR) decreases and the systemic vascular resistance (SVR) increases, the LV mass starts increasing as compared to the RV.
2. The heart is also structurally immature. There are fewer amounts of contractile proteins. The parasympathetic system is more dominant than the sympathetic system. Hence vagal response is more predominant. The vascular tone and the heart contractility is more dependent on exogenously administered catecholamines. Also exogenously administered calcium is required for its contractility as the sarcoplasmic reticulum is not well developed in premature hearts.
3. The compliance of the heart is also reduced. It becomes more sensitive to both volume as well as pressure overload. Also, the two ventricles are interrelated, such that dysfunction of any one ventricle leads to biventricular dysfunction. The neonatal heart depends on heart rate, contractility and rhythm to maintain its cardiac output.

CLASSIFICATION OF CONGENITAL HEART DEFECTS

1. **Increased pulmonary blood flow:**
   - Atrial septal defect
   - Ventricular septal defect
   - Patent ductus arteriosus
   - Endocardial cushion defects
   - *Transposition of great arteries*
   - Total anomalous pulmonary venous connection
   - *Truncus arteriosus*
   - *Single ventricle*
   - Anomalous origin of coronary arteries
2. **Decreased pulmonary blood flow:**
   - Tetralogy of Fallot
   - Pulmonary atresia
   - Tricuspid atresia
   - Ebstein anomaly
   - *Truncus arteriosus*
   - *Transposition of great arteries*
   - *Single ventricle with PS*
3. **Obstructive lesions**
   - Aortic stenosis
   - Pulmonary stenosis
   - Coarctation of aorta
   - Asymmetrical septal hypertrophy

The lesions in italics can fit into any of the two groups depending upon whether there is pulmonary obstruction or not.

It can also be broadly classified into two groups:

1. Those who have no cyanosis or **Acyanotic**
2. Those who have cyanosis or **Cyanotic**

Acyanotics usually have increased pulmonary blood flow and may be in congestive heart failure. Cyanotics, on the other hand, have decreased pulmonary blood flow causing hypoxaemia. One should note that a child may have increased pulmonary blood flow and still may be cyanotic and in congestive cardiac failure (TAPVC).

The PVR on the right side and the SVR on the left side play a vital role in the direction of these shunts. This is seen usually in large and non-obstructive shunts. The anaesthesiologist can manipulate the SVR and PVR by drugs, ventilation, thereby altering the shunt. This in turn helps to maintain better haemodynamics intra and postoperatively.

PULMONARY BLOOD FLOW

When the pulmonary blood flow is more than the systemic blood flow ($Q_p > Q_s$) as in ASD, VSD, there is increased lung water, increased airway pressure and resistance and decrease in pulmonary compliance. The lungs become stiffer with time. As the PVR drops gradually, the pulmonary blood flow (PBF) increases. This has a very damaging effect on the pulmonary vasculature. At some point of time, irreversible changes occur in the pulmonary vasculature with thickening of the vasculature. If left untreated, the PVR rises and the

Table 22.1 Normal pressures and saturations

	Pressure (mmHg)	Saturation (%)
SVC/IVC	—	70–75%
Right atrium	3–4	70–75%
Right ventricle	20/4	70–75%
Pulmonary artery	20/10	70–75%
Pulmonary capillary	7–9	—
Pulmonary vein	—	97%
Left atrium	7–8	97%
Left ventricle	100/8	97%
Aorta	100/60	97%

pulmonary artery pressures becomes more than the systemic pressures.

When the pulmonary blood flow is less than the systemic blood flow ($Q_p < Q_s$) as in TOF, there is mixing of venous (blue) and systemic (red) blood leading to hypoxaemia. In order to maintain oxygen transport, compensatory mechanisms like polycythemia, hyperventilation, increased blood volume, and development of Major Aorto-Pulmonary Collateral Arteries (MAPCAs) occur.

PREOPERATIVE ASSESSMENT

One should do a thorough preoperative assessment so as to get maximum information. One should be aware of the lesion and its pathophysiology. Like in olden days, History Taking and Physical Examination form the base of the preoperative assessment.

In CHD, associated other congenital anomalies may be present like macroglossia, micrognathia, cervical spine abnormalities. Down's babies have a large tongue. All these can cause difficulties during intubation.

Some of the kids present very early in life due to the complexity and severity of the lesion. The frequency of episodes (pneumonia/cyanotic spell) suggests the severity of the lesion.

Infants with increased pulmonary blood flow usually are in congestive cardiac failure. They may have failure to thrive, feeding difficulties, forehead sweating, suck-rest-suck cycle of feeding. They may have recurrent respiratory tract infections. They may have previous history of wheezing or hospitalization for the same (pneumonia). They may have tachycardia, tachypnoea, nasal flaring, subcostal/intercostal/suprasternal retractions, irritablility, cardiomegaly and hepatomegaly. Systemic hypoperfusion (due to increased PBF) results in pallor, feeble pulses and decreased capillary refill time. Any respiratory tract infection should be adequately treated before the child is taken up for surgery.[2] There is a higher incidence of respiratory and multiple postoperative complications. They stay longer in the ICU causing financial burden both on the parents as well as the hospital. Always optimise the child before taking up for surgery especially in elective and planned cases.

Infants with decreased pulmonary blood flow may be blue (cyanosis) or may become more blue with exercise, agitation or crying. They usually adapt themselves to the "squatting" position which helps to increase the SVR and thus increase the PBF by decreasing the right to left shunt. They may have episodes of loss of consciousness or seizures. They have increased tidal volume. Clubbing may be seen. They have exercise intolerance and have a blunted ventilatory response to hypoxia.

Wisdom Pearls

One should note that clinical cyanosis depends on the amount of de-oxygenated hemoglobin rather than on the oxygen saturation. For central cyanosis, more than 3 g/dL of arterial deoxygenated haemoglobin needs to be present.

Also cyanosis is less evident if a newborn has a very high proportion of foetal haemoglobin (Hbf).

Some of the children especially in developing countries like India, may present later in life. A child with a very large VSD may present with severe Pulmonary Arterial Hypertension (PAH) and significant cardiac dysfunction especially right ventricular dysfunction.

Talk to the paediatric cardiologist/surgeon/intensivist if you have any doubt.

PREOPERATIVE INVESTIGATIONS

Complete Blood Count

There is pallor or anaemia (nutritional) in patients with increased pulmonary blood flow like VSD due to poor feeding and congestive cardiac failure. High haemoglobin/haematocrit is an indicator of the severity of hypoxaemia and is seen in cyanotics (right to left shunts). Poor oral intake and iron deficiency can stop this increase in haematocrit and mislead the physician.

Increased WBC counts and a differential count may suggest of an ongoing/sub clinical infection. One needs to treat them with suitable antibiotics preoperatively so as to prevent postoperative respiratory and ventilatory complications.

PT/INR/aPTT/Bleeding Time/Clotting Time/Platelet Count and Smears

Those with polycythemia have coagulation abnormalities like thrombocytopenia, clotting factor deficiencies, fibrinolysis, DIC.[3] As blood is very thick, thrombosis is very common which may lead to cerebral, renal and pulmonary infarctions. Also dehydration due to long starvation periods may worsen the situation. Phlebotomy is indicated if the haematocrit is > 65%. This helps to reduce the viscosity and reduce the metabolic acidosis by improving tissue perfusion. There is less chance of bleeding in the postoperative period. Phlebotomy is usually performed in children > 5 years of age. 20 mL/kg body weight of patient's blood is replaced by plasma over a period of 1–2 hours.[4] In children less than 5 years of age, smaller volumes are replaced keeping a close watch on the haemodynamics. In adults, dextran can be used as a replacement solution in patients with heart failure.[5] **Consult a haematologist if required**. Ask for family history of bleeding tendencies.

Glucose and Electrolytes

Hypokalemia, hypocalcemia, hypoglycaemia, hypomagnesemia are very common. Hypocalcemia is common in children with DiGeorge syndrome. (DiGeorge-CHD with absent thymus with aortic arch abnormalities with left-sided obstructive lesions). Hypoglycaemia can aggravate heart failure.

Digoxin

Most of the patients are on Digoxin preoperatively. Intraoperative and postoperative rhythm issues have been seen in these patients and they are enhanced by hypokalemia, hypomagnesemia and increased S. creatinine. One may need to stop the drug preoperatively after checking the plasma drug levels.

Electrocardiography

Helps to know rhythm, chamber dilatation, hypertrophy, axis, electrolyte imbalance, heart blocks, etc.

Chest X-ray PA/Lateral

Gives valuable information about the pulmonary vascular congestion, pulmonary arterial hypertension, lung disease, airway compression, etc. Lateral X-ray is done in redo surgeries.

Sickling Test

Hypothermia, acidosis, anaemia as caused by CPB along with decreased perfusion pressures and the CPB circuit itself can cause sickling. Sickling occurs if haemoglobin S is present. If sickling test is positive, one needs to do a Hb electrophoresis. Exchange transfusion may be required.

Echo/Cardiac Cath/CT, MRI

Echocardiography (2D and Colour), Doppler assessments, cardiac catheterisation gives accurate information about the shunt size, gradients, cardiac function, vascular resistances and coronary anatomy.

NIL BY MOUTH AND PREMEDICATION

As per the standard guidelines, clear liquids can be given until 2–4 hours before surgery. Maintain hydration especially in cyanotics with a very high haematocrit. Keep the fasting period as low as possible. If required, an intravenous line may be placed and an infusion may be started.

Premedication is the first step towards a well-balanced anaesthesia. The arrival of a well sedated child in the operation room makes the induction of anaesthesia considerably smoother and stress free (Fig. 22.3). It reduces the dose of induction agents. In children with right to left shunts, consider a heavier premedication as crying and struggling during induction may precipitate a cyanotic spell.

Avoid premedication in neonates, prematures and sick children.

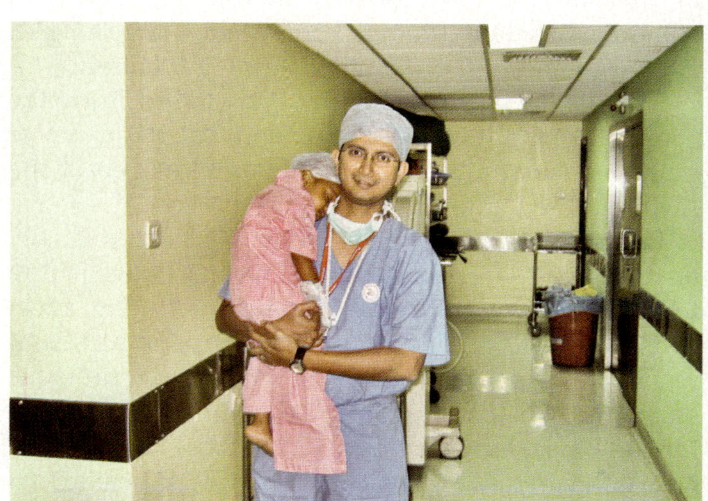

Fig. 22.3 Well sedated child

Some commonly administered premedication drugs are:

Syrup Pedichloryl	0.5 mL/kg
Injection Glycopyrrolate	5 μg/kg orally/IV
Midazolam	0.5 mg/kg orally
	0.2 mg/kg intranasally
Diazepam	0.2–0.4 mg/kg orally
Oral Transmucosal Fentanyl (Lozenge)	15–20 μg/kg[6]
Ketamine	5 mg/kg (IM/Intranasal)[7]

EQUIPMENT, POSITION AND MONITORING

Checklist

- Anaesthesia machine and circuit is checked.
- Intubation trolley is ready.
- All drugs are loaded in diluted form.
- All emergency drugs available in diluted form.
- OT ambient temperature adjusted to prevent hypothermia.
- Time out done.
- All lines (arterial/central) are available/IV fluids available.
- Fluid warmer/radiant warmer/heating blanket.
- Surgical instruments trolley prepared.
- Surgeon and perfusionist are inside the theatre, especially for sicker patients.
- External and internal defibrillator pads readily available and attached to mains.
- Blood is available and more so in redo surgeries.
- Heparin is loaded in case of redo surgeries.
- Femoral cannulation site marked in case of redo surgeries.
- Dual chamber pacemaker available.
- Coagulation analyzer in working condition.
- Infusion pumps 3–5 in number.
- Blood products—Whole Blood/Packed Cell/FFP/Platelets/Cryoprecipitate/Irradiated blood in patients with suspected absent thymus (DiGeorge) to prevent graft versus host reaction after transfusion.

Monitoring—Essential

- 12 lead ECG
- Invasive arterial and central venous lines
- Two pulse oximeters at two different places
- End tidal carbon dioxide
- Core/nasopharyngeal and skin temperature probes
- Trans-oesophageal echocardiography
- NIBP cuff
- Stethoscope.

Monitoring—Optional

- Cardiac output monitor
- Mixed venous oxygen saturation monitor
- Electroencephalography (EEG)
- Trans-cranial Doppler (TCD)
- Jugular venous saturation monitoring
- Near infra red spectroscopy (NIRS)

Air bubbles should be removed from the tubings of IV fluids. This should be done not only for patients with right to left shunts but for all patients. This is because even in patients with left to right shunts, there can be a transient reversal of shunt for a brief period in the cardiac cycle. Air filters can be used.

These small babies need to be positioned very carefully on the operating table. The operating table needs to be in working condition. All pressure points need to be padded to prevent pressure sores and brachial plexus injury especially in lateral thoracotomy positions. Prematures need to be handled very delicately.

Dosages

Inotropes infusions

Adrenaline	0.01–0.1 μg/kg/min
Nor-adrenaline	0.01–0.1 μg/kg/min
Isoprenaline	0.01–0.1 μg/kg/min
Dopamine	2–10 μg/kg/min
Dobutamine	2–10 μg/kg/min
Milrinone	50 μg/kg bolus followed by infusion of 0.375–0.8 μg/kg/min
Levosimendan	6–12 μg/kg bolus followed by infusion of 0.05–0.12 μg/kg/min

Vasodilator infusions

NTG	1–2 μg/kg/min
SNP	1–5 μg/kg/min
PGE_1	0.02–0.1 μg/kg/min

Antiarrhythmic drugs

Lidocaine	1–2 mg/kg bolus followed by 0.03 mg/kg/min infusion
Adenosine	0.15 mg/kg bolus (central line)
Procainamide	2 mg/kg over 5 mins

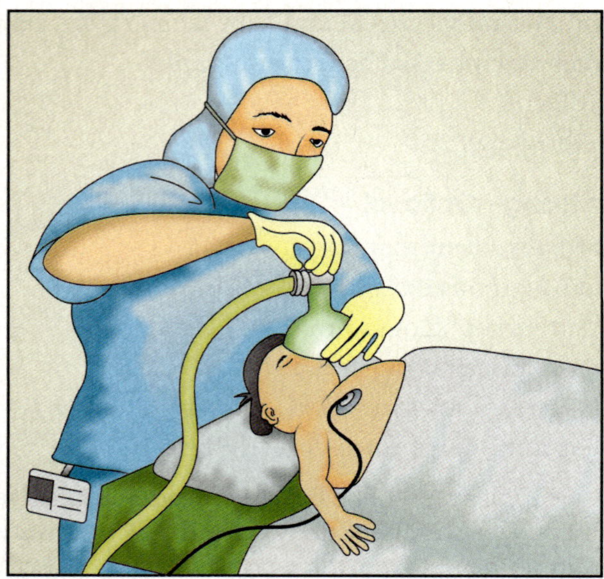

Fig. 22.4 Induction of anaesthesia

Amiodarone	5 mg/kg over 1 hr, then infusion of 5 mg/kg over 12 hrs
Beta blockers	
Propranolol	0.01–0.1 mg/kg
Esmolol	0.5–1 mg/kg bolus followed by 100–300 µg/kg/min infusion
Others	
Calcium chloride	10–20 mg/kg slowly
Sodium bicarbonate	1 mEq/kg
Phenylephrine	1–10 µg/kg
Heparin	3–4 mg/kg (1 mg = 100 units)
Protamine	3 mg/kg

INDUCTION OF ANAESTHESIA (Fig. 22.4)

Anaesthesia induction can lead to cardiac arrest especially in the sicker kids.[8–10] The arrest can occur in OT, Catheterisation Lab, or even during anaesthesia in remote locations.

If an intravenous line is not available, the child can be taken under anaesthesia with the help of inhalational agents.[11] One can immediately secure an intravenous line once the child is deep enough to allow it. In sicker kids, this should be preferably done by an experienced anaesthesiologist. If an intravenous line is available, one can do IV induction supported by inhalational induction. If the child is pre-medicated pretty well, it becomes very easy to separate the baby from the parents. A steal induction can also be performed in such patients. If the baby has a good cardiac reserve, there is a broad margin of safety. One should be very careful in sicker kids, especially in neonates and prematures, where there is a narrow margin of safety.

Intramuscular technique of induction is hardly used nowadays as it is very painful. It can be used in those children where intravenous line is difficult due to repeated prior surgeries or with history of long duration of hospitalisation. In sicker kids, it is preferable to put an intravenous line before induction, as they can be really unpredictable. They may not tolerate an inhalational induction.[12,13] They may crash on induction and may require inotropes or resuscitation drugs to be administered immediately.

In older children, one can put an intravenous line in the OR. One can apply Prilocaine cream at the site at least half hour before induction. Cyanotics usually have an IV line inserted so that IV fluids can be started preoperatively to maintain hydration.

Inhalational induction prolongs the induction in a right to left shunt[11] as the absorption of agent into the blood is delayed due to decreased pulmonary blood flow. In a left to right shunt, there is minimal effect on the speed of induction. Halothane is easily accepted by the child as it is non-irritant, causes smooth induction, bronchodilatation and relaxes the infundibular spasm (TOF). Halothane sensitizes the myocardium to the circulating catecholamines and can cause arrhythmias. It is now replaced with newer agents like isoflurane, sevoflurane[14–16] and desflurane. Isoflurane is irritant and can cause airway problems.[17]

Intravenous induction is faster in patients with right to left shunt as the pulmonary circulation is bypassed. In a left to right shunt, there is minimal effect on the speed of induction.

Dose of induction agents

Atropine	0.01–0.02 mg/kg
Glycopyrolate	5 µg/kg
Fentanyl	2–5 µg/kg
Midazolam	0.05–0.1 mg/kg
Sodium thiopental	3–5 mg/kg
Propofol	1–2 mg/kg
Ketamine	1–2 mg/kg
Scoline	1–2 mg/kg
Pancuronium	0.1 mg/kg
Vecuronium	0.1 mg/kg
Atracurium	0.5 mg/kg
Rocuronium	0.8 mg/kg

Nitrous oxide helps to maintain a stable plane of anaesthesia and prevent awareness especially in older kids. It can cause expansion of air emboli. One should not use nitrous oxide post cardio-pulmonary bypass. It has also been shown to have a negative inotropic and chronotropic effect.[18]

Most of the opioids cause bradycardia. Morphine if given rapidly can cause hypotension due to histamine release. To offset this, one can use muscle relaxants like pancuronium which causes tachycardia (cardiac output in smaller and sicker kids is rate dependent).

Pearls: Problems During Induction

1. Airway issues: Hypoxia, Hypercarbia.
2. Metabolic: Hypoxia and Hypercarbia can increase PVR. An existing left to right shunt may be reversed or a right to left shunt may worsen leading to metabolic acidosis and myocardial dysfunction.
3. Rhythm issues: Nodal, bradycardia, tachycardia, arrhythmias. A light plane of anaesthesia and electrolyte imbalance may worsen the situation.
4. Mechanical kinking of the endotracheal tube.
5. Difficult intubation, trauma while intubation, circuit leak or disconnection.

Induction Agents

Opioids

It can be used solely or in combination with other agents. They attenuate the stress response associated with intubation, surgical incision, sternotomy[19] and endotracheal tube suctioning. They are very useful in patients with severe pulmonary arterial hypertension (PAH) as they attenuate the pulmonary hypertensive response and help prevent what is known as pulmonary hypertensive crisis.

Opioids like morphine, fentanyl, alfentanil and sufentanil can be used.[20–24]

Propofol

It is a good induction agent with fast recovery.[25–27] It can be used in children more than 3 years of age. It can be used as a fast tracking agent.[28] It is said to have antioxidant and anti-inflammatory properties.

Etomidate

Dose is 0.3 mg/kg. It has a got a long duration of action. Decreased plasma cortisol levels are seen following induction of anaesthesia.[29]

Ketamine

It is useful in patients with right to left shunts like TOF where the drug bypasses the pulmonary circulation. It also causes increase in SVR, thereby reducing the magnitude of right to left shunt. It causes bronchodilation and secretions. Prior administration of glycopyrrolate can decrease the secretions. It also causes increase in PVR.[30]

Dexmedetomidine

It is an alpha 2 agonist. When used, it decreases the requirement of other agents like opioids and inhalational agents.[31] Bolus dose usually causes bradycardia. It is not to be used in patients who have rhythm disturbances or in patients with temporary or permanent pacemaker.[32] It is usually started as an infusion in the dose of 0.3–0.5 μg/kg/hr.[33]

MANIPULATION OF PVR AND SVR

Anaesthesiologist can to some degree manipulate the magnitude of intracardiac shunting by altering the PVR and SVR. As stated before, this is only possible in simple and unrestrictive shunts.

Pulmonary Vascular Resistance

Increase PVR

- Hypoxia
- Hypercarbia
- Acidosis
- Hyperinflation (PEEP)
- Atelectasis
- Sympathetic stimulation
- Hypothermia

Decrease PVR

- Hyperoxia
- Hypocarbia
- Alkalosis
- Normal FRC
- Drugs-NTG, SNP
- Milrinone (PDE_3 inhibitor)
- Sildenafil (PDE_5 inhibitor)
- Bosentan (endothelin receptor antagonist)[34]
- Prostaglandins (increase cAMP in vascular smooth muscle)[35]
- Levosimendan (Calcium sensitizer)
- Adenosine infusion (50 μg/kg/min)[36]
- Brain (or beta natriuretic peptide) secreted by ventricles of heart which increases cGMP[37]
- Inhaled nitric oxide—activates guanylate cyclase (Fig. 22.5)—cGMP-vasodilatation[38–40(a)]
- Inhaled NTG/SNP/Milrinone/Prostaglandin[41–43]

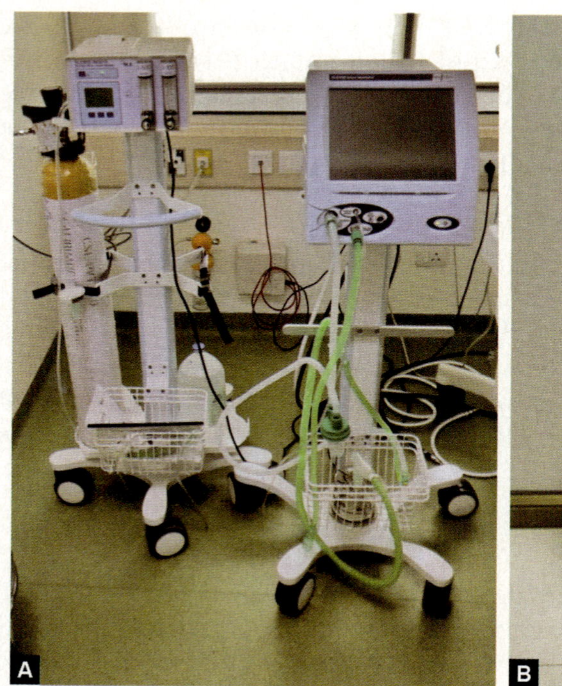
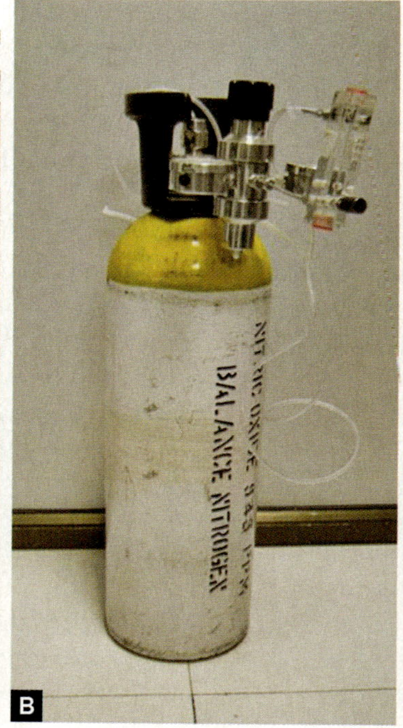

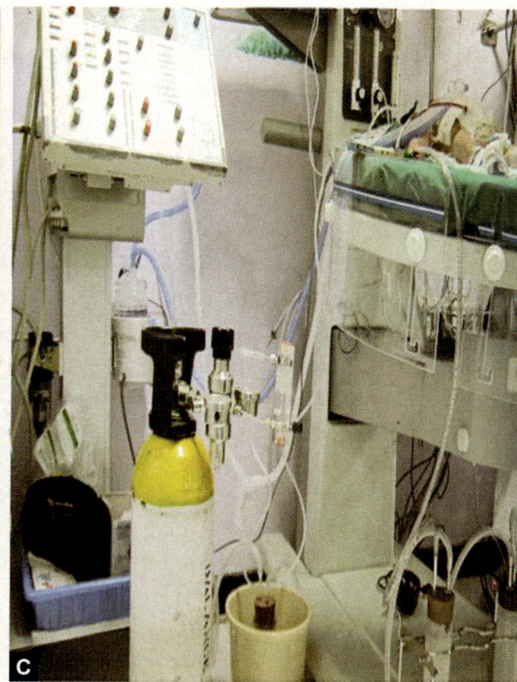

Fig. 22.5 (A) Nitric oxide and HFOV ventilator, (B) Nitric oxide cylinder and (C) Nitric oxide in progress

- Inhaled Prostaglandin I_2[44(b)]
- Inhaled Iloprost (Derivative of PGI_2[45]
- PGE_1

a. Disadvantages is that it can cause rebound pulmonary arterial hypertension, methhaemoglobin anaemia and NO_2 toxicity
b. Can cause bleeding due to platelet inhibition.

Systemic Vascular Resistance

In TOF, as the SVR increases, the right to left shunting decreases. One can use phenylephrine, ketamine, norepinephrine, manual external compression of abdominal aorta and squatting position.

MONITORING (Fig. 22.8)

There are some basic monitoring standards which are routinely followed in most of the paediatric cardiac surgeries. If facilities are available, some other advanced monitoring techniques can also be used.

Electrocardiogram (ECG)

A routine 5 lead ECG with ST analysis is used which helps to monitor the heart rate with the rhythm. One can detect arrhythmias, ischaemia, heart blocks or electrolyte imbalance with the help of ECG.

Invasive Blood Pressure Monitoring

Almost all of the surgeries require the insertion of an invasive arterial line. The advantages are that it is a continuous monitoring, beat to beat monitoring and one can do frequent blood sampling. Non-invasive blood pressure measurement can be done for some closed heart procedures like PDA especially in older kids. In some closed heart procedures like BT shunt, coarctation of aorta, PA banding, very large PDA (giant duct) invasive arterial line is a must as they cause a lot of variations in the blood pressure.

Arterial lines are usually inserted under strict aseptic precautions in neonates and small kids after general intubation. In older kids and adults, they can be inserted under sedation or local anaesthesia. The usual sites for insertion are radial and femoral and the not so usual sites are posterior tibial, axillary, dorsalis pedis and temporal arteries. A surgical cutdown may be required if one is not able to obtain an arterial line.

The site of insertion also plays an important role. In coarctation of aorta, one usually places the arterial catheter in the right radial artery and another one in the femoral artery. In a case of BT shunt, one usually places a radial artery catheter on the side opposite the shunt in redo surgeries, one of the femoral arterial site is kept exposed so as to go on an emergency bypass in case of any eventualities.

- < 5 kg—24 G cannula (Yellow)
- 5–20 kg—22 G cannula (Blue)
- > 20 kg—20 G cannula (Pink)

Central Venous Pressure (CVP)

It helps to monitor the right sided filling pressures, to give an infusion of vasoactive drugs and to give volume like crystalloid and colloids. They can be single, double, triple or five lumen catheters with a facility of placement of PA catheters or pacing catheters. The right internal jugular vein is the most preferred for cannulation. Other sites are left IJV, femoral vein. In surgeries like PDA and coarctation of aorta, it is better put the catheter in the left IJV as in a left thoracotomy position (right side down), there is a very high chance that the catheter can be kinked and get obstructed. In Glenn surgery, the catheter placed in the right IJV becomes a direct estimation of the pulmonary artery pressures once the superior vena cava is anastomosed to the right pulmonary artery.

Patient weight (kg)	Catheter size	Catheter length (cm)
< 2.5	3 F	5
2.5–6	4.5 F	6
7–20	5.5	8
> 20	7	12–15

Sometime, single lumen catheters are inserted into the left atrium or into the pulmonary artery. They are inserted by the surgeon intraoperatively. The catheter is placed into the LA/PA and it is then taken out subcutaneously through the skin and connected to the pressure transducer after meticulous deairing. This is very useful intra as well as postoperatively in surgeries like TAPVC, Truncus Arteriosus, Arterial Switch Operation, or in any conditions with a very reactive pulmonary vascular bed. The disadvantage is that they can cause bleeding and tamponade on removal especially if the child is crying. There is a very high chance of causing air embolism too.

It can also be inserted with a hybrid technique where the catheter is placed through a sheath into the superior vena cava and the surgeon then directs it into the PA intraoperatively just before coming off bypass. PA catheters with the facility to do mixed venous oximetry are also available in the market. The only disadvantage is that they require a 5F/6F sheath through which they can pass and hence it can be inserted only in older kids.

One can insert lines with the help of ultrasound too (Fig. 22.6).

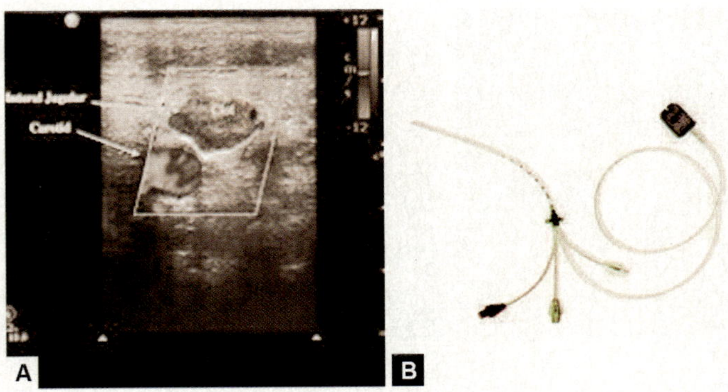

Fig. 22.6 (A) Ultrasound insertion of lines and (B) Mixed venous oxygen central venous catheter

Pulse Oximeter

It is a very useful monitoring tool in all cases. It is especially very useful in critical cases like BT shunt and PA band.

Temperature Monitoring

One can monitor brain, core and peripheral temperature with the help of nasopharyngeal, rectal and skin temperature. Even blood, esophageal, tympanic membrane and bladder temperature can be monitored. If there is a large gradient between core and peripheral temperature, it indicates inadequate perfusion. Also brain temperature is very important in cases which are done with deep hypothermic circulatory arrest (DHCA).

End Tidal CO_2

It is a very useful indicator of tracheal intubation. The values are not very reliable especially in cyanotic congenital heart disease. In surgery like PA band, a decrease in $ETCO_2$ is a good indicator of decrease in pulmonary blood flow after the placement of a band.

Transoesophageal Echocardiography (Fig. 22.7)

It is now available as adult, paediatric and neonatal (micro TEE) probes.

Probe	Weight (kg)
Adult	> 20
Paediatric	3–20
Neonatal(Micro TEE)	< 3

It ensures adequacy of surgical repair. It has a very crucial role in the operating room as well as in the ICU. Epicardial probes can also provide very valuable information. Always insert the probe with the bite guard so as to prevent damage to the probe. There are absolute and relative contraindications to the insertion of probe.

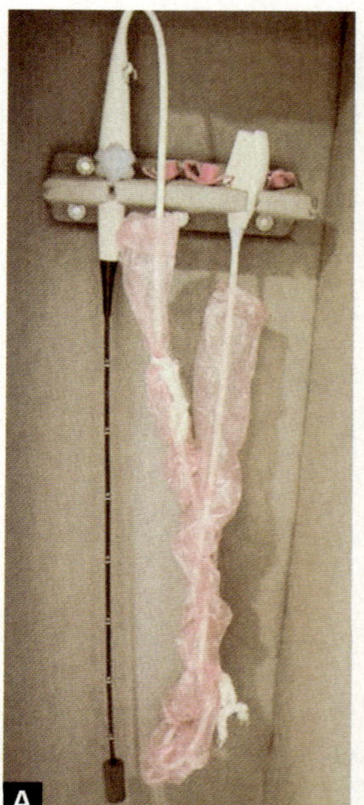

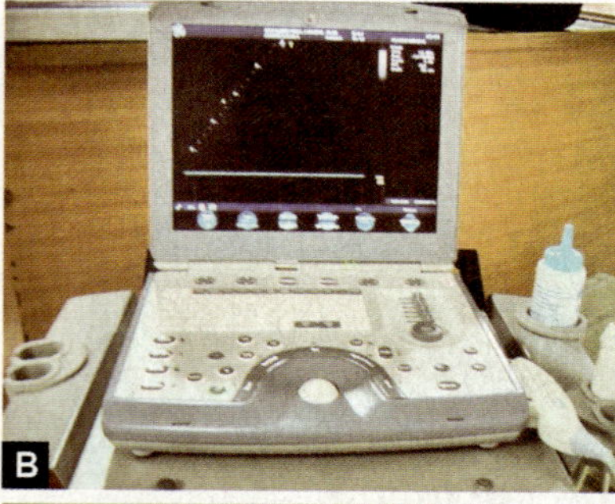

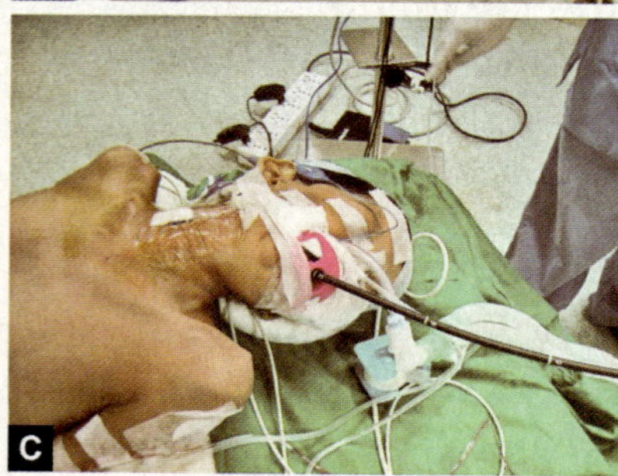

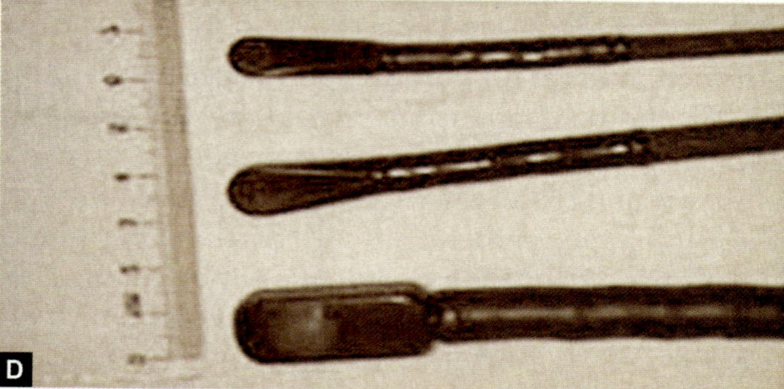

Fig. 22.7 (A) TOE probe, (B) Portable ECHO machine, (C) TOE probe *in situ* and (D) Different types of probes

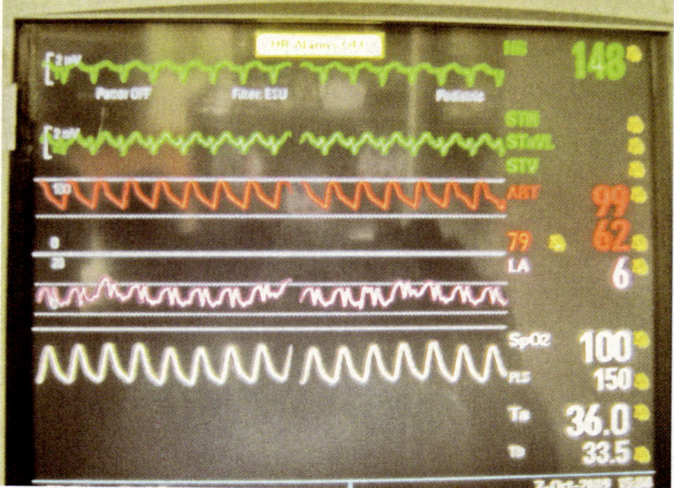

Fig. 22.8 Monitoring

Always remove the probe after protamine administration so as to prevent bleeding (Figs 22.7A to D).

Other Monitoring Modalities (Fig. 22.8)

- Continuous monitoring of cerebral saturation by Near Infrared Spectroscopy (NIRS).[46] It decreases at the commencement of CPB and increases after discontinuation.[47] In a study, values less than 45% for a long period of time were associated with significant psychomotor delays and MRI abnormalities.[48]
- Transcranial Doppler
- EEG, Computerised processed EEG
- Jugular venous blood saturation

CARDIOPULMONARY BYPASS (Fig. 22.9)

Almost all of the surgeries, except closed heart procedures are done with the help of cardiopulmonary bypass. There is a lot of difference in the CPB techniques in adults and paediatrics.

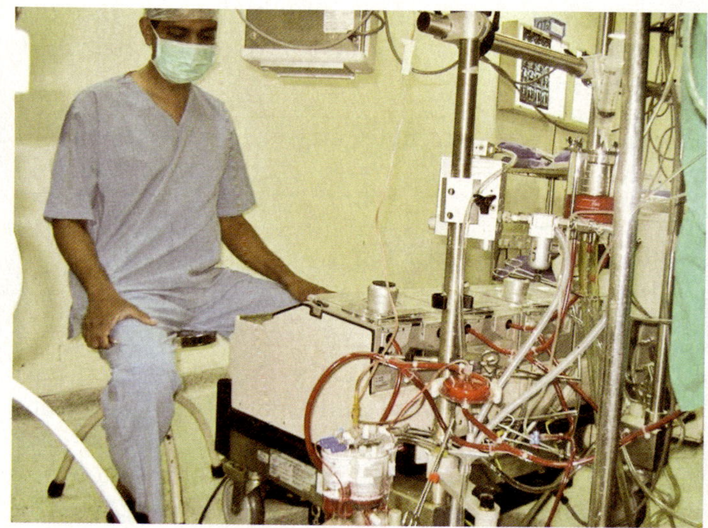

Fig. 22.9 CPB

In paediatrics, the circulating blood volume is less. So the blood is exposed to a relatively large artificial or prosthetic area (Tubings, Reservoir, Oxygenator). This can cause inflammation, oxidative stress, hemodilution, coagulation abnormalities and ischaemia reperfusion injury. This may all lead to low cardiac output, capillary leak and respiratory and pump failure in the post operative period.

The cannula sizes are very small. But even these small-sized cannulae can cause obstruction to the blood flow in the relatively small-sized vessels. The venous cannulae (SVC and IVC) can get obstructed or kinked during retraction of the heart or due to malposition leading to engorgement in the upper and lower extremity. After the patient is draped, one should always have a clear view of the forehead. The aortic cannula may also get dislodged or kinked which can be disastrous.

The CPB flow rates are higher in neonates and infants as compared to adults. The perfusion pressures are lower in children than in adults. The CPB flow rates need to be maintained for that particular temperature and body surface area. The perfusionist may flow at a lower rate which has a significant effect in the post-operative period. Hypoperfusion due to low flow rates may lead to low cardiac output and hyperlactatemia.[49]

In paediatrics a lot of surgeries are done under low to moderate hypothermia. This helps to provide organ protection. Also the pump flows can be reduced thus decreasing the trauma (to the blood) caused by CPB. Some surgeries may be done under deep hypothermic circulatory arrest.

Blood is usually added to the prime because a lot of hemodilution occurs on pump which decreases the oxygen carrying capacity. Anaerobic metabolism may take place if the circulating haematocrit is too low. With advances in perfusion technology, priming volume has considerably decreased. Newer circuits with priming volumes as low as 150–200 mL are now available in the market.

The ideal haematocrit accepted at most of the centres range between 21 and 25%.[50] Pre CPB filtration also reduces the priming volume.

All existing shunts like PDA/BT Shunt/MAPCAs must be ligated before going on pump so as to prevent systemic hypoperfusion.

Some patients have persistent left superior vena cava (LSVC) which usually drains into the coronary sinus. The LSVC in such cases has to be cannulated to ensure proper venous drainage.

CPB flow rates

Weight (kg)	CPB flow rates (mL/kg/min)
<3	150–200
3–10	125–175
10–15	120–150
15–30	100–120
30–50	75–100
50	50–75

Pre Bypass Checklist

- Baseline ABG after intubation.
- Aprotinin or tranexamic acid after confirming with the surgeon.
- Give heparin 3 mg/kg in acyanotics and 4 mg/kg in cyanotics (1 mg = 100 units).
- Check ACT after 3 mins and keep it above 480 secs.
- Maintain arterial blood pressure on the lower side of normal during aortic cannulation.
- If any pressures taken from any chamber of the heart, it has to be recorded in the anaesthesia sheet.
- Empty urine bag.
- Ventilate with 100% oxygen.
- Check for air bubbles in the aortic line after cannulation.
- Blood which is to added to the CPB prime to be double checked

Initiating Bypass

- Ensure all clamps removed
- Check aortic line pressure
- Check good venous return
- Clinically heart is empty
- Stop ventilation on full flows
- Record temperature to which patient is cooled
- If inotropes started prebypass, stop on bypass
- Bolus or continuous infusion of sedation and muscle relaxation
- Stop IV fluids
- Give any medications like phenoxybenzamine, lasix.

Monitoring on Bypass

- Pupillary size should be small and equal
- MAP should be 50–80 mmHg
- ABG done 5 mins after commencement of bypass and then every 30 mins
- Maintain ABG within normal limits
- Haematocrit maintained around 25% in children
- K^+ maintained around 4.00–5.00 meq/L
- ACT checked every hour and heparin administered to keep ACT > 450 secs.
- Cardioplegia every 20 mins unless requested otherwise
- Urine output 1–2 mL/kg/hr
- Blood sugar every hour. Up to 200 mg% acceptable in children
- Add insulin if sugars very high. Watch for potassium levels
- Record Aortic Cross Clamp time and CPB time
- Keep forehead open and watch for congestion

- SNP/Isoflurane/Sevoflurane continued on pump for uniform warming
- Rewarm slowly so as to keep an acceptable temperature gradient between the core and peripheral temperature.

Coming Of Bypass Checklist

- Is ABG satisfactory
- $S.K^+$ levels are acceptable
- Na^+, Cl^-, Ca^{++} and Mg^{++} levels are normal
- PCV >25%
- Nasopharyngeal temperature >37 °C
- Acceptable peripheral temperature
- Meticulous deairing done
- Ventilation with 100% oxygen and both lungs inflated
- No bleeding? Empty pleural spaces?
- Inotropes/vasodilators on flow if required and dose calculated
- ECG pattern
- Pacing box and cables available
- Blood and blood products available
- Urine bag empty
- Adequate surgical repair and myocardial function confirmed by TOE
- Watch for visual contractility of the heart
- Protamine and hydrocortisone loaded

In some patients, it may be difficult to wean them off from cardiopulmonary bypass. The reason may be pulmonary, cardiac or cardio-pulmonary. Such patients benefit from ECMO (Extra Corporeal Membrane Oxygenation). Recently a lot of patients are being put on ECMO and are also successfully weaned off.[51] Complications of ECMO include bleeding, tamponade and pulmonary haemorrhage.[52]

DEEP HYPOTHERMIC CIRCULATORY ARREST

Sometimes a very bloodless field may be required for the repair of complex lesions. At such times, DHCA provides ideal operating conditions. The patient is first cooled down gradually to 16°C and the circulation is arrested. A circulatory arrest time of 45 mins is well tolerated by the patient. If the surgeon is not able to complete the surgical procedure within 45 mins, DHCA is terminated and the surgery is then continued at very low flows. Many centres avoid DHCA and prefer low flows at deep hypothermia. The risk of developing neurological injury is very high after DHCA.[53,54] Some surgeons cannulate the innominate or the left common carotid artery for continuous cerebral perfusion.[55–57]

Surgeries done with the help of DHCA include:

a. Aortic arch reconstruction b. Norwood
c. Damus-Kaye-Stansel d. TAPVC

Steps

- Cooling the patient down to 16°C gradually with the help of CPB.
- Placing ice bags around the head of the patient.
- Ambient temperature of the OT is lowered.
- Barbiturates (Thiopental) before start of DHCA for cerebral protection.
- Methylprednisolone 30 mg/kg, 10 hrs preoperatively. attenuates the normal cerebral response to DHCA.[58]
- Avoid dextrose containing fluids or infusions.
- Sedation and muscle relaxation so as to decrease the metabolic rate.
- Calcium channel blockers and free radical scavengers prevent reperfusion injury.[59,60]
- Nasopharyngeal temperature probe to monitor brain temperature.
- Use of pH stat acid base management.
- EEG for brain activity.
- Correctly noting the DHCA time and warning the surgeon at the end of 45 mins.

MINIMALLY INVASIVE CARDIAC SURGERIES

With more emphasis now on cosmesis and with improvements in surgical techniques and the skill of the surgeon, many surgeries are now being performed with a very small incision. They include ASD, VSD, PDA, Partial AV canal, Sennings, etc. They are safe.[61] These patients are usually extubated in the operating room itself and can be shifted to the ward the very next day. As a result, the length of stay of the patient in the hospital is reduced. Video-assisted thoracoscopic PDA ligation is also being done.[62]

In the cardiac catheterisation lab too, most of the common heart defects like ASD,VSD and PDA are being closed by transcatheter "Amplatzer Devices"[63,64] (Fig. 22.10 A to C).

FAST TRACKING IN PAEDIATRIC CARDIAC SURGERY (Fig. 22.11)

With advances in surgical, anaesthesia and perfusion technology, a lot of patients are fast tracked and

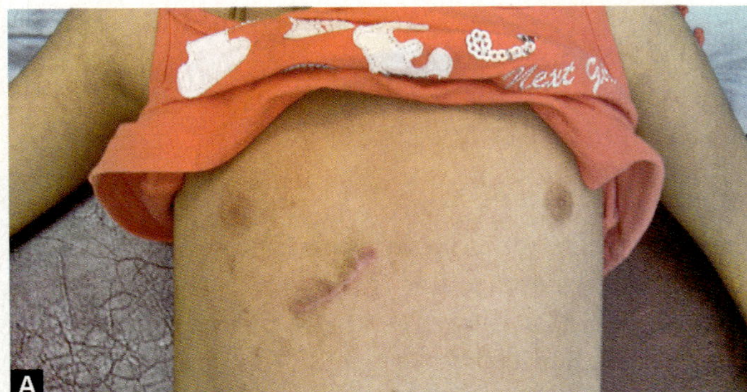
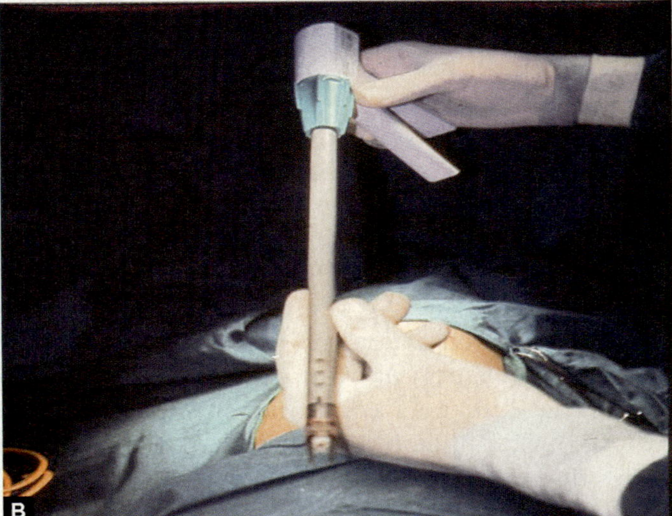
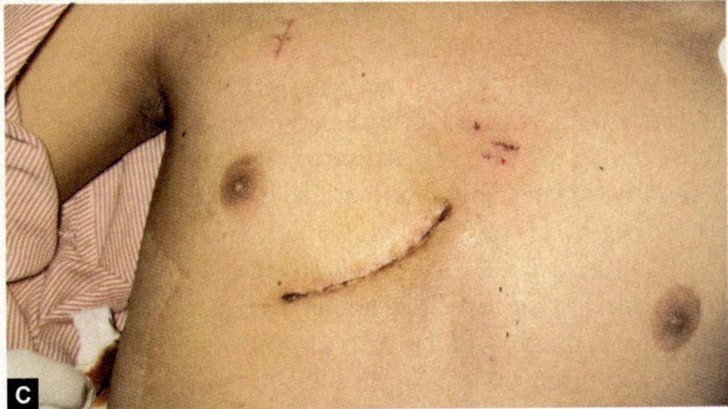

Fig. 22.10 (A) Scar of minimally invasive surgery, (B) Thoracoscopic PDA ligation and (C) Scar of minimally invasive surgery

extubated in the operating room itself. There has to be proper case selection and a lot depends on the skill of the anaesthesiologist. The anaesthesiologist has to reevaluate the patient at the end of surgery and depending upon the haemodynamic stability of the patient, take a decision to fast track and facilitate early extubation.[65]

Nowadays even infants with complex surgical procedures are being extubated on the operating table.[66]

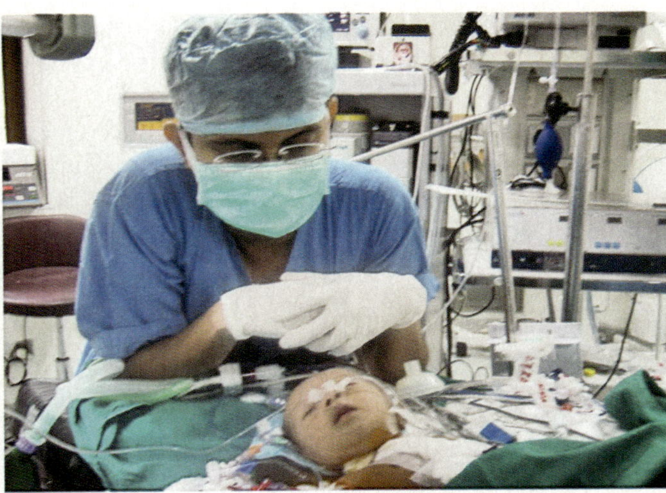

Fig. 22.11 Fast tracking in paediatric cardiac surgery

Fast Tracking—Risk Adjustment for Congenital Heart Surgery (RACHS)

1–2	Frequently eligible for fast tracking
3–4	Choose a fast tracking anaesthetic technique and re-evaluate them for early extubation at the end of the procedure
5–6	Not eligible

REGIONAL ANAESTHESIA

The main aim in combining regional with general anaesthesia is to fast track these patients and facilitate early extubation, provide good pain relief in the intra and postoperative period and thus maintain better haemodynamic stability of the patient. Opioids can be given intrathecally, epidural or as a single shot (caudal) with or without a local anaesthetic agent.

One should choose the right patient with no coagulation abnormalities and avoid postpuncture bleeding.[67–70]

Disadvantages is that it can cause vomiting, pruritus, urinary retention, respiratory depression leading to hypoxia and hypercarbia.[71]

ANAESTHESIA FOR CLOSED HEART PROCEDURES

Patent Ductus Arteriosus

Failure of the ductus arteriosus to close means that a left to right shunt exists from the aortic arch to the pulmonary artery. In premature, surgery is not advisable unless the patient is in gross congestive cardiac failure and is not able to wean from the ventilator. Medical management (Indomethacin/Ibuprofen) is usually tried before surgical closure is attempted. Medical management is rarely successful in very large ducts.

There is usually pulmonary congestion and oedema because of increased pulmonary blood flow. They are usually on digoxin and diuretics and may be on mechanical ventilation.

X-ray

- LA/LV dilatation
- RV dilatation
- Large pulmonary artery
- Large aorta
- Small aortic arch < PA diameter

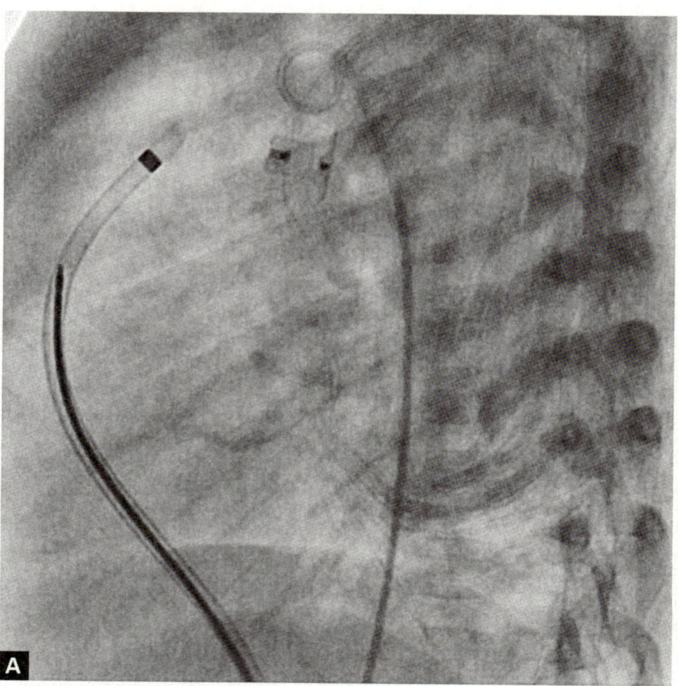

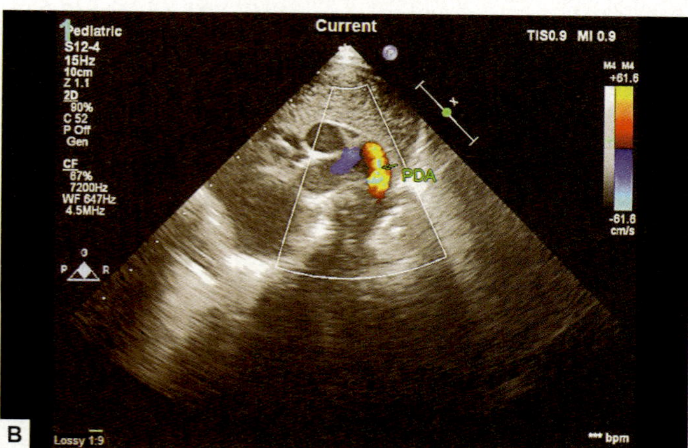

Fig. 22.12 **(A)** PDA device closure and **(B)** ECHO picture of PDA

ECG

- Left ventricular hypertrophy
- Left atrial enlargement
- Right ventricular hypertrophy

Surgical Procedures

1. Limited left thoracotomy with ligation of the duct
2. Clamped with vascular clips
3. Double ligation and division of the duct
4. Video assisted thoracoscopic PDA ligation
5. Catheter closure of PDA using disc devices, coils and buttons.

In premature, fractional inspired oxygen concentration should be as low as possible to prevent pulmonary oxygen toxicity and retrolental fibroplasia. Strict control of acid base status with electrolytes and prevention of hypothermia should be instituted. The OT ambient temperature should be kept at 24–26°C before the baby arrives. Strict fluid management as these patients are already in congestive cardiac failure. Some compromise in ventilation and pulmonary blood flow may occur with surgical manipulations like retraction of the lung. Judicious application of PEEP helps to improve oxygenation. But one needs to be very careful as this may injure the immature lungs. In premature, venous access can be difficult. Umbilical venous access can be used. A 22/24 G cannula may be inserted in the left internal jugular vein. Premature and neonates may be electively ventilated for some period of time till they become warm, haemodynamically stable, lungs are dry, all investigations are normal and acid base and electrolyte status is normalised. In neonates with a very large duct, one may feel the need to put an invasive arterial line. In such cases, the catheter is usually placed on the opposite side of the aortic arch. Umbilical artery can also be used. One should also rule out coarctation of aorta in such cases.

In older children, ECG, NIBP, pulse oximeter on right hand and foot, oesophageal stethoscope, $ETCO_2$ and peripheral temperature probe are useful monitoring tools. The importance of pulse oximeter on the foot is that there have been instances where the surgeon has accidentally ligated the descending aorta instead of the duct. After ligation of the PDA, the diastolic blood pressure increases. One can listen to the continuous machinery murmur of the PDA with the help of the bell of the stethoscope placed against the endotracheal tube. This murmur disappears after ligation. One should also be careful during patient positioning as it may cause pressure sores, brachial plexus injury.

Older patients can usually be extubated in the operating room itself. A good intercostal block along with intravenous pain killers and rectal suppository offers good pain relief in such patients.

Problems and Complications

- Ligation of the descending aorta or left pulmonary artery
- Bleeding
- Recurrent laryngeal nerve damage
- Ductal recanalization
- LV dysfunction caused by sudden increase in afterload

Co-arctation of Aorta (Fig. 22.13)

It is defined as the narrowing of the aorta which may be proximal, opposite or distal to the ductus arteriosus.

It accounts for 5–8% of congenital heart disease occurring in 1 in 3000 live births.

Symptoms	Signs
No symptoms	Hypertension
	Systolic murmur
	Feeble femoral pulse
	Radiofemoral delay

May be associated with bicuspid aortic valve, Turner syndrome, aortic stenosis and parachute mitral valve

In a preductal coarcatation, as the ductus arteriosus supplies the lower half of the body, collaterals do not form. The child is symptomatic with congestive cardiac failure due to increased LV afterload. PGE_1 infusion has to be started immediately to maintain the patency of the ductus.

In post ductal coarctation, collaterals are well formed in the foetal life. The child is asymptomatic. Systemic hypertension develops in the upper half of the body. There is decreased blood pressure distal to the coarctation.

Complications include sub-acute bacterial endocarditis (SABE), aortic dissection, and rupture, endarteritis, cerebral haemorrhage and LV failure.

X-ray

- Cardiomegaly
- Rib notching due to collateral circulation

ECG

- Left ventricular hypertrophy
- LV strain pattern

Surgical Procedures

- Left thoracotomy with resection and end-to-end anastomosis
- Subclavian flap angioplasty
- Patch augmentation
- Interposition graft
- Balloon dilatation/stenting in the cath lab.

Right radial and femoral artery are usually cannulated.[72] Femoral artery is cannulated to measure the perfusion of the distal aorta.

Blood loss should be anticipated especially in older kids where collaterals are well formed. Blood should be readily available in the OT. Two large bore venous access can be obtained after induction of anaesthesia. The perfusion pressure of the distal aorta should be maintained at around 40–50 mmHg. During the procedure, once the aorta is clamped, there is a sudden rise in the blood pressure in the upper half of the body. This surge in blood pressure can be controlled by the use of drugs like SNP, IV Labetalol and inhalational agents. One should not try to get down the blood pressure to near normal levels as the collateral circulation may be affected.

Of particular importance is the damage to the spinal cord which may occur during clamping of the aorta. The perfusion to the anterior spinal artery is compromised. This may result in paraesthesia and even paraplegia in the postoperative period. Monitoring somatosensory evoked potentials can be very useful. Other techniques like heparinised shunt, femorofemoral bypass and reimplantation of the intercostals arteries[73] can be done to improve the distal circulation. A small dose of steroid along with hypothermia are some of the strategies advocated for spine protection. Do not keep any warmer at the foot end of the patient. The heating blanket below the patient may also be switched off during the clamp.

After the clamp is released, the anaesthesiologist should anticipate some amount of blood loss. Also metabolic acidosis should be corrected by administration of sodium bicarbonate. SNP may be needed in the postoperative period to control hypertension.

Adequate pain relief may also help to control the hypertension. Thoracic epidural infusion of local anaesthetics along with narcotics, intravenous patient controlled analgesia, intravenous pain killers, rectal suppositories, intercostal block (with caution as collaterals are well formed and inadvertent intravenous instillation may occur). Older asymptomatic kids may

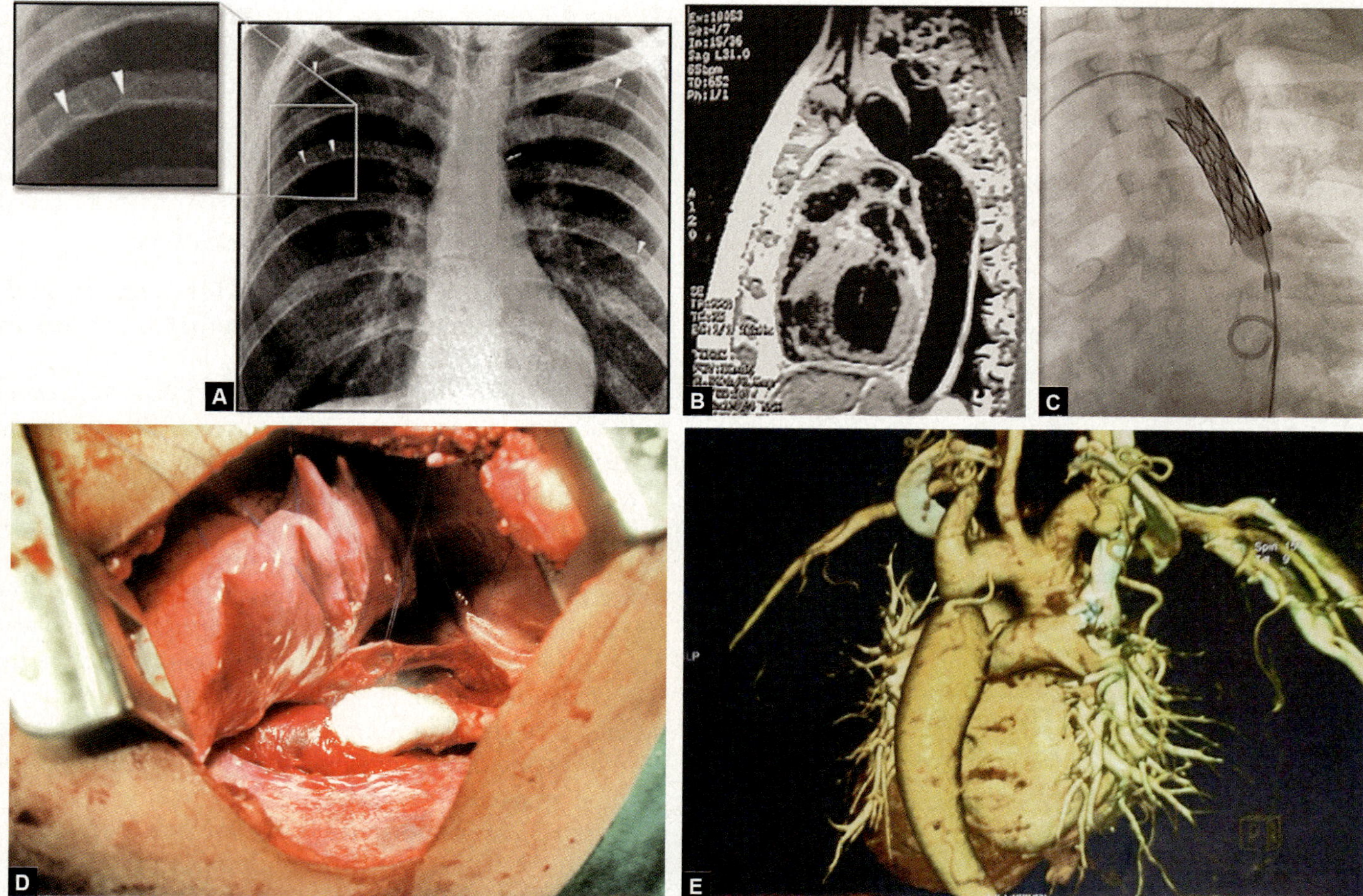

Fig. 22.13 (A) Rib notching, (B) Co-arctation of aorta, (C) Stenting, (D) Patch plasty and (E) Co-arctation of aorta (CT)

be extubated in the operating room itself. This also helps to get the blood pressure down to normal in the post-operative period. It also helps to perform a neurological examination in these patients. The smaller and sicker kids can be ventilated overnight.

Complications

- Paraplegia
- Bleeding
- Systemic hypertension
- Mesenteric arteritis
- Damage to left recurrent laryngeal nerve (vocal cord paralysis), phrenic nerve (diaphragm paralysis), thoracic duct (chylothorax) and sympathetic trunk (Horner syndrome).

Blalock-Taussig Shunt

This is a palliative procedure which is performed in conditions where the pulmonary blood flow is reduced and final or corrective surgery cannot be performed or is contraindicated. In developing countries due to financial constraints and inadequate facilities for open heart surgery, palliation in the form of shunts seems to be the only viable option.

Types

Shunt	Anastomosis
Classic B-T shunt	Right subclavian artery is ligated, disconnected and anastomsed to right pulmonary artery (end to side)
Modified B-T shunt	Interposition tube between right or left subclavian artery to right or left pulmonary artery (side to side)
Waterston shunt	Ascending aorta to right pulmonary artery

Contd...

Contd...

Shunt	Anastomosis
Potts shunt	Descending aorta to left pulmonary artery
Central shunt	Interposition tube between aorta and pulmonary artery.

Common defects for which a shunt is performed are Tetralogy of Fallot, tricuspid atresia, pulmonary atresia and single ventricle with pulmonary stenosis.

Radial artery cannulation should be done on the opposite side of the shunt. Midline sternotomy is usually preferred over the conventional thoracotomy.

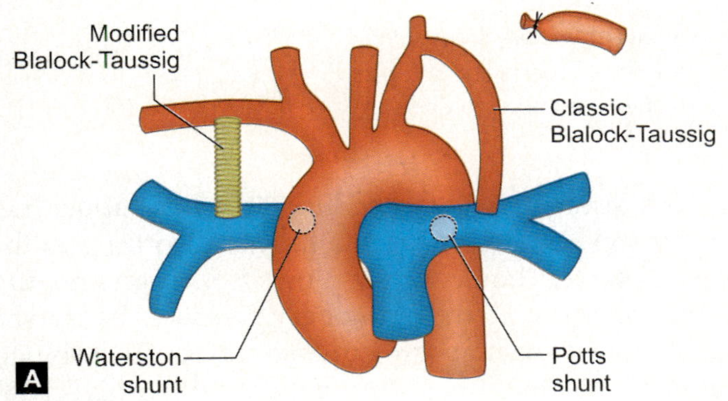

Fig. 22.14A Types of shunt

Retraction of the lung and a side clamp on the pulmonary artery may cause wide fluctuations in blood pressure and saturations. It is always empirical to ventilate with 100% oxygen. Bradycardia may occur. Inotropes may be needed in case of any myocardial dysfunction. Metabolic acidosis needs to be corrected promptly with sodium bicarbonate.

Some of the kids may have pulmonary blood flow which is totally dependent on the PDA. Care should be taken that the PGE_1 infusion should not be stopped but continued till the shunt is in place. Other kids may have a dynamic obstruction (TOF). A well balanced anaesthesia with an inhalational induction (halothane) relaxes the infundibular obstruction. One should use techniques to decrease the PVR so as to increase the pulmonary blood flow. Also the $ETCO_2$ underestimates the $PaCO_2$ because the pulmonary artery is clamped.

After the procedure the retracted lungs are re-expanded. One can hear the shunt murmur with the help of a bell of a stethoscope placed against the endotracheal tube (Fig. 22.15). On completion of surgery, there is increase in $ETCO_2$ (rise in pulmonary blood flow), decrease in diastolic blood pressure (run off) along with increase in saturations. The surgeon may decide to ligate the PDA or keep it open depending upon the final desired saturations.

The most common problems are given in Table 22.2.

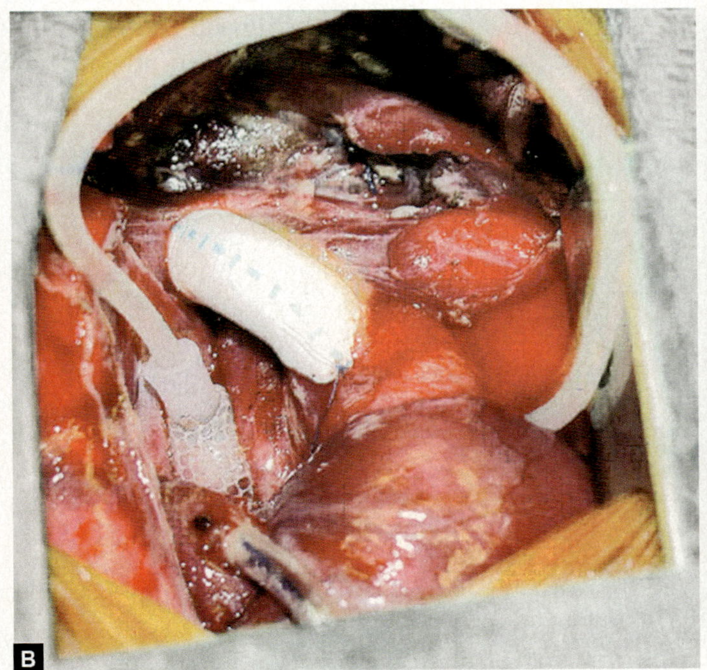

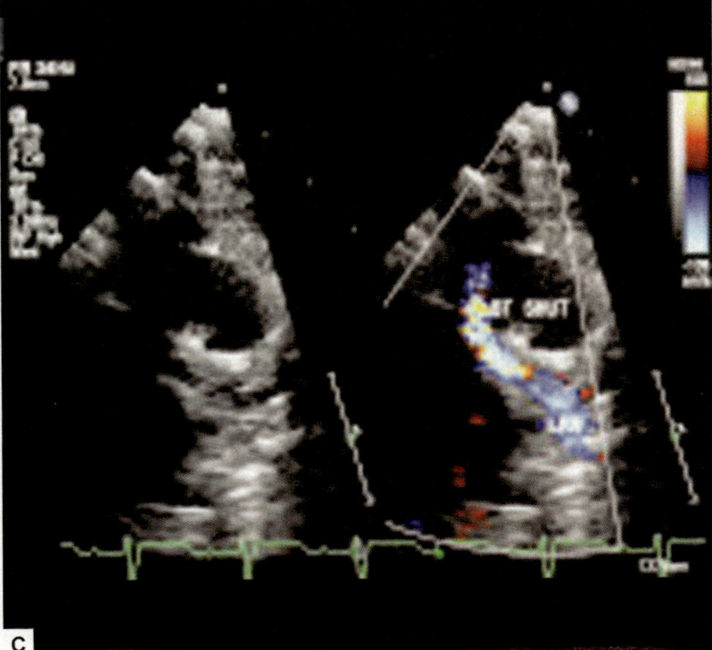

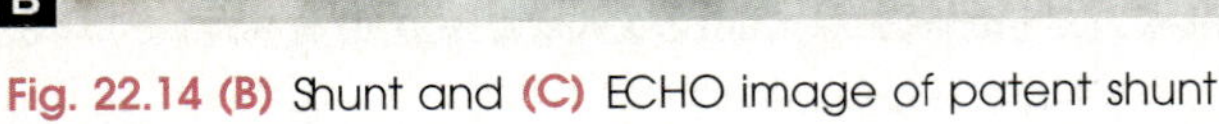

Fig. 22.14 (B) Shunt and (C) ECHO image of patent shunt

Table 22.2 Problems encountered in BT shunt

Shunt blockage	Shunt overflow
• Mechanical obstruction due to retraction, kinking or thrombosis • Shunt murmur not appreciated • Low saturations • Hypoxia eventually leading to cardiac failure	• Decrease in mean arterial blood pressure by 10 mmHg • Low diastolic blood pressure • Systemic hypoperfusion • Pulmonary edema • Metabolic acidosis • Very high saturations
Plan: • Get a 2D echo done immediately • High oxygen concentration • Heparin bolus followed by infusion • Keep ACT between 150 and 200 secs • No PEEP • Manoeuvres to decrease PVR • Inotropes may be required • Suitable corrective measures • Shunt revision if indicated	**Plan:** • Get a 2D echo done immediately • Keep FiO_2 as low as possible • PEEP • Manoeuvres to increase PVR • Diuretics • Inotropes may be needed • Correct metabolic acidosis • Shunt revision to decrease size of the shunt

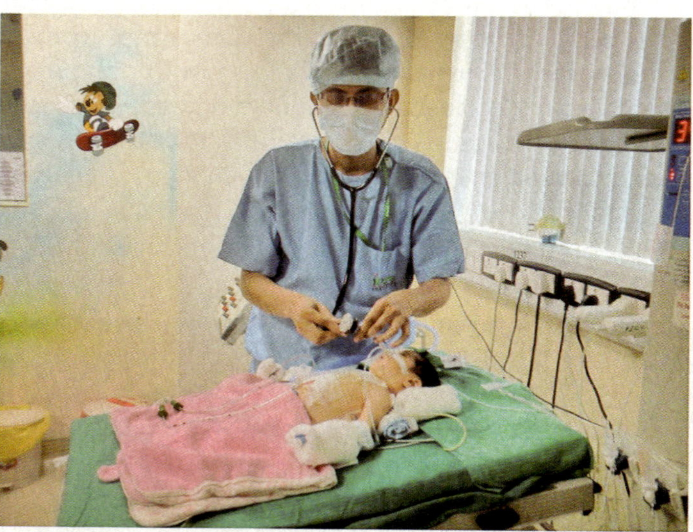

Fig. 22.15 Shunt murmur heard with bell of stethoscope

The older kids may be extubated in the operating room itself. The smaller and sicker ones can be ventilated overnight and extubated once they become stable.

Bidirectional Glenn Shunt

This is an end to side anastomosis between the superior vena cava (SVC) and the right pulmonary artery (RPA). The SVC-RA junction is completely transected and the SVC is then anastomosed to the RPA. It is usually done in patients who have a hypoplastic RV or LV and where two ventricular repair cannot be done.

As a result, deoxygenated blood from the upper half of the body is directed to the lungs. According to the law of physics, liquid always flows from high pressure to low pressure. So the pulmonary pressures have to be lower than the venous pressures so as to push the blood forward into the lungs. Any patient with a high PVR becomes unsuitable for surgery.

Manoeuvres to lower the PVR should be instituted postoperatively. The main pulmonary artery can be left alone (pulsatile Glenn) or can be ligated (non-pulsatile Glenn) depending upon the pulmonary artery pressures.

It can be done with or without the help of CPB[74] (Fig. 22.16).

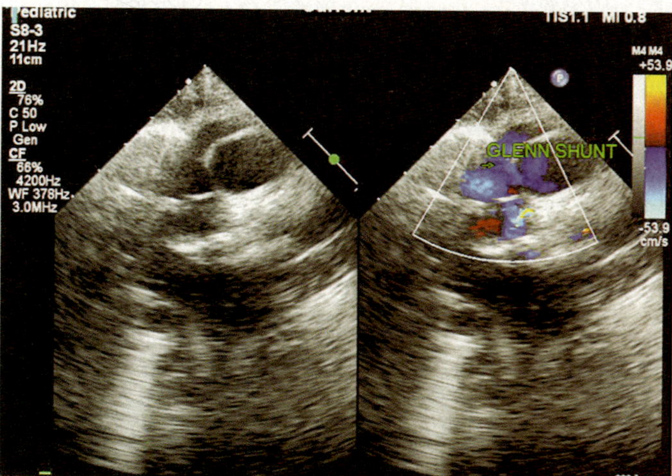

Fig. 22.16 ECHO picture of BDG

Advantages

- Increase in pulmonary blood flow
- Decreases the volume overload of the heart
- Less distortion of pulmonary artery
- Prevents development of pulmonary arterial hypertension

Complications

- Obstruction may cause venous congestion of the upper half of the body leading to SVC syndrome.
- Decreased pulmonary blood flow due to obstruction
- Arterio-venous fistula.

Pulmonary Artery (PA) Banding

In some defects, the pulmonary blood flow is very large like in univentricular hearts, truncus arteriosus, large VSD and multiple Swiss cheese VSD. In some of these cases, final or corrective repair may not be possible. If the pulmonary circulation is exposed to such high flows, irreversible changes occur in the pulmonary vasculature leading to pulmonary arterial hypertension. Hence PA banding is performed as a palliative procedure in order to protect the pulmonary vasculature in those cases where primary repair is not possible. Corrective and final surgery can then be performed at a later date when the child grows up. PA banding is also done so as to train the regressing left ventricle prior to Arterial Switch Operation.

A band is placed (mersilene tape) around the pulmonary artery. There are various formulas by which the PA band tightening is done. It also depends whether it is being performed for univentricular hearts or biventricular hearts or for transposition of great arteries for training the regressing left ventricle.

These kids are usually very sick and in severe congestive cardiac failure. Systemic hypoperfusion may occur due to increased pulmonary blood flow. The surgeon can manually occlude the PA by the finger. Keep the PVR high and SVR low. Do not use any agents which may cause myocardial depression. One should have a good working pulse oximeter placed at two positions. The surgeon places the band around the PA and tightens it slowly so that the pulmonary artery pressure falls to half or one-third of the systemic pressures. The systemic blood pressure increases with tightening of the band as more blood enters the systemic circulation.

End tidal CO_2 and pulse oximeter are very useful monitoring tools during the procedure.[75]

Problems

Too tight band	Too loose band
• Severe hypoxaemia • Severe RV dysfunction • Impending cardiac arrest • Right to left shunting • Migration of the band along with distortion or stenosis of branch PAs	• PBF still high • Objective of surgery not achieved

These kids are usually very sick and may be ventilated overnight.

An emergency debanding may be required in the operating room or in the ICU, if the band is too tight causing severe hypoxaemia and severe RV dysfunction with an impending cardiac arrest

ANAESTHESIA FOR OPEN HEART PROCEDURES

Atrial Septal Defect

There is a defect in the interatrial septum resulting in a communication between the right and left atrium. It is more common in females than in males.

Types

- Ostium secundum: Area fossalis, most common
- Ostium primum: Lower down in the septum and associated with a cleft in the anterior leaflet of the mitral valve.
- Sinus venosus defect: Junction of SVC and RA and associated with anomalous pulmonary venous return.
- Coronary sinus (Unroofed): Absent septation between the post wall of left atrium and coronary sinus. Usually associated with LSVC.

Pathophysiology

There is shunting of blood from the left atrium to the right atrium. The direction of flow depends on the pressures in the respective atria. This in turn depends on the end diastolic pressures of the respective ventricles. There is increased blood supply to lungs. In a moderate shunt, ($Q_p/Q_s = 1.5$). In large shunts ($Q_p/Q_s = 3$).

Q_p = Pulmonary flow

Q_s = Systemic flow

X-ray

- RA/RV Enlargement (Cardiomegaly)
- Increased bronchovascular markings
- Prominent pulmonary artery

ECG

- Right axis deviation
- RBBB
- Left axis deviation in primum defect
- Prolonged PR interval

Surgical Procedures

Surgery is usually advised before 4–5 years of age.

- Mid sternotomy ASD closure
- Minimally invasive ASD closure
- Robotic ASD closure
- Device closures of ASD in the cath lab

Anaesthesia Considerations

These patients are usually not sick. A good premedication with a balanced anaesthesia technique can be used successfully. The choice of muscle relaxants depends on the anaesthesiologist. Drugs like atracurium can be used as these patients can be fast tracked and early extubation facilitated. One can use more of inhalational agents and less of narcotics so as to achieve this goal.

As in all cardiac surgeries, one must avoid air in the intravenous lines, because even though the shunt is left to right, paradoxical air embolism can occur at some point in the cardiac cycle. Manoeuvres to increase the PVR can be employed pre-CPB so as to decrease the shunt fraction. One can decrease the PVR post-correction. The CPB time is usually very small and not much hypothermia is used. For small defects (direct closure), fibrillation can be used after the aorta is cross clamped.

Take Home Message

- Before the surgeon inserts the venous cannulae, the anaesthesiologist should put some PEEP on the ventilator so as to prevent air getting sucked into the right atrium through the cannula.
- The CVP is not a reliable indicator of right heart filling pressures in the postoperative period. The right atrium is dilated, especially in very large shunts. So, if one tries to rely on the CVP measurement to replace the volume and maintain a normal CVP of 6–8 mmHg, there is a very high chance that one can volume overload the patient.

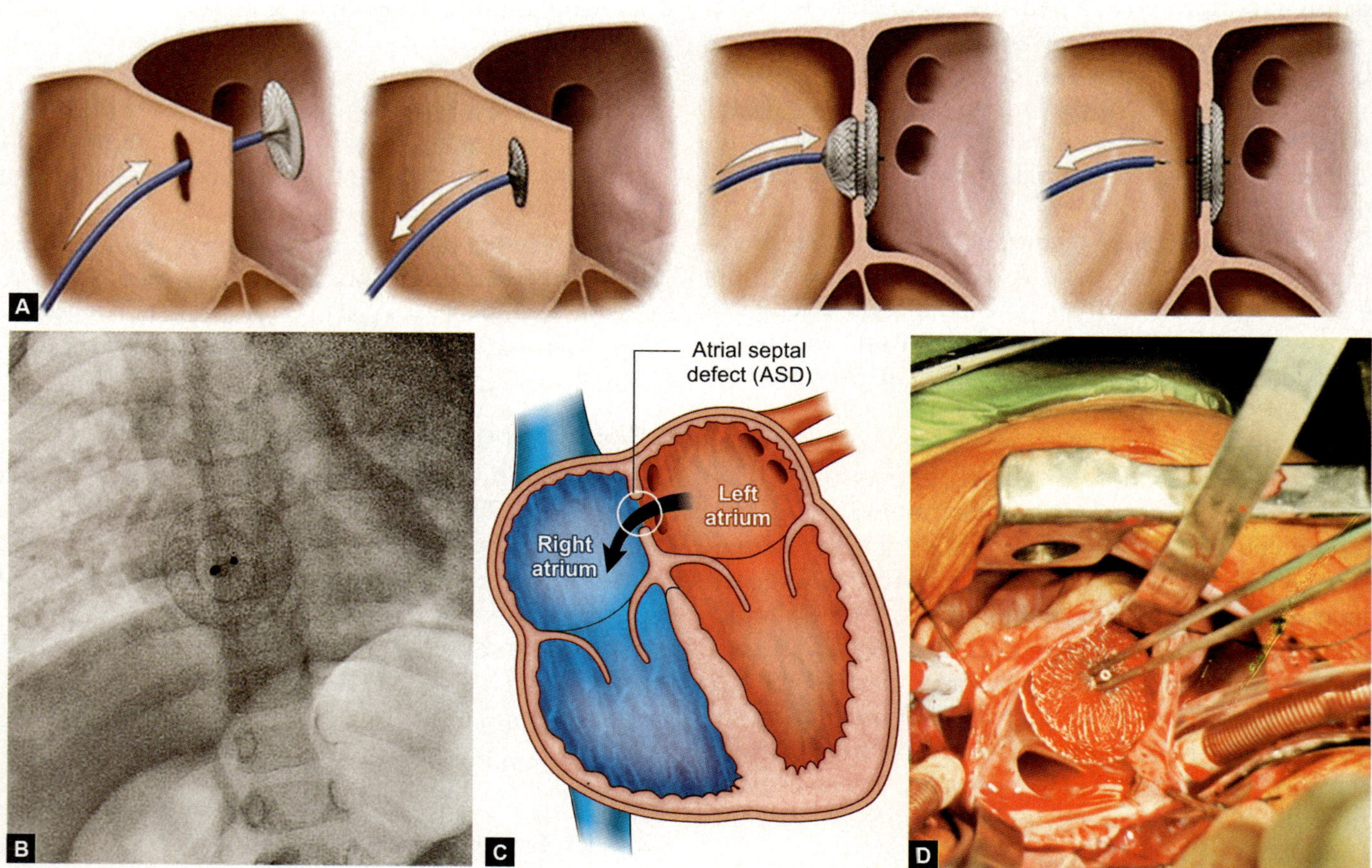

Fig. 22.17 (A) Steps of ASD device closure, (B) ASD device (amplatzer), (C) ASD and (D) Surgical removal of an ASD device which was embolised in cath lab

Problems and Complications

- Supraventricular arrhythmias like atrial flutter, atrial fibrillation
- Nodal or junctional rhythm
- Heart block and mitral regurgitation in Ostium primum repairs
- Residual defects
- Missed partial anomalous pulmonary venous return may result in residual left to right shunt
- Pulmonary edema if patient is overtransfused
- Device embolisation in the cath lab.

Ventricular Septal Defect

It is defined as a deficiency in the interventricular septum. The septum has a perimembranous, inlet, outlet and muscular extension.

Types

- Perimembranous/Infracristal/Subaortic VSD
- Subarterial/Supracristal/Subpulmonic VSD
- Inlet or canal type VSD
- Muscular VSD
- Apical VSD
- Multiple/Swiss Cheese VSD

In a small defect (restrictive VSD), there is a very high gradient across the VSD.

In a large defect (non-restrictiveVSD), there is a very small gradient across the VSD.

Note: So, higher the gradient across the VSD smaller is the defect and smaller the gradient, larger is the defect.

Pathophysiology

The blood is shunted from the left ventricle to the right ventricle. The PVR is about one-fifth of the SVR. Due to increased pulmonary blood flow, there is dilatation of the pulmonary artery, left atrium and left ventricle. If the defect is large or non-restrictive, the child develops symptoms by around one month of age when the PVR starts falling leading to increased pulmonary blood flow. There is tachycardia, tachypnoea, failure to thrive, forehead sweating, suck-rest-suck cycle and increased respiratory tract infections. There may be pallor. If this defect remains unrepaired, the high PBF causes irreversible changes to occur in the pulmonary vasculature. At one point of time, the pulmonary pressures become more than the systemic pressures. This causes the shunt to flow from right to left causing hypoxaemia.

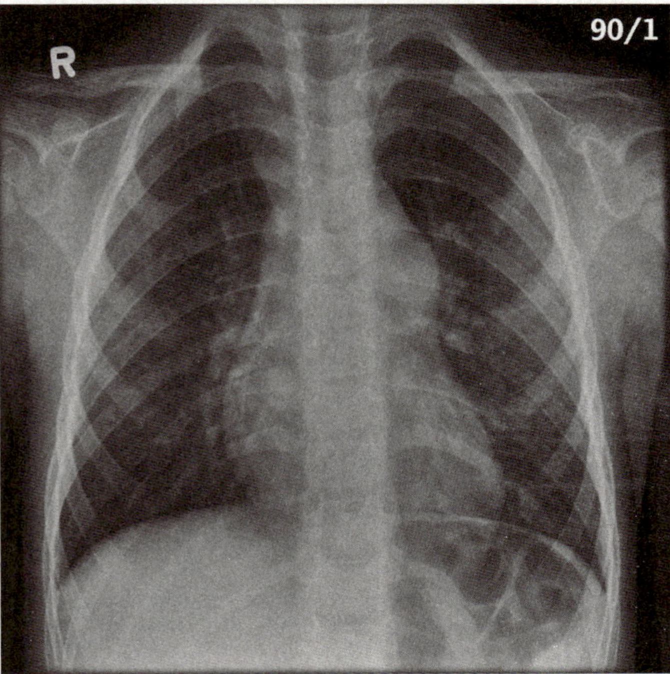

Fig. 22.18 X-ray picture in VSD

This is known as "Eisenmenger Complex". At this stage, surgery is not possible and the child can just be treated symptomatically so as to improve the quality of life.

X-ray (Fig. 22.18)

- Cardiomegaly
- LA/LV dilatation
- Dilated PAs and branch PAs
- Increased bronchovascular markings
- Normal heart and peripheral pruning in "Eisenmenger Complex".

ECG

- LVH
- RVH
- RBBB

Surgical Procedures

- VSD closure
- VSD device closure in cath labs
- Hybrid procedures (combined surgical and device closure in the operating room)
- PA banding as a palliative procedure in very sick neonates or infants with multiple VSDs so as to limit the pulmonary blood flow. Final corrective repair can be done at a later date when the child is old enough to take the stress of CPB.

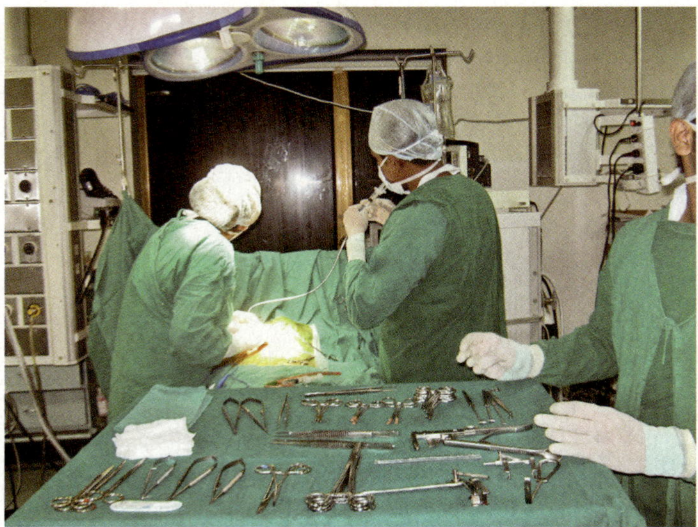

Fig. 22.19 Hybrid VSD closure

Anaesthesia Considerations

Patients with a very large defect, who are in congestive cardiac failure with severe failure to thrive and frequent respiratory tract infections (H/o hospital admission for pneumonia) may require surgery very early in life (around 3–4 months of age). These patients need to be optimised preoperatively. They are usually on digoxin, diuretics and Enalapril. Antibiotics may be started in the preoperative period if the child has an ongoing respiratory tract infection. These patients usually do not require much premedication preoperatively. It also depends on the clinical condition and the cardiac reserve of the patient.

Opioids can be used for induction if the kid is sick with limited cardiac reserve. Inhalational agents can be used in older kids. It is better to keep the fractional

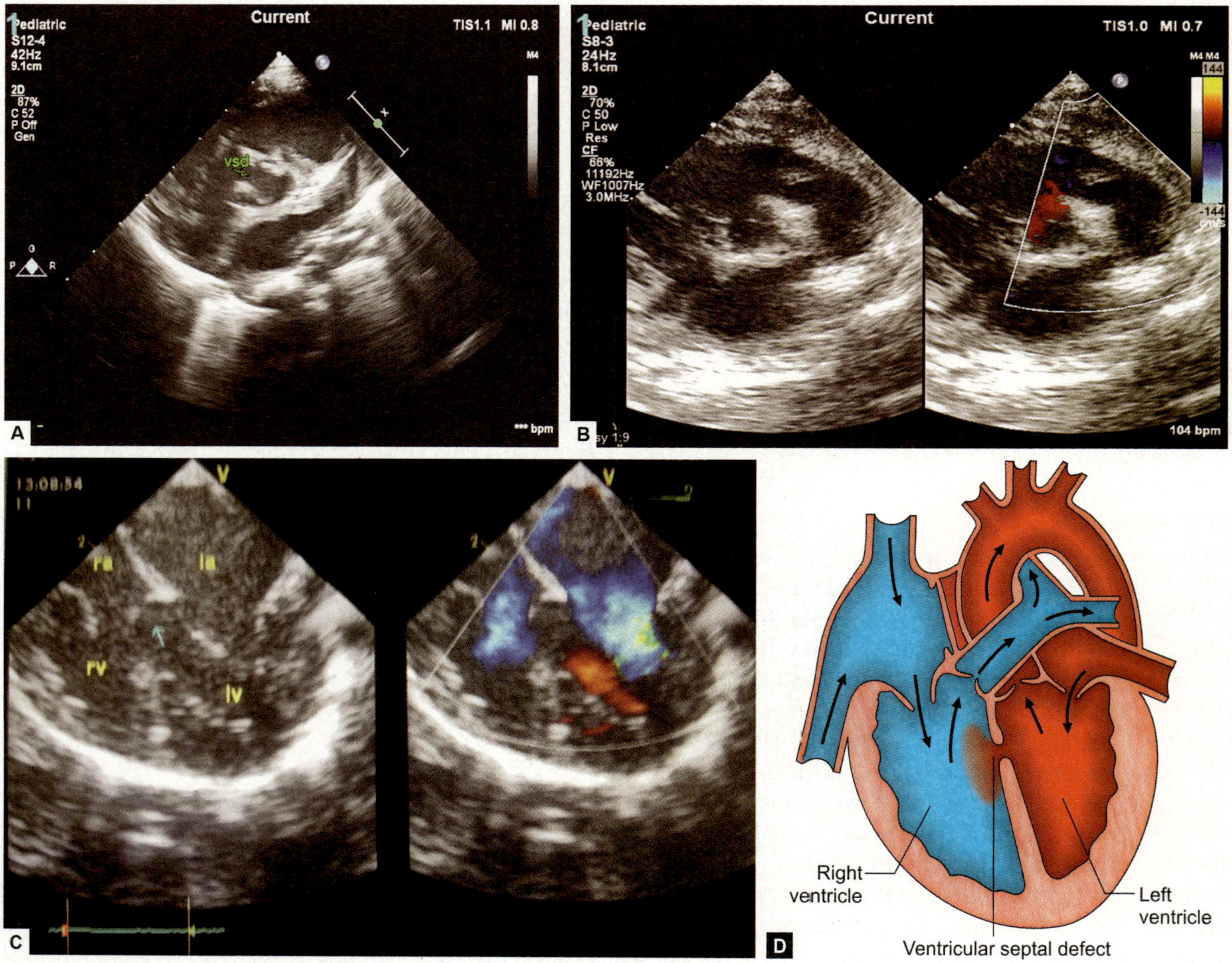

A
Current
TIS1.1 MI 0.8
vsd
B
Current
TIS1.0 MI 0.7
104 bpm
C
D
Right ventricle
Left ventricle
Ventricular septal defect

Fig. 22.20 (A) to (C) ECHO pictures of VSD and (D) VSD

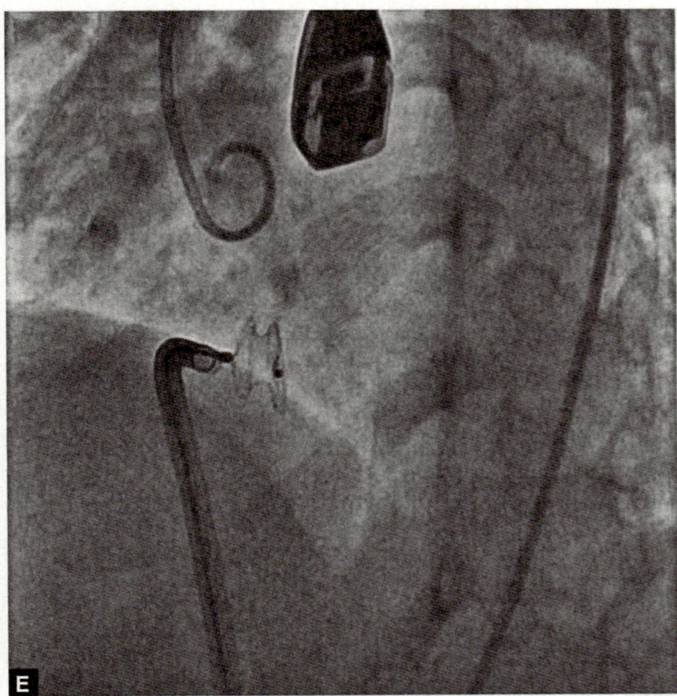

Fig. 22.20E VSD device closure

inspired oxygen concentration to as low as normal. One can maintain some degree of hypercarbia in the pre bypass period. This helps to decrease the left to right shunting across the VSD. One must be very meticulous in avoiding any air bubbles in the intravenous lines.

In patients with a reactive pulmonary vasculature or in patients with severe pulmonary arterial hypertension, one should hyperventilate in the post bypass period. Hypocarbia with hyperoxia without any PEEP helps to decrease the PVR and prevent pulmonary hypertensive crisis. Manoeuvres to decrease the PVR may be instituted in the postoperative period. Inotropes may be required. Inhaled nitric oxide along with Sildenafil and Bosentan may be required in the postoperative period to decrease the PVR.

In very small infants, DHCA at 18°C may be used. The older kids who have a relatively good cardiac reserve can be extubated within a few hours of surgery. Smaller and sicker kids may require prolonged ventilation.

Problems and Complications

- Residual VSD
- Pulmonary arterial hypertension and RV dysfunction
- LV dysfunction especially in LV ventriculotomy
- Ventricular outflow tract obstruction due to patch
- Heart block
- Low cardiac output
- Device embolisation in cath lab

Tetralogy of Fallot

It is defined as the cephaloanterior displacement of the conotruncal septum resulting in ventricular septal defect, overriding of aorta, right ventricular outflow tract obstruction and right ventricular hypertrophy.

The right ventricular tract obstruction may be subvalvar/valvar/supravalvar.

Associated Anomalies

- Right aortic arch
- Left superior vena cava
- ASD, PDA, CoA
- Abnormal distribution of coronary artery
- Coronary artery crossing right outflow tract
- Dextrocardia
- Abnormalities in the branch pulmonary arteries

Pink tets

They have mild stenosis of the right ventricular outflow tract with a large VSD with a left to right shunting across it. They usually have a smooth course in the postoperative period and respond well to intravenous volume.

Blue Tets

They have severe stenosis of the right ventricular outflow tract with a large VSD with a right to left shunting across it. They usually have a very stormy course in the postoperative period and respond well to inotropes.

Pathophysiology

As there is right ventricular outflow tract obstruction, there is reduced pulmonary blood flow and right to left shunting across the VSD. The severity of stenosis determines the degree of cyanosis and the occurrence of cyanotic spells. A decrease in SVR and increase in PVR results in worsening of right to left shunt.

Cyanotic spells are paroxysmal spells which usually occur when the child cries early in the morning resulting in deepening of cyanosis, tachypnoea and may lead to unconsciousness due to temporary cerebral ischaemia.

Treatment of Cynotic Spells

- Attach ECG, NIBP, pulse oximeter and call for help
- Immediate intravenous line
- 100% humidified oxygen

- Volume bolus which helps to open the RVOT. Rule out dehydration.
- Knee chest position or squatting position so as to increase the SVR. External compression of the abdominal aorta.
- Morphine/fentanyl to sedate the baby
- Phenylephrine 1–10 µg/kg which increases the SVR
- IV Propranolol 0.1 mg/kg
- Esmolol 100–200 µg/kg/min to slow the HR and relax infundibular spasm[76]
- Sodium bicarbonate to correct metabolic acidosis
- If it still persists, endotracheal intubation and ventilation

X-ray

- Boot-shaped heart due to the upward displacement of the RV due to right ventricular hypertrophy
- Oligemic lung fields
- Concave PA segment
- Small pulmonary artery
- Dilated aorta

ECG

- RAD (+120 to +150°)
- Tall R in V1

Surgical Procedures

- Palliative shunts like modified BT shunts.
- Intracardiac repair (ICR) which consists of VSD closure with infundibular resection of muscle bundle with or without a transannular patch with ligation of a previous B-T shunt if present.
- RV to PA conduit if there is pulmonary atresia or some branch (conal branch) of the coronary artery crossing the RVOT.

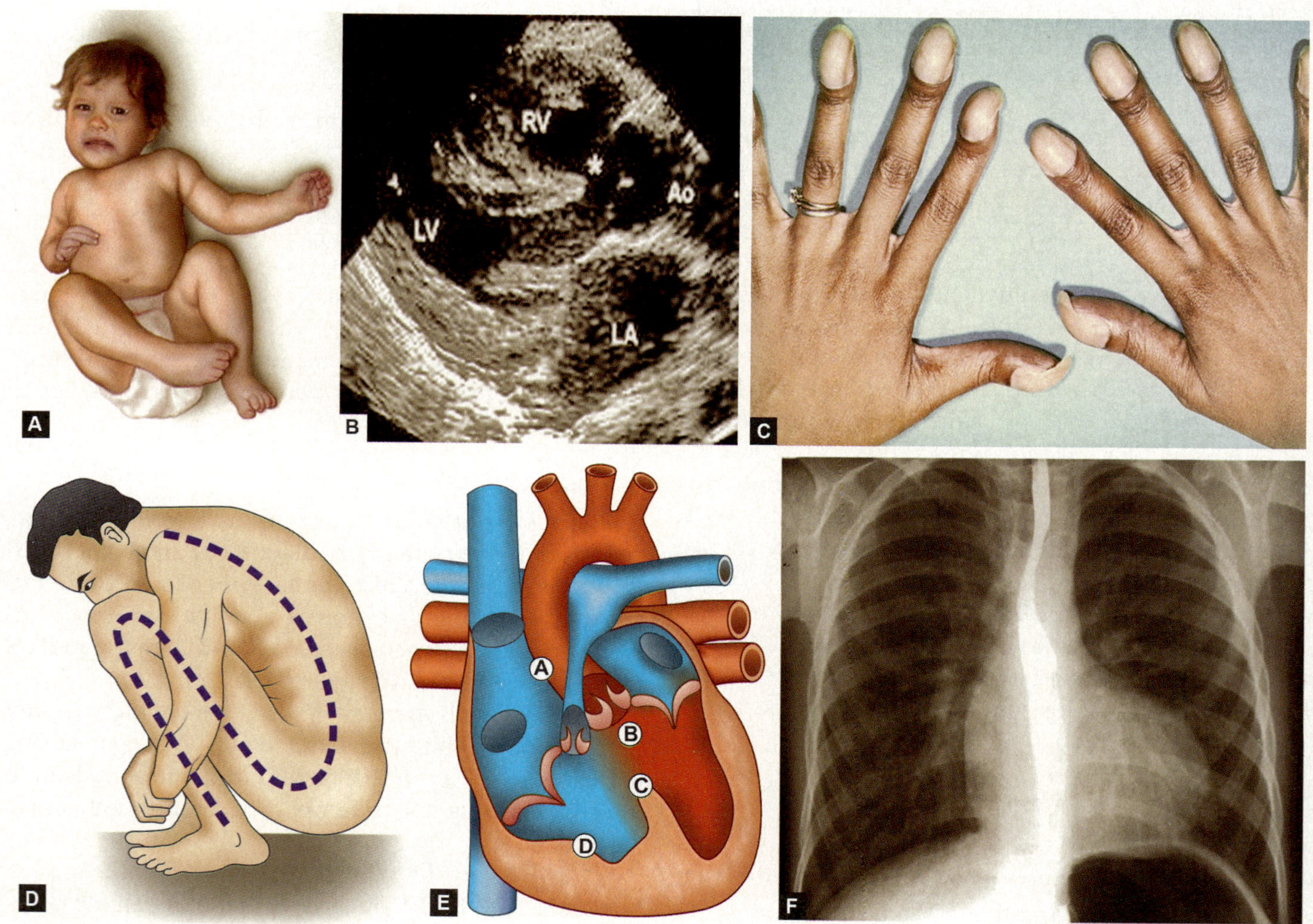

Fig. 22.21 (A) Cyanotic spell, **(B)** ECHO picture of TOF, **(C)** Clubbing, **(D)** Squatting position, **(E)** TOF and **(F)** X-ray picture of TOF

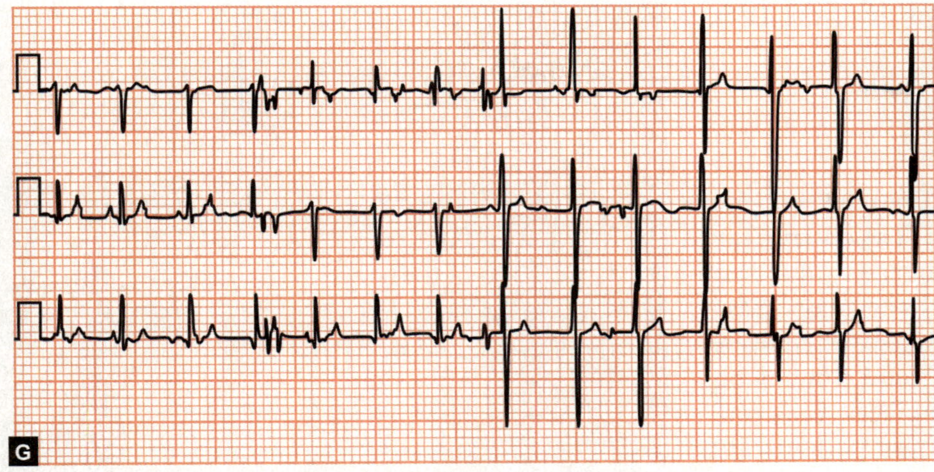

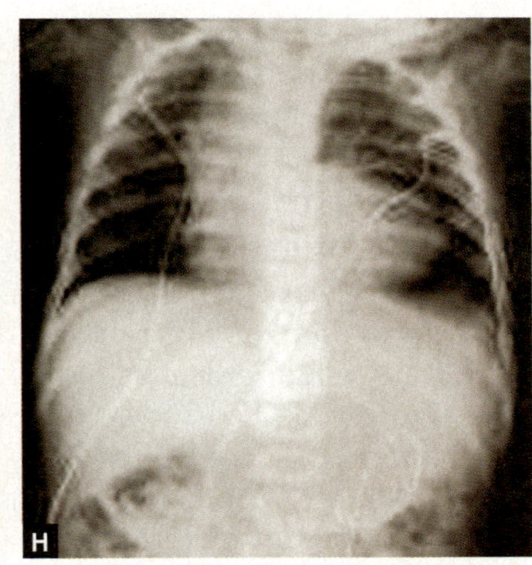

Fig. 22.21 (G) ECG picture of TOF and (H) X-ray picture of TOF

Anaesthesia Considerations

1. These patients are blue with cyanosis and clubbing. One should assess the frequency of cyanotic spells. The haematocrit may be very high depending upon the severity of the lesion. Polycythemia may cause metabolic acidosis due to inadequate tissue perfusion. Phlebotomy is indicated if the haematocrit is > 65 gm%. There is a very high chance of bleeding in the postoperative period due to deficiency in coagulation factors and structural defect in the platelets.
2. There should be no air bubbles in the intravenous lines.
3. It is important to keep the child well hydrated in the preoperative period. Long periods of fasting and dehydration can precipitate a cyanotic spell. A heavier premedication is advocated as a crying child is more prone to develop a cyanotic spell. Intravenous induction of anaesthesia is preferred. One can use an induction agent like Ketamine[77] which increases the SVR and decreases the right to left shunting. Hemodynamic goals include increasing the SVR and decreasing the PVR. Volume can be given liberally so as to keep the RVOT open. Also these patients require a higher CVP to maintain cardiac output due to the right ventricular hypertrophy and associated right ventricular diastolic dysfunction. Hypoxia, hypercarbia and metabolic acidosis should be prevented as it all can lead to increase in PVR. Halothane seems to be the best inhalational agent as it maintains the SVR, easily accepted by the patient and relaxes the infundibular spasm.
4. Adequacy of repair can be confirmed by transesophageal echocardiography. A decrease in RV systolic pressure with a ratio of RV/LV < 0.7 is acceptable. If the RV pressures are systemic or suprasystemic one may need to go back on CPB.

Problems and Complications

- Bleeding
- Residual VSD or RVOT obstruction
- RV/LV > 0.7
- RV failure, systolic and diastolic dysfunction
- Pulmonary regurgitation (free) due to transannular patch
- Heart block, RBBB
- Distal PAs may be small leading to increased RV afterload and RV failure
- Junctional ectopic tachycardia (JET). It is a very common arrhythmia after surgery. It usually responds to Amiodarone infusion and topical cooling of the patient
- Risk of sudden death

Total Anomalous Pulmonary Venous Connection

It comprises 1% of all congenital heart defects. In this, all the four pulmonary veins join together and form a confluence and then drain finally into the right atrium directly or indirectly. There is an ASD or PFO which is obligatory for the survival of the child.

Types

- Supracardiac: The confluence of the pulmonary veins drains into the innominate vein or SVC via a vertical vein.
- Cardiac: Coronary sinus or directly into the right atrium

- Infracardiac: Below the diaphragm into the IVC, hepatic or portal veins.
- Mixed: At two or more above locations

Pathophysiology

It mostly depends whether the pulmonary venous return is obstructed or non-obstructed. The obstruction can occur at any level like the confluence of the four pulmonary veins, vertical vein or at the level of ASD/PFO. Obstruction will lead to pulmonary venous hypertension. Increased pulmonary blood flow along with pulmonary venous hypertension leads to severe pulmonary arterial hypertension. These patients are usually very sick, cyanotic, in pulmonary edema and severely acidotic. Balloon atrial septostomy (BAS) can be performed as a palliative procedure to improve haemodynamics and saturations in kids with congestive cardiac failure.[78]

X-ray

- Cardiomegaly
- Pulmonary congestion
- "Figure of 8" or "snowman appearance" due to dilated supracardiac veins, right and left SVC and left innominate vein
- RA, RV and PA dilatation
- Small aorta

ECG

- Supraventricular tachycardia
- Bradycardia
- Sick sinus syndrome
- Ventricular ectopic beats

Surgical Procedures

It consists of redirection of pulmonary venous blood into the LA with closure of ASD.[79] Patients with obstruction need to be operated as soon as possible. The non-obstructed ones are usually less sick. It is usually done under moderate hypothermia. Occasionally, DHCA may also be employed.

Anaesthesia Considerations

Preoperatively, they may be intubated and on inotropic support. One can start an infusion of PGE_1 so as to decompress the hypertensive pulmonary artery system. One should avoid myocardial depression. Induction can be done with the help of narcotics and paralysing agents.

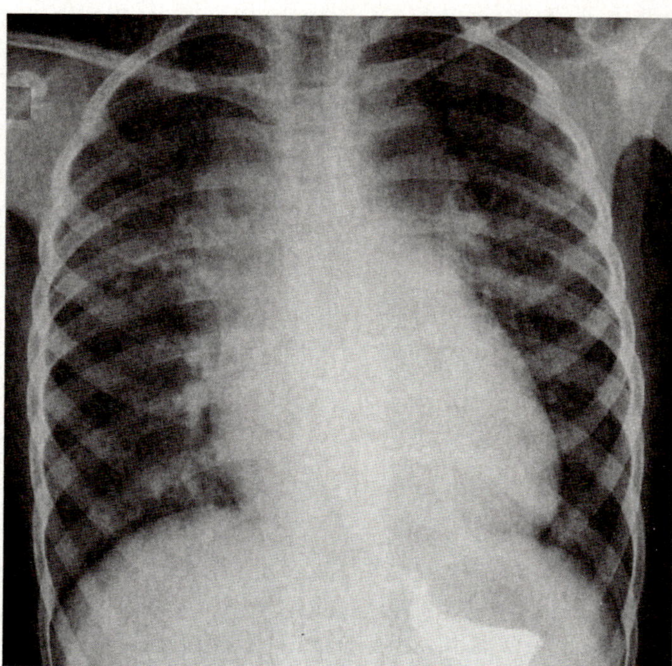

Fig. 22.22 X-ray picture of TAPVC

One should avoid hypoxia and hypercarbia as it may increase the PVR and clinically worsen the situation.

Two things of importance while coming off bypass are:

1. They may have a very reactive pulmonary vascular bed. There is a very high chance of pulmonary artery crisis. It is characterised by sudden vasoconstriction of the pulmonary vasculature in response to any sympathetic stimulation leading to hypoxaemia, desaturation, hypotension, bradycardia and severe RV failure. All manoeuvres and drugs to decrease the PVR may be employed while coming off bypass. Of particular mention is the use of inhaled nitric oxide, Milrinone, Sildenafil, Bosentan, Milrinone nebulisation, etc. Phenoxybenzamine may be given just before going on bypass. A pulmonary arterial line may be inserted by the surgeon intraoperatively. It gives a direct and continuous measurement of the pulmonary artery pressure. It is very useful while coming off bypass and also in the postoperative period in the ICU during weaning of such patients.
2. The left side of the heart is usually underfilled and may be non-compliant and poorly functional. After correction, as the LA and LV receives blood, there may be a significant amount of LV dysfunction. Inotropes may be required to support the failing ventricles.

Problems and Complications

- LV dysfunction
- Pulmonary hypertensive crisis
- Residual pulmonary venous obstruction
- RV failure
- Supraventricular arrhythmias

Transposition of Great Arteries

The aorta arises from the RV and the pulmonary artery arises from the LV. So there is atrio-ventricular concordance but ventriculo-arterial discordance. It is more common in males. The right and left circulation is in parallel rather than being in series. The deoxygenated blood from the upper and lower half of the body enters the right atrium which is then pumped into the aorta through the right ventricle. The oxygenated blood coming from the lungs is pumped into the pulmonary artery through the left ventricle. For the survival of the child, there has to be mixing of blood which is in the form of ASD/VSD (intracardiac) or PDA (extracardiac). It is for the same reason that PGE_1 infusion is started to keep the duct patent. Also Balloon atrial septostomy is done bedside under echo guidance or in the cath lab to facilitate adequate mixing. If mixing is inadequate, child is severely cyanotic and acidotic. If a large VSD is present, cyanosis is less severe and signs of congestive heart failure may be seen.

Also if there is a PDA, differential cyanosis is seen. Lower limb saturations are more than upper limb saturations. This is because oxygenated blood coming from the lungs is pumped from the LV into the PA and through the ductus arteriosus into the descending aorta.

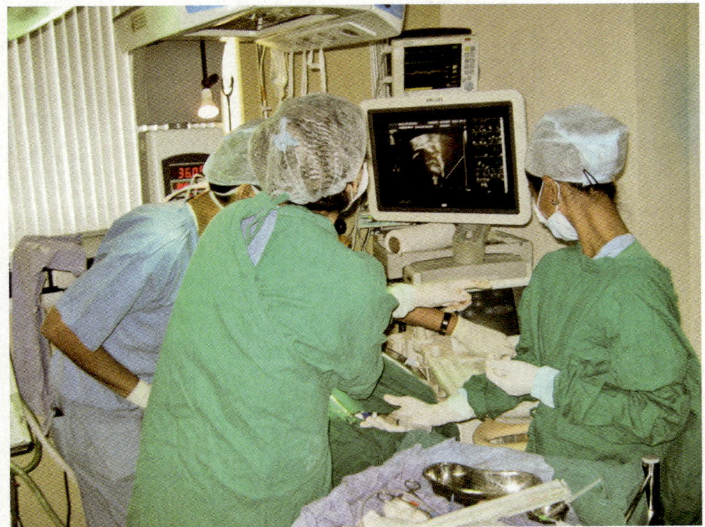

Fig. 22.23 Bedside BAS

Types

- D-LOOP
- L-LOOP

Surgical Procedures

- **Atrial switch operation (Senning/Mustard):** This is a physiological repair in which an intra atrial baffle is created in such a way that the systemic venous blood is routed into the left ventricle and the pulmonary venous blood is routed into the right ventricle. The RV continues to be the systemic ventricle pumping blood into the aorta while LV continues to be the pulmonary ventricle pumping blood into the pulmonary circulation.[80, 81] The Mustard procedure uses a pericardial baffle while Senning uses a right atrial flap.

  Complications include obstruction to systemic/pulmonary venous pathway causing SVC syndrome and pulmonary venous hypertension, atrial arrhythmias, RV failure and tricuspid insufficiency.

  It is the surgery of choice in the developing countries where patients present late after the LV has regressed and the mortality and morbidity after two stage repair (PA band followed by arterial switch operation) is very high.[82]
- **Arterial switch operation (Jatene):**[83] This is the surgery of choice[84] as it involves both anatomical as well as physiological correction. The two great arteries are disconnected and reattached to the respective ventricles.[85–87] Re-implantation of the coronary buttons to the neo aorta is also done. If the LV is regressed (as the LV gets used to pumping to low pressure pulmonary circulation), there is a lot of risk associated with the surgery. If such a regressed ventricle is then connected to the high pressure systemic circulation, it may not be able to take the load leading to ventricular dysfunction. Hence in patients with intact ventricular septum, there is a very high chance that the LV can regress early and hence ASO is performed as soon as possible within the first 10 days of life. It can also be done with a two-staged repair where the pulmonary artery is banded so as to increase the afterload of the LV and thereby prevent regression. In patients with VSD, due to equalisation of pressures between RV and LV, the LV does not regress early and corrective surgery can be performed even up to 2 months of age.

- **Rastelli procedure:** Usually done in patients with TGA, VSD, PS (LVOT obstruction). In this the VSD is closed in such a way that the LV blood is directed to the aorta and a conduit is placed from the RV to PA.

  Complications include conduit narrowing or obstruction and residual atrial shunt. Heart block may occur.

Anaesthesia considerations

Medical management includes starting PGE_1 infusion or doing a Rashkind BAS under echo guidance if mixing is inadequate. This stabilises the child preoperatively. The PGE_1 infusion needs to be infused continuously without any interruption until the child goes on CPB so as to maintain the patency of the ductus arteriosus. Premedication is usually avoided. An intravenous narcotic induction technique is used along with paralysing agent.

One must monitor ST segment intraoperatively while coming off bypass as coronary artery insufficiency and LV dysfunction can occur as a result of coronary reimplantation and long bypass and cross clamp times. NTG can be started so as to cause coronary vasodilatation. If there is kinking of the coronary vessels, revision may be necessary. Child may require inotropic support while coming off bypass. Bleeding can be an issue in the post bypass period due to CPB induced coagulopathy. Right heart dysfunction can also occur as majority of these patients are operated in the first two weeks of life when the neonatal PVR is very high. Prolonged mechanical ventilation may be required.

BNP levels can predict outcomes in the postoperative period.[88]

Narrowing of the neo PA and neo aorta can be a late complication especially when there is a discrepancy in the size of the aorta and pulmonary artery.

Congenitally Corrected Transposition of Great Arteries

In this condition, there is atrio-ventricular discordance (right atrium is connected to the left ventricle and left atrium is connected to the right ventricle) and ventriculo-arterial discordance (left ventricle is connected to the pulmonary artery and right ventricle is connected to the aorta). Although the physiological correction is done, blood enters the aorta and the pulmonary artery through the wrong ventricle. The AV valves are usually associated with the respective ventricle. RV is the systemic ventricle while LV is the pulmonary ventricle. The surgery done is Double

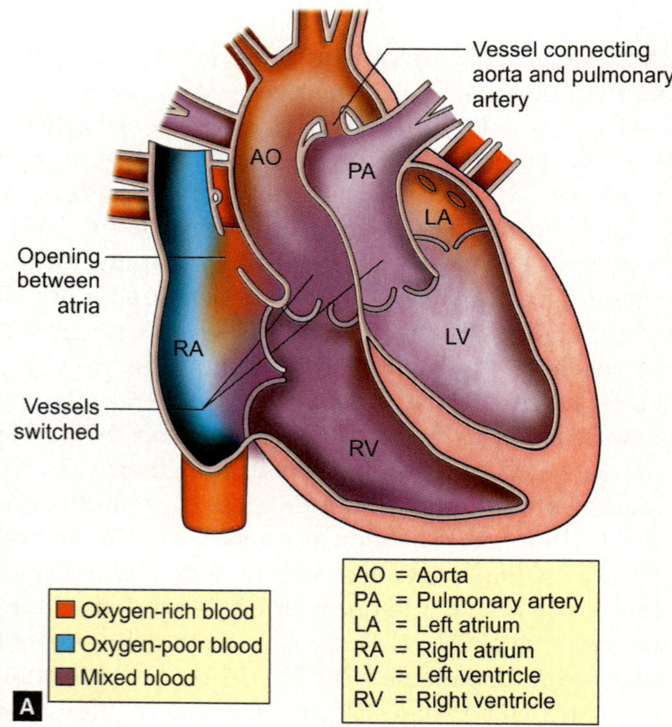

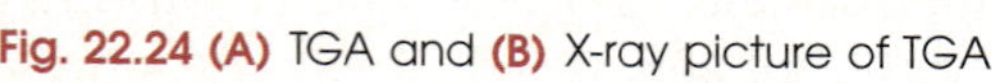

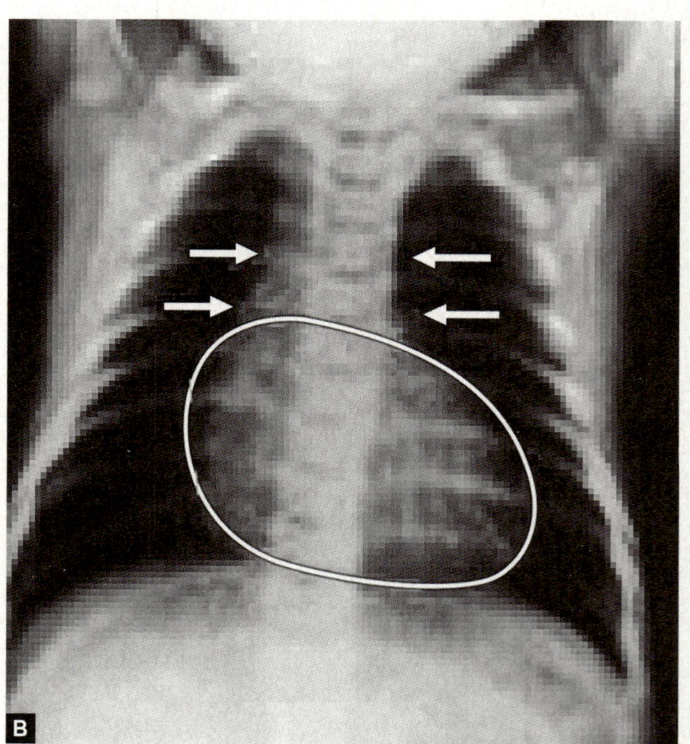

Fig. 22.24 (A) TGA and **(B)** X-ray picture of TGA

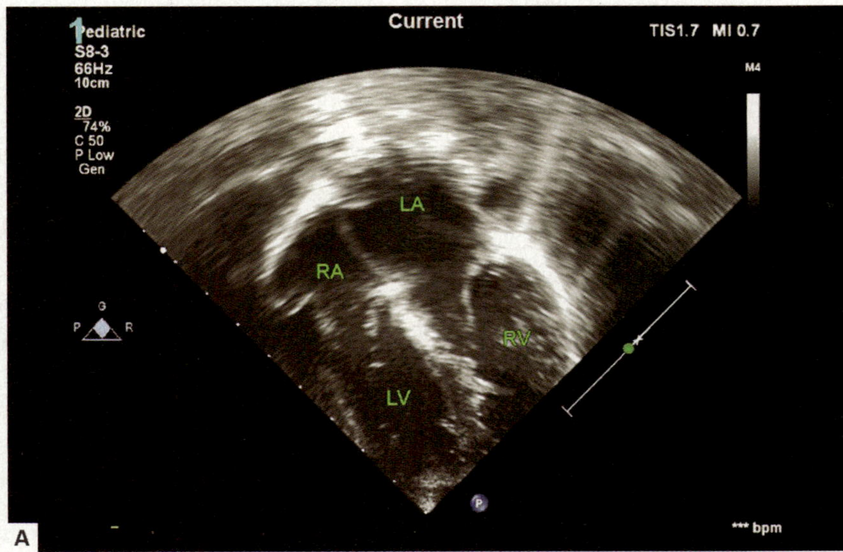

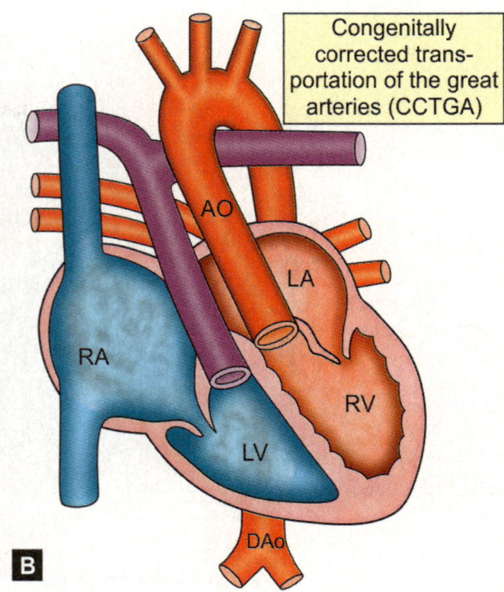

Fig. 22.25 (A) C-CTGA ECHO picture and (B) C-CTGA

Switch Operation (DSO) which includes Atrial Switch using Senning/Mustard + Arterial Switch Operation.

Tricuspid Atresia

There may be tricuspid atresia or stenosis. There is no communication between the RA and RV. It is usually associated with hypoplastic RV. Blood entering the RA is shunted to the left side through an ASD or PFO. VSD may also be present. Pulmonary stenosis/obstruction may also be present. There is volume overload of the left side of the heart as it receives both the systemic as well as pulmonary circulation.

The severity of pulmonary stenosis determines the degree of hypoxaemia in such patients.

Surgical Procedures

The surgeries for such patients are usually staged. In patients with decreased pulmonary blood flow with severe cyanosis, a modified BT shunt is usually done in the neonatal period as a palliative and emergency procedure. In tricuspid atresia associated with pulmonary atresia, PGE_1 infusion has to be started so as to maintain the patency of the ductus. This is because the duct is the only vessel supplying blood to the lungs. The PDA can then be ligated or left alone after the shunt is performed depending upon the saturations. In about 10–15% of the patients with tricuspid atresia, there is increased pulmonary blood flow. These may require a PA band so as to protect the pulmonary vasculature and make them suitable for the next stage of surgery.

At about 6–18 months of age, a bidirectional Glenn surgery is performed which reduces the volume overload of the heart.

At about 2–4 years of age, the Fontan procedure is performed.[89] In this the venous return from the lower half of the body is directed to the pulmonary circulation. IVC is connected to the RPA using a tube/graft. This can be intracardiac or extracardiac. Nowadays extra cardiac Fontan is routinely done. Total cavo-pulmonary connection (TCPC) as described by de Leval[90] is also widely practiced.

The PVR must be as low as possible for good results. The PVR should be less than 4 Wood units and the mean PA pressure should be < 15 mmHg.

In Glenn surgery the SVC is connected to the RPA and in Fontan surgery IVC is finally connected to the RPA. In this way the hypoplastic right heart is totally bypassed and physiological circulation is achieved. A fenestration is usually done which allows deoxygenated blood to enter the right atrium and thus left atrium (through ASD), thereby improving left heart filling. This may cause some amount of desaturation in the post-operative period. This fenestration can then be closed at a later date using a device.

If the ASD/PFO is small, Balloon atrial septostomy or a surgical septectomy may be required during the shunt/Glenn surgery.

Anaesthesia Considerations

- Optimise cardiac output.
- Manoeuvres to decrease the PVR should be instituted.

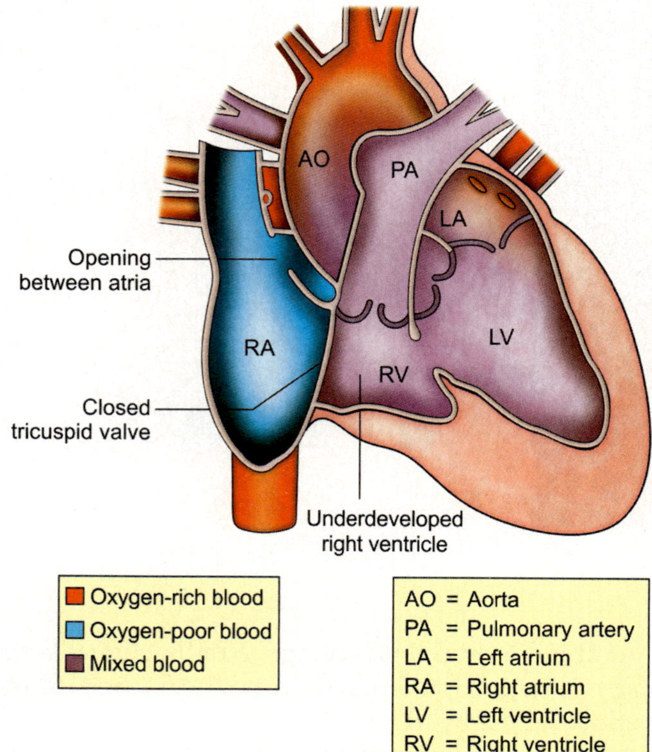

Fig. 22.26 Tricuspid atresia

- PEEP and high airway pressures are not well tolerated as it decreases the PBF.
- Extubate these patients, if haemodynamically stable, as soon as possible. Early return to spontaneous circulation increases the PBF.
- Fontan position (propped up position with legs placed above the pillow) help in the passive movement of blood towards the pulmonary circulation.
- Inotropic support may be needed in case of LV dysfunction. Increased LVEDP due to LV dysfunction results in high LA pressures. This causes the PVR to increase as a result of back pressure changes. Any increase in PVR is usually not well tolerated by the patient.
- Care should be taken to prevent long periods of fasting and dehydration.
- There should be no air bubbles in the intravenous lines and tubings.

Problems and Complications

- Systemic venous hypertension (Ascites, pleural effusion, pericardial effusion, puffiness of hands and legs)
- Low cardiac output
- Atrial arrhythmias
- Thrombosis of the conduit
- Pulmonary arterio-venous fistula
- Protein losing enteropathy

SUMMARY

Care of patients with congenital heart disease includes team work. A thorough understanding of the pathophysiology of the lesion along with the anticipated problems and complications go a long way in the treatment of these patients.

REFERENCES

1. Hoffmann JIE. Incidence of congenital heart disease: Postnatal Incidence. Pediatr Cardiol. 1995;16:103–113.
2. Malviya S, Voepel-Lewis T, Siewert M, et al. Risk factors for adverse postoperative outcomes in children presenting for cardiac surgery with upper respiratory tract infection. Anaesthesiology. 2003;98:628.
3. Tempe DK, Virmani S. Coagulation abnormalities in patients with cyanotic congenital heart disease. J Cardiothoracic Vascular Anaesthesia. 2002;16:752.
4. Maurer HM, McCue CM, Robertson LW, et al. Correction of platelet dysfunction and bleeding in cyanotic congenital heart disease by simple red cell volume reduction. Am J Cardiology. 1975;35:831.
5. Territo MC, Rosove MH. Cyanotic congenital heart disease: Hematologic management. J Am College Cardiology. 1991;18:320.
6. Friesen RH, Carpenter E, Madigan CK, et al. Oral transmucosal fentanyl citrate for preanaesthetic medication of paediatric cardiac surgery patients. Paediatric Anaesthesia. 1995;5:29.
7. Gharde P, Chauhan S, Kiran U. Evaluation of efficacy of intranasal midazolam, ketamine and their mixture as premedication and its relation with bispectral index in children with Tetralogy of Fallot undergoing intracardiac repair. Ann Card Anaesthesia. 2006;9:25.
8. Odegard KC, Dinardo JA, Kussman BD, et al. The frequency of anaesthesia related cardiac arrests in patients with congenital heart disease undergoing cardiac surgery. Anaesthesia Analgesia. 2007;105:335.
9. Flick RP, Sprung J, Harrison TE, et al. Perioperative cardiac arrests in children between 1998 and 2005 at a tertiary referral center: A study of 92881 patients. Anaesthesiology. 2007;106:226.
10. Ramamoorthy C, Haberkern CM, Bhananker SM, et al. Anaesthesia related cardiac arrests in children with heart disease: Data from the Pediatric Perioperative Cardiac Arrests (POCS) registry. Anaesthesia Analgesia. 2010; 110:1376.

11. Tanner GE, Angers DG, Barash PG, et al. Effect of left to right, mixed left to right and right to left shunt on inhalational anaesthetic induction in children. Anaesthesia Analgesia. 1985;64:101.
12. Friesen RH, Lichtor JL. Cardiovascular depression during halothane induction in infants: A study of three induction techniques. Anesth Analg. 1982; 61:42.
13. Friesen RH, Lichtor JL. Cardiovascular effects of inhalation induction with isoflurane in infants. Anaesthesia Analgesia. 1983;62:411;1983.
14. Lerman J, Davis PJ, Welborn LG, et al. Induction, recovery and safety characteristics of sevoflurane in children undergoing ambulatory surgery. Anaesthesiology. 1996;84:1332.
15. Delgado-Herrera L, Ostroff RD, Rogers SA. Sevoflurane: Approaching the ideal anaesthetic agent. CNS Drug Review. 2001;7:48.
16. Russel IA, Miller Hance WC, Gregory G, et al. The safety and efficacy of sevoflurane anaesthesia in infants and children with congenital heart disease. Anaesthesia Analgesia. 2001;92:1152.
17. Friesen RH, Lichtor JL. Cardiovascular effects of inhalation induction with isoflurane in infants. Anaesthesia Analgesia. 1983;62:411.
18. Hickey PR, Hansen DD, Stafford M, et al. Pulmonary and systemic hemodynamic effects of nitrous oxide in infants with normal and elevated pulmonary vascular resistance. Anaesthesiology. 1986;65:374.
19. Duncan HP, Cloote A, Weir PM, et al. Reducing stress responses in the prebypass phase of open heart surgery in infants and young children: A comparison of different fentanyl doses Br J Anaesthesia. 2000;84:556.
20. Robinson S, Gregory GA. Fentanyl-air-oxygen anaesthesia for ligation of PDA in preterm infants. Anaesthesia Analgesia. 1981;60:331.
21. Hickey PR, Hansen DH. Fentanyl and Sufentanil-oxygen–pancuronium anaesthesia for cardiac surgery in infants. Anaesthesia analgesia. 1984; 63:117.
22. Moore RA, Yang SS, McNicholas KW, et al. Haemodynamic and anaesthetic effects of sufentanil as the sole anesthetic for paediatric cardiovascular surgery. Anaesthesiology. 1985;62:725.
23. Davis PJ, Cook DR, Stiller RL, et al. Pharmacodynamics and pharmacokinetics of high dose sufentanil in infants and children undergoing cardiac surgery. Anaesthesia Analgesia. 1987; 66:203.
24. den Hollander JM, Hennis PJ, Burm AG, et al. Alfentanil in infants and children with congenital heart defects. J. Cardiothoracic Anesth. 1988;2:12.
25. Saint-Maurice C, Cockshott ID, Douglas EJ, et al. Pharmacokinetics of propofol in young children after a single dose. Br J Anaesthesia. 1989;63:667.
26. Patel DK, Keeling PA, Newman GB, et al. Induction dose of propofol in children. Anaesthesia. 1988;43:949.
27. Purcell-Jones G, Yates A, Baker JR, et al. Comparison of the induction characteristics of thiopentone and propofol in children. Br J Anaesthesia. 1987;59:1431.
28. Xia WF, LiuY, Zhou QS, et al. Protective effect of propofol and its relation to postoperation recovery in children undergoing cardiac surgery with CPB. Paediatric Cardiology. 2011;32:940.
29. Donmez A, Kaya H, Haberal A, et al. The effect of etomidate induction on plasma cortisol levels in children undergoing cardiac surgery. J Cardiothoracic Vascular Anaesthesia. 1998;12:182.
30. Hickey PR, Hansen DD, Cramolini GM, et al. Pulmonary and systemic haemodynamic responses to ketamine in infants with normal and elevated pulmonary vascular resistance. Anaesthesiology. 1985;62:287.
31. Klampt JG, de Andrade Vicente WV, Garcia LV, et al. Effects of dexmedetomidine–fentanyl infusion on blood pressure and heart rate during cardiac surgery in children. Anaesthesiology Res Pract. 2010;pii 869049.
32. Shepard SM, Tejman-Yarden S, Khanna S, et al. Dexmedetomidine related atrial standstill and loss of capture in pediatric patient after congenital heart surgery. Critical Care Medicine. 2011;39:187.
33. Koruk S, Mizrak A, Kaya Ugur B, et al. Propofol/dexmedetomidine and propofol/ketamine combinations for anaesthesia in paediatric patients undergoing transcatheter ASD closure: A prospective randomized trial. Clinical Ther. 2010; 32:701.
34. Raja SG, Dreyfus GD. Current status of Bosentan for treatment of Pulmonary Hypertension. Front Cardiovasc Drug Discov. 2010;1:1.
35. Friedman R, Mears JG, Barst RJ, et al. Continuous infusion of prostacyclin normalizes plasma markers of endothelial cell injury and platelet aggregation in primary pulmonary hypertension. Circulation. 1997;96:2782.
36. Fullerton DA, Jones SD, Grover FL, et al. Adenosine effectively controls pulmonary hypertension. Ann Of Cardiac Anaesthesia. 2008;11:6.
37. Ramakrishna H. Advances in the perioperative management of pulmonary hypertension. Front Cardiovascular Drug Discov. 2010;1:1.
38. Kadosaki M, Kawamura T, Oyama K, et al. Usefulness of nitric oxide treatment for pulmonary hypertensive infants during cardiac anaesthesia. Anaesthesiology. 2002;96:835.
39. Blaise G, Langleben D, Hubert B. Pulmonary arterial hypertension: Pathophysiology and anaesthetic approach. Anaesthesiology. 2003;99:1415.
40. Ichinose F, Roberts JD Jr, Zapol WM. Inhaled nitric oxide: A selective pulmonary Vasodilator: Current uses and therapeutic potential. Circulation. 2004; 109:3106.
41. Tempe DK. Perioperative management of pulmonary hypertension. Ann card Anaesthesia. 2010; 13:89.
42. Sablotzki A, Starzmann W, Scheubel R, et al. Selective pulmonary vasodilatation with inhaled aerosolized

milrinone in heart transplant candidates. Can Journal Anaesthesia. 2005;52:1076.

43. Denault AY, Lamarche Y, Couture P, et al. Inhaled milrinone: A new alternative in cardiac surgery? Semin Cardiothoracic Vasc Anaesthesia. 2006;10:346.
44. Mikhail G, Gibbs J, Richardson M, et al. An evaluation of nebulised prostacyclin in patients with primary and secondary pulmonary hypertension. European Heart Journal. 1997;18:1499.
45. Limsuwan A, Wanitkul S, Khosithset A, et al. Aerosolized iloprost for postoperative pulmonary hypertensive crisis in children with congenital heart disease. Int J Cardiology. 2008;129:333.
46. Edmonds HL Jr. Standard of care for central nervous system monitoring during cardiac surgery. J Cardiothoracic Vasc Anaesthesia. 2010;24:541.
47. Quarti A, Manfrini F, Oggianu A, et al. Noninvasive cerebral oximetry monitoring during cardiopulmonary bypass in congenital cardiac Surgery: A starting point. Perfusion. 2011;26:289.
48. Kussman BD, Wypij D, Laussen PC, et al. Relationship of intraoperative cerebral oxygen saturation to neurodevelopmental outcomes and brain MRI at one year of age in infants undergoing biventricular repair. Circulation. 2010;122:245.
49. Abraham BP, Prodhan P, Jaquiss RD, et al. Cardiopulmonary bypass flow rate: A risk factor for hyperlactatemia after surgical repair of secundum ASD in children. J Thorac Cardiovasc Surg. 2010; 139:170.
50. Jonas RA, Wypij D, Roth SJ, et al. The influence of hemodilution on outcome after hypothermic cardiopulmonary bypass: Results of a randomized trials in infants. J Thorac Cardiovascular Surg. 2003;126:1765.
51. Delmo Walter EM, Alexi-Meskishvii V, Huebler M, et al. Extracorporeal membrane oxygenation for intraoperative cardiac support in children with congenital heart disease. Interact Cardiovascular Thorac Surg. 2010;10:753.
52. Ye LF, Fan Y, Tan LH, et al. Extracorporeal membrane oxygenation for the treatment of children with severe haemodynamic alteration in perioperative cardiovascular surgery. World J of Pediatrics. 2010;6:85.
53. Ferry PC. Neurologic sequelae of open heart surgery in children. Am J Dis Child. 1990;144:369.
54. Bellinger DC, Wypij D, Kuban KC, et al. Developmental and neurological status of children at 4 years of age after heart surgery with hypothermic circulatory arrest or low flow CPB. Circulation. 1999;100:526.
55. McElhimney DB, Reddy VM, Silverman NH, et al. Modified Damus-Kaye-Stansel procedure for single ventricle, subaortic stenosis and arch obstruction in neonates and infants. Midterm results and techniques for avoiding circulatory arrest. J Thorac Cardiovasc Surg. 1997;114:718.
56. Asouk T, Kado H, Imoto Y, et al. Selective cerebral perfusion technique during aortic arch repair in neonates Ann Thorac Surg. 1996;61:1546.
57. Ohye RG, Goldberg CS, Donohue J, et al. The quest to optimise neurodevelopmental outcomes in neonatal arch reconstruction: The perfusion techniques we use and why we believe in them. J Thorac Cardiovascular Surg. 2009; 137:803.
58. Langley SM, Chai PJ, Jaggers JJ, et al. Preoperative high dose prednisolone attenuates the cerebral response to DHCA. Euro J Cardiothorac Surgery. 2000;17:279.
59. Steen PA, Gisvoid SE, Milde JH, et al. Nimodipine improves outcome when given after complete cerebral ischemia in primates. Anaesthesiology. 1985;62:406.
60. Werns SW, Shea MJ, Driscoll EM, et al. The independent effects of oxygen radical scavengers on canine infarct size. Reduction by superoxide dismutase but not catalase. Circ Res. 1985;56:895.
61. Sebastian VA, Guleserain KJ, Leonard SR, et al. Ministernotomy for repair of congenital cardiac disease. Interact Cardiovasc Thorac Surg. 2009;9:819.
62. Mukhtar AM, Obayah GM, Elnasry A, et al. The therapeutic potential of intraoperative hypercapnia during video assisted thoracoscopy in pediatric patients. Anaesthesia Analgesia. 2008;106:84.
63. Remadevi KS, Francis E, Kumar RK, et al. Catheter closure of ASD with deficient IVC Rims under TOE guidance. Catheter Cardiovascular Interv. 2009;73:90.
64. Huang TC, Hsieh KS, Lin CC, et al. Clinical results of percutaneous closure of large secundum ASD in children using the Amplatzer septal occlude. Heart Vessels. 2008;23:187.
65. Kin N, Weismann C, Srivastava S, et al. Factors affecting the decision to defer endotracheal extubation after surgery for congenital heart surgery: A prospective observational study. Anaesthesia Analgesia. 2011;113:329.
66. Original Article: Early extubation in pediatric patients after **cardiothoracic** surgery Yousef J Zureikat, Awni Al-Madani, Zeid Makahleh. **Heart Views**. 2007;8(2):40–42.
67. Finkel JC, Boltz MG, Conran AM, et al. Hemodynamic changes during high spinal anaesthesia in children having open heart surgery. Pediatric Anaesthesia. 2003;13:48.
68. Figueira Moure A, Pensado Castineiras A, Vazquez Fidalgo A, et al. Early extubation with caudal morphine after paediatric heart surgery Rev Esp Anestesiol Reanim. 2003; 50:64.
69. Peterson KL, De Campli WM, Pike NA, et al. A report of 220 cases of regional anaesthesia in pediatric cardiac surgery Anaesthesia Analgesia. 2000;90:1014.
70. Hammer GB, Ngo K, Macario A, et al. A retrospective examination of regional and general anaesthesia in children undergoing open heart surgery. Anaesthesia Analgesia. 2000;90:1020.
71. Peterson KL, De Campli WM, Pike NA, et al. A report of 220 cases of regional anaesthesia in paediatric cardiac surgery Anaesthesia Analgesia. 2000;90:1014.
72. Maddali MM, Valliattu J, al Delamine T, et al. Selection of monitoring site and outcome after neonatal co-arctation repair. Asian Cardiovasc Thorac Ann. 2008;16:236.

73. Cunningham JN Jr, Laschinger JC, Merkin HA, et al. Measurement of spinal cord ischemia during operations upon the thoracic aorta: Initial clinical experience. Ann Surg. 1982;196:285.
74. Murthy KS, Coelho R, Naik SK. Novel techniques of BDG Shunt without CPB. Ann Thorac Surg. 1999;67:1771.
75. Smolinsky AK, Shinfeld A, Paret G, et al. End Tidal CO_2 levels are a reliable indicator of band tightness in pulmonary artery banding. Ann Thorac Surg. 1995;60:523.
76. Nussbaum J, Zane EA, Thys DM. Esmolol for the treatment of hypercyanotic spells in infants with Tetralogy of Fallot. J Cardiothoracic Anesthesia. 1989;3:200.
77. Tugrul M, Camci E, Pembeci K, et al. Ketamine infusion vs isoflurane for the maintainance of anaesthesia in the prebypass period in children with Tetralogy of Fallot. J Cardiothoracic Vasc Anaesthesia. 2000;14:557.
78. Ward KE, Mullins CE, Huhta JC, et al. Restrictive interatrial communication in TAPVC. Am J Cardiol. 1986;57:1131.
79. Choudhary SK, Bhan A, Sharma R, et al. TAPVC: Surgical experience in Indians. Indian Heart Journal. 2001;53:754.
80. Senning A. Surgical correction of transposition of the great vessels. Surgery. 1959;45:966.
81. Otero Coto E, Norwood WI, Lang P, et al. Modified Senning operation for treatment of transposition of the great arteries. J Thorac Cardiovasc Surgery. 1979;78:721.
82. Pawade A. Recent advances in paediatric cardiac surgery. Ann Cardiac Anaesthesia. 2003;5:183.
83. Jatene AD, Fontes VF, Paulista PP, et al. Anatomic correction of the transposition of great arteries. J Thorac Cardiovascular Surgery. 1976;72:364.
84. Kirklin JW, Blackstone EH, Tchervenkov CI, et al. Clinical outcomes after the arterial switch operation for transposition. Patient support, procedural and institutional risk factors. Circulation. 1992; 86:1501.
85. Yacoub MH: The case for anatomic correction of transposition of great arteries. J Thorac Cardiovascular Surgery. 1976;72:364.
86. Jatene AD, Fontes VF, Souza LC. Anatomic correction of the transposition of great arteries. J Thorac Cardiovascular Surgery. 1982;83:20.
87. Castaneda AR, Norwood WI, Jonas RA, et al. Transposition of the great arteries and intact interventricular septum: Anatomical repair in the neonate. Thorac Surgery. 1984; 38:438.
88. Cannesson M, Bionda C, Gostoli B, et al. Time course and prognostic value of plasma B–type natriuretic peptide concentration in neonates undergoing arterial switch operation. Anaesthesia Analgesia. 2007;104:1059.
89. Fontan F, Baudet E: Surgical repair of tricuspid atresia. Thorax. 1971;26:240.
90. De Leval MR, Kilner P, Gewilling M, et al. Total cavopulmonary circulation: A logical alternative to atriopulmonary connection for complex Fontan—experimental studies and early clinical experience. J Thorac Cardiovascular surgery. 1988;96:682.

Anaesthesia for Paediatric Interventional Cardiology

Manish Kela

ABSTRACT

Anaesthetic management for paediatric cardiac catheterization can be uniquely challenging since these patients range in age from premature neonates to adolescents. Congenital cardiac anomalies can vary from relatively simple atrial septal defects to complex congenital cardiac anomalies such as hypoplastic left heart syndrome. Anaesthetic techniques used in these cases range from sedation and analgesia to general anaesthesia with endotracheal intubation.

This chapter reviews the general considerations, anaesthetic management for atrial septal defect, ventricular septal defect and patent ductus arteriosus device closure and for non-cardiac surgery.

GENERAL CONSIDERATIONS OF ANAESTHESIA FOR PAEDIATRIC INTERVENTIONAL CARDIOLOGY

Introduction

Congenital anomalies of heart and cardiovascular system occur in 7 to 10 per 1000 live births (0.7–1%).[1] Heart disease is the most common form of congenital disease and accounts for approximately 30% of the total incidence of all congenital diseases.

Presence of congenital heart disease in paediatric patients poses a greater challenge for anaesthetist as morbidity and mortality is quite high.[2,3]

Practical Concepts Regarding the Interpretation of a Catheterization Report[4]

1. **Normal intracardiac pressures (mmHg)** (Table 23.1):

Table 23.1 Normal intracardiac pressures (mmHg)

Location	Newborn	Child
Right atrium (mean)	0–4	2–6
Right ventricle	65–80/0–6	15–25/3–7
Pulmonary artery	65–80/35–50	15–25/10–16
Pulmonary wedge (mean)	6–9	8–11
Left atrium (mean)	3–6	5–10
Left ventricle	65–80/0–6	90–110/7–9
Aorta	65–80/45–60	90–110/65–75

Source: Carol L Lake, Peter D Booker. Paediatric cardiac anaesthesia. 4th edn.

2. **Shunt calculation:** Shunts are characterized in terms of their direction, i.e. left to right, right to left, bidirectional and the magnitude. Left-to-right shunts can be quantified based on the pulmonary (Qp) to systemic (Qs) blood flow ratio as follows:

$$Qp/Qs = (SaO_2 - MvO_2)/(PvO_2 - PaO_2)$$

where, SaO_2 = Systemic arterial saturation,
MvO_2 = Mixed venous O_2 saturation,
PvO_2 = Pulmonary venous O_2 saturation,
PaO_2 = Pulmonary arterial O_2 saturation,
Qp/Qs = Ratio more than 3:1 is considered to be a significant shunt.

3. **Vascular Resistance:** Resistance represents the change in pressure in the systemic or pulmonary circulation with respect to flow. This is expressed as mmHg/L/min (Wood units) and is usually normalized for body surface area. The systemic and pulmonary vascular resistance are derived as follows:

$$SVR = (MAP - RAP)/Qs$$

where, SVR is systemic vascular resistance, MAP is mean arterial pressure, RAP is right atrial pressure, and Qs is systemic blood flow

$$PVR = (Mean\ PAP - Mean\ LAP)/Qp$$

where, PVR is pulmonary vascular resistance, PAP is pulmonary artery pressure, LAP is left atrial pressure, Qp is pulmonary blood flow.

4. **Valve areas:** Valve areas of stenotic valve lesions are determined during cardiac catheterization using the Gorlin formula.

   The echocardiographic equivalent to this measurement is estimation of the valve area by the continuity equation.

$$A = CO/(K \times \sqrt{\Delta}\ P),$$

Where, A is valve area, CO is cardiac output, K is a constant specific for the specific valve (44.5 for aortic valve, 37.8 for mitral valve), and ΔP is (mean) pressure gradient.

5. **Gradients:** Pressure gradients across cardiac valves, great vessels, or conduits help quantify the severity of obstruction to flow across a stenotic lesion. Pressure readings are obtained with a catheter placed distal and proximal to the stenotic lesion and the gradient calculated.

Procedures Performed in Catheterisation Laboratory[4,5]

A. **Diagnostic:** To provide definitive anatomic and haemodynamic information about complex congenital heart diseases, to determine peak to peak pressure gradient, to assess pulmonary artery anatomy and major aortopulmonary collaterals (MAPCAS) in TOF, to measures right- and left-sided pressures.

B. **Interventional:**
   1. **Balloon dilation:** Atrial septostomy (Rashkind procedure)
      Valvular dilatation (pulmonary stenosis)
      Vessel dilatation (pulmonary artery stenosis, coarctation of aorta)
   2. **Device occlusion:** Patent ductus arteriosus, atrial septal defect, ventricular septal defect
   3. **Coil occlusion:** Patent ductus arteriosus, aorto-pulmonary collateral vessels
   4. **Retrieval of foreign bodies:** Embolized devices, fragments of central venous catheters, coiled and knotted central venous catheter.
   5. **Radio frequency ablation:** Accessory pathways, WPW syndrome, ectopic atrial tachycardia, ectopic ventricular tachycardia
   6. **Endomyocardial biopsy:** To confirm diagnosis of myocarditis or cardiomyopathy.

Physiological Consideration and Challenges

It is essential that the anaesthesiologists caring for CHD children have a comprehensive understanding of the underlying physiology of cardiovascular and non-cardiac system and its impact on the delivery of anaesthesia. This includes:

Cardiovascular system	Non-cardiac system
• Complex cardiac physiology· • Less cardiovascular · reserve • Intracardiac or extra-cardiac shunting of blood	• Difficult airway due to congenital syndrome· • Other associated anomalies, e.g. tracheo-esophageal fistula, omphalocele, etc. • Anomalies of trachea, bronchi and lungs
• Obstruction or regurgitation of blood flow	• Limited respiratory reserve

Preoperative Assessment:[4–6]

It should encompass detailed information about the cardiac lesion, altered physiology and its implications. In addition presence of associated other systemic anomalies should be excluded. This includes:

1. Complete understanding of the anatomical changes due to cardiac defect or palliative procedure.
2. Direction and amount of shunting.
3. Presence and severity of pulmonary hypertension.
4. Extent of reduced or increased pulmonary flow in the neonatal age, complex congenital heart diseases might have persistence of foetal circulation for survival
5. Degree of hypoxaemia, polycythaemia: Fatigue, headache, visual disturbances, depressed mentation and paraesthesia of toes and fingers are presenting symptoms of polycythaemia. It leads to thrombosis and infarction in cerebral, renal and pulmonary region. Paediatric patient might not present with these symptoms. They may have cyanotic spells, squatting episodes, suck-rest-suck cycle, fatiguability, failure to thrive and central or peripheral cyanosis.
6. Coagulation abnormalities: Due to hypofibrinogenaemia and factor deficiencies.
7. Functional status of the patient: Fatigue and dyspnoea on feeding and irritability indicate poor functional status.
8. Respiratory reserve: Presence of increased respiratory rate, diaphoresis, intercostal muscles

retraction, nasal flaring, and use of accessory respiratory muscles indicate poor respiratory reserve.

9. Congestive heart failure: May show signs like tachycardia with low volume pulse, a gallop rhythm, tachypnoea, difficulty in feeding, excessive perspiration, jugular venous distention, pulmonary congestion or hepatomegaly.
10. Associated anomalies or syndromes: Include musculoskeletal abnormality (8.8%), neurological defects (6.9%), and genitourinary irregularities (5.3%). Down's syndrome is one of the most common syndromes associated with congenital heart anomaly.
11. Medication history must be elicited. Patients with CHD might be on aspirin, warfarin, diuretics, angiotensin converting enzyme (ACE) inhibitors, and antiarrhythmic. In current practice, all cardiac medications should be given on the morning of surgery with exemption of ACE inhibitors due to their hypotensive effects during anaesthetic induction.

Investigations

- **Complete blood count:** Polycythaemia is very common which increases blood viscosity. Consider phlebotomy in patients with symptomatic hyperviscosity and haematicrit >65%.[4,5]
- **Coagulation profile:** Platelet count, prothrombin time and partial thromboplastin time should be done in all patients.
- **Serum electrolytes:** Should be done in patients who receive diuretics, digitalis and parental nutrition.
- **Chest X-ray:** For confirming position of the heart (dextrocardia) and to confirm cardiomegaly, atelectasis, acute respiratory infection, vascular markings and elevated hemidiaphragm. Increased pulmonary flow leads to pulmonary congestion which causes prominent bronchopulmonary markings. While decreased pulmonary flow causes oligaemic lung fields.
- **ECG** may show ventricular strain or chamber hypertrophy.
- **Echocardiography** for doppler and colour flow mapping.
- **Catheterization** for information about pressures in different chambers, magnitude of shunt and coronary anatomy.
- **Blood gas analysis** in patients with cyanotic defects.

Monitoring

Standard American Society of Anaesthesiologist monitoring for the children with CHD undergoing cardiac cathetarisation laboratory procedure includes electrocardiogram, noninvasive blood pressure, pulse oximetry, end tidal carbon diaoxide, temperature and airway pressure.

Additional invasive monitoring, like invasive blood pressure, central venous pressure, transesophageal echocardiography and urinary catheter may be warranted on an individual basis when either the child's presentation or proposed intervention or anaesthetic management predicts the likelihood of circulatory instability.

Caution: In the presence of right to left shunt, the end-expiratory CO_2 consistently underestimates the true arterial CO_2 level.

Preoperative Preparation in Cath Lab

A fully equipped anaesthesia work station with airway and intubation equipment and emergency cardiorespiratory resuscitative drugs should be available. Pacemaker with external pacing pads and a defibrillator with the appropriate-sized paediatric paddles should be confirmed.

A chart that will enumerate the calculated dosages, volume and the infusion rate of the anaesthetic, resuscitative and vasoactive agents as well as the maintenance fluid in a closed system using programmable syringe pumps should be ready.

All intravenous tubings and syringes should be free of air bubbles to prevent paradoxical embolism. Consent and nil by mouth status should be confirmed.

Anaesthesia for Catheterization Laboratory Procedures

Catheterization procedures should only be performed in centres where facilities for paediatric heart surgery are available. The aim of the anaesthesia management is to facilitate cardiac catheterization under physiological conditions in a spontaneously breathing, deeply sedated pain free patient.

Polycythaemic patient must be well hydrated before induction and prolonged fasting periods should be avoided. Antibiotic prophylaxis should be administered as per the international guidelines.

Catheterization procedures can be performed under local, sedation, monitored anaesthesia care (MAC) and general anaesthesia.

Airway management may range from sedation with spontaneous respiration, to mask, laryngeal mask airway or endotracheal anaesthesia. Sevoflurane is preferred due to its better haemodynamic stability in CHD patients.[7]

Maintenance of Anaesthesia and Analgesia

Techniques include total intravenous anaesthesia using ketamine, with or without midazolam, high-dose opioids (when postoperative ventilation is planned), inhalational agents, muscle relaxation and combinations of the above. High doses of analgesia is not required and only local anaesthetic infiltration at access site is sufficient.

Active warming strategies are essential to prevent hypothermia during catheterization which may result in delayed recovery from sedation and anaesthesia.

Intraoperatively glucose containing fluid should be given as children have low glycogen stores which make them vulnerable to hypoglycemia.

Advantages of General Anaesthesia

- Ventilation can be controlled to optimize gas exchange.
- Interventions performed to assess reversibility of pulmonary hypertension (high FiO_2, inhaled nitric oxide) can be easily performed.
- Positive pressure ventilation reduces risk of air entering through large bore delivery sheaths, thereby preventing air embolism.
- Precise device placement is also facilitated with muscle relaxants that eliminate patient movements.
- A secured airway allows the anaesthesiologist to concentrate on hemodynamic issues.

Disadvantages of General Anaesthesia

- Positive pressure ventilation can alter the intra-cardiac pressures, shunt fraction as well as reduction in gradient across the valve in stenosis cases.
- Produce drug induced alterations in rate and rhythm.

Sedation for Children undergoing Cardiac Catheterization

Ketamine: It is the anaesthetic agent used most frequently.[8,9] The combination of sedation and analgesia with maintenance of respiratory drive and airway reflexes makes it a preferable choice.

- **Dose:** Initial bolus 1–2 mg/kg IV, followed by, an infusion of 25–100 µ/kg/min

Propofol: It has rapid onset, predictable level of sedation, rapid recovery and a low incidence of nausea and vomiting with minimal adverse effects.[9]

- **Dose:** 1.5–2.5 mg/kg followed by 50–200 µg/kg/min infusion. It decreases the blood pressure and heart rate by 10–30% and systemic vascular resistance by 15–20% which can have serious consequences in patients with severe aortic stenosis, cyanotic heart disease and compromised myocardial function.

Dexmedetomine: It is a unique and selective alpha 2-adrenoceptor agonist, which results in hypotension, bradycardia and sedation.[10]

- **Dose:** Loading dose of 1 µg/kg dexmedetomidine administered over 10 min followed by an infusion rate of 0.5–1 µg/kg/hr.

  Dexmedetomidine does not depress respiratory drive.

Benzodiazepines: Produce dose-dependent respiratory depression, which is more marked in patients with respiratory disease, congenital heart disease and when combined with opioids. Midazolam is the most commonly used.

Opioids: Newer opioids like fentanyl, alfentanil and remifentanil have rapid onset of action, shorter duration and provide better haemodynamicstability.

Remifentanil: Loading dose of 1 µg /kg followed by an infusion of 0.5–0.6 µg kg/hr.

Considerations for general anaesthesia: All commonly used induction agents are well tolerated depending on the rate and dose of the drug. Systemic vascular resistance (SVR) and peripheral vascular resistance (PVR) balance should be considered when using intravenous agents. Inhalation induction is acceptable in CHD patients with uncomplicated cardiac lesion. Patients with poor cardiac function, who require inotropes preoperatively, may not tolerate inhalational induction, and favour the use of ketamine.

Procedural Complications

- Dislodgement or malposition of the device or coil resulting in embolization or obstruction or regurgitation.
- Blood loss.
- Hypothermia.
- Vascular injury.
- Air embolism.
- Pericardial effusion and tamponade.
- ST segment changes, arrhythmias, complete heart block, atrial fibrillation.
- Failure of the procedure and need for urgent surgical intervention.
- Brachial plexus neuropathy due to stretching of nerve plexus during positioning.

Challenges Faced by Anaesthesiologist in Cath Lab

- Usually located away from operating room.
- Transfer of critically ill patient from intensive care to catheterisation laboratory or vice versa can be difficult.
- Rooms are usually not properly illuminated.
- Access to patient's airway is difficult.
- Monitoring interference with catheterisation laboratory equipment.
- Use of contrast media and its complications like anaphylaxis; contrast induced nephrotoxicity and vasovagal reaction.
- Radiation exposure.

Anaesthesia for Device Closure

Endovascular devices are available for the closure of ASDs, VSDs and PDAs.[4]

General anaesthesia with endotracheal intubation is required for ASD and VSD device closure as procedure require TEE probe *in situ*. PDA device closure can be done under intravenous sedation as the procedure does not require TEE but general anaesthesia is preferred as procedures can be of unpredictable duration and patient must be immobile to allow accurate catheter deployment across the orifice of the PDA.

The main aim is to avoid acute and persistent increase in systemic vascular resistance or decrease in pulmonary vascular resistance as these changes will increase the magnitude of left to right shunt.

1. Most patients with L–R shunt tolerate anaesthesia well without hemodynamic compromise.
2. Heparin should be administered for these procedures to minimise the risk of thrombus formation. (75–100 IU/kg).
3. Meticulous de-airing of all fluid lines should be undertaken to reduce the potential of paradoxical embolization.
4. Antibiotic prophylaxis to prevent infective endocarditis as per international guidelines is required.
5. Standard ASA monitors including ECG, non-invasive blood pressure, pulse oximetry, and capnography are essential during the procedure.
6. Analgesic requirements are minimal following these procedures.
7. In view of interventional treatment, VSD is much more complicated and takes longer time than ASD or PDA. Placement of ASD/PDA device is usually associated with minimal haemodynamic disturbances, whereas VSD device placement is usually associated with profound hemodynamic instability, arrhythmias and blood loss. Therefore, invasive monitoring and inotropic support with the placement of external defibrillator pads is recommended in these patients.
8. Attention must be given towards the blood loss during repeated blood sampling and also the heparin level before shifting the child out of the catheterization laboratory.
9. Vagal stimulation can occur during device placement and may require treatment with atropine.
10. Post-procedural medication includes: Aspirin 75 to 100 mg/day for six months: Clopidogrel 75 mg/day for 4 weeks and endocarditis prophylaxis for one year.

ASD DEVICE CLOSURE[11, 12]

ASDs account for approximately 10% of congenital cardiac defects.

ASDs are classified into four types anatomically (Fig. 23.1).

Spontaneous closure occurs by 18 months in almost all patients born with ASDs <3 mm diameter and in 80% of those with defects 3–8 mm. Defects with diameters >8 mm rarely close spontaneously and may require surgery later in life.[10]

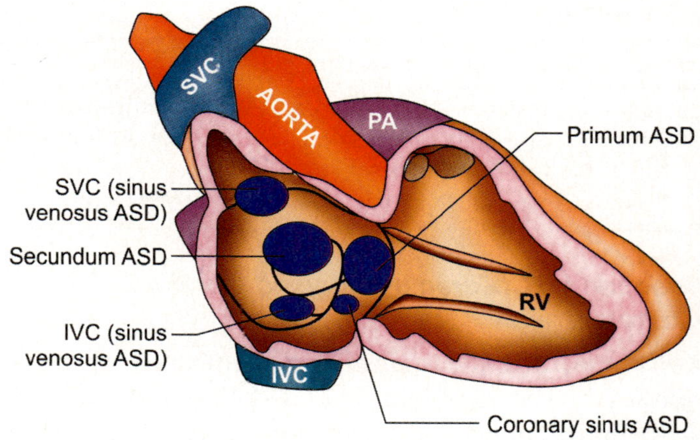

Fig. 23.1 ASDs are classified into four types anatomically—(1) Ostium secundum ASD (60–70%), (2) Ostium primum ASD (15–20%); a defect of the endocardial cushion, often associated with mitral regurgitation due to an anterior leaflet cleft. (3) Sinus venosus ASD (5–15%) nearly always associated with anomalous pulmonary venous drainage and (4) Coronary sinus ASD

Source: www.learnonly.com

Indications of ASD Closure

1. Isolated secundum ASD with a diameter of less than 40 mm
2. Presence of a left-to-right shunt exceeding 1.7:1 or signs of right ventricular overload (defined as a dilated right atrium and right ventricle on echocardiography).
3. Clinical symptoms: Frequent respiratory infection (more than six events per year), failure to thrive.

Contraindications

1. Secundum ASD associated with complex congenital cardiac malformations
2. A single defect too large for occlusion (more than 3 cm)
3. Multiple ASDs
4. Multifenestrated ASDs within the interatrial septum
5. A defect too close to the superior vena cava, inferior vena cava, pulmonary veins, atrioventricular valves, or coronary sinus.
6. No adequate rims for the device to sit.
7. Ostium primum ASD.

Preoperative Investigation

- Transthoracic echocardiography (TTE): It defines the size position and morphology of ASD and ventricular size and function.
- Positive bubble test: A small PFO can only be demonstrated by a positive bubble test (air bubbles seen in both right and left atria) during a valsalva manoeuvre.
- Colour Doppler: Defines the direction of blood flow and its velocity, to assess the relative left and right atrial pressure.
- Preoperative TEE: For confirmation of the defect, accurate sizing, and determination of adequacy of rim for appropriate percutaneous closure.

Other investigations include ECG, coagulation studies (if on warfarin), full blood count, and blood biochemistry.

Choice of Device

There are a variety of devices available for ASD closure.

Amplatzer septal occluder (Fig. 23.2)

The most established device is made from a double nitinol disk with a polyester coat. The nitinol (nickel titanium alloy) has the ability to return to its original conformation after deformation. This permits delivery of the device through a sheath and re-conformation across the ASD. This device is strong, self-centres in the ASD, and is easily recaptured and redeployed. Alternatively, the HELEX septal occluder may be used. It is more suitable for the closure of smaller ASDs (www.eplabdigest.com).

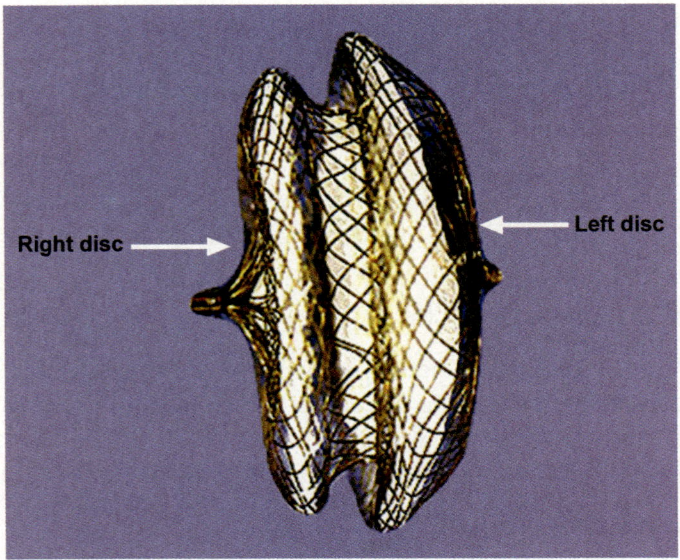

Fig. 23.2 Amplatzer septal occluder

Placement of Septal Occlusion Device

The closure of both PFOs and ASDs involves the placement of catheter-deployed closure devices that usually is advanced from the femoral vein into the right atrium and across the septal defect. Fluoroscopy and TEE or intracardiac echocardiography (ICE) is used to guide the positioning and deployment of the device and to confirm the adequacy of closure.

Complications

Major complications include the following.

1. **Air embolism:** During deployment, air embolism can cause transient myocardial ischaemia, leading to ST–T changes on ECG and demonstrable regional wall motion abnormalities on TEE. Intervention is not required, and cardiac function usually recovers spontaneously. Cerebrovascular episode/stroke can also occur due to air embolism.
2. **Arrhythmias:** Atrial fibrillation or flutter is relatively common during placement of the device due to atrial manipulation. It is self-limiting and rarely causes haemodynamic compromise.
3. **Thrombus formation on device or applicator:** Full anticoagulation should be commenced immediately.

4. **Embolization of the device:** This is extremely rare, but can embolise in RA or RV causing RVOT obstruction or in LA causing obstruction of mitral valve.
5. **Pericardial haemorrhage and tamponade:** This is caused by damage to a cardiac structure by a wire. A pericardial drainage catheter or sternotomy may be required if the bleeding is severe or continuous.

VSD DEVICE CLOSURE

Ventricular septal defect is the most common form of congenital heart defect accounting for about 20% of all forms of defects. A large number of VSDs close spontaneously by the time child reaches 2 years of age.

Classification[13]

1. Perimembranous VSD: The most common type (80%)
2. Muscular VSD: Account for the 5 to 20% of all the VSDs.
3. AV canal defect (5%)
4. Infundibular/Subpulmonary VSD (5–7%)

Indications for Percutaneous Closure of Congenital VSDs

1. Clinical evidence of significant left-to-right shunt with congestive heart failure.
2. Poor weight gain.
3. Cardiomegaly on chest X-ray.
4. Dilated left-sided cardiac chambers on echocardiography.

The main objective of closing these defects is to avoid further development of pulmonary hypertension and to prevent pulmonary vascular disease.

Investigations

- Transthoracic (TTE) and transesophageal (TEE) echocardiography: To determine the type and diameter of VSD, left ventricular size, pulmonary artery pressure and the distance and relationship of the defects with the aortic, mitral and tricuspid valves.
- Cardiac catheterization: To measure the shunt ratio.
- Ventriculography: To assess the VSD diameter and the relationship between VSD and aorta.

Several devices have been used for percutaneous closure of VSDs: Rashkind PDA Occluder (Bard), Lock's Clamshell (Bard), Sideris buttoned device, and Amplatzer Muscular VSD Occluder (AGA).

Procedure

The selected device size is usually 1 to 2 mm larger than the size of the defect. It involves crossing the VSD, mostly from the left ventricular side, forming an arteriovenous loop and positioning the delivery sheath in the left ventricle either from the femoral vein or jugular vein depending upon the location of the VSD. Angiographic and TEE monitoring of the device position during implantation is necessary for accurate device placement.

Complications

Arrhythmias: Ventricular arrhythmias, transient atrial fibrillation and conduction defects including complete

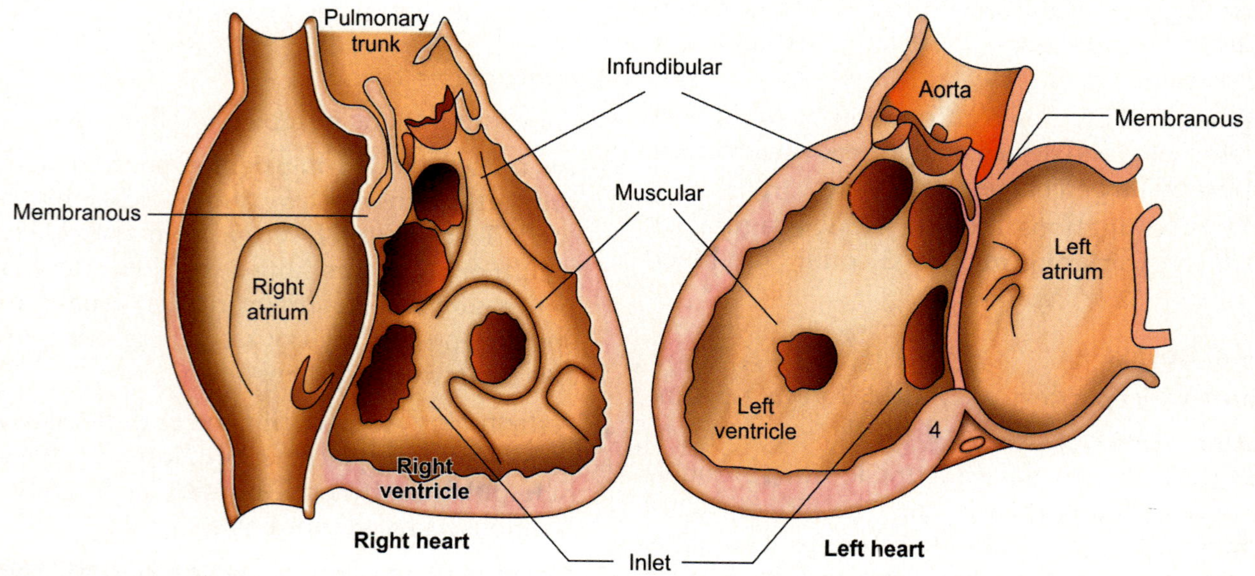

Fig. 23.3 Types of VSD
Source: annals.org

atrioventricular (AV) block. Conduction defects may be transient or permanent. This complication is associated with the proximity of VSD to the conduction system. Complete AV block is suggested to occur due to direct trauma from the device or due to the development of inflammatory reaction or scar tissue in the conduction system associated with the procedure.[14]

Device embolizations: The devices can migrate to the left or right ventricles and be subsequently embolized to the ascending aorta or pulmonary artery.

Air embolism: Meticulous techniques of catheter and wire exchanges can minimize this complication.

Haemolysis: This is a rare complication usually associated with residual shunt. If haemolysis is severe and the patient requires multiple blood transfusions, device removal is recommended.

Valvular regurgitation: Tricuspid, mitral and aortic valve regurgitation may occur due to impingement of the device or part of it on the tricuspid/mitral subvalvular apparatus or if the device is too close to the aortic valve leaflets.

Pericardial effusion: May result from catheter irritation or minute wire perforation during the procedure.

PDA DEVICE CLOSURE[15, 16]

PDA is a common form of congenital heart defect with an incidence of one in 2500 to 5000 live births.

Ductus arteriosus is an intrauterine vessel connecting proximal pulmonary artery segment to the anterior descending aorta at the level where main pulmonary artery comes closer to the left pulmonary artery. Normally, it closes spontaneously within the first 24–48 hours after birth as a result of muscular contractions. If ductus arteriosus fails to close physiologically after the second postnatal month, it is termed patent ductus arteriosus (PDA).

Indications

1. Volume overloading of the left atrium and left ventricle.
2. The risk of endocarditis, aneurysm of PDA, and pulmonary vascular disease.

Contraindications

1. Irreversible pulmonary vessel disease (Eisenmenger syndrome)

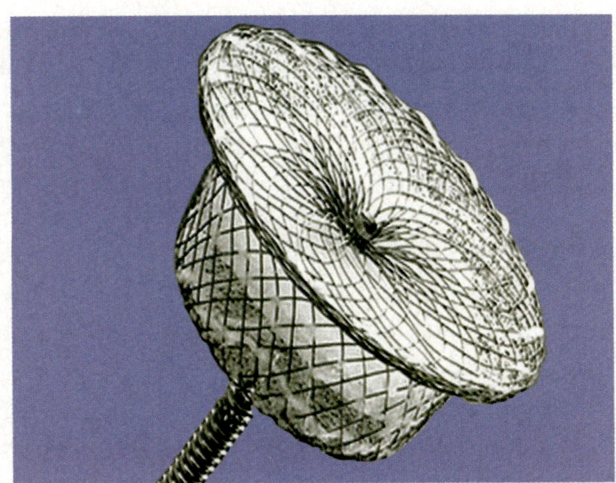

Fig. 23.4 Amplatzer duct occluder
Source: www.medint.sk

2. Pulmonary/systemic pressure or resistance ratio above 2/3
3. Restrictive PDA.

Devices

Several devices have been used for percutaneous closure of VSDs: Amplatzer duct occluder (ADO): Most commonly used—Rashkind PDA umbrella, Button device, PDA coils.

Amplatzer occluder is used for a PDA with a diameter of more than 3 mm, while coils are used for small PDA with diameter less than 3 mm.

Transcatheter closure of small to moderate PDA is now an established method of treatment for most patients with PDA.

Procedure

The customary approach is to perform an aortogram to define the size and geometry of PDA. The device then can be inserted by using either tranvenous (antegrade) or transarterial (retrograde) approach.

Complications

1. Embolization during release of the device is one of the important complications of the procedure. Embolization can occur in systemic, and generally in pulmonary artery
2. Residual shunt: Due to improper size of device.
3. Hemolysis: Believed to be as a result of mechanical injury to the red blood cells.
4. Infective endocarditis
5. Narrowing of descending aorta and pulmonary artery

Caution: Do not inject any air bubble in circulation.

General anaesthetic Considerations for Children with Congenital Heart Disease for Non-cardiac Surgery

In general, children with CHD undergoing non-cardiac surgery have an increased risk of morbidity, perioperative cardiac arrest, and a higher 30 days mortality.[17,18]

Major Consequences of CHD

- **Cyanosis** is a response to chronic hypoxia because of decreased pulmonary blood flow (PBF) and/or mixing.
- **Congestive heart failure** is due to increased PBF resulting from shunt lesions, obstructive lesions and impaired ventricular contractility.
- **Pulmonary hypertension (PHT)** occurs in left to right (L to R) shunts with increased PBF. PHT also develops with prolonged pulmonary venous obstruction [e.g. total anomalous pulmonary venous drainage (TAPVD)], high left atrial pressure [e.g. hypoplastic left heart syndrome (HLHS)] and in mixing lesions with increased PBF (e.g. truncusarteriosus). PHT is not usually a feature of the R to L shunts.
- **Arrhythmias** may be part of the presenting pathology but often occur as a result of surgery.

Risk classification of children with heart disease undergoing non-cardiac surgery (Table 23.2)[19]

Non-cardiac Features of CHD[20]

Lungs

- Decreased lung compliance from chronically increased PBF (L to R shunting, pulmonary venous congestion).
- Airway compression by vascular structures.
- Haemoptysis, phrenic nerve or recurrent laryngeal nerve injury (during previous surgery) may be present. Phrenic nerve damage with diaphragmatic dysfunction will have an impact on respiratory mechanics. Recurrent laryngeal nerve injury may result in chronic aspiration and lung disease.
- CHD patients might have a blunted response to hypoxia.

Haematological

- Polycythaemia is a compensatory mechanism to hypoxemia and cyanosis.
- Hyperviscosity syndrome results from polycythaemia.
- Haemostatic abnormalities correlate with the degree of hypoxemia and erythrocytosis. Problems include either qualitative or quantitative platelet abnormalities, decreased fibrinogen, increased fibrinolysis, and clotting factor deficiencies.

Neurological

- CNS signs and symptoms may include headache, depressed mentation, transient ischaemic attacks, cerebrovascular accidents with permanent neurological sequelae, dizziness and blurred vision.
- Paradoxical emboli to CNS
- Brain abscesses
- Cerebral thrombosis

Preoperative Assessment

1. To understand the underlying lesion, type and knowledge of the circulation.
2. Evidence of long-term complications and other features that put children into a high-risk category.
3. Evidence of recent upper or lower respiratory tract infections which may cause changes in airway reactivity and PVR which may be poorly tolerated in children with poor pulmonary compliance or PHT.
4. Venous access: May be problematic. Many children may have had multiple peripheral and central venous lines in the past.

Table 23.2 Risk classification of children with heart disease undergoing non-cardiac surgery[19]

High risk	Intermediate risk	Low risk
Physiologically poorly compensated and/or presence of major complications	Physiologically normal or well compensated	Physiologically normal or well compensated
Complex lesions	Simple lesions	Simple lesions
Major surgery (intraperitoneal, intrathoracic, anticipated major blood loss requiring transfusion)	Major surgery (intraperitoneal, intrathoracic, anticipated major blood loss requiring transfusion)	Minor (or body surface) surgery
Under 2 years old	Under 2 years old	Over 2 years old
Emergency surgery	Emergency surgery	Elective surgery
Preoperative hospital stay more than 10 days	Preoperative hospital stay more than 10 days	Preoperative hospital stay less than 10 days
ASA status IV or V	ASA status IV or V	ASA status I–III

5. Routine drug therapy: Most cardiac medications should be continued before operation. Some anaesthetists prefer to omit full form ACE inhibitors based on adult literature, but evidence in children is lacking reference. Aspirin should be continued to prevent shunt thrombosis, and children on warfarin need admission for monitoring and switching to intravenous heparin.
6. Endocarditis prophylaxis: International guidelines must be followed.
7. Associated non-cardiac congenital anomalies must be ruled out.
8. Preoperative fasting: Starvation time should be minimised. Alternatively, an intravenous line can be placed for fluid replacement from the time of starvation. Preoperative phlebotomy is performed in children with symptomatic hyperviscosity and in those with haematocrit more than 65%.
9. Investigations: As discussed in general considerations.

Haemodynamic Principles of Anaesthetic Management of Shunts[4–6]

Aim is to improve oxygenation and myocardial function by the manipulation of flow through the shunt:

1. **In patients with Left to right (L → R) shunt**
   Minimal effect on inhalation or intravenous induction:
   - Avoid increasing SVR: May benefit from afterload reduction.
   - Avoid negative inotropes
   - Beware of fluid overload, or worsening congestive heart failure (CHF)
   - Oxygenate well, ventilate early and monitor appropriately.
2. **In patients with right to left (R → L) shunt**
   Prolonged inhalational induction, faster IV induction
   - Maintain high SVR: Adequate fluid administration; pharmacologically—ketamine, phenylephrine; physically—knees to chest, pressure on groin, and occlusion of femoral arteries.
   - Maintain adequate (or increased) intravascular volume and good blood pressure.
   - Avoid increase in PVR.
   - Minimise intrathoracic pressure: Normal to low ventilatory pressures, low PEEP, complete neuromuscular blockade.
   - Oxygenate well and monitor appropriately until full recovery.
   - Meticulous attention to air bubbles in the intravascular lines is crucial.

All commonly used induction agents are well tolerated depending on the rate and dose of the drug. SVR and PVR balance should be considered when using intravenous agents. Inhalation induction is acceptable in CHD patients with uncomplicated cardiac lesion. Patients with poor cardiac function, who require inotropes preoperatively, may not tolerate inhalational induction, and favour the use of ketamine.

Hypercyanotic "*tet*" Spell under Anaesthesia[4,5]

Sudden fall in saturation, hypotension and bradycardia suggest hypercyanotic spell.

Management

1. Hyperventilation with 100% oxygen
2. Increase depth of anaesthesia
3. IV fluid (5–10 mL/kg) to maintain right ventricle filling
4. β-blocker to relieve infundibular spasm: Inj propranolol 0.02–0.2 mg/kg is preferred over other β-blockers as it decreases heart rate, increases SVR (uninhibited alpha action) and stabilizes vascular reactivity of systemic arteries, hence decrease in SVR is prevented.
5. Phenylephrine: 5–10 μg/kg to increase SVR
6. Morphine: 0.1–0.2 mg/kg.
7. Inj sodabicarb: 1 mEq/kg IV to treat acidosis.
8. Inj ketamine: Sedates patient and also increases SVR

Pulmonary Hypertension

It is defined as an increase in the mean pulmonary arterial pressure of more than 25 mmHg at rest or 30 mmHg with exercise.[21]

It is more commonly considered to occur when systolic PA pressure > half systolic systemic pressure.

The anaesthetic goals in managing such a patient are to prevent increase in PVR and depression of myocardial function.

Pulmonary HTN crisis intervention measures[21]

1. 100% oxygen: Potent pulmonary dilator.
2. Nitric oxide: Administered by inhalation only, starting dose of 20 ppm, increase to 40 ppm if no response, maximum dose 80 ppm.
3. Phosphodiesterase inhibitors: Sildenafil is a selective pulmonary vasodilator given orally. Dose: 0.25–1 mg/kg, given three to four times a day
4. Prostacyclin analogues: Epoprostenol requires a continuous infusion and has a short half-life

(< 6 minutes). The starting dose is 2 ng/kg/min with increments of 2 ng/kg/min every 15 minutes until desired effects occurs.

5. Non-selective endothelin receptor antagonist: Bosentan, oral dose 31.25 mg twice a day for children less than 20 kg.
6. Inotropes to maintain cardiac output and pulmonary blood flow
7. Extra corporeal membrane oxygenation

Factors affecting PVR[4,5]

Increase PVR	Decrease PVR
• High airway pressure	• Low airway pressures
• PEEP	• No PEEP
• High airway resistance·	• Low airway resistance·
• Atelectasis·	• High FiO_2
• Hypoxia·	• Hypocarbia
• Hypercarbia	• Low haematocrit·
• Acidosis	• Ablated stress response
• Increased haematocrit	• Alkalosis
• Catecholamines	

Postoperative Considerations

Patients with CHD should be observed in high-dependency bed or intensive care unit to detect arrhythmia, cardiac ischaemia, dehydration, pain, ventilator issues at the earliest.

Postoperative Analgesia

For major surgery, intravenous opioid infusions are commonly used. Regional techniques have been used but reports are rare. High spinal blocks are well tolerated in healthy children and are not associated with adverse hemodynamic effects seen in adults.[22] Epidural with general anaesthesia is reported in neonates with complex cardiac defects undergoing general surgery.

Regional Anaesthesia in CHD

Regional anaesthetic techniques serve as useful adjuvants to general anaesthesia in children with CHD.[22] With possible exception of the presence of a coagulopathy, children with CHD should be considered for regional anaesthesia with the following cautions:

1. Because the lungs may absorb up to 80% of the local anaesthetic in the first passage, the risk of local anaesthetic toxicity is theoretically increased in children with right-to-left shunts.
2. Vasodilatation resulting from central axis blockade may be hazardous in patients with significant aortic stenosis or other left-sided obstructive lesions. It may cause an increased right-to-left shunt in susceptible children.

On the other hand, peripheral vasodilatation in patients with polycythemia may have benefit of improved microcirculatory flow and decreased venous thrombosis.

SUMMARY

The safe anaesthetic management of children with CHD during cardiac intervention requires familiarity with the principles of paediatric anaesthesia, and a thorough understanding of the specific cardiac lesion. The anaesthesiologist must understand the underlying pathophysiology, the purpose of the study and the anaesthesia-induced changes in the hemodynamic parameters. Fully equipped catheterization laboratory, surgical backup, and ECMO support should be available in any centre planning interventional cardiac catheterization.

Anaesthetic management of the procedures in the cardiac catheterization laboratory must include the same level of preparation and strict vigilance that would apply in the operating room settings.

One Fact to Remember/Paediatric Anaesthesia Pearls

Ketamine is the best induction agent in patient with R–L shunt.

Take Home Messages

- Congenital heart disease is the commonest birth defect.
- Four major consequences of CHD: cyanosis, congestive heart failure, pulmonary hypertension, and arrhythmias.
- Dehydration is detrimental in cyanotic heart disease.

Key Points

- Evaluate the airway
- Improve or optimise oxygenation
- Preserve myocardial function.
- Optimise balance between systemic and pulmonary vasculature resistances.
- Be prepared: Resuscitation drugs, equipment, analgesia and postoperative care (ensure an ICU bed for ill or unstable patients).

FAQs with Answers

Q. How will you recognise the intraoperative cyanotic spell? How will you treat it?

A. Sudden fall in saturation, hypotension and bradycardia suggest hypercyanotic spell.

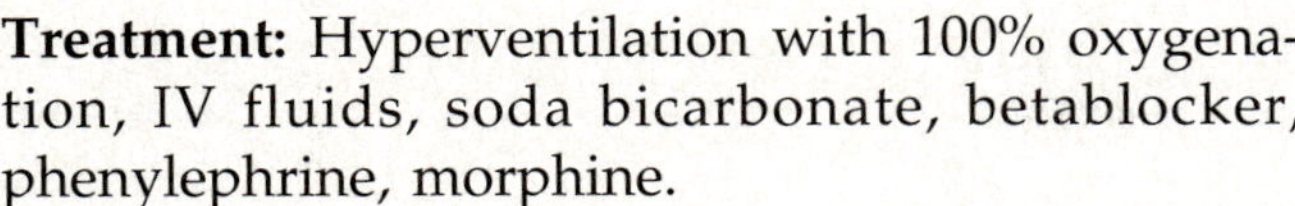

Treatment: Hyperventilation with 100% oxygenation, IV fluids, soda bicarbonate, betablocker, phenylephrine, morphine.

Q. What is the important precaution will you take while taking the IV line in CHD?

A. Avoid injecting any air bubble while taking the IV line to prevent paradoxical embolism.

(*Acknowledgement for inputs from*: Dr. Vidhi Shah and Dr. Amarja Nagre)

REFERENCES

1. Mohindra R, Beebe DS, Belani KG. Anaesthetic management of patients with congenital heart disease presenting for non-cardiac surgery. Ann Card Anesth. 2002;5(1): 15–24.
2. Sp Ark Celok Lek. Anaesthesia for noncardiac surgery in children with congenital heart disease. 139(1–2):107–15.
3. Swiatnicka-Lucinska M, Markiewicz M, Moszura T, et al. Complications during anesthesia for diagnostic and interventional cardiac procedures in children with congenital heart defects. Anestezjol Intens Ter 2009; 41(3):130–4.
4. Carol L Lake, Peter D Booker. Paediatric cardiac anaesthesia. 4th edn.
5. Joel A Kaplan. Kaplans Cardiac Anesthesia. 6th edn.
6. Hines and Marschall. Stoeltings Anesthesia and Coexisting diseases. 5th edn.
7. Russell IA, Miller Hance WC, Gregory G, et al. The safety and efficacy of Sevoflur anaesthesia in infants and children with congenital heart disease. Anesth Analg. 2001;92(5): 1152–8.
8. Singh A, Girotra S, Mehta Y, et al. Total intravenous anesthesia with ketamine for pediatric interventional cardiac procedures. J Cardiothorac Vasc Anesth. 2000;14:36–9.
9. Kogan A, Efrat R, Katz J, et al. Propofol-ketamine mixture for anesthesia in pediatric patients undergoing cardiac catheterization. J Cardiothorac Vasc Anesth 2003;17:691–3.
10. Munro HM, Tirotta CF, Felix DE, et al. Initial experience with dexmedetomidine for diagnostic and interventional cardiac catheterization in children. Paediatr Anaesth. 2007;17:109–12.
11. Bedford D. The anatomical types of atrial septal defect, their incidence and clinical diagnosis. Am J Cardiol 1960;6:568.
12. Patrick A Calvert, Andrew A Klein. Anesthesia for percutaneous closure of atrial septal defects. Continuing eduction in Anesthesia, Critical care and Pain. 2008;1:16–20.
13. Soto B, Becker AE, Moulaert AJ, et al. Classification of ventricular septal defects. Br Heart J. 1980;43(3):332–343.
14. Yip WC, Zimmerman F, Hijazi ZM. Heart block and empirical therapy after transcatheter closure of perimembranous ventricular septal defect. Catheter Cardiovasc Interv. 2005;66(3):436–44.
15. Gournay V. The ductus arteriosus: Physiology, regulation, and functional and congenital anomalies. Arch Cardiovasc Dis 2011;104:578–85.
16. Moore JW, Levi DS, Moore SD, et al. Interventional treatment of patent ductus arteriouses. Catheter Cardiovasc Interv. 2005;64:91–101.
17. Baum VC, Barton DM, et al. Influence of congenital heart disease on mortality after noncardiac surgery in hospitalized children. Pediatrics. 2000;105:332–5.
18. Hennein HA, Mendeloff EN, Cilley RE, et al. Predictors of postoperative outcome after general surgical procedures in patients with congenital heart disease. J Pediat Surg. 1994;7:866–70.
19. Michelle C White, James M Peyton. Anaesthetic management of children with congenital heart disease for non-cardiac surgery. Contin Educ Anaesth Crit Care Pain. 2012;12(1):17–22.
20. Greenwood RD, Rosenthal A, Parisi L, et al. Extracardiac abnormalities in infant's with congenital heart disease. Pediatrics 1975;55:485–92.
21. Friesen RH, Williams GD. Anesthetic management of children with pulmonary arterial hypertension. Paediatr Anaesth. 2008;18:208–16.
22. Imbelloni LE, Vieira EM, Sperni F, et al. Spinal anesthesia in children with isobaric local anesthetics: report on 307 patients under 13 years of age. Pediatr Anesth 2006;16: 43–48.

Anaesthesia for Children with Congenital Heart Disease Undergoing Non-cardiac Surgery

Raveendra US

INTRODUCTION

Children with congenital heart disease (CHD) requiring non-cardiac procedures present unique set of challenges to the anaesthesiologist. Decision making regarding the anaesthetic management is as crucial as the other aspects of patient care. The various related issues are discussed in this chapter.

Background

CHD is known to have a incidence of about 1 in 125 live births. With modern treatment modalities 90% of them survive into adulthood. About 30% of the children with CHD undergo surgery for extra cardiac anomaly in the first year of life.[1] When a child with CHD comes for non-cardiac surgery, the cardiac defect may be symptomatic or asymptomatic and surgically corrected or uncorrected. Surgical procedure can be corrective or palliative. The procedure can be anatomical or physiological repair. Residual effects after the correction and multiple drug therapy further complicate the clinical situation. More complex the lesion, more extensive is the pathophysiological changes and more challenges for the anaesthesiologist.

Available data from the studies and case reports indicate that the mortality and morbidity in these children are higher compared to those without CHD.[2] Also, many of these children require extensive and often prolonged multi-disciplinary care, particularly in the postoperative period. In a review of perioperative anaesthesia related cardiac arrests in children, it was found that majority of the arrests took place during non-cardiac surgery and children less than 2 years accounted for 75% of the incidents.[3] Aortic stenosis, cardiomyopathy and single ventricle accounted for 75% of the cardiac arrests in the same review. In another series, mortality of 19% was reported in children less than 2 years and with hypoplastic left heart syndrome (HLHS) undergoing non-cardiac surgery.[4] Overall, CHD is associated with increased morbidity, perioperative cardiac arrest and 30 days mortality.

EMBRYOLOGY

Heart is the first functional organ to appear in embryo, the critical stages of development occurring between 2nd and 8th week of gestation. Various cardiovascular structures are derived from mesoderm, beginning with the formation of a cardiogenic crescent on 15th day of embryonic life. Different stages of development and embryologcal basis of different lesions are listed in Tables 24.1 and 24.2A and B.

Mechanisms underlying the development of CHD have not been completely understood. In less specific terms, these could include abnormalities in one or more of the multiple processes involved in normal cardio genesis such as cell migration, haemodynamic function, cell death and extracellular matrix formation, all of which involve poorly understood multiple genetic pathways.[5]

TYPES OF CHD AND PATHOPHYSIOLOGY

Congenital cardiac defects can range from simple lesion with minimal or no complications to complex lesions with multiple defects, extensive pathophysiological changes and severe functional limitations. Broadly, they can be classified into lesions with left to right shunt, right to left shunt, obstructive lesions, single ventricle

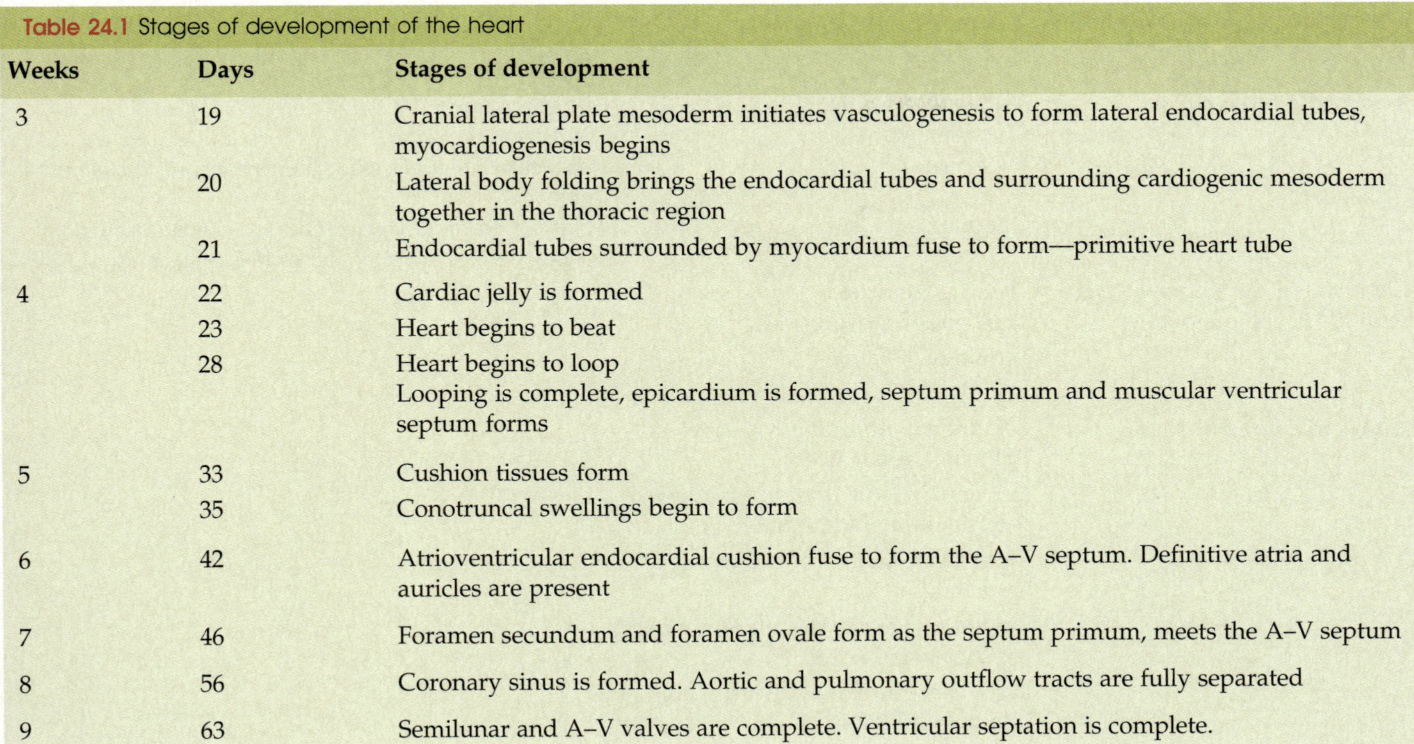

Table 24.1 Stages of development of the heart

Weeks	Days	Stages of development
3	19	Cranial lateral plate mesoderm initiates vasculogenesis to form lateral endocardial tubes, myocardiogenesis begins
	20	Lateral body folding brings the endocardial tubes and surrounding cardiogenic mesoderm together in the thoracic region
	21	Endocardial tubes surrounded by myocardium fuse to form—primitive heart tube
4	22	Cardiac jelly is formed
	23	Heart begins to beat
	28	Heart begins to loop Looping is complete, epicardium is formed, septum primum and muscular ventricular septum forms
5	33	Cushion tissues form
	35	Conotruncal swellings begin to form
6	42	Atrioventricular endocardial cushion fuse to form the A–V septum. Definitive atria and auricles are present
7	46	Foramen secundum and foramen ovale form as the septum primum, meets the A–V septum
8	56	Coronary sinus is formed. Aortic and pulmonary outflow tracts are fully separated
9	63	Semilunar and A–V valves are complete. Ventricular septation is complete.

Table 24.2A Defects during the stages of development

Defects		Remarks
Cardiac repositioning	Dextrocardia	Dextrocardia with situs solitus (isolated dextrocardia) is seen with severe cardiac anomalies like heterotaxy syndrome, transposition of great arteries. Dextrocardia with situs inversus is less likely to be accompanied with cardiac defect
Atrial septation	Patent foramen ovale Ostium secundum defect Sinus venosus defect Common atrium	Ostium secondum is most common type Ostium primum seen in up to 20% of children with Down's syndrome
Atrioventricular camal (also called endocardial cushion defects) or A–V septal defects	Atrial communication, ventricular communication, and abnormal development of A–V valves. Complete form has all three of these components	Commonly associated with Down's syndrome
A–V valves	Tricuspid and mitral valve defects, Ebstein anomaly	Isolated mitral valve anomalies are rare in children

physiology lesions, defects of conduction and myocardial diseases. CHD can be cyanotic or acyanotic which are further subdivided based on pulmonary blood flow (Table 24.3). In addition, there can be associated extra cardiac defects and also, CHD can be part of syndromes with well defined clinical and genetic features. Down's syndrome is an example (Table 24.4).

Pathophysiological consequences of CHD include changes in the pattern of circulation, arrhythmia, hypoxia and cyanosis, pulmonary arterial hypertension, shunting, ventricular dysfunction, ventricular outflow

Table 24.2B Defects related to the stages of development

Defects		Remarks
Ventricular septation	• Membranous type	Most common
	• Muscular type·	2nd most common
	• Inlet type·	Defects in inlet are associated endocardial cushion defects.
	• Outlet type	Outlet defects also referred to as conal, supracristal, sub-arterial or doubly committed defects
Conotruncal development and semi-lunar valve formation	• Truncus arteriosus	
	• Transposition of great arteries·	
	• Tetralogy of Fallot·	
	• Aortopulmonary window	
Aortic arch development	• Left aortic with retroeosophagel right subclavian artery·	
	• Left aortic arch with retroesophageal diverticulum of kommerell·	
	• Right aortic arch with mirror image branching·	
	• Right aortic arch with retroesophageal left subclavian artery	
	• Right aortic arch with diverticulum of Kommerell·	
	• Double aortic arch	

Table 24.3 Classification of congenital heart disease (CHD)

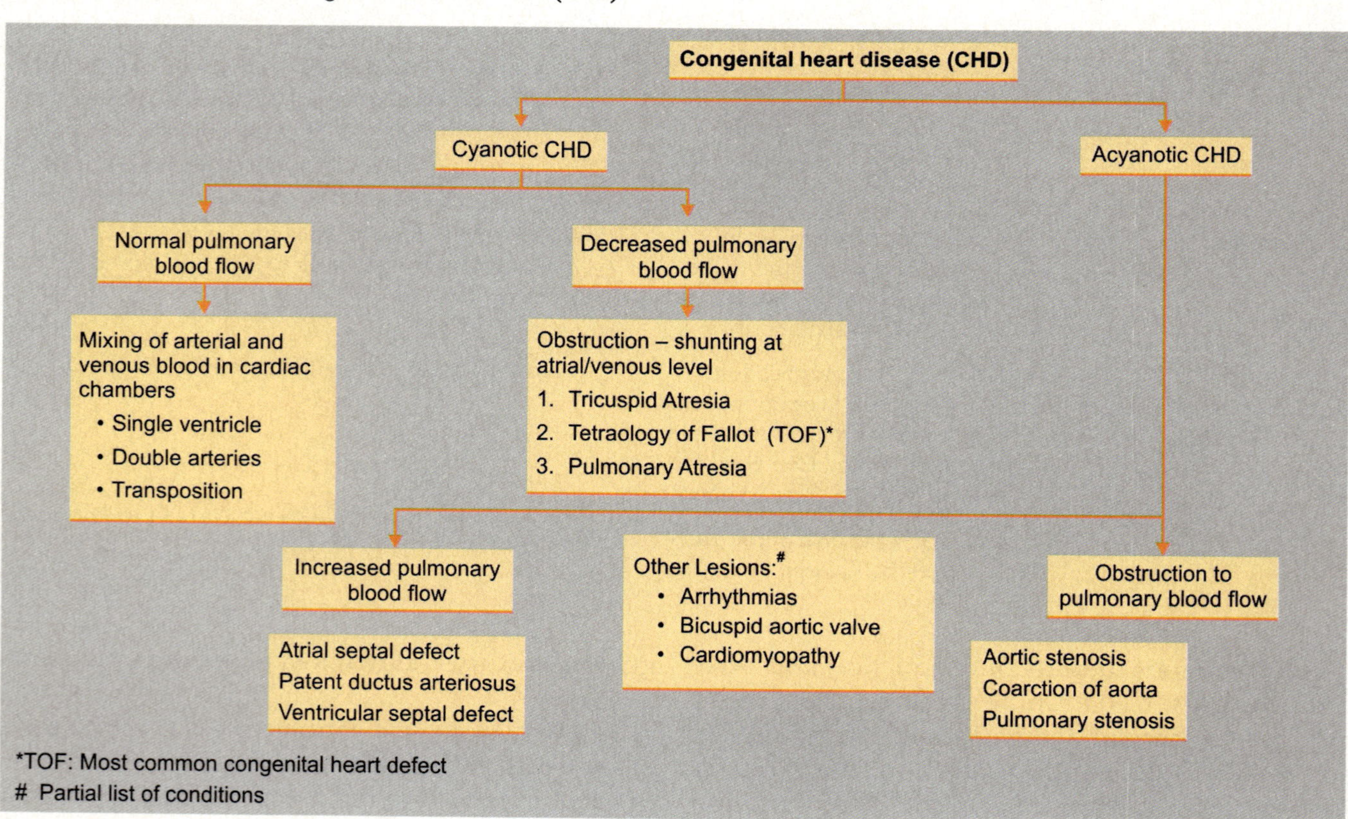

Table 24.4 Syndromes and associated CHD

Syndormes	Salient features	Cardiac defects
Digeorge syndrome	• Hypoparathyroidism • Hypoplastic thymus· • Conotruncal heart defects • Cleft lip/palate	Conotruncal heart defects (TOF, interrupted aortic arch, VSD, vascular ring)
Eisenmenger's syndrome		VSD, with pulmonary hypertension, right to left shunt with enlarged left ventricle
Marfan syndrome	• Deficiency of fibrillin • Scoliosis, deformities of breast bone • Joint contractures • Unusual arm span • Long fingers and toes· • Dislocation of lens in the eyes	Mitral valve prolapsed, arrhythmia, aortic regurgitation, aortic dissection
Noonan syndrome	• Behavioural problems, learning difficulties· • Distinct facial appearance· • Webbed neck· • Low hair line in the back of head· • Short stature • Widely set eyes • Drooping of upper eyelids, small jaw, low nasal bridge	Pulmonary valvular stenosis, malformation of certain blood and lymph vessels, blood clotting and platelet deficiencies
William syndrome	• Characteristic facial appearance· • Heart and blood vessel problems • Hypercalcemia • Low birth weight, feeding problems, irritability • Dental abnormalities, hernias· • Hyperacusis, musculoskeletal problems· • Excessively social type of personality • Developmental delay	Narrowing of aorta (supra valvular aortic stenosis), pulmonary stenosis and increased risk for blood vessel narrowing
Cayler syndrome	• Hypoplasia of depressor angulioris muscle with cardiac defects	Ventricular septal defects, atrial septal defects and/or tetralogy of Fallot
Ehler-Danlos syndrome	• Joint hypermobility, skin fragility, easy bruising, osteoarthritis· • Collagen gene disorder	Aortic root dilatation, mitral valve prolapse
Ellis-van Creveld syndrome	• Cleft lip or palate, epispadiasis or undescended testis • Polydactyly, deformed nails, short arms and legs· • Tooth abnormalities	Atrial septal defect
Holt-Oram syndrome	• Skeletal abnormalities of hands and arms	Atrial septal defect, ventricular septal defect, cardiac conduction abnormalities
Ebstein's anomaly	• Seen in infants of mother taking lithium during first trimester	Abnormality of the anterior leaflet of tricuspid valve, atrialization of right ventricle, associated with either an atrial septal defect or patent foramen ovale

obstruction, myocardial ischemia, congestive cardiac failure, end organ pathology and infective endocarditis. These changes are often interrelated in a particular CHD or can be the consequence of the primary defect or repair. In addition, significant extra cardiac anomalies could be associated.

Table 24.5 Pathophysiology of congenital heart disease

Congenital heart disease

Injury necrosis ablation

Arrhythmia (atrial and ventricular) heart block

Multiple drug treatment

Sequelae after palliation/partial correction

Congestive cardiac failure

Ventricular outlet obstruction ventricular dysfunction

Pressure and volume overload ischaemia PVOD

Shunting VSD, ASD, PDA

Left – right Right – left

Shunt reversal and hypercyanotic episodes

Cyanosis and hypoxia

Hyperviscosity polycythemia

End organ damage ↑ Thrombosis ↑ Stroke ↑ SVR

Patterns of Circulation

Any CHD can be associated with a normal (in "series") physiological *or* balanced (or "parallel") circulatory pattern *or* single ventricle physiology.[6] Small isolated defects like atrioventricular defect (ASD), ventricular septal defect (VSD), etc. can have normal circulation while large unrepaired ASD and VSD and Blalock Taussing (B–T) shunt are considered to have a parallel or "balanced circulation". In this group, the pulmonary and systemic circulation function in parallel and communicate with each other. It implies that relation between the pulmonary vascular resistance (PVR) and systemic vascular resistance (SVR) maintain the balance between the two circulations. These patients are at risk of worsening of cyanosis following high inspired oxygen concentration (FiO_2) due to pulmonary vasodilatation. Similarly, any reduction in SVR leads to increase in right to left shunt and worsens hypoxia. Last category of circulation is single ventricle physiology. These defects are not amenable to anatomically complete biventricle corrections.

Arrhythmia

Arrhythmias of different types can complicate the anesthetic management of children with CHD. They could be present preoperatively due to anatomical proximity of the defect to the conduction system or as a sequel of previous corrective (post ASD or VSD repair) or palliative (Mustard or Senning procedure, Fontan procedure) surgery.[7] Chronic hypoxemia and persistent haemodynamic stress also predispose to arrhythmia. Necrosis or progressive fibrosis extending into the conducting system and damage to atrioventricular node or Bundle of His are some of the underlying mechanisms for development of arrhythmia.[8] Clinically, these children can be asymptomatic or can be associated with haemodynamic instability and are at risk of sudden death. Different types of arrhythmia include atrial arrhythmia, ventricular ectopics (VE), primary malignant arrhythmia, brady-tachy syndrome, symptomatic bradycardia, 2nd or 3rd degree atrioventricular block, long QT syndrome, bundle branch block and complete heart block. Some of these require placement of permanent pacemaker or internal cardioverter defibrillator.

Hypoxia and Cyanosis

Presence of unrepaired or partially palliated CHD is likely to be associated with cyanosis due to hypoxia. It can be present in the settings of right to left shunt and with both increased and decreased pulmonary blood flow. Co-existing cardiac failure and arrhythmia worsen hypoxia and significantly increase the risk of complications.

The consequences of persistent hypoxia include end organ ischaemia and increase in erythropoietin levels which in turn increase the haematocrit, haemoglobin and viscosity. Hyperviscosity with haematocrit, more than 65% and haemoglobin more than 20 g% increase red cell rigidity and affect oxygen delivery, more so when superimposed iron deficiency is present. Hyperviscosity is associated with high SVR, increased risk of stroke due to cerebral and renal thrombosis.[9] The risk of stroke is increased by dehydration, fever, iron deficiency and age less than 5 years. Abnormalities in laboratory tests of haemostasis include prolonged prothrombin time and partial thromboplastin time. Thrombocytopenia, platelet dysfunction, decreased platelet survival, hypofibrinogenemia and accelerated fibrinolysis are the other haematological abnormalities.

Cyanotic lesions include tricuspid atresia, pulmonary atresia, Tetralogy of Fallot's, transposition of great arteries (TGA) and truncus arteriosus.

"Tet spells" or cyanotic attacks are seen in children with TOF, especially with obstruction to right ventricle outflow, precipitated by infundibular spasm. This forces right to left blood flow through VSD resulting in cyanosis. The precipitating factors include stress like crying, feeding, defecation, awakening or pain, light plane of anaesthesia and sympathetic stimulation. The "Tet spells" initiates a vicious cycle of prohypoxemic events causing further cyanosis and hypoxia leading to convulsions.

Treatment of the cyanotic attacks is described in the Table 24.6.

Table 24.6 Treatment of Tet spells (cyanotic or hypercyanotic attack)*

1. Improve preload with 15–30 mL/kg crystalloid
2. Ketamine (1–2 mg/kg) IV to increase systemic vascular resistance (SVR)
3. Relieve infundibular spasm with proponolol 0.1 mg/kg IV or esmolol 0.5 mg/kg bolus followed by infusion 50–30 µg/kg/min
4. Manage persistent hypoxemia with phenylephrine 0.5–2 mg/kg (increase SVR)
5. Correct metabolic acidosis if present with 1–2 meq of $NaHCO_3$ (increase SVR and PVR)
6. Mechanical ventilation with FiO_2 of 1, low inspiratory pressure and prolonged I: E ratio
7. Manual compression of abdominal aorta (if feasible)
8. Cardiopulmonary bypass or extra corporeal membrane oxygenation (ECMO)

***Comments:** Inhalation agents may help to decrease right ventricle outflow obstruction Inj Morphine Sulphate 0.05–0.1 mg/kg IV or IM can be used to decrease the stress in awake children along with knee chest position.

Pulmonary Artery Hypertension

Pulmonary artery hypertension (PAH) is one of the predictors of outcome after non-cardiac surgery in children with CHD and is defined as mean pulmonary arterial pressure of 25 mmHg at rest or 30 mmHg on exercise.[10] Most important etiological factors are increased pulmonary blood flow due to left to right shunt, prolonged pulmonary venous obstruction and high PVR due to high left atrial pressure. Initially, PHT is reversible. Structural changes with progressive and persistent PAH include medial hypertrophy of pulmonary vascular bed progressing to necrotizing vasculitis. This condition is called pulmonary vascular occlusive disease (PVOD). The time course, severity and consequences of PAH and PVOD depend on whether there is volume or pressure overload or both, duration of the CHD before repair and size of the shunt. PAH due to volume overload, as in case of large VSD is reversible if the repair is done in infancy. PAH due to pressure overload is of insidious onset. A popularly used clinical classification of PAH was proposed in 1998 which incorporated clinical presentations, therapeutic options and pathophysiological mechanisms.[11]

PAH can lead to haemodynamic deterioration by several mechanisms such as rapid rise in PVR, pulmonary hypertensive crisis and right heart failure.[12] PVR increases in response to multiple stimuli such as alveolar hypoxia, hypoxemia, hypercarbia, metabolic acidosis and pain. PVR is more sensitive to changes in hydrogen ion concentration than changes in carbon dioxide.

Pulmonary hypertensive crisis is life threatening and develops when the PAP exceeds systemic pressure due to rapid rise in PVR. This leads to acute reduction in right ventricular output and failure. In the absence of inter atrial communication, pulmonary blood flow further decreases which leads to reduced cardiac output ultimately causing biventricular failure. If there is a communication between the atria, left ventricular output and consequently coronary blood flow may be maintained. Hypoxia can result from right to left shunt, ventilation perfusion mismatch and intrapulmonary shunting.

Echocardiographic findings suggestive of PAH are tricuspid regurgitation, doppler velocity of more than 2.5 ms^{-1} or estimated systolic pulmonary arterial pressure 50% more than the systemic systolic arterial pressure.

Pulmonary vasodilators used for treatment of PAH include inhaled nitrous oxide (iNO), phosphodiesterase 5 inhibitors (PDE-5) like sildenafil and dipyridamole, prostacyclin analogs like epoprostenol (intravenous) and iloprost (inhaled drug), endothelium antagonist, bosentan and calcium channel blockers like diltiazem.

Shunting

It is the communication between the systemic and pulmonary circulation at the atrial or ventricular levels or between great vessels. The size and direction of shunt blood flow are determined by the size of the defect, pressure gradient between the two chambers or vessels, relation between the PVR and SVR, compliance of the ventricles and viscosity of blood.[13] A shunt could be left to right, right to left or bidirectional, resulting in changes in total systemic flow (Q_s) and total pulmonary blood flow (Q_P). Total pulmonary blood flow is equal to the sum of effective pulmonary blood flow and recirculated pulmonary blood flow. Similarly, total systemic flow is the sum effective systemic flow and the recirculated systemic flow. Thus, in presence of a shunt, the two circulations are not equal in terms of blood flow and the ratio, (Qp/Qs) is used to quantify a left to right shunt. Normally, in the absence of blood flow through the shunt, (Qp/Qs) is 1. A value up to 1.5 is considered as small, 1.6–2 as moderate and more than 2 as severe shunt. Common left to right shunt lesions are uncomplicated ASD, VSD, atrioventricular canal defects and Blalock-Taussig shunt (performed for the 1st stage repair of HLHS).

Left to right shunt causes oxygenated blood to flow into the pulmonary circulation, gradually overloading the pulmonary vascular system. At the same time, the systemic blood flow decreases. A persistent increase in pulmonary blood flow increases PVR and leads to PAH, increase in left atrial volume/pressure, pulmonary edema and volume overload. Volume overload can lead to biventricular failure. Increased PBF causes impairment of pulmonary function, small airway obstruction, air trapping, left main stem airway obstruction, increased in interstitial lung water content and pulmonary vascular occlusive disease. Prolonged left to right shunt can lead to Eisenmenger's syndrome due to shunt reversal.[14]

Complications of a shunt include reversal of the shunt and hypercyanotic attacks. Reversal occurs in a left to right shunt when the SVR decreases due to effect of drugs or hypovolemia or when the PVR increases as a result of increased airway pressure. Factors precipitating a hypercyanotic episode include surgical stimulation, dynamic right heart outflow obstruction, reduced pulmonary blood flow due to hypovolemia, increased airway pressure and reduced SVR.

Ventricular Dysfunction

CHD is associated with varying degrees of ventricular dysfunction. Progressive dysfunction is due to various factors such as primary disease causing chronic pressure and volume overload, remodeling of cardiac structure, effect of surgical repair (faulty procedure, complications of the procedure, injury to coronary artery, etc), chronic hypoxemia and arrhythmias.[15]

Volume overload induced ventricular dysfunction develops relatively early in the chronology of CHD unless surgical correction takes place in the first year of life. Pressure overload also results in progressive deterioration of ventricular function, but at a slower rate and symptoms develop later in the course. Children with cardiomyopathy also can present with severe ventricular dysfunction.

Ventricular Outflow Obstruction

Obstruction to outflow from the ventricles develops due to obstruction to ventricular outflow at the valvular, sub valvular or supra valvular levels leading to persistent pressure overload. The obstruction could be residual or recurrent, fixed or dynamic. Causes of right ventricular outflow obstruction are pulmonary stenosis, TOF, hypoplastic pulmonary artery, some types of double outlet right ventricle and Rastelli's procedure. When RV pressure exceeds systemic pressure, inter ventricular septal shift leads to left ventricular dysfunction, reduction in systemic circulation and even left ventricular outflow obstruction.[16] Aortic stenosis (AS), coarctation of aorta, some types of HLHS and Shone's anomaly produce pressure effects on left ventricle and result in dysfunction of the ventricle.

Ventricular outflow obstruction could be asymptomatic preoperatively and the first sign of dysfunction may be hypotension in response to a volatile agent during anaesthesia.

Myocardial Ischaemia

Children with CHD are prone to develop varying degrees of myocardial ischaemia from anatomical abnormalities of coronary arteries (e.g. anomalous origin from pulmonary artery), sequel of arterial switch operation and imbalance between myocardial oxygen demand and supply. Persistent load over the ventricle can induce abnormalities of coronary angiogenesis resulting in underdevelopment of capillaries, disproportionate to ventricular mass. Subendocardial perfusion is the first to be affected resulting in ischaemia. Underlying mechanism of ischaemia is interaction between the factors influencing the subendocardial perfusion, namely diastolic blood pressure, ventricular end diastolic pressure and heart rate (HR). HR determined the diastolic period during which coronary filling takes place. Tachycardia, is one of the factors which can precipitate myocardial ischaemia.

Congestive Cardiac Failure

Congestive cardiac failure (CCF) could be present pre-operatively and is a result of persistent pressure or volume overload. In children, cardiac failure invariably means biventricular failure. Often, even if there are no obvious signs of failure in the preoperative phase, stress imposed by anaesthesia, effect of drugs like propofol and compounding factors like hypovolemia can precipitate cardiac failure. Presence of or predisposition to cardiac failure requires that invasive monitoring (blood pressure and central venous pressure) should be considered even for apparently minor surgical procedures, requiring sedation or anaesthesia.

Cardinal features of congestive cardiac failure are tachycardia, tachypnoea, hepatomegaly and cardiomegaly.

End Organ Pathology

CHD is often associated with significant changes in respiratory system, neurological, renal, hepatic systems and psychology of the patient. The underlying mechanisms include alterations in lung mechanics, airway compression, chronic hypoxia, cyanosis, low perfusion, sequel of surgery and genetic factors. Decreased lung compliance and increased airway resistance result in requirement for higher airway pressure during mask ventilation increasing the risk of aspiration. Neurological changes include changes in cognitive function, hyperactivity, speech and language disabilities, seizures, stroke and choreoathetosis. Cerebral and venous thrombosis can be a consequence of plycythemia and hyperviscocity. Renal and hepatic dysfunction may be subclinical and even routine laboratory tests may be normal. Perioperative dysfunction can develop following compromise in oxygen supply or perfusion of liver or kidney.

Extracardiac anomalies

Important ones from anaesthesiologist's point of view are those involve the airway, cleft lip and palate, tracheoesophageal fistula, congenital diaphragmatic hernia, pyloric stenosis, craniofacial anomalies, etc. Many of these require surgical correction early in childhood. More than one anomaly may be present. Underlying mechanisms include genetic, teratogenic and other unknown causes.

Preanaesthetic Assessment

Detailed preanaesthetic evaluation (PAE) is crucial for understanding the nature and extent of the cardiac defect and to plan for the anaesthetic management. *An asymptomatic child with CHD does not always imply a healthy child.* High degree of suspicion is required to "unearth" potentially life threatening complications. The cornerstones of PAE are history, clinical examination, investigations and review of past medical records.

History: Carefully elicited history gives valuable information regarding the functional status of the child. An asymptomatic child with CHD with normal clinical examination may not require further evaluation for minor to moderately invasive procedures and risk due to CHD is minimal. Presence of symptoms like dyspnoea, wheeze, easy fatigability, delayed milestones, syncope, cyanotic attacks (tet spells), etc indicate poor cardiac reserve and possibility of complex CHD. Recent or recurrent respiratory tract infection can increase PVR and worsen the PAH.

Clinical examination: Should focus on vital signs, examination of cardiovascular and respiratory system, airway and other systems as relevant, to corroborate the historical findings. History and clinical examination should also help to uncover potentially dangerous complications like pulmonary hypertensive crisis (PHTC). Level of activity is a good indicator of cardiac reserve, with a normal level of activity appropriate to the age indicating a good cardiac reserve. On inspection, presence of tachycardia, irregular pulse and cyanosis are indicators of poor cardiac reserve. Bradycardia is an ominous sign, which along with dyspnoea, syncope, pallor, cyanosis, right ventricular heave and bronchospasm are the features of PHTC. Blood pressure should be measured in both the upper and lower limb if coarctation of aorta is suspected. Jugular venous distention and palpable liver can be present in children with congestive heart failure.

Evaluation of the cardiovascular system should begin with the auscultation of the first and second heart sounds, evaluation of the murmurs, if present and examination of the lungs. Any murmur, if present, should be evaluated for its characters, location, intensity, radiation and associated click. Following general rules can be used for interpretation of murmurs: (a) all systolic murmurs, other than pan systolic are benign, (b) all pan systolic murmurs are pathological and commonly are due to VSD and tricuspid regurgitation, (c) in VSD, louder the murmur, smaller the defect, (d) all diastolic murmurs are pathological and (e) all murmurs which radiate are pathological.

Some children with congenital complete heart block could present with an implanted pacemaker or internal cardioverter defibrillator devices. The anaesthesiologist should hold consultation with the paediatric cardiologist to know the indication for pacemaker and its settings, type and functional details, in addition to consulting the manufacturer's instructions.[17]

Investigations

These are ordered based on the findings of history, clinical examination and anaesthetic implications of the proposed surgery. A child with CHD which is asymptomatic, has been corrected early and completely, undergoing minimal to moderately invasive procedures need not require extensive investigations. Broadly, in every patient, the need for each of the following tests should be considered carefully.

1. Routine haematological tests: To detect anemia, polycythemia and hyperviscosity.
2. Tests of coagulation: Bleeding time, clotting time, prothrombin time and international normalized ratio (INR).
3. Blood grouping and cross matching
4. Platelet count
5. Electrocardiogram: Can provide useful information in a child with CHD. It should be evaluated for rate, rhythm, presence of ectopics, chamber enlargement, ischemia and QTc interval.
6. X-ray chest helps to diagnose cardiomegaly, congestive cardiac failure, pulmonary hypertension, respiratory infection, etc.
7. ECHO: Echocardiography helps in assessing CHD in terms of size, flow and pressure gradient, myocardial function, dilatation of cardiac chambers and valvular function.
8. Holter monitoring and stress testing
9. Arterial blood gas analysis and electrolytes
10. Cardiac catheterization
11. Cardiovascular magnetic resonance imaging (MRI)
12. Liver function tests
13. Other tests as dictated by specific clinical findings or surgical needs.

It should be remembered that echocardiography, transesophageal echo (TEE) and cardiovascular MRI require either sedation or anaesthesia. The choice depends on age, type of CHD, clinical findings, duration of the procedure, anxiety levels of the child, parental consent and cognitive development of the child. Children less than 7 years, mentally challenge children, those requiring TEE, extremely anxious children, those with poor anaesthetic risk, etc. require general anaesthesia with endotracheal intubation.

Risk Stratification

Risk assessment depends on multiple factors as shown in Table 24.7. More complex the lesion, higher the risk. Similarly, major surgical procedures, presence of complications related to defect, previous repair and co morbid conditions indicate a higher risk. Based on the available evidence, risk can be low, intermediate and high depending on various aspects of the defect, pathophysiological changes and other patient and surgery related factors.

Table 24.7 Factors associated with high risk of perioperative morbidity

- ASA PS ≥ 4
- Birth in a tertiary hospital
- Complex lesions (including single ventricle physiology, cardiomyopathy, aortic stenosis)
- Less than 2 years old
- Low ejection fraction
- Left ventricle outflow tract obstruction
- Major surgery
- Presence of long term sequeale (arrhythmia, cardiac failure, pulmonary hypertension, cyanosis)
- Prehospital stay > 10 days
- Preoperative arrhythmias

Low risk children are the ones whose defect is single or simple, have normal circulation with no significant shunt or other pathophysiological consequences, age more than 2 years, undergoing minor or minimally invasive elective surgery, belong to American Society of Anaesthesiologists (ASA) physical status 1–3 and who do not require prolonged preoperative stay in the hospital. Classical example can be an active child of 5 years, with a small ASD, with room air saturation more than 95%, posted for elective herniotomy.

Intermediate risk is when the physiology is well compensated, lesion is simple, age less than 2 years, elective major surgery (intrathoracic or intra abdominal) with anticipated blood loss, ASA physical status of 4–5, requiring pre-procedure hospital stay of more than 10 days.

High risk category include children with complex CHD with congestive heart failure, PHTC, arrhythmia or cyanosis, age less than 2 years, major or emergency surgery, prehospital stay of more than 10 days and ASA 4 and 5. Risk of major complications related to anaesthesia during non-cardiac surgery has been reported to be 3–16%.[18]

Contents of PAE are shown in Table 24.8.

Preoperative Preparation, Instructions and Premedication

Preoperatively, discussions are held with the child, surgeon and parents regarding the risk status, anaesthetic plan, anticipated complications and postoperative management. It is also the time to decide about the need for consultation with the paediatric cardiologist and other specialists as required. Children with complex CHD and significant complications should be evaluated by paediatric cardiologists. However, the anaesthesiologist should have final responsibility of accepting the patient for anaesthesia or sedation based on the facilities available, complexity of the condition, adequacy of the optimization and his/her experience. Specific preparations in a child with CHD include correction of dehydration, continuation or discontinuation of pre-existing drug therapy, clear instructions regarding the fasting time, infective endocarditis prophylaxis and ordering premedication.

Adequate hydration, ensured by preventing excessive fasting and intravenous fluids, is important in children with cyanotic CHD with hyperviscosity. Clear liquid can be given up to 2 hours prior to surgery towards this goal. Young children with cyanotic CHD should be posted early in the morning to prevent excessive fasting. It also provides for longer periods of observation after the surgery.

Children with CHD could be on multiple drugs for either maintaining of the surgical correction, cardiac function, rhythm or for management of complications. Common drugs and their implications are described in Table 24.9.

When a child is on pacemaker, it should be set to asynchronous mode before the surgery to prevent the influence of the cautery and defibrillation function also should be deactivated.

Finally, some children with complex CHD may require preoperative medical stabilization (e.g. maintenance of ductal patency with prostaglandins), palliative shunts, balloon atrial septostomy, interventional cardiac catheterization, etc. before elective non-cardiac surgery.

Premedication helps in smooth separation from the parents and having a quiet and cooperative child at the time induction. Crying in a child with cyanotic CHD

Table 24.8 Components of preanaesthetic evaluation

- Airway examination
- Co-morbidity and its impact
- Drug therapy, pre existing
- Implanted devices like pacemaker
- Investigations, as relevant
- Presence of complications due to defect or repairs (arrhythmias, cardiac failure, pulmonary hypertension, hypoxia)
- Room air saturation
- Understanding the defect(s); anatomy, physiology and type of circulation
- Vascular access

Table 24.9 Medications and indications in children with CHD

Drug	Indication
ACE inhibitors	Management of hypertension
Antibiotics	I:E prophylaxis
Aspirin	Maintaining shunt patency
Beta blockers	Treatment of 'tet' spells, control of heart rate
Bosentan	Pulmonary hypertension
Epoprostenol	Pulmonary hypertension
Ilioprost	Pulmonary hypertension
Indomethacin	PDA
PGE_1	PDA
Sildenafil	Pulmonary hypertension
Warfarin	Anticoagulation

can precipitate hypercyanotic spells. Midazolam in the dose of 0.5 mg/kg oral, 30 minutes prior to surgery produces good anxiolysis without significant sedation.[19] Patient should be administered oxygen supplementation with a nasal cannula or face mask and monitored after sedative premedication. Use of a cardiac grid describing the nature of defects and physiological goals of anaesthetic management helps to minimize errors of judgement and enhance the safety.

Appropriate infective endocarditis (IE) prophylaxis should be provided as per AHA guidelines. According to 2013 guidelines of American Heart Association, the categories of children with CHD requiring IE prophylaxis are: (a) history of IE, (b) unrepaired cyanotic CHD including palliative shunts and conduits, (c) completely repaired CHD with prosthetic mesh or device in the first six months and (d) repaired CHD with residual defects at the site of repair.[20]

Not all procedures require IE prophylaxis. Minor procedures such as injection of local anaesthetic for dental treatment, removal of deciduous teeth, bronchoscopy and most of the diagnostic gastrointestinal and urological procedures do not require IE prophylaxis. IE prophylaxis is required in procedures in which there is manipulation of gingival tissue or periapical region of teeth, perforation of oral mucosa or breach of mucus membrane such as tonsillectomy, adenoidectomy, etc. Prophylaxis is against endocarditis produced by *Streptococcus viridans* and the recommended dose in children is oral amoxicillin 50 mg/kg, not exceeding 2 g 60 min before the procedure. In case the patient is unable to take orally, ampicillin in the same dose can be given intravenously on the table in theatre. Clindamycin can be used as a substitute in patients allergic to penicillin, in the dose of 20 mg/kg, both oral and intravenous. In these children ceftriaxone or cefazolin 50 mg/kg, IM or IV can also be used.

Anaesthetic Management

Just like CHD is not a single entity, there is no single anesthetic technique or a combination of drugs which "suites all" children with CHD. Almost all known anaesthetic techniques and drugs have been used in these patients. The choice depends on multiple factors such as effects of premedicants, effects of anaesthetics, analgesics and adjuvants on volume status, blood pressure, PVR, SVR, rheological properties of blood, heart rate and myocardial contractility. Anaesthetic goal is to maintain the haemodynamic and other physiological parameters within the normal limits to prevent worsening of the cardiac function due to hypoxia, myocardial dysfunction, arrhythmia, outflow obstruction or congestive cardiac failure. Effects of individual anaesthetics are discussed in the following sections.

Table 24.10 Anaesthetic management: Factors to be considered in decision making

- Type of defect and repair (palliation versus correction)
- Presence of Shunt: Type, extent, pulmonary blood flow
- Pulmonary artery hypertension
- Ventricular dysfunction
- Cyanosis and hypoxia
- Arrhythmia
- Co-morbid conditions and extra cardiac anomalies
- Proposed surgical procedure
- End organ dysfunction and injury
- Effect of anaesthetic drugs and techniques

Induction

In general, choice of method of induction, intravenous or inhalational depends more on the presence or ease of venous access and preference of the anaesthesiologist than the particular type of defect. Maintenance of stability of various physiological variables like heart rate (HR), PVR, SVR, etc. is more important than individual drug.

Inhalational induction is preferred in children with CHD without intravenous access, children with difficult airway and those with certain type of CHD. All the available volatile agents have been used safely. Halothane is now replaced by sevoflurane, with or without nitrous oxide. Desflurane can also be used, but QTc interval prolongation on ECG is a concern. Halothane has been shown to decrease QTc in children in a study.[21] Speed of induction with volatile anaesthetics depend on PBF, solubility of the agent and the magnitude and direction of the shunt. In case of right to left shunts, induction may be slightly prolonged, more so with an agent with higher solubility like halothane. With these drugs, high inspired concentration and positive pressure ventilation increase the speed of induction. However, one should be cautious that high concentration of halothane with positive pressure breaths for induction can cause severe myocardial depression causing bradycardia and hypotension, progressing even to cardiac arrest. Also, the volatile anesthetics themselves can adversely affect the shunting pattern and lastly, with very large right to left shunt, increase in FiO_2 does not increase the partial pressure of oxygen (PaO_2). Time for inhalational induction, with left to right shunt is usually unchanged compared to normal children. Nitrous oxide hastens the induction with volatile agents but has the disadvantages of risk of enlargement of air bubble (can cause paradoxical air embolism in intracardiac shunts) and inability to provide high FiO_2.

All the four known induction agents, propofol, thiopentone, ketamine and etomidate have been used in CHD.[22,23] Presence of a left to right shunt does not have significant affect on intravenous induction, whereas right to left shunt can result in dramatic effects during intravenous induction as the drugs reach the site of action faster. Propofol, when used for induction, decreases SVR and mean arterial pressure (MAP) with no effects on PAP and PVR. Ketamine, on the contrary, increased MAP without effect on SVR. It is the induction agent of choice in cyanotic CHD and is also used for treatment of cyanotic attacks. Ketamine also has been safely used for procedures not requiring endotracheal intubation.[24] Intramuscular ketamine in the dose of 4–8 mg/kg intramuscular has been used for induction in uncooperative children with CHD. Etomidate is cardio stable and the only concern is the adrenal suppressive effects, which is not clearly proven in the context of its use for induction of general anaesthesia. In presence of cardiac failure, both intravenous and inhalational induction (as in case of emergency procedures in children with CHD) can be slow and one needs to wait for sufficient time before the drug effects are evident.

Airway management technique is decided on the basis of the surgical needs and postoperative concerns regarding the need for intensive care support. Supraglottic airway devices are acceptable if there is no contraindications.

Maintenance of Anaesthesia

Balanced anaesthesia with a combination of opioid analgesic, oxygen and nitrous oxide and sevoflurane or isoflurane, with or without muscle relaxant has been observed to result in stable clinical conditions. Circulatory effects of volatile agents are dose dependent and titratable. In children with single ventricle lesions neither sevoflurane nor fentanyl—midazolam combination causes significant depression of myocardial contractility. Both sevoflurane and isoflurane have been extensively used during general anaesthesia in children with CHD.[25,26] Experience with desflurane is limited and the experience of the concerned anaesthesiologist is important in choosing the volatile anaesthetic. High concentrations of volatile agents can cause myocardial depression which is poorly tolerated by most of the children with CHD.

Major goals during maintenance phase are prevention of deterioration in the clinical condition of the patient by maintain volume status, normal ratio of SVR to PVR, adequate analgesia, early diagnosis and management of complications, use of appropriate FiO_2 and intensive monitoring of the patient.

Specific Anaesthetic Goals Based on the Preoperative Pathophysiology

Severe PHT: Further rise under anaesthesia can result in low cardiac output, right ventricular failure and hypoxemia. Anaesthetic goals are to maintain oxygentation, adequate ventilation with normocarbia and depth of anaesthesia. Use of pulmonary vasodilators like nitric oxide may be required. Acidosis, systemic hypertension should be avoided.

Left Ventricular Outflow Obstruction

Intraoperatively, coronary ischemia and low cardiac output can result from tachycardia, arrhythmia, hypotension and severe myocardial depression. Anaesthtic goals are to maintain ventricular filling pressure, SVR, sinus rhythm and normal myocardial contractility.

Single Ventricle Physiology

Postsystemic to pulmonary artery shunt: Pulmonary to vascular resistance ratio determines the pulmonary and systemic circulation both of which are supplied by a functional single ventricle. Avoiding hyperoxygenation and hyperventilation and maintaining ventricular function are the anaesthetic goals.

Dilated Cardiomyopathy

It is associated with low ejection fraction and heart cannot compensate for reduction in SVR, reduced preload or contractility. Hence, the anaesthetic goals are to maintain normal preload and SVR. Severe myocardial depression should be avoided.

Specific issues related to some common CHD are mentioned in glossary.

Monitoring: Standard monitoring includes pulse oximeter, non-invasive blood pressure, electrocardiogram and end tidal carbon dioxide measurements. In addition, as the complexity of the procedure and/or CHD increase, the extent of monitoring also needs to be increased. The additional monitors that may be required are: (a) invasive blood pressure monitoring for a better control of blood pressure, (b) arterial blood gas measurements, (c) temperature monitoring, (d) central venous pressure monitoring, (e) transoesophageal echocardiogram and (f) urine output. Recently, non invasive and continuous monitoring of haemoglobin has been introduced into clinical practice. Similarly, continuous cardiac output monitoring is also possible with an arterial cannula in place.

Interpretation and significance of monitored values are important and must be in the context of preoperative findings and intraoperative anaesthetic goals. SpO_2 values should be interpreted based on the type of CHD and preoperative room air saturation. In a cyanotic CHD the difference between end tidal carbon dioxide ($ETCO_2$) and $PaCO_2$ is widened, and increases 2–3 mmHg for every 10% drop in SpO_2.[27]

Recently, transesophageal echocardiography has been suggested[28] as intraoperative monitor of cardiac function and to guide fluid management. This is particularly useful because conventional monitoring of filling pressure and blood pressure, etc. may not reliably detect the complications in the early stages of development during the surgery.

Complications and Management

Some of the important complications include hypotension, arrhythmia, reversal of shunt, hypercyanotic attacks, cardiac failure, sudden cardiac arrest, stroke and hypothermia.

Hypotension could result from various causes such as hypovolemia, blood loss, vasodilatation, reduction in SVR, cardiac failure, arrhythmia and anahylaxis. Maintenance of normal range of MAP is achieved with fluids, titration of anaesthetic agents, early replacement of blood loss, vasopressors (phenylephrine, noradrenaline or adrenaline) and management cardiac dysfunction with onotropes as appropriate. Hypovolemia has been found to be an important *preventable* cause of intraoperative hypotension.

Changes in PVR can induce changes in the direction and magnitude of shunt and quantity of PBF, cause PHTC, precipitation of cardiac failure or severe hypoxemia in the perioperative period. Hypoxia, hypercarbia, acidosis, hyperinflation, hyperviscosity and sympathetic stimulation increase PVR, whereas oxygen, hyperventilation, normal functional residual capacity, haemodiluation and sympathetic block prevent rise in PVR. Management of PHTC is with 100% oxygen, hyperventilation, pulmonary vasodilation, support and analgesic supplement.

Arrhythmia in the perioperative period can be atrial, ventricular or conduction blocks. It could be continuation of preoperative arrhythmia or fresh changes induced by surgery or anaesthesia related events. In presence of significant CHD, arrhythmias can be potentially life threatening and contribute to congestive cardiac failure, hypotension and sudden cardiac arrest. All efforts should be made to anticipate, early diagnosis and aggressive treatment. Defibrillation or cardio version may be required for arrhythmia management.

Other complications reported include sudden cardiac arrest in a child with valvular AS undergoing laparoscopic procedure and report of renal failure and multi organ dysfunction in a series of children with Fontan circulation undergoing non-cardiac surgery.[29,30]

MANAGEMENT OF "TET SPELLS"

Management includes intravenous fluids to improve the right ventricular stroke volume, increase the depth of anaesthesia, sedation, increasing FiO_2, increasing the SVR to improve PBF by increasing the left to right shunt and avoiding exogenous catecholamines. Summary of treatment is shown in Table 24.6.

At the end of surgery, early extubation should be the goal, unless contraindicated. This helps to minimize the postoperative agitation which could lead to changes in PVR and also may reduce the need for deep sedation.

Postoperative Care

Level of care is commensurate with the severity of the pathophysiological changes preoperatively and at the end of surgery, perioperative complications and type of surgery. High risk children requiring care in the paediatric intensive care include those who had perioperative complications, cardiac failure, those requiring intense monitoring and requiring intense analgesia.

Intravenous opioids have been safely used for postoperative analgesia, both as infusions and bolus. Intravenous dexmedetomedine has been used without loading dose in a series of children for congenital cardiac surgery, as a postoperative analgesic without significant respiratory events or need for reintubation. 15% of patients had hypotension. Many types of regional analgesia, alone or in combination with general anaesthesia have been used in children with CHD. Uneventful epidural analgesia in neonates with complex defects undergoing non-cardiac surgery is reported.[30]

Other Issues

Care to avoid air bubbles in the system is very important, especially when there is a communication at the atrial and ventricular levels. If there is any complication, surgeon should be informed early and included in decision making.

Spinal anaesthesia has been safely used in normal infants and small children for many surgical procedures and they tolerate up to 20% fall in MAP without adverse clinical features. Recently, Ludmya et al. in a retrospective review, compared the effect of awake spinal anaesthesia in children with CHD and normal children.[31] They observed no significant differences in the incidence of complications in both the groups. However, the choice of spinal anaesthesia depends on the type and pathophysiological changes in particular CHD.

Higher FiO_2 is not always beneficial in all children with CHD. Those who are used to chronic hypoxia can have a further reduction in PBF due to vasodilators effects of oxygen resulting in worsening of hypoxia. Children with Fontan physiology are safe at PaO_2 of 40–45 mmHg or SpO_2 of 70–75%.

PROCEDURAL SEDATION IN CHILDREN WITH CHD

Large number of procedures are being done under sedation in children and those with CHD are no exception. The choice of sedation as an alternate to general anaesthesia depends on the complexity of the CHD, experience of the anaesthesiologist and the set up. The procedures include cardiac imaging in MRI suite, dental procedure, or change of some devices like ventricular assist device, etc.

Similar to general anaesthesia, thorough PAE should be performed with relevant investigations. Patient should be fasting as per standard guidelines. Those who belong to ASA 3 or 4 and above need to undergo sedation in a hospital based set up with all facilities for intensive post operative care. Ideal drugs include propofol, ketamine and recently dexmedetomedine. Opioids like fentanyl and benzodiazepine like midazolam also can be safely used for sedation. Titration of the drug to the response needed and avoiding poly pharmacy are the key to safe sedation.

Recent Advances

Dexmedetomedine is a popular addition to the anaesthesiologists armamentarium. It has been safely used in children with CHD for procedural sedation as well as an adjunct to general anaesthesia.[32] Its unique advantages are stable haemodynamics, ability to prevent tachyarrhythmia, blunting of sympathetic stimulation, reduction in anaesthetic requirements, analgesic property, neroprotective effects, proneuroapoptic activity and minimum effects on respiratory system and airway.

Paediatric patients with severe left ventricular failure or structural abnormalities of the heart and who are waiting for cardiac transplant, may be on ventricular assist devices and may come for other procedures. A knowledge of these devices is essential in such cases.[33]

Clevidipine is a new non-anesthetic drug used in the management of perioerative hypertension in children with CHD. It belongs to dihydropyridine group of calcium channel blocker, with a half life of 1–3 min. It is administered intravenously and is suitable for infusion. Clevidipine is metabolized by blood and tissue esterases. It reduces mean arterial pressure by vasodilatation.

FEATURES AND ANAESTHETIC IMPLICATIONS OF SPECIFIC DEFECTS

Aortic Stenosis (AS)

- Can be supravalvular or subaortic. Bicuspid aortic valve (most common CHD) may be associated with coarctation of the aorta.
- Critical neonatal AS is a ductal dependent lesion
- Shone's anomaly is AS with mitral stenosis and aortic coarctation
- Supravalvular AS is associated with Williams syndrome

Anaesthesia: Ventricular outflow obstruction and dysfunction could be present. Tachycardia, hypotension, arrhythmia should be avoided. Dehydration should be prevented preoperatively by minimal fasting period. Titrate and slow induction and low concentration of inhaled agents help maintain haemodynamic stability.

Atrial Septal Defect (Fig. 24.1)

- One of the common defects, with three different types based on location.
- Osteum primum defect (primum ASD), usually associated with atrioventricular canal defect. Surgical repair at less than 5 years of age.
- Osteum secundum defect (secundum ASD), can be asymptomatic, usually managed by device closure.
- Sinus venous defect, can be asymptomatic, device closure is used.

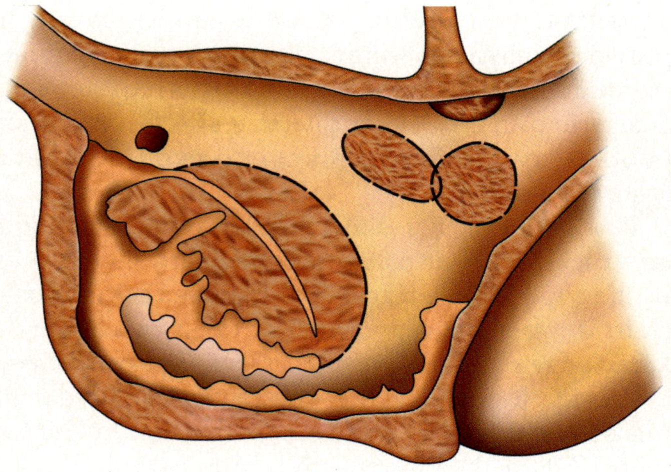

Fig. 24.1 Atrial septal defect

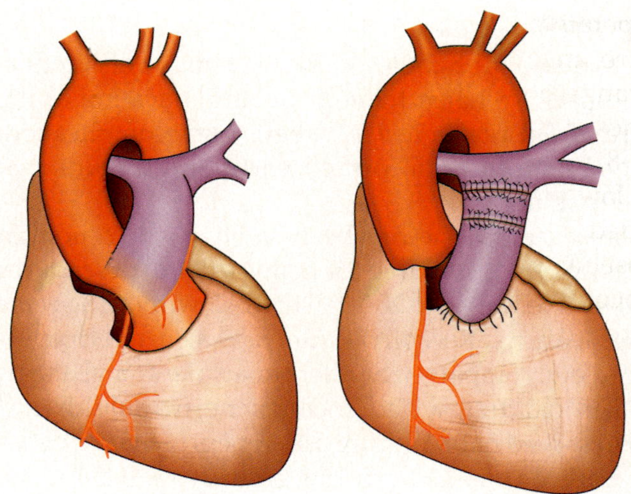

Fig. 24.2 D-transposition of great arteries

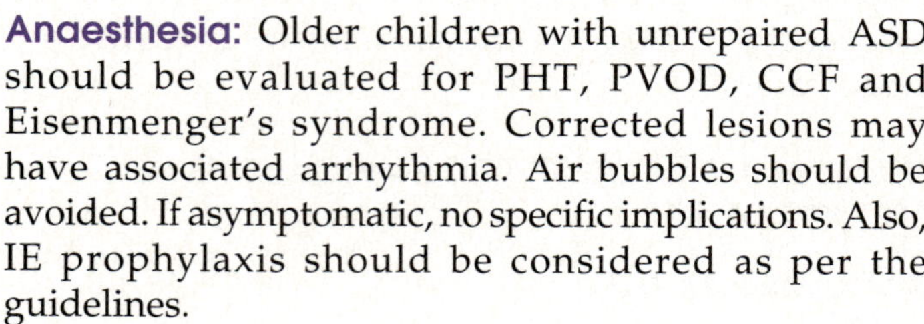

Anaesthesia: Older children with unrepaired ASD should be evaluated for PHT, PVOD, CCF and Eisenmenger's syndrome. Corrected lesions may have associated arrhythmia. Air bubbles should be avoided. If asymptomatic, no specific implications. Also, IE prophylaxis should be considered as per the guidelines.

Coarctation of Aorta

- Could be preductal, ductal or post ductal. Preductal can be part of *Turner's Syndrome*
- Can be associated with ventricular hypertrophy and hypertension.
- Can be a medical emergency in neonatal period requiring maintenance of ductal patency

Anaesthesia: Blood pressure monitoring in pre- and post-ductal levels with arterial line on the right hand or femoral artery. Ketamine should be avoided. Volatile anaesthetics should be avoided in high concentrations neonates and small infants. High dose fentanyl with midazolam is well tolerated. Intraoperatively, beta blockers or vasodilators may be required.

D-Transposition of Great Arteries (Fig. 24.2)

- Aorta arises from right ventricle and pulmonary artery (PA). A VSD is associated in 15% of these patients. In the absence of any type of shunt (ASD, VSD or PDA), there can be severe hypoxia and cyanosis. In such cases, atrial septostomy is done as an emergency procedure.
- These children might have undergone Mustard or Senning procedure.

Anaesthesia: Depends on the age, whether surgically corrected or not, and extent of pathophysiological changes. After arterial swith operation most of these children can be treated as structurally normal heart. Interventional catheterization may be required to treat severe pulmonary stenosis preoperatively. Pacemaker may be present. Maintenance of haemodynamic stability is the key anaesthetic goal. Inotopic support should be started early in ventricular dysfunction.

Single Ventricle Physiology (Including HLHS)

- Also called univentricular heart, functionally there is only one ventricle with two atrioventricular valves, resulting complete mixing of the two circulations and predisposing for cyanosis, hypoxia, myocardial dysfunction and congestive cardiac failure.
- Single ventricle physiology is seen in HLHS, severe tricuspid stenosis or atresia, double outlet right ventricle, etc. Some of them may be dependent on PDA for survival. Only palliative procedures are possible. Usually, three stage repair is done for this condition, most common final palliative procedure being Fontan procedure.
- Patients with HLHS undergo Norwood or Hybrid procedures. In these patients, PBF and consequently oxygenation can be compromised by peak airway pressure, controlled ventilation and positive pressure ventilation. They can come for non-cardiac procedures before or after complete palliative or in between the different stages.

Anaesthesia: In unoperated children, drugs required to maintain the ducal patency should be continued.

Preoperatively, they should be evaluated for cardiac failure and arrhythmia. Baseline SpO_2 can be in the range of 70–75% only. Low FiO_2 of 0.21, maintenance of hypercarbia to pH of 7.30 with tidal volume of 6–8 mL/kg and respiratory rate of 8–10/min with low positive end expiratory pressure are recommended.

Post Fontan, the ventricle is hypertrophic, dilated and hypocontractile. Prone for precipitation of cardiac failure under anaesthesia, arrhythmia may require cardio version. Air bubble should be avoided.

Ketamine or etomidate for induction and muscle relaxants with high dose of opioids and midazolam have been safely used. Care should be exercised with volatile agents.

Tetralogy of Fallot (Fig. 24.3)

- Cyanotic CHD with pulmonary stenosis, VSD, over riding of aorta and RVH. Usually undergo a palliative shunt in early infancy and complete repair by 6–12 months.
- PBF depends on systemic blood pressure. Increased SVR improves oxygenation. Increased PVR increases right to left shunting.

Anaesthesia: SVR and blood pressure should be maintained, rise in PVR should be prevented, so also the infundibular spasm to prevent cyanotic attacks. They should be treated early and aggressively. Uptake and elimination of inhalational agents is slow and IV agents have faster onset of action. Ketamine is a useful drug in these children. Hypervolemia should be avoided to prevent precipitation of RV failure.

Ventricular Septal Defect (Fig. 24.4)

- Isolated or part of complex CHD such as TOF, Truncus arteriosus, etc.
- Single, small defects and repaired ones are asymptomatic.
- Large defects can cause increase PBF leading to RV overload and consequences.
- Presence of multiple defects is called "Swiss Cheese septum".

Anaesthesia: Small defects, minimal shunts and those with anatomical repair and younger age have no additional risk. Air bubbles should be avoided. In larger defects, RV overload, increased PVR and PHT should be looked for and included in formulating anaesthetic goals. Reversal of shunt should be prevented by maintaining SVR PVR relationship.

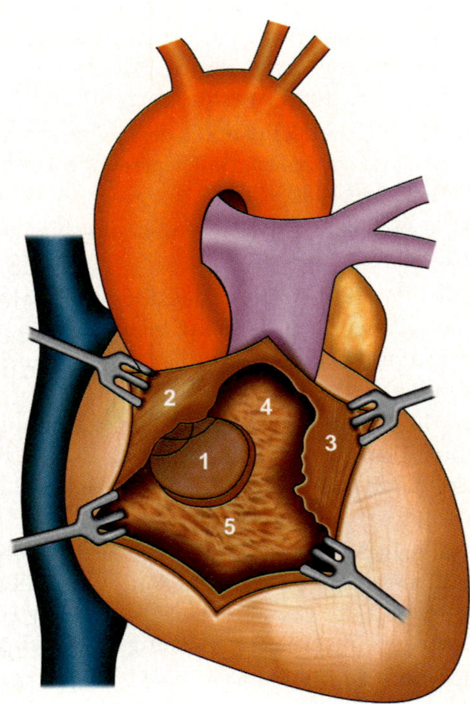

Fig. 24.3 Tetralogy of Fallot
1-VSD with overriding aorta, 2-parietal RV hypertrophy, 3-septal RV hypertrophy, 4-infundibular septum, 5-papillary muscle conus

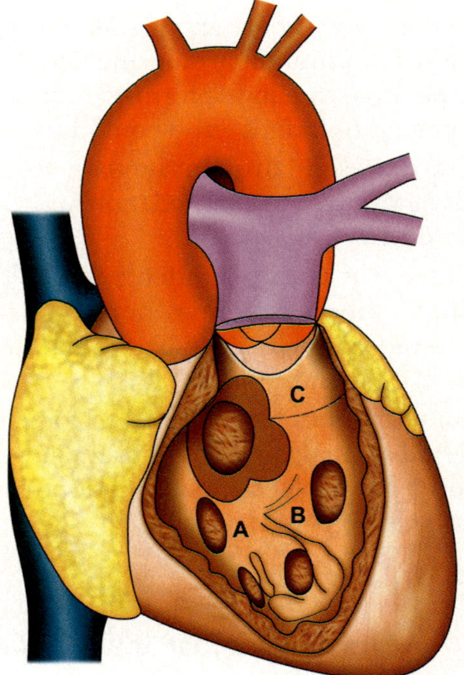

Fig. 24.4 Ventricular septal defect
A-Membranous, B-Trabecular, C-Infundibular

SUMMARY

- Children with CHD represent a heterogenous population undergoing a variety if non-cardiac procedures requiring sedation or general anaesthesia.
- The CHD could be simple, complex, single or multiple, cyanotic or acyanotic, repaired or unrepaired and corrected or palliated. They can have extra cardiac anomalies requiring surgery or can be part of recognized syndromes. Bicuspid aortic valve, ASD and VSD are among the more common CHDs.
- Preanaesthetic evaluation should focus on the anatomical nature of the defect, pathophysiological consequences such as shunting, arrhythmia, cardiac failure, ventricular dysfunction, PAH, etc. and also the presence of complications like cardiac failure, pulmonary hypertensive crisis, etc.
- Preoperative preparation and should aim for optimization of hydration status, anxiolysis, management of cardiac failure, if present, management of PAH if severe and development of an anaesthetic plan. A cardiac grid incorporating the goals is useful.
- All the available drugs and techniques have been used in anaesthetizing these patients. It is the management of pre-defined physiological goals through proper dosing, and titration of the drugs and appropriate monitoring including invasive ones, which determines the outcome.
- High-risk category of patients should be identified in advance and appropriate arrangement for higher level of perioperative care in the form of support services, additional consultations, etc. should be made.
- Ketamine is a useful drug for intravenous and intramuscular induction and for sedation in children with cyanotic CHD.
- Intraoperatively, particular attention should be given to maintain normovolemia, normothermia, preoperative saturation limit, analgesia and to minimize changes in PVR and SVR.
- Regional techniques have been used for surgery and postoperative analgesia. Opioid analgesics can be safely used for analgesia, both intraoperatively and in postoperative period.

GLOSSARY

Anatomic repair implies that morphological left ventricle is connected to aorta and right ventricle to pulmonary artery resulting in circulation in series. Anatomic repair can be simple or complex. A simple repair is done in a structurally normal heart, like in PDA, ASD and VSD without PHT. Complex repair is performed for TGA, TOF, aortic stenosis, pulmonary stenosis and truncus artrisus.

Physiological repair refers to surgical correction following which circulation is in series, but patient still has a univentricular physiology, anatomically either univentricular or biventricular (where RV is systemic ventricle and LV is pulmonary ventricle), e.g. following Mustartd or Senning procedure for TGA.

Rastelli procedure is performed for D-TGA when arterial switch is contraindicated. After the procedure LV functions as systemic ventricle.

Common surgical procedures for different CHD are shown in Table 24.11.

REFERENCES

1. Greenwood RD, Rosenthal A, Parisi L, et al. Extracardiac abnormalities in infants with congenital heart disease. Pediatrics. 1975;55(4): 485–92.
2. Baum VC, Barton DM, Gutgesell HP. Influence of congenital heart disease on mortality after non-cardiac surgery in hospitalized children. Pediatrics. 2000; 105(2):332–5.
3. Ramamoorthy C, Haberkern CM, Bhananker SM, et al. Anesthesia-related cardiac arrest in children with heart disease: data from the Pediatric Perioperative Cardiac Arrest (POCA) registry. Anesth Analg. 2010;110(5):1376–82.
4. Torres A Jr, DiLiberti J, Pearl RH, et al. Noncardiac surgery in children with hypoplastic left heart syndrome. J Pediatric Surg 2002;37:1399–1403.
5. Witt C. Cardiac embryology. Neonatal Network 1997; 16(1):43–49.
6. Michelle CW, James MP. Anaesthetic management of children with congenital heart disease for non-cardiac surgery. Contin Educ Anaesth Crit Care Pain. 2012;12(1): 17–22.
7. Frank Ville D. Anesthesia for children and adults with congenital heart disease. In: Lake CL, Booker PD (Eds). Pediatric Cardiac Anesthesia. Philadelphia: Lippincott Williams and Wilkins, 2005;601–632.
8. Diaz LK, Hall S. Anesthesia for non-cardiac surgery and magnetic resonance imaging. In: Andropoulos DB, Stayer SA, Russel IA (Eds). Anesthesia for congenital heart disease. Massachussets: Blackwell Publishing, 2005;427–452.
9. Phornphutkul C, Rosenthal A, Nadas AS, et al. Cerebrovascular accidents in infants and children with cyanotic congenital heart disease. Am J Cardiol. 1973;32(3):329–34.
10. Galie N, Rubin LJ. Introduction: new insights into a challenging disease. A review of the Third World

Table 24.11 Common surgical procedures for different CHD

Surgical procedures	Palliation/correction	Indications	Age	Remarks
Arterial switch (Jantene) Atrial switch* (Mustard and Senning)	Anatomical repair Physiological repair	Transposition of great arterires (TGA)[€]	After birth	Atrial switch is replaced byArterial switch
Blalock-Taussig shunt[$]	Palliation	Tetraology of Fallot (TOF)	<2 weeks, if tet spells are present	Complete correction by 2 years of age
Fontan procedure (Total Cavo Pulmonary Correction)[¥]	Palliative (Final stage correction)	Single ventricle including HLHS[#]	2 years	Presence of high pulmonary vascular resistance is a contraindication
Glenn shunt (Hemi-Fontan)[^]	Palliative	Tricuspid atresia	2 years	Also part of the surgical treatment path for HLHS
Hybrid procedure (Trans catheter and surgical palliation)	Correction	HLHS	Neonates	Avoids major surgery and improves neurological and cardiac outcome
Norwood procedure (Stage 1 single ventricle palliation)	Palliative	HLHS and variants	Neonates	Ductus arteriosus patency maintained with prostaglandin therapy High risk surgery

*Post procedure, patient can have sinus node dysfunction, ventricular dysfunction and arrhythmia

$BT shunt is also done for pulmonary atresia, severe pulmonary stenosis and tricuspid atresia

^Performed after the removal of BT shunt or pulmonary artery banding in staged correction of single ventricle CHD

#HLHS—Hypoplastic left heart syndrome

€ Also called D-TGA

¥TAPVC

Symposium on Pulmonary Arterial Hypertension. J Am Coll Cardiol 2003;43:1S.

11. Simonneau G, Galie N, Rubin LJ, et al. Clinical Classification of pulmonary hypertension. J Am Coll Cardiol 2004;43:5S–12S.
12. Carmosino MJ, Friesen RH, Doran A, et al. Perioperative complications in children with pulmonary hypertension undergoing noncardiac surgery or cardiac catheterization. Anesth Analg. 2007;104(3):521–7.
13. Ziayd M, Hiojazi MD, et al. Paediatric cardiac intervention. J AM Coll Cardiol Intv 2008;1(6):603–611.
14. Rossouw B. Balancing the heart and lungs in children with large cardiac shunts. Continuing medical education 2013;31(1).
15. Lynch J, Pehora C, Holtby H, et al. Cardiac arrest upon induction of anesthesia in children with cardiomyopathy: an analysis of incidence and risk factors. Paediatr Anaesth 2011;21:951–957.
16. Friesen RH, Williams GD. Anesthetic management of children with pulmonary arterial hypertension. Pediatr Anesth 2008;18:208–216.
17. Navaratnam M, Dubin A. Pediatric Pacemakers and ICDs: how to optimize perioperative care. Pediatric Anesth. 2011;21:512–521.
18. van der Griend BF, Lister NA, McKenzie IM, et al. Postoperative mortality in children after 101 885 anesthetics at a tertiary pediatric hospital. Anesth Analg 2011;112: 1440–1447.
19. Levine MF, Hartley EJ, Macpherson BA, et al. Oral midazolam premedication for children with congenital cyanotic heart disease undergoing cardiac surgery: a comparative study. Can J Anesth 1993;40:934–938.
20. AHA guidelines: Prevention of Infective endocarditis 2013.
21. Ebru A, Ayse HK, Sema O, et al. The effects of sevoflurane and desflurane anaesthesia on QTc interval and cardiac rhythm in children. Pediatr Anesth 2007;17:563-567.
22. Williams GD, Jones TK, Hanson KA, et al. The haemodynamic effects of propofol in children with congenital heart disease. Anesth Analg 1999;89: 1411–1416.
23. Sarkar M, Laussen PC, Zurokowski D, et al. Hemodynamic responses to etomidate on induction in pediatric patients. AnesthAnalg 2005; 101:645–650.
24. Morray JP, Lynn AM, Stamm SJ, et al. Haemodynamic effects of ketamine in children with congenital heart disease. Anesth Analg 1984;63:895–899.
25. Rivenes SM, Lewin MB, Stayer SA, et al. Cardiovascular effects of sevoflurane, isoflurane, halothane and fentanyl/ midazolam with 100% oxygen in children with congenital

heart disease: an echocardiography study of myocardial contractility and haemodynamics. Anaesthesiology 2001;94:223–229.

26. Laird TH, Stayer SA, et al. Pulmonary to systemic blood flow ratio effects of sevoflurane, isoflurane, halothane and fentanyl/midazolam with 100% oxygen in children with congenital heart disease. Anesth Analg 2002;95:1200–1206.

27. Lazzell VA, Burrows FA. Stability of the intraoperative arterial to end tidal carbon dioxide partial pressure difference in children with congenital heart disease. Can J Anaesth. 1991;38: 859–865.

28. Komal K, Isobel R, Wanda C, et al. Role of transesophageal echocardiography in the management of paediatric patients with congenital heart disease. Pediatr Anesth. 2011; 21(5):479–493.

29. Groenewald CB, Latham GJ. An expected cause of cardiac arrest during laparascopy in an infant with supravalvular aortic stenosis. Pediatr Anesth. 2013;23(1):91–93.

30. Rabbits JA, Groenewald CB, Mauermann WJ, et al. Outcomes of general anesthesia for non-cardiac surgery in a series of patients with Fontan palliation. Pediatr Anesth. 2013;23(2):180–182.

31. Ludmyla K, Einat B, et al. Spinal anesthesia for non-cardiac surgery in infants with congenital heart diseases. Pediatr Anesth. 2012;22:647–653.

32. Tobias JD, Gupta P, Naguib A, et al. Dexmedeto medine applications for pediatric patient with congenital heart disease. Pediatr Cardiol. 2011;32: 1075–1087.

33. Miller SP, Mcqullen PS, Hamrick S, et al. Abnormal brain development in newborn with congenital heart disease. N Engl J Med. 2007;357:1928–1938.

25

Paediatric Neuroanaesthesia

Anita Shetty, Ruchi Jain and Jimmy John

INTRODUCTION

Developing and maturing neurological and physiological status pose inherent challenges in paediatric patients. Essential concepts of neuro-anaesthesia are almost same in all age groups. In this chapter, we will emphasize the important distinguishing features in management of paediatric neurosurgical patients.

GENERAL CONSIDERATIONS

Neurophysiology

The data on paediatric neurophysiological values is limited and has been deduced from human adult and animal studies.

Cerebral Blood Flow

Cerebral blood flow (CBF) is an important determinant of intracranial pressure. CBF is defined as the difference between the mean arterial pressure (MAP) and intracranial pressure (ICP). CBF is regulated by cerebral metabolic rate ($CMRO_2$), cerebral perfusion pressure (CPP), arterial blood carbon dioxide ($PaCO_2$) and oxygen (PaO_2) tensions, the influence of various drugs, and intracranial pathology. CBF is normally auto-regulated or is constant over a given range of CPPs. The values increase with age. In premature infants it is 12 mL/100 g/min, 23–40 mL/100 g/min in full term neonates, 90 mL/100 g/min from 6 months to 3 years of age and 100 mL/100 g/min from 3 to 12 years of age. CBF is higher in children as compared to adults (50 mL/100 g/min).[1]

Cerebral Metabolic Rate

The CBF is coupled with the metabolic requirements of the developing brain. The $CMRO_2$ and CBF increase proportionally after birth. In children, the $CMRO_2$ is higher at 5.2 mL/100 g/min than the adults (3.5 mL/100 g/min). Therefore, children are less to lerant to hypoxia. Neonates have a lower $CMRO_2$ (2.3 mL/100 g/ min) and are comparatively tolerant to hypoxaemia.[2]

Cerebral Auto-regulation

The auto-regulatory range of blood pressure in a neonate is between 20 and 60 mmHg.[3] This is probably due to lower metabolic requirements of the perinatal brain. The curve of cerebral auto-regulation is shifted to the left in neonates. Also, its slope is significantly steep at the lower and upper limits of the curve. This narrow range of auto-regulation puts neonates at a higher risk of cerebral ischemia and intra-ventricular haemorrhage secondary to hypotension and hypertension respectively.

Arterial Carbon Dioxide/Oxygen Tension ($PaCO_2$/PaO_2)

In adults, increase in $PaCO_2$ causes a linear increase in CBF. In a neonate, the cerebrovascular response to changes in $PaCO_2$ is partially developed. Hence, CBF does not increase significantly until hypercapnia is severe. In contrast, the neonatal brain is more sensitive to changes in PaO_2 as compared to adults and the CBF increases in response to smaller decreases in PaO_2.

Intracranial Pressure

The Monro-Kellie doctrine states that the skull is a closed box with brain tissue, blood and cerebrospinal fluid (CSF) as its contents. An increase in volume of one of these components with increase in ICP will result in a compensatory reduction of other components. The posterior fontanelle closes at about 6 months of age, the anterior fontanelle at around 1 year–1½ years, and final cranial suture closure may be as late as 10 years. In the infant, before cranial suture fusion, an increase in the contents of the cranium is compensated by an increase in skull size. However, this accommodation is possible only if the change is gradual. Acute increases, such as after traumatic brain injury, will still result in raised ICP as in adults. As a result of increased compliance of cranium, infants do not present with features of raised ICP until significant disease progression.

Other Physiological Differences

The brain receives a greater percentage of cardiac output (CO) in children as compared to adults. CBF is 10% to 20% of the CO during the first 6 months and peaks at 55% between the second and fourth years. Cerebral blood flow settles to the adult levels of 15% by 7 to 8 years.[4] The larger heads of the infants and children constitute a large percentage of the body surface area and blood volume. Hence, children are at a greater risk for significant haemodynamic instability during neurosurgical procedures (Table 25.1).

PREOPERATIVE EVALUATION

Many neurosurgical conditions in paediatric patients are 'emergencies' and a detailed preoperative evaluation may not always be possible. The signs and symptoms of raised ICP in neonates and infants are different from older children and adults. Neonates and infants present with irritability, bulging fontanelles and increased head circumference. Older children may complain of headache, diplopia and vomiting. The Glasgow Coma Scale has been modified for paediatric patients (Table 25.2).

One must look for craniofacial anomalies, congenital heart diseases, respiratory tract infections, congenital anomalies and bleeding disorders in all cases. Patients with supra-sellar pathologies like craniopharyngiomas must have an endocrine evaluation. A two-dimensional echocardiography (2D-ECHO) may be needed to rule out congenital heart diseases especially in neonates. 2D-ECHO is also indicated in children with arteriovenous malformations as they can have features of congestive cardiac failure.

Patients may be on long term anticonvulsant therapy which may lead to hepatic, haematological and metabolic disturbances. Phenytoin and phenobarbital are

Table 25.1 Effect of anaesthetic agents and other drugs on cerebral physiology[4,5]

Anaesthetic	CBF	$CMRO_2$	ICP	CO_2 reactivity	Cerebral auto-regulation
Thiopental	↓	↓	↓	0	0
Etomidate	↓	↓	↓	0	—
Propofol	↓	↓	↓	0	0
Fentanyl	0/↓	0/↓	0/↓	0	0
Alfentanil	0/↓/↑	0/↓	0/↓/↑	0	0
Sufentanil	0/↓/↑	0/↓	0/↓/↑	0	0
Remifentanil	0/↓	0/?↑	0/↓	0	0
Ketamine	↑	0/↑	↑	0	0
Midazolam	↓	↓	0/↓	↑	↑
Nitrous oxide	↑	0/↑	↑	0	0
Isoflurane	↑	↓	↑	0	0
Desflurane	↑	↓	↑	0	0/↓*
Sevoflurane	↑	↓	↑	0	0
Succinylcholine	0	0	↑	—	—
Vecuronium	0	0	0	—	—
Atracurium	0	0	0	—	—
Rocuronium	0	0	0	—	—
Pancuronium	0	0	0	—	—
Dexmedetomidine	↓	↓	0/↓	0	0

CBF: cerebral blood flow; $CMRO_2$: cerebral metabolic rate for oxygen consumption; ICP: intracranial pressure; 0: no effect, ↓: decreased, ↑: increased, –: no effect, *: at ≤ 1 MAC, + in adult patients

Table 25.2 Modification of the Glasgow Coma Scale for paediatric patients

Type of response	Score	Age related responses		
		>1 year	<1 year	
Eye-opening response	4	Spontaneous	Spontaneous	
	3	To verbal command	To shout	
	2	To pain	To pain	
	1	None	None	
Motor response	6	Obeys commands	Spontaneous	
	5	Localizes pain	Localizes pain	
	4	Withdraws to pain	Withdraws to pain	
	3	Abnormal flexion to pain (decorticate)	Abnormal flexion to pain (decorticate)	
	2	Abnormal extension to pain (decerebrate)	Abnormal extension to pain (decerebrate)	
	1	None	None	
		0–2 years	2–5 years	>5 years
Verbal response	5	Babbles, coos appropriately	Appropriate words, phrases	Oriented and converses
	4	Cries but is consolable	Inappropriate words	Confused conversation
	3	Persistent crying or screaming to pain	Persistent crying or screaming to pain	Inappropriate words
	2	Grunts or moans to pain	Grunts or moans to pain	Incomprehensive sounds
	1	None	None	None

enzyme inducers and hasten the metabolism of non-depolarizing muscle relaxants and anaesthetic agents, increasing the requirement of these drugs. Valproic acid may cause thrombocytopenia and hepatic dysfunction. Phenytoin may also lead to gingival hyperplasia which may result in bleeding during airway manipulation.

Platelet count, prothrombin time and thromboplastin time help rule out most bleeding disorders. Electrolyte imbalance is frequently seen in patients with vomiting and in dehydration due to poor oral intake as a result of impaired consciousness. Cross matched blood units should be available before all craniotomies in paediatric patients.

Anaesthesia Management

Routine preoperative fasting guidelines have to be followed.

Premedication

Crying leads to an increase in ICP. Hence, sedative premedication may be required in infants beyond 9 months of age to allow easy separation from parents. Oral premedication with midazolam is associated with lesser respiratory depression as compared to opioids. If an intravenous (IV) line is present, midazolam can be given IV as well in titrated doses. Ketamine increases ICP and is usually contraindicated in neurosurgical patients. Sedative premedication should be avoided in patients with raised ICP as even minor decrease in respiratory drive can lead to hypercapnia and worsen the ICP.

Vascular Access

Two 'good' peripheral intravenous lines are required for most neurosurgeries. Central venous cannulation may be required in many cases especially in surgeries done in sitting position. Subclavian and jugular venous cannulations have a risk of pneumothorax but are extremely useful in the setting of venous air embolism. In infants and smaller children aspiration of air from multi-orificed catheters may not be easy due to the small lumens of individual ports.[6] Peripherally inserted central lines via the ante cubital veins may be used in older children. Access to femoral vein is easier and does not interfere with venous drainage from the head like the jugular venous catheters. However, air cannot be aspirated via this route. Intra-arterial blood pressure can be monitored via the radial artery. Other alternative sites preferred are dorsalis pedis, femoral and posterior tibial artery.

MONITORING

Electrocardiography, pulse oximetry, non-invasive blood pressure, urine output and temperature need to be monitored in all patients. Temperature may be monitored by using nasopharyngeal or rectal temperature probes. Intra-arterial blood pressure is preferably monitored for all craniotomies and prolonged spine surgeries. CVP monitoring may be required in cases where prolonged operative time, major surgical haemorrhage or diabetes insipidus is anticipated to guide fluid therapy. Neuromuscular monitoring may be required if muscle relaxants are given by infusions or to rule out causes for delayed recovery. Special neurological monitoring is required for some cases.

Neuro-monitoring help in early detection and correction of any injury to brain and spinal cord. It also helps in modifying the surgical technique as per patient's physiology.

Neurophysiologic Monitoring[4,7]

Neurophysiologic monitoring is important in surgeries that may place the cortico-spinal tracts, dorsal columns, cranial nerves (CNs), or nerve roots at risk of intra-operative insult. Surgeries where neuro-monitoring may be used are anterior and posterior spinal fusions, tethered cord release, dorsal rhizotomies, and craniotomies for tumour and posterior fossa decompressions.

Different modalities are electromyography (EMG), somatosensory-evoked potentials (SSEPs), motor-evoked potentials (MEPs), electroencephalography (EEG), brainstem auditory-evoked potentials (BAEP), and other specific CN (VII, IX, X, XII) EMG.

EMG

EMG activity may occur by surgical manipulation of the nerve, inadvertent irritation of nerves by retractors or stretch pressure on the nerve from positioning. Neuromuscular-blocking agents must not be used when EMG is to be monitored.

SSEPs

Monitoring SSEPs gives valuable information concerning the integrity of the sensory tract (ascending sensory pathway) from the periphery to the primary sensory cortex. Anaesthetics can alter the amplitude and latency of the cortical potentials in a dose-dependent manner. SSEPs are not affected by neuromuscular-blocking drugs.

MEPs

Motor deficits can occur without any sensory deficit. Hence, it is necessary to monitor the functional integrity of the motor tracts (descending motor pathways) of the spinal cord by MEP. Desflurane at 0.5 MAC levels can be used for monitoring of MEPs. Total intravenous anaesthetic (TIVA), accomplished by propofol and remifentanil or sufentanil infusions is ideal. Muscle relaxants must not be used during MEP monitoring. Low dose dexmedetomidine (0.2 mg/kg/hr) without initial loading dose does not affect MEP.

SSEPs and MEPs are Used During Spine Surgeries

Other evoked potential monitoring modalities are visual evoked potentials to assess the visual system and brainstem auditory evoked potentials to assess cranial nerve VIII and brainstem pathways.

EEG

EEG records the electrical activity of the brain. It is used when drug induced metabolic suppression is required and cerebral hypo-perfusion is present. Low levels of inhalation anaesthetic can be used.

Monitors of Cerebral Oxygenation

EEG, transcranial Doppler ultrasonography (TCD) and cerebral oximetry are used to monitor cerebral ischemia in infants and children.

Systemic arterial hypotension, when accompanied by intracranial hypertension, can cause cerebral ischaemia. Routine use of these monitoring modalities is often not feasible due to the proximity of the surgical field.[4]

Detection of Seizure Foci

Epileptogenic activity is documented by electrographic seizures or EEG spike activity. Electro-corticography (ECoG) is recorded via electrodes placed on the surface of the brain after the dura is opened. If epileptogenic foci are in close proximity to cortical areas controlling speech, memory, motor, or sensory function, electrophysiologic monitoring is utilized to minimize injury to these areas. Low concentrations of volatile anaesthetics and opioids alone do not depress ECoG and EEG signals. Neuromuscular blockade should be used cautiously, if cortical stimulation of the motor strip in a child under general anaesthesia requires either EMG or direct visualization of muscle movement. Most intravenous and inhalational anaesthetics depress EEG activity and may degrade mapping. Hence, switchover to a nitrous oxide and narcotic based technique before mapping with enough time to eliminate agents that affect EEG activity is commonly practised.

POSITIONING

General considerations for positioning in neuro-anaesthesia

1. Neurosurgical procedures are lengthy with limited access to head and airway.
2. Anaesthesiologist should be able to access the IV lines and visualise the child under drapes.
3. Pressure points should be properly padded and airway well secured.
4. Pins in paediatric patients can cause skull fracture, dural tear and subdural haematoma.
5. Tachycardia and hypertension due to pins should be attenuated by deepening the plane of anaesthesia or with local anaesthetics.
6. Excess rotation of head can cause compression of internal jugular vein leading to raised ICP.
7. Excessive neck flexion can cause endo-bronchial migration of the tube as well as obstruction of lymphatic and venous drainage resulting in macroglossia. Hyperflexion of the head and neck may decrease bloodflow in vertebral and carotid arteries, leading to brainstem and cervical spine ischemia, resulting in quadriparesis and quadriplegia.
8. Eyes should be lubricated and protected from cleansing solutions and external pressure to prevent postoperative visual impairment.
9. Vital parameters should be monitored while giving position.
10. Avoid extreme stretching of nerves.
11. Head up tilt improves venous drainage but increases the chance of venous air embolism

Supine Position is Used for Frontal, Temporal or Parietal Access

Lateral position is used for posterior parietal and occipital access. An axillary roll, inflatable pillow or a gel pad should be placed under the upper chest to prevent arm ischemia, brachial plexus injury and compartment syndrome. It is not used commonly in paediatric patients.

Prone position is used for spinal, occipital and posterior fossa procedures. Patients are induced on the trolley and then log rolled onto the chest rolls or special frames placed on the operating table. The head should be kept in neutral position while turning. Keeping the abdomen free improves the excursion of the diaphragm resulting in improved oxygenation and ventilation and decreased intra-abdominal pressure. This improves venous return and reduces surgical bleeding. The head may be fixed on pins, horseshoe headrest or head rests with mirror system. Eyes, nose, and ears should be protected against pressure.

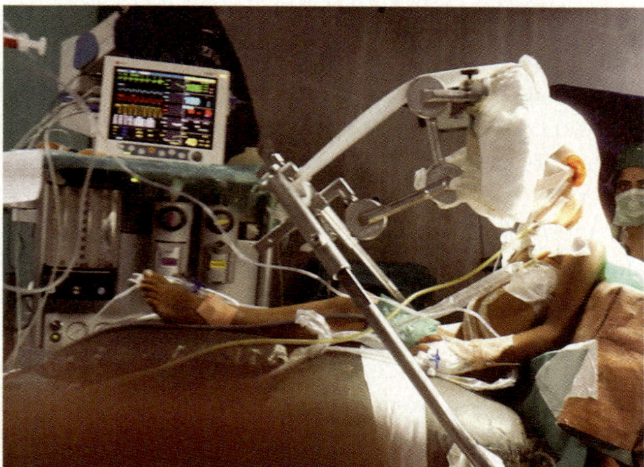

Fig. 25.1 Sitting position is used for posterior fossa and cervical spine surgery

Sitting position (Fig. 25.1) is used for posterior fossa and cervical spine surgery. This position provides better venous and CSF drainage and better surgical access. Decreased venous return and hypotension can cause cerebral ischaemia. Venous air embolism, macroglossia, upper airway obstruction, pneumo-cephalus, subdural hematoma and quadriplegia can occur.

Airway Management

Differences in the paediatric and adult airway have to be kept in mind. Manual inline stabilization is required during intubation in patients with traumatic brain injuries, cervical spine trauma, atlanto-axial dislocations and Chiari malformations. As the airway is inaccessible during the intraoperative period in most neuro-surgeries, the endotracheal tube should be meticulously fixed to avoid displacement during and after positioning. Careful auscultation can help detect accidental endo-bronchial intubation after flexion of head. Extreme flexion of neck can lead to kinking of endotracheal tube at base of tongue. Significant airway oedema can develop in prone position which may necessitate delaying extubation at the end of surgery. In such cases the patient should be nursed in a head high position and ventilated electively till airway oedema settles.

Induction and Maintenance of Anaesthesia

The goal of anaesthesia in neurosurgical patients is maintenance of CPP and avoidance of increase in ICP.

In the absence of an IV line, or in case of difficult IV access, induction with sevoflurane is favoured as crying can result in increased ICP. If an IV line is in place, IV induction is preferred over inhalational induction as the latter results in cerebral vasodilation and increase in ICP. Thiopental (3–5 mg/kg) and propofol (2–3 mg/kg) can be selected. Muscle relaxation can be achieved with non-depolarizing muscle relaxants (NDMR) like rocuronium, atracurium or vecuronium. Succinylcholine is to be avoided as it leads to fasciculations and can increase ICP. However, in anticipated difficult airway, securing the airway takes priority over controlling ICP. In such situations, a defasciculating dose of NDMR may be given prior to succinylcholine. Rapid sequence induction needs to be carried out in patients at increased risk of aspiration. A total intravenous technique may be used for maintenance with target controlled infusions of propofol and remifentanil. Inhalational agents can be used for maintenance in concentrations <1 MAC.

Fluid Management

Glucose containing solutions should be avoided as hyperglycaemia worsens cerebral oedema and reperfusion injury. Premature babies, neonates and infants are at greater risk of hypoglycaemia and should be given dextrose containing fluids (5–6 mg/kg/min of dextrose infusion)[4] with sugar monitoring. Isotonic saline and Ringer's lactate are commonly used fluids. However, too much of normal saline (>60 mL/kg) can lead to hypernatremia and hyperchloremic metabolic acidosis. The administration of large volumes of Ringer's lactate solution can reduce plasma osmolality and increase brain water content and ICP as approximately 114 mL of free water is given for each litre of lactated Ringer's solution. The paediatric brain is unable to adapt to excess free water. Hence, hyponatremia results in cerebral oedema more rapidly in paediatric patients.[8] Safety and effectiveness of PLASMA-LYTE A™ in paediatric patients have not been established by adequate and well-controlled trials, however, the use of electrolyte solutions in the paediatric population is referenced in the medical literature. In the Cochrane database review of colloids versus crystalloids for fluid resuscitation in critically ill adult patients, the authors concluded that there is no evidence to support the use of colloids over crystalloids in the resuscitation of patients with burns, trauma, or after surgery, Colloids which are significantly more expensive are not associated with improved survival.[9] There is no evidence to suggest the utility of one colloid over the other.[10]

Temperature Management

Mild hypothermia (34–35ºC) may help in reduction of $CMRO_2$; however, severe hypothermia should be avoided. Fluid warmers, warm air devices and heated mattresses are required to prevent hypothermia and warm the patient prior to extubation.

Management of intraoperative raised ICP/"Tight brain"

1. Confirm adequate venous drainage by giving head elevation and correcting extreme flexion or rotation of neck.
2. Control airway pressure: If airway pressure is increased, rule out obstruction, bronchospasm, inadequate muscle relaxation, endo-bronchial intubation and pneumo-thorax.
3. Diuresis by mannitol (0.25–1 gm/kg) and/or furosemide.
4. Titrate $PaCO_2$ to ≥ 25 mm of Hg
5. Reduce mean arterial blood pressure.
6. Reduce metabolic rate of brain by giving adequate analgesia (opioids) and deepen the plane of anaesthesia (barbiturates/propofol). Anti-seizure drugs may be given.
7. Potential vasodilators like N_2O, inhalational agents, nitroglycerine, nitroprusside or calcium channel blockers need to decreased or stopped.
8. CSF drainage by ventriculostomy or lumbar drain.
9. Persistent raised ICP after all these measures should raise suspicion of intracranial haemorrhage.

VENOUS AIR EMBOLISM

Venous air embolism (VAE) is a commonly encountered problem in neurosurgery as the operative site is frequently above the level of the heart. In children, the bigger size of the head as compared to the body puts them at higher risk of VAE as the head remains above the level of heart even in supine position. Posterior fossa tumours constitute a large chunk of all childhood intracranial tumours and these are frequently operated in sitting position which has a higher incidence of VAE.

Massive air embolism is rare and slow entrainment of air is more common. The presence of a patent foramen ovale (PFO) or septal defects increase the risk of paradoxical air embolism. Pre-cordial doppler ultrasonography and trans-oesophageal echocardiography (TEE) along with $ETCO_2$ help in detection of VAE. TEE can detect as little as 0.02 mL/kg of air, whereas doppler can pick 0.05 mL/kg of air.[11] Fall in $ETCO_2$ is not specific for VAE as hypotension due to any cause will result in decrease in $ETCO_2$. Aspiration of air through the central line is diagnostic as well as therapeutic in VAE. The problem of VAE is compounded by technically difficult central venous access, smaller size of neck veins leading to obstruction of venous drainage from head and smaller lumens of multi orifice catheters making aspiration of air difficult. Patients may undergo elective closure of PFO prior to undergoing neurosurgery. Maintaining normo-volemia helps in preventing VAE.

Once VAE is suspected steps should be taken to prevent further entrainment of air, to relieve right heart obstruction and to support haemodynamics. The surgeon should be alerted to flood the field with saline. Bilateral jugular vein compression may be tried. The head may have to be lowered below the level of the heart. However, this may not be easy with the head fixed by pins. N_2O should be discontinued and air aspirated from the right heart catheter. 100% O_2 should be administered and haemodynamics should be supported by volume replacement and inotropes as required.

Reversal and Extubation

The goals for extubation in neurosurgery are to have a rapid awakening to permit quick neurological assessment, maintenance of haemodynamic stability and minimal straining on endotracheal tube. Smooth emergence from anaesthesia is desirable as coughing can increase intracranial pressure and blood pressure which can lead to intracranial haemorrhage. Fentanyl 0.5–1 µg/kg or lignocaine 1 mg/kg can be given to reduce coughing. Esmolol, labetalol and dexmedetomidine may be used for controlling haemodynamic responses. The patient should be extubated only after confirming adequacy of spontaneous ventilation in an awake patient as postoperative respiratory depression can lead to raised ICP. Caution should be exercised prior to extubation in patients with surgical manipulation of the brainstem and lower cranial nerve nuclei as they may have respiratory dysfunction due to damage to the respiratory centre. Prolonged surgery in prone and sitting position may lead to airway oedema and airway obstruction postextubation. Patients with preoperative poor GCS and those with delayed recovery from anaesthesia due to a variety of causes may require postoperative ventilation.

Common Causes of Delayed Recovery from Anaesthesia after Neurosurgery

1. Residual effect of anaesthetic drugs
2. Respiratory failure—hypoxia, hypercarbia
3. Surgical
   a. Surgical insult to respiratory centre, hypothalamus
   b. Cerebral oedema
   c. Intracranial haemorrhage
   d. Thrombosis
4. Paradoxical air embolism
5. Pneumo-encephalus
6. Hypothermia
7. Endocrine/metabolic
   a. Hypothyroidism
   b. Fluid and electrolyte imbalance—diabetes insipidus
   c. Hypoglycaemia
8. Haemodynamic instability
9. Seizures
10. Raised ICP due to any cause

Postoperative Analgesia

Paracetamol given intravenously or as a suppository provides adequate analgesia for most intracranial surgeries. Tramadol causes nausea and vomiting and hence should be used after pre-emptive anti-emetics like ondansetron. Patients undergoing complex spine surgeries may require opioids like fentanyl or morphine to control postoperative pain. However, close monitoring is required while using opioids since respiratory depression may occur. Non-steroidal anti-inflammatory drugs may be added 24 hours after surgery when risk of bleeding decreases.

Postoperative Nausea and Vomiting

Postoperative nausea and vomiting is common in neurosurgical patients and is treated with $5HT_3$ antagonists like ondansetron and dexamethasone.

> **Key Point: Seizure Prophylaxis**
>
> Seizures are common in postoperative period. Patients may be given a loading dose of phenytoin 10–15 mg/kg followed by maintenance dose of 2 mg/kg 8 hourly. Levitracetam may be required in some cases. Hypoglycaemia, electrolyte imbalance, intracranial haemorrhage, cerebral ischaemia are usual causes of postoperative seizures.

SPECIFIC PROCEDURES IN NEUROSURGERY

Meningocoele or Meningomyelocoele

Failure of the neural tube to fuse by 28 days postconception causes herniation of the meninges or meninges with neural elements, resulting in meningocoele or meningomyelocoele (Fig. 25.2). If the neural tube defect occurs

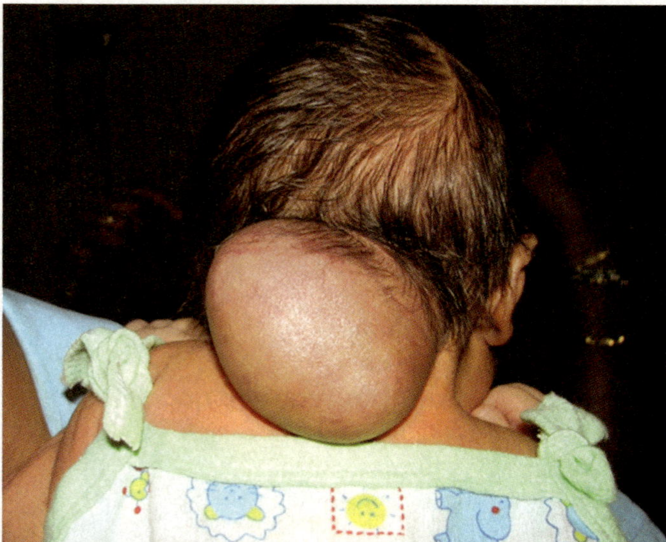

Fig. 25.2 Meningocoele or meningomyelocoele

in the cranium, it will result in encephalocoele. Meningomyelocoele may be associated with Chiari II malformation, hydrocephalus, intestinal malformation, renal anomalies, cardiac malformation and tracheo-esophageal fistula.[12]

Chiari II malformation causes caudal displacement of cerebellum, tonsils and medulla. Hydrocephalus occurs due to obstruction of fourth ventricular outflow. These children may present with brainstem dysfunction like apnoea, vocal cord palsy resulting in stridor, autonomic instability, depressed gag-reflex with risk of aspiration.[1]

Anaesthesia Considerations

1. Surgery is carried out in the first 24 to 48 hours to reduce the risk of infection. Anaesthesia challenges of neonate should be kept in mind.
2. If there are large exposed lesions, there may be increased risk of fluid loss, dehydration and electrolyte abnormalities.
3. During induction and endotracheal intubation, care should be taken to avoid pressure on the herniated sac by padding or placing on soft gel.
4. If the meningomyelocoele is large, lateral position can be used.
5. Brainstem compression during laryngoscopy and intubation in Chiari II malformation can cause bradycardia.[13]
6. Latex allergy is common in these patients.
7. If spinal cord below the meningomyelocoele is tethered, detethering of cord will require EMG monitoring. Muscle relaxant should not be used.
8. In the postoperative period, these children are prone to hypoventilation and apnoea due to brainstem dysfunction.
9. Complications arising from prone position.

Craniosynostosis[14,15]

Craniosynostosis occurs due to premature closure of one or more cranial sutures (Fig. 25.3). Syndromes such as Apert's, Crouzon's, Pfeiffer's are associated when multiple sutures are involved. If untreated, it can lead to intracranial hypertension and abnormal neurologic or intellectual development.

Surgical approaches can be minimally invasive like endoscopic strip craniectomy to open procedures like total calvarial reconstruction and fronto-orbital advancement.

Anaesthesia Implications

1. Airway may be difficult in patients with syndromes.
2. Hydrocephalus and increased ICP may be present.
3. Major blood loss may occur due to proximity to major venous sinuses as well as from the surgical site.
4. Venous air embolism.
5. Corneal injury if the eyes are in the surgical field and they are not protected. Lubricating ointment may be applied to lubricate the eyes.
6. Manipulation may lead to occulo-cardiac reflex. Treatment is by removal of stimulus and administration of anti-muscarinic drugs.

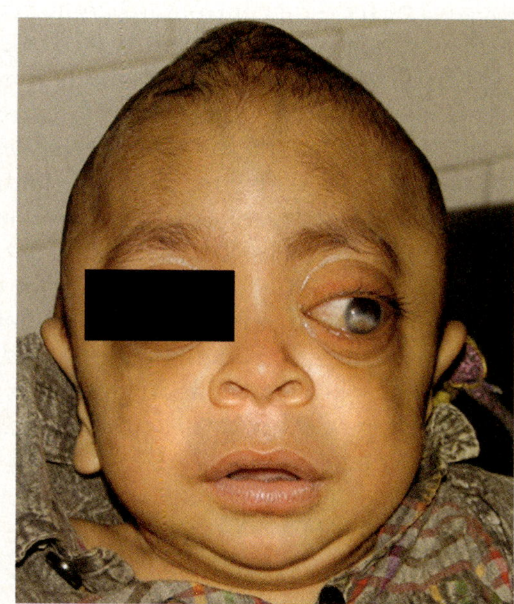

Fig. 25.3 Craniosynostosis

7. If surgery is below the orbital ridge, post-operative facial oedema can occur and cause airway obstruction.
8. Hypothermia due to prolonged surgical time.

Brain Tumours[4]

Brain tumours in children most commonly occur in the posterior fossa. Surgeries are done in the sitting or prone position.

Anaesthesia considerations for posterior fossa tumours

1. Hydrocephalus may be present due to obstruction to flow of CSF leading to raised ICP.
2. Problems related to sitting and prone position have to be kept in mind.
3. Complications such as VAE, massive haemorrhage may occur.
4. If Mayfield head frame is used, complications due to pin fixation can occur.
5. Sudden changes in intra-operative blood pressure and pulse rate may indicate manipulation of brainstem.
6. Postoperative apnoea, airway obstruction and aspiration can occur if brainstem or lower cranial nerves are damaged during surgery.

Most common supra-tentorial tumours are craniopharyngiomas.

> **Take Home Message**
> Brain tumours in children most commonly occur in the posterior fossa. Surgeries are done in the sitting or prone position.

Anaesthesia Considerations

1. May be associated with hypothalamus and pituitary dysfunction. Hence, perioperative steroid administration may be required.
2. Endocrine abnormalities can occur. Hence, thyroid and adrenal functions must be evaluated.[4] In the postoperative period, diabetes insipidus (DI) can occur. It may cause hypovolemia and hypernatremia. Diabetes insipidus is treated with IV fluids and synthetic vasopressin.

FAQ with Answer

Q. Which is the most common CNS supra-tentorial tumour in children?

A. They are craniopharyngiomas.

Hydrocephalus

Hydrocephalus is a condition with enlarged ventricles due to increased CSF production or decreased CSF absorption or obstruction to CSF drainage (Fig. 25.4).

Hydrocephalus can be congenital or acquired.

Congenital causes are aqueductal stenosis, Dandy-Walker syndrome, Chiari malformations, meningomyelocele, etc. Acquired causes are posterior fossa lesions, intra-ventricular haemorrhage, infection, etc. Management of hydrocephalus is diverting the CSF from ventricles to peritoneum, pleura or atrium. Pleura or atrium are used if the peritoneum is infected. Endoscopic third ventriculostomy may also be used to drain CSF.[1]

Anaesthesia Considerations

1. Shunt procedures require exposure from head to toe. Hence, patients are prone to hypothermia.[1]
2. Children may be dehydrated due to vomiting or reduced intake. Rehydration is necessary prior to induction.
3. Large dilated scalp veins in infants with hydrocephalus can be used for induction of anaesthesia if required.[4]
4. Intubation is difficult if the head is large. Lateral position or bolsters can be placed below the shoulders during intubation.
5. During ventriculo-peritoneal (VP) shunt tunnelling is very stimulating. Hence, plane of anaesthesia should be deepened during the same.

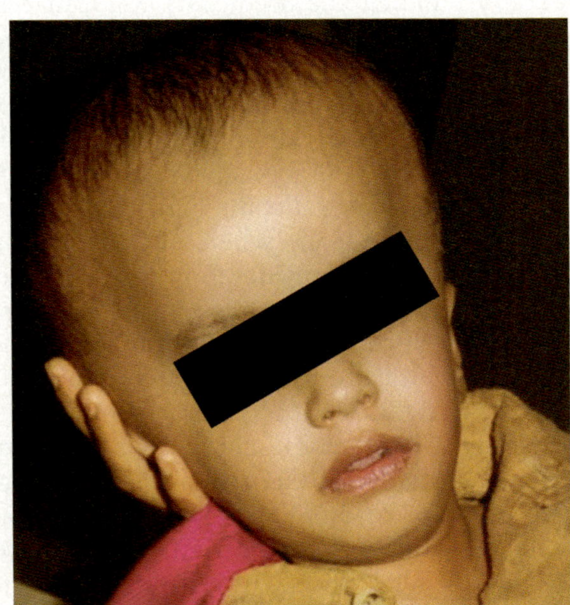

Fig. 25.4 Hydrocephalus

6. During ventricular atrial shunt, arrhythmias and VAE can occur.[4]
7. Rapid drainage of CSF from ventricles can cause arrhythmias due to cephalad movement of brain and pressure on hypothalamus.[16]
8. The third ventricle is close to the midbrain CVS centres. Hence, irrigation and manipulation of the floor of the 3rd ventricle during endoscopic ventriculostomy can lead to bradycardia and arrhythmias.[14]
9. In children with altered mental status, there is an increased risk of aspiration of gastric contents in the postoperative period due to handling of peritoneum during VP shunt.[1]

Traumatic Brain Injury[17,18]

In traumatic brain injury (TBI), it is important that the treatment strategies are aimed at primary injury as well as reduction of secondary injuries.

Causes of primary injury are skull fractures, brain contusions, and intracranial haematomas and diffuse axonal injury.

Two major causes of secondary injury in TBI are hypotension and hypoxia.

Large head to toe ratio and immature neck can cause a more diffused injury due to acceleration and deceleration injury. Severity of cerebral oedema in paediatric patients is more as compared to adults.

Anaesthesia Considerations

Perioperative management consists of rapid assessment, ongoing resuscitation and early surgical intervention. Evaluation includes assessment of airway, breathing, circulation, neurological status and extracranial injuries. Basic Life Support algorithm should be instituted. All TBI patients should be considered to have a full stomach and cervical spine injury. Endotracheal intubation should be done when GCS <9. The 2012 Guidelines recommend consideration of craniectomy in paediatric patients who are showing early signs of neurologic deterioration or herniation, or are developing intracranial hypertension refractory to medical management. The 2012 Guidelines recommend both bolus therapy 3% saline and continuous infusion 3% saline for treatment of ICH in paediatric patients. Effective doses for bolus therapy range from 6.5 to 10 mL/kg/ L after TBI for paediatric patients with elevated ICP. The 2012 Guidelines recommend maintaining $PbtO_2 \geq 10$ mmHg, based on level III evidence of brain oxygenation monitoring. In critically ill patients, thiopentone and propofol can cause vasodilation and hypotension. Hence, etomidate and ketamine can be used for induction. Succinylcholine is not contraindicated and is probably safer than high-dose rocuronium when there is concern for a difficult airway. Succinylcholine may be used for difficult intubation. Rocuronium is a good alternative when succinylcholine is contraindicated.

> **One Fact to Remember**
>
> Two major causes of secondary injury in Traumatic brain injury are hypotension and hypoxia.

Rapid sequence induction and manual in-line stabilisation is used during intubation

Intraoperative goals are:

1. Maintain $PaO_2 \geq 60$ mmHg and $PaCO_2$ at 35–40 mmHg. Hyperventilation with a $PaCO_2 < 30$ mmHg is not recommended except for the treatment of imminent herniation or for temporary surgical relaxation of the brain.
2. Hypotension should be avoided as even a single episode of hypotension is associated with poor outcome. Vasoactive agents (phenylephrine) may be used to treat hypotension. Maintain CPP at 40–70 mmHg.
3. Mannitol (0.25–1 gm/kg) is used to treat elevated ICP. Hypertonic saline can be used to treat raised ICP that is refractory to mannitol. A reduction in the brain volume may cause relief of the tamponade, which prevents ongoing bleeding. Hence, mannitol should be administered after blood has been evacuated.
4. Glucose containing fluids should be avoided unless serum glucose is < 70 mg/dL.
5. There is no role for routine therapeutic hypothermia but hyperthermia should be avoided.
6. Corticosteroids have no role in TBI.
7. In small children, evacuation of an extradural or subdural haematoma can cause considerable blood loss. Blunt abdominal trauma and long bone fractures can also be a source of bleeding. Hence, cross matched blood and blood products should be available. Maintain haemoglobin at 7–10 g/dL.
8. No significant difference has been found in outcomes comparing intravenous and inhalational anaesthetic agents. N_2O may be avoided to prevent increase in ICP.
9. The 2012 Guidelines recommend consideration of external ventricular drains (EVD) to manage ICP.

10. The 2012 Guidelines recommend barbiturate therapy in haemodynamically stable patients when maximal medical and surgical therapy has failed to control ICP.
11. Prophylactic use of anti-seizure therapy is not recommended for children with severe TBI for preventing late posttraumatic seizures. Prophylactic anti-seizure therapy may be considered as a treatment option to prevent early posttraumatic seizures in young paediatric patients and infants at high risk of seizures after head injury.

Vascular Anomalies[4]

Arterio-venous malformations are not common in paediatric population. Children may present with haemorrhagic seizures and hydrocephalus.[1] Treatment of AVM consists of intravascular embolization in a radiology suite or surgical excision.

Anaesthesia Considerations

1. In neonates, large AVMs such as Vein of Galen malformation may present with congestive heart failure requiring haemodynamic support.
2. Surgery may be associated with major blood loss.
3. Excision of AVM may cause hypertension and hyperaemic cerebral oedema requiring treatment with vasodilators such as labetalol and nitroprusside.[4]

Moya Moya Disease[19]

Moya Moya disease is a chronic cerebrovascular disorder present in children as well as adults. There is progressive stenosis or occlusion of terminal portion of internal carotid artery. Formation of collaterals between internal carotid artery and external carotid artery gives the characteristic 'puff of smoke' appearance on angiogram. Children may present with ischaemic stroke, intra-cranial haemorrhage, headache, seizures or TIA.

Medical management does not halt progression. Surgical treatment consists of revascularisation procedures to promote neovascularisation. Revascularisation procedures are indirect bypass procedures such as Encephalo-Duro-Arterio-Synangiosis or direct revascularisation procedures such as, superficial temporal artery to middle cerebral artery bypass.

Anaesthesia Considerations

1. Anaesthesia goal is to maintain a balance between oxygen supply and demand.
2. Cerebral blood flow is maintained by maintaining normovolemia, normotension, normothermia and normocapnoea.[19] Hypercapnoea and hypocapnoea can result in steal phenomenon from the ischaemic region, hence there is a greater risk of cerebral ischaemia.[4]
3. Avoid increase in $CMRO_2$, associated with laryngoscopy, tracheal intubation and surgical events, by adequate depth of anaesthesia.

Intra-operative goals to maintain cerebral perfusion should be continued in the postoperative period.[4]

KEY POINTS

1. The differences in myelination, cerebral blood flow and metabolic requirements of paediatric brain need to be kept in mind while anaesthetizing paediatric patients.
2. The narrow range of auto-regulation in neonates puts them at higher risk of ischaemia and intracerebral haemorrhage.
3. Young children are able to compensate for intracranial hypertension by increasing the skull volume prior to suture fusion.
4. The goals of anaesthesia in paediatric neurosurgical patients are maintenance of cerebral perfusion pressure (CPP), cerebral oxygenation, brain relaxation, preservation of neurological function and rapid neurological recovery.
5. The principle of neuro-anaesthesiais maintenance of normal ventilation, normothermia, normovolemia, normoglycemia and avoidance of electrolyte imbalance.

SUMMARY AND CONCLUSION

Though basic concepts of neuro-anaesthesia are same in adults and paediatrics, there are anatomical and physiological differences which pose a challenge to the anaesthesiologist. The provision of safe anaesthesia requires understanding of cerebral physiology in paediatric patients and the influence of various anaesthetic agents on the brain.

REFERENCES

1. Rath GP, Dash HH. Anaesthesia for neurosurgical procedures in paediatric patients. Indian J Anaesth. 2012;56:502–10.
2. Yungfang JH, Krass IS. Physiology and metabolism of brain and spinal cord. In: Newfield P, Cottrell JE, (Eds).

Handbook of Neuroanaesthesia. Philadelphia: Lippincott Williams and Wilkins. 2007;p.120.
3. Pryds O. Control of cerebral circulation in the highrisk neonate. Ann Neurol 1991;30:3219.
4. Soriano SG, McManus ML. Paediatric neuroanaesthesia and critical care. In: Cottrell JE, Young WL (Eds). Cottrell and Young's neuroanaesthesia. Philadelphia: Mosby Elsevier. 2010;p.327–341.
5. Sakabe T, Matsumoto M. Effects of anaesthetic agents and other drugs on cerebral blood flow, metabolism, and intracranial pressure in: Cottrell JE, Young WL (Eds). Cottrell and Young's neuroanaesthesia. Philadelphia: Mosby Elsevier. 2010;p.78–94.
6. Cucchiara RF, Bowers B. Air embolism in children undergoing suboccipital craniotomy, Anesthesiology 1982;57:338–339.
7. Francis L, Mohamed, Patino M, et al. Intraoperative Neuromonitoring in Paediatric Surgery. International Anaesthesiology Clinics. 2012; 50(4):130–143.
8. Bailey AG, McNaull PP, Jooste E, et al. Perioperative crystalloid and colloid fluid management in children: where are we and how did we get here? Anaesthesia & Analgesia. 2010;10:375–390.
9. Perel P, Roberts I. Colloids versus crystalloids for fluid resuscitation in critically ill patients. Cochrane Database Syst Rev2007:CD000567.
10. Bunn F, Trivedi D, Ashraf S. Colloid solutions for fluid resuscitation. Cochrane Database Syst Rev 2008:CD001319.
11. Mirski MA, Lele AV, Fitzsimmons L, et al. Diagnosis and Treatment of Vascular Air Embolism. Anesthesiology 2007;106:164–77.
12. Singh D, Rath GP, Dash HH, et al. Anesthetic concerns and perioperative complications in repair of myelomeningocele: A retrospective review of 135 cases. J Neurosurg Anesthesiol. 2010;22:11–5.
13. Chand MB, Agrawal J, Bista P. Anaesthetic Challenges and Management of Myelomeningocele Repair. Postgraduate medical journal of NAMS.2011;11:41–46.
14. Furay C, Howell T. Paediatric neuroanaesthesia. Cont Educ Anaesth Crit Care Pain. 2010;10:172–6.
15. Stricker PA, Fiadjoe JE. Anaesthesia for Craniofacial Surgery in Infancy. Anaesthesiology Clinics. 2014;32: 215–235.
16. Alfery D, Shapiro H, Gagnon R. Cardiac Arrest Following Rapid Drainage of Cerebrospinal Fluid in a Patient with Hydrocephalus. Anesthesiology. 1980;52:443–444.
17. Bhalla T, Dewhirst E, Sawardeka A, et al. Perioperative management of the paediatric patient with traumatic brain injury. Paediatric Anaesthesia. 2012;12:627–640.
18. Hardcastle N, Benzon HA, Vavilala MS. Update on the 2012 guidelines for the management of paediatric traumatic brain injury—information for the anaesthesiologist. Paediatric Anaesthesia. 2014;24:703–710.
19. Parray T, Martin TW, Siddiqui S. Moyamoya Disease: A Review of the Disease and Anaesthetic Management. J Neurosurg Anaesthesiol. 2011;23: 100–109.

26

Paediatric Thoracic Anaesthesia

Sandeep Sahu, Hemlata and Indu Lata

INTRODUCTION

Providing anaesthesia to paediatric patients undergoing thoracic surgery is very challenging. As has already been discussed in previous chapters, the anatomic and physiologic differences as well as the differences in responses to pharmacologic agents in paediatric population place them at higher risk of anaesthetic complications than the adults. Special ventilatory requirements during thoracic anaesthesia and the need for single lung ventilation (SLV) further adds to the complexity of administering anaesthesia to these patients. The anaesthesiologist practicing thoracic anaesthesia needs to have a clear understanding of the physiology of SLV, the techniques of lung separation, and the technical skill necessary to apply these techniques. The focus of this chapter will be intra-operative anaesthetic care of infants and children undergoing non-cardiac thoracic surgery including monitoring and anaesthetic techniques and pain management techniques. Common disorders of neonatal period, infancy and childhood that require thoracic surgery involving thoracotomy and thoraco-scopy will be discussed. Management of anaesthesia during video assisted thoracoscopic surgery (VATS) in children will also be discussed.

GENERAL ANAESTHETIC CONSIDERATIONS

The indications for thoracotomy in the infant or child can be congenital abnormalities (cysts), tumours (mediastinal masses), infective lesions (bronchiectasis), or trauma (gunshot wounds). Any paediatric patient scheduled for thoracic surgery should undergo a thorough preoperative evaluation and appropriate imaging and laboratory studies according to the lesion involved. Fasting guidelines, choice of premedication, and operating room preparation are done as for other infants and children scheduled for major surgery. Arterial catheterization should be performed for most patients undergoing thoracotomy as well as those with severe lung disease undergoing thoracoscopic surgery. This allows continuous arterial blood pressure monitoring during manipulation of the lungs and mediastinum as well as blood gas analysis during SLV. Arterial catheterization is not required for thoracoscopic procedures of relatively short duration in patients without severe lung disease. Central venous catheter is generally not required if there is adequate peripheral intravenous access for projected fluid and blood administration. Maintenance of anaesthesia is generally done with inhaled anaesthetic agents administered in 100% O_2. Isoflurane is preferred as it causes less attenuation of hypoxic pulmonary vasoconstriction (HPV) compared with other inhaled agents, although this has not been studied in children.[1] Nitrous oxide is avoided. Use of intravenous opioids helps to reduce the concentration of inhaled anaesthetics used and thereby limiting impairment of HPV. Use of total intravenous anaesthesiais also an option. For thoracotomy, general anaesthesia should be combined with regional anaesthesia and postoperative analgesia, especially when thoracostomy tube drainage is used following surgery as it is a source of significant postoperative pain.

Most of the thoracic surgeries, including diagnostic thoracoscopy and VATS, require SLV as it provides improved exposure of the surgical field, and possibly a diversion of ventilation from the damaged airway or lung. At the same time, SLV requires manipulation of the airways resulting in significant physiological changes and potential hypoxemia. Because of the rarity of SLV procedures, limited airway size, and limited techniques available for lung isolation especially in infants, the complexity of the challenge of SLV is further increased in paediatric patients. Positioning of the patient has often been used as a means to minimize spillage of lung contents because DLTs cannot be used in very small patients[2] and suction through the ETT may not be adequate to control large quantities of pus freed during surgical manipulation. Positioning can also cause significant ventilatory changes in children.

VENTILATION AND PERFUSION DURING THORACIC SURGERY

For adults and children, both ventilation (V) and perfusion (Q) are higher in the more dependent portion of the lungs as compared to the less dependent parts due to pressure gradient and gravitational pull. Therefore, V and Q are normally well matched. However, the gravitational gradient of blood flow exceeds the gradient of ventilation, resulting in a higher V/Q ratio at the apices than the bases, with a mean value of 0.8 as explained in Fig. 26.1A and B.[3] During thoracic surgery, the V/Q mismatch is increased by several factors that apply equally to infants, children and adults:[3]

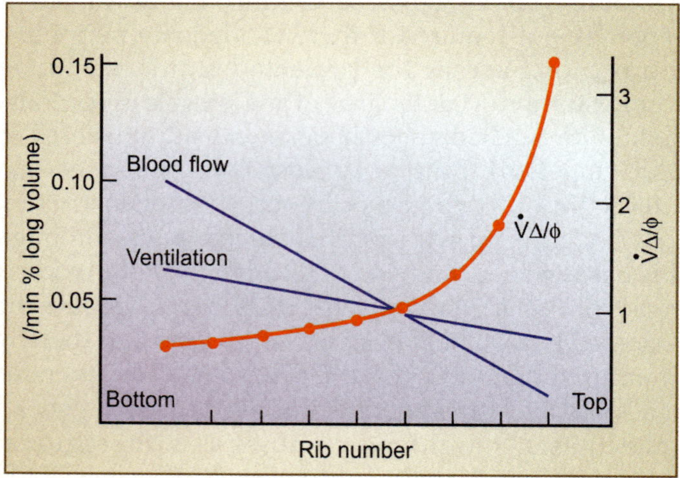

Fig. 26.1A Distribution of ventilation, blood flow and ventilation-perfusion ratio in the normal, upright lung. (Straight lines have been drawn through the ventilation and blood flow data. Because blood flow falls more rapidly than ventilation with distance up the lung, ventilation-perfusion ratio rises, first slowly, then rapidly.)

Source: West JB: Ventilation/blood flow and gas exchange. 4th edn. Oxford, England, Blackwell Scientific, 1985.

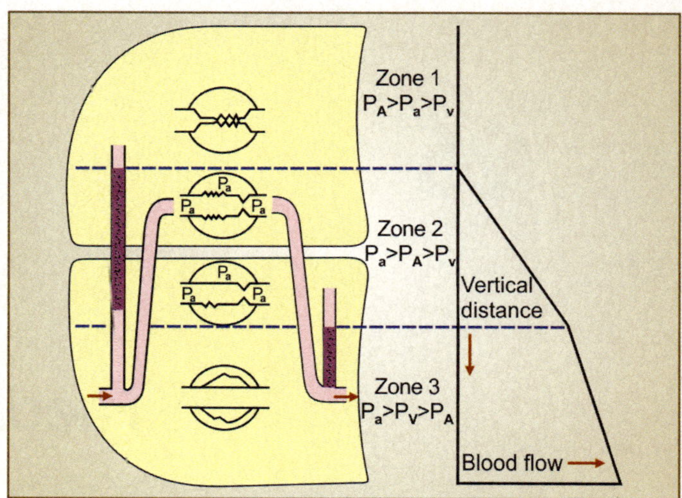

Fig. 26.1B Effects of gravity on the distribution of pulmonary blood flow in the lateral decubitus position. Vertical gradients in the lateral decubitus position are similar to those in the upright position and cause the creation of west zones 1,2 and 3 consequently pulmonary blood flow increases with lung dependency and is largest in the dependent lung and least in the nondependent lung. (P_a, pulmonary artery pressure, P_A, alveolar pressure, P_v, pulmonary venous pressure.

Source: Benumof JL. Physiology of the open chest and one lung ventilation. In: Thoracic Anaesthesia, New York, Churchill Livingstone, 1983; p. 288.

1. Decrease in FRC of both lungs caused by general anaesthesia, neuromuscular blockade and mechanical ventilation.
2. Atelectasis caused by compression of dependent lung in the lateral decubitus position.
3. Collapse of the operative lung resulting from surgical retraction or SLV.
4. Decrease in HPV caused by inhaled anaesthetics and other vasodilating drugs.

PHYSIOLOGY OF LATERAL DECUBITUS POSITION

During spontaneous respiration, the ventilation of the dependent lung is favoured by a greater excursion of the dependent diaphragm (doming effect) than the nondependent lung. This doming effect is abolished by muscle paralysis and Intermittent Positive Pressure Ventilation (IPPV) resulting in increased ventilation of the nondependent lung. Compression of the dependent hemithorax by the mediastinum and abdominal contents also impedes ventilation of the dependent lung as in Fig. 26.2.[4] However, the overall impact of lateral decubitus position on V/Q mismatch is different in infants as compared with older children and adults. In adults, oxygenation is better with the healthy lung in

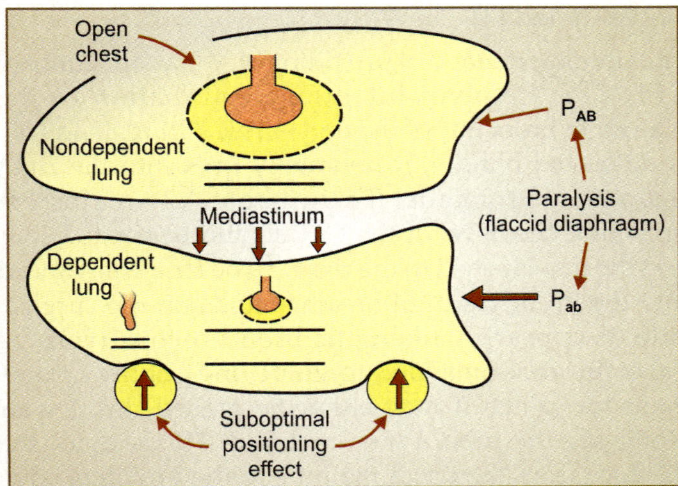

Fig. 26.2 V–Q relationship in the anesthetized patient in the lateral decubitus position with an open chest, paralyzed. The nondependent lung is well ventilated (indicated by large dashed lines) and poorly perfused (small perfusion vessel), and the dependent lung is poorly ventilated (small dashed lines) because of compression by the mediastinum (down arrows), pressure of the abdominal contents (P_{AB}), and suboptimal positioning, but it is well perfused (large perfusion vessel)

Source: Benumof JL, Alfrey DD. In: Miller RD (Ed) 2nd edn. *Textbook of anaesthesia.* 1994; p.1662–1755

the dependent position. This is due to an increase in blood flow to the dependent healthy lung and a decrease in blood flow to the nondependent diseased lung caused by the gravitational pull and hydrostatic pressure gradient between the two lungs.[5] Unlike in adults, in infants with unilateral lung disease, oxygenation is improved with the healthy lung nondependent and the diseased lung dependent.[6] Several factors are responsible for this difference between adults and infants: First, infants have a soft, easily compressible rib cage that cannot fully support the underlying lung. Therefore, FRC in infants is closer to the residual volume. This makes airway closure likely in the dependent lung even during normal tidal ventilation.[7] Second, in the lateral decubitus position in infants, there is a significant loss in patient's mechanical advantage to ventilation caused by loading of the dependent diaphragm by abdominal hydrostatic pressure gradient due to their small size. Third, the infant's small size results in reduced hydrostatic pressure gradient between nondependent and dependent lungs. Consequently, there is only a small increase in perfusion to the dependent ventilated lung. Lastly, higher oxygen requirement coupled with a smaller FRC in infants predisposes them to hypoxemia. Baseline oxygen consumption in infants is 6–8 mL/kg/min, compared with 2–3 mL/kg/min in adults.[8] For all these reasons, infants are susceptible to more oxygen desaturation during SLV while placed in lateral decubitus position.

PHYSIOLOGY OF SINGLE LUNG VENTILATION

With the initiation of SLV, there is significant change in the distribution of V and Q. Ventilation of the dependent lung increases while that of the nondependent lung stops. Once ventilation of the non-dependent lung ceases, the V/Q matching becomes almost entirely dependent on the amount of blood flowing through the apnoeic non-dependent lung. The partial pressure of oxygen (PaO_2) value drops to almost 50% (from 400 mmHg up to 200 mmHg) within half-an-hour of initiation of SLV with an inspired oxygen fraction (FiO_2) of 1.0.[3] This is mainly caused by the pulmonary arteriovenous shunt of the deoxygenated blood through the upper nonventilated lung.[9] Also, the blood supply to the nondependent lung decreases with the initiation of SLV and consequent nondependent lung atelectasis and alveolar hypoxia. This redirection of blood flow is primarily caused by HPV.[10] HPV is believed to be the most important determinant of blood flow through the non-ventilated lung. It causes a reduction in blood flow through the non-ventilated lung from 40–50% of cardiac

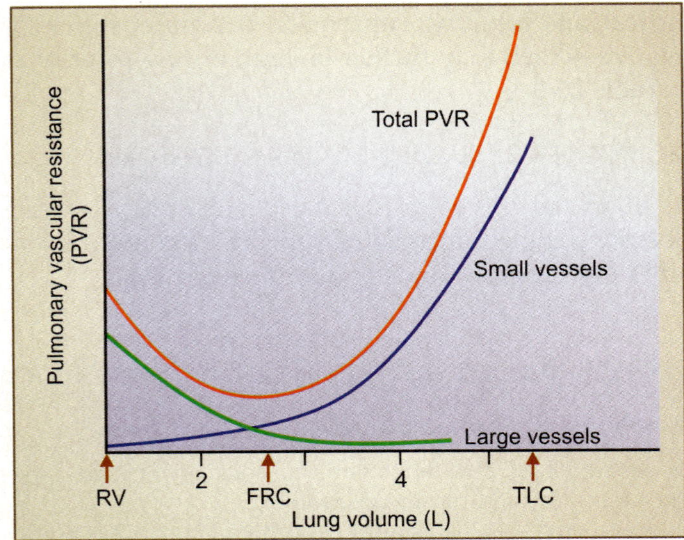

Fig. 26.3 The relationship between pulmonary vascular resistance (PVR) and lung volume. PVR is lowest at functional residual capacity (FRC) and increases as the lung volume decreases toward residual volume (RV), owing primarily to increase in resistance of large pulmonary vessels. PVR also increases as lung volume increases above FRC toward total lung capacity (TLC) because of an increase in the resistance of small interalveolar lung vessels

Source: Peter D Slinger, Campos JH, Miller's Anaesthesia 7th edn. 2010; p. 1847

output to 20–30% of cardiac output. The phenomenon of HPV starts immediately on initiation of SLV, with little potentiation over time. Pulmonary vascular resistance (PVR) is minimal at FRC, so a small reduction in pulmonary blood will occur when the non-ventilated lung collapses towards residual volume as in Fig. 26.3. Surgical manipulation of the lung is also likely to reduce its blood flow either by distorting and so occluding pulmonary vasculature or by direct clamping of pulmonary vessels as part of the surgical procedure.

Both alveolar and mixed venous PO_2 influence HPV. A fall in mixed venous PO_2 mildly increases HPV, and an abnormally high mixed venous PO_2 may decrease HPV as oxygen diffuses from the alveolar capillary blood into the non-ventilated alveoli and the HPV is maximal when alveolar PO_2 is approximately 20–40 mmHg.[11] Alveolar carbon dioxide tension and the blood pH level also influence the HPV response. Hypercapnia and metabolic acidosis increase HPV, whereas hypocapnia and alkalosis decrease HPV. The aim of ventilation during OLV is to maintain arterial PO_2 and PCO_2 as near normal as possible and is achieved by maintaining adequate alveolar ventilation while minimising the amount of shunt through the non-ventilated lung.

Indications for SLV: As in an adult patient, the indications for lung separation can be absolute or relative, which may further be high or low priority as in Table 26.1.

TECHNIQUES OF SLV IN INFANTS AND CHILDREN

As in adults, there are four basic techniques for lung isolation: Single-lumen ETT, bronchial blockers, univent tubes and double-lumen endobronchial tubes.

Single-lumen ETT

The simplest method of providing SLV is a conventional ETT. This involves intentional intubation of the mainstem bronchus of the non-surgical lung. If an ETT is advanced blindly, it invariably goes into the right mainstem bronchus. To intubate left mainstem bronchus, the bevel of the ETT should be rotated 180° and the head turned to the right.[12] The ETT is advanced into the bronchus until breath sounds on the surgical side disappear. A fiberoptic bronchoscope (FOB) is generally recommended to guide and confirm placement for which it may either be passed through or alongside the tube. When a cuffed ETT is used, the distance from the tip of the tube to the proximal edge of the cuff must be shorter than the length of the mainstem bronchus so that the cuff is entirely in the bronchus.[13] This technique is simple and requires no special equipment other than a FOB, and can be performed quickly in emergency situations such as pulmonary haemorrhage and contralateral tension pneumothorax. Disadvantages are as follows:

1. Inability to suction the operative lung,
2. Inadequate and slow collapse of the unventilated nonoperative lung as there is no port for the egress of trapped gases,
3. An inadequate seal of the ventilated lung, especially if a smaller uncuffed ETT is used, and
4. Hypoxaemia due to obstruction of the upper lobe bronchus, especially when the short right mainstem bronchus is intubated.

Balloon-tipped Bronchial Blockers

The balloon-tipped bronchial blockers (BB) remains the 'technique of choice' in paediatric patients, under the

Table 26.1 Indications for lung separation

Absolute indications	Relative indications
1. Separation of each lung to prevent spillage of normal lung • Pus or blood from an infected lung • Bleeding source or during bronchopulmonary sepsis, pneumonia and massive atelectasis. 2. Control of distribution of ventilation to only one lung • Bronchopleural and bronchocutaneous fistulae • To avoid rupture of giant U/L cysts or unilateral bullae under positive-pressure ventilation can be avoided by SLV. 3. Video-assisted thoracoscopic surgery (VATS) 4. U/L lung lavage 5. Minimally invasive cardiac procedures require lung collapse.	1. Surgical exposure high priority • Upper lobectomy, pneumonectomy • Thoracic aortic aneurysm repair 2. Surgical exposure low priority • Lower or middle lobectomy • Esophageal resection • Thoracoscopy

age of 6 years.[14] Commonly used bronchial blockers are Fogarty embolectomy catheter and Arndt bronchial blocker. These devices have a balloon at the end that is inflated to occlude the main bronchus of the operative lung and they are placed under direct vision with a FOB.

Fogarty Embolectomy Catheter

The Fogarty embolectomy catheter (Edwards Life Sciences, Irvine, CA, USA) (Fig. 26.4) is a through-lumen catheter which may be placed with or without FOB guidance.[15] To facilitate its placement, the tip of its stylet can be bent at the distal end to allow directing it laterally into the desired main bronchus. The catheter can be placed either alongside the ETT or through the ETT. To place a BB outside the ETT, two techniques have been described. In one technique, the bronchus on the operative side is initially intubated with an ETT.[13] Through this ETT, a guidewire is then advanced into the bronchus and the ETT is removed. The blocker is then advanced over the guidewire into the bronchus. An ETT is then reinserted into the trachea along the blocker catheter. Alternatively, the blocker can be directly introduced through the trachea using direct laryngoscopy, keeping its concavity forward. Once inside the trachea, the tip of the blocker catheter is rotated 90° to the right or left and then it is advanced into the desired mainstem bronchus. After that, an ETT is placed into the trachea alongside the blocker catheter. FOB visual guidance is used to confirm the position of catheter balloon in the proximal mainstem bronchus. Tan and Tan-Kendrick have suggested that the age, but not the weight, of the patient is a good predictor of the main bronchial diameters (Table 26.2).[16] It provides a better airway seal and more predictable lung collapse and better operating conditions as compared to an ETT in the bronchus.[17]

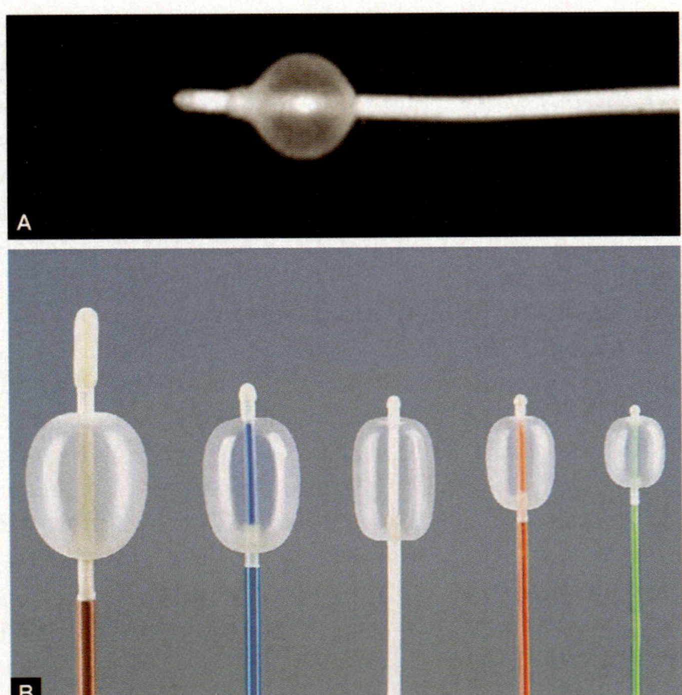

Fig. 26.4 Fogarty embolectomy catheters

Source: www.edwards.com

Table 26.2 Fogarty catheter size as per Tan and Tan-Kendrick

Age (years)	FG size for girls	FG size for boys
0–1	3	3
1–2	3	3
2–4	3	3
4–6	4 or 5	4 or 5
6–8	4 or 5	4 or 5
8–10	4 or 5	4 or 5
10–12	5	4 or 5
>12	6	5 or 6

Arndt Bronchial Blocker

The Arndt Endobronchial Blocker (Cook, WEB, Critical care, Bloomington, IN, USA) (Fig. 26.5), also called wire-guided endobronchial blocker (WEB), is an end-hole, balloon wedge catheter. It also contains a flexible wire loop that passes from the proximal end and emerges at

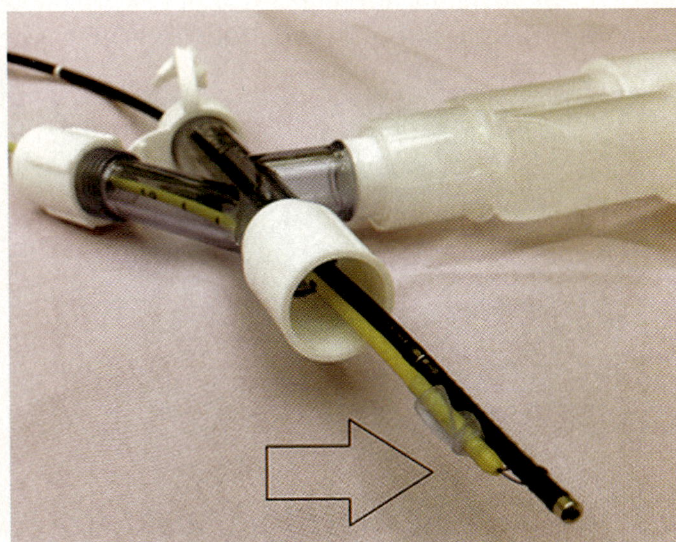

Fig. 26.5 **Arndt endobronchial blocker:** Wire loop is coupled with FOB to direct the blocker to the mainstem bronchus

Source: Fabila TS, Menghraj SJ. One lung ventilation strategies for infants and children undergoing video assisted thoracoscopic surgery. Indian J Anaesth 2013;57:339–44.

the tip of the blocker. The Arndt Multiport Adaptor, a special three-port adaptor, is an invaluable component of the blocker kit that allows uninterrupted ventilation at the time of placement of the blocker with the FOB. This adaptor has one port for the introduction of FOB, a second port for the balloon-tipped BB and a third port for ventilation circuit (Fig. 26.6).[18] First of all the blocker is inserted through the blocker port of multiport connector which locks the catheter in place and maintains an airtight seal. It is advanced until the guide loop is within the body of the adapter. Then, the FOB is inserted through the bronchoscopy port until it passes through the loop (Fig. 26.5). The coupled FOB and endobronchial blocker is then advanced into the trachea and further on to the desired mainstem bronchus after correct identification.[19] Once the blocker enters the bronchus and it is in position, the FOB is slowly withdrawn. The cuff is then inflated under direct FOB visualization with incremental introduction of air until total bronchial blockade is achieved.[20] Then the FOB is removed and the bronchoscope port tightened to permit proper ventilation.[21] After successful placement, the wire loop is withdrawn and the lumen can be used as a suction port to expedite lung collapse and for oxygen insufflation to the unventilated lung. However, the lumen is too small for suctioning to clear the lung of secretions.

This blocker is available in three sizes (5, 7 and 9 Fr) and is only suitable if the ETT to be used has an ID of at least 5.0 mm, generally limiting the use of this technique to children over the age of 2 years. The 5 Fr WEB has an outer diameter of 2.5 mm and requires a small bronchoscope of at least 2.2 mm for positioning.[22] However, if the ETT is too small to accommodate the smallest available WEB and FOB simultaneously, this blocker may be placed outside the ETT using a technique that has already been described above for the placement of Fogarty embolectomy catheter. The balloon of the blocker is low-pressure, high-volume and is 1.0 cm long which corresponds to the length of the right mainstem bronchus in children approximately 2 years old. This allows catheter balloon to remain entirely in the mainstem bronchus without obstructing the right upper lobe bronchus. The FOB visualisation is enhanced by the presence of the blue balloon on a yellow catheter. Disadvantages of the Arndt blocker are its high cost and the inability to reinsert the wire once it has been pulled out, making it impossible to redirect the blocker if required. Dislodgement of the blocker balloon into the trachea is a potential problem associated with this technique. This may result in blockage of ventilation to both lungs by the inflated balloon. The balloons of most BB catheters currently used have low-volume, high-pressure properties. So, overdistension can damage or even rupture the airway.[23] However, Guyton et al have recently reported that bronchial blocker cuffs produced lower cuff to tracheal' pressures than double lumen tubes.[24]

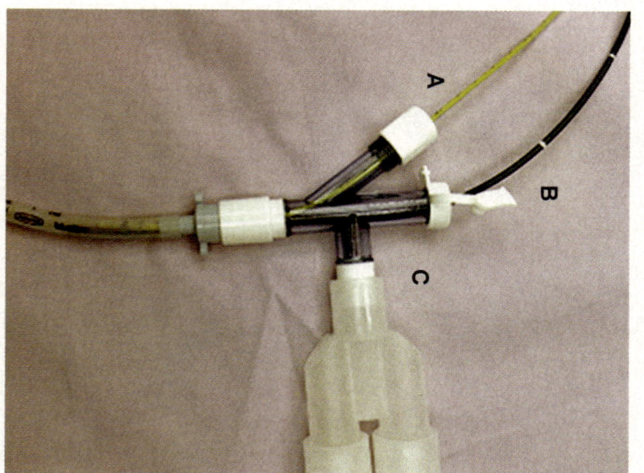

Fig. 26.6 Arndt Multiport adaptor for Arndt endobronchial blocker® by Cook. A–blocker port, B–FOB port, C–ventilation port

Source: Fabila TS, Menghraj SJ. One lung ventilation strategies for infants and children undergoing video assisted thoracoscopic surgery. Indian J Anaesth. 2013;57:339–44.

Double-lumen Tubes

All DLTs are essentially two tubes of unequal length moulded together. The shorter tube ends in the trachea and the longer tube in the bronchus. DLTs have cuffs located on the tracheal and bronchial lumens. When tracheal cuff is inflated, it allows positive pressure ventilation. The bronchial cuff, when inflated, allows ventilation to be diverted to either or both lungs, and protects each lung from contamination from the contralateral side (Fig. 26.7A to C). Conventional DLTs were earlier available only in adult sizes (35, 37, 39, and 41 Fr). Now, they are also available in smaller sizes (26, 28 and 32 Fr). The smallest cuffed DLT is a 26 Fr (Rusch, Duluth, GA, USA) which can be used in children 8 to 10 years old. DLT sizes 28 and 32 Fr (Mallinckrodt Medical, Inc., St. Louis, MO, USA) are suitable for children 10 years of age and older. For infants, a special DLT named "Marraro paediatric bilumen tube" has been described.[25]

The advantages of DLTs include:

1. Ease of insertion and rapid separation of the two lungs,

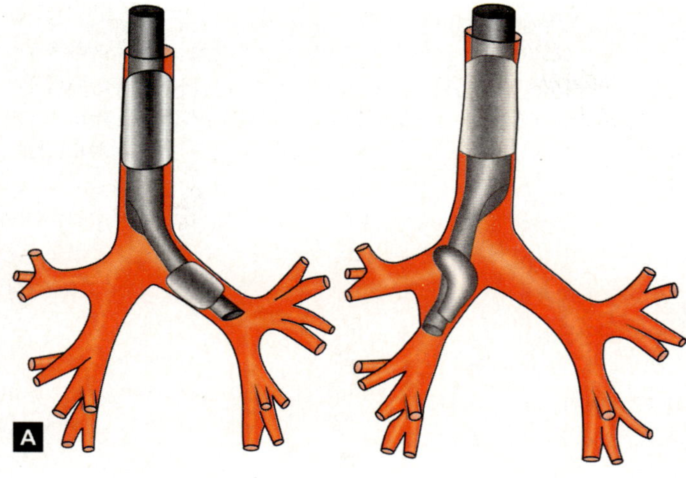

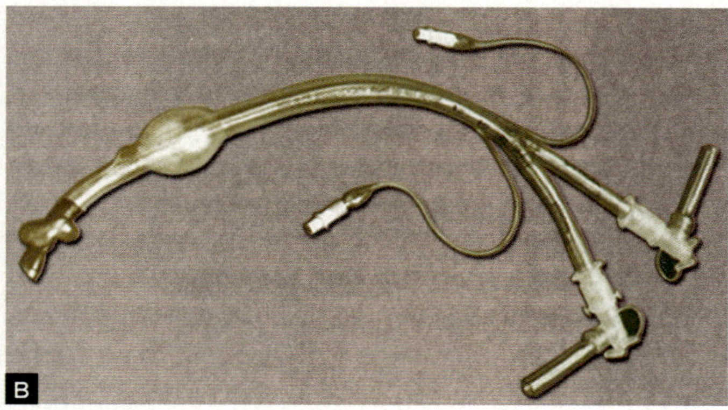

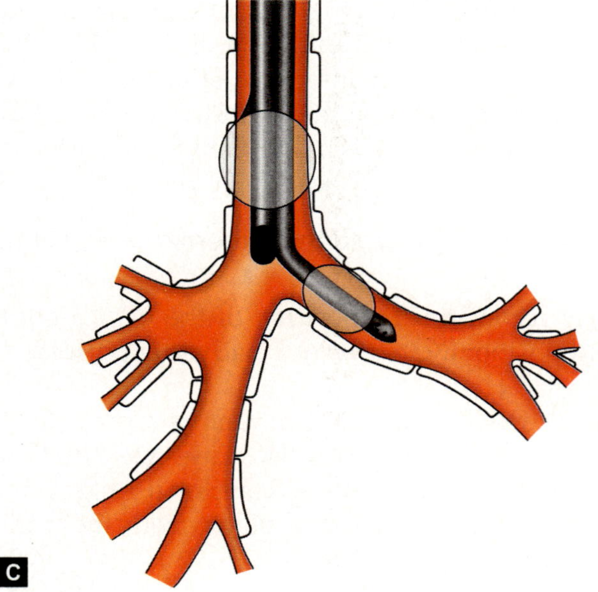

Fig. 26.7A to C (A) Robertshaw left and right DLTs in place, (B) Broncho-cath right DLT and (C) Left sided DLT

Source: Dorsch and Dorsch 5th edn., 2009; p. 636–638

2. Ability to suction either side of the lung individually,
3. Ability to switch to two lung ventilation rapidly as the need arises, and
4. Ability to improve oxygenation by applying CPAP to the operative lung and PEEP to the non-operative lung.

In children, left sided DLTs are preferred over right sided DLTs because they are easier to place and eliminate concern of obstruction of right upper lobe bronchus because of the shorter length of the right main bronchus. However, the only absolute contraindication for right sided DLTs is the presence of an anomalous right upper lobe take-off from the trachea, which probably occurs in 1 in 250 cases.[26] DLTs are unsuitable for patients with abnormal tracheobronchial anatomy and for children requiring postoperative mechanical ventilation. DLTs cannot be used in children less than 8 years of age as 26 Fr DLT is the smallest commercially available. DLTs are safe and easy to use. The high volume/low pressure properties of the bronchial cuff reduces the risk of ischaemic pressure damage to airway if they are not overinflated with air or distended with nitrous oxide while in place. There are very few reports of iatrogenic airway injury from DLTs in adults and none in children.[27] Direct measurement of bronchial diameter is more accurate method of choosing a correct size DLT for children rather than relying on age, gender, height or weight.[28] This can be done either directly from chest radiograph or can be computed from tracheal width (WT) using the formula [WLB (width of left bronchus) = (0.4 × WT) + 3.3]. The technique of insertion of DLT in children is the same as in adults. The tip of the tube is inserted just beyond the vocal cords and the stylet is withdrawn. The tube is then rotated through 90° to the desired side and then advanced into the bronchus. This method of placement of DLT without any visual assistance may result in intubation of the wrong bronchus initially in 14 to 30% cases.[29] FOB can be used to confirm tube placement as in adults. However, for this purpose, a bronchoscope with a small diameter and sufficient length must be available.

Univent Tubes

The Univent tube (Fuji Systems Corporation, Tokyo, Japan) is a conventional ETT with a second lumen containing a small tube that can be advanced into a bronchus. A balloon located at the distal end of the smaller tube, when inflated, serves as a blocker (Fig. 26.8). Paediatric-sized univent tubes are now

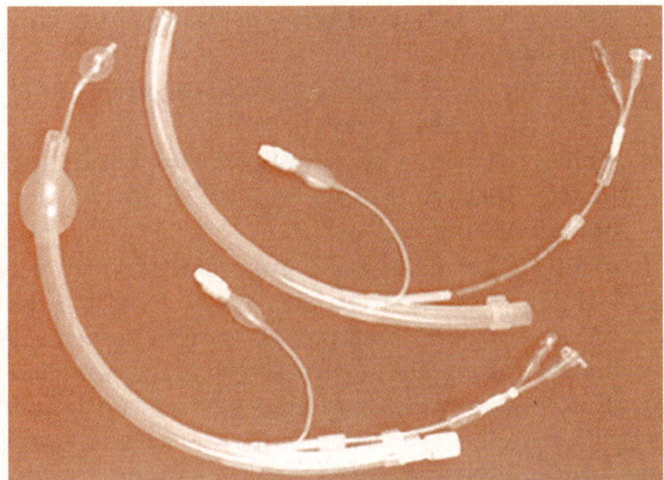

Fig. 26.8 Univent bronchial-blocking tubes. Top: The bronchial blocker is retracted. Bottom: The bronchial blocker is advanced, and the cuff is inflated

Source: Dorsch and Dorsch, 5th edn. 2009; p. 649

available in sizes as small as 3.5 mm and 4.5 mm internal diameter for use in children over 6 years of age.[30] The univent tube with a 3.5 mm internal diameter has an external size of 7.5–8.0 mm while univent tube size 4.5 mm internal diameter has an outer diameter of 8.5–9 mm. Thus, the 3.5 mm tube can be used for older children between 6 and 8 years of age for whom even the smallest DLTs (26 Fr) are not appropriate.[30]

For proper placement, the univent tube is inserted orotracheally similar to a conventional ETT and rotated 90° so that the blocker lumen is on the thoracotomy side. After inflating the balloon and securing the tube, the bronchial blocker shaft is pushed out of the tracheal tube pocket. For successful placement of univent tube, FOB assistance may be required, wherein the bronchial blocker shaft is pushed away under direct vision.[31] Because of the firm attachment of the blocker tube to the main ETT, displacement of the Univent blocker balloon is less likely than with other blocker techniques. When compared to double-lumen EBT, Zheng H et al. have reported a higher incidence of intraoperative malposition but reduced airway injury and improved compliance during SLV.[32] However, because of the low-volume, high-pressure characteristics of their blocker balloon, mucosal injury can occur during normal inflation.[33] There is a small lumen in the blocker tube which allows egress of gas and can be used to insufflate oxygen or suction the operated lung. Univent tubes have a disproportionately high resistance to gas flow[34] and a large amount of cross-sectional area is occupied by the blocker channel.

Table 26.3 Size according to age for selecting appropriate tubes or catheters for SLV in infants and children

Age (years)	Endotracheal tube (ID)	Bronchial blocker (Fr)	Univent tube (ID)	Double lumen tube (Fr)
0.5–1	3.5–4.0	2–3		
1–2	4.0–4.5	3		
2–4	4.5–5.0	5		
4–6	5.0–5.5	5		
6–8	5.5–6.0	5	3.5	
8–10	6.0 cuffed	5	3.5	26
10–12	6.5 cuffed	5	4.5	26–28
12–14	6.5–7.0 cuffed	7	4.5	32
14–16	7.0 cuffed	7	6.0	35
16–18	8.0–8.5 cuffed	7–9	7.0	35

Guidelines for selecting appropriate tubes or catheters for SLV in infants and children are shown in Table 26.3. These recommendations are based on average values for airway dimensions and we can safely use larger DLTs in large teenagers.

STRATEGIES FOR AVOIDING AND TREATING HYPOXEMIA DURING SLV

After achieving lung isolation and collapse, it is equally important to ensure that the oxygenation of the patient is well maintained. Normally there is a fall in arterial oxygenation during SLV that reaches its maximum 20 to 30 minutes after the initiation of SLV; then the saturation stabilizes or may rise slightly as HPV increases over time. Desaturation mostly occurs within the first 10 minutes of SLV and in the vast majority of cases, hypoxemia responds readily to treatment.

General Measures to Avoid Hypoxaemia During SLV Include

1. Always reconfirm the position of the device after patient positioning to rule out inadvertent displacement.
2. Always ventilate with 100% oxygen as it provides a higher margin of safety and also causes vasodilation of vessels in the dependent ventilated lung, thus promoting redistribution of blood from the non-dependent unventilated lung.
3. The inspired concentration of inhaled anaesthetics should be kept to less than 1 MAC to minimise inhibition of HPV and decrease in cardiac output.
4. Use a tidal volume of 5 to 10 mL/kg body weight. If inflation pressure is high, the respiratory rate may

be increased at lower tidal volume to avoid excessive airway pressures.

5. Maintain adequate cardiac output to ensure good tissue perfusion. This helps in maintaining high mixed venous oxygen content and decreases the effect of shunted blood in causing desaturation. This is very helpful in paediatric patients as they have a large shunt fraction (20 to 30%).

Once Hypoxaemia Develops, a Stepwise Approach Should be Followed to Treat it

1. Resumption of two-lung ventilation. This is necessary in case of severe desaturation though it necessitates interruption of surgery. After obtaining an adequate level of oxygenation, a search for the cause of desaturation can be made and prophylactic measures instituted before attempting another trial of SLV.
2. Increase FIO_2 to 1.0 and ensure that it is delivered. However, this measure should be avoided in those patients who have received bleomycin or similar therapies that potentiate pulmonary oxygen toxicity.
3. The position of the device used for SLV should be rechecked to rule out any obstruction in the ventilated lung.
4. Ensure that there is no hypotension or decrease in cardiac output. Accidental compression of the inferior vena cava during pulmonary resections may cause fall in blood pressure and cardiac output leading to rapid desaturation during OLV. Inotropes or vasopressors may be used as indicated. MAC of volatile anaesthetics should be decreased to less than 1 MAC and vasodilator administration should be stopped
5. A recruitment maneuver of the ventilated lung should be performed. The lung should be inflated to 20 cm H_2O or more for 15 to 20 seconds to eliminate any atelectasis.
6. Application of CPAP to the nondependent lung improves oxygenation by preventing total collapse of the alveoli.[35] CPAP should be commenced only after lung inflation. CPAP commenced from a fully deflated lung is not very effective because the opening pressure of collapsed alveoli is higher than the CPAP pressure. Higher level of CPAP (>10 cm H_2O) should be avoided as it may cause excessive inflation of the operative lung thus interfering with the surgical procedure.
7. Application of 5 to 10 cm H_2O PEEP to the ventilated lung is helpful in some patients. It is necessary to perform a recruitment maneuver before applying PEEP to get the maximal benefit. PEEP raises the end-expiratory volume of the ventilated lung toward the FRC in patients with normal lung mechanics and in those with restrictive disease. Unlike CPAP, application of PEEP does not require reinflation of the nonventilated lung and interruption of surgery. PEEP and CPAP have been shown to be equally effective for increasing PaO_2 levels during SLV in patients with normal lung function.[36]

MONITORING AND ANAESTHETIC TECHNIQUES

These had already been discussed under "general considerations" at the beginning of this chapter.

PAIN MANAGEMENT TECHNIQUES

A variety of regional anaesthetic techniques have been used successfully for intraoperative anaesthesia and postoperative analgesia, including epidural anaesthesia, intercostal blocks, paravertebral blocks and intrapleural infusions. Out of these, thoracic epidurals are very effective but its safety in anaesthesized patients has been questioned.[37] In infants and young children, a caudal epidural catheter can reliably be advanced cephalad to thoracic segments for achieving pain relief.[38] However, in older children, epidural catheter may directly be inserted at thoracic levels T6 to T8. Intercostal nerve blocks may either be performed prior to skin incision or at the end of surgery prior to chest closure. There is an overlap of sensory dermatomes, which necessitates blockage of nerves above and below the area of surgery. Intercostal catheter placement for post-thoracotomy pain relief is also an option in children.[39] Paravertebral blocks are equally effective as intercostal blockade, though it has not been reported for post-thoracotomy pain in children.

SURGICAL LESIONS OF THE THORAX

Surgical intervention is required for a variety of congenital and acquired thoracic conditions in the paediatric age group. Congenital lesions manifesting in neonates and infancy are: tracheal stenosis, pulmonary sequestrations, lung hypoplasia, pulmonary AV fistulas, congenital lobar emphysema, and congenital cystic lesions of thorax, CDH, TEFs, PDAs, COTAs and vascular rings. The acquired and congenital lesions manifesting in childhood are: pectus excavatum, empyema, neoplasms and scoliosis.

THORACOSCOPIC SURGERIES

Video assisted thoracoscopic surgery (VATS) is a less invasive approach for thoracoscopic surgery. Compared with thoracotomy, it offers the advantages of smaller chest incisions, reduced postoperative pain, fewer postoperative complications and more rapid postoperative recovery resulting in shortened hospital stay. This makes VATS favourable for paediatric patients.[40,41] During the past two decades, the use of VATS has dramatically increased in children and is being used extensively for lung biopsy, thymectomy, hiatal hernia repair, Heller's myotomy, spinal fusion, CDH repair, PDA repair,[42] pleural debridement in patients with empyema and sometimes for metastatic lesions or mediastinal masses.[44] For thoracoscopy, SLV is usually preferred over ventilation of both the lungs as it improves visualization of thoracic contents and reduces the chance of lung injury being caused by the use of retractors. A thorough understanding of the underlying pathology and severity of pulmonary disease as well as the ability to tolerate lateral decubitus position and PPV is must for providing anaesthesia for thoracoscopic surgeries. Nitrous oxide should not be used. In most cases, arterial line is not mandatory though it may help in monitoring the hemodynamic responses to positive pressure. Hypovolaemia should be avoided and fluid and blood therapy should be monitored. $ETCO_2$ monitoring may not be reliable in these cases, and use of arterial blood gas or transcutaneous CO_2 monitoring may be helpful. The procedure may not be tolerated very well in certain patients especially in very small infants. In such situation, reinsuflation of the lungs, PEEP to the dependent lung or CPAP to the operative lung may be required to allow the surgery to be continued but with decreasing visualization.

Decortications

Thoracic empyema is a life-threatening condition in paediatric surgical practice and the most common indication for decortication. However, appropriate management of paediatric empyema thoracis remains controversial and the most appropriate therapy depends on the stage of the disease at presentation.[45] Anaesthetic management for thoracotomy requires a thorough understanding of the severity of disease, its underlying pathology and the degree of lung restriction due to the pleural thickening and abscess formation and is guided by the patient's condition and the extent of thoracotomy and decortications. Hypovolemia may exacerbate the hemodynamic responses to positive pressure, so it should be avoided by adequate monitoring and proper management of blood and fluid therapy. Postoperative pain relief should be adequate to allow early mobilization and compliance with physiotherapy. Hypoventilation and hypoxaemia resulting from incisional pain of thoracotomy can be deleterious in such already compromised child.

Lung Cyst Excision

Most of these cysts are congenital in origin, although acquired postpneumonic lung cysts are known to be fairly common in children. True congenital bronchial cysts arise from the trachea or bronchus and may press upon them from outside and cause obstruction. Cysts occurring at the periphery of the lung are more problematic for the anaesthesiologists where a flap valve mechanism seems to operate which may result in localized lobar emphysema. Severe bronchiectasis resulting in honeycomb cysts in the lung occurs mostly in older children and presents distinct anaesthetic problems. In patients undergoing surgical excision of infected pulmonary cyst, the healthy lung must be isolated in order to protect it against transbronchial spillage should inadvertent rupture of the cyst occur during its dissection and exposure. Although SLV is recommended for cystic lesions of the lung, in case of bilateral lesions conventional two-lung ventilation would be safer in view of possible rupture of the cyst on the ventilated side.[46]

Lobectomy and Pneumonectomy

In children, pneumonectomy is done for various congenital abnormalities, tumours and inflammatory lesions, such as bronchiectasis. Atelectasis and pneumonia occur following lobectomy and pneumonectomy but may be less of a problem in latter case due to the absence of residual parenchymal dysfunction on the operative side. However, the mortality rate following pneumonectomy is much higher because of postoperative cardiac complications and acute lung injury.[47] Immediately after pneumonectomy, the ventilator function decreases and there is an increase in pulmonary artery pressure and pulmonary vascular resistance resulting in right ventricular dysfunction. Perioperative management differs dramatically, depending on the indication for surgery. Airway compression and physiologic compromise may worsen with induction of anaesthesia as sympathetic and muscular tones are reduced. Those patients who are in poor general condition may require postoperative ventilatory support, especially if they had only marginal compensation before surgery. For pneumonectomy, it is desirable to use a device that does not interfere with the ipsilateral airway (i.e. for left pneumonectomy, a right-sided DLT) or else the device (DLT or bronchial blocker) must be withdrawn prior to stapling the bronchus in order to avoid accidental inclusion into the suture line. Intraoperative tidal volume and acute lung injury post-surgery are important areas of concern in the management of patients undergoing pneumonectomy. So, in the pneumonectomy patient, it is advised to use lower tidal volumes (i.e. 5–6 mL/kg, ideal body weight) and limit peak and plateau inspiratory pressures (i.e. <35 and 25 cm H_2O, respectively) during SLV.[48] In patients undergoing major lung resections, intraoperative fluid administration should be restricted while preserving renal function. Inotropes/vasopressors may be required to maintain hemodynamic stability. Patients with adequate predicted postoperative respiratory function can usually be extubated in the operating room.

CDH Repair

Congenital diaphragmatic hernia (CDH) is a defect in the diaphragm caused by failure of a portion of the foetal diaphragm to develop. It results in extrusion of abdominal contents into the thoracic cavity, causing impairment of lung growth and is associated with varying degrees of bilateral lung hypoplasia. It is a life-threatening condition with an incidence between 1:2000 and 1:4000 live births and it constitutes 8% of all congenital anomalies.[49] The most common defect (90% of cases) is posterolateral (through foramen of Bochdalek) out of which 80% are left-sided. Others are anteromedial (Morgagni) and paraesophageal hernia and eventrations. Besides pulmonary hypoplasia, there can be pulmonary hypertension, arteriolar reactivity and left ventricular dysfunction. About 40% of patients with CDH have associated major congenital anomalies (cardiac, skeletal, CNS and genitourinary) with a much poorer outcome.[50] Degree of lung hypoplasia and the severity of symptoms depend on the gestational age at which herniation occurred. Cyanosis, dyspnoea, and apparent dextrocardia constitute the classic triad of CDH. Physical examination reveals tachypnea, scaphoid abdomen, bulging chest, decreased breath sounds, apparent dextrocardia or right-displaced heart sounds, and bowel sounds in the chest. Radiographic examination of the chest shows bowel in the left hemithorax, mediastinal shift and compression of the right lung (Fig. 26.9A and B). Right-sided hernias occur late and signs and symptoms are milder. CDH is often diagnosed prenatally and foetal surgical repair is an option. The goal of the initial management of CDH is to stabilize the cardiorespiratory status by improving oxygenation, correcting metabolic acidosis, reducing the right-to-left shunting, and increasing pulmonary perfusion.[51] Any surgical intervention should be avoided when the infant is hypoxic and acidotic.[52] Instead, medical management is directed at reducing

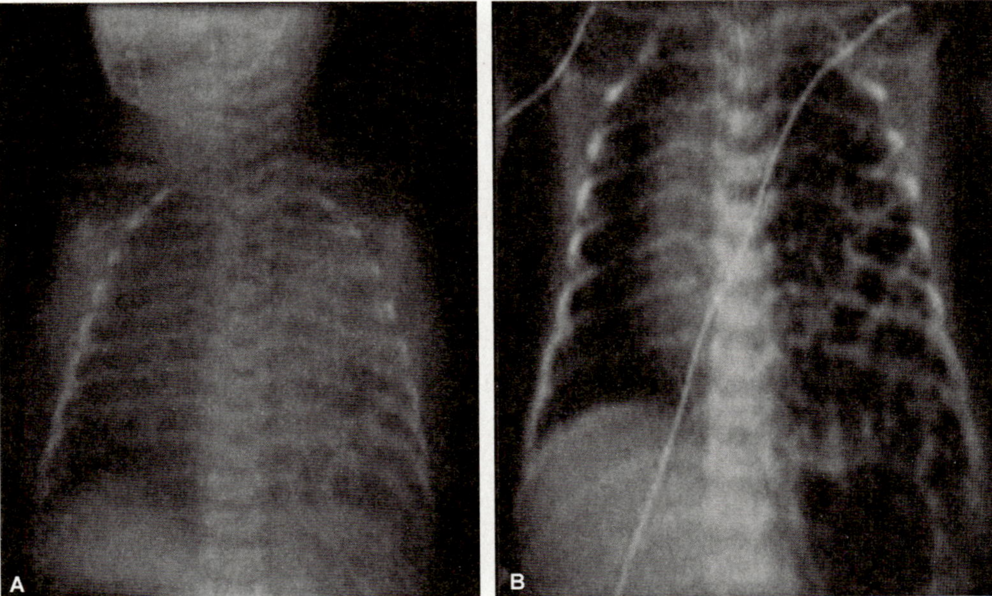

Fig. 26.9A and B Chest X-ray in CDH showing bowel in the left hemithorax, mediastinal shift and compression of the right lung
Source: Ali Hekmatnia, Kieran McHugh emedicine. medscape.com. updated 24 July 2013

pulmonary hypertension and right-to-left shunting for which various vasodilators have been used such as prostacyclin,[53] nitric oxide,[54] dipyridamole and tolazoline.[55] Positive pressure ventilation by bag and mask is very dangerous for infants with CDH, because this may distend the stomach and intestines present in the left hemithorax, further decreasing chest compliance. Early tracheal intubation and decompression of the stomach helps in preventing further distention of the displaced abdominal viscera and subsequent pulmonary compression. In cases of severe lung hypoplasia and refractory pulmonary hypertension, extracorporeal membrane oxygenation (ECMO) is recommended immediately at birth to avoid progressive lung injury.[56] A particularly poor prognosis is predicted if the patient was born at less than 33 weeks' gestation, weighs < 1000 g or requires endotracheal intubation immediately after birth, there is associated cardiac deformities, preoperative alveolar-to-arterial oxygen gradient is greater than 500 mmHg, or there is severe hypercarbia despite vigorous ventilation.[57] Pulmonary compliance and radiographic findings also predict prognosis.[58] Surgical correction is usually performed through an abdominal subcoastal incision, but a transthoracic or thoraco abdominal approach is also possible. In infants with large defects, a silastic pouch is used for primary closure of the abdomen after the hernia is reduced. Surgical correction through a subcostal incision with ipsilateral chest tube placement may be performed prior to or during ECMO.[59] Pulmonary vascular resistance is decreased by administering 100% oxygen. Hyperventilation is used to induce a respiratory alkalosis. Sympathetic discharge should be minimized (e.g. using a high-dose opioid technique). Small tidal volumes and low inflating pressures should be used during ventilation to avoid pneumothorax on the contralateral (usually right) side. Both nitrous oxide[60] and high frequency oscillatory ventilation (HFOV)[61] have been used during surgical repair. A high index of suspicion of right-sided pneumothorax should be maintained, and in the event of acute deterioration of respiratory or circulatory function, a thoracostomy tube should be placed. Intravascular volume, acid–base status and a normal body temperature should be maintained. Hypothermia may cause an increase in pulmonary vascular resistance, which may increase right-to-left shunting through a patent ductus arteriosus (PDA) or the foramen ovale. Hypothermia increases oxygen consumption, and in patients with poor cardiorespiratory functions, it may result in inadequate oxygen delivery and acidosis, which then further increases pulmonary vasoconstriction and worsens arterial desaturation. Nitrous oxide is avoided in infants with CDH because it can diffuse inside the viscera and exaggerate lung compression. Low concentrations of inhalation anaesthetics (sevoflurane or isoflurane) can be administered. In most cases, high-dose narcotics are administered and are continued into the postoperative period. Mechanical ventilation is continued postoperatively in nearly all cases.

SUMMARY

The management of paediatric patients for high-risk thoracic surgery remains to be one of the most difficult challenges for the anaesthesiologist. Need of SLV adds to the complexity of the anaesthetic technique. Various investigators have agreed that no single variable has the sufficient power to predict pulmonary complications or death in a thoracic surgical population. Even though some variables correlate with complications; overall, none of them predict pulmonary complications successfully in high-risk patients. Analyzing the nature of the primary lung pathology and manipulating the anaesthetic technique accordingly may improve the perioperative outcome. Thus proper understanding of the basic lung pathology, its impact on lung function, the corrective nature of surgery and physiology of SLV is necessary for optimum management of such seemingly complicated pulmonary surgical cases.

REFERENCES

1. Benumof JL, Augustine SD, Gibbons JA. Halothane and isoflurane only slightly impair arterial oxygenation during one-lung ventilation in patients undergoing thoracotomy. Anaesthesiology. 1987;67:910–914.
2. Conlan AA, Moyes DG, Schutz J, et al. Pulmonary resection in the prone position for suppurative lung disease in children. J Thorac Cardiovasc Surg. 1986;92:890.
3. Hammer GB. Paediatric thoracic anaesthesia. Anesth Analg. 2001;92:1449–64.
4. Dinesh K Choudhry. Single-Lung Ventilation in Paediatric Anaesthesia. Anesth Clin N Am. 2005; 23: 693–708.
5. Sommer N, Dietrich A, Schermuly RT, et al. Regulation of hypoxic pulmonary vasoconstriction: Basic mechanisms. Eur Respir J. 2008;32:1639–51.
6. Heaf DP, Helms P, Gordon MB, et al. Postural effects on gas exchange in infants. N Engl J Med. 1983;28:1505–8.
7. Mansell A, Bryan C, Levison H. Airway closure in children. J Appl Physiol. 1972;33:711–4.

8. Dawes GS. Fetal and Neonatal Physiology. Chicago, Yearbook Medical. 1973.
9. Shaffer TH, Wolfson MR, Panitch HB. Airway structure, function and development in health and disease. Paediatr Anaesth. 2004;14:3–14.
10. Benumof JL. One-lung ventilation and hypoxic pulmonary vasoconstriction: implications for anesthetic management. Anesth Analg. 1985;64: 821–33.
11. Domino KB, Wetstein L, Glasser SA, et al. Influence of mixed venous oxygen tension (PVO_2) on blood flow to atelectatic lung. Anesthesiology. 1983;59; 428–34.
12. Kubota H, Kubota Y, Toshiro T, et al. Selective blind endobronchial intubation in children and adults. Anesthesiology. 1987;67:587–589.
13. Hammer GB, Manos SJ, Smith BM, et al. Single lung ventilation in paediatric patients. Anesthesiology. 1996;84:1503–1506.
14. Campos JH. Progress in lung separation. Thoracic Surg Clin. 2008;15:71–83.
15. Lin YC, Hackel A. Paediatric selective bronchial blocker. Paediatr Anaesth. 1994;4:391–392.
16. Tan GM, Tan-Kendrick AP. Bronchial diameters in children—use of the Fogarty catheter for lung isolation in children. Anaesth Intensive Care. 2002;30:615–8.
17. Mohan VK, Darlong VM, Kashyap L, et al. Fiberoptic-guided Fogarty catheter placement using the same diaphragm of an adapter within the single-lumen tube in children. AnesthAnalg. 2002;95:1241–1242.
18. Campos JH. Update on lung separation techniques: Double-lumen tubes and bronchial blockers. Revista Mexicana de Anestesiologia. 2011;34:S270–7.
19. Campos JH, Kerstine KH. A comparison of left sided broncho-cath with the torque control blocker univent and the wire guided blocker. Anesth Analg. 2003;96:283–9.
20. Campos JH. Which device should be considered the best for lung isolation: Double-lumen endobronchial tubes versus bronchial blockers. Curr Opin Anesthesiol. 2007;20:27–31.
21. Rothenberg SS. Thoracoscopy in infants and children: State of the art. J Pediatr Surg. 2005;40: 303–6.
22. Wald SH, Mahajan A, Kaplan MB, et al. Experience with the Arndt paediatric bronchial blocker. Br J Anaesth. 2004;94:92–4.
23. Borchardt RA, LaQuaglia MP, McDowall Wilson RS. Bronchial injury during lung isolation in a paediatric patient. Anesth Analg. 1998;87:324–325.
24. Guyton DC, Besselievre TR, Devidas M, et al. A comparison of two different bronchial cuff designs and four different bronchial cuff inflation methods. J Cardiothorac Vasc Anesth. 1997;11:599–603.
25. Marraro G. Selective bronchial intubation in paediatrics: the Marraro paediatric bilumen tube. Paediatr Anaesth. 1994;4:255–8.
26. Stene R, Rose M, Weinger MB, et al. Bronchial trifurcation at the carina complicating use of double-lumen tracheal tube. Anesthesiology. 1994; 80:1162–4.
27. Massard G, Rouge C, Dabbagh A, et al. Tracheobronchial lacerations after intubation and tracheostomy. Ann Thorac. Surg 1996;61:1483–7.
28. Brodsky JB, Lemmens HJ. Left double-lumen tubes: Clinical experience with 1,170 patients. J Cardiothorac Vasc Anesth. 2003;17:289–98.
29. Klein U, Karzai W, Bloos F, et al. Role of fiberoptic bronchoscopy in conjunction with the use of double-lumen tubes for thoracic anaesthesia: a prospective study. Anesthesiology. 1998;88:346–50.
30. Hammer GB, Brodsky JB, Redpath J, et al. The Univent tube for single lung ventilation in children. Paediatr Anaesth. 1998;8:55–57.
31. Inoue H, Shohtsu A, Ogawa J, et al. New device for one-lung anaesthesia: Endotracheal tube with movable blocker. J Thorac Cardiovasc Surg. 1982; 83:940–1.
32. Zheng H, Duan Y, Geng WM, et al. A comparison of double-lumen endotracheal tube with univent blocker during thoracic surgical anaesthesia. Zhonghua Yi Xue Za Zhi. 2012;92:2481–4.
33. Benumof JL, Gaughan SD, Ozaki GT. The relationship among bronchial blocker cuff inflation volume, proximal airway pressure, and seal of the bronchial blocker cuff. J Cardiothorac Vasc Anesth. 1992;6:404–408.
34. Slinger PD, Lesiuk L. Flow resistances of disposable double-lumen, single-lumen, and Univent tubes. J Cardio thorac Vasc Anesth. 1998;12:142–144.
35. Capan LM, Turndorf H, Patel C, et al. Optimization of arterial oxygenation during one-lung anaesthesia. Anesth Analg. 1980;59:847–51.
36. Fujiwara M, Abe K, Mashimo T. The effect of positive end-expiratory pressure and continuous positive airway pressure on the oxygenation and shunt fraction during one-lung ventilation with propofol anaesthesia. J ClinAnesth. 2001;13:473.
37. Bromage PR, Benumof JL. Paraplegia following intracord injection during attempted epidural anaesthesia under general anaesthesia. Reg Anesth Pain Med. 1998;23: 104–107.
38. Gunter JB, Eng C. Thoracic epidural anaesthesia via the caudal approach in children. Anesthesiology. 1992;76: 935–938.
39. Cooper MG, Seaton HL. Intraoperative placement of intercostal catheter for postthoracotomy pain relief in a child. Paediatr Anaesth. 1992;2:165–167.
40. Shah R, Reddy AS, Dhende NP. Video assisted thoracic surgery in children. J Minim Access Surg. 2007;3:161–7.
41. Oak SN, Parelkar SV, Satish Kumar KV, et al. Review of video-assisted thoracoscopy in children. J Minim Access Surg. 2009;5:57–62.
42. Nezafati MG, Nahmoodi E, Hashemian SH, et al. Video-assisted thoracoscopic surgical (VATS) closure of Patent

Ductus Arteriosus: report of three-hundred cases. Heart Surg Forum. 2002; 5:57–59.

43. Cohen G, Hjortdal V, Ricci M, et al. Primary thoracoscopic treatment of empyema in children. J Thorac Cardio vasc Surg. 2003;125:79–83.
44. Hammer GB. Single-lung ventilation in infants and children. Paediatr Anaesth. 2004;14:98–102.
45. Lemenseg P Strangec, Sahns A. Empyema thoracis, therapeutic management and outcome. Chest. 1995;107:1532–7.
46. Ramnath N, Demmy TL, Antun A, et al. Pneumonectomy for bronchogenic carcinoma: Analysis of factors predicting survival. Ann Thorac Surg. 2007;83:1831–1836.
47. Keon TP. Death on induction of anaesthesia for cervical node biopsy. Anesthesiology. 1981;55:471.
48. Zeldin RA, Normadin D, Landtwig BS, et al. Post-pneumonectomy pulmonary edema. J Thorac Cardiovasc Surg. 1984;87:359–364.
49. Keijzer R, Liu J, Deimling J, et al. Dual-hit hypothesis explains pulmonary hypoplasia in the nitrofen model of congenital diaphragmatic hernia. Am J Pathol. 2000;156: 1299–306.
50. Bedoyan JK, Blackwell SC, Treadwell MC, et al. Congenital diaphragmatic hernia: associated anomalies and antenatal diagnosis. Outcome-related variables at two Detroit hospitals. Pediatr Surg Int. 2004;20:170–6.
51. Hazebroek FWJ, Tibboel D, Bos AP, et al. Congenital diaphragmatic hernia: Impact of preoperative stabilization. A prospective pilot study in 13 patients. J Pediatr Surg. 1988; 23:1139.
52. Levin DL. Congenital diaphragmatic hernia: A persistent problem. J Pediatr. 1987;111:390–392.
53. Kaapa P, Koivisto M, Ylikorlaka O, et al. Prostacyclin in the treatment of neonatal pulmonary hypertension. J Pediatr. 1985;107:951–953.
54. Mariani G, Barefield ES, Carlo WA. The role of nitric oxide in the treatment of neonatal pulmonary hypertension. Curr Opin Pediatr. 1996;8:118–125.
55. Ivy DD, Ziegler JW, Kinsella JP, et al. Dipyridamole attenuates rebound pulmonary hypertension after inhaled nitric oxide withdrawal in postoperative congenital heart disease. J Thorac Cardiovasc Surg. 1998;115:875–882.
56. Frenckner B, Ehren H, Granholm T. Improved results in patients who have congenital diaphragmatic hernia using preoperative stabilization, extracorporeal membrane oxygenation, and delayed surgery. J Pediatr Surg. 1997;32: 1185–1189.
57. Geary MP, Chitty LS, Morrison JJ. Perinatal outcome and prognostic factors in prenatally diagnosed congenital diaphragmatic hernia. Ultrasound Obstet Gynecol. 1998;12:107–111.
58. Donnelly LF, Sakurai M, Klosterman LA. Correlation between findings on chest radiography and survival in neonates with congenital diaphragmatic hernia. Am J Roentgenol. 1999;173: 1589–1593.
59. Truog RD, Schena JA, Hershenson MB, et al. Repair of congenital diaphragmatic hernia during extracorporeal membrane oxygenation. Anesthesiology. 1990;72:750–753.
60. Leveque C, Hamza J, Berg AE, et al. Successful repair of a severe left congenital diaphragmatic hernia during continuous inhalation of nitric oxide. Anesthesiology. 1994; 80:1171–1175.
61. Bouchut JC, Dubois R, Moussa M, et al. High frequency oscillatory ventilation during repair of neonatal congenital diaphragmatic hernia. Paediatric Anaesth. 2000;10:377–379.

Anaesthesia for General Abdominal and Urosurgical Procedures

Rakesh Garg and Uma Hariharan

ABSTRACT

The perioperative anaesthetic management of children is quite challenging. Apart from age related concerns, the anaesthetic concerns for abdominal surgical procedures appears similar to adults. However, association of congenital anomalies may require modifications for the perioperative care. The risk of aspiration, and need of rapid sequence induction and tracheal intubation is required to prevent aspiration even for children. The awake versus under anaesthetic airway management needs to be individualized based on child general status and cooperativeness. The major abdominal surgical procedures have a major fluid shift and thus fluid management needs to be cautiously and judiciously managed in the perioperative period. The use of regional anaesthesia may be considered for providing optimal pain relief in the perioperative period.

GENERAL ABDOMINAL PROCEDURES

GENERAL CONSIDERATIONS

The abdominal procedures in children are challenging not only because of the age but also depends to pathology and surgical procedure planned for correction of the anomaly.[1] Balanced general anaesthesia with inhalational agents, opioids and muscle relaxants is commonly used for paediatric abdominal surgeries. Endotracheal intubation, supraglottic airway device insertion or even face mask ventilation can be utilized, depending upon the type and duration of surgery. Regional anaesthesia, in the form of paediatric spinal or caudal block can be used as the sole anaesthetic technique in cooperative children. Upper abdominal procedures affect pulmonary function more and can cause postoperative pulmonary complications (PPCs), especially if pain relief is inadequate. Heat loss via radiation, conduction and evaporation is major problem in abdominal operations. To prevent the deleterious complications of hypothermia, all fluids (skin preparation, irrigation and intravenous) should be warmed. Active measures in the form of heated mattress, warm operation theatre environment, warming blankets, covering exposed body parts with cotton or plastic sheets (specially the head with its large surface area), humidified closed anaesthesia circuits and radiant incubators for neonates, should be used. All possible means must be utilized in preventing and treating postoperative shivering. Some children may be on preoperative chemotherapy for cancer leading to anaemia, pancytopenia, renal, hepatic, cardiac and pulmonary toxicity. A thorough preoperative evaluation of all the possible systems involved, along with strict asepsis during all procedures, is important in these children. Gastrointestinal cancers may be associated with hypercoagulability, which also has regional anaesthetic implications. Postoperative pain management in paediatrics is a challenging field, especially as assessment of severity is difficult for the novice. Regional techniques, especially ultrasound guided peripheral nerve blocks, can be advantageous in ensuring a smooth postoperative course as well as quench parental anxiety. Patient controlled analgesia (PCA) or nurse controlled analgesia (NCA) for small children can be utilized for preventing breakthrough pain and decrease postoperative opioid requirements. Postoperative nausea vomiting (PONV) is a complication which can delay discharge from the post-anaesthesia care unit (PACU) and hence has important cost implications in day care surgery.[2] Antiemetics like droperidol, ondansetron and dexamethasone are recommended for paediatric abdominal surgeries.

ABDOMINAL EMERGENCIES

Children may present with acute abdomen due to various causes and sometimes a diagnostic laparoscopy may be required to clinch the diagnosis. The anaesthetic principles include restoration of circulating blood volume and prevention of pulmonary aspiration of gastric contents.[3] The latter can be achieved by giving oral non-particulate antacid (0.3 mL/kg of 0.3 mol/L of sodium citrate 30 min prior) and systemic metoclopramide (gastric hurrying agent). This can be followed by passage of nasogastric tube if there is gastric distension and rapid sequence induction with cricoid pressure to secure the airway. The former can be achieved by securing a reliable venous access (preferably above the diaphragm), volume resuscitation according to the degree of hypovolemia, arranging for blood and using anaesthetic agents that do not depress the myocardium further. Intestinal obstruction in the newborn period is mostly due to congenital atresias: Ileal and duodenal. They may be associated with Down's syndrome and cardiac anomalies. Other causes of obstruction include: Malrotation, volvulus and meconium ileus.[4] Intussusception is the commonest cause of obstruction in infants over 2 months of age, followed by Meckel's diverticulum. The clinical features of obstruction include vomiting, distension, constipation/obstipation, abdominal pain and pallor. Dehydration, hypochloremic metabolic acidosis, electrolyte imbalance and hypotension may also be the presenting features. It is important to correct the above problems and achieve a definite trend towards improvement, before induction of anaesthesia. In some cases, blood supply to the involved bowel may be compromised leading to bowel resection and considerable blood loss. In the event of gut perforation, the child may present in a state of shock and appropriate antibiotics must be given along with fluid resuscitation and rapid sequence induction with cricoid pressure. Anaesthetic considerations for perforation peritonitis are similar to that for intestinal obstruction. Unexpected blood loss, problems due to bowel resection, heat and third space loss must be anticipated.

Exomphalos is caused by an incomplete return of gut contents to the abdominal cavity during foetal life. Intestine, liver or spleen can herniated into the umbilical cord. Most of these children are premature with associated congenital anomalies. Gastroschisis is herniation of intestinal contents through a defect in the lateral abdominal wall (right side), not covered with a membrane. In both conditions, the child can be posted for replacement of gut into the abdominal cavity. Large evaporative heat and water loss along with predisposition to infection are the problems encountered. Significant fluid and protein loss from the bowel can lead to higher than normal fluid requirements. Good muscle relaxation with controlled ventilation is required for primary surgical closure of the abdomen. Postoperative respiratory embarrassment must be managed with elective ventilation until the abdominal pressure and distension diminish. Starting of enteral nutrition may be delayed due to ileus and total parenteral nutrition (with its attendant complications) may be required to tide over the crisis.

Necrotizing enterocolitis is a serious disease especially of the premature infants. There is hypoperfusion of the bowel resulting in mucosal ischaemia, hyperosmolar damage and increased susceptibility to infection, with a high mortality rate. 50% patients have Gram negative septicemia. Most of these babies may have history of birth asphyxia and hyaline membrane disease. The clinical features include abdominal distension, bloody stools, ileus, pnematosis intestinalis (gas in the bowel wall), septicemia, acidosis and shock. Apart from medical management, surgery is required for resection of necrotic bowel or repair of perforation. Correction of hypovolemia, acidosis and infection (removal of umbilical catheters) must be undertaken prior to surgery. Blood should be arranged and invasive monitoring may be required in most cases. Nitrous oxide must be avoided and the child may require postoperative ventilatory support. Strict asepsis, parenteral nutrition and systemic narcotics for pain should be ensured.

Meconium ileus occurs in 10–15% patients with cystic fibrosis, where the distal ileum is obstructed with inspissated meconium. It may be complicated by perforation, gangrene, volvulus and meconium peritonitis. Anaesthetic problems are related to the degree of obstruction, the presence of complications, preoperative pulmonary function and infection control. Use of humidified gases and avoidance of atropine help improve clearance of respiratory secretions.

Incision and drainage of infective pathology in the abdomen (abscess, cysts) can also present as a semiemergency. The child may be febrile with tachycardia and tachypnea. Fluid requirements may be more than normal and sudden release of infective material (bacteremia) may cause postoperative septicemia. Temperature control, antibiotic cover, maintaining adequate urine output and complete asepsis must be ensured, apart from following rapid sequence induction for airway control.

Paediatric trauma can present as acute abdomen (either accidental or as a part of child abuse). Irrespective of whether it is blunt or penetrating injury, the child must be thoroughly examined for signs of injury to other body organs. If there are signs of raised intracranial tension, then head down position must be avoided during surgery. The child must be managed according to the protocols of advanced trauma life support (ATLS). Rapid sequence induction with airway and cervical spine protection must be ensured, along with correction of shock and arranging for blood. Focused assessment sonography in trauma (FAST) can help in faster diagnosis and no time should be wasted in taking the child to the operating room for emergency laparotomy, where indicated.

ABDOMINAL ENDOSCOPIC AND LAPAROSCOPIC SURGERIES

The availability of smaller laparoscopic equipment and increased expertise, the endoscopic and laparoscopic procedures are attempted in children by paediatric surgeons.[5–10] These procedures are increasingly being done because of the proposed benefits including smaller incisions, decreased intraoperative surgical stress, lesser tissue trauma, lesser perioperative pain, faster recovery including bowel function and thus earlier hospital discharge. These procedures usually have lesser respiratory morbidity especially for upper abdominal procedures. The procedures include not only for diagnostic but also definitive surgical interventional procedures. The commonly performed laparoscopic surgeries include appendicectomy, cholecystectomy, herniorraphy, orchidopexy, orchiectomy, cancer staging, biopsies, tumour abalation, diaphragmatic repair, liver procedures, and splenectomy. Laparoscopic interventions are useful for trauma child assessment, abscess drainage. Laparoscopic fundoplication for GERD (gastro-esophageal reflux disease) and laparoscopic bariatric surgery for adolescent obesity are also being done.[11]

Laparoscopy requires insufflation of the gas (usually carbon dioxide) in the abdomen (which may be intraperitoneal or extraperitoneal depending upon proposed surgical intervention) using a Veress needle. Gasless laparoscopy is well described in adults and in future may be well accepted for paediatric laparoscopic surgical intervention as well.[12,13] The impact of pneumoperitoneum depends on age of the child, respiratory pathology, head down tilt, anaesthetic technique (volatile agents), and mode of ventilation. Hypercarbia is more commonly observed in infants.[14] It also leads to compromised perfusion of abdominal organs including splanchnic, hepatic, and renal blood flow.[15]

Anaesthetic Management

The general anaesthesia is the most preferred anaesthetic technique for endoscopic and laparoscopic procedures in children. The endotracheal intubation with controlled ventilation is standard technique for laparoscopy. The use of supraglottic airway devices, like LMA, LMA-Proseal, Igel, etc. have been reported equally effective in adults but definitive evidence is absent in children specially in infants. The need of regional anaesthesia is usually not required when general anaesthesia has been administered for laparoscopic procedures. Suctioning of the stomach with a naso- or oro-gastric tube is recommended to decrease risk of visceral injury during trocar insertion and facilitate surgical access. Particular attention must be paid during positioning of the child in Trendelenburg or reverse Trendelenburg position. Adequate padding and support must be provided to prevent movement of the child off the table as well as to prevent neuro-vascular stretching or compression. Intra-abdominal pressures must be kept below 15 mmHg. Inadvertent endobronchial intubation may occur due to abdominal gas insufflation or cephalad movement of the diaphragm in Trendelenberg position. Airway pressure monitor, end tidal carbon dioxide measurement and precordial stethoscope (over left chest) are routinely recommended in such cases. The use of nitrous oxide is controversial, as it is associated with bowel distension, postoperative nausea vomiting (PONV) and aggravating air embolism (expanding air spaces).[16] During laparoscopy the risk of hypothermia due to dry and cold gases may be reduced by warming of the gases being insufflated and also be reducing the gas flow to less than 2 L/min. The child should be properly covered and other warming techniques like blankets should be used during the procedure. The increased occurrence of PONV after laparoscopic procedures may be managed prophylactically using antiemetics. Pain following laparoscopy occurs due to residual air, vascular traction, nerve stretching, visceral manipulation and can be minimized with systemic agents and local anaesthetic (like bupivacaine) infiltration of incision site or intraperitoneal local anaesthetic instillation. The oral analgesics (like acetaminophen, nonsteroidal anti-inflammatory agents) may also be suitable in the postoperative period for pain management.

ANAESTHESIA FOR PAEDIATRIC LIVER TRANSPLANTATION

A detailed review of the above topic is beyond the scope of this chapter. Hence, a brief overview is presented. Conditions causing end-stage liver disease in the paediatric population and amenable to transplant include: Biliary atresia, Wilson's disease, Liver tumours, Hemochromatosis, Alpha1 antitrypsin deficiency, tyrosinemia, Crigler-Najjar syndrome, etc. Majority of liver transplants is orthotopically performed, meaning the new liver is placed in the same location as the diseased liver.

A thorough pre-anaesthetic evaluation of both the donor and the recipient must be done. Concurrent problems like infection, ascites, varices, coagulopathy and encephalopathy must be managed prior to induction of anaesthesia. Modified Child-Pugh's grading and PELD (Paediatric Endstage Liver Disease) score as per UNOS criteria for organ procurement should be utilized.[1] Candidates with fulminant hepatic failure (status 1) are allocated organs ahead of all other waiting patients. The stratification of deceased organ donation was formulated by the United Network for Organ Sharing (UNOS). This system uses a risk determination based on a 3-month pretransplant assessment risk profile to assign priority and organ allocation to the most severely ill patients.

PELD score = 0.480 × Log_e (bilirubin mg/dL) + 1.857 × Log_e (INR) – 0.687 × Log_e (albumin g/dL) + 0.436 if patient is < 1 year (scores for patients < 1 year listed for liver transplantation; continue to include the value assigned for age of < 1 year until the patient is actually aged 2 year) + 0.667 if the patient has growth failure (< –2 standard deviation) 10 (then round to the nearest whole number).

Anaesthetic concerns depend on the stage of liver transplant:

1. **Pre-anhepatic stage:** This is associated with massive blood loss due to coagulopathy and difficult dissection. Anaesthetic goals include maintenance of hemodynamic stability (adequate fluid and blood administration), correction of coagulation abnormalities (Cryoprecipitate and FFP transfusion), and glucose homeostasis and temperature control.
2. **Anhepatic stage:** This begins with clamping of the IVC (inferior vena cava) and portal vein, which is associated with significant reduction in preload. This is tolerated well by paediatric patients due to better development of collateral blood flow. Anaesthetic goals include treating the metabolic derangements due to the absent liver, like correction of hypocalcemia, metabolic acidosis, hyperlactatemia, hyperkalemia and glucose homeostasis. Reperfusion with removal vascular clamps completes this stage.
3. **Neohepatic stage:** The postanhepatic stage is heralded by the completion of hepatic artery anastomosis and completion of biliary drainage. Anaesthetic goals include treatment of reperfusion syndrome, calcium supplementation, avoiding congestion of the new graft and maintaining adequate urine output. Children less than 10 kg weight usually require elective ventilation for 24 hours. There is restriction of lung function due to proportionately larger liver graft, pre-existing intrapulmonary shunts, pleural effusion, postoperative pulmonary oedema and decrease in pulmonary diffusing capacity.

ANAESTHESIA FOR COMMON SURGICAL PROBLEMS

Herniotomy, Orchidopexy, Appendicectomy, Hirschsprung disease, Cholecystectomy, Pyloromyotomy

Herniotomy/Herniorrhaphy (Inguinal, Umbilical): The processus vaginalis is a peritoneal covering enclosing the testicles during their descent from the abdomen through the inguinal wall into the scrotum. It usually closes at birth in term infants. In premature neonates, the hernia incidence is more common based on gestational age. The continued patency of this structure is the principal factor in the development of congenital hernias and hydroceles. The reported risk factors include prematurity, respiratory pathologies, and intraperitoneal fluid. Males are more frequently affected than females, right side more than left, incidence highest in the first year of life and in premature babies. The surgical procedure is usually an open technique but laparoscopic procedures have also been reported. The hernia repair is usually a planned elective procedure but at times, it may be taken as urgent procedure where incarceration or bowel obstruction occurs. Anaesthesia may be induced using volatile agents or intravenous induction agents depending upon child cooperation and presence of intravenous line. Induction of anaesthesia can be done with inhalational agents (sevoflurane) and then deepened after securing of intravenous access. Endotracheal intubation is usually unnecessary, except in premature child or with difficult airway or associated cardio-respiratory problems. In cases of bowel obstruction, rapid-sequence induction along with cricoid pressure is done. Availability of smaller size LMA's (size 0, 1, 1.5, 2, 2.5) has improved postoperative outcome as most of these procedures are done as day-care surgeries. The child must be sufficiently anaesthetized during manipulation of the spermatic cord to avoid laryngospasm or bradycardia. Maintenance of spontaneous respiration and supplementation of general anaesthesia with caudal (0.75–1 mL/kg of 0.25% bupivacaine) or ilioinguinal-iliohypogastric nerve block are usually practiced. For umbilical hernia repair, rectus sheath block can be given to supplement general anaesthesia.

Appendicectomy: Appendicitis is more commoner in age group of 10–19 years but the risk of perforation is more commoner in infants to the extent of 80%. Appendectomy can be done either as an elective procedure (interval appendicectomy) or as an emergency procedure. It is increasingly being done laparoscopically these days. Preoperatively, these children have issues related to fluid and electrolyte imbalance due to vomiting and dehydration and thus require adequate resuscitation. Endotracheal intubation after intravenous rapid sequence induction with cricoid pressure is the standard. However, in a fasting child, supraglottic device can also be used. If higher dose of bupivacaine in caudal block (1–1.25 mL/kg of 0.25% plain bupivacaine) is a concern, transversus abdominis plane (TAP) block and port-site infiltration with local anaesthetics can be used for pain management. Muscle relaxation with controlled ventilation is usually required for better surgical access, especially if done laparoscopically.

Cholecystectomy: The incidence of gall stones is increasing, especially in teenage children. Several factors are implicated, like diet, obesity, infections, presence of haemolytic tendencies or enzyme defects.[17] Anaesthesia for cholecystectomy is along standard principles. Usually it is performed laparoscopically.[18] Care must be taken to rule out active hepatitis, as any surgery in this phase can lead to liver cell failure. Obstructive jaundice must also be ruled out, if the bilirubin levels are high. Proseal-LMA with controlled ventilation, supplemented with TAP block can be utilized. Other issues related to laparoscopic procedures have been detailed elsewhere in this chapter.

Hirschsprung's disease: Hirschsprung's disease is the commonest cause of functional intestinal obstruction in the newborn due to gangliosis or absence of ganglion cells in the intrinsic nerve supply gastrointestinal tract.[19] It usually presents with delayed passage of meconium, irritability, failure to thrive and distension of the abdomen. In the past, a colostomy was created to relieve the obstruction, followed later by a formal pull-through before stoma closure. As it is associated with high morbidity and mortality, nowadays pull-through is done without creating a stoma. It is due to lack of ganglion in the distal colon and rectum. There is vomiting, reluctance to feeds and abdominal distension within 48 hours of birth. Diagnosis can be made by failure to pass meconium, multiple air-fluid levels on erect X-ray, Barium enema studies, anorectal manometry and rectal suction biopsy. Neonatal problems during anaesthesia are related recurrent intestinal obstruction, development of potentially fatal complications like necrotizing enterocolitis, prolonged surgery, blood loss, prevention of hypothermia and fluid and electrolyte balance. The surgical intervention usually takes longer time (6–8 hours) as it involves explorations of perineum and abdomen. Both open and laparoscopic surgical techniques have been reported. Anaesthesia may be induced either using inhalational agent or intravenous induction agent. Rapid sequence induction with cricoid pressure is recommended with endotracheal intubation and controlled ventilation. The nitrous oxide should be avoided and may be discontinued after induction. The general principle of temperature homeostasis and fluid management is of utmost important for these procedures.

Pyloromyotomy: Pyloromyotomy is required for child with pyloric stenosis which occurs due to gross thickening of the circular muscles of the pylorus.[20] It may be associated with other congenital disorder like cleft palate and esophageal reflux.[21] It presents between 2 and 8 weeks of age. The classical picture is of hypochloraemic, hypokalaemic, metabolic alkalosis, followed by hypoventilation; fall in cardiac output and urine output, leading to metabolic acidosis, hypoxia and shock. Jaundice may also be seen and is related to caloric deprivation and hepatic gluconyltransferase deficiency. The surgery may be either laparoscopically or as an open intervention. The major issues are dehydration, acid–base abnormalities and risk of aspiration. This surgical intervention is usually not an emergency and thus child may be optimized prior to surgery. This procedure requires injection of air to evaluate for any surgical leak. Rehydration with saline and electrolyte replacement (5% dextrose in 0.45% saline with 40 mMol/L potassium infused at 3 litre/m^2 per hour) must be done prior to surgery (which may take 24–48 hours). Rapid sequence induction with properly applied sellicks and controlled ventilation is the usual practice. Gastric evacuation through a ryles tube prior to induction does not completely eliminate the possibility of aspiration. There are chances of postoperative respiratory depression. Hence, extubation should be carried out once the child is wide awake with good muscle power and neuromuscular monitoring is desirable. Other complications reported in the postoperative period include hypoglycaemia, apnoea, convulsions and cardiac arrest. Subcostal TAP (transversus abdominis plane) block (preferably ultrasound guided) is found to be very effective in pain relief after pyloromyotomy and gastrostomy.

ANAESTHESIA FOR SURGERY ON ABDOMINAL SOLID ORGANS

Biliary Atresia: Kasai Procedure

It is a surgical palliation for biliary atresia and involves hepatic portoenterostomy.[22] It is a congenital condition characterized by disappearance of biliary structures and their replacement by fibrous tissue.[23,24] There are three main types: Type 1—atresia of common bile duct; Type 2— atresia of common bile duct+ common hepatic duct; Type 3—atresia of the entire extra hepatic duct system. The main problems include cholestasis, cirrhosis, portal hypertension and liver failure. Infants present before 6 weeks of age with progressive jaundice, pale stools, dark urine, coagulopathy, failure to thrive, hepatosplenomegaly and ascites.[25] Apart from medical and nutritional management, surgical treatment is the standard of care achieved by portoenterostomy. Pre–operative preparation involves investigations, intramuscular vitamin K, oral neomycin, arrangement of blood and fresh frozen plasma (FFP), adequate hydration and atropine premedication (0.05–0.1 mg given 30–60 min preop). An intravenous access, invasive monitoring (especially with associated sepsis, pneumonia, cholangitis, and severe cirrhosis), temperature maintenance and adequate urine output is desirable. Anaesthesia induction may be inhalational or intravenous technique. Inhalational induction may be by sevolfurane and propofol may be used for intravenous induction. Isoflurane is preferable for maintenance as it has been reported to maintain hepatic blood flow. The nitrous oxide is avoided to prevent bowel distension. Neuromuscular blocking agents may include cisatracurium or atracurium. The fluid of choice is lactated Ringer's solution but 1–5% dextrose may be added to prevent hypoglycemia. During surgery, cardiac output may fall because of decreased venous return due to inferior vena cavae kinking during liver manipulation. Surgery may have blood loss and fluid and blood management should be done judiciously. Some infants with preexisting multi-organ failure, sepsis and pneumonia may require postoperative ventilatory support. The child should be monitored in an intensive care setting. Postoperative analgesia can be achieved with systemic opioid infusion (morphine 0.5–1 mg/kg/day) or electronic patient controlled analgesia (PCA) pumps. In the follow up, child may have cholangitis, portal hypertension and deficiency of fat-soluble vitamin and will be of concern when such child is scheduled for revision surgery or other incidental surgical intervention.

Hepatic Resection

Hepatic resection may be required for liver tumours, predominantly hepatoblastoma and hepatocarcinoma.[26–30] These tumours occur either under 4 years of age or between 12 and 15 years of age. These may be associated with cirrhosis, Wilson's disease, von Gierke's disease, glycogenesis (type I), cystinosis, extrahepatic biliary atresia, α_1-antitrypsin deficiency and Solo's syndrome. The basic management is similar as described for biliary atresia. Abdominal surgery reduces total hepatic blood flow. Volatile anaesthetics alter portal venous and hepatic arterial vascular resistance. Intravenous anaesthetics have not demonstrated significant effect on postoperative liver function. Xenon is an ideal anaesthetic agent having no effect on organ perfusion and no changes in hepatic arterial flow. There is an impending risk of perioperative haemorrhage, hepatic failure and coagulopathy in children undergoing liver resections in the presence of preoperative liver dysfunction. A thorough preoperative evaluation with arrangement of adequate blood and blood products must be ensured. Drainage of ascitic fluid, treatment of esophageal varices, prevention of kernicterus and maintenance of renal function must be done concurrently. Caution must be exercised in children on preoperative chemotherapeutic agents as they may further compromise liver function and may be associated with cardiomyopathy (adriamycin and anthracycline). Pulmonary function may be impaired due to diaphragmatic splinting or presence of shunts. Intraoperatively, attempts must be made to decrease liver congestion to facilitate surgery and minimize blood loss. Central venous pressure (CVP) is preferably maintained between 3 and 5 cm H_2O so as to decrease bleeding and reducing need for blood transfusion. Major or extended liver resections may be prolonged surgeries with massive fluid shifts and these children may require liver transplantation in the future. Invasive monitoring and securing large bore intravenous access can be challenging in small children. Fluid and electrolyte balance especially of potassium must be maintained in the perioperative period. Children with benign liver tumours usually have preserved liver function. Malignant tumours include hepatoblastomas and hepatocarcinomas. Meticulous attention must be paid by the surgeon in dissection to prevent damage to biliary ducts and canaliculi. Hypothermia prevention is of prime importance by using active warming measures, which must be continued in the postoperative period. Pain management is usually multimodal with use of opioid PCA pumps. Ultrasound guided TAP blocks can be given in older children if equipment and expertise exist.[31,32] Some children may require postoperative elective ventilation and all must be cared for in a dedicated paediatric intensive care unit. The extent of liver resection affects the magnitude and duration of coagulation defect, necessitating close monitoring of prothrombin time and platelets postoperatively.

Splenectomy

Indications for splenectomy in the paediatric population include thalassemia major, Kala azar and lymphoproliferative disorders. The main anaesthetic concerns include anticipation and management of blood loss. Strict asepsis must be ensured. Pneumococcal vaccine must be preferably given a week preoperatively. When splenectomy is done as part of trauma care in abdominal injuries, availability of blood may be difficult and fluid resuscitation must proceed as per ATLS protocol.[33] Pain management can be done both by systemic agents and by epidural analgesia.

UROSURGICAL PROCEDURES

GENERAL CONSIDERATIONS

Urologic surgeries are quite common in the paediatric population, with an increase in diagnostic modalities.[34] The anaesthetic considerations are unique as the child will have to be positioned away from the anaesthesia circuit and various irrigating solutions would be used for the procedure.[35,36] Usually these surgeries are performed in lithotomy position. It is difficult to place infants and newborns in lithotomy for prolonged periods. Apart from the risk of neurovascular injury in lithotomy position, the availability of miniature lithotomy poles and its fixation in operating room tables is also a major task, especially in the developing world. In newborns, plastic-covered thick cotton rolls can be placed below both the thighs and legs may be kept in abducted position gently by an assistant for short procedures. For infants, plastic saline or irrigation bottles can be placed below both the thighs and legs fixed in the desired position by non-irritating tapes. High lithotomies must be limited for a short period of time. Care must also be taken in changing head position, especially in steep Trendelenburg or reverse Trendelenburg position. Cardiovascular changes which occur with different positions must be kept in mind in managing these children. Particular attention must be given in preventing tube or airway displacement and falling-off the patient in this scenario. Anaesthesia circuit must be long enough to reach the child from the workstation. It must be remembered that this can increase the dead space, which can be deleterious in paediatric patients. Difficult airway cart, including working suction and other resuscitative equipment must be readily available. Hypothermia and its prevention is a concern in all paediatric surgeries, more so in urologic procedures. This is because a large amount of cold irrigating solutions is used. The temperature of the fluid, its quantity, height of the pole from which irrigation fluid is flowing and type of fluid used must be noted and constantly assessed. Core temperature monitoring is a mandatory requirement. Active measures in the form of forced air heaters, fluid warmers, covering the exposed areas of the child with cotton or plastic sheet, keeping the operating environment warm and use of warming blankets, must be undertaken for maintaing normothermia. Caution must also be taken in preventing the electro-surgical equipment and the drapes from wetting by the irrigation fluid. Pain management is also a prime area of importance.[37] Regional techniques like penile blocks, caudal blocks and epiduals are advantageous, not only in decreasing intra-operative anaesthetic requirements, but also in ensuring a smooth postoperative course.[38] Multi-modal analgesia with paracetamol suppositories, NSAIDS (avoided in patients with renal dysfunction) and opioids (systemic and neuraxial) can also be utilized for better postoperative pain management.

Preoperative Assessment

Genitourinary problems affect the fluid balance, electrolyte concentrations, kidney functions and the cardiovascular system. It is important to remember that they may be associated with serious congenital anomalies in the paediatric population. Anaemia may result from chronic infection or renal failure. Reduction in glomerular filtration rate and rise in plasma urea and creatinine levels will cause sodium and water retention, leading to hypertension, metabolic acidosis, failure to thrive and electrolyte imbalance. These children may also be on several drugs of significance to the anaesthesiologists, like diuretics, steroids, chemotherapeutic agents and antihypertensives. Hypertensive children should also be evaluated for presence of catecholamine-secreting tumours and reno-vascular disease.

CONGENITAL ANOMALIES

These anomalies can either occur in isolation or in association with other congenital defects, like cardiac or abdominal anomalies (which may go undetected).[1] They can either affect the kidney or the urinary tract or appear as an external defect. It must be remembered that children with congenital urological abnormalities are at greater propensity to develop latex allergy, which can sometimes be fatal.

Congenital renal anomalies include polycystic kidneys, complete renal agenesis, renal dysplasia, Potter's syndrome, renal artery stenosis, ectopic kidneys and malrotations. Horseshoe kidneys may present as an incidental finding, which can impede surgical access and is prone to trauma. Anaesthetic considerations include, excluding other associated congenital anomalies, control of hypertension, preservation of renal function and infection control.

Congenital anomalies of the urinary tract can present as intra-uterine urinary obstruction, causing renal dysplasia, hydronephrosis and oligohydramnios. Distal urinary tract obstruction can be due to posterior urethral valves (commonest), urethral strictures or diverticuli. Children with ureteric reflux may need to undergo diagnostic cystoscopy, retrograde pyelogram, urodynamic studies, urethral reimplantation and strictureplasty. These children may develop renal parenchymal damage and hypertension, secondary to infection and urinary backflow.

Reimplantation of ureters is required for vesicoureteral reflux and the surgical procedure may take 2 to 5 hours. The anaesthetic technique is usually general anaesthesia along with endotracheal intubation for airway management. The caudal or lumbar epidural catheter not only provides optimal perioperative analgesia bit also prevents postoperative bladder spasm. The urine output measurement is difficult as it leaks in the surgical field, so other markers of haemodynamic need to be assessed during long surgical procedure.

Prune-belly Syndrome

It can occur as a part of urethral obstruction malformation complex.[39] It may be associated with cryptorchidism, volvulus, pulmonary stenosis, deafness and mental retardation.[40] Abdominal skin is wrinkled, with no abdominal musculature, which hinders clearing of respiratory secretions. Causes of death in the neonatal period include renal or pulmonary failure. Anaesthetic considerations include avoiding aspiration of gastric contents, choice of drugs not excreted by the kidney, intensive chest physiotherapy, fluid management, postoperative elective ventilation and appropriate antibiotics.

Bladder Exstrophy

It occurs due to failure of the infraumbilical mesenchyme to migrate into the area of cloacal membrane, preventing midline fusion of the anterior abdominal wall. Early surgical closure in the neonatal period is recommended to prevent infection, urinary obstruction and squamous metaplasia. Repeated surgeries and anaesthesia exposure is required for both diagnostic and therapeutic purposes. In addition to invasive monitoring (arterial and central venous line), obtaining a good intravenous access to tackle blood and fluid loss during surgery is of paramount importance. Anaesthesia must be planned keeping in mind that most of these surgeries are prolonged. Arranging adequate blood, absolute infection control, maintaining normothermia, fluid and electrolyte balance, positioning considerations and good postoperative pain management must be ensured in all cases.

Adrenogenital Syndrome

It can occur due to deficiency of C-21 hydroxylase enzyme (causing masculinization in the female) or deficiency of C-11 hydroxylase (causing hypertension). Apart from medical management, surgical genitoplasty may be required early (at 6 months of age). Anaesthetic concerns include good venous access, difficult airway, adequate steroid cover (dose of hydrocortisone supplementation according to body weight), fluid and electrolyte balance and caudal analgesia for pain management.

COMMON GENITAL SURGERIES

Hypospadias

Hypospadias may be repaired in single stage or multiple stages based on multstaged procedure depending upon the defect severity. Severe degree of hypospadias may require major surgeries, like Duckett procedure or bladder mucosal graft operations. Mild to moderate degree of hypospadias can be repaired under general anaesthesia (with or without muscle relaxants) plus caudal analgesia or penile block. Spontaneous respiration with LMA (laryngeal mask airway) insertion can beneficial, especially as these are done as day-care procedures. Maintenance of anaesthesia can be by inhalation or a balanced technique. Caution must be excised in premature infants (gestational age less than 44 weeks post-conception), as they are prone for postoperative apnoea. Anaesthetic management involves controlled ventilation, adequate blood and fluid replacement, reliable intravenous access, temperature maintenance and multi-modal postoperative analgesia.

Orchidopexy/Orchidectomy

The undescended testis may occur in 0.8% of 1-year-old boys and may be associated with hernia. The testes may lie in abdomen, inguinal canal or above the scrotum at external ring. These abnormally located testes require either inguinal canal exploration or even exploration of the posterolateral surface of the peritoneal cavity. Orchidopexy is recommended in the early childhood to prevent infertility and development of testicular malignancy. These testis is either remover or there are released and placed in the scrotal sac and sometimes requires stages surgical intervention. These interventions may be done via open surgical technique or by laparoscopic approach. The perioperative anaesthetic management is similar as described for hernia repair. However, the incidence of intraoperative bradycardia and laryngospasm is more due to nerve supply of spermatic cord and testicle which gets activated during their manipulation (strong vagal stimulant) and thus requires deeper plane of anaesthesia. Even use of regional anaesthesia may prevent activation of such responses. Analgesia can be provided with either caudal block or ilioinguinal-iliohypogastric nerve block. Ultrasound guidance for performing these blocks can be sought where facilities exist, to improve efficacy and minimize complications. The use of prophylactic antiemetics (ondansetron, 0.1 mg/kg) is suggested.

Torsion testes can present as an emergency, whereby orchidectomy may be required if vascular supply is compromised for prolonged periods. Urgent surgical exploration is warranted in all cases of acute scrotum. Anaesthesia must aim at preventing gastric aspiration (full stomach precautions and rapid sequence induction) and fluid resuscitation, apart from other routine considerations, especially pain management. Testicular manipulation is associated with high incidence of vagal stimulation and postoperative nausea vomiting.

Circumcision

Circumcision can usually be performed under general anaesthesia with spontaneous ventilation supplemented with caudal block.[41,42] Anaesthesia must be deepened when the foreskin is clamped. While giving penile blocks, absolute care must be taken to avoid adrenaline containing local anaesthetics. Most of these children can be sent home the same day in the soothing comfort of their parents/guardians company.

Cystoscopy

Cystoscopy is required in children primarily for evaluation for abnormalities of the urethra, bladder, and ureters. Cystoscopies can also be done as day-care procedure. The anaesthetic technique may vary from mask ventilation to use of laryngeal mask airway. Care must be taken in lithotomy positioning, long anaesthesia circuit for mask ventilation away from the anaesthesia workstation and temperature control. During cystoscopy, urethral stimulation may lead to laryngospasm which has been described as Breuer-Lockhart reflex. Use of irrigation fluid may hamper accurate blood loss estimation as well as predispose to hypothermia. The child may be exposed to repeated anaesthetics to check cystoscopies being performed for various urogenital problems.

WILMS' TUMOUR

Wilms' tumour, also known as nephroblastoma, is the commonest abdominal tumour of children and may be bilateral or associated with other renal anomalies (extopic and solitary kidneys), ureteral duplications and hypospadias. Other associated conditions include Beckwith-Wiedemann syndrome and neurofibromatosis. It usually presents between 1 and 3 years. Children can present for surgical resection, chemotherapy or radiotherapy. Preoperative evaluation should exclude anaemia, hypertension (seen in 60% of patients), renal failure and metastasis (commonly lung and liver). If child has received peroperative chemotherpay, then evaluation for side effects of chemotherapeutic agents needs to be assessed. Sedation under monitored anaesthesia care may be required for radiotherapy or for various diagnostic procedures. Staging of the tumour has important prognostic implications. Its size may be large enough to impinge on the diaphragm and compromise lung function. Rapid sequence induction for airway protection is recommended. Nitrous oxide should not be used to prevent bowel distension. Analgesia may be provided by intravenous opioids which also reduces anaesthetic requirements. Use of epidural analgesia is also an optimal option. Tumour may also invade the renal vein or inferior vena cava, which can either embolise during handling or impede venous return. Blood loss during surgery can be extensive, warranting adequate venous access, invasive monitoring and early transfusion. It is imperative to maintain renal function and normothermia, both during intra- and post-operative periods.

OTHER ABDOMINAL TUMOURS

Other related tumours, which can present during childhood, include neuroblastomas (retroperitoneal tumour arising from neural crest tissues) and phaeochromocytoma (adrenal or extra-adrenal tumours arising from cromaffin cells).[43] Anaesthetic concerns include control of hypertension, management of blood loss, excluding other organ involvement, invasive monitoring and adequate pain management.[44] Adequate alpha-blockade must be ensured before starting beta-blocker therapy. Drugs or events stimulating catecholamine release must be avoided and postoperative course must be managed in a dedicated paediatric intensive care unit.

SURGERY ON THE FEMALE GENITAL ORGANS

Ovarian cyst, especially dermoid cyst is common and can present acutely following a twist or cyst rupture. Anaesthesia must aim at preventing gastric aspiration, airway protection, providing adequate muscle relaxation, estimation of fluid/blood loss and pain relief. Rarely, there may be congenital anomalies of the utero-vaginal canal, leading to bicornuate uterus or absent uterus. This may go undetected till the time the child attains the age of menarche. She can present for emergency draining of hematometra. Anaesthetic considerations are similar as stated above and blood transfusion may be required. Plastic reconstructive procedures of the malformed genital tract are also undertaken in some centers. They are usually long or staged operations, with its attendant anaesthetic implications.

PAEDIATRIC RENAL TRANSPLANTATION

Kidney transplant is being increasingly performed these days in children and adolescents, for end-stage renal disease.[45] Donor availability, cost, legal issues, cross-matching and graft uptake are key issues which need to be addressed. Preoperative evaluation is usually extensive and adequate blood and blood products must be arranged. Preoperatively, child may be on regular dialysis and on multi-drug therapy, including steroids.[46] Pre-existing chronic renal failure and chronic dialysis-induced patho-physiological changes in the child must be considered in the anaesthetic management.[47] Immunosuppressive therapy and antibiotics need to be started at induction. Reliable peripheral and central intravenous line, as well as arterial catheter needs to be inserted before induction under mild sedation and local anaesthesia. Apart from CVP (central venous pressure), other monitors of intravascular volume status and its responsiveness may be utilized in special cases (like stroke volume variation, pulse variation index and extravascular lung water). Existing arterio-venous shunts must be protected for future use in dialysis. Preferably, the left arm should not be used for obtaining any vascular access. Renal function, body weight, electrolyte and acid-base status must be evaluated, especially if dialysis is done preoperatively. Transplantation of a large donor kidney (from an adult or adolescent) into a small recipient (child) requires anastomoses to the aorta and inferior vena cava, rather than the iliac vessels. This can cause severe hypotension during cross-clamping as well post-transplant (larger kidney draws greater amount of the cardiac output for its perfusion). It may also cause problems during abdominal closure. Metabolic acidosis and electrolyte imbalance can be deleterious in the re-perfusion phase. Adequate renal perfusion must be maintained to ensure good urine output. A high-normal CVP is usually maintained just prior to unclamping. At least 2 mL/kg/hour of urine output is desirable post-transplantation. Mannitol, loop diuretics and fenoldopam have been advocated for renal protection. Maintaining a good mean arterial pressure is imperative for adequate renal function. Great care must be taken to identify signs of graft rejection, early. Complete asepsis must be ensured during pre-, intra- and post-operative periods. Nephrotoxic agents must be avoided. Children may develop postoperative pulmonary oedema and may require short-term elective ventilation in a dedicated intensive care unit. Drug interaction between immunosuppressive and anaesthetic agents must be kept in mind. Diligent charting of intake-output and vitals must be ensured. Pain management is usually multi-modal. Ultrasound guided tranversus abdominis plane block or rectus sheath block can be utilized, if possible. Clear communication between the nephrologists, paediatrician, anaesthesiologist and the surgeon is mandatory for a better outcome. With modern immunosuppressive agents, better donor selection and advanced surgical techniques, the incidence of acute graft rejection has been minimized significantly. Chronic graft rejection and persistent renal dysfunction is still a problem, leading to the recipient children returning back to dialysis, emphasizing preservation of fistula sites.

ANAESTHESIA FOR ROBOTIC SURGERIES IN PAEDIATRICS

With the advancement in technology, surgery has become minimally invasive and multi-dimensional for most procedures.[48] Robotic surgery, though common in the developed world, is still in its infancy in India, especially in paediatric population. Not only it is cosmetically better, but also it is associated with improved postoperative recovery and less pain.[49] The da Vinci Surgical System is used, where smaller instruments (5 mm size as opposed to 8 mm for adults) are used in children. As the working space is limited and the abdominal wall is thinner, proper introduction and positioning of ports and manipulation instruments is paramount. Robotic radical nephrectomies and cystectomies (with neobladder formation) are being done for malignancies.[50] Anaesthetic considerations include positioning issues of steep trendelenberg position, restricted intravenous fluid therapy and physiological changes associated with pneumoperitoneum.[51] These surgeries may be prolonged, especially due to learning curve of this new procedure.[52] It must be remembered that absolute muscle relaxation is required after docking of the robotic assembly, as even slight movement of the patient can cause devastating complications. Balanced anaesthesia with controlled ventilation (preferably pressure controlled ventilation in extreme head down position to avoid barotraumas) after endotracheal intubation is the preferred technique.[52,53] Adequate padding, soft shoulder supports to prevent falling down of the child, prevention of deep vein thrombosis, gentle lithotomy positioning, slow insufflation and de-sufflation, cushioning of bony prominences and maintaining normothermia are the pillars of a successful robotic surgery program. Protocols for monitoring in such cases must be established in each institution. Apart from routine monitors, airway pressure, tracheal tube cuff pressure, bispectral index, neuromuscular monitoring and multigas monitor is desirable for better outcome. Systemic analgesics, including opiods and port infiltration with local anaesthetics can be used for pain management. Special drills for emergency de-docking in the event of a crisis situation must be regularly done for all personnel working in a robotic theatre.

SUMMARY

The paediatric anaesthesia is challenging due to anatomical and physiological concerns. The abdominal and urological surgical interventions are associated with special issues which requires care during the perioperative management. These include use of laparoscope and associated concerns; risk of regurgitation and aspiration; perioperative analgesia; prolonged duration surgical procedures and associated comorbidities.

REFERENCES

1. Hammer G, Hall S, Davis PJ. Anaesthesia for general abdominal, thoracic, urologic and bariatric surgery in Smith's anesthesia for Infants and Children. 7th edn. Motoyama EK, Davis PJ. Elsevier, Philadelphia. 2006; 695–7.
2. Tramer M, Moore A, McQuay H. Omitting nitrous oxide in general anaesthesia: Meta-analysis of intraoperative awareness and postoperative emesis in randomized controlled trials. Br J Anaesth 1996;76:186–190.
3. Cote CJ, Goudsouzian NG, Liu LMP, et al. Assessment of risk factors related to the acid aspiration syndrome in pediatric patients—gastric pH and residual volume. Anesthesiology. 1982;56: 70–72.
4. Peña A, Hong A. Advances in the management of anorectal malformations. Am J Surg. 2000;180:370.
5. Tomicic JT, Luks FI, Shalon L, et al. Laparoscopic gastrostomy in infants and children. Eur J Pediatr Surg. 2002;12:107–110.
6. Esposito C, Van Der Zee DC, Settimi A, et al. Risks and benefits of surgical management of gastroesophageal reflux in neurologically impaired children. Surg Endosc. 2003; 17:708–710.
7. Hirvonen EA, Poikolainen EO, Pääkkönen ME, et al. The adverse hemodynamic effects of anesthesia, head-up tilt, and carbon dioxide pneumoperitoneum during laparoscopic cholecystectomy. Surg Endosc. 2000;14: 272–277.
8. Park A, Heniford BT, Hebra A, et al. Pediatric laparoscopic splenectomy. Surg Endosc. 2000; 14:527–531.
9. Esposito C, Gonzalez Sabin MA, Corcione F, et al. Results and complications of laparoscopic cholecystectomy in childhood. Surg Endosc. 2001; 15:890–892.
10. Bourne MC, Wheeldon C, MacKinlay GA, et al. Laparoscopic Nissen fundoplication in children: 2–5 year follow-up. Pediatr Surg Int. 2003;19:537–539.
11. Wyner J, Brodsky JB, Merrell RC. Massive obesity and arterial oxygenation. Anesth Analg. 1981; 60:691–695.
12. Lukban JC, Jaeger J, Hammond KC, et al. Gasless versus conventional laparoscopy. N J Med 2000; 97:29–34.
13. Canestrelli M, Canni M, Mori R, et al. The new techniques of gynaecologic laparoscopy: Gasless, open Hanson, optic trocar. Panminerva Med. 1999; 41:371–377.
14. Sprung J, Whalley DG, Falcone T, et al. The impact of morbid obesity, pneumoperitoneum, and posture on respiratory system mechanics and oxygenation during laparoscopy. Anesth Analg. 2002;94:1345–1350.
15. Steiner CA, Bass EB, Talamini MA, et al. Surgical rates and operative mortality for open and laparoscopic cholecystectomy in Maryland. N Engl J Med. 1994;330:403–405.
16. Taylor E, Feinstein R, White PF, et al. Anesthesia for laparoscopic cholecystectomy: Is nitrous oxide contraindicated?. Anesthesiology. 1992;76:541–546.
17. Soper NJ, Barteau JA, Clayman RV, et al. Comparison of early postoperative results for laparoscopic versus standard open cholecystectomy. Surg Gynecol Obstet. 1992;174:114.
18. Yu HP, Hseu SS, Yien HW, et al. Oral clonidine premedication preserves heart rate variability for patients undergoing laparoscopic cholecystectomy. Acta Anaesthesiol Scand. 2003;47:185–190.
19. Wulkan ML, Georgeson KE. Primary laparoscopic endorectal pull-through for Hirschsprung's disease in infants and children. Semin Laparosc Surg. 1998;5:9–14.
20. Vanderwinden JM, Mailleux P, Schiffman SN, et al. Nitric oxide synthase in infantile hypertrophic pyloric stenosis. N Engl J Med. 1992; 327:511.
21. Sorensen HT, Skriver MV, Pedersen L, et al. Risk of infantile hypertrophic pyloric stenosis after maternal postnatal use of macrolides. Scand J Infect Dis. 2003;35:104–107.
22. Wildhaber BE, Coran AG, Drongowski RA, et al. The Kasai Portoenterostomy for biliary atresia: A review of a 27 year experience with 81 patients. J Pediatr Surg. 2003;38: 1480–1485.
23. Green DW, Howard ER, Davenport M. Anesthesia, perioperative management and outcome of correction of extrahepatic biliary atresia in the infant: A review of 50 cases in the King's College Hospital series. Pediatr Anaesth. 2000;10:581–589.
24. Hartley JL, Davenport M, Kelly DA. Biliary Atresia. Lancet. 2009;374:1704–13.
25. Popovic L, Batinica S, Mestrovic T, et al. The value of cholinesterase activity after Kasai operation. Pediatr Surg Int. 2003;19:605–607.
26. Borland LM, Roule M, Cook DR. Anaesthesia for pediatric orthoptic liver transplantation. Anaesthesia and Analgesia. 1985;64:117–124.
27. Carmichael FJ, Lindop MJ, Farman JV. Anaesthesia for hepatic transplantation: Cardiovascular and metabolic alterations and their management. Anesthesia and Analgesia. 1985;64:108–116.
28. Owen CA, Rettke SR, Bowie EJW, et al. Hemostatic evaluation of patients undergoing liver transplantation. Mayo Clinic Proceedings. 1987;62:761–772.
29. Yudkowitz FS, Chietero M. Anesthetic issues in pediatric liver transplantation. Pediatr Transplant. 2005;9:666–672.
30. Hammer GH, Krane EJ. Anaesthesia for liver transplantation in children. Paed Anaes. 2001;11:3–18.
31. Ross AK, Eck JB, Tobias JD. Pediatric regional anesthesia-beyond the caudal. Anesth Analg. 2000;91:16–26.
32. Willschke H, Marhofer P, Bosenberg A, et al. Ultrasonography for ilioinguinal/iliohypogastric nerve blocks in children. Br J Anaesth. 2005;95:226–330.
33. Wesson DE, Filler RM, Ein SH, et al. Ruptured spleen—when to operate? Journal of Pediatric Surgery. 16:324–326.

34. Cramolini GM. Diseases of the renal system. Anesthesia and Uncommon Pediatric diseases. In Katz J and Steward DJ (Eds). Philadelphia: Saunders. 1987;pp 155–221.
35. Shukis A, Merola C. Anesthesia for pediatric urological surgery. Int Anesthesiol Clin. Winter. 1993;31:109–117.
36. Monica G, Rita V. Anaesthesia for paediatric urology. Contin Educ Anaesth Crit Care Pain. 2010;10:152–157.
37. Whitrock K. Pain management for pediatric urological surgery. Int Anesthesiol Clin. 1993;31:119–40.
38. Bhalla T, Sawardekar A, Dewhirst E, et al. Ultrasound-guided trunk and core blocks in infants and children. J Anesth. 2013;27:109–123.
39. Henderson AM, Vallis CJ, Sumner L. Anaesthesia in the prune-belly syndrome: a review of 36 cases. Anaesthesia. 1987;42:54–60.
40. Woodhouse CRJ, Ransley PG, Innes-Williams D. Prune-belly syndrome: Report of 47 cases. Arch Dis Child. 1982; 57: 856.
41. White J, Harrison B, Richmond P, et al. Postoperative analgesia for circumcision. Br Med Journal. 1983;286: 1934–1937.
42. Yeoman PM, Cooke R, Hain WR. Penile block for circumcision? A comparision with caudal blockade. Anaesthesia. 1983;38:862–866.
43. Kaufman BH, Telander RL, van Heerden JA, et al. Phaeochromocytoma in the pediatric age group; current status. Journal of Pediatric Surgery. 1983;18:879–884.
44. Weinblatt ME, Heisel MA, Siegel SE. Hypertension in children with neurogenic tumours. Pediatrics. 1983;71: 947–1951.
45. Potter D, Feduska N, Melzer J, et al. Twenty years of renal transplantation in children. Pediatrics. 1986;77:465–470.
46. Fernando ON. Renal transplantation in children. In Williams DI, Johnston JH, (Eds). Pediatric Urology. Buttersworth, London. 1982;pp 49–56.
47. Della RG, Costa MG, Bruno K, et al. Pediatric renal transplantation: Anesthesia and perioperative complications. Pediatr Surg Int. 2001;17:175–179.
48. Goedele VH, Susan L, Winifred H. Pediatric Robotic Surgery: Early Assessment. Pediatrics. 2009;124:1642–1649.
49. Volfson IA, Munver R, Esposito M, et al. Robotic-assisted urologic surgery: Safety and feasibility in the pediatric population. J Endourol. 2007;21:1315–1318.
50. Klein MD, Langenburg SE, Kabeer M, et al. Pediatric robotic surgery: Lessons from a clinical experience. J Laproendosc Adv Surg Tech A. 2007;17:265–271.
51. Jeong RL. Anesthetic considerations for robotic surgery. Korean J Anesthesiol. 2014;66:3–11.
52. Najmaldin A. Pediatric telerobotic surgery: Where do we stand. Int J Med Robot. 2007;3:183–186.
53. Mariano ER, Furukawa L, Woo RK, et al. Anesthetic concerns for robotic-assisted laparoscopy in an infant. Anesth Analg. 2004;99:1665–1667.

Anaesthesia for Plastic and Reconstructive Surgery

Vibhavari Naik

GENERAL CONSIDERATIONS

Providing anaesthesia for children needing plastic and reconstructive surgeries can be often very challenging. The fact that one congenital anomaly is often associated with the presence of another, it is important to examine these children in detail during the preoperative evaluation. Many of these kids would be posted for multiple or sequential procedures and hence talking to them and their parents to allay their anxiety is as important as planning a good anaesthetic technique. Expertise in regional anaesthesia techniques always helps the anaesthesiologist to give very good pain control after some of these surgeries. Some of these procedures are day care procedures and hence additional care to avoid postoperative nausea and vomiting is vital.

CLEFT LIP AND PALATE REPAIR

Introduction

Occurrence

The incidence of clefts varies from 1 : 1,000 to 1 : 500 live births across various ethnic populations. Cleft lip can be incomplete or complete; unilateral or bilateral; associated with or without cleft palate. Bilateral cleft lip with palate is associated with a protruding premaxilla (Fig. 28.1) predicting a difficult airway. Isolated cleft palate is more often associated with systemic syndromes and these kids need to be carefully evaluated.

Embryology

Face development takes place from 4th to 12th week in the embryo. Two maxillary and two mandibular processes unite in the midline anteriorly to form facial features along with medial and lateral processes of frontonasal prominence that encroach superiorly. Cleft lip and anterior palatal defect arises due to partial or complete non-fusion of frontonasal and maxillary processes. Whereas, cleft palate arises due to partial or complete non-fusion of palatal processes from the mandibular prominence on either side.

Surgical Repair

Traditionally, Rule of 10s for planning cleft lip surgery has been described by Wilhelmmessen and Musgrave in 1969 suggesting at least 10 weeks age, 10 pounds weight and 10 gm haemoglobin. Cleft lip can be operated as early as within a few days after birth; though most plastic surgeons like to wait till the child is 2–3 months old. Similarly, there is a controversy regarding the ideal age for operating cleft palate, which

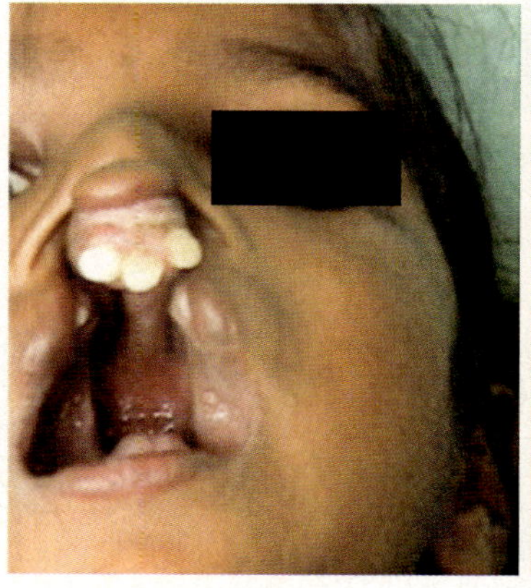
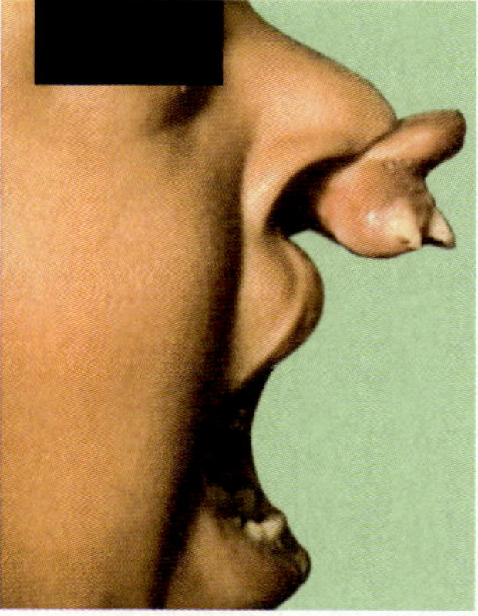

Fig. 28.1 Three years old girl with Protruding premaxilla
Source: Prof D Mukunda Reddy and the Department of Plastic Surgery, Nizam's Institute of Medical Sciences, Hyderabad

is usually operated between 9 and 12 months of age. Some of the other procedures that these children can be posted for are: Total correction (combined lip and palate repair), palatoplasty, VPI (velopharyngeal incompetence) repair, CLND correction (cleft lip nasal deformity correction), orthodontic procedures like palatal spacer insertions and alveolar bone grafting.

Preoperative Evaluation

General

A comprehensive evaluation of the child is required particularly when the child is coming for the first time. We have to look for other congenital anomalies along with any syndromic features. The list of syndromes associated with clefts is exhaustive, but the most common ones include—Pierre Robin's syndrome, Treacher Collins syndrome, Apert's syndrome, VACTERYL. To cover the details of these syndromes is out of scope of this chapter.

Most children with clefts have a running nose due to nasal regurgitation of feed. It is imperative to distinguish an infective upper respiratory tract infection from a benign nasal regurgitation. Presence of fever, cough, and raised white blood cell counts point towards infective origin and may require rescheduling the surgery. Some centers prefer to preoperatively start these kids on antibiotics in an attempt to reduce respiratory complications. There is insufficient evidence for this practice. Postoperative respiratory complications are more common in palate surgeries than in lip and again more when the procedure is bilateral as compared to unilateral.

Anaemia and malnutrition is a common occurrence particularly in developing countries, more so in these babies due to social stigma. Cleft surgery is an elective surgery and hence the child should be adequately optimized before taking up for surgery.

Airway

Assessment of airway is always difficult in children and is more of clinician's intuition than objective parameters, which can be measured as in adults. Breathing difficulty at birth, obstructive sounds in sleep, nursing in lateral and prone position, apnoea during feeding, high arched palate, retrognathia, facial asymmetry should caution us towards a difficult airway.

Systemic

Cardiac evaluation is required to rule out congenital heart disease. The incidence of association of cardiac anomalies in these children is around 15%. Frequent respiratory tract infections are often found in kids with left to right circulation defects. The priority of cardiac repair over cleft repair should be considered in haemodynamically significant cardiac defects. For anomalies that do not deserve repair, e.g. small ASDs or VSDs, perioperative management should be in consideration with the physiological changes due to these defects.

Investigations

Investigations required for cleft surgeries include complete blood count (CBC), prothrombin time (PT, INR) to rule out coagulation disorders and viral screening as per the institute's protocols. Other investigations like ECG, 2D Echo may be required if suspecting cardiac anomaly. Chest X-ray should not be ordered routinely for cleft cases as a part of preoperative assessment. A child with multiple congenital anomalies or syndromes may require appropriate investigations as per systemic involvement.

Anaesthetic Management

Introduction

Cleft surgeries are done under GA with endotracheal intubation. Cleft lip repairs in adults and older children may be considered for local anaesthesia with sedation in resource-restricted centers. The type of anaesthesia does not affect outcomes, though some literature suggests more emergence delirium and nausea, vomiting with sevoflurane as compared to propofol-based anaesthesia.

Fasting Guidelines

Fasting as per ASA NPO guidelines. Clear liquids allowed up to 2 hours (glucose water, honey water). Breast milk up to 4 hours and formula feeds or solids up to 6 hours preoperatively may be allowed.

Premedication

Premedication is an essential part of paediatric anaesthesia. Many routes like oral, nasal, per rectal have been used successfully, but the most reliable and convenient is oral route. Similarly many drugs have been tried, e.g. midazolam, trichlofos, clonidine, dexmedetomidine, ketamine, phenargan, etc. Detailed discussion about premedication is out of scope of this chapter. One can use any of these as per availability and experience. But, we need to remember to be careful in children with obstructive syndromes where it may be best avoided.

Induction

Inhalational induction is preferred to take the control of the airway. IV line can be placed after the child drifts off to sleep. Intravenous induction may also be used if IV line is secured before hand. Propofol 2–4 mg/kg or Thiopentone 5–7 mg/kg can be used for induction followed by a muscle relaxant. Atracurium 0.5 mg/kg or Vecuronium 0.1 mg/kg is more commonly preferred than the long acting NDMR (non-depolarising muscle relaxant) like pancuronium. Many anaesthesiologists would prefer Suxamethonium for intubation too. The choice between Suxamethonium and NDMR is a debatable topic. Children with obstructive syndromes need careful planning for induction and intubation. Anaesthesia is maintained with appropriate inhalational agent—halothane (lesser used due to increased arrhythmogenicity with adrenaline infiltration), isoflurane, sevoflurane or desflurane.

Intubation

Airway management can be difficult in some kids—difficult laryngoscopy is more common than difficult mask ventilation in these kids. A difficult airway cart comprising of LMAs, oral and nasal airways, different sizes of curved and straight blade laryngoscopes, paediatric bougie, video laryngoscope and fiberoptic bronchoscope is desirable. Gentle handling is advocated to prevent trauma to the cleft structures during laryngoscopy. A moist, soft-rolled gauze piece tucked in the groove often provides support while avoiding mucosal injury during laryngoscopy. Nasal intubation is not routinely preferred and is also contraindicated in patients with previous pharyngoplasty. Oral intubation with a preformed South Pole endotracheal tube like RAE (Ring Adair Elwyn) tube is preferred to keep the breathing circuit out of surgeons field. Small-rolled gauze may be required to help fixing the RAE tube to the lower lip. Red rubber L-shaped Oxford tubes earlier designed for these surgeries are now replaced by disposable South Pole tubes. A disadvantage with preformed tubes is that they could be too long or too short depending on the height of the patient. Some centers have used flexometallic LMAs to secure the airway without significantly increased complications. Throat pack with small wet gauze helps further protect the airway. It is important to monitor the airway pressure while the Dingman mouth gag is opened. A wrongly placed tongue blade or excessive opening of gag can compress and kink the endotracheal tube reflecting in raised airway pressures. Sometimes opening the gag may cause migration of tube inside leading to endobronchial intubation.

Maintenance

Anaesthesia is maintained with inhalational agents. Multimodal approach to analgesia is used. Local blocks are often added to opioids for analgesia. PONV prophylaxis is essential for these surgeries—either as dexamethasone 0.15 mg/kg at the beginning of surgery or ondansetron 0.15 mg/kg 30 mins prior to extubation. Adrenaline infiltration by the surgeon is common in these surgeries. The maximum dose of adrenaline needs to be limited to 2 μg/kg with halothane, 5 μg/kg with isoflurane as well as with sevoflurane to avoid the risk of arrhythmias.

Local Blocks

Local blocks of relevant nerves along with local infiltration of incision with adrenaline with or without local anaesthetic is an important adjunct to GA and helps not just to reduce bleeding intraoperatively, but also in reducing the postoperative pain. The maximum dose of lignocaine is 7 mg/kg when used with adrenaline and for sensorcaine is 2.5 mg/kg.

Infraorbital Nerve Block

Infraorbital nerve emerges from the infraorbital foramen and provides sensory innervation to the area of face between lower eyelid and upper lip including the lateral aspect of the nose. There are two ways of blocking it—the external approach and the mucosal approach. One must remember to block the nerves on both sides even if operating for unilateral cleft defect as the sensory supply on the medial part of cleft lip arises from contralateral nerve.

Extraoral approach: Palpate the infraorbital foramen on or below the inferior orbital margin as a depression in bone. This point usually falls on an imaginary line passing through the center of pupil vertically down to the angle of mouth. Clean the skin with betadine skin prep lotion and inject 1–3 mL around the infraorbital foramen. Aspirate to rule out accidental vascular injection as infraorbital vessels run close to the nerve.

Intraoral approach: Anaesthetise the mucosa of upper sulcus with 4% lignocaine pellet, if not under general anaesthesia. Palpate the infraorbital foramen from

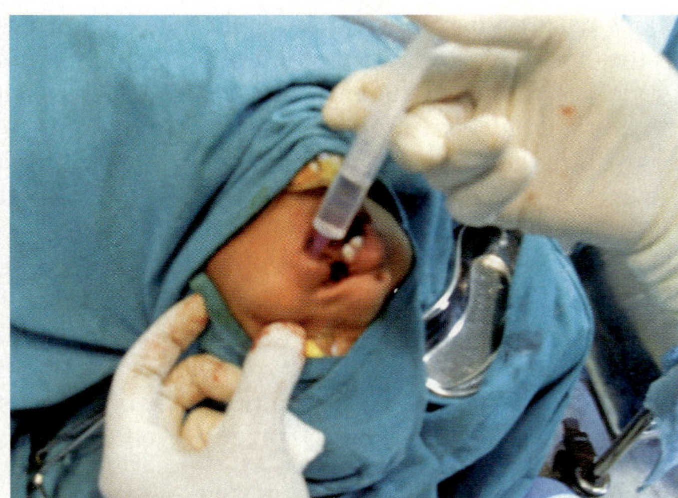

Fig. 28.2 Intraoral infraorbital block before cleft repair

Source: Prof D Mukunda Reddy and the Department of Plastic Surgery, Nizam's Institute of Medical Sciences, Hyderabad

outside, while a puncture is made intraorally in the gingival sulcus and the needle is guided below the subcutaneous tissue till the tip is close to infraorbital foramen and 1–3 mL of local anaesthetic is deposited (Fig. 28.2).

Palatal Nerve Block

Palate is innervated by 3 nerves—greater palatine nerves, lesser palatine nerves, nasopalatine nerves on both sides. Palatal nerve block involves blocking all the 3 pairs of nerves bilaterally (Fig. 28.3). Hence, palatal nerve block involving all these nerves, is complex and is replaced by infiltration of adrenaline with or without local anaesthetic along the palatal defect by many surgeons.

Extubation

At the end of surgery, it is necessary to check the haemostasis with near normal blood pressure and remember to remove the throat pack. Nose, nasopharynx and oropharynx should be cleared of blood and blood clots. Suctioning should be gentle and under vision. If anticipating airway obstruction, be prepared with nasopharyngeal airway and/or tongue stitch. Nasopharyngeal airway can be prepared using uncuffed endotracheal tube and cutting it at appropriate length. The tip of the nasopharyngeal airway should be adjusted to lie below the soft palate and above the tip of epiglottis, which can be confirmed before the mouth gag is removed. Tongue stitch placed close to posterior third of the tongue, helps to pull away tongue from the posterior pharyngeal wall if the child is obstructing after extubation (Fig. 28.4). The depth at extubation should be titrated to achieve a calm and comfortable/sedated child without respiratory obstruction. A crying child postoperatively is more likely to bleed from the palatal raw areas and create more anxiety amongst parents. In syndromic children, check the depth of neuromuscular blockade with nerve stimulator before extubation to avoid residual blockade, as even small amount of residual paralysis can compromise the airway significantly. Older children undergoing cleft rhinoplasty need to be reminded to breathe through the mouth after waking up as the nose is often packed with dressings.

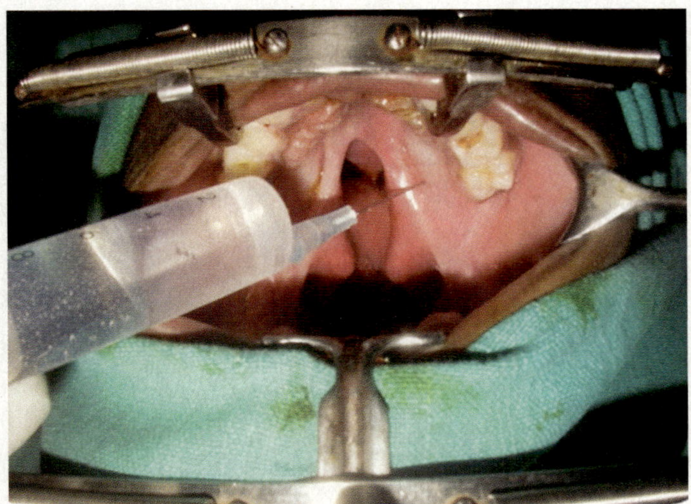

Fig. 28.3 Palatal nerve block

Source: Prof D Mukunda Reddy and the Department of Plastic Surgery, Nizam's Institute of Medical Sciences, Hyderabad

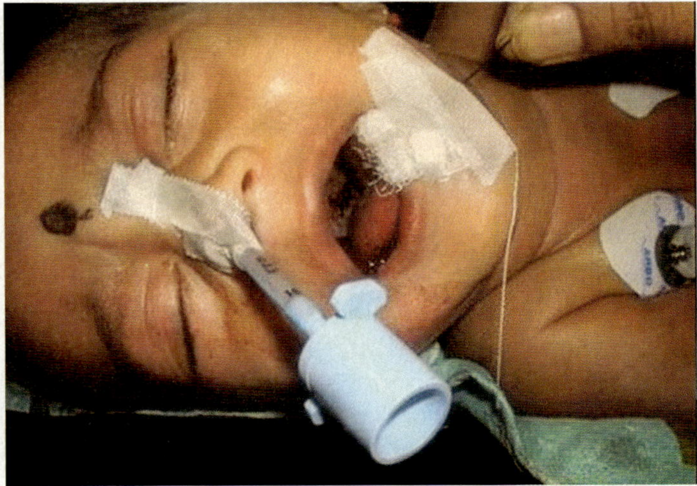

Fig. 28.4 Tongue stitch and nasopharyngeal airway in a child with retrognathia after palatoplasty.

Source: Prof D Mukunda Reddy and the Department of Plastic Surgery, Nizam's Institute of Medical Sciences, Hyderabad

Perioperative Adverse Airway Events

The incidence of perioperative adverse airway events is up to 40% in patients undergoing cleft surgeries. They are more common after palate repair than lip repair. Airway events can vary from benign snoring, mild stridor to laryngospasm, bronchospasm and respiratory obstruction, based on the etiology. Steroids might have a preventive effect though routine use is not justified.

Postoperative Care

These kids should be nursed in lateral position in the early postoperative period, so that blood stained saliva can easily trickle out. Parents should be counselled well about what to expect in the postoperative period. Avoid heavy sedative medication in the postoperative period. Start orals as early as the child is awake and is able to swallow. Analgesics like paracetamol along with NSAIDs like ibuprofen is often adequate. Syndromic children should be kept in ICU on the first postoperative day to observe the airway obstruction, which might worsen following palate closure surgeries, particularly with oedematous tissues. Such kids might benefit from steroids for first 3–5 days.

Key Points

1. Running nose is common in children posted for cleft repair. It is essential to rule out infective origin.
2. 'Rule of 10' in cleft surgery is no longer followed by many.
3. Oral intubation with preformed South Pole tube is used to keep the breathing circuit out of surgical field.
4. Remember to block infraorbital nerves on either side even for unilateral cleft lip repair.
5. Nasopharyngeal airway and/or tongue stitch help prevent postoperative respiratory obstruction in high risk cases.
6. Early postoperative care should be given in lateral position to allow blood stained saliva and secretions to trickle out of mouth till children are fully awake and able to swallow.

CRANIOFACIAL SURGERY

Introduction

Craniofacial surgery involves correction of major craniofacial anomalies most of which are congenital. Craniofacial surgery includes craniosynostosis, syndromic facial anomalies including hemifacial microsomias, clefts and post traumatic facial deformities. Anaesthesia for cleft surgeries is discussed separately. Craniosynostosis is next commonest cause for craniofacial reconstruction. Incidence of craniosynostosis is 1 : 3000–4000 children. It is caused by early fusion of cranial sutures causing compensatory abnormal growth of cranium leading to skull deformity. In the case in which the growth of skull lags behind the growth of the brain, there would be raised intracranial pressure. Craniosynostosis can be simple or complex, based on whether a single cranial suture or multiple sutures are involved. Skull shape types are based on the cranial suture involved—e.g. trigonocephaly (Fig. 28.5) involving metopic suture, brachycephaly (Fig. 28.6) involving bicoronal suture, scaphocephaly involving coronal suture or a combination of these. It may or may not be a part of syndrome. There are many syndromes associated with craniosynostosis, the most common ones being—Apert, Crouzon, Pfeiffer, etc.

Embryology

Cranium is formed of two paired—frontal and parietal bones and one unpaired occipital bone which are joined

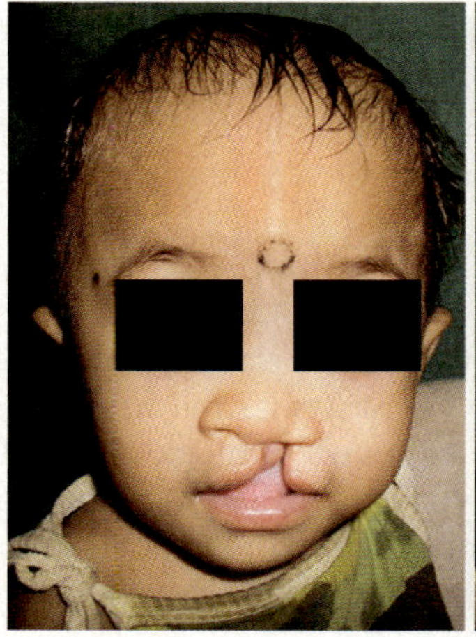
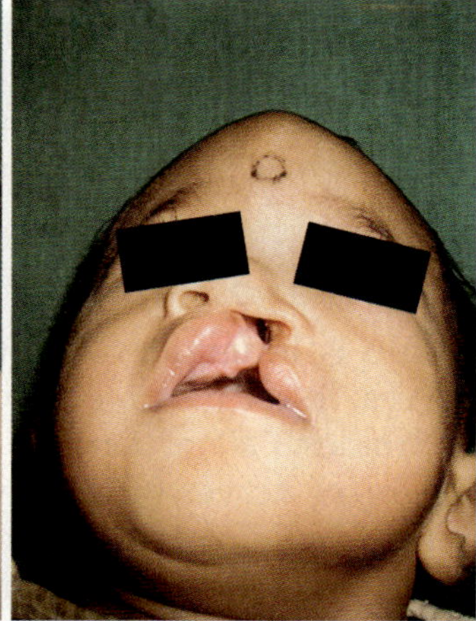

Fig. 28.5 Ten months old child with Trigonocephaly and cleft lip
Source: Prof D Mukunda Reddy and the Department of Plastic Surgery, Nizam's Institute of Medical Sciences, Hyderabad

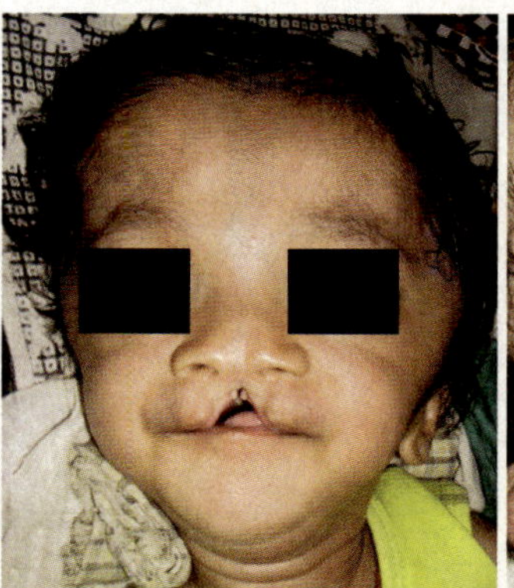
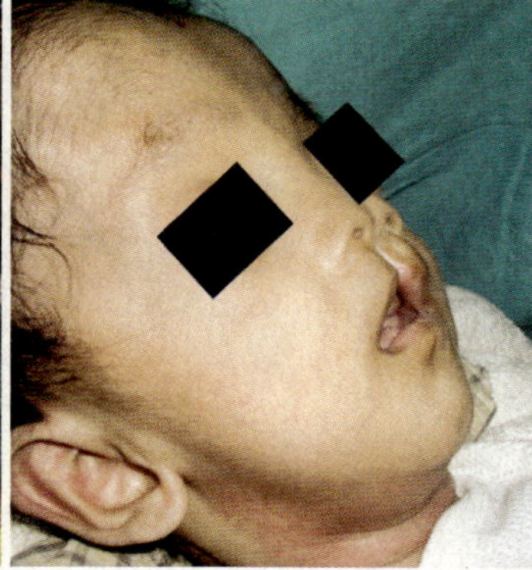

Fig. 28.6 Six months old child with Brachycephaly and cleft lip
Source: Prof D Mukunda Reddy and the Department of Plastic Surgery, Nizam's Institute of Medical Sciences, Hyderabad

to each other with sutures. The growth of skull occurs at these suture lines to accommodate for the increasing brain size. Premature closure of these sutures lead to a change in the growth vector of these skull bones effecting to abnormal growth patterns and unnatural shapes of the cranium. Anticonvulsant intake by the mother in early pregnancy has been linked to craniosynostosis in the child.

Surgical Repair

Many kids are getting operated in their infancy or early years of their life. In kids where brain development or vision, may get affected, or there is evidence of increasing intracranial pressure, it is essential to operate early. The earlier the child is operated, it is easier to mould the skull bones, but with a small chance of resurgery after the child grows up to correct residual defects. Operating late allows older kids to tolerate the procedure and the blood loss better, but with the limitation of harder bones, making remodeling difficult. Many centers would consider around 1year of age for elective primary surgery.

In craniosynostosis, surgical technique depends on the cranial suture involved. Usually an incision is made ear to ear and the scalp, is reflected off the skull. Skull repair is done by wedge removals, bony incisions, bone grafts and or frontal orbital advancements, whichever is relevant. Remodeling may be done with bio-absorbable plates and screws (Fig. 28.7). Strip craniectomy is sometimes done as a rescue where the child may not tolerate an extensive procedure. Many centers involve the paediatric neurosurgeon as a part of the surgical team.

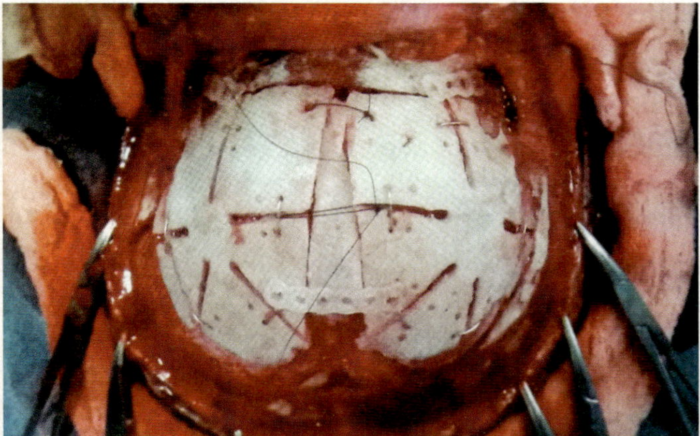

Fig. 28.7 Intraoperative cranial vault remodeling with bioabsorbable plates and screws

Source: Prof D Mukunda Reddy and the Department of Plastic Surgery, Nizam's Institute of Medical Sciences, Hyderabad

Mid-face hypoplasia and hypertelorism is usually corrected between 6 and 10 years of age. Le fort osteotomy and advancements are done as single stage procedure or with distraction osteogenesis. Orthodontic jaw surgeries are often done after 15 years of age. Mandibular advancements may be required for retrognathia. Otoplasty may be indicated for ear deformities.

Anaesthetic Management

Overview

Anaesthesia for kids posted for craniosynostosis is challenging due to the associated airway difficulties, massive blood loss, risk of air embolism, hypothermia and coagulopathy. Apert's and Crouzon's syndromes are the frequently associated syndromes. Adequate planning is required for these cases and it is usually posted as the first and the sole case on the list.

Preoperative Assessment

Careful preoperative evaluation includes airway assessment, ruling out syndromes and associated systemic comorbidities. Raised ICT is present in around half of the syndromic kids and hence essential to evaluate and treat. History of headache, seizures and developmental delay often suggest raised ICT. Mid-face hypoplasia and enlarged tongue as in Apert's, is often associated with airway difficulties and history of obstructed breathing in sleep should be asked for. Associated cleft palate may aggravate difficulties in intubation and associated syndactyly may increase difficulty for intravenous access. Rule out cervical vertebral fusion that may limit extension. Other issues like vision and hearing abnormalities should also be recorded and included in the care. Adequate blood and blood products need to be cross matched and kept ready. Blood loss in the range of 20–40 mL/kg can be expected in these surgeries, though it often depends on the surgeon's experience and techniques. Talking to the child's parents regarding the magnitude of the procedure and the related comorbidities is vital. Postoperative stay in the ICU for a day or two needs to be informed.

Investigations

Complete blood count, coagulation screen, blood grouping and cross matching, viral screen (as per hospital protocol). Surgeons order CT or CT reconstruction of the skull to quantify the defect and may ask for CT venogram to delineate sinuses.

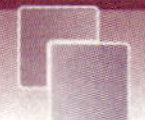

Premedication

Premedication in kids with raised ICT and difficult airway is best avoided. For others, it may be used to calm the child depending on the anaesthesiologist's choice and plan.

Induction

Induction technique can be based on comorbidities and the institute specific protocols. Both inhalational and intravenous inductions are acceptable. Airway cart should be kept ready. Kids with anticipated difficult airway may require fiberoptic intubation. Wire reinforced tubes—nasally or orally can be used to prevent kinking under the drapes. South Pole RAE tube is often used in fronto-orbital advancements. Securing the endotracheal tube with sutures or water-resistant plasters along with tube securing device is suggested. Else a gauze roll intraorally to stabilize the tube can be used. Endotracheal tube should be further supported by a tube rest. Spending some extra time in meticulous securing of endotracheal tube is essential as it is often inaccessible after the surgery starts. Surgical position can be semi-sitting with neck flexed or prone position. Adequate padding and support to prevent damage to eyes, nose should be checked. Excessive flexion may increase ICT by impeding venous return.

Monitoring

Apart from the routine monitoring, temperature monitoring and invasive blood pressure monitoring needs to be planned. Central venous access helps in volume replacement, volume status assessment and the use of inotropes if required. Additional wide bore peripheral line may also be placed.Active vigilance and high index of suspicion should be exercised to monitor venous air embolism.

Maintenance

Maintenance of anaesthesia is usually inhalational with supplemental opioids and muscle relaxants. Hypothermia should be actively prevented by the use of warm air blankets and fluid warmers. Intraoperative blood loss can often be severe, more than 40–50% of blood volume. Strategies to reduce blood loss should be planned in collaboration with the surgical team, e.g. use of skin clips on the cut ends of skin flaps or bone wax for bony edges. Tranexamic acid bolus (5 mg/kg) followed by infusion (1 mg/kg/hour) has been shown to help reduce blood loss. Desmopressin has been used with effectiveness in some centers. Intraoperative haemodynamic support with vasopressors should be started as and when required.

Postoperative Care

All patients require postoperative care in the ICU. Warming the child, transfusion of blood and blood products, correction of coagulation abnormalities, correction of metabolic derangements and stabilization of hemodynamics should be the goal of care. Some of the known complications in these children are—DIC, post-extubation croup, infections, CSF leak, hyponatremia and renal failure.

Key Points

1. Craniosynostosis is a major procedure and requires meticulous planning and coordination with the surgical team.
2. Evaluation of associated anomalies and raised intracranial pressure is essential.
3. Anticipate and plan for major blood loss.
4. Plan postoperative ICU care.

SYNDACTYLY

Introduction

Syndactyly is fusion of digits. Incidence of syndactyly is 1:2000 to 1:3000 across ethnicities with a male:female ratio of 2:1. It can be isolated malformation or as a part of syndrome. Around 1/3rd of children with syndactyly are associated with syndrome and around 2/3rd have other hand malformations. Syndactyly is associated as a part of more than 28 syndromes including—Apert syndrome, Holt-Oram, Poland, Down, etc. Constriction band syndrome (or Amniotic band syndrome) can also be associated with syndactyly. It is necessary to rule out anomalies related to heart, gastrointestinal and urogenital systems.

Embryology

Embryologically, syndactyly is non-separation of digital appendages due to failure of mesenchymal differentiation, which usually occurs between 6th and 8th week in utero.

Surgical Repair

Type and complexity of syndactyly varies from patient to patient and hence each child needs individualised approach. Syndactyly can be simple where only soft tissue fusion is present, or complex where bony fusion is also encountered (Fig. 28.8). Simple syndactyly correction is short, minor procedure requiring web space creation with local skin flaps and Z plasty.

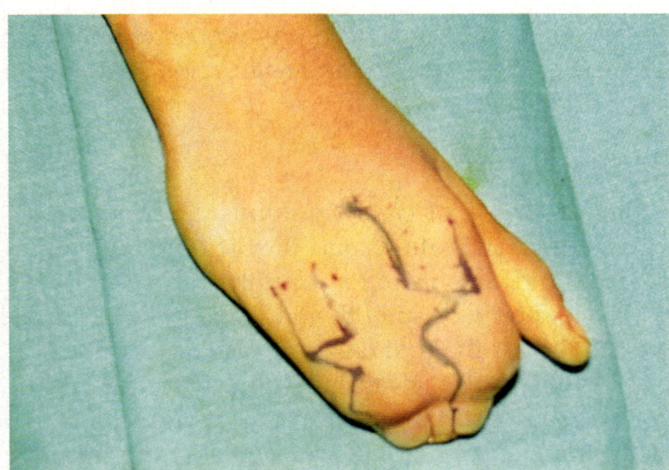

Fig. 28.8 Hand of child with complex syndactyly

Source: Prof D Mukunda Reddy and the Department of Plastic Surgery, Nizam's Institute of Medical Sciences, Hyderabad

Whereas complex syndactyly is usually seen in syndromic children—Apert (Fig. 28.9) and Poland being the commonest. It requires more complex repairs, full thickness skin grafts, or even free flaps for web space creation when tissue available is very less. Complex syndactyly repairs are often staged procedures—usually thumb is released first to improve functionality. The first dressing after syndactyly repair often requires immobility and hence done under sedation or short general anaesthesia by many plastic surgeons.

There is wide variation in the ideal age for syndactyly release, which is based on the anatomical complexity, functional requirement, differential growth rate of the involved digits and available soft tissue for coverage. While simple releases can be performed soon after birth, most surgeons prefer waiting for a couple of months. For complex syndactyly release, it is usually performed as staged procedure, the earliest being after six months of age. By and large, it is better to operate before school going age if possible, to allow development of writing skills.

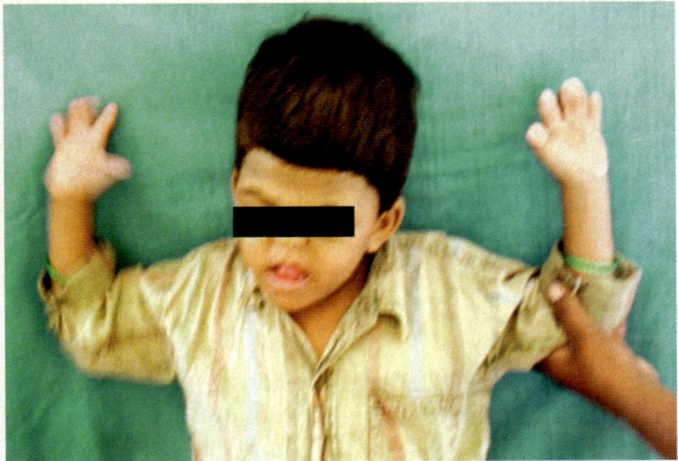

Fig. 28.9 Child with Apert's syndrome and syndactyly

Source: Prof D Mukunda Reddy and the Department of Plastic Surgery, Nizam's Institute of Medical Sciences, Hyderabad

Preoperative Evaluation

Syndactyly repairs are elective procedures and hence time should be spent in completely evaluating a syndromic child and optimisation if required. Apert syndrome is often associated with craniosynostosis and raised ICP, requiring neurology consultation and optimisation. It is also associated with mid-facial hypoplasia which may pose difficulty in intubation. Holt-Oram syndrome is associated with cardiac septal defects and require cardiology consultation to define priorities in correction. Poland syndrome is unilateral absence or hypoplasia of pectoralis muscle and the associated hand with syndactyly. It could be associated with dextrocardia, diaphragmatic hernia, rib cage defects, liver and gastrointestinal tract anomalies. All associations should be ruled out to plan safe anaesthesia.

Investigations

Routine investigations as per institute's protocol, and specific cross consultations or evaluations of specific syndromes are required. Hand and leg imaging is done as per surgeons requirement, to prepare a plan for surgical correction.

Anaesthetic Management

Most of the time, syndactyly release can be done as a day care procedure, unless associated as a part of complex syndrome, in which case, child may require overnight admission for cardiorespiratory monitoring. Also infants and preterm children should not be preferred for discharge on the same day.

Multiple limb syndactyly release can be operated in the same sitting, but involves planning of intravenous access, NIBP cuff and pulse oximeter probe placement. Some larger defects may need full thickness skin grafting to cover the defect. Full thickness skin grafts are harvested from the ipsilateral cubital fossa or the groin. Rarely a major procedure like free flap is performed when local tissue is deficient. Free flap procedure is a long duration surgery and requires large bore IV access, regulation of body temperature, meticulous calculation of fluid deficits and blood transfusion wherever necessary.

Anaesthetic planning should be meticulous, in consideration with the associated syndrome and systemic involvement. Anaesthesia plan should be a combination of GA and regional block techniques. Children with anticipated airway problems should have an airway plan ready. Children with normal airway receive supraglottic airway along with local/regional block. Axillary block is commonly performed as it covers hand well and also provides postoperative analgesia. Ultrasound and or nerve stimulator guided techniques often improve the quality and duration of the block. Many additives like opioids, ketamine, alpha-2 agonists have been used with variable results and depend of the choice and comfort of the anaesthesiologist. Spinal or caudal block can be used when correcting syndactyly in lower limb.

Tourniquets

Use of tourniquets is very common in plastic and orthopaedic surgeries. Tourniquet helps reduce blood loss but its inappropriate use may result in complications. Tourniquet related problems and complications include—hemodynamic responses to inflation and deflation, bleeding due to improper application, tourniquet pain, nerve injury or tourniquet palsy, post tourniquet syndrome progressing to compartment syndrome, pressure sores and soft tissue injury, other ischemic or thrombotic complications. These complications are preventable and can be avoided by limiting the tourniquet pressure as well as duration of occlusion. Selecting the widest cuff suitable for the patient and adding a layer of cotton roll or gauze between the tourniquet and skin, further protects the limb from mechanical injury. Skin around the edges of tourniquet should be watched for pinching during inflation and corrected if necessary. Ideal tourniquet pressure varies from patient to patient and should be calculated using the limb occlusion pressure technique. Limb occlusion pressure (LOP) is the lowest pressure required to completely occlude the arterial blood flow to the limb. This can be calculated manually or using a doppler. Torniquet pressure is usually set at LOP plus a safety margin of 50, 75 or 100 mmHg respectively, for LOP <130 mmHg, LOP between 130 and 190 mmHg and LOP >190 mmHg. Thus for most paediatric patients, tourniquet pressure can be around 50–75 mmHg more than the highest recorded systolic blood pressure.

Tourniquet deflation is required every 60–90 mins for upper limb and every 90–120 mins for lower limbs. Deflation time of 15 mins or more may be required for adequate revascularization and restoration of adequate muscle ATP levels.

Postoperative Care

Postoperative use of casts or splints can often make younger children irritable and they should be padded well to avoid any iatrogenic injury. Postoperative emergence should be smooth and younger kids may be kept sedated for the first few hours, to avoid excessive movement of the surgical limb. Older kids should be explained the importance of immobilization of limb. An effective regional block usually provides good analgesia for a couple of hours, helping smooth awakening of the child. Later, paracetamol and NSAIDs can be added to the multimodal analgesia. Opioids should be used carefully in syndromic children, anticipating airway problems.

Key Points

1. Complex syndactyly are mostly associated with syndromes.
2. Plan for multimodal analgesia including regional blocks wherever feasible.
3. During multiple limb syndactyly release, discuss with surgeons before hand, to plan the placement of IV line, NIBP and pulse oximeter probes.
4. Free flap is rarely required, but when planned, needs meticulous planning as required for major surgery.
5. Tourniquet inflation pressure should be calculated by the limb occlusion pressure (LOP) technique.
6. Take all precautions to avoid tourniquet related injuries. Monitor the tourniquet pressure and duration.

POST-BURNS RECONSTRUCTION SURGERY

Introduction

Children suffering from burns may require surgical intervention and care both during the acute and the chronic phases of burns. Discussion regarding care during the acute phase is out of scope of this chapter. Anaesthetic management in the delayed phase is discussed.

Surgical Repair

Acute phase usually requires anaesthesia for wound dressings, debridements and/or escharotomies. While reconstructive plastic surgery like contracture release, Z plasty, scar excision, skin grafting, tissue expansion, local, rotational or free flaps, etc. are required in the chronic phase.

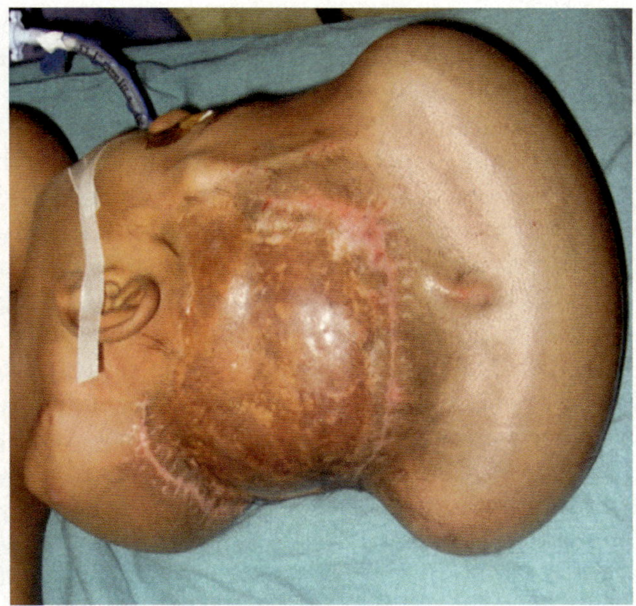

Fig. 28.10 Two tissue expanders placed to cover up skin loss on the lateral side of head.

Source: Prof D Mukunda Reddy and the Department of Plastic Surgery, Nizam's Institute of Medical Sciences, Hyderabad

Tissue expanders are increasingly used in the recent years, to generate extra normal skin required to cover the defect (Fig. 28.10). It is a two-staged procedure—first stage requires placement of the tissue expander implant, and the second stage involves removal of implant and using the newly generated skin for reconstruction. Impending rupture of the skin over tissue expander is considered a surgical emergency.

Preoperative Assessment

Children with history of burns are often anxious and need to be scheduled for multiple procedures. Hence, a good communication should be established with the child and his parents. The focus of preoperative assessment should be on the location and type of surgery. Post-burn contractures in neck can be associated with multiple airway abnormalities like microstomia, restriction of neck extension, nose block due to scar and/or tight scar over neck (Fig. 28.11). Similarly, post-burn contractures on the hand and axilla could be associated with difficulty in finding venous access, positioning and placement of monitors like blood pressure cuff (Fig. 28.12).

Investigations

Standard investigations as per institute's protocol is advised.

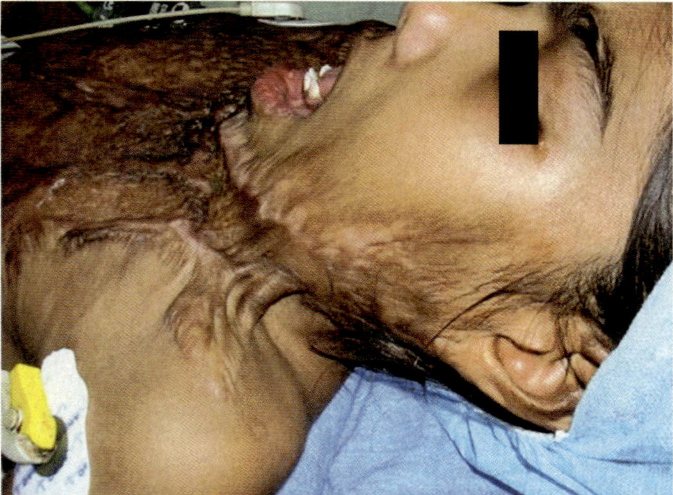

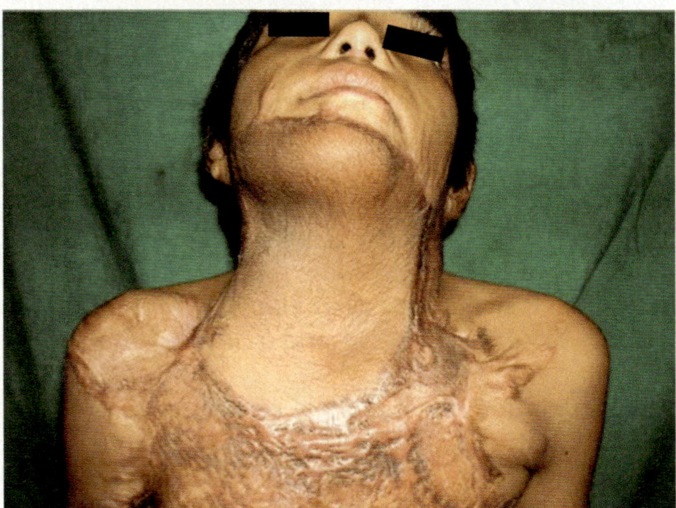

Fig. 28.11 Nine-year-old girl with severe post-burns neck contracture and after release of neck contracture

Source: Prof D Mukunda Reddy and the Department of Plastic Surgery, Nizam's Institute of Medical Sciences, Hyderabad

Anaesthetic Management

Planning the airway management is crucial in burn contractures of neck. In these cases, mask ventilation as well as laryngoscopy can be difficult. Surgical airway like tracheostomy is often impossible due to contractures over neck. Fiberoptic intubation can be an option in centers with the equipment and expertise. For other centers, use of low doses of intravenous ketamine along with local tumescent infiltration to release the neck extension limiting contracture has been reported. Once the contracture is released, the patient is intubated and further procedure continued. Some anaesthesiologists prefer to maintain spontaneous respiration and use inhalational induction till airway is secured. Laryngeal mask or any other supra glottis airway is an alternative

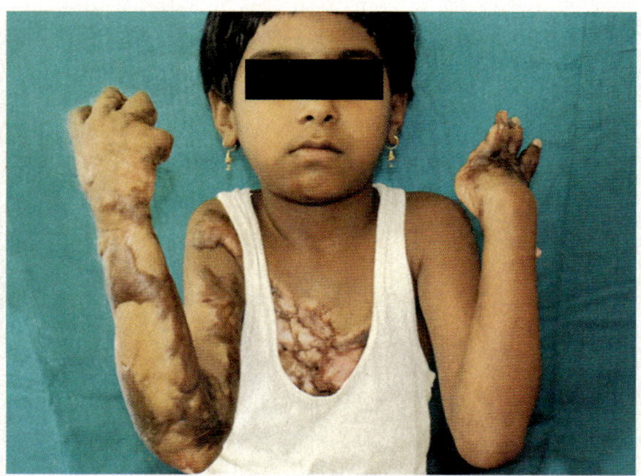

Fig. 28.12 Six years old girl with post-burn contractures of both hands

Source: Prof D Mukunda Reddy and the Department of Plastic Surgery, Nizam's Institute of Medical Sciences, Hyderabad

plan to manage airway in spontaneously breathing sedated child till the neck contracture is released to allow for intubation. Awake intubation has been documented in adults, but is often impossible in kids due to lack of cooperation. Also airway blocks may not be possible due to scarred tissues. A child with difficult airway needs a primary plan along with an alternate plan, two anaesthesiologists and a difficult airway cart ready.

Adequate documentation of airway difficulty will help in planning anaesthesia for the subsequent procedures.

Premedication

Premedication should be avoided in children with anticipated airway difficulty and can be otherwise used as per institute's policy.

Induction

Intravenous access can be difficult in children with extensive burn areas. Central lines may be planned appropriately. Induction to be planned based on airway difficulty anticipated.

Monitoring

Routine monitoring as per institutes protocol, which includes the minimum monitoring standards. Temperature control is important for large area burns debridement as children tend to become hypothermic. Many a times in extensive burns debridement, placement of ECG leads, pulse oximeter probes and blood pressure cuff may be challenging. Prevent drying of eyes in scars over lids.

Maintenance

Muscle relaxants have an altered behavior in burn patients. In the acute phase, depolarising muscle relaxant like succinyl choline should be avoided due to its hyperkalemic response. This effect translates to the development of extrajunctional receptors, particularly in denervation and extensive burn injuries. Literature suggests avoiding succinyl choline in burn patients after the initial 24 hours until 1–2 years later. On the contrary, the need for non-depolarising muscle relaxants is increased in the chronic phase. This is reflected by delayed onset of action, higher doses needed for paralysis as well as faster recovery from neuromuscular blockade. Good analgesia should be provided for debridements as it is a very painful procedure. A combination of opioids, NSAIDS, and small dose intravenous ketamine 0.25–0.5 mg/kg can be used. Skin harvest site on thigh should be covered with supplemental femoral nerve block. If the contracture release is done on hand, appropriate brachial plexus block should be used.

Local Anaesthesia

Tumescent local anaesthesia has been tried in older children with difficult airway and in resource limited centers. This solution is injected subcutaneously after giving mild sedation. This technique provides good analgesia, allowing incision and release of the scar under local anaesthesia and also helps to reduce blood loss. Tumescent solution is prepared by adding 30 mL of 2% lignocaine, 20 mL of 8.4% sodium bicarbonate and 1 mg of adrenaline to 450 mL of Ringers lactate solution. The dose of tumescent solution that can be used is up to 7 mg/kg body weight of lignocaine. This technique also provides good postoperative analgesia.

Postoperative Care

Most of the procedures require immobilization of the repaired area necessitating the use of splints or casts. These can make the child irritable and hence smooth recovery should be planned.

Key Points

1. Children with burns require anaesthesiologists care in both acute and chronic phases of treatment.
2. Difficult airway should be assessed and anaesthetic management planned accordingly.
3. Succinyl choline should be avoided in the acute phase care until a year later.
4. Burn patients develop tolerance to non-depolarizing muscle relaxants.

TEMPOROMANDIBULAR JOINT ANKYLOSIS

Introduction

Temporomandibular (TM) joint ankylosis is relatively more common in older children and young adults, in females 3 times more common than males. It can be fibrous or bony ankylosis. Etiology is multi factorial and traumatic, inflammatory or congenital seem to be common in younger children. TM joint ankylosis can be associated with mandibular and maxillary hypoplasia, reduced mouth opening, inability to protrude jaw—all these contributing to difficult intubation (Figs 28.13 and 28.14).

Surgical Repair

TM joint ankylosis is surgically released by discectomy with or without coronoidectomy followed by gap arthroplasty using temporalis muscle or costochondral reconstruction of the excised joint. Some times, the joint is replaced with prosthesis. In patients with significant mandibular hypoplasia, distraction osteogenesis may also be planned.

Preoperative Assessment

Preoperative evaluation should focus on airway abnormalities and its implications. Ruling out associated congenital anomalies should be done in younger children.

Investigations

Preoperative surgical tests as per institute's protocol are advised. Often 3D reconstruction images of TM joint is ordered by the surgeon. In patients with anticipated difficult airway and retrognathia, lateral X-ray of face and neck may help assess tongue size, retrognathia and anterior larynx.

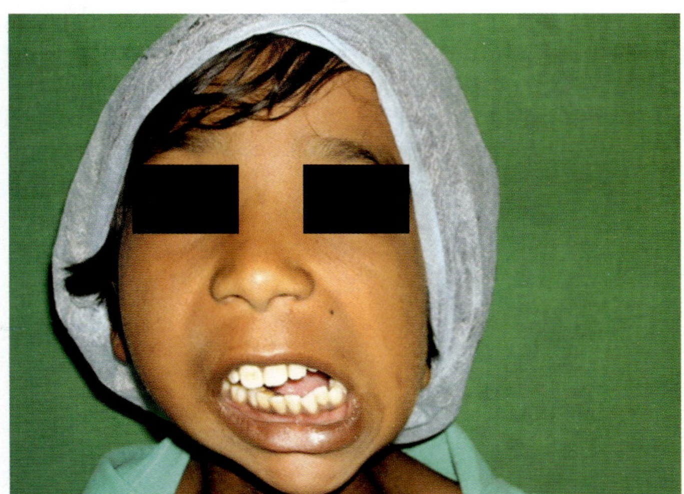

Fig. 28.13 Child with Temporomandibular joint ankylosis

Source: Prof D Mukunda Reddy and the Department of Plastic Surgery, Nizam's Institute of Medical Sciences, Hyderabad

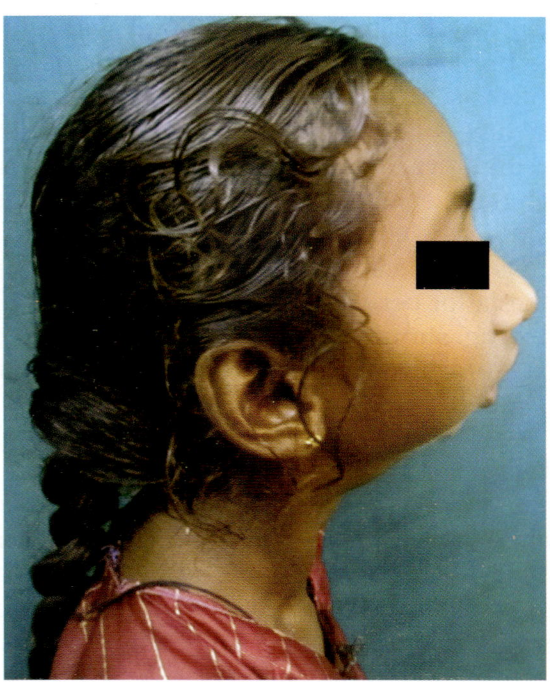

Fig. 28.14 Girl with Temporomandibular joint ankylosis with mandibular hypoplasia

Source: Prof D Mukunda Reddy and the Department of Plastic Surgery, Nizam's Institute of Medical Sciences, Hyderabad

Anaesthetic Management

The mask ventilation is not very difficult generally, unless associated with significant retrognathia. Difficult intubation due to inadequate mouth opening should be anticipated. Various techniques have been described in the literature like blind nasal intubation, nasal fiberoptic intubation, retrograde intubation and rarely elective tracheostomy. Detailed description of these techniques is out of the scope of this chapter. Some case reports have described the use of LMA and LMA guided intubation or molar laryngoscopy and intubation in patients with limited mouth opening. Another group has used blind oral intubation guided by air bubbles when mouth opening was adequate enough to slip in a tongue depressor. These techniques are operator dependent and each institute should have a protocol based on the available resources and expertise. Many institutes do not have paediatric flexible fiberoptic bronchoscope or only have a single size, which may not be appropriate for the child. Many techniques in literature have been described to intubate using adult flexible bronchoscope, either nasally or orally. After visualization of the glottis, appropriate size endotracheal tube is slipped through the opposite nostril and guided under vision or a long metal guide wire passed through the suction port of bronchoscope and used for rail roading the endotracheal tube. Mandibular nerve block has been described as an adjuvant to general anaesthesia for perioperative analgesia. Intraoperative monitoring should be performed as per routine standard of care. Antiemetic prophylaxis should be considered.

Postoperative Care

Extubation should be performed after the child is awake and able to maintain an open airway. Though the mouth opening will improve at the end of surgery, active manipulation at the repaired TM joint is discouraged to prevent disturbance at the surgical repair.

Key Points

1. Restricted mouth opening in TM joint ankylosis makes laryngoscopy difficult.
2. Blind nasal intubation is commonly practiced in these cases, unless associated with other airway anomalies.

Take Home Message

Child with craniofacial anomaly can surprise you anytime—never be unplanned and unprepared!!

FAQ with Answer

Q. What is the Rule of 10 in cleft surgery?

A. Rule of 10 for planning cleft lip surgery has been described by Wilhelmmessen and Musgrave in 1969 suggesting that the child should satisfy the following three criteria—at least 10 weeks age, 10 pounds weight and 10 gm haemoglobin.

Only One Fact to Remember

A child with one congenital anomaly is likely to have more—search for them!

REFERENCES

1. Nargozian C. The airway in patients with craniofacial abnormalities. Paediatr Anaesth review. 2004 Jan;14(1): 53–9.
2. Jackson O, Basta M, Sonnad S, et al. Perioperative risk factors for adverse airway events in patients undergoing cleft palate repair. Cleft Palate Craniofac J. May, 2013; 50(3):330–6.
3. Stricker PA, Fiadjoe JE. Anesthesia for craniofacial surgery in infancy. Anaesthesiol Clin. Mar, 2014;32(1):215–35.
4. Thomas K, Hughes C, Johnson D, et al. Anesthesia for surgery related to craniosynostosis: A review. Part 1. Paediatr Anaesth. Aug, 2012;p. 29.
5. Hughes C, Thomas K, Johnson D, et al. Anesthesia for surgery related to craniosynostosis: A review. Part 2. Paediatr Anaesth. Jan, 2013;23(1):22–7.
6. Anderson TA, Fuzaylov G. Perioperative anesthesia management of the burn patient. Surg Clin North Am. Aug, 2014;94(4):851–61.
7. Fuzaylov G, Fidkowski CW. Anesthetic considerations for major burn injury in pediatric patients. Paediatr Anaesth. Mar, 2009;19(3):202–11.
8. Barnett S, Moloney C, Bingham R. Perioperative complications in children with Apert syndrome: A review of 509 anesthetics. Paediatr Anaesth. Jan, 2011;21(1):72–7.
9. Sporniak-Tutak K, Janiszewska-Olszowska J, Kowalczyk R. Management of temporomandibular ankylosis—compromise or individualization—a literature review. Med Sci Monit. May, 2011;17(5):RA111–6.
10. Rastogi A, Gyanesh P, Nisha S, et al. Comparison of general anaesthesia versus regional anaesthesia with sedation in selected maxillofacial surgery: A randomized controlled trial. J Cranio maxillofac Surg. Apr, 2014;42(3):250–4.
11. Bates SJ, Hansen SL, Jones NF. Reconstruction of congenital differences of the hand. Plast Reconstr Surg. Jul, 2009; 124(1 Suppl):128e–143e.

Anaesthesia for Paediatric Orthopaedic and Spine Surgery

Amit Padvi, Deepa Kane and SK Srivastva

GENERAL CONSIDERATIONS IN PAEDIATRIC ORTHOPAEDIC SURGERY

1. Isolated orthopaedic conditions are commonly seen in majority of children but only a few are associated with syndromes and neuromuscular disorders.
2. Frequent exposure to general anaesthetics due to certain surgical procedures, viz. plaster application, plaster changes and removal of metal work.
3. Application of tourniquet is common and hence awareness and understanding of associated problems is very important.
4. Regional anaesthetic techniques in many surgeries ease the perioperative and postoperative period.
5. Postoperative analgesia promotes early ambulation that gives good patient compliance and better post surgical results.
6. Scoliosis surgery: Importance should be given on proper patient positioning, controlled haemodynamics, and intraoperative neurophysiological monitoring.

Significant disability and deformity due to some common congenital anomalies, bone and cartilage diseases, or connective tissue disorders can affect the lives of many children. Proper anticipation of risk factors and optimization of health before surgery can lead to an uneventful anaesthetic course. This chapter will discuss anaesthetic management of common orthopaedic procedures in healthy children with comorbidities as well as more complex procedures and spine surgeries.

Congenital Malformations

Amniotic Band Constriction (ABS)

It is a congenital disorder caused by entrapment of foetal parts (usually a limb or digits) in fibrous amniotic bands while in utero. The early detection of the ABS and an early fetoscopic release can offer a better prognosis in limb functionality, trophicity, preventing amputation and intrauterine foetal demise.

Congenital Talipes Equinovarus (Clubfoot)

1. Common congenital orthopaedic abnormality requiring surgery during infancy.
2. Incidence is 0.9% live births in India[1]
3. Clubfoot can occur in either one or both feet—bilateral cases of clubfoot account for around 50% of cases. It is almost twice as common in males as in females.
4. Although many children apparently look healthy; a few of them have associated neuromuscular disorders or arthrogryposis or cerebral palsy.
5. Conservative management requires serial plasters depending on the criteria applied for better results.

Treatment

6. Corrective surgery and repeated changes of plaster with manipulation:
   a. **This is a staged surgery which involves:** Stage 1 or primary operation is usually performed between 3 and 9 months of age. Certain amount of medial soft tissue release and tendon lengthening to bony correction with or without application of K-wire.

> **Note:** Patient is positioned supine or prone depending on the surgical approach and technical expertise and usually takes about an hour for unilateral limb surgery.

b. In about 25% of patients further surgeries (tendon transfers and osteotomies) are required.

During preoperative assessment special attention should be given for abnormalities in lumbar and sacral spine if caudal anaesthesia is considered. There may be the possibility of associated congenital neuromuscular disease.

Clinical Pearls

- Venous access may be difficult; take IV access in the upper limb. It is mandatory to take IV access in upper body during bilateral procedures.
- Endotracheal intubation with IPPV is recommended in infants and if the child is to be positioned prone, ETT should be taped properly as accidental extubation may occur in prone position.
- Tourniquets: Simultaneous bilateral tourniquet inflation may contribute to decrease preload, hyperthermia (reduced heat loss distal to the tourniquet). Bilateral tourniquet deflation at the same time can expose to metabolite surge from the ischaemic limbs. It should be released sequentially.
- Regional analgesia techniques can be used for perioperative and postoperative analgesia. Caudal block (0.3–0.5 mL/kg of 0.25% bupivacaine or equivalent with or without additives), a lumbar epidural with catheter or a sciatic nerve block may be used.
- During postoperative period maintenance fluid is essential until the infant resumes feeding.

Postoperative Pain Management

Bilateral or extensive procedures can lead to severe pain. Multimodal analgesia can be obtained by epidural infusion or intravenous opioids combined with a NSAID and paracetamol. Combination of paracetamol, NSAID and oral opioid is effective in less extensive procedures.

Developmental Dysplasia of the Hip (DDH)/ Congenital Dislocation of the Hip

Ideally, this condition is detected in the neonatal period by screening. In India there is late presentation of children with developmental dysplasia of the hip. Neonatal hip instability is in the order of 2 per thousand live births.[2] It is common in females than in males, can either be congenital or acquired.[3] The left hip is affected most commonly. There is variable incidence in different parts of the world. For the treatment Pavlik harness or gallows traction is applied before undergoing an arthrogram and closed reduction is done under general anaesthesia. The hip is manipulated into a reduced position with the femoral head aligned with the acetabulum. This procedure is often combined with a percutaneous adductor tenotomy. A lower body plaster cast (hip spica) is applied and is changed (under general anaesthesia) at roughly monthly intervals for a period of 2–3 months. Older children will often require an open reduction of the hip followed by a series of hip spicas. Later on, a pelvic and/or femoral osteotomy is required.

Clinical Pearls

- There may be other associated congenital anomalies.
- Arthrogram and closed reduction of dislocated hip is normally performed in infants detected at screening, and takes about an hour.
- An inhalational induction is commonly used. Venous access must be restricted to the upper limbs.
- Analgesia is required for an adductor tenotomy. Local anaesthetic can be infiltrated at the operative site.
- Open reduction may be required if the hip cannot be reduced manually. Caudal block with (0.5–0.75 mL/kg of 0.25% bupivacaine) is generally performed preoperatively.

Open Reduction of Dislocated Hip

- Usually performed in older children.
- Premedication is essential to allay anxiety since, the child will present for repeated anaesthetics.
- Generally venous access can be secured under inhalational induction.
- Venous access must preferably be in the upper extremity.
- Endotracheal intubation and IPPV is commonly practiced. LMA with spontaneous ventilation combined with a caudal or epidural block can be used.
- Frequent changes in patient position during the procedure are anticipated, so anaesthesiologist must be vigilant while securing the ETT or LMA and IV cannula.
- Caudal epidural injection (0.75–1 mL/kg of 0.25% bupivacaine) will block the inguinal dermatomes.
- Lumbar epidural injection (0.3–0.5 mL/kg of 0.25% bupivacaine will provide a dense block) which can be combined with a NSAID or an opioid.
- Window in the back of the hip spica allows access for an epidural catheter if it is left *in situ*.
- Day care procedure as it generally involves removing the current hip spica, washing the lower body,

application of another spica, and a check pelvic radiograph to ensure that the hip remains reduced. The whole procedure takes 40–60 min.

Femoral Osteotomy

Indications

1. Perthes disease.
2. As a part of the treatment of late DDH.
3. Cerebral palsy where it is usually combined with reduction of a dislocated hip and often a pelvic osteotomy to reshapen the acetabulum.

> **Clinical Pearls**
>
> 1. Children with Perthes disease are usually healthy.
> 2. Children with late DDH are anxious or uncooperative.
> 3. In cerebral palsy there are many issues like gastroesophagel reflux, postoperative upper airway obstruction, epilepsy, and associated medications.
> 4. An inhalational induction may be easier in young children or in children with cerebral palsy. In older children, IV induction is preferred.
> 5. Endotracheal intubation with IPPV is common and maintenance is with volatile anaesthetic agent in oxygen and air or nitrous oxide.
> 6. In Perthes disease, being operated for an isolated femoral osteotomy, a LMA with spontaneous ventilation might be considered.
> 7. Blood loss is variable and usually replaced with crystalloid or colloid. Occasionally blood transfusion is needed if pelvic osteotomy is performed simultaneously.
> 8. Options for 'single shot' regional analgesia include:
>   a. Caudal epidural block in younger children.
>   b. Lumbar epidural block.
>   c. Psoas plexus block.
>   d. A three in one block (this has a significant failure rate for this operation).
>   e. The fascia iliaca compartment block.
> 9. Lumbar epidural catheter should be inserted in children with severe cerebral palsy where the femoral osteotomy is combined with pelvic surgery as postoperative muscle spasm may be extremely painful.

Postoperative care

1. Maintenance fluids are usually required overnight.
2. Intravenous infusion of opioids or PCA should be instituted after regional block wears off and combined with paracetamol and a NSAID.
3. Intravenous or epidural analgesia is usually required for 24–72 hours depending on the extent of surgery.

Pelvic Osteotomy

Indications

1. As a part of the treatment of late DDH.
2. An irreducible dislocated hip where anatomical reduction cannot be achieved (Chiari medial displacement osteotomy).
3. A hip dislocation associated with severe cerebral palsy (Dega or Pemberton procedures).

> **Clinical Pearls**
>
> 1. Children are anxious or uncooperative due to frequent anaesthesia experiences.
> 2. In cerebral palsy challenging anaesthesia concerns include possible impairment of protective airway reflexes, convulsions, and associated drugs. Blood transfusion may be required if patient has to undergo combined surgical procedures.
> 3. Endotracheal intubation and IPPV are the standard norms.
> 4. Anticipating significant blood loss; two wide bore IV access should be secured to replace the ongoing volume loss.
> 5. In certain cerebral palsy patients, with poor venous access, an internal jugular catheter may be required to provide adequate access.
> 6. A urinary catheter is helpful in monitoring urine output for the assessment of circulating volume. Many patients may suffer from urinary retention postoperatively due to epidural anaesthesia.
> 7. Excessive blood loss can lead to anaemia. Children are also prone to hypothermia due to prolonged surgical duration.

Postoperative care

1. Active warming in the recovery area is required if patient is hypothermic.
2. Maintenance fluids are required for 24–48 hours.
3. For postoperative pain relief epidural analgesia is a choice for 48–72 hours, supplemented with paracetamol and regular NSAID if no contraindications.

Other congenital malformations like Klippel-Feil syndrome may have restricted C-spine mobility, cardiac defects and scoliosis. Acquired conditions like osteomyelitis, septic arthritis can present in emergency hours. The major concern is systemic bacterial infection leading to septic shock. A benign and malignant tumour may lead to pathologic fracture that requires excision, curettage, radical excision and amputation. Blood loss, metastasis, chemotherapy are the major concerns.

Patients requiring surgical intervention for polydactyly, syndactyly repair may have associated syndromes like Apert's syndrome, Ellis-van Creveld syndrome, Holt-Oram syndrome, Moebius sequence. They occasionally may have cardiac defects (ASD, VSD), micrognathia, cleft palate, cranial nerve palsy.

SCOLIOSIS

A complex deformity of the spine resulting in lateral curvature and rotation of the vertebrae is called scoliosis. Depending on the severity, children can have restrictive lung disease with ventilation-perfusion mismatch and hypoxemia. Cardiovascular involvement might be in the form of increased right heart pressures or mitral valve prolapse. There might be associated congenital heart diseases. Thus a thorough understanding of the pathophysiology of the disease is very important.

Normal Curvatures of Spine

1. **Primary curves of spine:** Present since birth, e.g. thoracic and sacral concave anteriorly
2. **Secondary curves:** Acquired after birth, e.g. cervical and lumbar convex anteriorly

Idiopathic (genetic) Scoliosis

1. Accounts for 70% of cases[4]
2. Early onset or infantile (< 5 years of age) or late onset adolescent types.
3. Occurs mainly in adolescents with severe curves, more predominant in girls.
4. With severe curvature, the chest cavity can become narrowed resulting in a restrictive lung defect. This is rarely significant for curves < 65°. Severe respiratory compromise probably only occurs in curves > 100°.

Congenital Scoliosis (probably not genetic)

1. Open posterior spinal defect with neurologic deficit (e.g. myelomeningocele)[5]
2. Closed defect with neurological deficit (e.g. diastematomyelia with spina bifida) and without neurological deficit (e.g. hemivertebra, unilateral unsegmented bar).
3. Extravertebral causes like congenital rib fusions.

> **Note:** Congenital malformations like Klippel-Feil syndrome may have restricted C-spine mobility, cardiac defects.[6]

Neuromuscular Scoliosis[7]

1. Associated with myopathies, e.g. Duchenne and upper and lower motor neuron diseases, e.g. cerebral palsy, spinal muscular atrophy, poliomyelitis. Respiratory function may be further compromised by inability to cough, bulbar palsy (Werdnig-Hoffmann disease) causing poor secretion handling leading to recurrent aspiration, and reduced ventilatory capacity.
2. Scoliosis tends to involve most of the thoracolumbar spine.

> **Note:** There is a higher incidence of complications including perioperative haemorrhage and respiratory failure than in idiopathic scoliosis.

Others

1. Neurofibromatosis may be associated with CNS tumours, occasional pheochromocytoma
2. Mesenchymal diseases, e.g. dwarfism, Marfan's, rheumatoid arthritis, osteogenesis imperfect leads to C-spine fusion causing poor cervical mobility, restrictive lung disease.
3. Trauma such as vertebral fracture or irradiation.
4. Arthrogryposis multiplex may be asoociated with TMJ ankylosis, C-spine immobility, GE reflux, and postoperative upper airway obstruction.

Measurement of severity: Curve magnitude is determined by the Cobb's angle on radiograph of spine.[8]

Three steps: X-ray spine: AP view

1. A perpendicular drawn from the bottom of the lowest vertebra whose bottom tilts towards the concavity of the curve.
2. Another perpendicular is drawn from the top of the upper vertebra whose tip tilts towards the concavity.
3. The angles at which these perpendiculars intersect is the Cobb's angle (Fig. 29.1).
   a. Surgery is indicated when Cobb's angle > 40°°
   b. With neuromuscular diseases even, when Cobb's angle > 20°°

Factors Determining the Severity

1. Etiology itself is detrimental of the severity.
2. Site of spinal curve involved
3. Measuring the grade of Cobb's angle
4. Number of vertebrae involved
5. Progression speed of the scoliosis.
6. Female gender

Surgical correction is aimed to prevent the progression and preserve respiratory and neurologic function, allay pain and improve cosmetic appearance.

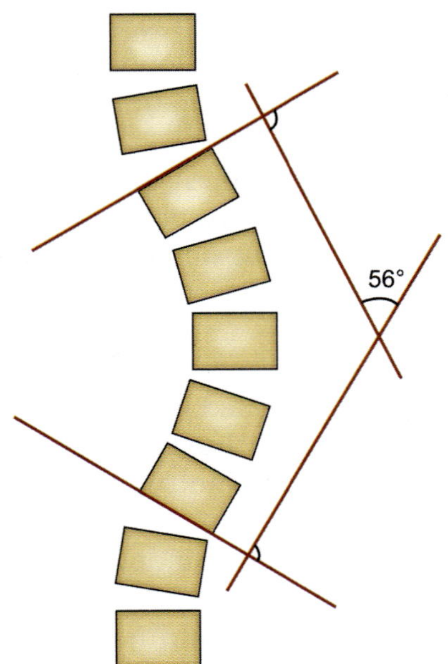

Fig. 29.1 Cobb's angle

Surgery can be done by the following approaches:

a. Posterior approach (most common)
b. Anterior approach
c. Anterior and posterior or combined approach
d. Single or follow-up operations
e. Video assisted thoracoscopic surgery

Posterior Approach

1. Most common approach.
2. Posterior spinal fusion is done with bone grafting.
3. The patient is positioned in prone position and the spinous processes and interspinous ligaments are removed and the facet joints are destroyed.
4. Fixation of spine is done with internal fixation devices such as Harrington's rods.
5. Pedicle screws or laminar hooks are used for multilevel fixation and two contoured rods are used to correct the deformity in all planes.
6. For smaller children or those with bones unable to support laminar hooks (most patients with neuromuscular curves), Luque rods and sublaminar wires are used.
7. Bone graft is applied to the entire fusion area after instrumentation and correction of the deformity.
8. The instrumentation provides stability enabling early postoperative mobilization before bony fusion is complete.
9. Risk of a thoracotomy is avoided.
10. Blood loss is reduced.
11. In the absence of anterior release, the degree of correction obtained is less than combined approach.

Combined Approach

1. A combined anterior and posterior approach is used in more severe and rigid curves or where there is a need to prevent anterior growth.
2. The two procedures may be staged over 1–2 weeks or done as one operation.
3. Staged approaches are associated with less morbidity and mortality in high-risk patients.
4. For the anterior approach a large thoraco-abdominal or flank incision is made followed by retroperitoneal dissection. Surgical access may be aided by single lung ventilation especially in older children.

Anterior Approach

1. For some congenital curves, an anterior approach alone is used.
2. Used for anterolat thoracotomy or thoracoscopy
3. Decompression with or without instrumentation
4. Rib bump is also treated at the same time.

Complications: Complications of scoliosis surgery include major neurological injury, blood loss, coagulopathy, venous air embolism and postoperative visual loss.

Clinical Pearls

1. A multidisciplinary approach is ideal.
2. Preoperative assessment should focus on cardiorespiratory function, fatiguability, ability to cough, and frequency, severity of respiratory infections.
3. Spirometry may show a moderate restrictive defect.
4. Postoperative ventilation is rarely indicated unless the defect is severe (FVC < 30% predicted) or two-stage surgery is undertaken on the same day.
5. Neurological assessment should be done to assess tingling, numbness, paraesthesia, pain and its nature, motor function, muscle spasm and bladder-bowel changes.
6. Arterial blood gases are indicated in severe cases as child may require chronic ventilatory support postoperatively and is usually seen in patients with severe early onset idiopathic scoliosis or a myopathy.
7. Associated cardiac abnormalities may complicate conditions associated with scoliosis, e.g. cardiomyopathy and dysrhythmias in Duchenne muscular dystrophy or aortic and mitral valve abnormalities in Marfan's syndrome.
8. Preoperative ECG, echocardiogram, and review by a cardiologist is essential in these children.

Contd...

Clinical Pearls *(Contd...)*

9. Assessment is practically difficult in some patients, e.g. a patient with severe cerebral palsy unable to perform spirometry.
10. Full blood count, platelet count, prothrombin time/index, partial thromboplastin time should be checked. Blood group and cross-matching should be done.
11. Airway difficulties should be anticipated when the upper thoracic or cervical spine is involved. Some disorders like Duchenne muscular dystrophy, mucopolysaccharoidosis may lead to hypertrophy of tongue.
12. We soak the throat pack with Betamethasone valerate 0.1% cream and apply it also over tongue and lips in patients who go prone for long overs to avoid oedema of pharynx, tongue and lip. This facilitates on table extubation.

Anaesthetic Management

1. Anaesthesia management involves multi-tasking team approach involving patient, parent, anaesthesiologist, orthopedician, paediatrician, nurses, physiotherapist and occupational therapist. Their combined efforts can only provide excellent results.
2. A holistic approach to patient care should be followed. Queries of the patient's parents should be addressed and the surgical outcome of earlier similar cases should be demonstrated. This helps to encourage and positively motivate the patient and parent.
3. Good nutrition, optimisation of general condition and autologous blood donation should be considered preoperatively.
4. In the absence of contraindications, sedative premedication with oral, nasal or intravenous route may be used to facilitate a smooth induction.
5. Antibiotic prophylaxis should be administered if associated cardiac anomaly is present. Drugs to prevent aspiration and antisialagogues should be given. Antisialogogues help by reducing secretions which tend to cause soaking and loosening of tape securing the endotracheal tube.
6. Corticosteroids might be given, if preexisting neurological deficit is present, as per the recommendations.
7. Following inhalational or IV induction routine monitoring is initiated.
8. Patients with difficult airway are best intubated preserving their spontaneous respiration either by inhalational anaesthetics or awake fibreoptic intubation.
9. Non-kinking armoured ETTs are usually preferred for posterior approach. Double lumen tubes or endobronchial blockers may be needed for anterior fusions in older children.
10. Maintenance of anaesthesia with volatile anaesthetic in air and oxygen combined with an infusion of propofol. The choice depends on requirements for monitoring evoked potentials and personal preference.
11. Large bore venous access is required. Central venous access is indicated in patients with difficult peripheral access, those having combined procedures, or where inotropic support may be needed.
12. An arterial line for gas monitoring and blood sampling is sited.
13. Particular attention should be given to patient positioning by adequately padding pressure points and properly securing the eyes. Patients undergoing thoracotomy for anterior release are placed in the lateral position while for posterior fusion prone position is used. The arms should be positioned in not more than 90° of abduction or forward flexion. Avoid compression of the axilla, ulnar nerve at the elbow, and lateral cutaneous nerve in the upper thigh. Free movement of the abdomen is needed to allow for adequate ventilation and to avoid elevated venous pressure, which can contribute to bleeding. Eyes must be protected and free from external pressure.
14. Temperature should be maintained by using warming mattress, forced warm air blanket, and warm IV fluids with monitoring of core temperature.
15. Haemorrhage and coagulation abnormalities:
    a. It depends on duration and approach to the surgery, the number of segments fused, the underlying pathology, and the surgical technique.
    b. Patients with neuromuscular diseases are at high risk of bleeding because they often have longer, more complex procedures with osteopenic bones.
    c. Blood conservation strategies to reduce perioperative loss include ensuring free abdominal movement, the use of antifibrinolytics and cell salvage.
    d. Deliberate hypotension and haemodilution (to reduce blood loss) may be used but are not pursued vigorously because of concerns about spinal cord perfusion.

e. Cell salvage is used in high-risk patients although in small patients allogenic transfusion is often needed before there is enough processed blood from cell salvage.
f. Aprotinin (proteolytic enzyme inhibitor acting on plasmin and kallikrein to inhibit fibrinolysis) can be used in high-risk patients.

Spinal Cord Monitoring

The risk of spinal cord injury is 0.3–0.6%. Straightening of the deformity, contusion, decreased blood flow, distraction and haematoma leads to compression of spinal cord. Motor pathways supplied by the anterior spinal artery are most vulnerable for ischaemia.

Stagnara Wake-up Test

It involves sufficient emergence from anaesthesia by lightening the depth to test lower limb motor function. Loss of function may be irreversible and if the test is positive, the surgeon is obliged to remove all the implants. Patient movement during emergence may result in accidental extubation or loss of IV access. Preoperative instructions and rehearsal is necessary.[9]

Ankle Clonus Test

This involves elicitation of clonus; based on the fact that lower motor neuron function returns first, with inhibitory (cortical) impulses returning later. Thus the clonus is initiated early when patient is under light plane of anaesthesia and unable to move or unresponsive to verbal stimuli. Absence of clonus is suggestive of injury to the spinal cord.

Note

Under anaesthesia inhibitory (cortical) functions are lost first resulting in excitatory state of lower motor neurons and the appearance of ankle clonus, but it disappears once the deep plane of anaesthesia is achieved.

Somatosensory evoked potentials (SSEPs)[10]

1. This involves stimulation of a peripheral nerve (usually the posterior tibial) and the detection of a spinal response with epidural electrodes or a cortical response with scalp electrodes.
2. It tests the functional integrity of the pathway from the periphery via the posterior columns to the cerebral cortex.
3. It only monitors the dorsal sensory pathways and not the vulnerable anterior motor pathways. An amplitude fall of more than 50% is usually regarded as significant.
4. There is an incidence of false negative recordings, i.e. spinal cord damage occurs despite the detection of SSEPs, e.g. use of electrocautery equipment and electric drills, anaemia, hypothermia.
5. Anaesthesia drugs like thiopentone, N_2O and volatile anaesthetic agents decrease the amplitude and increase the latency. Propofol and midazolam do not interfere with SSEPs. Ketamine, etomidate and pethidine increase the signal amplitude.

Motor Evoked Potentials (MEPs)

1. This involves stimulating the motor cortex with transcranial electrical impulses and signal detection from muscles as a compound muscle action potential (CMAP) or at spinal level with epidural electrodes.
2. The technique monitors the anterior cord.
3. Compound muscle action potentials can also be generated by surgical manoeuvres that result in irritation of nerve roots or cord concussion.
4. Compared to SSEPs, MEPs are markedly depressed by almost all anaesthetic agents.

Clinical Pearls

1. Volatile anaesthetics depress SSEPs and MEPs in a dose dependent manner.
2. Ketamine and etomidate may enhance recordings.
3. Nitrous oxide profoundly depresses SSEPs and MEPs unless epidural recordings are used.
4. Muscles relaxants reduce background noise and enhance SSEP recordings. Profound muscle relaxation abolishes CMAPs but not epidural MEPs.
5. Bite blocks are recommended when using CMAP monitoring to prevent biting on the endotracheal tube and tongue lacerations.
6. A typical anaesthetic for MEP monitoring is sevoflurane (0.4–0.7 MAC).

Postoperative Care

1. Most common complication post operatively is lung atelectasis.
2. A chest tube is essential after anterior surgery to drain the resulting pneumothorax and haemothorax.
3. Admission to intensive care for IPPV may be required depending on the preoperative and intraoperative respiratory dynamics.
4. Careful intravascular fluid maintenance is required with hourly urine output measurements, assessment

of central venom pressure and appropriate replacement of ongoing losses.

5. Effective analgesia facilitates aggressive physiotherapy, incentive breathing and early mobilization.
6. Multimodal pain management can be provided for postoperative analgesia with:
   a. Intravenous opioids, paracetamol and NSAID.
   b. For posterior fusions an epidural catheter placed by the surgeon under direct vision and tunneled subcutaneously from the surgical wound can be used for a continuous infusion of local anaesthetics.
   c. For anterior corrections an epidural catheter can be placed in the paravertebral space underneath the reconstituted parietal pleura.

FRACTURES IN CHILDREN

1. Fractures are common in children.
2. Most of these fractures are closed and involve the upper extremity.
3. Treatment generally involves a closed reduction of the fracture.
4. Most fractures are simple and treated without the presence of an anaesthesiologist. But to perform satisfactory treatment of musculoskeletal injuries in emergency hours, safe and effective levels of sedation and analgesia are essential to minimize pain and allay the anxiety of the child.[11]
5. Factors to consider for administering general anaesthesia include: the ease of administration, efficacy, safety, amnestic effects, analgesic effects, sedative effects, duration of effects, reliability, patient and parent acceptance, and cost.[12]
6. Regional or general anaesthesia can be considered. But it is impossible to evaluate motor function even if dilute concentration of local anaesthetics are used for regional blockade. Ultrasonography is now been increasingly used to administer regional blocks in paediatric patients.
7. When using general anaesthesia, "full stomach" precautions should be used to minimize the risk of vomiting and pulmonary aspiration of gastric contents. This necessitates the use of rapid-sequence induction and airway protection with an endotracheal tube.

FAT EMBOLISM SYNDROME (FES)

It is a collection of respiratory, hematologic, neurologic, and cutaneous symptoms and signs associated with trauma and other disparate surgical and medical conditions such as sickle cell acute chest syndrome and acute pancreatitis.[13,14]

Pathophysiology

It is caused by an inflammatory response to embolized fat globules. Fat and marrow elements are embolized into the bloodstream during acute long bone fractures or intramedullary instrumentation like:

a. Intramedullary nailing
b. Hip and knee arthroplasty

Two theories regarding the causes of fat embolism include:

1. **Mechanical theory:** Embolism is caused by droplets of bone marrow fat released into venous system.
2. **Metabolic theory:** Stress from trauma causes changes in chylomicrons which result in formation of fat emboli.

Diagnostic Criteria for Fat Embolism Syndrome

Major Criteria

1. Pulmonary insufficiency: $PaO_2 < 60$ mmHg
2. Neurologic dysfunction:
   a. Confusion
   b. Disorientation
   c. Lethargy
   d. Focal deficits
   e. Seizures
   f. Coma
3. Petechiae

Minor Criteria

1. Fever
2. Thrombocytopenia
3. Anaemia
4. Tachycardia
5. Elevated erythrocyte sedimentation rate
6. Retinal changes

Additional

1. $PaCO_2 > 55$ mmHg
2. pH < 7.3
3. RR > 35
4. Dyspnea
5. Anxiety

Note

End-tidal CO_2 monitoring does not seem to be as sensitive to fat emboli, as it is in other embolic states. It has not been as effective as echocardiography in detecting smaller emboli.[15]

Prevention

Early fracture stabilization (within 24 hours) of long bone fracture is most important factor in prevention of FES. Use of external fixation for definitive fixation of long bone fractures in medically unstable patients decreases the risk.

Treatment

Medical Management

It consists of early resuscitation and stabilization, administration of 100% oxygen, mechanical ventilation with high PEEP (positive end expiratory pressure). An adequate intravascular volume must be maintained and inotropic infusion and red blood cell transfusion are often required. Intravenous heparin, low-molecular-weight dextran, and steroids can be used. Early administration of methylprednisolone may decrease the incidence of FES.[16]

FAQs

Q. What are the anaesthetic challanges in a child with cerebral palsy for femoral osteotomy?

Q. How to measure Cobb's angle?

SUMMARY

Anaesthesia for paediatric orthopaedic surgery challenges the anaesthesiologist. Varies from a simple procedure to complex surgery, healthy patients to syndromic or with underlying neuromuscular diseases. Associated anomalies, pathophysiology, and surgical procedure creates challenging anaesthetic dilemmas to decide the anaesthetic plan. Thus, meticulous planning for anaesthetia, a thorough preoperative evaluation and seeking the help of superspeciality care from cardiology, pulmonary, neurology, and/or genetics specialists ease the anaesthesia course for small orthopaedic patients. In the future, the continued advances in our specialty will allow for complex, more extensive, and more innovative operations on small and miniatures than was possible in the past.

REFERENCES

1. Mittal R, Sekhon A, Singh G, et al. The presence of congenital orthopaedic anomalies in a rural community. International Orthopaedics. 1993;17(1):11–12.
2. Rebello G, Joseph B. Late presentation of developmental dysplasia of the hip in children from southwest India—Will screening help? Indian J Orthop. 2003;37:210–4.
3. Sherilyn WD, Joline S. Musculoskeletal Complications of Neuromuscular Disease in Children. Phys Med Rehabil Clin N Am. 2008;19:163–194.
4. Marc AA, Douglas CB, Adolescent idiopathic scoliosis: natural history and long term treatment effects. Scoliosis 2006,1:2 doi:10.1186/1748–7161–1–2.
5. Radulescu M, Ulmeanu EC. Prenatal ultrasound diagnosis of open spinal dysraphism in the cervical verterbrae. Case report. Med Ultrason. 2012 Sep; 14(3):254–6.
6. Madhoo and the fat embolism syndrome. A double-blind therapeutic study. The Journal of Bone and Joint Surgery. 1987.

30

Anaesthesia for Paediatric Ear, Nose and Throat Surgery

Nirav Kotak

GENERAL ANAESTHETIC CONSIDERATIONS IN PAEDIATRIC ENT SURGERY

1. The airway is often shared with the surgeon permitting only limited access during the procedure. The shared airway requires excellent communication between surgeon and anaesthetist.
2. The anaesthetist is often remote from the airway.
3. Many procedures are scheduled as day care cases.
4. Large numbers of paediatric ENT procedures are performed, mostly in general hospitals rather than paediatric centres.
5. Requires sound knowledge of anatomy, physiology, and pathology of the paediatric airway.
6. Requires awareness of unusual conditions or syndromes associated with airway and intubation difficulties.
7. The reinforced laryngeal mask airway offers a suitable alternative to the tracheal tube for airway management in adenotonsillectomy.
8. Obstructive sleep apnoea syndrome (OSA) is increasingly an indication for adenotonsillectomy in young children and is a risk factor for increased perioperative respiratory complications.
9. Postoperative nausea and vomiting can be a major cause of morbidity in patients undergoing adenotonsillectomy and ear surgery.
10. Children account for approximately one-third of all patients undergoing ear, nose, and throat (ENT) surgery. Procedures range from simple day-case operations, such as myringotomy, to complex airway reconstruction surgeries.

ANAESTHESIA FOR ADENOTONSILLECTOMY

Tonsillectomy is one of the most frequently performed surgical operations in children.

The tonsils and adenoids are lymphoid tissues forming part of the Waldeyer's ring encircling the pharynx. They appear in the second year of life, are largest between 4 and 7 years of age and then regress.

Indications

1. Recurrent throat infections (recurrent tonsillitis)—if they have had five or more episodes of sore throat per year because of tonsillitis, or if symptoms have persisted for at least 1 year and are disabling.

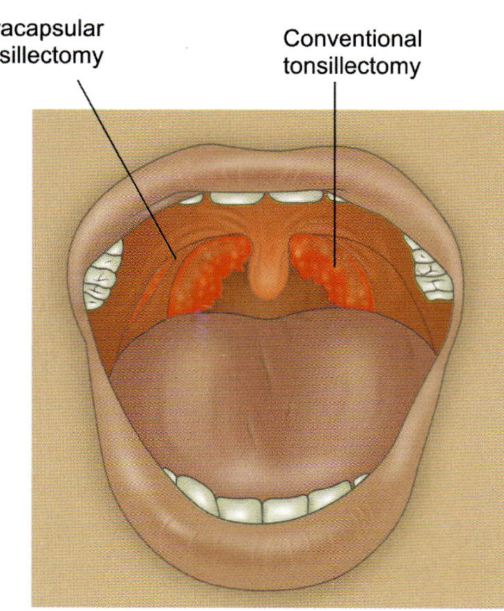

Fig. 30.1 Tonsillectomy surgeries

2. Other indications for tonsillectomy include chronic tonsillitis, peritonsillar abscess.
3. Adenoidectomy is indicated when there is evidence of enlarged adenoids causing nasal obstruction, OSA, or hearing loss.
4. Preexisting conditions that may predispose to upper airway obstruction: Congenital or acquired craniofacial abnormalities, e.g. Pierre Robin, Treacher Collins, Down's syndrome and neuromuscular disease, e.g. cerebral palsy.

Children with Obstructive Sleep Apnoea (OSA)[1]

1. Children with OSA have history of an abnormal sleep pattern with restlessness, snoring, and apnoeic pauses, extended neck position during sleep, and daytime hypersomnolence. This can chronically lead to neurocognitive impairment and behaviour problems.
2. These children may have failure to thrive and develop facial abnormalities.
3. Sleep studies show the frequency and duration of apnoea and associated decrease in arterial oxygen saturation.
4. In severe chronic OSA, chronic hypoxia can result in pulmonary hypertension, cor pulmonale, and right heart strain pattern on ECG.
5. The gold standard test for diagnosis of OSA is nocturnal polysomnography; but it is expensive. Overnight oximetry to score the frequency and depth of desaturation events may be useful.
6. In children with long-standing OSA, a full blood count will reveal polycythaemia.
7. Children with adenotonsillar hypertrophy can present with nasal obstruction, recurrent infections, secretory otitis media and deafness (secondary to Eustachian tube dysfunction), and OSA.

Anaesthetic Concerns

A. Airway management considerations

1. Sharing the airway with the surgeon
2. Remote access
3. Need to prevent soiling of the respiratory tract

B. Anaesthesia techniques:

1. The endotracheal tube

Advantages:

- The tracheal tube provides a definitive airway.
- South-facing RAE tube positioned in the midline provides good surgical access.

Disadvantages:

- Muscle paralysis or a deep plane of anaesthesia is required.
- Endobronchial intubation or accidental extubation can occur with surgical movement of the neck.
- There is a dilemma of whether to extubate the patient when fully awake and being able to protect the airway or still deeply anaesthetized to avoid a stormy emergence and bleeding.

2. The reinforced LMA

Advantages:

- Avoidance of the use of neuromuscular blocking agents.
- Smooth emergence.

> **Note**
> 1. To avoid soiling the laryngeal inlet, the LMA should be removed with the cuff still inflated.
> 2. To ensure best surgical access:
>   a. The smallest size LMA should be used
>   b. When positioned correctly, the cuff should not be visible once the Boyle-Davis gag has been opened to its fullest extent.

Disadvantages:

- An incorrectly sized LMA, or too large a blade on the mouth gag, can cause obstruction.
- It does not offer the definitive airway compared to a endotracheal tube.
- It may restrict surgical access in younger patients.

However, with both the endotracheal tube and the LMA, dislodgement or compression can occur during positioning of the mouth gag, and airway patency must be re-confirmed before surgery proceeds. Intravenous induction with propofol, tracheal intubation with succinylcholine, and spontaneous ventilation with sevoflurane is the commonest anaesthetic technique used. However, there is a concern about the danger of succinylcholine-induced hyperkalaemic cardiac arrest in children with undiagnosed muscle disease. Alternative techniques for intubation include deep inhalation anaesthesia, combinations of propofol with a short-acting opioid, or the use of a intermediate acting non-depolarizing neuromuscular blocking agent. Meticulous attention should be paid to hemostasis. Extubation is preferred when child totally awake. The patient is nursed in tonsillar position in the recovery room. The placement of a throat pack as well as its removal at the end of surgery is very important.

Analgesia

Adequate postoperative analgesia is best provided with a combination of simple analgesics and small doses of opioids. Paracetamol and NSAIDs have a morphine-sparing effect. NSAIDs, with the exception of ketorolac, do not cause increased bleeding. Hence ketorolac should be avoided.[2] Administering the simple oral analgesics before operation is safe and ensures effectiveness by the end of surgery. Alternatively, the rectal route can be used after induction of anaesthesia. However, this route may not achieve therapeutic levels by the end of surgery.

A single dose of dexamethasone 0.1–0.2 mg/kg^{-1} reduces the postoperative analgesic requirements. Local anaesthetic infiltration of the tonsillar bed has not been found to be superior to placebo.[3]

Prevention of PONV—multimodal approach is indicated:

1. Minimizing starvation,
2. Avoiding the use of nitrous oxide (N_2O). Adequate analgesia and prophylactic administration of antiemetics. A combination of ondansetron 0.1–0.2 mg/kg^{-1} and dexamethasone 0.1–0.2 mg/kg^{-1} intraoperatively is effective.
3. Intraoperative fluid administration
4. Rescue antiemesis can be given with further doses of ondansetron with or without cyclizine 0.5–1 mg/kg^{-1}.

SPECIAL CONSIDERATIONS

OSA

Moderate or severe OSA includes at least two of the following:[1]

1. Hourly apnoeas 10–20 or more in number.
2. Minimum saturation below 90%.
3. Transcutaneous carbon dioxide ($TcCO_2$) measurement elevated 10–15 mmHg or more.

Recommendations for the Postoperative Care of These Patients

1. Patients requiring postoperative endotracheal intubation will be admitted to an intensive care bed.
2. The following will be admitted to a high dependency bed:
   a. Patients with syndromes potentially affecting the airway (e.g. Down's, Treacher Collins, Pierre Robin) and moderate or severe OSA.
   b. Patients requiring an artificial airway such as a nasopharyngeal airway.
   c. Patients aged ≤12 months. The tonsillectomy might not be indicated at less than 1 year.
   d. Patients with marked obesity or malnourishment (body mass index (BMI) more than or less than two standard deviations from the mean) and moderate or severe OSA.
3. Patients without a recognized syndrome affecting the airway but with a diagnosis of moderate or severe OSA will be admitted to a high acuity monitored bed in the ward.
4. Patients with mild OSA will be admitted to a general ward bed, with the ability to monitor the patient as required.

Anaesthesia Considerations

1. Sedative premedication and long-acting opioids should be avoided in patients with severe OSA.
2. Inhalational induction is preferred, as airway obstruction commonly occurs during induction, and children with associated craniofacial anomalies may prove to be difficult to intubate. Airway obstruction is alleviated with CPAP or insertion of an oral airway, when depth of anaesthesia is sufficient. Children with OSA are at an increased risk of desaturation, laryngospasm, and developing airway obstruction during induction of anaesthesia.
3. They have increased sensitivity to the respiratory depressant effects of sedatives and opioids and a diminished ventilatory response to CO_2 compared with normal.
4. Small dose of fentanyl as analgesia is preferred as this is associated with less postoperative respiratory depression.
5. Close postoperative monitoring and the availability of an ICU bed is mandatory because children with OSA are at risk of postoperative apnoea and hypoxia. Severe cases may require supplemental oxygen or a nasopharyngeal airway or nasal CPAP or intubation.
6. Obstructive symptoms do not resolve immediately after surgery.

Day-care Tonsillectomy

The guidelines for children to undergo such procedure[4]

1. 5 years of age or older.
2. No significant history of respiratory obstruction.
3. Indication for surgery: Recurrent tonsillitis.

4. ASA class I or II
5. No intercurrent illness.
6. Family should have a 30 minutes road access to a hospital and should be able to communicate.

Exclusion criteria:

1. <2–3 years of age
2. Associated with OSA
3. Patient with craniofacial abnormalities
4. Patients with failure to thrive or significant obesity
5. Patients with hypotonia
6. Patients with chronic medical problems.
7. Living at a distance of more than one hour drive from the hospital or having no private transport.

Anaesthesia Pearls

1. Risk of early haemorrhage and the management of postoperative pain and PONV should also be considered.
2. Majority of early postoperative bleeds occur within the first 4 hrs after surgery, hence an extended observation period of 4–6 hrs before discharge is recommended.
3. A multimodal analgesic and antiemetic regime is very important, as the main reasons for overnight admission are PONV, pain, and poor oral intake.

BLEEDING TONSIL

Haemorrhage is the most serious complication after tonsillectomy and can occur within the first 24 hrs (primary haemorrhage) or up to 28 days after surgery (secondary haemorrhage).

Factors influencing haemorrhage rates:

1. Age (lower rates in children than adults)
2. Indication for surgery (highest rates with quincy and recurrent tonsillitis, lowest with obstructive symptoms)
3. Surgical technique (higher rates with use of diathermy and disposable equipment, lower with blunt dissection).

Anaesthetic Considerations in Bleeding Tonsil

1. **Hypovolaemia:** Blood loss is because of venous or capillary ooze from the tonsillar bed and is difficult to measure, as it occurs over several hours and is partly swallowed. Excessive blood loss may lead to the child spitting the blood. The child is likely to be seriously hypovolaemic and anaemic. Early indicators of hypovolaemia are tachycardia, tachypnoea, delayed capillary refill, and decreased urine output, whereas hypotension and altered sensorium are indicators of advanced volume depletion.
2. Preoperative resuscitation includes establishing a good vascular access and if required insertion of an interosseous line. Haemoglobin, coagulation profile and blood grouping, cross-matching should be done. Child should be adequately resuscitated with intravenous fluids and blood, blood products as deemed necessary. This is essential as induction of anaesthesia in a hypovolaemic child can precipitate cardiovascular collapse. Rapid sequence induction with endotracheal intubation and controlled ventilation should be done. Controlled ventilation provides good conditions for haemostasis. The main aim is to maintain haemodynamic stability with intravenous fluids, blood and blood-products.
3. **Risk of pulmonary aspiration** (swallowed blood with or without oral intake). All these patients must be considered as full stomach. Preoxygenation and rapid sequence induction with slight head-down positioning of the patient ensures rapid control of the airway and protection from pulmonary aspiration. Consideration should be given to adopting the left lateral position if there is excessive bleeding.
4. **Potential for a difficult intubation** because of excessive bleeding obscuring the view with or without oedema after earlier airway instrumentation. A selection of laryngoscope blades, smaller than expected tracheal tubes, and two suction catheters should be immediately available. Endotracheal intubation should be done by the seniormost person in the anaesthesia team.
5. **Stress to both child and parents.**
6. Once haemostasis is achieved, a large-bore stomach tube is passed and the stomach emptied. Neuromuscular block is antagonized and the trachea is extubated, with the child fully awake, in the recovery position. Postoperatively, the child should be monitored closely for any recurrence of bleeding.

Postoperative Care

1. Oral intake usually resumes in the early postoperative period.
2. A combination of paracetamol 15 mg/kg oral 4 hourly, ibuprofen 10 mg/kg oral 6 hourly, and codeine phosphate 1 mg/kg oral 4 hourly is commonly given for postoperative analgesia.

EAR SURGERY

The commonly performed ear surgeries are mastoidectomy, myringotomy, myringoplasty and tympanoplasty.

Mastoidectomy

It is performed to remove infected air cells within the mastoid bone usually caused by cholesteatoma. Cholesteatoma arises from migration of squamous epithelium into the middle ear and comprises keratinizing squamous epithelium and accumulated desquamated epithelium that accumulates in the middle ear as a result of chronic middle ear infection. It erodes middle ear structures and remains a source of ongoing infection. Otitis media is the secondmost prevalent illness of childhood. This is because of a combination of factors including eustachian tube dysfunction and an increased susceptibility to upper respiratory tract infection in early childhood. The short eustachian tube in young children predisposes to reflux of nasopharyngeal secretions into the middle ear space and thus to recurrent infections. Oedema of the eustachian tube mucosa secondary to recurrent URTI, and mechanical obstruction of the eustachian tube orifice by enlarged adenoids, leads to a negative pressure in the middle ear and a transudative effusion (secretary otitis media). Children with otitis media present with deafness and complications such as perforation, ossicular chain damage, and cholesteatoma.

Surgery is performed to improve hearing and to eradicate middle-ear disease.

Types of Surgeries

1. **Simple (or partial) mastoidectomy:** The operation is performed through the ear or through an incision behind the ear. The surgeon opens the mastoid bone and removes the infected air cells. The eardrum is incised to drain the middle ear.
2. **Radical mastoidectomy:** The eardrum and most middle ear structures are removed, but the innermost small bone (the stapes) is left behind so that a hearing aid can be used later to offset the hearing loss.
3. **Modified radical mastoidectomy:** The eardrum and the middle ear structures are saved, which allows for better hearing than is possible after a radical operation. The wound is stitched around a drain, which is removed a day or two later.

Tympanoplasty

It is performed to repair a persistent perforation in the tympanic membrane. Tympanoplasty is performed when there is extensive middle-ear damage and involves reconstruction of the tympanic membrane and the ossicular chain. The approach to the ear can be per meatal or postaural, the latter providing better surgical access. Two surgical techniques of tympanic membrane grafting are used, the underlay and the overlay. The underlay technique involves elevation of a tympanomeatal flap and placing the graft material underneath (or medial to) the eardrum. The overlay technique involves stripping the lateral epithelium of the eardrum and placing the graft material on the outer side of (or distal to) the eardrum. Various graft materials may be used, the most common being temporalis fascia, tragal perichondrium, and fat.

Anaesthetic Considerations

1. **Anxiety:** These procedures are performed in the older child or teenager and can be of prolonged duration. They will often have had many anaesthetics and may be anxious.
2. **Effect of N_2O on the middle ear:** As the relative solubility of N_2O in blood is 34 times that of nitrogen, it diffuses across into the non-compliant middle-ear cavity much more rapidly than nitrogen can leave. This can lead to pressures as high as 350 mm H_2O within 30 min of commencing N_2O, especially in the presence of eustachian tube dysfunction. Displacement of tympanoplasty grafts, worsening of deafness, rupture of the tympanic membrane, and increased PONV are associated with elevated middle-ear pressures. Also, after discontinuation of N_2O, rapid re-absorption of the gas leads to negative pressures in the middle ear and this can lead to lifting off the underlay tympanic membrane graft. As the middle ear remains open until the surgeon places the graft over the tympanic membrane, N_2O can be used up to 10–15 min before graft placement and then discontinued. However, it is best to avoid its use in middle-ear surgery completely.
3. **Bloodless operative field:** Bleeding during middle-ear surgery distorts the view through the operating microscope and can make the procedure difficult. Venous ooze can be minimized by a head-up tilt of 10–15° and ensuring unimpeded venous drainage. Epinephrine infiltration by the surgeon, relative hypotension (mean arterial pressure 10–20% < normal), and avoidance of tachycardia minimize arterial bleeding.
4. **Use of facial nerve monitoring by the surgeon:** The facial nerve runs through the middle ear in close relation to the ossicles and through the mastoid before emerging from the stylomastoid foramen. Therefore, it is vulnerable to damage during middle-ear surgery, especially as the disease process can

distort the anatomical relationship of the nerve to the ear structures and make identification difficult. Intraoperative facial nerve monitoring is useful for identification and preservation of the nerve during ear surgery. A single dose of a short-intermediate-acting relaxant can be used to aid tracheal intubation; its effects should have worn off sufficiently before the stage in the operation when facial nerve monitoring is required. However, it may be prudent to avoid the use of relaxants altogether by using other agents to facilitate intubation or by avoiding intubation. For either technique, maintenance of anaesthesia with propofol or sevoflurane offers many advantages. They allow controlled ventilation without neuromuscular blocking agents, thus permitting unimpeded facial nerve monitoring. The use of TIVA is also associated with a lower incidence of PONV.

5. **High associated incidence of PONV:** Routine prophylactic ondansetron and dexamethasone are indicated because of the emetogenic potential of middle-ear surgery. Avoiding prolonged starvation, adequate hydration, avoiding N_2O, use of TIVA, and balanced analgesia also help decrease PONV.
6. **Immobility:** Whether using a tracheal tube or an LMA, the patient requires controlled ventilation for this procedure. Much of the surgery is performed using an operating microscope; therefore, if paralysis is to be avoided, a deep plane of anaesthesia is required to guarantee immobility. Controlled ventilation also allows control of the end-tidal CO_2, which helps to minimize bleeding.

   Airway management can be achieved with a tracheal tube or a reinforced LMA. The advantages of a tracheal tube over an LMA are a secure airway and ease of controlled ventilation, though a stormy emergence contributing to graft displacement is a disadvantage. Smoother emergence can be ensured by tracheal extubation in a deep plane of anaesthesia. A reinforced LMA has the advantages of less airway stimulation and smooth emergence, but care must be taken to limit airway inflation pressures in order to prevent gastric distension during controlled ventilation.
7. **Analgesia:** Oral paracetamol and NSAIDs can be given before surgery to older children or these can be given rectally or intravenously during surgery. A greater auricular nerve block reduces the postoperative opioid requirement. Postoperative analgesia is provided by a combination of paracetamol 15 mg/kg oral 4 hourly, ibuprofen 10 mg/kg oral 6 hourly, and an oral opioid—codeine phosphate 1 mg/kg oral 4 hourly.

Myringotomy and Grommets

It is one of the commonest paediatric operations in India.

1. Myringotomy refers to an incision in the tympanic membrane and suction of the middle ear secretions. This may be combined with placement of grommet (tympanostomy/pressure-equalizing tubes). Myringotomy and insertion of grommet are used to improve middle-ear aeration and hearing in chronic otitis media.
2. Most commonly performed in infants and toddlers.
3. Usually a short procedure in the supine position with the head turned to the opposite side.
4. Usually bilateral.
5. An operating microscope is used and the magnified field of view requires an immobile patient.
6. Most procedures are performed as day cases.

Preoperative Assessment

There is a high incidence of respiratory symptoms in this patient group. The preoperative assessment should elicit features of URTI, as otitis media is associated with recurrent URTI and these children can consequently have increased airway irritability. A small percentage of this population may also display symptoms of OSA secondary to adenoidal hypertrophy. The anaesthetic technique usually involves the patient breathing spontaneously via a facemask or LMA, with the head

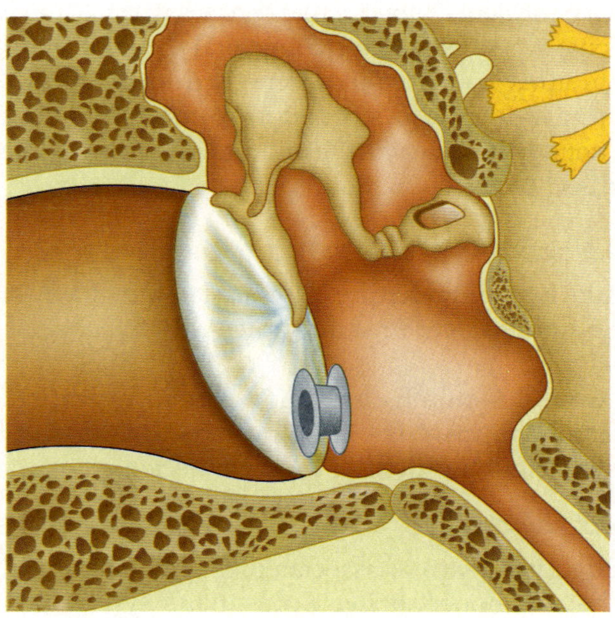

Fig. 30.2 Myringotomy with grommet

positioned to one side. In most cases the procedure is uneventful but there is an incidence of laryngospasm and hypoxia associated with it. A significant minority of patients have an underlying congenital condition notably Down's syndrome, which may present additional considerations.

Anaesthetic Technique

1. Method of induction as indicated or requested. There is a high incidence of inhalational induction because of the age of patients and difficult venous access.
2. Airway management is with a face mask or LMA.
3. Anaesthesia is maintained with volatile agent in oxygen and air or nitrous oxide.
4. Spontaneous ventilation is the norm.

Postoperative Care

Postoperative pain is unpredictable and variable ranging from no apparent distress to a howling, inconsolable child. Pain mainly results from trauma to the external auditory meatus and possibly acute pressure changes in the middle ear. Simple analgesics such as paracetamol and NSAIDS are sufficient. Some anaesthetists premedicate with analgesics—paracetamol or ibuprofen.

Myringoplasty

It involves repair of a tympanic membrane perforation in a dry ear.

Insertion of Bone-anchored hearing aid (BAHA)

Indication

It is a treatment of conductive deafness in children with chronic ear infections or congenital external auditory canal atresia who cannot benefit from conventional hearing aids. It allows sound to be conducted through the bone rather than via the middle ear, a process known as direct bone conduction.

The Procedure is Done in Two Steps

Firstly, a titanium fixture is implanted into the mastoid bone and this over time integrates with the bone of the skull.

Around 6 months later, at a second operation, an external abutment is placed over the fixture and this allows a sound processor to be connected.

Specific Problems

1. High incidence of associated congenital anomalies, the commonest being Goldenhar's syndrome and Treacher Collins syndrome.
2. High incidence of congenital heart disease and craniofacial anomalies.
3. The main anaesthetic concern is difficult intubation. In most cases, after inhalation induction, the airway can be safely and easily maintained using a reinforced LMA. However, equipment for fibreoptic intubation should be available. Analgesia is provided with a combination of paracetamol, NSAID, and a small dose of opioid. Routine antiemetics are indicated, as PONV is common.

COCHLEAR IMPLANTS

Introduction

It is a therapeutic option for patients with irreversible hearing loss and deaf mutism. Cochlear implants are extremely expensive computerised electric prosthesis that partially replace the functions of the cochlea. The operative technique is complicated and necessitates preservation of functional integrity of the facial and cochlear nerve.

Contraindications

Uncontrolled otitis media, autism, severe intellectual disability, and central nervous system disorders which are likely to affect the auditory pathways and compromise speech perception.

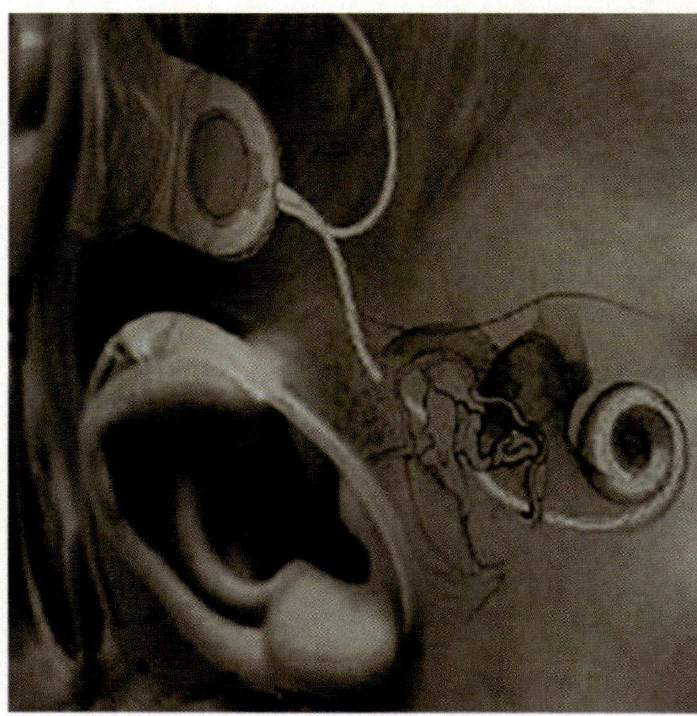

Fig. 30.3 Cochlear implant

Indications

Approximately 50% of the cases have acquired hearing loss mostly because of perinatal infections with TORCH group of organisms. Various syndromes as Usher, Pendred, Waardenburg, Treacher Collins, Klippel Feil, Jervel and Lange-Neilsen, Refsum, Albers-Schonberg, Cockayneand trisomy 13 and 18 syndromes may be involved.

Common Postoperative Complications

These problems are related to flap, delayed facial nerve palsy, dizziness, PONV.

Intraoperative Complications

Severe bleeding, perilymph leakage because of inner ear abnormalities. Perilymph leak can be managed by letting the fluid drain off before inserting the electrode and then sealing around entry point with muscle or connective tissue. In addition injection mannitol and re-positioning of head are also useful.

Type of Anaesthesia

Cochlear implants have been successfully done under local anaesthesia, however, general anaesthesia is preferred due to evolving experience, time consuming surgery and local anaesthesia requires co-operation from the patients, which is difficult in this category of patients, particularly the children.

Preoperative Evaluation

It should include assessment of the development milestones and evaluating neurological deficits. The general appearance of the skull suggests the presence of macrocephaly, microencephaly or craniosynostosis. The head and neck region examination may reveal features of cerebral palsy, congenital syphilis, microphthalmia, cataract and cranial nerve palsies. The whorl patterns of hair may reveal the presence of cerebral malformation, whereas abnormal palmer creases should alert the anaesthesiologist of Down's syndrome. Complete haemogram and blood grouping are done. However, in presence of syndromal illnesses, specific investigations such as ECG or renal function tests should be done. In case of congenital deafness, there may be presence of a variety of syndromes, each having specific anaesthetic significance. Abnormalities in facial appearance with a difficult airway may indicate Treacher Collins syndrome. Eye disorders could be a part of Usher syndrome. Klippel-Fiel anomaly is associated with fusion of the cervical vertebrae making the intubation difficult. Alport syndrome is associated with renal failure and endocrinal abnormalities. Goiter and metabolic disorders indicate Pendred syndrome. Jervell and Lange-Nielsen syndrome is usually associated with a history of syncopal attacks, prolonged QT interval on the ECG which may lead to dangerous ventricular arrhythmias. These patients should be treated with beta blockers prior to surgery.

General Anaesthesia

Parental presence is desirable during induction of anaesthesia to avoid separation anxiety. Oral midazolam can be used as a premedicant or induction with the child in mother's lap with 3 mg/kg of thiopentone can be done except in cases of anticipated difficult intubation. In order to reduce intraoperative bleeding, mild hypotension and mild hypocapnia can be maintained. Mild hypotension can be maintained with the help of inhalational agents or injection clonidine. Air warming blanket device should be used for prevention of hypothermia. Inj. ondansetron 0.1 mg/kg should be given prior to skin closure to decrease incidence of PONV. During the surgery, the facial nerve is identified with the help of a nerve stimulator. Therefore, muscle relaxants should be avoided during these period and anaesthesia should be maintained with local or IV anaesthetics. Cautery should not be used at all once the cochlear implant is in place. At the end of surgery, BERA testing of the electrode array is done or electrically evoked stapedius reflexes are evaluated to confirm proper functioning of the implant. During this procedure, low concentrations of inhalational anaesthetics should be continued and no fluctuations in $ETCO_2$ should occur.

Precautions for Patients with Cochlear Impant

1. Monopolar electrosurgical instruments should not be used on the head and neck as this can permanently damage the implant. Bipolar electro-surgical instruments can be used but direct use over the implant is to be avoided.
2. Electro convulsive therapy should not be used.
3. Radiotherapy should not be given directly over the implant as it will cause serious damage to the implant.
4. MRI is contraindicated in patients with cochlear implants. However, with the advent of newer implants the magnet can be removed by a simple surgery and then MRI can be undertaken and the magnet then can be replaced after the procedure is complete.[5]

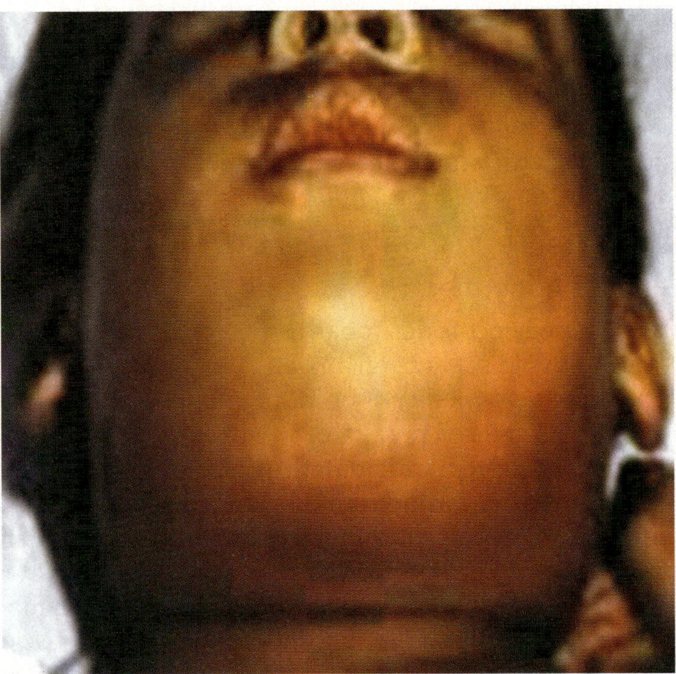

Fig. 30.4 Ludwig angina

LUDWIG'S ANGINA

Ludwig angina is defined as a potentially lethal, rapidly spreading cellulitis, involving the sublingual and submandibular spaces.

Etiology: Recent dental extraction, dental caries, compromised host, co-morbidities (diabetes), Streptococcus, Staphylococcus, mixed aerobic/anaerobic infection, *B. fragilis*.

Clinical features: Brawny bilateral board like oedema, suprahyoid induration, tender swelling in the floor of the mouth, and elevation and posterior displacement of the tongue, trismus.

Complications: Upper airway obstruction, reinfection, asphyxiation, descending mediastinitis, spread to other spaces, death.

Treatment: Incision and drainage of associated spaces, teeth extraction, antibiotics, steroids.

1. Antibiotics: Extended spectrum penicillins, Clindamycin + Ciprofloxacin, Flagyl (*B. fragilis*)
2. Steroids: To reduce oedema especially when airway compromise is suspected.
3. Prompt airway management is critical, but the presence of swelling on the neck, glottic oedema, elevation of the tongue, trismus, or pharyngeal oedema can create problems.
4. Blind nasal intubation with topical anaesthesia or GA is not advisible as unexpected bleeding, spread of oedema may occur. Pus may come out due to trauma. These all may lead to further airway compromise.
5. Fibreoptic guided nasal intubation (awake) by an experienced person.
6. Elective tracheostomy under local anaesthesia However, cellulitis of the neck with involvement of the tracheostomy site makes it a more difficult procedure. Also, surgical dissection of the fascial planes in the neck may open and contaminate the pathways, leading to life-threatening mediastinal invasion.
7. Cricothyroidotomy with jet insufflation should always be ready.
8. Superficial cervical plexus block with inferior alveolar nerve block, i.e. intraoral mandibular nerve block with conscious sedation maintained by fractionated doses of midazolam has a high success rate, low complication rate and high patient acceptance rate. Complications include infection, hematoma, phrenic nerve blockade, local anaesthetic toxicity, nerve injury and spinal anaesthesia.
9. Incision and drainage under local anaesthesia in an awake patient.[6]

Oesophagoscopy

1. Rigid oesophagoscopy is performed for the removal of an ingested foreign body.
2. History of ingestion, dysphagia, and odynophagia are the usual presenting symptoms, whereas a previous stricture is a predisposing factor for obstruction.
3. The commonest site of impaction of the foreign body is at the level of the cricopharyngeus muscle.
4. Oesophagoscopy should be performed in all cases of suspected impacted foreign body to prevent complications of perforation, mediastinitis, and fistula formation.

Anaesthetic Consideration

Factors to be considered

1. **Management of the shared airway:** The tracheal tube should be secured on the left side to allow easier access for the endoscopy.
2. **Risk of pulmonary aspiration:** A rapid sequence induction protects against pulmonary aspiration and ensures rapid control of the airway.
3. **Risk of oesophageal perforation during the procedure:** Adequate depth of anaesthesia and muscle

relaxation during the procedure is essential to reduce the risk of oesophageal perforation. Analgesia is provided by a combination of intravenously or rectally administered simple analgesics and a small dose of opioid. The patient is extubated when fully awake. If oesophageal perforation is suspected, oral intake should be withheld, IV antibiotics commenced, and the patient closely observed for features of mediastinitis, such as severe chest pain, pyrexia, and subcutaneous emphysema.

Bronchoscopy

Indications

Diagnostic	Therapeutic
1. Recurrent pneumonia	1. Foreign body removal
2. Tracheo-oesophageal fistula	2. Mucus plugs, e.g. cystic fibrosis
3. Airway obstruction	3. Lobar collapse
4. Laryngomalacia	4. Refractory atelectasis
5. Haemoptysis	5. Balloon dilatation
6. To obtain biopsy or brushings	6. Stent insertion
7. Failure to wean from ventilator	7. Laser treatment

Most patients have some degree of respiratory compromise. Signs and symptoms include stridor, wheeze, hoarseness, recurrent infection, cyanosis, persistent cough, dyspnoea, and tachypnoea.

Types of Bronchoscopes

Rigid bronchoscope

Rigid ventilating bronchoscope (Fig. 30.5) is the most common bronchoscope used in paediatrics. It consists of a metal tube with a removable optical telescope. Holes in the wall allow ventilation of the contra-lateral lung when the distal end of the bronchoscope is positioned in a bronchus. The side arm has a 15 mm attachment for an anaesthetic T-piece circuit. Ventilation occurs between the lumen of the bronchoscope and the outer surface of the telescope. The telescope occupies most of the internal diameter of smaller bronchoscopes and impedes ventilation in infants. With the telescope in place, a closed system exists and allows controlled ventilation but the cross sectional area of lumen through which the infant can breathe is reduced. Using too large a bronchoscope leads to compression of tracheal mucosa and postoperative oedema with the risk of stridor.

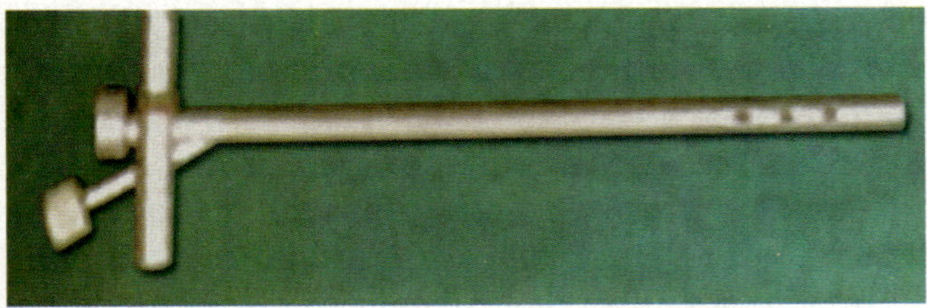

Fig. 30.5 Ventilating rigid bronchoscope

Venturi bronchoscopes

It is commonly used in adults but in paediatrics should be limited to patients weighing >40 kg because of the risk of barotrauma. Ventilation occurs via jet insufflation with oxygen and entrained air using a Sanders injector. Anaesthesia is maintained with IV agents. CO_2 retention is a greater problem with this method.

Fibreoptic bronchoscopes

Fibreoptic bronchoscopes have a greater field of vision than rigid scopes and their smaller diameter allows access to the distal airways. The smallest diameter of fibreoptic bronchoscope has an ED 1.8 mm distally and 2.2 mm proximally.

Preoperative Assessment

Previous anaesthetic charts provide useful information regarding laryngoscopy, airway obstruction, size of ETT and any difficulties encountered. Careful history and examination focusing on airway and respiratory system, e.g. how do symptoms change with position, crying, and feeding is required. Specific investigations may be indicated, e.g. CXR for suspected foreign body aspiration, CT for lower airway obstruction.

Anaesthesia Technique

Rigid Bronchoscopy

Premedication

1. Avoid sedative premedication if there is evidence of airway obstruction or respiratory compromise.
2. An anticholinergic (atropine 10–20 mcg/kg or glycopyrronium bromide 5–10 mcg/kg) is given intravenously at induction for an antisialogogue effect and to prevent bradycardia from airway manipulation.

Induction

1. Inhalational induction with sevoflurane or halothane in 100% oxygen.
2. Sevoflurane provides a more rapid induction but causes more depression of ventilation than halothane.

3. Application of CPAP will help overcome upper airway obstruction.
4. When the depth of anaesthesia is adequate topical lidocaine (up to 4 mg/kg) should be sprayed on the epiglottis, larynx, and between the vocal cords which will help avoid coughing, breath holding, and laryngospasm during the examination.
5. The patient is positioned supine with a support beneath the scapulae to extend the neck and push the trachea anteriorly.
6. Spontaneous ventilation is maintained in children with possible airway obstruction and in diagnostic procedures where functional assessment of the upper airway is required
7. Anaesthesia is maintained with volatile anaesthetic agent with 100% oxygen given through a T-piece circuit attached to the side port of the bronchoscope. Alternatively, total IV anaesthesia (TIVA) can be used for maintenance. Propofol suppresses airway reflexes, provides rapid emergence, and decreases pollution of the operating theatre atmosphere with anaesthetic agents.
8. When the telescope is introduced, the cross sectional area of the bronchoscope is reduced and the work of breathing may be significantly increased. This is a significant problem in infants where narrow bronchoscopes are used. Adequate gas exchange may require intermittent removal of the telescope from the bronchoscope to allow a period of uninterrupted ventilation.
9. If assisted ventilation is used, a long time constant may be needed to avoid air trapping.
10. Dexamethasone (250 mcg/kg IV) may be given to reduce postoperative airway oedema.

Fibreoptic Bronchoscopy

1. Generally as for rigid bronchoscopy.
2. The method of airway management depends on the indications for the examination. If the laryngomalacia is suspected, then a facemask (fitted with an angle piece modified for passage of a bronchoscope) with spontaneous ventilation is required to allow examination of the larynx during normal breathing. Under these circumstances, an LMA will distort the larynx and may impede movement of the vocal cords.
3. When a facemask or LMA is used, spontaneous ventilation is maintained and CPAP used to aid management of airway obstruction. An appropriately sized LMA allows the passage of a larger fibrescope than with a tracheal tube.
4. If a spontaneous ventilation technique is used, then LA is applied to the larynx via the injection port of the fiberscope to provide topical anaesthesia before the fibrescope passes through the larynx.
5. Examination of the bronchial tree and/or broncho-alveolar lavage allows the use of an ETT if indicated.

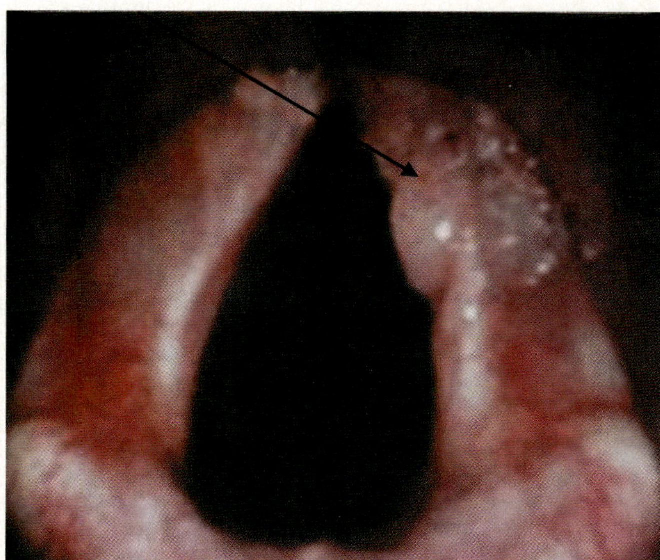

Fig. 30.6 Laryngeal papilloma

Postoperative care

Oral paracetamol and NSAID will provide adequate analgesia. Patients should remain nil by mouth for 2 hours after topical anaesthesia to the larynx. Further doses of steroid and nebulized adrenaline may be necessary if the patient has postoperative stridor.

MICROLARYNGEAL SURGERY

Indications

1. Laryngeal papillomatosis
2. Congenital or acquired anatomical laryngeal lesions such as laryngomalacia and laryngeal web.

Anaesthetic Technique

1. Performed using a suspension laryngoscope and operating microscope.
2. Often involves laser surgery to the airway and the relevant precautions that go with this.
3. Camera and video display allow the anaesthetist to observe the airway and surgical field.
4. Patients often present for repeated procedures and may have significant airway obstruction and may

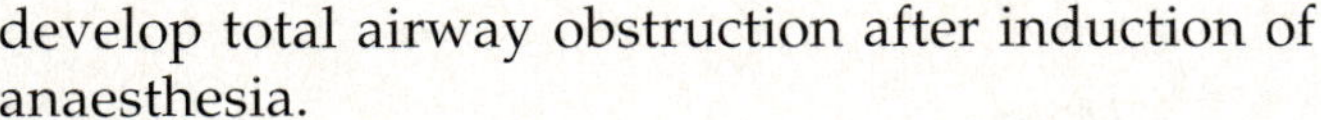

develop total airway obstruction after induction of anaesthesia.

5. If the child has a tracheostomy, then a standard anaesthetic technique is used with induction. The tracheostomy is connected to the anaesthetic circuit and spontaneous ventilation or IPPV used.
6. If there is no tracheostomy, then sedative premedication is avoided. An inhalational induction with sevoflurane or halothane in 100% oxygen is performed. The larynx is sprayed with lidocaine (up to 4 mg/kg) to ensure dense topical analgesia.
7. Options for maintenance include:
   a. Endotracheal intubation and IPPV. A narrow ETT is used to allow visualization of the larynx. However, the view of the larynx is impaired.
   b. Spontaneous ventilation with volatile anaesthetic in oxygen through an ETT (placed through the nose or via dedicated channel in the suspension laryngoscope) with the distal end in the oropharynx above the laryngeal inlet so as not to obscure the surgical field.
   c. Apnoeic insufflation where the child is paralyzed and volatile anaesthetic and oxygen insufflated through an ETT placed as above. Arterial CO_2 rises during apnoea and during prolonged procedures surgery is interrupted to allow a period of IPPV. There is also pollution of the operating theatre atmosphere with volatile agent.
   d. A propofol infusion can be used to supplement anaesthesia and reduce pollution.
   e. Jet ventilation combined with TIVA in a paralyzed patient. This has a risk of barotrauma.

Postoperative Care

Oral paracetamol and NSAID will provide adequate analgesia. Patients should remain nil by mouth for 2 hours after topical anaesthesia to the larynx. Further dose of steroid and nebulized adrenaline may be necessary if the patient has postoperative stridor. Patients require arterial oxygen saturation monitoring for at least 2 hours to detect hypoxia secondary to hypoventilation.

SUMMARY

ENT surgeries are one of the commonest surgeries performed and comprise approximately one-third of all paediatric surgeries. Procedures vary from simple ear operations to complex airway reconstruction surgeries. Sharing of airway with surgeon limits access to the patient's airway. Many procedures such as adenotonsillectomy and ear surgery are scheduled as day care procedures. Postoperative nausea and vomiting are the major concerns in these surgeries. A thorough understanding of the anatomy and physiology of paediatric airway along with associated airway manifestations of syndromes plays a key role in the successful anaesthesia management of these surgeries.

FAQs with Answers

Q. The gold standard test for diagnosis of OSA?
A. Nocturnal polysomnography.

Q. The commonest site of impaction of the foreign body?
A. At the level of the cricopharyngeus muscle.

Facts to Remember

1. Prevention of PONV—multimodal approach is indicated.
   a. Minimize starvation.
   b. Avoiding the use of nitrous oxide (N_2O).
   c. Adequate analgesia and prophylactic administration of antiemetics and dexamethasone 0.1–0.2 mg/kg^{-1} intraoperatively is effective.
   d. Intraoperative hydration.
2. Haemorrhage is the most serious complication after tonsillectomy and can occur within the first 24 hrs (primary haemorrhage) or up to 28 days after surgery (secondary haemorrhage).

REFERENCES

1. Schwengel DA, Sterni LM, Tunkel DE, et al. Perioperative management of children with obstructive sleep apnea. Anesth Analg 2009;109:60–75.
2. Splinter WM, Rhine EJ, Roberts DW, et al. Preoperative ketorolac increases bleeding after tonsillectomy in children. Can J Anaesth. Jun, 1996;43(6):560–3.
3. Radha R, Tanya H. Anaesthesia for paediatric ear, nose, and throat surgery. Continuing Education in Anaesth Crit Care Pain 2007;7:143–147.
4. Nandana S, Darshinder S. The guidelines for children fit to undergo such procedures. Paediatric anaesthesia for day surgery anaesthesia tutorial. Nov, 2010;1–10.
5. Ashish C, Tarneja VK, Singh VK, et al. Cochlear implant: Anaesthesia challenges. Medical Journal Armed Forces India. 2004 Oct;60(4):351–356.
6. Marple BF. Ludwig angina: A review of current airway management. Arch Otolaryngol Head Neck Surg. 1999;125:596–599.

Anaesthesia for Paediatric Ophthalmic Surgery

Namita Padvi, Amit Padvi and Nitin Padvi

GENERAL CONSIDERATION

Ophthalmic surgery frequently deals with the extremes of ages from paediatric to geriatric patients. A practical approach to anaesthesia for paediatric patient with ophthalmic problem can present a real challenge to the anaesthetist. An understanding of some basic anaesthetic principles for paediatric ophthalmic surgery is very important for clinical practice.

Fears of operation, injections, physicians and peculiar operation theatre environment where the children are separated from their parents prior to anaesthesia invariably produce traumatic experiences in the tender mind of the young children.[1] Therefore, children do not tolerate the use of sedation and local anaesthesia technique; they almost always require general anaesthesia. Most patients are healthy, only a few patients do have certain syndromes, which affects their anaesthetic management. Many times these surgeries are performed on day care basis.

Indications for Ophthalmic Surgery

Anaesthesia management changes with the urgency of surgery. The most common cause for emergency ophthalmic surgery is trauma and the incidence is higher in children and young adults. Ocular trauma has to be dealt with immediately, usually within 1st hour of presentation. Ophthalmological surgeries can be classified as extraocular and intraocular. Extraocular conditions include naso-lacrimal duct obstruction and strabismus. Intraocular conditions include glaucoma, cataract, retinoblastoma and retinopathy of prematurity.

Syndromes with Ophthalmic Manifestations

1. Down's syndrome (Trisomy 21)
2. Alport syndrome (progressive hereditary nephritis)
3. Marfan syndrome
4. Ehlers-Danlos syndrome/Homocystinuria
5. Mucopolysaccharidoses
6. Craniofacial syndromes:
   a. Crouzon's
   b. Apert
   c. Pfeiffer
7. Phakomatoses
8. Fetal alcohol syndrome
9. Galactosemia,
10. Hypercalcaemia
11. Sturge-Weber syndrome
12. Prematurity
13. Fabry disease
14. Tay-Sachs disease
15. Osteogenesis imperfecta
16. Infections like:
    a. Herpes simplex
    b. Cytomegalovirus (CMV)
    c. Rubella
17. Others:
    a. Congenital myotonic dystrophy
    b. Sickle cell disease

Physiological Considerations

Intraocular Pressure (IOP)

An understanding of the physiologic and pharmacologic control of IOP is of prime importance to the anaesthesiologist. The ability to avoid fluctuations in

IOP is the guiding principle to provide satisfactory anaesthesia for all intraocular procedures and especially in children with glaucoma and traumatic injury to the globe.

The normal range of IOP varies between 10 and 20 mmHg and may differ by as much as 5 mmHg between the two eyes. Normal pressure in neonates is somewhat lower (average, 9.5 mmHg) but approximate adult pressure is reached by 5 years of age (Pensiero et al. 1992).[2] A pressure above 25 mmHg at any age is considered abnormal (Johnson and Forrest, 1994).

The three primary factors governing IOP:

1. External pressure,
2. Venous congestion, and
3. Changes in intraocular volume.

IOP is normally maintained in the normal eye by the volume and evectional pressure of the aqueous humor. Overall the volume of the vitreous humor is usually constant.

1. Coughing, vomiting, and Valsalva maneuver may increase IOP up to 40 mmHg or more.
2. Respiratory acidosis increases IOP
3. Metabolic acidosis decreases IOP
4. Respiratory alkalosis decreases IOP
5. Metabolic alkalosis increases IOP
6. Hypoxia is capable of increasing IOP by dilating intraocular vessels
7. Hyperoxia appears to decrease IOP

The three important ophthalmic reflexes which are elicited by pressure/torsion on the extraocular muscles are:

1. The oculocardiac reflex (OCR)
2. The oculorespiratory reflex (ORR)
3. The oculoemetic reflex (OER)

General anaesthesia affects IOP as below:

1. Most induction and maintenance agents decrease IOP by 20–30% (3–6 mmHg).
2. Ketamine probably increases IOP, may be in dose dependent manner over 5 mg/kg.
3. Opioids have no effect or small decrease in IOP.
4. Non-depolarizing neuromuscular blockers have no effect or small decrease in IOP.
5. Succinylcholine causes increase in IOP of about 8 mmHg for 5–7 min.
6. Face mask, laryngoscopy, endotracheal intubation, and insertion of a Laryngeal Mask Airway [LMA] can increase IOP. Coughing and upper airway obstruction also increases IOP.

The Oculocardiac Reflex (OCR)

Manipulation of the eye ball, causing torsion of extraocular muscle leading to bradycardia is termed oculocardiac reflex (OCR). This may lead to the fatal life threatening complications like cardiac arrest which may go unnoticed. It was first described by Ashner (1908) (Fig. 31.1).[4]

The afferent pathway: Ophthalmic division of the trigeminal nerve to the vagal centre

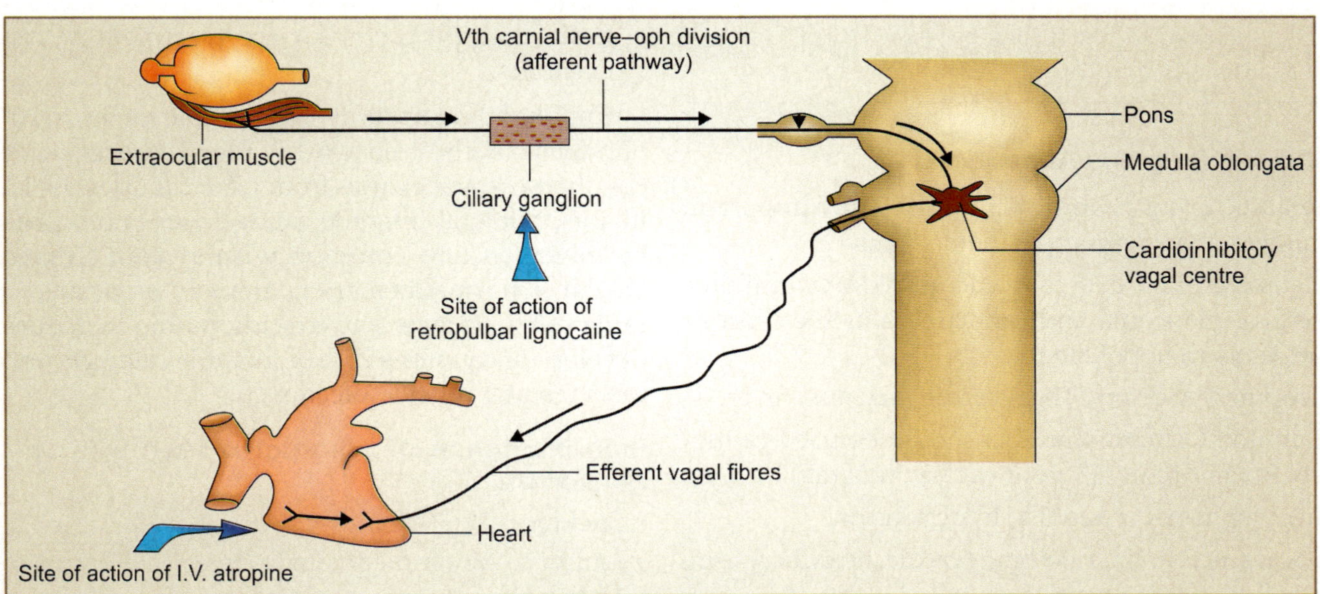

Fig. 31.1 Oculocardiac reflex (OCR)

The efferent pathway: Vagal nerve to the heart.

It is a trigeminal-vagal reflex triggered due to:

a. The traction on the extraocular muscles (especially the medial rectus which has up to six times the mass the lateral rectus)
b. Manipulation of the globe increases the intraocular pressure
c. More commonly due to sudden or strong traction compared to gentle progressive traction on the muscles particularly common during strabismus (squint) surgery.

The response is:

a. Usually a sinus bradycardia
b. Junctional rhythms, atrioventricular block, atrial and ventricular ectopics can also occur

The reflex weakens with repetition of the stimulus or the application of topical local anaesthetic.

Treatment

1. Prevention: Avoiding aggressive and non-physiological manipulations.
2. Pretreatment with Anticholinergic agents like Atropine 0.01 mg/kg, Inj. Glycopyrrolate 0.004 mg/kg. Their role is controversial. In certain conditions atropine may transform severe bradycardia into serious ventricular arrhythmias.
3. Ask surgeon to temporarily stop manipulation.

> **Pearls in Paediatric Anaesthesiology**
> Oculocardiac reflex (OCR) may lead to fatal life threatening complications like cardiac arrest.

Ophthalmic Drug and Anaesthesia

Ophthalmic drugs have systemic effects and important drug interactions with anaesthetic drugs.

1. Acetazolamide: Is a carbonic anhydrase inhibitor used for glaucoma and can cause alkaline diuresis that leads to hypokalemia.
2. Atropine eye drops: Tachycardia, dryness, fever.
3. Mannitol: Osmotic diuretic; should be used cautiously in children with poor cardiac function.
4. Phenylephrine: α agonist; hypertension.
5. Pilocarpine; cholinergic; bradycardia, bronchospasm.
6. Timolol maleate: β blocker, bradycardia, bronchospasm, precipitates congestive cardiac failure.

Preoperative Evaluation

This should include:

1. General health evaluation including blood pressure measurement.
2. Note of current medication.
3. Record of allergies.
4. Assessment of hearing and understanding.
5. Assessment of patients' ability to co-operate with the procedure and lie reasonably supine during surgery.
6. Identification of social problems.
7. Instruction on eye drop instillation.
8. Clear explanation of the procedure and effects on the patient.
9. Opportunity for patient to ask questions.

ANAESTHESIA FOR VARIOUS SURGERIES

Cataract

White opacification of lens is called cataract. Paediatric cataract is a common and one of the most treatable causes of lifelong visual impairment found in children. Blindness is because of opacification of lens that interferes with the focus of light on the retina. It is estimated that globally, 20 million children under the age of 16 suffer from cataract, and among these, 200,000 (15%) are severely visually impaired or blind.[5,6] According to etiology, paediatric cataract can be classified as:

1. **Congenital:** Idiopathic or associated with some syndrome (present at birth), infantile (develops during the first 2 years), or juvenile (late onset).
2. **Acquired:** Post traumatic or as a complication of radio therapy given for the treatment of retinoblastoma.

Childhood cataracts are responsible for 5% to 20% of blindness in children worldwide. The prevalence of childhood cataract varies from 1.2 to 6.0 cases per 10,000 infants. Bilateral infantile cataracts are more likely to be inherited and common with systemic diseases. Ocular abnormalities are commonly associated with unilateral cataracts and are idiopathic in nature. In developing countries 25% of infantile cataracts are due to congenital rubella infection.

High incidence of cataract is seen with several syndromes:

- Stickler
- Laurence-Moon-Biedl syndrome
- Hallermann-Streiff
- Marfan

- Lowe
- Cerebrotendinous xanthomatosis.
- Metabolic diseases: Galactosamia
- Chromosomal abnormalities: Down's (Trisomy 21)

Early cataract surgery allows photo-stimulation of retina. Cataract surgeries in children can be performed on day-care basis. Consideration of associated congenital comorbidities is important. General anaesthesia with LMA or endotracheal intubation is commonly done. The main anaesthesia aim is to avoid drugs and manoeuvres that can cause rise in IOP.

Etiology

1. Hereditary (most common): Autosomal dominant, Lowe's oculo-cerebro-renal syndrome (X linked recessive), Down's syndrome (Trisomy 21), Edwards syndrome, cri du chat syndrome.
2. Metabolic: Glucose-6-phosphate dehydrogenase (G6PD) deficiency, galactosaemia, hypoglycaemia, hypocalcaemia in infancy.
3. Trauma: Blunt or penetrating, usually unilateral.
4. Inflammation: Uveitis (juvenile chronic arthritis).
5. Tumour: (retinoblastoma).
6. Intrauterine infection: Rubella, CMV, toxoplasmosis, toxocariasis.
7. Radiation exposure, e.g. total body for leukaemia.
8. Steroids: Chronic use.

Treatment

Surgery for cataract comprises extra capsular cataract extraction (ECCE) with intra ocular lens (IOL) implantation. Surgical time usually varies between 45 and 60 minutes.

Anaesthesia Management

1. The aim of anaesthesia is to provide complete akinesia and avoiding rise in IOP.
2. Deep plane of anaesthesia is required especially after globe incision to avoid expulsion of vitreous humor and other globe contents.
3. A smooth induction and emergence without coughing is desirable.
4. Intravenous or inhalational induction is appropriate.
5. Use of succinylcholine after globe incision should be avoided as it can cause increase in intraocular pressure.
6. Usually endotracheal intubation with intermittent positive pressure ventilation (IPPV) is advocated to avoid hypercapnia which can cause further rise in IOP.
7. Maintenance of anaesthesia is usually done with inhalational anaesthetic using oxygen and air. The risk of postoperative nausea and vomiting [PONV] is more with nitrous oxide, hence it is avoided.
8. Avoid a high concentration of oxygen in premature neonates as it causes retinopathy.
9. Antiemetics should be given to minimize the effects of vomiting on IOP. Mostly two agents with different mechanisms of action, e.g. ondansetron 100 mcg/kg and dexamethasone 100–200 mcg/kg are used.
10. Extubation should be done smoothly in deep plane to avoid postoperatively coughing and excessive crying.
11. Analgesia is provided with topical tetracaine drops, a nonsteroidal anti-inflammatory drug [NSAID] or rectal paracetamol.

Postoperative Care

1. Early resumption of oral intake is important in postoperative period.
2. A combination of paracetamol, nonsteroidal anti-inflammatory drugs [NSAID] is used for analgesia.
3. Postoperative nausea and vomiting [PONV] may require a further antiemetic of a different class from the one(s) given during anaesthesia, e.g. metoclopramide 0.1 mg/kg IV if ondansetron and dexamethasone are already used.
4. Specific care for an underlying syndrome related to airway management should be taken in consideration.

SQUINT OR STRABISMUS

Divergence of visual axes is termed strabismus or squint. A corrective surgery for strabismus is one of the most common paediatric eye operations performed. One or two extraocular muscles to the globes are detached and reattached.

1. The prevalence of strabismus in Indian population is estimated to be 3–4%[8]
2. Male : female ratio 1:1

Aetiology

1. Usually idiopathic, occasionally secondary to trauma, infection, inflammation (neuromuscular disorders).

2. Familial, prematurity, associated with cerebral palsy, meningomyelocele, hydrocephalus.

Treatment

1. Surgery comprises recession (lengthening), resection (tightening or shortening) or transposition of any, or combinations of the extra-ocular muscles (four recti and two obliques).
2. An adjustable suture is sometimes used in older children to reduce the incidence of malposition. The final position is achieved at 24–48 hours after surgery, using local anaesthetic eye drops.

Preoperative Assessment

Most patients are healthy children. Associated syndromes should be taken in consideration before giving anaesthesia.

Anaesthetic Technique

1. Generally performed under general anaesthesia with controlled ventilation.
2. Major anaesthetic concerns: OCR, PONV, Malignant hyperthermia (MH).
3. Inhalational or intravenous induction can be used.
4. Endotracheal tube or a Laryngeal Mask Airway [LMA] can be used to secure the airway.
5. Maintenance of anaesthesia: Volatile anaesthetic in oxygen and air.
6. Total intravenous anaesthesia [TIVA] may reduce the incidence of postoperative nausea and vomiting [PONV].
7. Topical adrenaline used to produce conjunctival vasoconstriction and reduce bleeding, may get absorbed systemically. Electrocardiogram [ECG] should be observed closely for this period.
8. Forced duction test: It is used to evaluate mechanical limitation. It is used to distinguish a paretic muscle from one with restricted motion. It involves intraoperative manipulation of the eye into the normal axis by traction on the sclera. The test is contraindicated if succinyl choline is given in the previous 20 minutes, which causes contraction of extraocular muscles. Non-depolarizing muscle relaxants can be used safely as they do not interfere with testing.
9. Oculocardiac reflex (OCR): Traction on the extraocular muscles during surgery can produce vagal stimulation via the trigemino-vagal reflex. It can be prevented by delicate surgical handling.

   While giving the retrobulbar block, if moderate pressure is applied to the eye, OCR can be triggered. Once the block works, it prevents the reflex by blocking its afferent limb. It is common during any surgery in which there is traction on the rectus muscle or eyelid or pressure on the eyeball or empty globe. It is common during strabismus surgery, enucleation and endoscopic sinus surgery. OCR leads to a variety of dysrhythmias including sinus or junctional bradycardia, atrioventricular block, bigeminy, multifocal premature ventricular contractions, ventricular tachycardia or sinoatrial arrest. Intraoperatively the changes in rhythm may decrease as the reflex may fatigue with continued intermittent traction. Once the surgeons remove the traction on the rectus muscles or pressure on the eye, the signs usually disappear. Treatment includes premedication with anticholinergic agents like glycopyrrolate or atropine 10–20 μg/kg to reduce the frequency, intensity, and duration of this reflex.
10. Analgesia: Topical tetracaine, rectal or intravenous paracetamol, intravenous fentanyl 1–2 mcg/kg.
11. Postoperative nausea and vomiting [PONV] occurs in 50–75% of patients following strabismus surgery which further increases the postoperative hospital stay. The exact mechanism of nausea and vomiting following strabismus surgery is not known. It may be due to an altered visual perception and a different afferent input postoperatively or secondary to an oculoemetic reflex. More than one prophylactic antiemetics are clearly indicated by society for ambulatory anaesthesia.[9] Metoclopramide decreases nausea and vomiting to a much lesser degree as compared to ondansetron, in patients following strabismus surgery. Therefore, serotonin antagonists are frequently used in conjunction with dexamethasone. Use of nitrous oxide and opioids increases the risk of PONV. Propofol reduces the chances of PONV.
12. In the past, children operated for strabismus were thought to be at an increased risk of developing malignant hyperthermia (MH).[10] It may be because of the association between patients with MH and associated musculoskeletal disorders, including strabismus and ptosis. Today malignant hyperthermia is not considered to be a risk for children with strabismus.
13. Children undergoing strabismus surgery are also more susceptible to develop Masseter muscle

spasm (MMS), especially those receiving halothane and succinylcholine. Thus if MMS is suspected, it is important to recognize that this patient may be susceptible to developing MH. Hence a detailed family history should be elicited in the pre-anaesthesia examination.

BLOCKAGE OF PUNCTUM OF NASOLACRIMAL DUCT

Nasolacrimal duct obstruction (NLDO):

1. Obstruction of nasolacrimal duct may be either congenital or acquired.
2. Obstruction of the nasolacrimal duct leads to the excess overflow of tears called epiphora.
3. Symptomatic epiphora responds to surgical probing of the entire lacrimal drainage duct. For complete NLD obstruction a dacryocystorhinostomy (DCR) is considered.

Anaesthesia Management

General anaesthesia is preferred. TIVA can be administered for probing of the duct as it can be done in 5–10 minutes. Patency of the nasolacrimal duct might require irrigation with saline or fluorescein. To prevent excessive pooling, possible laryngospasm, and aspiration, suctioning and Trendlenburg position might be required.

Nasolacrimal stent placements, dacryocystorhinostomy are procedures, which may require more time and can be complicated by appreciable blood loss. They are generally managed with general anaesthesia and endotracheal intubation in children. Postoperative analgesia can be provided with acetaminophen, ketorolac, or small doses of opioids.

RETINOPATHY OF PREMATURITY

It was previously known as retrolental fibroplasia (RLF).[11] It is a vasoproliferative disorder that may result in blindness. Both oxygen toxicity and relative hypoxia can contribute to the development of ROP. 15 to 20% of premature infants weighing below 1500 g develop variable degrees of acute retrolental fibroplasia (RLF). Approximately 5% of those infants who develop RLF can be expected to become blind.[12]

1. Hyperoxia suppressed vascular endothelial growth factor that results in arrest of normal retinal vascularization.
2. Hypoxia-triggered stimulation of vascular endothelial growth factor results in vascular proliferation.
3. The incidence of ROP has reduced with the practice of decreasing the concentration of supplemental oxygen and thereby a corresponding reduction in acceptable baseline oxygen saturation levels to 95% in neonates. It is now an accepted practice to maintain oxygen saturation at or around 95% in premature infants having surgery.

Following stages describe the ophthalmoscopic findings at the junction between the vascularized and avascular retina in retinopathy of prematurity.

1. Stage 1 is a faint demarcation line
2. Stage 2 is an elevated ridge
3. Stage 3 is extraretinal fibrovascular tissue
4. Stage 4 is sub-total retinal detachment
5. Stage 5 is total retinal detachment.

Treatment

1. Laser photocoagulation: Peripheral retinal ablation is the mainstay of ROP treatment. The destruction of the avascular retina is performed with a solid state laser photocoagulation device which is portable.
2. Cryotherapy: Regional retinal destruction is done using a probe to freeze the desired areas.
3. Scleral buckling and/or vitrectomy surgery: For severe ROP (stages 4 and 5) for eyes that progress to retinal detachment.
4. Intravitreal injection: Injection of bevacizumab (avastin) has been reported as a supportive measure in aggressive posterior retinopathy of prematurity.

Anaesthetic Management

1. Challenges: Multiple medical comorbidities which may be associated
   a. Apnoea of prematurity
   b. Bronchopulmonary dysplasia
   c. Congenital cardiac anomalies
   d. Others: Low birth weight, prematurity, neonatal oxygen exposure, recurrent apnoea, exchange transfusion, and vitamin E deficiency.
2. Anaesthetic goal is to provide minimal cardio-respiratory compromise and a quiet surgical field.
3. Infants with ROP may require anaesthetic care for non-ocular procedures also. ROP is of particular interest to the paediatric anaesthesiologist because the routine management of the infant at risk may alter the development or progression of the disease itself.

4. For children on ventilator, general anaesthesia with mechanical ventilation is commonly administered. LMA can be used.
5. Opioids: Cautiously administered, co-existing apnoea may be exacerbated.
6. Extubation: Only after regular respiratory pattern without apnoea is achieved; caffeine citrate 10 mg/kg IV may be effective in significant apnoea.
7. Mechanical ventilation: Patients may require 12–24 hrs after the procedure, especially if any opioid is required for pain management.

ENUCLEATION

Eye removal can be of three types:
1. **Evisceration** removal of the iris, cornea, and internal eye contents, but with the sclera and attached extraocular muscles left behind.
2. **Enucleation** removal of the eyeball, but with the eyelids and adjacent structures of the eye socket remaining. An intraocular tumor excision requires an enucleation, not an evisceration.
3. **Exenteration** removal of the contents of the eye socket, including the eyeball, fat, muscles, and other adjacent structures of the eye. The eyelids may also be removed in cases of cutaneous cancers and unrelenting infection. Exenteration is sometimes done together with maxillectomy (removal of the maxilla).

Indications

1. Cancer of the eye, such as retinoblastoma and uveal melanoma.
2. Severe injury to the eye when the eye cannot be saved or attempts to save the eye have failed.
3. End stage glaucoma.
4. Painful blind eye.
5. In cases of sympathetic ophthalmia (inflammation of the eye) to prevent affection of other eye, which if untreated can cause blindness.
6. Congenital cystic eye
7. The cornea from a deceased person, can be used for a living person who needs a corneal transplant by a surgical operation called keratoplasty.
8. Constant infection in a blind or otherwise useless eye.

Retinoblastoma

1. Retinoblastoma is the most common intraocular malignancy in the paediatric population.[13] Patients generally present by 3 years of age.
2. These patients require frequent examinations until the age of 5 years.
3. Treatment involves combinations of enucleation, external beam radiation, localized radiotherapy, laser ablation, thermotherapy, cryotherapy, and chemotherapy (Uusitalo and Wheeler, 1999).[14] External beam radiotherapy is advocated in children with bilateral disease requiring enucleation of the more involved eye and in those with diffuse vitreous and subretinal seeding.
4. Anaesthetic management for enucleation consists of general anaesthesia with controlled ventilation. The procedure carries risk of OCR-mediated dysrhythmias, hence appropriate prophylaxis with atropine or glycopyrrolate is warranted. Intraoperative blood loss can be significant, and controlled hypotension should be provided (Johnson and Forrest, 1994).[15]
5. External beam radiotherapy may require multiple sessions. The session requires the child to be akinetic for a few minutes. For safety of medical personnel from excessive radiation, during the session, patients may be unattended for some time. Anaesthesia modalities can vary from intravenous or intramuscular ketamine or intravenous Propofol or brief inhalation anaesthetics by face mask, laryngeal mask airway or endotracheal intubation. Some patients might pose problems with difficult veins because of concomitant chemotherapy and multiple sessions. These patients might have a central venous catheter in place for adjuvant chemotherapy.

GLAUCOMA

Paediatric glaucoma is generally a congenital abnormality inherited in an autosomal recessive pattern as described by Shaffer and Weiss.[16] Some are associated with systemic diseases, congenital disorders, or other ocular abnormalities. It is characterized by elevated IOP causing reduced capillary blood flow to the optic nerve with eventual loss of optic nerve tissue and function.

1. Primary congenital glaucoma is due to failure of development of trabecular drainage channels for aqueous humour.
2. Secondary glaucoma is due to blockage of existing drainage channels secondary to infection, inflammation or trauma. Some rare syndromes like Axenfeld-Reiger and Sturge-Weber syndrome may also lead to glaucoma.

The definitive diagnosis is established by tonometry, corneal examination, funduscopy, and gonioscopy.

Surgical Treatment

1. Examination under anaesthesia and measurement of IOP: Surgery is of brief duration and can be managed under TIVA.
2. Goniotomy is done to visualize the anterior chamber. An incision is made in the trabecular meshwork to allow for aqueous drainage.
3. Trabeculectomy: A new drainage channel is created to drain aqueous from the intraocular anterior chamber to extraocular sub-Tenon's space.
4. Trabeculotomy: A fine probe inserted into Schlemm's canal creates a new drainage channel.
5. Laser treatment aimed at the ciliary body can help to reduce the production of aqueous.

Preoperative Assessment

These children might present for multiple short anaesthesia procedures. Underlying any congenital syndromes should be ruled out. Concurrent medical therapy to reduce IOP and their anaesthetic implications should be considered.

Anaesthetic Technique

1. To avoid any rise in intraocular pressure (IOP). A smooth induction and emergence without coughing is desirable.
2. Intravenous or inhalational induction is appropriate. Ketamine and Succinyl choline should be avoided.
3. IOP is usually measured post-induction and before airway manipulations, i.e. usually before endotracheal intubation.
4. Anaesthesia is maintained with volatile anaesthetic in oxygen and air. Nitrous oxide is often avoided to reduce the risk of postoperative nausea and vomiting [PONV]. Antiemetics are given to minimize the effects of vomiting on IOP. It is common to use two agents with different mechanisms of action, e.g. ondansetron 100 mcg/kg (max 4 mg), dexamethasone 100–200 mcg/kg.
5. Analgesia can be provided with topical tetracaine drops, a nonsteroidal anti-inflammatory drugs [NSAID], paracetamol, opioids like fentanyl 1–2 mcg/kg.

Postoperative Care

Oral intake is usually resumed early in the postoperative period.

VITRECTOMY

Retinopathy of prematurity is the major cause of retinal tear and detachment, but may also result from trauma and vitreous degeneration common to certain syndromes. Small tears can be managed by laser therapy or cryopexy; more significant tears and detachment often require complex surgical management. Surgical modalities include scleral buckling (in combination with cryopexy), closed vitrectomy, and open-sky vitrectomy.

Anaesthetic management is the same as for other major ophthalmic procedures. General anaesthesia with endotracheal intubation and controlled ventilation is generally done. Prophylaxis for OCR should be given during such procedures as the extraocular muscles are often bridled to permit optimal positioning. IOP also needs to be controlled and lowered with agents such as mannitol and acetazolamide.

Open Globe Injuries in a Patient with a "Full Stomach"

1. Traumatic eye injuries are to be operated urgently in children to salvage the eye. After penetrating trauma the intraocular pressure is atmospheric. External pressure on the eye or an increase in internal pressure can prolapse the lens, iris or vitreous and markedly reduce the chances of saving the eye.
2. The major anaesthesia concern preoperatively and during the induction of anaesthesia is to prevent any rise in IOP. Coughing, crying, straining and vomiting increase the intraocular venous blood volume and hence IOP, which causes the ocular contents to extrude.
3. Preoperatively, the child should remain quiet, and should be sedated for easy separation from the parents. Eyes should be patched to minimize eye movements.
4. Child can be premedicated with oral or nasal midazolam or oral clonidine. For painless IV insertion EMLA (eutectic mixture of local anaesthetics) cream should be applied. After proper preoxygenation, rapid–sequence induction of anaesthesia should be done in all such cases. After complete neuromuscular blockade with a non-depolarizing muscle relaxant, gentle laryngoscopy and endotracheal intubation should be attempted. To minimize the pressor response a dose of lidocaine (1–1.5 mg/kg) or fentanyl (2–3 μg/kg) can be given.
5. For neuromuscular blockade, rocuronium (0.8–1.5 mg/kg) offers advantages over atracurium,

vecuronium, pancuronium and succinyl choline. It causes rapid onset of paralysis and a decrease in IOP without side-effects. Rocuronium (1.2 mg/kg) provides intubating conditions comparable to succinylcholine within 60 seconds. (Mazurek et al., 1998;[17] Perry et al., 2002[18]). Rocuronium is probably the most effective alternative to succinylcholine, especially for patients where the later is contra-indicated. A gastric tube should be placed to aspirate the stomach contents after the airway is secured.

Key Points

Postoperative nausea and vomiting is one of the most common complications following strabismus surgery, which can prolong postoperative hospital stay. It can be managed with combination of anti-emetic drugs.

FAQs with Answers

Q. Which are three important ophthalmic reflexes?

A. 1. The oculocardiac reflex (OCR)
   2. The oculorespiratory reflex (ORR)
   3. The oculoemetic reflex (OER).

Q. How to prevent PONV?

A. Use oxygen and air, avoid use of nitrous and do not use single antiemetic drug, instead use combinations.

REFERENCES

1. Beeby DG, Morgan Hughes JO. Behaviour of unsedated children in the anaesthetic room. Br J Anaesth. 1980;52: 279–281.
2. Pensiero S, Da Pozzo S, Perissutti P, et al. Normal intra-ocular pressure in children. J Pediatr Ophthalmol Strabismus, Slack Inc.© 1992;29:79–84.
3. Renu S. Anaesthesia for ophthalmic surgery, Journal of postgraduate medical education, training and research Sept, 2005;2(5):19–20.
4. Ashner B. Concerning a hitherto not yet described reflex from the eye on circulation and respiration, Wien, Klin, Woschanschr, 1908;21:1529–30.
5. Johnson GJ, (Ed). The epidemiology of eye disease. 2nd edn. London: Arnold; 2003.
6. Foster A, Gilbert C, Rahi J. Epidemiology of cataract in childhood: A global perspective. J Cataract Refract Surg. 1997;23:601–4 [PMID: 9278811].
7. http://www.vision2020india.org/pdfs/ceh_17_ 50_s.pdf
8. Vijayalakshmi P, Nirmalan P, Kothari MT. Paediatric ophthalmology and strabismus in India. J aapos. 2004;8: 18–9.
9. Gan, Tong J (MD), Meyer, Tricia A (PharmD). Society for Ambulatory Anaesthesia Guidelines for the Management of Postoperative Nausea and Vomiting Anaesthesia and Analgesia: Dec. 2007; 105(6):1615–1628. doi: 10.1213/ 01.ane.0000295230. 55439.f4
10. Hoffman GM, Ghanayem NS, Postoperative Two-Site NIRS Predicts Complications and Mortality after Stage 1 Palliation of HLHS. Anesthesiology 2007;107:A234–41.
11. http://retinopathyofprematurity.org/Babyblindinglights 01.htm
12. Sira Bi, Grunwald Ine, Yassur Y, et al. Treatment of acute retrolental fibroplasias by cryopexy, British Journal of Ophthalmology, 1980;64:758–762.
13. Abramson DH. Retinoblastoma. Pediatr Emerg Casebook. 1985;3:3–15.
14. Uusitalo AU M, Wheeler M, O'Brien S, et al. New approaches in the clinical management of retinoblastoma, Ophthalmol Clin. 1999;12:255.
15. Johnson R, Forrest F. Local and general anaesthesia for ophthalmic surgery. Butterworth-Heinemann Medical Oxford, UK, 1994.
16. Shaffer RN, Weiss DI. Congenital and Paediatric glaucomas. CV Mosby: St Louis, 1970, quoted by Krishnadas R, Ramakrishnan R, Congenital Glaucoma, A Brief Review Journal of Current Glaucoma Practice, http://www.jaypeejournals. com/eJournals/ShowText.aspx?ID=159&Type= FREE&TYP=TOP&IN=_eJournals/images JPLOGO.gif&IID=19&isPDF=NO.
17. Mazurek AJ, Rae B, Hann S, et al. Rocuronium Versus Succinyl choline: Are They Equally Effective During Rapid-Sequence Induction of Anaesthesia? Anaesthesia and Analgesia:December 1998;87(6): 1259–1262.
18. Perry JJ, Lee J, Wells G. Are Intubation Conditions Using Rocuronium Equivalent to Those Using Succinylcholine? Academic Emergency Medicine. Aug. 2002;9(8):813–823.

32

Anaesthesia for Paediatric Dentistry

Indrani Hemantkumar Chincoli

ABSTRACT

It is important to ensure that children receive safe and effective pain control during dental procedures. A range of techniques are available, comprising four overlapping categories: Behavioural techniques, local anaesthesia (LA), conscious sedation, and general anaesthesia (GA). Most dental procedures in children are completed using local anaesthesia. However, very young, uncooperative children may require sedation. Close vigilance and certification in paediatric resuscitation is mandatory for those practicing sedation. General anaesthesia is not without risk and should be given in a hospital setting by a trained personnel only. The standards of general anaesthesia for dentistry should be the same as those in any other setting.

Key Words

Conscious sedation, Deep sedation, Maxillary block, Mandibular block, Palatine block, Mental nerve block, Dental chair anaesthesia.

INTRODUCTION

Dental treatment is one of the most common reasons for providing anaesthesia services to children. Paediatric patients are most often anxious, fearful, uncooperative and difficult to handle. In children, these procedures are often associated with a significant amount of pain, fear of the unknown, surprises, "shots", and physical restraint, for which pharmacological behavior management is required. Many adults carry the trauma of their dental treatment they received as children. Most procedures can successfully be completed under adequate local anaesthesia. However, a few may need sedation or general anaesthesia.[1]

HISTORY

The first general anaesthetic was administered for a dental extraction by a Connecticut dentist, **Horace Wells** (Fig. 32.1). He observed at a travelling show that laughing gas induced anaesthesia. He began experimenting with the gas himself. On the 11th December 1844, he underwent extraction of one of his own wisdom teeth by a colleague whilst under the influence of nitrous oxide. In the

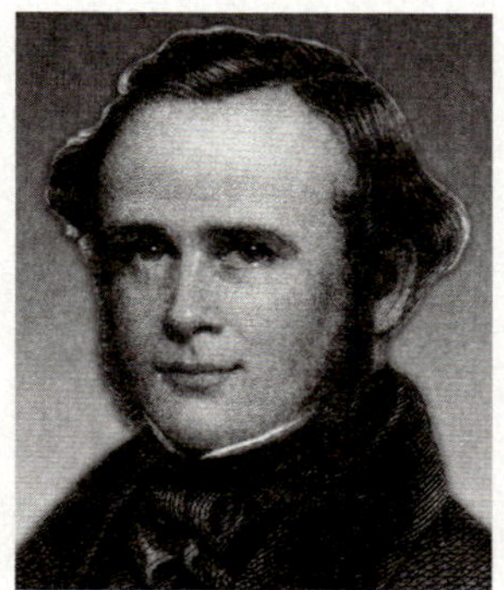

Fig. 32.1 Horace Wells

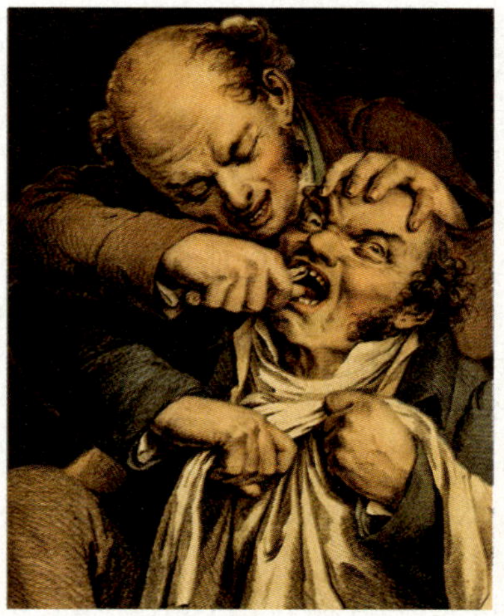

Fig. 32.2 Dental anaesthesia by Horace Wells

following year, he demonstrated this technique in Harvard. Unfortunately, his patient cried in pain during the procedure and Wells was laughed out of the lecture theatre. However, on December 30, 1845, a pupil of Wells, William Morton, exploited the properties of ether to facilitate dental extraction. This agent was subsequently demonstrated successfully to the public in Massachusetts on 16th October 1846. The concept of general anaesthesia was thus born. This development facilitated the expansion of the dental profession, enabling increasing emphasis on restorative and conservative work.

Around the turn of the century, local anaesthesia was introduced. It remained an experimental technique until the introduction of lidocaine in the 1940s. In the 1970s and 1980s , there were many deaths in the dental chair which were due to various reasons like substandard monitoring and absence of resuscitative equipment. Professor David Poswillo[2] made recommendations in 1990 for the safe provision of general anaesthesia in dentistry outside hospital. The key recommendations were:

1. Avoid general anaesthesia where possible;
2. The same standards of personnel, monitoring and equipment should apply whether anaesthesia is administered in a hospital or in a dental surgery clinic; and
3. Dental surgeries should be inspected and registered.

In the late 1990s the General Dental Council and the Royal College of Anaesthetists issued further guidance.[3,4]

General Anaesthesia (GA) was misused for anxiety control. It was hence recommended that general anaesthesia should only be administered where no alternative existed such as the following:

1. Situations in which it would be impossible to achieve adequate local anaesthesia and so complete treatment without pain;
2. Patients who, because of problems related to age/ maturity or physical/learning disability, are unlikely to allow safe completion of treatment; and
3. Patients in whom long-term dental phobia will be induced or prolonged.

Recommendations were also made that administration of dental anaesthesia should only be carried out by:

1. Anaesthetists on the specialist register of the General Medical Council (Qualified Anaesthestists)
2. Trainees working under supervision in programmes accredited by the Royal College of Anaesthetists (Residents doing Postgraduate course in Anaesthesia working under supervision); or
3. Non-consultant career grade doctors working under the responsibility of a named consultant anaesthetist (Qualified anaesthesiologists working under a consultant).

PERCEPTION OF PAIN IN CHILDREN

The perception of pain in children is related to their cognitive development. Other factors which interfere with the perception of pain include fear, family, learning, and previous experiences of pain. Children who are over the age of 10 years have the ability to think abstractly and respond appropriately to explanations. They may cooperate with dental treatment performed under local anaesthesia, with or without sedation. Up to 2 years of age, they are unable to distinguish between pressure and pain and may require sedation or GA. Between the ages of 2 and 10 years, they understand pain and differentiate it from other sensations such as pressure or vibration but still may require GA. Children over the age of 10 years may cooperate with dental treatment performed under local anaesthesia, with or without sedation. GA may be needed in patients with specific medical illness or if the procedure is complex.

Common Paediatric Dental Problems for which Anaesthesia Services is Required[5–8]

- Caries—dental treatment may involve the filling, restoration of teeth especially if it is extensive, extraction or surgical removal of teeth that cannot be restored.
- Scaling of teeth to prevent periodontal problems.
- Mentally challenged patients
- Allergy to local anaesthetics
- Dental phobia especially if a child has undergone a painful dental treatment earlier

Problems of Dental Anaesthesia

The problems of dental anaesthesia are related to both patient and surgical factors.

Patient Factors

Since most of the cases are between the age group of 6 months and 6 years, the children will have all attendant problems of Paediatric Anaesthesia. They may present with adenotonsillar hypertrophy, respiratory tract infections with an associated increased risk of airway problems, cardiac disease, seizures, learning disability/ syndromes/retardation/ADHD, etc. These patients may be uncooperative and communication may be challenging. Individuals from institutions are at higher risk of hepatitis B. These patients are often uncooperative and impossible to communicate. Parental separation and procuring an intravenous line are difficult. They have a high vagal tone and the needle phobia by itself can trigger arrhythmias in them. Awake patients often gag too much during the procedure making it difficult for the dental surgeons to work on them. Titrating the levels of sedation during the procedure so that they meet discharge criteria can be a challenge to the anaesthesiologist.

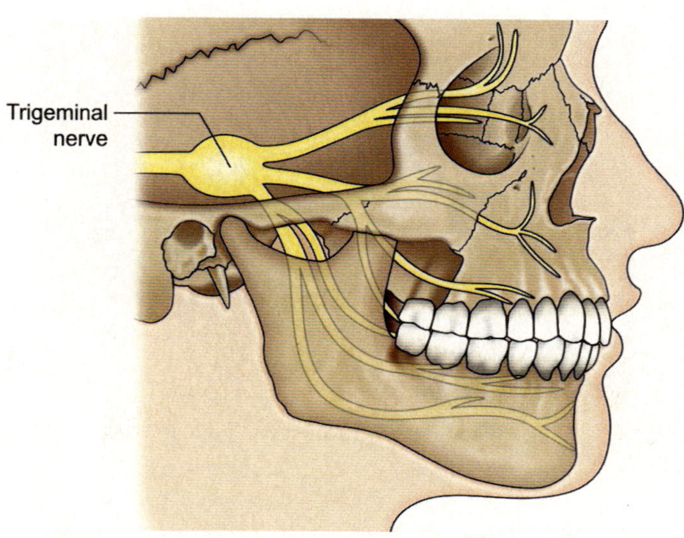

Fig. 32.3 Innervations of the teeth

SURGICAL FACTORS

The anaesthesiologists and the dental surgeon share the airway. The airway can become soiled with blood and debris triggering a laryngospasm. The trigeminal nerve, if not blocked, can trigger arrhythmias. Arrhythmias can also occur by the use of halothane or by any degree of hypoxia or hypercarbia.

Paediatric Dentistry Anaesthesia

This is usually provided as:
- Office dentistry with local anaesthesia
- Outpatient dentistry with oral sedation/infiltration anaesthesia or nerve block, and N_2O–O_2 mixture
- Office/outpatient dentistry with general anaesthesia
- Inpatient dentistry with general anaesthesia

LOCAL ANAESTHESIA

This is the anaesthesia of choice in older children. Infiltrative anaesthesia is sufficient for most of the procedures. Nerve blocks are given when there is extensive work. Lidocaine and prilocaine in cartridges containing 2.2 mL with or without epinephrine/ felypressin is available. Smaller volumes can produce faster onset of action with shorter duration of effect. One needs to be careful in the presence of reduced bone density of the maxilla and mandible as it causes rapid diffusion and absorption of LA. There can be failure or delay in the action of local anaesthetics in the presence of infection.

Maxillary Anaesthesia

Innervation of maxillary teeth is by the anterior, middle, and posterior superior alveolar (dental) nerves, which are branches of the maxillary nerve. Local infiltration to the apical foramina of the teeth should be given in addition. Injection of LA solution in the sulcus adjacent to the tooth requiring treatment is usually effective. This block provides anaesthesia to the buccal and labial soft tissues. Anaesthesia of the hard and soft palate requires injection directly into the palate by means of the Palatine nerve block. The infra-orbital nerve, a terminal branch of the maxillary nerve can be blocked from the upper labial sulcus opposite the canine tooth. The branches of the anterior superior alveolar nerve provides anaesthesia to the anterior maxilla and upper lip.

Mandibular Anaesthesia

The lower teeth are innervated by the inferior alveolar (dental) nerve. It is blocked before it enters the bone at

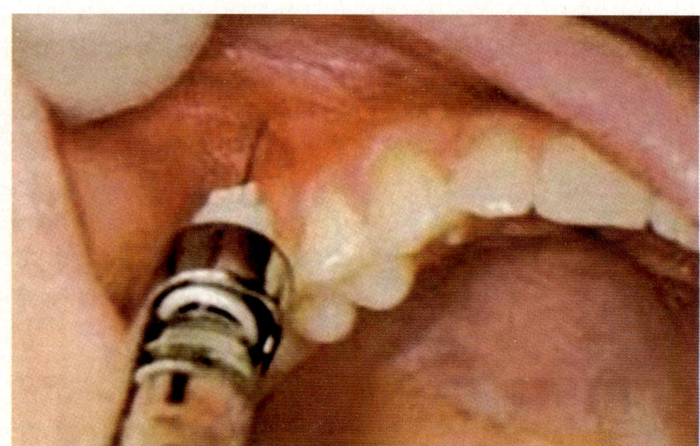

Fig. 32.4 Maxillary block—insert needle for anterior superior alveolar (ASA) nerve block in muco-buccal fold over maxillary first premolar

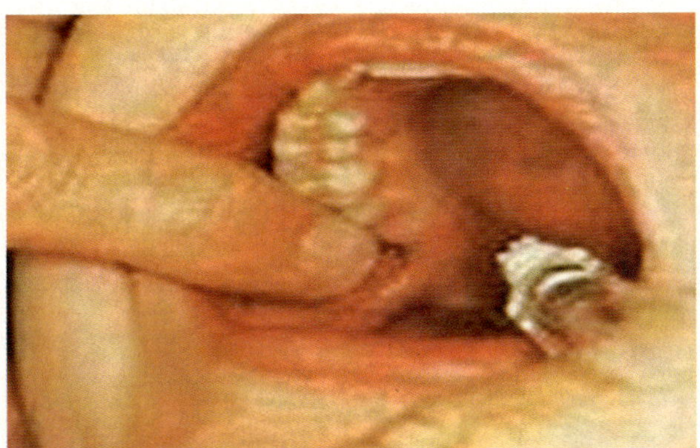

Fig. 32.5 Palatine block—maxillary nerve block, greater palatine approach

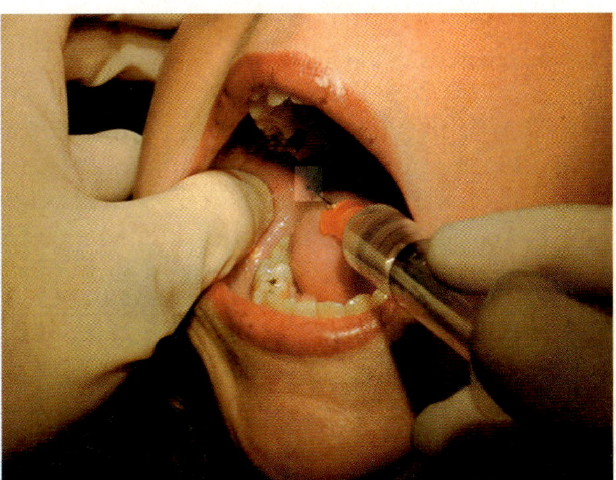

Fig. 32.6 Mandibular block

the **mandibular foramen** on the medial aspect of the ramus, just behind the lingula. This block provides anaesthesia to the bone of the mandibular body and the pulps of all the teeth on that side of the mouth, except central incisor where there may be some cross-over supply from the inferior dental nerve on the opposite side. Labial cortex of the mandible in the incisor region is very thin. This allows the diffusion of sufficient local anaesthetic solution, providing anaesthesia to the pulps of the teeth. In older children, a **periodontal ligament injection** may be required to achieve adequate pulpal anaesthesia of each mandibular tooth.

Mental Nerve Anaesthesia

Mental nerve anaesthesia is provided by injection of LA at the mental foramen. This anaesthetizes the soft tissues of the labial gingiva, the lower lip, and chin. The local anaesthetic solution will also diffuse via the mental foramen to reach the incisive branch, which supplies

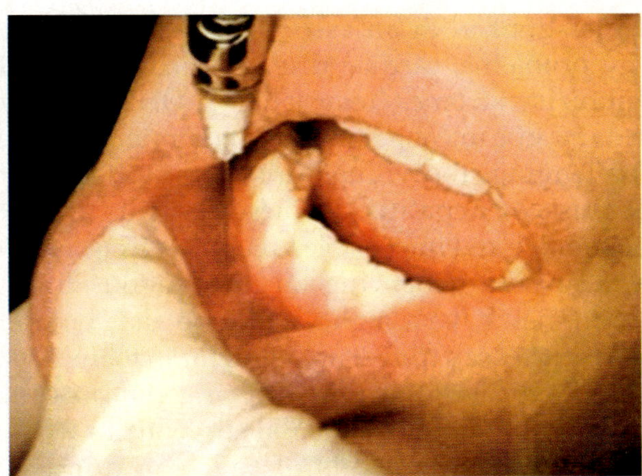

Fig. 32.7 Mental nerve block

the pulps of lower teeth, namely the first premolar, the canine, and incisor teeth.

Local anaesthetic solution	Maximum dose
2% lidocaine/1:80 000 epinephrine	4.4 mg kg^{-1}
3% prilocaine/felypressin 0.03 IU/mL	6.6 mg kg^{-1}
4% prilocaine	5 mg kg^{-1}
0.25–0.5% Bupivacaine	2 mg/kg

Complications of LA

Local Complications

1. Failure of the block, infection, intravascular injection, haematoma, nerve damage, facial nerve palsy, and needle fracture.
2. Risk of trauma to the anaesthetized region of the face caused by biting and chewing.

Systemic Complications

1. Dose-related toxicity of the local anaesthetic agent
2. Hypersensitivity reactions.
3. Children >6 months of age absorb local anaesthetic agents more rapidly—**toxicity** well below toxic levels in adults
4. Cardiovascular effects: Arrhythmias (LA and vasoconstrictor)
5. Central nervous system: Seizures, unconsciousness, and respiratory arrest.

Sedation

The first monitoring guideline for sedation was written by Dr Charles Coté and Dr Theodore Striker in 1983 (published in 1985) while working on behalf of the

American Academy of Paediatrics (AAP) Section on Anaesthesiology. This guideline was written in response to reports of three deaths in a single dental office and other concerns primarily involving dental sedation.[9] Written with the cooperation of the American Academy of Paediatric Dentistry and the American Society of Anaesthesiologists (ASA), the purpose of the guidelines was to develop a framework from which improved safety could be developed for children requiring sedation to perform a required procedure.[10,11]

The guideline emphasized on issues, such as the need for informed consent, appropriate fasting before sedation, frequent measurement and charting of vital signs, the availability of age and size appropriate equipment, the use of physiologic monitoring, the need for basic life support skills, and proper recovery and discharge procedures. The presence of an independent observer whose only responsibility was to monitor the patient was introduced for deeply sedated paediatric patients. Advanced airway and resuscitation skills were encouraged but not required. Finally, these original guidelines defined three terms for depth of sedation, viz. conscious sedation, deep sedation, and general anaesthesia.

CONSCIOUS SEDATION

Conscious sedation is defined as a technique in which the use of a drug or drugs produces a state of depression of the central nervous system enabling treatment to be carried out, but during which *verbal contact with the patient is maintained.*

Children who cannot tolerate dental procedures with local anaesthesia alone may be managed using a **conscious sedation** technique, resulting in a moderately depressed level of consciousness. **The patient must retain their protective airway reflexes, and be able to respond to and understand verbal communication.**

Deep or Procedural Sedation

For procedural sedation, analgesia usually must be ***deeper*** than that given to adults. Due to physiologic differences, children are at ***higher*** risk for respiratory depression and life-threatening hypoxia. Technically, providers with the intent to practice "moderate sedation" may be closer to the definition of "general anaesthesia" because children can easily slip from one level to another.

In 1992, the Committee on Drugs of the AAP (primary author Dr Coté) revised the 1985 guideline.[9] This guideline stated that a patient could easily progress from one level of sedation to another and that the practitioner should increase vigilance and monitoring. Pulse oximetry was made compulsory for all patients undergoing sedation. This new guideline also discouraged the practice of administering sedation at home by parents—a practice that was not infrequent in dental and radiologic sedation at that time. An amendment to this guideline was produced by the same Committee on Drugs of the AAP 2002. It eliminated the use of the term "conscious sedation" and clarified the fact that these guidelines apply to any location where children are sedated, including in or out of the hospital. The current guidelines use the terminology of minimal sedation, moderate sedation, deep sedation, and general anaesthesia. This language is consistent with that used by the ASA and the Joint Commission on Accreditation of Healthcare Organizations (JCAHO).

Children who are uncooperative, physically or mentally compromised or need long procedures, e.g. impacted tooth/four quadrant restorations, need sedation. Intramuscular, intravenous, oral or inhalational route are used for sedation more often. The drugs and techniques used for sedation must carry a margin of safety wide enough to make loss of consciousness unlikely.[12]

Dental practitioners should be trained in the safe provision of sedation. All members of the dental team providing sedation must have received theoretical, practical and clinical training before undertaking independent practice. They must also be trained to deal with sedation-related complications, including cardiorespiratory arrest. Patients should be carefully selected and medically pre-assessed, and consent must be obtained. Moderate and deep sedation should preferably be practiced in a secondary or a tertiary centre. The anaesthesia machine should be well serviced and checked. Standard resuscitative (Defibrillator) and monitoring equipment like Multipara monitor (Cardioscope/Precordial/$ETCO_2$/SpO_2/NIBP/Temp) should be available. The suction should be a good working one. The patients need to be assessed properly in the preoperative period and clear instructions about fasting, i.e. allowing clear fluids 2 hours before as in general anaesthesia should be explained. The option of having the parent during sedation should be left to them.

Aim of sedation: Reducing fear and anxiety, augmenting pain control, and minimizing movement.

Grades of Sedation

- **Mild**
- **Moderate**
- **Deep**

There is no clear demarcation from one level to another.

1. **Mild and moderate sedation is provided** by qualified dental surgeons who are certified by state board.
2. **Deep sedation should be provided by** anaesthesiologists

Current AAPD Sedation Guidelines

There are 5 functional levels of sedation

- **I :** Anxiolysis
- **II:** Interactive
- **III :** Non-interactive, arousable with mild/moderate stimuli
- **IV:** Non-interactive, arousable with intense stimuli
- **V:** GA

Levels of sedation are considered to be on a continuum because a sedated child can go in and out of an intended level quite rapidly.

Sedation Methods

1. **Inhalation**
2. **Oral**
3. **Transmucosal**
4. **Intravenous**

The standard technique for intravenous sedation by Dental Surgeons is a titrated dose of a **single agent** (e.g. Midazolam/Propofol). Only qualified anaesthesiologists should provide moderate or deep sedation using multiple drugs.

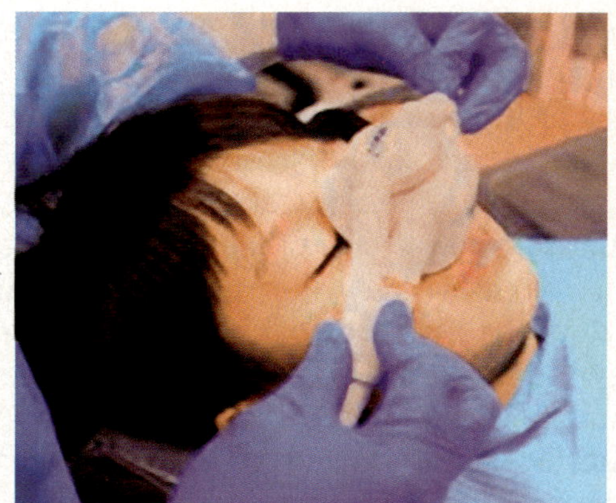

Fig. 32.8 Inhalation sedation

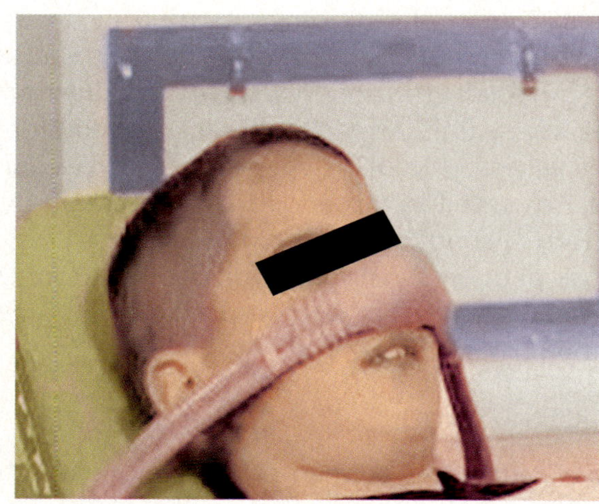

Fig. 32.9 Nasal mask

Methods other than Intravenous Routes

Inhalational sedation is achieved using a titrated mixture of up to a maximum of 70% nitrous oxide in oxygen or Sevonox. It is the first choice for paediatric dental patients who have a sufficient level of understanding to cooperate with the procedure but who are not able to tolerate local anaesthesia alone. Oral sedation is commonly achieved using midazolam or sodium trichlofos. Transmucosal routes are also equally useful and achieved by the nasal, sublingual or rectal routes using midazolam, ketamine, sufentanil.

Intravenous Sedation

This is achieved using titrated doses of inj. ketamine/propofol with or without inj. midazolam/dexmeditomidine. Inj. dexmedetomidine has been successfully used for dental sedation. Short acting agents are preferred so that discharge is faster. Inj. Propofol can be given in intermittent boluses or by target controlled infusion. Since there is a narrow margin of safety, providers should be competent and experienced and be able to manage any potential complications, e.g. airway obstruction or even cardiac arrest. Oxygen, resuscitation equipment and reversal agents (flumazenil/naloxone) should be available. Narcotics like inj. fentanyl or remifentanil are used only if the procedure is painful and local anaesthetic blocks are not given. Lytic cocktail is discouraged. The surgeon uses a pharyngeal pack to prevent any debris or blood soiling the airway. A gag or bite-block is then positioned on the side opposite the extractions to open the mouth. Downward pressure by the dentist during extraction of mandibular teeth has the potential for airway obstruction. This can be partially prevented if the dentist uses the non-extracting hand to pull up on the patient's mandible.

General Anaesthesia

General anaesthesia for dentistry is not without risk and should not be undertaken as a first-line means of anxiety control. General anaesthesia should now only be performed in the hospital setting and requires a trained anaesthetist. Complications of modern anaesthesia may be minimal, but skilled team work is required to prevent any catastrophe. Dental facility may be in a different location that easy access for emergency services may be difficult.[7]

Equipment, Monitors and Drugs

All standard equipment gadgets, monitors and drugs for anaesthesia and resuscitation should be available and checked before administering anaesthesia. This includes the anaesthesia machine with vaporizer, oxygen, nitrous oxide, paediatric breathing circuits, nasal and facial masks, oral and nasal airways, various laryngoscopes with all sizes of blades, all range of nasal and oral tracheal tubes, independent suction apparatus, etc. Difficult intubation cart should be available while dealing with various syndromic children with airway issues. Short acting and fast emergence agents are preferable as almost all patients get discharged on the same day. Defibrillator should be immediately available. The anaesthesiologist should be adequately trained in paediatric resuscitation. The modern dental chair should be capable of head-down tilt with hydraulic capability so that it may be tilted in the Trendelenberg position in the event of power failure. The anaesthesiologist must check all equipment before use and there should be immediate access to spare another apparatus in the event of failure.

Consent

Written and informed consent by the parent/ guardian is mandatory

DENTAL CHAIR ANAESTHESIA

Even though the nomenclature is dental chair anaesthesia, children are almost always made to lie flat on the dental chair which has capability of a head low position while providing general anaesthesia. Only ASA physical status class I and II patients should be administered Dental Chair Anaesthesia or Office-Based anaesthesia care. Patients with compromised airway requiring advanced airway management devices, haemodynamic instability requiring invasive monitoring and those who require prolonged postoperative care should be operated on an in-patient setting. Congenital cardiac anomalies and syndromes (predisposing to difficult airway, unstable spine, etc.) should be specifically looked for in paediatric patients.[5,6,13,14]

Preanaesthetic Preparation

The parent is explained about the anaesthetic and dental procedure and clear fluids are allowed up to 4 hours preoperatively. The older child may be psychologically prepared before the procedure.

Conduct of General Anaesthesia

Preoperative Assessment

Patients must be assessed completely as in any other case, particularly regarding their medical, social and surgical suitability for day-case anaesthesia. The feasibility of performing the procedure under local anaesthesia with or without sedation should always be considered first. If general anaesthesia needs to be given, the risks of general anaesthesia should be explained to the patient, and consent obtained.

Premedication

Premedication is rarely required, although the highly anxious or uncooperative child may benefit from a short acting benzodiazepine. EMLA cream is used to facilitate intravenous cannulation.[14] Chloral hydrate (50–100 mg/ kg^{-1}), trimeprazine (2 mg/kg^{-1}) or midazolam (0.5–0.75 mg/kg^{-1}) may be given orally mixed with a small quantity of juice to make the drug palatable. Intranasally (midazolam 0.2–0.3 mg/kg^{-1}) or inj. sufentanil or inj. ketamine are used.[14,15]

Monitoring

Minimum monitoring standards must be met for all cases undergoing sedation or general anaesthesia. This includes capnography in cases where endotracheal intubation is employed. A full range of resuscitation equipment must be available, and all equipment should be of a standard equal to that used for the administration of anaesthesia in any other setting.

Induction of Anaesthesia

The principles of day care anaesthesia should be adhered to as these patients get discharged within a few hours of their treatment. Hence ultra short acting drugs are used in these patients. In small children, gaseous induction using sevoflurane (with parental presence) is often easiest. Halothane was a popular gas for inhalational induction but has been thrown into disrepute due to its cardiovascular side effects.[16] Sevoflurane may either be introduced in 2% increments every 2 to 3 breaths to a maximum of 8%, with maintenance of anaesthesia up to 4%, or it may be introduced as a single breath induction at a concentration of 8%, with maintenance up to 4%. However, if sevoflurane is not available, halothane is preferred over isoflurane as the later is an irritant and can lead to coughing or laryngospasm. Desflurane offers the advantage of reduction in recovery time but is not a preferred gas for induction due to its pungency.[16–19]

A cannula must be inserted for all procedures unless it is for single tooth or easy extraction which takes a few seconds. Older children may have a gaseous or intravenous induction. Propofol is the agent of choice as it ensures quick recovery and good anti-emesis. However, thiopentone or ketamine can also be used.

Airway for Extractions

The choice depends on the surgery planned. Hence it is important to discuss the procedure with the surgeon. Extraction of a few easy baby teeth is done using a transparent neonatal mask over the nares. The surgeon inserts a gauze pack from one buccal sulcus to the other in order to prevent too much mouth breathing and aspiration of tooth fragments. A gag or bite-block is positioned on the side opposite the extractions to open the mouth. Total intravenous anaesthesia using propofol will be adequate for most extractions. However, the nasal mask is still used by some dental anaesthetists. Adenotonsillar hypertrophy can compromise the nasal airway and the use of nasopharyngeal airways have been shown to significantly improve airway patency and reduce episodes of airway obstruction.[20]

Laryngeal mask airway (LMA) is safe in most procedures. It provides some barrier to aspiration when compared to mask. The armoured LMA is better as it has a narrower shaft and hence occupies less space in the mouth and its flexibility makes it easier to keep out of the field. It is important to hold the LMA firmly in place during the surgery because it has a tendency to move.[21]

The airway is shared by the anaesthesiologist and dentist.[22] The operating position is semi-reclined or supine. Traditionally, dental chair anaesthesia was administered in the sitting position which caused postural hypotension and collapse of the patient. This position is not used anymore. In the supine position, the incidence of airway obstruction due to tongue fall and pharyngeal soiling of blood is high.

Airway for Restorations/Conservations

Operations for dental conservation and periodontal procedures are prolonged and involves water being squirted into the mouth. General endotracheal anaesthesia (GETA) should be given. A cuffed endotracheal tube should be preferably used and throat packing done to prevent aspiration. Nasal intubation is preferred if there is no contraindication for the same. An LMA makes the surgery difficult because it leaves a little space for the dental drill and suction. A gag or bite-block is then positioned on the side opposite the extractions to open the mouth.

Maintenance

For short procedures, spontaneous respiration using inhalational agent (sevoflurane), nitrous oxide and 50% oxygen gives flexibility and rapid recovery. Incremental doses/continuous/target controlled infusion of propofol can be used for maintenance of anaesthesia. For extensive and complicated restorations, it is better to paralyse and ventilate the patient.

Recovery

The tooth sockets may bleed after extraction especially in the presence of infection. Initially, patients are best nursed in left lateral position with a degree of head-down tilt to encourage drainage of any blood and secretions away from the larynx and administered 100% oxygen. After gentle oropharyngeal suctioning, the LMA or endotracheal tube should be removed after the return of cough reflex and consciousness. Oxygen supplementation ameliorates the severity of desaturation if extubation or LMA removal is done when the child is deep but may not prevent it. The patients are monitored in the recovery area for at least 30 minutes before returning to dental clinic. No oral fluids are given for 2–3 hours to avoid vomiting and aspiration.

Postoperative Analgesia

Extraction of baby teeth is not painful. Four quadrant restorations may be painful and the child may need Inj. paracetamol 10–15 mg/kg. Analgesia may be given rectally using paracetamol or diclofenac suppositories. Ibuprofen or paracetamol may be given orally if needed.

Fitness for Discharge

Patients should be clinically observed to be alert, oriented, and breathing adequately. Older children should be able to walk unassisted, and should be haemodynamically stable. There should be no obvious surgical complications. Simple scoring systems, like Aldrete postanaesthetic recovery score (colour, respiration, circulation, consciousness and activity) as criteria can be applied.

In-patient Anaesthesia

Oral surgical and maxillofacial surgical procedures (temporo-mandibular joint ankylosis release, fixation of maxillary, mandibular and nasal fractures, mandibular setback, maxillary advancement, osteotomies and removal of tumours) need children to be admitted in the hospital.

Pre-anaesthetic Evaluation

It is same as for any other major operation. However, it is pertinent to note that these patients can have swelling of face, missing or loose teeth, pain and trismus limiting mouth opening, etc. Thorough airway and radiographic evaluation (e.g. antero-posterior and lateral views of neck) should be done. The nasal patency should be determined to facilitate nasal intubation. Such patients may have polytrauma and complete radiological and biochemical evaluation is necessary. Children with congenital temporo mandibular joint ankylosis should have a complete sleep study and thyroid profile done preoperatively. They are susceptible to obstructive sleep apnoea and may present with hypothyroidism. Neurological evaluation is necessary in patients with co-existing head injury. Their fluid and electrolyte status must be assessed because these patients do not eat or drink well.[5]

Difficult airway trolley must be kept ready at all times. Fibre-optic intubation is the gold standard in the presence of anticipated difficult intubation. Anaesthesiologists should be capable of awake nasotracheal intubation or retrograde intubation if a paediatric fiberscope is not available.[23]

All anaesthesiologists should be trained to perform an emergency cricothyrotomy or a mini tracheostomy if the need arises. Neuromuscular blocking drugs should not be given until mask ventilation is possible. Inter-dental wires are placed in the end following fracture mandible surgeries, etc. The throat pack should be removed and patient extubated only when complete consciousness is regained. A wire cutter should always be present by the patients side in case airway obstruction occurs in the postoperative period. Steroids are administered in the postoperative period as children may have airway/facial oedema.

Clinical Pearls

1. The anaesthesiologist and the dental surgeon share the airway.
2. Uncooperative and crying children pose a great challenge .

Contd...

Clinical Pearls *(Contd...)*

3. Presence of cardiac disease, seizures, learning disability/ syndrome/retardation/ ADHD increase the risk of GA.
4. Presence of adenotonsillar hypertrophy or respiratory tract infections are associated with airway problems.
5. The airway can become soiled with blood and debris triggering a laryngospasm.
6. High vagal tone, stimulation of trigeminal nerve, needle phobia, hypoxia and hypercarbia can trigger arrhythmias.
7. Children can easily slip from one level of sedation to a deeper level easily and complete vigilance and monitoring is necessary.
8. Training in advanced airway and paediatric resuscitation is required by all those who provide sedation.
9. General anaesthesia is indicated only in a select group of patients in whom sedation cannot be given and the highest standards of anaesthesia should be maintained.
10. Principles of day care anaesthesia should be followed.

COMPLICATIONS OF DENTAL ANAESTHESIA

Hypoxaemia

There is high potential for airway obstruction resulting in hypoxaemia following dental anaesthesia. This can result from inhalation of teeth, crowns, portions of filling, etc. This obstruction is accentuated by coexisting rhinitis and hypertrophied adenoids and tonsils in young children. Airway closure occurs at lung volumes well above functional residual capacity (FRC) producing a large intrapulmonary shunt. General anaesthesia can further exacerbate the reduction in FRC and intrapulmonary shunt with resultant hypoxia.[24–26] Increasing fractional inspired oxygen concentration to 0.5 reduces intraoperative desaturation. Application of 5 cm H_2O continuous positive airway pressure (CPAP) can result in significant reduction in incidence and severity of peroperative arterial desaturation by increasing FRC and overcoming partial airway obstruction.[27]

Arrhythmias

There is a high incidence of cardiac arrhythmias due to vagal dominance in children. This can get exacerbated especially with the use of halothane.[28] They occur following light anaesthesia, elevated levels of catecholamines and trigeminal nerve stimulation. They are increased in the presence of hypercarbia or hypoxia. The arrhythmias usually occur during extraction of teeth but are transient, seldom require treatment and respond to cessation of operative stimulus.

Subcutaneous Emphysema

Subcutaneous emphysema of face and cervical areas, though rare can occur due to the use of air driven, ultra-high speed dental instruments. The air enters along the mandibular periosteum. Nitrous oxide should be discontinued on detection of emphysema and respiratory parameters closely monitored.[29]

Dislocation of Temporo-mandibular Joint

It can occur in children if mouth is opened too wide. Airway obstruction due to alteration in position of tongue is possible. The dislocation can be reduced at the end of surgery.

Operating Room Pollution

Air pollution due to anaesthetic gases is very common in dental anaesthesia areas as scavenging systems and efficient ventilation of the operating room with more than 12–15 air changes per hour are not usually present.

Hyperthermia

Tissue destruction, environmental temperature during surgery, administration of certain drugs like atropine, dehydration and bacteraemia have all been implicated in fever following dental anaesthesia. Procedures provoking bacteraemia (extractions) can be managed by routine administration of antibiotics.[30]

CONCLUSION

Children receiving general anaesthesia or sedation for dentistry should be dealt in the most safe, effective and efficient manner by a qualified anaesthesiologist trained from time to time for paediatric resuscitation. Dental treatment under general anaesthesia can be carried out in a day care facility with a high level of patient and parent satisfaction.

SUMMARY

1. The first ever general anaesthetic was administered for a dental extraction by a Connecticut dentist, Horace Wells.
2. Most dental procedures in children can successfully be completed under adequate local anaesthesia with or without sedation.
3. Paediatric patients are uncooperative, impossible to communicate and may present for dental treatment under general anaesthesia with adenotonsillar hypertrophy, respiratory tract infections with an associated increased risk of airway problems, cardiac disease, seizures, learning disability/ syndrome/ retardation/ADHD, etc.
4. Excessive gagging, high vagal tone, arrhythmias, laryngospasm increases their anaesthetic risk during deep sedation or general anaesthesia. Hence GA should never be their first-line means of anxiety control.
5. The same standards of personnel, monitoring, equipment or conduct of sedation or general anaesthesia should apply whether anaesthesia services are provided in a hospital or in a dental surgery clinic.

Multiple Choice Questions

1. The following factors predispose to arrhythmias during anaesthesia for dentistry:

A. Adenotonsillar hypertrophy
B. I.V. induction
C. Sevoflurane anaesthesia
D. Hypercarbia
E. Stimulation of the facial nerve

2. Conscious sedation:

A. Is adequate once verbal contact with the patient is lost
B. May be achieved via the trans-nasal route
C. Is most safely achieved using a combination of two different drugs in order to achieve a synergistic effect
D. May only be administered by an anaesthetist on the specialist register of the General Medical Council
E. Should only be considered where general anaesthesia is contraindicated.

3. The following may increase the chance of aspiration under a general anaesthetic for dental extraction:

A. The supine position
B. Placement of an oropharyngeal pack
C. The use of a gag or bite-block
D. Extreme patient anxiety
E. Recovery from anaesthesia in a head-up tilt position

4. Dental extraction may be most appropriately performed under conscious sedation in the following patients:

A. A patient with known allergy to local anaesthetic
B. A cooperative patient for extraction of four impacted wisdom teeth
C. An ASA class I young adult
D. A 3-year-old child for extraction of a single tooth
E. A severely mentally handicapped adult.

REFERENCES

1. Joseph A Giovannitti Jr, DMD. Dental Anaesthesia and Paediatric Dentistry. pp 95–99.
2. Poswillo D. General Anaesthesia, sedation and resuscitation in dentistry. Report of an expert working party for the standing dental advisory committee. London: Department of Health, 1990.
3. General Dental Council. Maintaining Standards. Guidance to Dentists on Professional and Personal Conduct. London: General Dental Council, 1998.
4. The Royal College of Anaesthetists. Standards and Guidelines for General Anaesthesia for Dentistry. London: The Royal College of Anaesthetists, 1999.
5. Cantlay K, Williamson S, Hawkings J. Anaesthesia for dentistry. Cont Edu Anaesth Crit Care Pain 2005;5:71–5.
6. Bajaj P. Anaesthesia and analgesia in dentistry. India:Paras Medical Publisher, 2005.
7. The Royal College of Anaesthetists. Standards and guidelines for general anaesthesia in dentistry. London: The Royal College of Anaesthetists, 1999.
8. American Academy of Paediatric Dentistry. Guidelines for the elective use of conscious sedation, deep sedation and general anaesthesia in paediatric patients. Ped Dentistry 1985;7:334.
9. Goodson JM, Moore PA. Life-threatening reactions after pedodontic sedation: An assessment of narcotic, local anesthetic, and antiemetic drug interaction. J Am Dent Assoc. 1983;107:239–45.
10. Committee on Drugs, Section on Anesthesiology, American Academy of Paediatrics. Guidelines for the elective use of conscious sedation, deep sedation, and general anaesthesia in paediatric patients. Paediatrics 1985;76:317–21.
11. American Academy of Paediatric Dentistry. Guidelines for the elective use of conscious sedation, deep sedation, and general anaesthesia in paediatric patients. ASDC J Dent Child 1986;53:21–2.
12. Standards in Conscious Sedation for Dentistry. Report of an independent expert working group. London: Society for the Advancement of Anaesthesia in Dentistry, 2000.
13. UK National Clinical Guidelines in Paediatric Dentistry. Guidelines for the use of general anaesthesia (GA) in paediatric dentistry. London, 2008.
14. Stanford J. General anaesthesia for dentistry. Anaesth Int Care Med 2008;9:344–7.
15. Flynn PJ, Strunin L. General anaesthesia for dentistry. Anaesth Int Care Med. 2005;6:263–5.
16. Paris ST, Cafferky M, Yate PM, et al. A comparison of sevoflurane and halothane for outpatient dental anaesthesia in children. BJA. 1997;79:280–4.
17. Blayney MR, Malins AF, Cooper GM. Cardiac arrhythmias in children during outpatient general anaesthesia for dentistry: A prospective randomised trial. Lancet. 1999; 354:1864–6.
18. McAteer PM, Carter JA, Cooper GM. Comparison of isoflurane and halothane in outpatient paediatric dental anaesthesia. BJA. 1986;58:390–3.
19. Loan PB, Mirakhur RK, Paxton LD, et al. Comparison of desflurane and isoflurane in anaesthesia for dental surgery. BJA. 1995;75:289–92.
20. Bagshaw ON, Southee R, Ruiz K. A comparison of the nasal mask and the nasopharyngeal airway in paediatric chair dental anaesthesia. Anaesthesia. 1997;52:786–9.
21. Quinn AC, Samaan A, McAteer EM. The reinforced laryngeal mask airway for dento-alveolar surgery. BJA. 1996;77:185–8.
22. Woodcock BJ, Michaloudis D, Young TM. Airway management in dental anaesthesia. Eur J Anaesthesiol. 1994;11:397–401.
23. Zmyslowski WP, Maloney PL. Naso-tracheal intubation in the presence of facial fractures. JAMA. 1989;262:
24. Lanigan CJ. Oxygen desaturation after dental anaesthesia. BJA 1992;68:142–5.
25. Bone ME, Galler D, Flynn PJ. Arterial oxygen saturation during general anaesthesia for paediatric dental extractions. Anaesthesia. 1987;42:879–82.
26. Fairley HB. Airway closure. Anesthesiology. 1972;36: 529–32.
27. Suresh D, Purdy G, Wainwright AP, et al. Use of continuous airway pressure in paediatric dental extraction under general anaesthesia. BJA. 1991; 66:200–4.
28. Plowman PE, Thomas WJW, Thurlow AC. Cardiac dysrhythmias during anaesthesia for oral surgery. Anaesthesia. 1974;29:571–3.
29. Rosenberg MB, Wunderlich BK, Reynolds RN. Iatrogenic subcutaneous emphysema during dental anaesthesia. Anesthesiology. 1979;51:80–1.
30. Holan G, Kadari A, Engelhard D, et al. Temperature elevation in children following dental treatment under general anaesthesia with or without prophylactic antibiotics. Ped Dentistry. 1993;15:99–103.

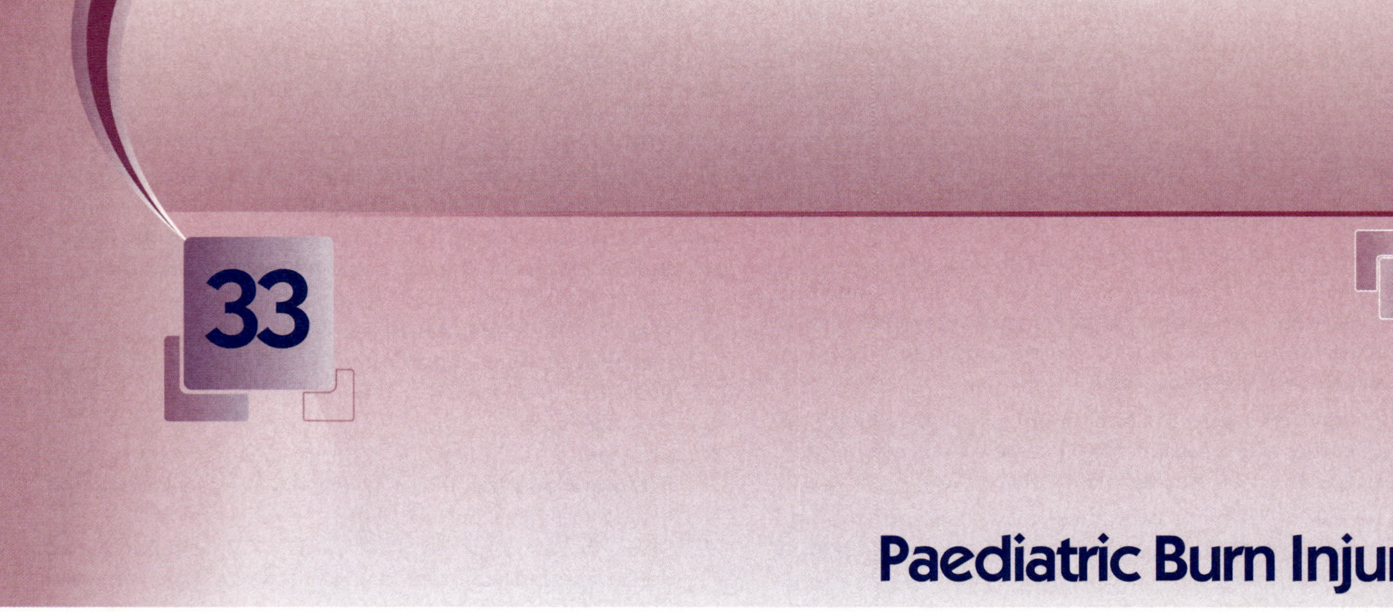

33 Paediatric Burn Injury

Rochana G Bakhshi

INTRODUCTION

Burn injuries are a major cause of mortality and morbidity, as well as a significant drain on limited health care resources. Worldwide mortality due to thermal injuries has reduced due to advances in resuscitation, critical care, protective ventilator strategies and aggressive treatment of burn wound sepsis.[1] This is also augmented by community education and prevention campaigns.

EPIDEMIOLOGY

World Health Organization (WHO) estimates show approx 1 million children sustain burn each year in the USA. Moreover fire associated burns were responsible for 3,20,000 deaths worldwide in 2002.[1]

Burn profile usually depends on the socioeconomic flux of a country. Developed nations have better prevention policies, safe kitchen technology and fuel; hence incidence of burn has reduced. In developing nations burns continue to be endemic because of slums and large scale use of stoves and fuels. A study by Ahuja et al showed that an economic uplift and shift from kerosene to LPG stoves brought down the annual burn admission in Delhi burn unit by about 43%.[2]

The at-risk paediatric population has a bimodal distribution of age. Toddlers are unaware of risk posed by heat sources, hot water, barbeque plates, etc. Older children knowingly have risk taking behavior associated with flames. Mortality also follows a bimodal pattern of early and late death. Early death occurs due to refractory shock, inability to secure airway, carbon monoxide poisoning, coexisting trauma, etc. Late deaths are due to sepsis, wound infection and multiple organ failure.[3,4] In the developed world 70% of burnt children are 4 years of age and belong to impoverished backgrounds.

INITIAL MANAGEMENT

At the scene priority is to isolate the patient from the source, once secured patient is provided with 100% oxygen and is examined for associated trauma.

Airway, breathing and circulation should be rapidly assessed while administering high flow oxygen and establishing monitors. Airway may be affected by inhalation of smoke or direct thermal injury to the face.[5] Cervical spine care is a must with immobilisation with collar, sandbags, tape or manual inline stabilisation.

History is important regarding burning in an enclosed space or explosion and whether consciousness was lost. Examine for soot around the nose, mouth, in sputum, burnt eyelashes, nasal hair, etc. Dysphonia, dysphagia, stridor should be looked for.

Hot dry gases causes supraglottic injury, steam inhalation results in deeper parenchymal injury. Blast injuries can be to chest in form of barotrauma and contusion of lung.

Airway oedema may develop quickly in such patients. Carbonaceous particles along with a variety of toxins are carried up to alveolar level. This may lead to bronchospasm, pulmonary oedema, degranulation and autolysis of pulmonary macrophages which lead to hypoxemia.

Indications for endotracheal intubation in patients with inhalation injury and burns are:

1. Decreased mental status
2. Airway obstruction due to generalised post-burn oedema

3. Pulmonary failure due to subglottic inhalation injury
4. Direct thermal injury to upper airway including tongue and mouth, larynx oropharynx causing oedema formation which may quickly progress to complete airway obstruction within minutes to hours.

Facial and airway oedema warrant that an experienced anaesthesiologist performs the intubation. Use of paralytic agents should be guarded so as to avoid the 'cant ventilate, cant intubate' situation. Short acting agents such as fentanyl, propofol or midazolam may be used with caution.

In patients requiring intubation following **considerations to be kept in mind:**

1. Smaller tube may have to be used due to airway oedema.
2. Practice of cutting the endotracheal tube should not be routinely done in cases as facial swelling may increase dramatically and 'bury' the end of an inappropriately short tube somewhere within the mouth.
3. Tube should be sufficiently in so that the distal end is not drawn out of the trachea by effects of mucosal oedema.
4. Neck burns may make tracheotomy difficult though it may be ideal for the patient.

During transport there can be accidental extubation and catastrophic loss of airway. Thus cotton tape is used to secure the tube. Tube may be obstructed due to copious mucous production.

In burns >10%, nasogastric tube for gastric decompression should be put.

Circulation

Hypovolemic shock occurring in the first few hours after a significant burn may be due to other injury which should be ruled out.

Large venous access should be obtained in at least two unburnt sites.

Skin creases over the femoral vessels often spare this site.

Blood samples should be sent for full blood count, electrolytes, glucose and cross-match.

Haematocrit rises initially due to plasma loss but anaemia may follow due to hemolysis, recurring surgical blood loss and sepsis induced marrow suppression.

Burnt epidermis permits large evaporation fluid losses of up to 200 mL/m^2/hr. These and other fluid losses cause hypoalbuminaemia and shock.

Inadequate fluid replacement leads to hypoperfusion and renal failure, while excessive fluid will lead to tissue oedema and increasing burn depth. Monitoring includes heart rate (HR), blood pressure (BP), oxygen saturation, urinary output (UO), complete blood count, albumin and lactate levels. Urine output in children should be >2 mL/kg/hr.

The 6 'c' approach should be applied for wound care[6]

- Remove nonsticking Clothing
- Cooling with water
- Cleaning with chlorhexidine
- Chemoprophylaxis
- Covering with layer of gauze impregnated with petroleum jelly wrapped with absorbent gauze
- Pain Cure

FLUID CALCULATION IN BURNS

The parkland formula (ringer lactate at the rate of 4 mL/kg/TBSA% burn/24 hours, with 50% given during first 8 hours, is based on the amount of fluid necessary to replace sodium loss.[7]

The Evans formula (RL 1 mL/kg/TBSA% burns + D5W at 2 L/m/24 hrs is suitable for children. When burns are more than 50% TBSA, they are treated at 50% TBSA rates, on day 2, 50% day 1 requirement are used.[8] In very small children (i.e. <10 kg), it may be necessary to add glucose to their IV fluids to avoid hypoglycaemia.

After 48 hours, fluids are given for maintenance and replacement of evaporative losses.

Evaporation losses = (25 mL + TBSA% burn) × (m^2)/hr

After 12–24 hrs, if Albumin is <2 gm/dl, Alb 5% at 15 mL/hr or 25% at 3 mL/hr is given.[9]

PATHOPHYSIOLOGY OF BURNS IN CHILDREN

Before understanding the management and assessment, we should know the pathophysiology of burns and assessment in paediatric population.

Fluid loss from the burnt area begins immediately and lasts for about 36 hours. Fluid shifts and loss occur due to microvasculature and cell membrane.[7] Plasma loss may be more than 4 mL/kg/hr and sodium loss 0.5 meq/kg/% total body surface area (TBSA).

Children may go into hypovolemic shock even with 10% TBSA burn.

Coagulation, stasis and hyperaemia are the three recognized zones of burn injury.[10]

Zone of coagulation is an area where irreversible coagulation of tissue protein has occurred and is almost unsalvagable.

Decreased tissue perfusion characterizes the zone of stasis. So initial treatments aims at improving blood flow to this area so as to prevent extension of injury.

The third hyperaemic zone which is outermost is least at risk unless infection ensues (Fig. 33.1).

Illustration of zones of burn injury. The centre part (zone of coagulation shown in red) is the worst affected and the one surrounding it (orange zone of stasis) is characterized by decreased tissue perfusion. The burn depth in this zone can be prevented from worsening by appropriate first aid and adequate initial fluid resuscitation. The body surface area in children is different from adults due to large head as shown in Fig. 33.2.

Burnt epidermis permits large evaporative fluid losses of up to 200 mL/m^2/hr. These and other fluid losses cause hypoalbuminaemia and shock.

Inadequate fluid replacement leads to hypoperfusion and renal failure, while excessive fluid will lead to tissue oedema and increasing burn depth. Monitoring includes heart rate (HR), blood pressure (BP), oxygen saturation, urinary output (UO), complete blood count, and albumin and lactate levels. Urine output in children should be >2 mL/kg/hr.

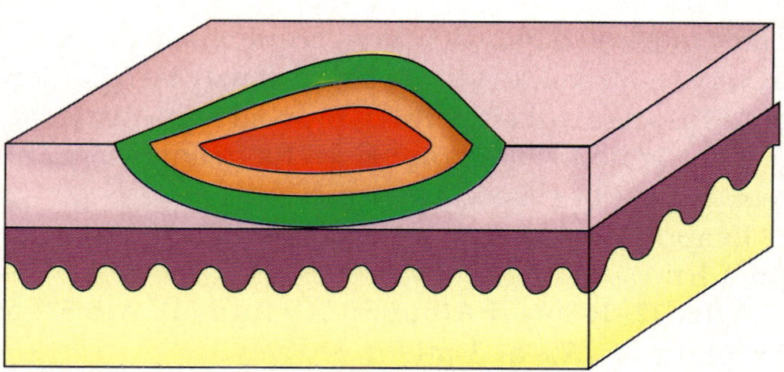

Fig. 33.1 Third hyperaemic zone

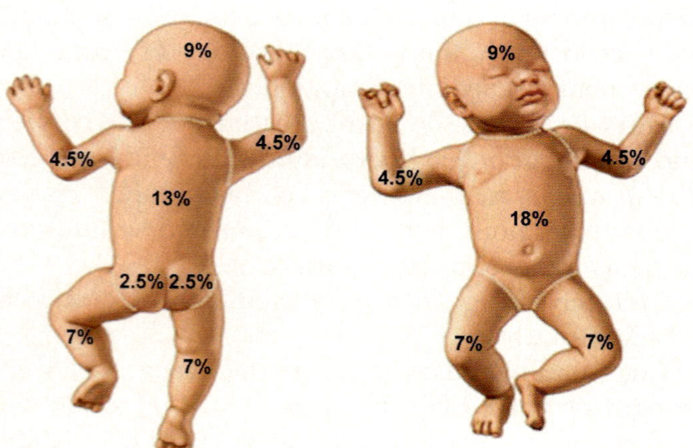

Fig. 33.2 Body surface area in children

Burn injury leads to a state of hypermetabolism and protein hypercatabolism that persists till skin remains uncovered. Early excision and skin cover can reduce this hypermetabolic state but protracted protein loss can occur up to a year after burn injury. So caloric and protein requirements are increased to two to 2.5 times the normal.

Caloric Requirements

Caloric requirements in children can be calculated using Galveston formula:

(1800 Kcal/m^2) + (1300 Kcal/m^2 burnt)

Calories should be provided as 60% carbohydrates, 25% protein and 15% fat.[11]

Proteins are provided as per body weight, i.e. 1.2–2 gm/kg/day or the calorie/nitrogen ratio (CNR).

A CNR of 150 for minor burns and 100 for major burns.[12,13]

- A positive nitrogen balance of 0–4 gm/day is the goal.
- Nitrogen balance = [protein intake (gm) × 16%] mg/dL
- Water deficit = 0.6 × (kg) × {(plasma Na/140) –1}
- Water Excess = 0.6 × (kg) × {1– (plasma Na/140)}

Systemic effects of burn injury

Haematologic alterations: Initially there is a red cell (RBC) loss in proportion to the degree of burns. RBCs get directly destroyed due to burns and due to loss into capillary thrombi produced by complement and coagulation cascade activation. Oxygen free radicals and proteases also destroy RBCs. In the first 24 hours RBC loss may be up to 20% and later on at a rate of 1% to 2% per day till the wounds are grafted.[14] Increased haemoglobin during burn resuscitation indicates hemoconcentration and the need for more fluid to be infused. During recovery phase bone marrow remains hyporesponsive probably due to high circulating levels of cytokines and other inflammatory mediators. Platelets decrease immediately after burns due to increased aggregation, consumption during formation of microemboli and dilution due to fluid resuscitation. Platelet count will increase after 10 to 14 days. One has to keep in mind the likelihood of disseminated intravascular coagulation (DIC) due to activation of fibrinolytic and thrombotic pathways.[15]

In children, during recovery phase, factor V, VII and VIII and fibrinogen may be elevated for several weeks to months.

Renal effects: Renal function impairment may be due to hypotension, hypovolemia, hypoxemia, haemoglobinuria, myoglobinuria, etc. Inadequate resuscitation exacerbates renal damage due to decreased renal blood flow. Oliguria during resuscitation is due to decrease in renal blood flow.[16] Goal is to maintain a urine output of 0.5 to 1 mL/kg/hr. Increased circulating glucose levels may induce an osmotic diuresis which may give a false sense of well-being that renal blood flow is adequate. Children with more than 40% burns may have tubular dysfunction and inadequate response to antidiuretic hormone (ADH) and aldosterone. Renal failure may set in 5 days after burns. The kidneys may be affected by nephrotoxic antibiotics, stress hormones and circulating free haemoglobin.

In spite of fluid resuscitation pharmacology of drugs excreted by kidney may be unpredictable.

Hepatic effects: Liver may also be affected due to factors like hypovolemia, hypotension, hypoxemia, hypoperfusion due to release of cytokines such as interleukin 1 and tumor necrosis factor, etc. Hepatic oedema with release of liver enzymes may occur.[17] Once burn shock has resolved, liver blood flow increases due to the hyper metabolic phase and metabolism of glucose and fats also increases. Hepatic protein synthesis is affected with a drop in formation of constitutive proteins such as albumin, prealbumin and transferrin.

Burn Shock

Children with major burns may exhibit systemic inflammatory response syndrome (SIRS) which manifests as tachycardia, tachypnoea, fever, and leucocytosis with refractory hypotension. In the worst form, multiple organ dysfunction syndromes (MODS) may develop. Tumor necrosis factor alpha is released from macrophages in response to local or systemic injury. It activates an antimicrobial defence mechanism and tissue repair, but in turn leads to release of other mediators such as interleukins; IL-1, IL-6, and interferon gamma (IFN gamma). Interleukins potentiate the destructive effects of TNF and IFN stimulates cytokine secretion, phagocytosis and the respiratory burst activity of macrophages thus amplifying the inflammatory response.[18]

Chemokines such as IL-8 play a role in tissue destruction. Non-cytokine factors such as platelet activation factor, eicosanoids, leukotrienes and thromboxane A_2 also contribute to SIRS and MODS. Complement activation also causes leucocyte attraction and activation leading to cellular destruction through the release of reactive oxygen intermediates and proteases.[19]

A child with inadequate resuscitation may not be able to increase his cardiac output to the extent needed to maintain arterial pressure in presence of excess vasodilatation with signs of shock and hypotension. Once adequately resuscitated, there is hyperdynamic circulation with low systemic vascular resistance and high cardiac output.

Anaesthetic Considerations

Pharmacologic Considerations

In the early or resuscitative phase of burn injury several factors such as increased blood viscosity, hypovolemia, and decreased cardiac function lead to decreased blood flow to organs and tissues.

In the second stage of burn injury, known as hypermetabolic phase, hypermetabolism and increased blood flow to all major organs are predominant. It is still unclear if drug metabolism is increased.[20]

Acidic drugs such as benzodiazepines and antiepileptics are bound to albumin and basic drugs such as muscle relaxants and tricyclic antidepressants are bound to alpha-1 acid glycoprotein.

In the early or acute phase albumin may critically fall and drugs bound to albumin have an increased free component, whereas drugs bound to alpha-1 acid glycoprotein have a decreased free component. Therefore, muscle relaxants have lower free fractions. Resistance to atracurium, vecuronium and pancuronium have been noted. It may also be attributed to increased number of receptors on muscle membranes. This effect begins about sixth day, peaks at 15 to 40 days and may decrease by day 70. Some resistance has been seen even at 500 days after burns. Despite all this, serum half life is unchanged and reversal of neuromuscular blockade is not a problem.

The well known hyperkalemic response of succinylcholine warrants word of caution against this drug. Onset of hyperkalemia is as early as 24 to 48 hours post burns and may continue for 2 years after.[21]

Airway Problems

Child with Scalds and Inhalation Injury

Children with scald injuries without inhalation injury, younger than 3 years old and more than 19% burns, may require endotracheal intubation. One should avoid high peak inspiratory pressures and high cuff pressures.

Thoracic eschar syndrome: Patients with circumferential deep burns of the chest often develop respiratory compromise, whether or not inhalation injury is present. The cause of this syndrome is progressive oedema formation beneath the tight, inelastic skin which generates a straight jacket like impediment to respiratory excursion. Decreased compliance during bag ventilation, increasing peak airway pressures when on ventilator, and rising end tidal carbon dioxide ($ETCO_2$) and partial arterial pressure of carbon dioxide ($PaCO_2$), one must rule out kinking, dislodged or obstructed endotracheal tube or tension pneumothorax. Once ruled out, bedside escharotomy has to be done as rapidly as possible.

Other causes of impaired ventilation in these patients include severe bronchoconstriction, which responds to inhaled bronchodilators. Recent pharmacologic option for treating airway inhalation injury is inhaled heparin. Desai and colleagues reported a reduction in reintubation rates and mortality in burnt children who were treated with inhaled heparin and N-acetylcysteine in adults with smoke inhalation injury.[22]

Children have smaller airways and endotracheal tubes, hence more vulnerable to airway obstruction.[23] Obstructing clots and casts are common life threatening problems during acute phase of burn injury and hence some authors routinely recommend nebulized heparin to all patients with smoke inhalation injury.

CHRONIC AIRWAY PROBLEMS

Managing the difficult airway in the burns is most challenging due to deranged pathophysiology. Facial burns can cause severe airway compromise a restricted mouth opening, distorted anatomy of neck, making the larynx more anterior, limited extension which contribute to a difficult laryngoscopic view. The loss of airway can prove to be disastrous and lead to permanent neurological damage due to cerebral anoxia or intra-cerebral haemorrhage.

Simple manoeuvres like putting a one inch thick layer of padding beneath the infant's or toddler's entire torso will preserve the neutral alignment of spine and maintain a patent airway as shown in Fig. 33.3.

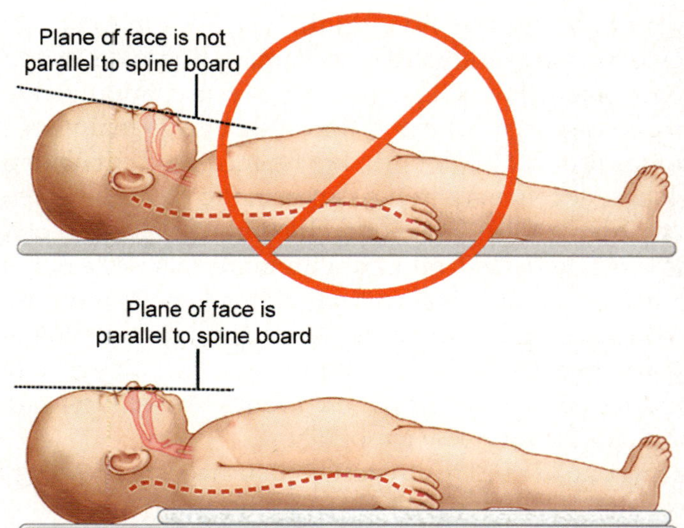

Fig. 33.3 Neutral alignment of spine

Mortality from difficult airway management is very high in neonate and young children and is estimated at 30–40% deaths related to anaesthesia practice.

In addition to above, the differing anatomy from adult airway, such as relatively large head size which flexes the neck, large size of tongue, short neck, anteriorly located larynx, small oral aperture adds to the difficulty.

Any blind intubation can make the endotracheal tube lodge in the anterior commissure as the vocal cords are angled in this age group.

Due to difficult airway anatomy preoperative sedation in a child is not always feasible. Predicting difficult airway in the children between age of 0 and 15 years has invariably proved inaccurate in spite of applying Samsoon and Young modification of airway assessment.

Excessive crying due to separation from the parents and generalized restlessness due to unfamiliar atmosphere are the other issues of concern of anaesthesiologist.

CARBON MONOXIDE POISONING (CO)

Combustion of organic material in oxygen depleted environments results in formation of carbon monoxide and cyanide. Inhaled CO has 200 times affinity to haemoglobin as compared to oxygen, forming carboxy Hb. Pulse oximeter cannot distinguish oxy Hb from carboxy Hb giving erroneously high readings. If carboxy haemoglobin is between 5 and 20%, the child should be on high flow oxygen which hastens the dissociation of carboxy Hb. If levels exceed 20%, metabolic acidosis and coma can ensure hyperbaric oxygen therapy is the treatment of choice, if not available at least endotracheal intubation and 100% oxygen should be instituted.

Cyanide poisoning can also occur as incomplete combustion of household plastics in presence of low oxygen can give rise to cyanide formation. Cyanide poisoning results in metabolic acidosis, coma and unusually high venous oxygen saturation as cyanide prevents cells from using oxygen.

Carbon monoxide also impairs mitochondrial function and carboxyhaemoglobin (coHb) causes brain injury as a result of oxidative stress, inflammation and excitatory amino acids. The standard 2-wave length pulse oximeter will falsely provide a high peripheral saturation of oxygen reading (SpO_2), even when coHb is in the lethal range >50, as it cannot discriminate between coHb and oxygenated Hb. An arterial saturation of oxygen (SaO_2) reading derived from an arterial blood gas sample and analysed using a co-oximeter will show depressed haemoglobin oxygen saturation. The half life of coHb using 100% oxygen was 7.4 min + 25 but ranged from 26 to 148 mins.[24]

Hyperbaric oxygen therapy (HBOT) is the mainstay of treatment in carbon monoxide poisoning. HBOT accelerates carbon monoxide clearance beyond that achieved using 100% oxygen at 1 atmosphere; the main rationale for its use is prevention of delayed neurocognitive syndrome. This syndrome produces memory loss and other cognitive defects, with onset from 2–28 days after exposure.[25]

The Cochrane group reviewed 6 randomised controlled trials of HBOT prevention of neurologic sequelae and concluded that the efficacy of HBOT in this setting is uncertain.[26] Patients with smoke inhalation injury, burns and carbon monoxide poisoning may not always benefit with HBOT.[27]

Cyanide (HCN) is the other metabolic asphyxiant. It is produced by combustion of plastics, foam, paints, wool and silk. It impairs cellular use of oxygen by binding to the terminal cytochrome on the electron transport chain, causing lactic acidosis and an elevated mixed venous saturation. Rapid assay of cyanide is not available. Half life of cyanide in are available for cyanide poisoning. An antidote kit available in the US contains amyl nitrite for inhalation and sodium thiosulphate for IV injection.

The nitrites oxidise haemoglobin to methaemoglobin, which chelates HCN. Sodium thiosulfate combines with HCN to form thiocyanate which inhalation injury and suspected cyanide poisoning is discouraged. The nitrates can cause severe hypotension and the methaemoglobin does not transport oxygen; particularly in patients with burn shock and impaired transport and use of oxygen resulting from carbon monoxide and HCN poisoning.[8] So without knowing CoHb and methaemoglobin levels, nitrites should be restricted. Sodium thiosulfate is safer, but of slow onset.

Recently hydroxocobalamin (a form of vitamin B_{12}) is available as intravenous injection in the US, this drug is well tolerated and rapidly chelates HCN.[29]

SEPSIS

Infection is the leading cause of death in patients who survive the acute phase of burn injury.

Patients with extensive thermal or smoke inhalation injury are prone to develop pneumonia, secondary to gram negative invasion, e.g. *Pseudomonas aeruginosa or klebsiella pneumoniae* or gram positive such as *Staphylococcus aureus*. Indiscriminate antibiotic use can predispose to colonisation with multidrug resistant organisms.

Burnt skin produces a toxic lipid protein complex (LPC) cutaneous burn toxin (CBT) that is highly immunosuppressive. There is suppression of humoral and cellular specific immune functions and neutrophil and macrophage non-specific immune functions.[30] Burns increase bowel permeability and translocation of bacteria and absorption of endotoxins.[31] The other sources of infection commonly are Intravenous catheters; burn wound infection, endotracheal intubation, urinary catheters, etc. In children the most common infections are burn wound infection and catheter associated septicaemia. Wound biopsy in order to quantify organism count (>100,000/gm), stage the invasive process and to identify type of infection, bacterial, fungal or viral, could be done. Bacterial or fungal infections need wound debridements and appropriate systemic and topical antibiotics. Candidial infections may follow, if there is delayed wound closure or extensive use of broad spectrum antibiotics. Tetanus prophylaxis has to be given to all patients.

PAIN MANAGEMENT

Despite major advances in burn wound management and survival, burn pain is inadequately treated globally. This is because of its complexity and lack of specific education in healthcare professionals. Burns are classified by thickness and area affected, yet pain does not always correlate accordingly. Afferent nerve destruction associated with deeper burns theoretically reduces the amount of pain experienced, but in clinical practice this is not a reliable predictor.

Pain is perceived at the time and site of burn, due to stimulation of local nociceptors and transmission of the nerve impulse in Aδ and C fibres, thereby relaying the pain message to the dorsal horn of the spinal cord.

During initial phase of burns there is decreased blood flow to the organs and subsequent decrease in drug clearance. Later on the metabolism increases so clearance of drug increases. One has to be cautious about drugs with high protein binding as in more than 20% burns there is large amount of capillary leakage and loss of interstitial proteins.

Four patterns of pain have been observed in burn patients. There may be constant pain at rest and in motion (background pain), aggravated by episodes of intense and sudden pain (breakthrough pain), pain during procedures and pain in postop period. There are various pain scales available for pain assessment but for young children behavioural observational scales are in use such as the FLACC score.

A major contributing factor to poor pain management is the difficulty children have in expressing their pain and problems that the health professionals may have in interpreting and assessing this information correctly.

FLACC tool:[32] (Face, Legs, Activity, Cry and Consolability)

FLACC is a behavioural assessment tool. It has five categories where each has a score of 0–2. The overall score lies between 0 and 10. The child is observed for 2–5 minutes and body activity, face, and cry noted according to the scale.

Faces/Ladder Scale

Children as young as three years old can communicate and make judgements about their pain.[33] Wong-Baker FACES Pain Rating Scale can be used for children ≥3 years of age.[34] The faces/ladder scale should be explained to the child, telling him that, the smiling face indicates no pain and the distressed face indicates severe pain. The wording can be read by the older child and he states the degree of pain either by using the numbers or faces on scale of 0–10 (Fig. 33.4).

0 : no pain
1 : very little pain
2 : tingling
3 : little bit sore
4 : aching
5 : stinging
6 : banging
7 : feels awful
8 : really hurts
9 : pain going out of control
10 : worst pain ever

Pharmacotherapy

An ideal analgesic in a child should have the following characteristics:

i. easy to administer
ii. well tolerated

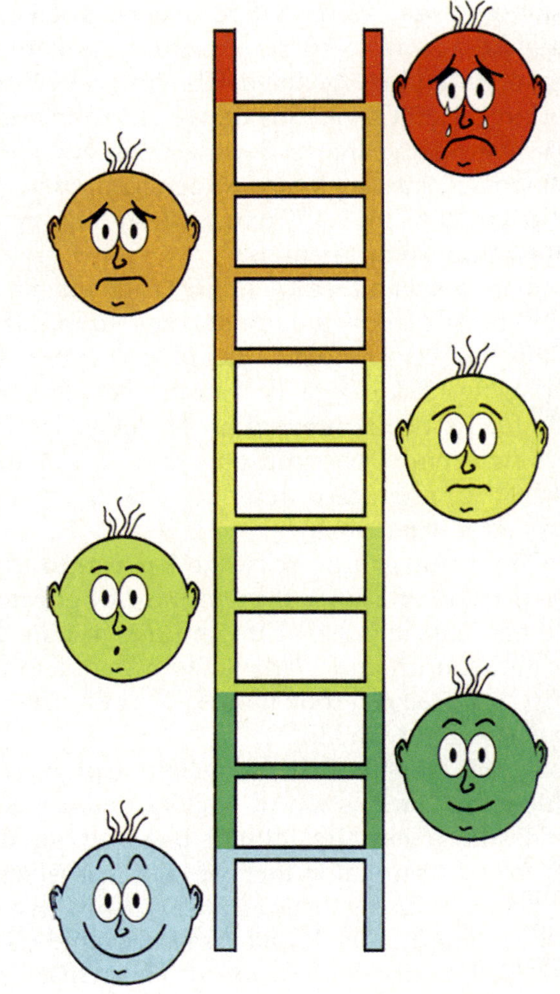

Fig. 33.4 Pain ladder

iii. rapid onset of analgesia with short duration of action
iv. minimal side-effects

In acute setting drugs should be given by the IV route. Intranasal route is a good alternative as it avoids painful injection, has rapid onset and good bioavailability.

Paracetamol: A p-aminophenol derivative that exhibits antipyretic and analgesic activity. It has both central and peripheral analgesic action. The IV route allows rapid passage in the systemic circulation and hence rapid onset of action. Used along with opiods it has a synergistic effect. Meyer et al described its use in the treatment of background pain in children after acute burn injury.

NSAIDS have analgesic and anti-inflammatory properties. They act via nonselective inhibition of prostaglandin and thromboxane synthesis via inhibition of cyclooxygenase enzyme (inhibits platelet aggregation and renal prostaglandin production). Side effects may limit the use of NSAIDS.

Opioids: Pain at rest is moderate and should be treated with moderate potency drugs. Opioids have a good flexibility regarding potency, route of administration and duration of action tailored to every patient.

Morphine has the lowest lipid solubility of all the opioids, which accounts for its slow entry into the brain and subsequent delayed onset of clinical effect. Its peak analgesic effect occurs 10–20 minutes after IV administration of a bolus dose of 0.1 mg/kg. Children should be managed in a High Dependency or Intensive Care area. (Dosage for children < 6 months of age is 0–12.5 μg/kg/hour and for children > 6 months of age is 0–25 μg/kg/hour.) Rate and dosage should be adjusted according to child's pain and sedation scores.

Morphine can be delivered by NCA (nurse controlled analgesia)—usually in a high dependency setting. Bolus dose is 20 μg/kg with a background infusion of 0–20 μg/kg/hour and a lock out interval of 20–60 minutes. Criteria for administration of a bolus dose are if the pain score is seven or more on a scale of 0–10 and the sedation score no greater than one. Respiratory rate should be above minimum rate for the age of the child and oxygen saturation must be monitored by continuous pulse oximetry.

Fentanyl: A synthetic, potent narcotic analgesic with potency up to 100 times that of morphine is highly lipid soluble and has a rapid onset of action (1–2 min). The duration of analgesia is about 60 minutes. Possible side effects include hypotension, bradycardia, apnoea, chest wall spasm, muscle rigidity, and respiratory depression. Fentanyl lozenges are a solid formulation of fentanyl citrate on a stick in the form of a lollipop that dissolves slowly in the mouth for transmucosal absorption. Doses around 15–20 μg/kg seem satisfactory and provide rapid onset (10 min) of pain relief.[35,36] In children, 10 μg/kg is equianalgesic to Oxycodone 0.2 mg/kg.[37]

Intranasal fentanyl has been shown to be equivalent to oral morphine in the provision of analgesia for burn wound dressing changes in children. Intranasal fentanyl may be a suitable analgesic agent for use in paediatric burns dressing changes either alone or in combination with oral morphine as a top up agent.[38]

Remifentanil: A novel, ultrashort-acting esterase metabolized synthetic opioid. It is a selective "mu" opioid agonist and has an ester linkage rendering it susceptible to rapid metabolism by nonspecific blood and tissue esterases. Remifentanil has been used for postoperative analgesia in neonates and has been found to have a similar pharmacological profile in neonates to that of older children and adults. Le Floch et al.[39] identified Remifentanil on its own to be a useful agent for undertaking dressing changes in spontaneously breathing, nonintubated burn patients.

Ketamine: Acts both in the central and peripheral nervous system. It exerts strong adjuvant analgesic properties by inhibiting the binding of glutamate to the NMDA-R receptor. This mode of action is different to the action of opioid drugs such as morphine and therefore the use of ketamine in combination with morphine can improve pain relief. Ketamine in combination with morphine reduces the need for high dose of morphine to be used and therefore minimises side effects.[40,41]

Entonox: A homogenous gas made of 50% nitrous oxide and 50% oxygen, is a potent analgesic that may be used for changing the burn dressing in some conscious children.[42] It is self-administered using a demand apparatus that safeguards against inadvertent overdose. Entonox is quick acting due to the insoluble nature of nitrous oxide and wears off rapidly once administration ceases. It can either be used alone or in conjunction with other analgesics. Entonox is contraindicated in situations such as decreased consciousness, pneumothorax or air embolism (where expansion of the air trapped within the body might be dangerous), or gross abdominal distension.

Newer Agents

Alpha 2 Adrenergic Antagonists. Maintaining appropriate sedation and analgesia in children with burns can be quite challenging and often requires high doses of analgesics and anxiolytics because tolerance develops quickly. Escalating doses of opioids and benzodiazepines provide a little additional benefit while increasing the incidence of side effects. Clonidine acts by augmenting descending inhibitory spinal cord pathways. The dose used in paediatric practice is 1–3 μg/kg three times a day orally or IV.[43] Clonidine is known to reduce the need for morphine in the management of postoperative pain. The addition of clonidine to the pharmacological treatment of burn pain offers a possible adjunct to the standard opioid and benzodiazepines regimen. When clonidine is no longer required the dose must be reduced gradually to avoid withdrawal and rebound hypertension.

Dexmedetomidine is a novel alpha 2-adrenergic agonist that provides sedation, anxiolysis, and analgesia with much less respiratory depression than other sedatives.[44]

Gabapentin has established efficacy in the reduction of burn-induced hyperalgesia. It binds to presynaptic calcium channels involved in pain hypersensitivity and indirectly inhibits NMDA receptor overactivation.[45] Gabapentin is started at 10 mg/kg and titrated up to 40–50 mg/kg/day. Recent studies have found gabapentin to be useful in the management of neuropathic pain following burn injury but further research is required to define its precise usage.[46] On a different role, Gabapentin has also been found to be effective in the management of itch in children (common after burn injury) unresponsive to simple anti-itch medications such as chlorpheniramine and trimeprazine.[47]

Non-pharmacological Treatments

Various non-pharmacological strategies such as education (understanding of the condition), distraction, relaxation, cutaneous stimulation, acupuncture, biofeedback, hypnosis, imagery, cognitive, and behavioural techniques can be employed to treat the pain associated with burns. Distraction techniques such as talking, singing, praying, describing photographs, listening to music, and playing games reduces the perception of pain by stimulating the descending control system that leads to painful stimuli being transmitted to the brain.[48] Used in conjunction, these modalities help reduce analgesic requirements.[49]

SUMMARY

Paediatric burn patients are best managed by a multidisciplinary team comprising of physicians, nurses, physical therapists, blood bank and laboratory services and social workers. Patients need to be catered to not just in acute phase but also long term over the years when they come for repeated surgeries. The anaesthetic approach should be geared to the constantly changing physical condition of the patient.

REFERENCES

1. Fraser JF,Venkatesh BS. Recent advances in management of burns. Australasin Anaesthesia, 2005;pp. 23–33.
2. Ahuja RB, Bhattacharya S. An analysis of 11, 196 burns admissions and evaluation of conservative management techniques. Burns. 2002;28:555–61.
3. Housinger TA, Brinkerhoff C, Warden GD. The relationship between platelet count, sepsis, and survival in pediatric burn patients. Arch Surg. 1993;128(1):65-6; discussion 6–7.
4. Sheridan RL. Sepsis in pediatric burn patients. Pediatr Crit Care Med. 2005;6(3):S112–119.
5. Cancio LC. Airway management and smoke inhalation injury in the burn patient. Clin Plastic Surg. 2009;36: 555–67.
6. Morgan ED, Bledsoe SC, Barker J. Ambulatory management of burns. Am Fam Physician. 2000;62:2015–26,2029–30,2032.
7. Demling RH. Fluid resuscitation after major burns. JAMA. 1983;250:1438–40.
8. Latarjet J. A simple guide to burn treatment. International Society for Burn Injuries in collaboration with the World Health Organization. Burns. 1995;21:221–5.
9. Sheridan RL, Prelack K, Cunningham JJ. Physiologic hypoalbuminemia is well tolerated by severely burned children. J Trauma. 1997;43:448–52.
10. Hettiaratchy S, Dziewulski P. "ABC of burns: pathophysiology and types of British Medical Journal. 2004; 328(7453):1427–1429. Erratum appears in British Medical Journal. 2004;329(7458):148.
11. Garrel DR, Razi M, Lariviere F, et al. Improved clinical status and length of care with low-fat nutrition support in burn patients. JPEN J Parenter Enteral Nutr. 1995;19: 482–91.
12. Larsson J, Lennmarken C, Martensson J, et al. Nitrogen requirements in severely injured patients. Br J Surg 1990; 77:413–6.
13. Matsuda T, Kagan RJ, Hanumadass M, et al. The importance of burn wound size in determining the optimal calorie: Nitrogen ratio. Surgery. 1983;94:562–8.
14. Deitch EA, Sittig KM. A serial study of the erythropoietic response to thermal injury. Ann Surg. 1993;217:293.
15. Kowal-Vern A, Gamelli RL, Walenga JM, et al. The effect of burn wound size on hemostasis: A correlation of the hemostatic changes to the clinical state. J Trauma. 1992; 33:50.
16. Aikawa N, Wakabayashi G, Ueda M, et al. Regulation of renal function in thermal injury. J Trauma. 1990;30:S174.
17. Jeschke MG, Low JFA, Spies M, et al. Cell proliferation, apoptosis, NF-KappaB expression, enzyme, protein and weight changes in livers of burned rats. Am J Physiol Gastrointest liver Physiol. 2001;280:G1314.
18. Tominaga K, Yoshimoto T, Torigoe K, et al. IL-1 synergizes with IL-8 or IL-1β for IFN-γ production from human T cells. Int Immunol. 2000;12:151.
19. Czermak BJ, Sarma V, Pierson CL, et al. Protective effects of C5a blockade in sepsis. Nature Med. 1999;5:788.

20. McCall JE, Fischer CG. Anesthesia for children with burns in Smith's Anesthesia for Infants and Children; 7th edn. Mosby Elsevier. 2006;975–90.
21. Martyn JA. Succinylcholine hyperkalemia after burns. Anesthesiology. 1999;91:321.
22. Desai MH, MlCak R, Richardson J, et al. Reduction in mortality in pediatric patients with inhalation injury with aerosolized heparin/N acetylcysteine therapy. J Burn Care Rehab. 1998;19:210–2.
23. Canciol C. Airway management and smoke Inhalation Injury in Burn Patients; Clin Plastic Surg. 2009;36;555–67.
24. Weaver LK, Howe S, Hopkins R, et al. Carboxy hemoglobin half life in carbon monoxide—poisoned patients treated with 100% oxygen at atmospheric pressure. Chest. 2000; 117:801–8.
25. Piantadosi CA. Carbon monoxide poisoning. N Engl JMed. 2002;347:1054–5.
26. Juurlink DN, Buckley NA, Stanbrook MB, et al. Hyperbaric oxygen for carbon monoxide poisoning. Cochrane Database Syst Rev. 2005;CD002041.
27. Grube BJ, Marvin A, Heimbach DM. Therapeutic hyperbaric oxygen: help or hindrance in burn patients with carbon monoxide poisoning. J Burn Care Rehabil 1988; 9:249–52.
28. Kirk MA, Gerace R, Kuliq KW. Cyanide and methhemoglobin kinetics in smoke inhalation victims treated with the cyanide antidote kit.Ann Emerg Med. 1993;22:1413–8.
29. Borron SW, Baud FJ, Barriot P, et al. Prospective study of hydroxocobalamine for acute cyanide poisoning in smoke inhalation. Ann Emerg Med. 2007;49;794–801.
30. Stratta RJ, Warden GD, Ninnerman JL, et al. Immunologic parameters in burned patients: Effect of therapeutic interventions. J Trauma. 1986;26:7–17.
31. Ziegler TR, Smith RJ, O'Dwyer ST, et al. Increased intestinal permeability associated with infection in burn patients. Arch Surg. 1998;123:1313–9.
32. Merkel S, Volpel-Lewis T, Shayevitz J, et al. "The FLACC: a behavioural scale for scoring postoperative pain in young children," Paediatric Nursing. 1997;23(3)293–297.
33. Rømsing J, Møller-Sonnergaard J, Hertel S, et al. "Postoperative pain in children: comparison between ratings of children and nurses," Journal of Pain and Symptom Management. 1996;11(1):42–46.
34. Wong DL, Hockenberry-Eaton M, Wilson D, et al. Wong's Essentials of Pediatric Nursing, CV Mosby, St. Louis, Mo, USA, 6th edn. 2001.
35. Stanley TH, Leiman BC, Rawal N, et al. "The effects of oral transmucosal fentanyl citrate premedication on preoperative behavioral responses and gastric volume and acidity in children," Anesthesia and Analgesia. 1989; 69(3):328–335.
36. Schechter NL, Weisman SJ, Rosenblum M, et al. "The use of oral transmucosal fentanyl citrate for painful procedures in children," Pediatrics. 1995;95(3)335–339.
37. Sharar SR, Carrougher CJ, Selzer K, et al. "A comparison of oral transmucosal fentanyl citrate and oral oxycodone for pediatric outpatient wound care," Journal of Burn Care and Rehabilitation. 2002;23(1)27–31.
38. Borland ML, Bergesio R, Pascoe EM, et al. "Intranasal fentanyl is an equivalent analgesic to oral morphine in paediatric burns patients for dressing changes: a randomised double blind crossover study," Burns. 2005;31(7): 831–837.
39. Le Floch R, Naux E, Pilorget A, et al. "Use of remifentanil for analgesia during dressing change in spontaneously breathing non-intubated burn patients," Annals of Burns and Fire Disasters. 2006;19(3).
40. Visser E, Schug SA. "The role of ketamine in pain management," Biomedicine and Pharmaco therapy. 2006;60(7): 341–348.
41. Schulte H, Sollevi A, Segerdahl M. "The synergistic effect of combined treatment with systemic ketamine and morphine on experimentally induced windup-like pain in humans," Anesthesia and Analgesia. 2004;98(6)1574–80.
42. Powers PS, Cruse CW, Daniels S, et al. "Safety and efficacy of debridement under anesthesia in patients with burns," Journal of Burn Care and Rehabilitation. 1993;14(2)part 1:176–180.
43. Richardson P, Mustard L. "The management of pain in the burns unit," Burns. 2009;35(7):921–936.
44. Walker J, Maccallum JM, Fischer C, et al. "Sedation using dexmedetomidine in paediatric burn patients," Journal of Burn Care and Research. 2006;27(2):206–10.
45. Simonnet G. "Preemptive antihyperalgesia to improve preemptive analgesia,"Anesthesiology. 2008;108(3): 352–354.
46. Gray P, Williams B, Cramond T. "Successful use of gabapentin in acute pain management following burn injury: A case series," Pain Medicine. 2008;9(3):371–376.
47. Mendham JE. "Gabapentin for the treatment of itching produced by burns and wound healing in children: a pilot study," Burns. 2004;30(8)851–853.
48. Kamel AH, Abd El-Latif Z, El-Rahim JA, et al. "A comparative study of three modalities of pain relief during wound dressing of burn children," Annals of Burns and Fire Disasters. 2003;16(1):2003.
49. Ashburn MA. "Burn pain: The management of procedure related pain." Journal of Burn Care and Research. 16(3): 365–371.

Perioperative Management of Paediatric Trauma Patient

Sandeep Sahu, Prem Raj Singh and Indu Lata

ABSTRACT

The understanding of the pathophysiology of resuscitation and trauma is evolving and changing day by day. The haemodynamic response to haemorrhage may be changed by the type of injury and patient age or sex. Paediatric patients are unique as per there anatomy, physiology, psychology and pharmacology of drugs, resuscitation needs and its responses. If facility available, they should be treated in dedicated paediatric trauma centre, if not, then an adult trauma centre with experience of handling and separate policies for paediatric patients. Most of the aspect of paediatric anatomy, physiology and pharmacology had been described in other chapters of this book. This chapter focuses principles of trauma resuscitation and its perioperative management in paediatric patients. For better understanding of subject we had divided the chapter in two sections; resuscitation and perioperative challenges and its management.

INTRODUCTION

Data from developed countries who have well stabilised trauma system shows that traumatic injuries are major cause (about 45%) of death in 1 to 14 years age in the US. Road traffic accidents (59% mortality, in age group 5–14), pedestrian and bicycle accidents, falls, burns, sports injuries and physical assault are the most common causes of injury.[1] As per the UK data, > 80% of injuries are caused by blunt trauma. Head injury is present in the majority of cases and accounts for 75% of deaths. Injury mechanisms vary with age. In infants, non-accidental injury is most common, whereas, for toddlers, falls are the predominant injury mechanism.[2]

The anaesthesiologists may play the following important roles for paediatric patients:

1. Prevention and prehospital care of trauma victim
2. Initial stabilization and resuscitation in the emergency department (ED)
3. Providing procedural sedation and analgesia for diagnostic and therapeutic purposes
4. Emergent surgery for life saving in operation room (OR)
5. Semi-elective surgeries and procedures after initial stabilization like fractures and dislocations
6. Management in paediatric intensive care unit (PICU)
7. Pain management in hospital and rehabilitation care

RESUSCITATION OF PAEDIATRIC TRAUMA

Basic requirement is a coordination and networking of a trauma system so that one can get right care at right place by right persons.

ORGANIZATION OF A TRAUMA SYSTEM

A need for specialized trauma care facilities for paediatrics has become increasingly evident over the past years. Trauma causing tremendous increase in morbidity and mortality, economic burden not only in the developed countries but also in developing countries. Paediatric trauma management requires a coordinated team approach of different specialty where anaesthesiologists can play a leadership role. Paediatric trauma deaths have a trimodal pattern with 50% dying at the scene from either severe head injury or major haemorrhage. A further 30% die within first few hours from head injury, haemorrhage or airway emergencies, late death due to organ failure and sepsis are often due to inadequate initial resuscitation. Up to 30% deaths are preventable by rapid identification of problems and early aggressive treatment and transfer at right hospital within times.[3] The clinical components of trauma system are to ensure the continuum of care from pre-hospital, effective triage and resuscitation to rehabilitation. The elements of an effective trauma system includes:[4]

Prevention: Prevention is always better when there are falsies in providing care. Unlike adults in paediatric they cannot understand and follow rules. Parents or guardians should be with them, all the times even while sleeping so one can take preventions on their behalf. It includes the following:

- Commitment for dedicated better care of paediatric trauma care patients.
- Public education regarding automobile safety, firearm safety, and burn prevention.
- Paediatric life-support courses for providers and prehospital personnel.
- Legislation regarding establishment and enforcement of traffic rules and establishment of trauma registry.

Prehospital care: Resuscitation should be tailored to each child and should begin in the field. One can take an unstable patient to nearest ED for stabilization if paediatric trauma patient facility is far away. A better prehospital service in continuation of hospital care and integrated communication is the key of success that is helpful in:

- Prevent further injury
- Timely transport of the injured patients to most appropriate centre
- Well-developed communication and triaging system
- Education and training.

Important information as mnemonics, **MIST**: mechanism of injury, injuries sustained, and vital signs baseline or during transport, treatment received and response should be given by prehospital paramedics/EMT during transfer to hospital where patient will get definitive treatment.[5]

Trauma/hospital care: Trauma care is provided from trauma centre are of level I-III depend on the facilities, trauma unit or a separate area acute care facilities as per the local needs including the emergency department. There should be a separate place for paediatrics for resuscitation and stabilization, a dedicated paediatric ICU and dedicated team for definitive surgical and medical care and referral facilities.[6]

REHABILITATION

Trauma system ensures that a life goes back to its right place right time back to society and perform and contributes for self and society. So there is always need of good rehabilitation centre where care is not with the sympathy but with the empathy.

In-hospital management: Whenever possible, children should be transferred by dedicated paediatrics pre- or inter-hospital transfer team. In-hospital management of the injured requires combined effort of all aspects. This include ready availability of relevant specialists and smooth transition between the emergency department, operating room, PICU, and other sites where care is delivered. Procedure must exist for coordination of the various surgical and non-surgical specialists, not only in the initial assessment and early definitive care phase, but also in the PICU, surgical and medical wards and discharge.

Resuscitation: It should be as per paediatric advance trauma life support (PATLS) and advanced trauma life support (ATLS) principles of American College of Surgeons, USA.[3,4] These include, initial assessment and resuscitation of trauma patient. The components are:

- **Primary survey and initial resuscitation and its adjuncts**
- **Secondary survey and its adjuncts**
- **Emergency treatment and definitive care**
- **Transfer as per need and protocols**

The primary survey follows the 'ABCDE' sequence and involves a rapid physiological assessment to identify immediate threats to life that compromise oxygenation and circulation and its immediate management in a structured order as per priority. The Broselow Paediatric Emergency Tape is a useful guide to the management of injured paediatric patient. It is ready reference for ED or prehospital personnel for selection of resuscitative drugs doses, amount of fluids and equipment as per paediatric patient height.[7]

A-Airway with C-spine control (it kills first within seconds like laryngeal-tracheal injuries)

B-Breathing and Ventilation (identify and manage life threatening pneumothorax, haemothorax, pericardial tamponed, flail chest)

C-Circulation and haemorrhage control (because paediatrics blood volume reserve is less, so try to stop bleeding along with volume resuscitation is the best approach in trauma)

D-Disability assessment (detailed neurological examination)

E-Environment (prevention of hypothermia) and Exposure (to examine in detail to prevent missing the injuries)

Airway

Maintaining a patent airway should be the first priority in managing a child with acute trauma. Anatomical differences in children airway require special considerations. The larger head and relatively smaller mid-face make airway obstruction more common in children than in adults. The classic sign of upper airway partial obstruction is inspiratory stridor. Respiratory effort with no air flow indicates the complete airway obstruction. It is also important to include the possibility of cervical spinal injuries, head injury, and the presence of a full stomach in peadiatric patients. Traumatic brain injury (TBI) is more common in children (75%) in comparison with adults and the cervical spine injury is about <2% of trauma cases. There can be 30–40% of patients, who have traumatic myelopathy, have spinal cord injury without radiological abnormality (spinal cord injury without radiological abnormalities, SCIWORA).[8] Need of drugs and its dose depend on consciousness level, intubating conditions, haemodynamic condition and associated injuries. Modified RSI (rapid sequence induction) should be used with cricoid pressure for intubation. One should use low dose of thiopentone or etomidate to avoid hypotension, especially in TBI to prevent decrease in CPP. The need to avoid a further hypoxic insult to the child with TBI while protecting the C-spine remains particularly challenging. The modified jaw thrust maneuver is the best way to open the airway and protect the cervical spine. One should prepare and ready to face the difficult airway in paediatric patients with trauma. Videolaryngoscopes may be useful in emergency and trauma settings. The oral cavity can be suctioned with a Yankauer catheter to remove secretions, but with caution to avoid stimulating the gag reflex. We should identify the threatened airway clinically by seeing signs of airway obstructions like: restless, wheeze, stridor, use of assess or muscles, respiratory distress, cyanosis, high end tidal CO_2 and low SPO_2.[9]

Orotracheal intubation with manual in-line immobilization (MILS) after RSI should be used to secure the airway in trauma. The alignment of cervical spine should be maintained, and the patient's heart rate and oxygen saturation, $ETCO_2$ should be monitored during the intubation. If intubation fails, then immediate consider for plan-B and prepare for surgical airway.[9]

Criteria for intubation/ventilation with definitive airway are similar to that of adult:

1. Airway obstruction despite supraglottic device
2. Inadequate ventilation with bag and mask ventilation
3. Glasgow Coma Scale (GCS) <8 or raised intracranial pressure (ICP)
4. Shock unresponsive to fluid resuscitation
5. Suspected raised need for prolonged ventilation
6. Need for transport to higher centre of haemodynamically unstable patient (better to have prophylactic secured airway).

Breathing

Adequacy of breathing and ventilation need to be rapidly assessed. Assessment includes respiratory rate (RR), depth and effort, auscultation of breath sounds, and visualizationof the chest movements for asymmetry and expansion. Anticipate respiratory failure if:[10]

- increased RR, particularly with signs of distress (e.g. increased respiratory effort including nasal flaring, retractions, see saw breathing, or grunting);
- an inadequate RR, effort, or chest excursion (e.g. diminished breath sounds or gasping), especially if mental status is depressed;
- Cyanosis with abnormal breathing despite supplementary oxygen.

As paediatric patients have greater oxygen consumption, smaller functional residual volume, and increased chest wall compliance so they are predispose to airway collapse and hypoxia. Life-threatening thoracic injuries should be immediately identified and treated, as pneumothorax by niddle placement in 2nd intercostal space followed by intercostal drainage (ICD), haemothorax by ICD, open pneumothorax (by 3-side cover dressing and ICD), and pericardial tamponed by niddle thoracentesis.[3]

Circulation

It is useful to label the shock into clinical categories: compensated shock, decompensated shock, and cardiopulmonary failure in order to prioritize the resuscitation strategies. Adequacy of circulation should be assessed by evaluating heart rate and rhythm, capillary refill time, skin colour, temperature, arterial pressure (AP) and heart sound quality, mental status.

It is also important to identify any visible haemorrhage like on extremities and nonvisible haemorrhage sites like chest, abdomen and pelvis to confirm the above clinical features. Actual blood volume is small, therefore, even small blood loss can cause circulatory compromise. AP is well maintained until hypovolaemia is quite severe, >25–40% of blood volume loss.[11] Hypotension is a late and preterminal sign of decompensated shock in children and may be abruptly followed by bradycardia. Tachycardia is a more useful sign of hypovolemia, but may also reflect pain and fear and anxiety.[12]

Management of circulation in bleeding trauma patient:[13]

1. Ensure adequate vascular access, IV access is often easier in the hands and feet than in the antecubital fossae. If failure to have IV access is achieved within 90 sec in a severely injured child <6 year of age, interosseous access is recommended.
2. Obtain blood specimens for investigations, blood grouping (takes 15 min) and cross-match (1 hr), so O –ve blood (universal donor) can be given if immediately transfusion need.
3. Assess the grade and severity of shock and do early haemorrhage control.
4. Euvolemic fluid resuscitation (isotonic 0.9% NS preferred over RL) should be administered in 20 mL/kg^{-1} boluses guided by heart rate and peripheral perfusion. If failure to improve with >40 mL/kg^{-1} of crystalloid, then blood 10 mL/kg^{-1} boluses should be given followed by frequent reassessments as per response (large volume crystalloid resuscitation in uncontrolled haemorrhage may be detrimental, early use of blood products PRBC, FFP and platelets as 1:1:1).
5. Avoid hypothermia, hyperglycemia and hypoglycemia maintain euglycemia.
6. Reassessment frequently clinically and investigation for coagulation (TEG, PT/INR).

Disability

A brief neurological assessment is done to determine changes in level of consciousness. Conscious level is rapidly assessed using the mnemonic AVPU score:

A: Alert
V: Responds to voice
P: Responds to pain
U: Unresponsive

A baseline GSC scale (best Eye opening, Motor and Verbal response) and pupillary (sign and size) assessment is also important. Neurological status should be monitored frequently throughout the care of the patient. Changes in level of consciousness are an early indication of decreased oxygenation and perfusion, or significant head injury.[12]

Exposure

A detailed inspection and examination of the body to rule out missed injuries is required. The assessment should be thorough but done quickly, to reduce the chance of hypothermia. Make the environmental temperature of ED/OR 25–30°C to avoid surface cooling. Switch off the air conditioning and make all possible efforts to external warming by use of overhead heaters, blankets; warmed and humidified ventilation or patient's body warmer.

Pain management: It is important to give analgesics after neurological examination if not given earlier after or during primary survey as per policies. IV route will be preferred because of responses can be predicted as compared to other routes. Acetaminophen or fentanyl may be good options. If intubated then morphine is the drug of choice and should be given in a dose of 0.1–0.2 mg/kg^{-1}.

Secondary Survey

The secondary survey is only commenced after primary survey and resuscitation has been completed and child is stable. If any time patient condition or vitals worsen go back to primary survey. It consists of a detailed from head to toe and back and front examination of the child to get the all possible injuries depend on mechanism of injury. During secondary assessment, the mnemonic FGHI is most commonly used.[14]

F: Full set of vital signs; Family presence
G: Give comfort
H: Head-to-toe assessment; History
I: Inspect posterior surfaces

Head and face: The scalp and face should be inspected for lacerations, depressions, or foreign bodies, and palpated for pain and tenderness. TBI is a major cause of morbidity and mortality in paediatric trauma victims. A neurological assessment should be performed consisting of a GCS, neurological examination, pupillary reflexes, and examination of fundus. The primary goal of management is similar like of adults with prevention of secondary insults (hypoxia and hypotension), control of ICP, maintenance of adequate cerebral perfusion pressure (CPP), osmolar therapy, and identification

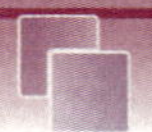

of mass lesions requiring emergency surgical evacuation. A brain computed tomographic (CT) scan is indicated after secondary survey if the GCS <12, loss of consciousness at time of injury, skull fracture, retrograde amnesia, neurological symptoms/signs, or severe injury. The ears and nose should be checked for blood or cerebral spinal fluid.[9] The nose should be examined for any deformities, bleeding and nasal septal haematoma. Inspect the neck to look for pain, tenderness, lacerations, swelling, deformities, and jugular vein distension.Trachea should be examined for any deviation, crepitus. Larynx injury can be suspected by any change of voice, cry and additional sound.

Chest: Thoracic injuries occur in about 3% of children with blunt trauma. Identify the life threatening injuries as described above. The sternum and ribs of a small child are soft and compliant. They are not easily broken, but the viscera of the chest are at risk for compression injury, even without rib fracture. Pulmonary contusion are common even without rib fractures. Palpate the clavicle and chest wall for crepitus and fracture and observe for symmetrical chest wall movement and expansion, and assess for pain during respirations. Lung and heart sounds should be auscultated.

Abdomen: Paediatric abdomens have thin body wall and have closely spaced organs. Abdominal trauma accounts for about 10% of trauma in children. It is second only to airway problems as the most frequent cause of preventable death. A physical examination can detect 97% of abdominal injuries. Splenic injury is the most common followed by hepatic, renal, intestine, and pancreatic. The abdomen should be inspected for distension, bruising, and lacerations. Palpation of the abdomen should be done for tenderness and pain. Nowadays FAST (focused assessment sonography in trauma patient) is bedside USG, work as point of care in blunt or penetrating abdomen and chest injury in haemodynamically unstable patients to immediately detect solid organ injuries that should be managed in OR.[15] Ultrasound had a sensitivity of 80% (76–84%) and a specificity of 96% (95–97%) for the identification of haemoperitoneum.[16] CT scan abdomen should be performed if any doubt persists in abdominal injuries. In paediatric trauma 95% of the abdominal injuries are managed non-operatively by conservative treatment, only 5% need to go OR.[17,18]

Extremity: Skeletal injury may occur in 10–15% of the paediatric victims. Inspect all the limbs and joints, palpate for area of tenderness and check joint movement, stability and muscular power. Examine sensory and motor function of any nerve or peripheral nerves that may have been injured. Pelvic fractures are uncommon in children. Long bone fractures may cause significant blood loss and lead to hypovolaemic shock and therefore should be immobilized in splints as soon as possible. Splint help to reduce the pain, further bleeding and neurovascular compromise.

Tertiary survey: A routine head to toe examination of patients should take place within 24 hrs of the injury, to document any missed injuries and re-evaluate existing injuries and their treatment. This is particularly important in non-ambulant children.

DAMAGE CONTROL RESUSCITATION (DCR)

Any trauma patients may have severe metabolic, coagulation, and physiological derangement. DCR is a recent concept in trauma management that involved: time limited permissive hypotension, early control of bleeding, use of massive haemorrhage protocols to correct the haemorrhagic shock and acute coagulopathy of trauma (PRBC, FFP, platelet as 1:1:1) and damage control surgery (DCS) done basically for haemorrhage control and use of tranexamic acid. DCS is all the early efforts to stop bleeding by laparotomy and packing than delaying the definitive surgery, till then patient is physiologically and metabolically restored in ICU or by angioembolization of selective bleeders if facility available. Time to surgery and haemorrhage control is a key determinant of outcome and the transfer to surgery should only be delayed for key, life-saving interventions.[19,20]

Damage Control Surgery or Early Total Care (ETC)/ Definitive Surgery

DCS is rapid, emergency essential surgery to save life or limb while delaying the time consuming reconstruction surgery later on after pit stop resuscitation and catch up in OR/ICU. The priority is short-term physiological recovery over anatomical reconstruction in the seriously injured and compromised patient. It has following aims and components:

1. Haemorrhage control.
2. Decompression of compartments: Cranium, thorax, abdomen and limbs.
3. Decontamination of wounds and ruptured viscera.
4. Fracture splintage.

The aim is to render the patient resuscitable, by stopping haemorrhage, and prevent further damage whilst minimizing the surgical stress insult. The ETC is definitive fixation of all long bone fractures within 24 h of injury, but only once the patient is physiologically and metabolically normalizing and stabilizing. The decision is taken under leadership of anaesthetic, surgical, and critical care clinician's team, and it is guided by clinical, physiological and metabolic parameters taken frequently and informed the protocols to everyone involved in the continuum care. Alternative surgical strategies and stop points should be identified for default in the event of patient deterioration.[21]

Perioperative Management of Paediatric Trauma Patient

Anaesthesiologist should know the principles of resuscitation of unstable paediatric trauma patients. They should also know the management when these unstable patients undergo DCS or emergency life saving procedures or surgery and definitive surgery or their postoperative care in NICU (neonatal intensive care unit)/PICU. Anaesthesiologist, surgeons, and other personnel should work as a coordinate team when managing children with trauma. This combined effort will help in better outcome and reliable identification of suspected injuries and its management. So that anaesthesiologist can more effectively anticipate the bleeding and its physiologic effect and during surgical procedure can give best in physiological restoration perioperatively and in PICU.[22]

Preoperative evaluation: If the child condition permits, the preoperative evaluation should include a complete assessment. Vital sign should be stable and appropriate for age. Sensorium, urine output, skin turgor can be used to evaluate and estimate the child's preoperative volume status. However, in urgent procedures only brief history outlined by AMPLE mnemonic may be feasible.[22]

A: Allergies
M: Medications taken or taking
P: Past medical history
L: Last oral intake, last tetanus immunization
E: Events related to the injury

The OR should be prepared according with age-appropriate equipment, rapid-infusion devices, fluid warmers and infusion pumps, diluting and labeling the medications in age-appropriate dose. Temperature should be closely monitored because the potential for both iatrogenic hypothermia and hyperthermia. Hypothermia can be prevented by maintaining a warm operating room environment, using warming blanket and warming lights and warming all intravenous fluids.[23] Assessment should include review of essential and available laboratory reports, such as haemoglobin, electrolytes, coagulation studies and ABG determination. Diagnostic imaging studies including X-rays (only chest and pelvic X-ray in unstable patient) and CT scans should be obtained only once patient stabilized and urgent need for further management as per need and recommendations.[24]

Airway management: Thorough airway examination is crucial in paediatric patients. The anaesthesiologist should be prepared to encounter the following anatomical and physiological features of paediatric airway as described in another chapter. The following are important red flags for paediatric trauma patients:[25]

1. Most of the paediatric victims may have already intubated when reached ED. The anaesthesiologists duty is to assess the airway and tube (tube size, cuffed/incuffed, presence and magnitude of air leak if uncuffed tube, depth of the tube, breath sounds, ventilation and oxygenation). A chest X-ray may be done to review the correct position of the tube.
2. Before intubation, their lungs should be denitrogenated with 100% O_2 for several breaths. So O_2 reserves are increased so can tolerate longer period of apnea during intubation.
3. For emergency surgery always assumed to be full stomach and rapid sequence induction is preferred.
4. ET tube of the appropriate size should be chosen either cuffed or uncuffed, the general opinion, however, is cuffed tubes, even in the prehospital settings.
5. The choice of agent for induction of anaesthesia depends on the haemodynamic, neurological and airway status. For haemodynamically stable patients, low dose thiopentone or propofol can be used. Etomidate 0.1–0.2 mg/kg^{-1} is a preferable induction agent in hypovolemic patients with a head injury. Fast muscle relaxation could be achieved with succinylcholine or rocuronium.
6. If difficult airway with failed laryngoscopy, one can use different video laryngoscope like GlideScope[25] and laryngeal mask airway.[26]

INTRAOPERATIVE MANAGEMENT

Balanced general anaesthesia should be used for maintenance. No agent proven better than other.[27]

Isoflurane, sevoflurane, and continuous intravenous infusion of propofol and opioids have all been used safely.[28] Although total intravenous anaesthesia technique is more popular in neurosurgical procedures.[29] With taken care of standard recommended monitoring as per the procedure needs like SPO_2, $ETCO_2$, ECG, temperature, urine out, serial ABG and invasive monitoring (CVP, arterial pressure) and coagulation tests.

Intraoperative fluid management: Most of the important points had been raised under resuscitation. The other issues are: Children have small blood volumes to loose. It is difficult to identify and classify shock classically as in adults.[30] All intravenous fluids should be prewarmed to 37°C to avoid hypothermia. Resuscitation should start with isotonic non-dextrose containing crystalloids. However, hypoglycemia is harmful for TBI, and should be avoided.[31] Hypertonic saline in adult trauma had showed some good results with less fluid requirement with no difference in mortality. However, more evidence for use is needed in paediatrics.[32] Although colloids are not preferred now a days during resuscitation as per recent protocols. Hydroxyethyl starch and albumin have also been used in paediatrics with no significant adverse effects.[33] The end-points of fluid resuscitation is usually include normalization of pulse rate and urine output >1 mL/ kg^{-1}/h^{-1}. Under resuscitation with crystalloids and blood may lead to impending shock and multiple organ failures, whereas supranormal resuscitation may lead to heamodilution, lethal traid (hypothermia, coagulopathy, and acidosis) and transfusion-related complications.

Guidelines for use of blood products are not well established in paediatric trauma. Clinical decisions either follow adult protocols, or are made per individual clinical judgement. In general, blood loss less than 10% of blood volume can be replaced by crystalloids. Losses between 10% and 20% can be replaced by crystalloids or blood but losses over 20% must be replaced by blood.[34] Massive transfusions may be required in paediatric cases with severe trauma as like of adults.[35] In all paediatric patients, the use of blood products to treat coagulation disturbances should be based on laboratory parameters including the prothrombin time (PT), INR, partial thromboplast in time, and platelet count. Antifibrinolytic agents (tranexamic acid) and procoagulant drugs such as recombinant factor VII have been used in trials and case series in patients with TBI.[36] Investigations like serial haematocrits, lactate, and base deficit had proven useful to guide fluid and blood product administration; there is no clear haemoglobin thresholds for paediatric patients other than those extrapolated from studies looking at adult outcomes.[37]

Temperature control: Paediatric patients due to large surface area relative to body weight, immature thermoregulation mechanism, effects of general anaesthesia and ambient temperature of OR can lead to rapid development of hypothermia.[38] One should be aware of risk of hyperthermia with all warming techniques, therefore, monitoring of core temperature is necessary.[39]

Therapeutic hypothermia: Hypothermia has been shown to reduce intracranial pressure in adult and paediatric patients by reducing the cerebral swelling in animal models. Induced hypothermia has also been shown to decrease mortality and improve outcome in neonates with hypoxic-ischemic injury. In addition, early unintentional hyperthermia in paediatric TBI and has been associated with worse outcomes. Finally, although a large, randomized controlled trial in adults following TBI found no benefit to moderate (33°C) cooling within 8 hours of injury. This evidence fueled hope for a potential role of early hypothermia therapy in paediatric TBI in past.[40] Recent Cochrane systematic review was done to assess the effectiveness of the application of therapeutic hypothermia to reduce death and disability when administered to adult patients who have been admitted to hospital following TBI. This review found some evidence to suggest that therapeutic hypothermia may be of benefit in the treatment of TBI.[41] Recently Cool kid trail shows that hypothermia for 48 hrs with slow rewarming does not reduce mortality of improve global functional outcome after paediatric severe traumatic brain injury.[42]

Postoperative pain management: It is well stabilized that all paediatric patients perceive pain. Pain management not only reduces anxiety and fear but also essential for better outcome and shorter stay in ICU. Multimodal analgesia technique should be used to avoid side effects of one drug. Acetaminophen is a commonly used drug with dosage 10–15 mg/kg, every 4–6 hours, intravenously for mild to moderate pain. Rectal administration produces delayed and variable uptake.[43] The opioid analgesics like fentanyl, morphine can be used for severe pain in young children. Regional anaesthesia techniques like epidural, paravertebral block and femoral nerve block are quite effective in pain management in trauma patient.[44] Nowadays USG guided regional nerve or plexus block proves more effective, reduces opioid consumption and side effects.[45]

Postoperative care and extubation: Most of the polytrauma patients after resuscitation and surgery will require monitoring and further stabilization in ICU. There can be significant fluid shift, acidosis, and soft tissue swelling because of massive blood loss and aggressive fluid resuscitation. Airway swelling due to trauma or prolong dependent position and abdominal compartment syndrome are usually found that may require mechanical ventilation in the ICU.[46] Upper airway obstruction is the single most common cause of extubation failure in facial trauma and burn.[47]

The decision to extubate polytrauma patient in the OR must be considered carefully. The success of extubation depend on cardiovascular stability, normal acid–base balance, presence of intact airway reflexes, ability to clear secretions, an intact central inspiratory drive, ability to exchange gases efficiently, and respiratory muscle strength to meet the work associated with respiratory demand.[48]

Transfer: Trauma patients may need to several intrahospital to OR, ICU and imaging or interhospital transfer for better patient care to higher centre. There are higher chances of mishaps with physiologic deterioration during transport.[49] Before transport, anaesthesiologist should reassess patient for haemodynamic stability, adequate oxygenation, and functionality of the monitors. Intraoperative monitoring should be continued during transport, and keep ready the resuscitation drugs. A detailed written and verbal report of perioperative events and management must be given to the handling team, ensuring the continuity of care and patient safety.[50]

SPECIAL TRAUMA SITUATIONS

Child Abuse

The diagnosis of child abuse is made by finding an acute injury that may have a plausible explanation and signs of frequently past trauma. There may be multiple healing bruises, contusions, and fractures. It may be psychological or sexual abuse and failure to meet a child's need for food, clothing, shelter, hygiene, medical care, education, or supervision.

Suspicion of child abuse begins with an inappropriate or inadequate explanation for injuries or when the degree of trauma more than that it should. Multiple hospital admissions, emergency department visits, doctor or hospital "shopping," and a history of previous trauma should be of concern. Certain clinical features are common to child abuse, story regarding the injury changes over time but they are by no means pathognomonic. Most abused children are older than 3 years with poor hygiene and delayed somatic or psychological development.[51]Abused child may develop post-traumatic stress disorders. One should identify this preventable cause of child trauma, report it and take necessary legal action to minimize this and manage abused child in ED and Trauma centre as per above descriptions.

SUMMARY

Paediatric trauma management is a multidisciplinary team work to help patients and their families to overcome its after-effects. It is important to understand anatomical and physiological challenges in paediatric trauma patients manage with good skills of resuscitation and acute care. Anaesthesiologists' can play a vital role for care of paediatric patient's right from admission in ED, during surgical intervention, and postoperative care to discharge.

REFERENCES

1. Heron M, Hoyert DL, Murphy SL, et al. Deaths: Final data for 2006. Natl Vital Stat Rep. 2009;57:1–134.
2. Guice KS, Cassidy LD, Oldham KT. Traumatic injury and children: A national assessment. J Trauma 2007;63:S68–80.
3. Advanced Paediatric Life Support. The Practical Approach. 4th edn. London: BMJ Publishing Group; 2004.
4. Advanced Trauma Life Support, 12th edn. American College of Surgeons 2012.
5. D'Amours S, Sugrue M, Russell R, Nocera N (Eds). Clinical Guidelines: Pre-Hospital Information and Hand—Over. Handbook of Trauma Care, 6th edn. Sydney: University of New South Wales, 2002. Available from http://www.sswahs.nsw.gov.au/liverpool/trauma/handbook1.html (accessed 1 August 2014).
6. Statement of American Academy of Paediatrics and Paediatric Orthopedics society of North America. Management of paediatric trauma. Paediatrics 2008;121;849.
7. Avarello JT, Cantor RM. Paediatric major trauma: An approach to evaluation and management. Emerg Med Clin North Am. 2007;25:803–36.
8. Pang D. Spinal cord injury without radiographic abnormality in children, 2 decades later. Neurosurgery. 2004;55: 1325–42.
9. Brain Trauma Foundation Guidelines for acute medical management of severe TBI in infants, children and adolescents. Paediatric Critical Care Medicine 2003;4(3 Suppl): S1–490.

10. Kleinman ME, Chameides L, Schexnayder SM, et al. Part 14: Paediatric advanced life support: American heart association guidelines for cardiopulmonary resuscitation and emergency cardiovascular care. Circulation. 2010; 122(18 Suppl 3):S876–908.
11. Pauline M Cullen. Paediatric Trauma. Continuing Education in Anaesthesia, Critical Care and Pain. BJA. 2012: 1–5.
12. Paediatric Trauma Care Guidelines 2011 available at www.mc.uky.edu/trauma services/Paediatric Trauma Care Guidelines 2011.pdf (assessed on 20 July 2014).
13. Rossaint R, Bouillon B, Cerny V, et al. Management of bleeding following major trauma: An updated European guideline. Crit Care. 2010;14:R52.
14. Grant McFadyen J, Ramesh Ramaiah, Sanjay M Bhananker. Initial assessment and management of paediatric trauma patients. Int J Crit Illn Inj Sci. 2012 Sep–Dec;2(3):121–127.
15. Scaife ER, Fenton SJ, Hansen KW, et al. Use of focused abdominal sonography for trauma at paediatric and adult trauma centres: A survey. J Pediatr Surg. 2009;44:1746–9.
16. Holmes JF, Gladman A, Chang CH. Performance of abdominal ultrasonography in paediatric blunt trauma patients: A meta-analysis. J Pediatr Surg. 2007;42:1588–94.
17. Fenton SJ, Hansen KW, Meyers RL, et al. CT scan and the paediatric trauma patient—are we overdoing it? J Pediatr Surg. 2004;39:1877–81.
18. Holmes JH (4th), Wiebe DJ, Tataria M, et al. The failure of nonoperative management in paediatric solid organ injury: A multi-institutional experience. J Trauma. 2005;59: 1309–13.
19. McCullough AL, Haycock JC, Forward DP, et al. Early management of the severely injured major trauma patient. British Journal of Anaesthesia 2014;113(2):234–41.
20. Midwinter MJ. Damage control surgery in the era of damage control resuscitation. J R Army Med Corps 2009;155:323–6.
21. Lamb CM, MacGoey P, Navarro AP, et al. Damage control surgery in the era of damage control resuscitation. British Journal of Anaesthesia 2014;113(2):242–9.
22. Jeffery C Metzger, Alexander L Eastman, Paul E Pepe. Year in review 2008: Critical Care–trauma. Critical Care 2009; 13(5):226–231.
23. Ramesh Ramaiah, Sam Sharar. Anaesthetic management of the paediatric trauma patient (Ch-20). Essentials of Truama Anaesthesia. Cambridge Medicine editor Albert J Varon, Charles E Smith. pp. 263–274.
24. Tarun Bhalla[1], Elisabeth Dewhirst, Amod Sawardekar, et al. Perioperative management of the paediatric patient with traumatic brain injury. Paediatric Anaesthesia 2012;22: 627–640.
25. Sagarin MJ, Chiang V, Sakles JC, et al. Rapid sequence intubation for paediatric emergency airway management. PediatrEmerg Care. 2002;18:417–23.
26. Fonte M, Oulego-Erroz I, Nadkarni L, et al. A randomized comparison of the Glide Scope video laryngoscope to the standard laryngoscopy for intubation by paediatric residents in simulated easy and difficult infant airway scenarios. PediatrEmerg Care. 2011;27:398–402.
27. Levy RJ, Helfaer MA. Paediatric airway issues. Crit Care Clin. 2000;16:489–504.
28. Yulia Ivashkov, Sanjay M Bhananker. Perioperative management of paediatric trauma patients. Int J Crit Illn Inj Sci. 2012;2(3):143–148.
29. Engelhard K, Werner C. Inhalational or intravenous anaesthetics for craniotomies. Pro inhalational? Curr Opin Anaesthesiol. 2006;19:504–8.
30. Hans P, Bonhomme V. Why we still use intravenous drugs as the basic regimen for neuro surgical anaesthesia. CurrOpinAnaesthesiol. 2006;19:498–503.
31. Schwaitzberg SD, Bergman KS, Harris BH. A paediatric trauma model of continuous hemorrhage. J Pediatr Surg. 1988;23:605–9.
32. Cochran A, Scaife ER, Hansen KW, et al. Hyperglycemia and outcomes from paediatric traumatic brain injury. J Trauma. 2003;55:1035–8.
33. Bulger EM, May S, Kerby JD, et al. Out-of-hospital hypertonic resuscitation after traumatic hypovolemic shock: A randomized, placebo controlled trial. Ann Surg. 2011;253:431–41.
34. Sumpelmann R, Kretz FJ, Gabler R, et al. Hydroxyethyl starch 130/0.42/6:1 for perioperative plasma volume replacement in children: Preliminary results of a European Prospective Multicentre Observational Postauthorization Safety Study (PASS) Paediatr Anaesth. 2008;18:929–33.
35. Barcelona SL, Thompson AA, Cote CJ. Intraoperative paediatric blood transfusion therapy: A review of common issues. Part II: Transfusion therapy, special considerations, and reduction of allogenic blood transfusions. PaediatrAnaesth. 2005;15:814–30.
36. Spinella PC, Holcomb JB. Resuscitation and transfusion principles for traumatic haemorrhagic shock. Blood Rev. 2009;23:231–40.
37. Nathaniel Greene, Sanjay Bhananker, Ramesh Ramaiah. Vascular access, fluid resuscitation, and blood transfusion in paediatric trauma. Int J Crit Illn Inj Sci. 2012;2(3): 135–142.
38. Cassey JG, Armstrong PJ, Smith GE, et al. The safety and effectiveness of a modified convection heating system for children during anaesthesia. PaediatrAnaesth. 2006;16: 654–62.
39. Bernardo LM, Gardner MJ, Lucke J, et al. The effects of core and peripheral warming methods on temperature and physiologic variables in injured children. Pediatr Emerg Care. 2001;17:138–42.
40. Clifton GL, Drever P, Valadka A, et al. Multicentre trial of early hypothermia in severe brain injury. J Neurotrauma. 2009;26:393–397.
41. Samantha Crossley, Jenny Reid, Rachel McLatchie, et al. A systematic review of therapeutic hypothermia for adult

patients following traumatic brain injury. Critical Care 2014;18(2):R75. Published online Apr 17, 2014. doi:10.1186/cc13835

42. David P Adelson, Stephen R Wisniewski, John Beca, et al. Comparison of hypothermia and normothermia after severe traumatic brain injury in children (Cool Kids): a phase 3, randomised controlled trial. The Lancet Neurology 2013;129(6): 546–553.
43. Stephanie Dowden, Maria McCarthy, George Chalkiadis. Achieving organizational change in paediatric pain management. Pain Res Manag. 2008;13(4):321–326.
44. Todd KH, Ducharme J, Choiniere M, et al. Pain in the emergency department: Results of the pain and emergency medicine initiative (PEMI) multicentre study. J pain. 2007;8:460–6.
45. Oberndorfer U, Marhofer P, Bosenberg A, et al. Ultrasonographic guidance for sciatic and femoral nerve blocks in children. Br J Anaesth. 2007;98:797–801.
46. Mittnacht AJ, Thanjan M, Srivastava S, et al. Extubation in the operating room after congenital heart surgery in children. J Thorac Cardiovasc Surg. 2008;136:88–93.
47. Thiagarajan RR, Bratton SL, Martin LD, et al. Predictors of successful extubation in children. Am J Respir Crit Care Med.1999;160:1562–6.
48. Newth CJ, Venkataraman S, Willson DF, et al. Weaning and extubation readiness in paediatric patients. Pediatr Crit Care Med. 2009;10:1–11.
49. Paret G, Ben Abraham R, Yativ O, et al. Intrahospital transport of critically ill children Harefuah. 1999;136:609–11.
50. Wallen E, Venkataraman ST, Grosso MJ, et al. Intrahospital transport of critically ill paediatric patients. Crit Care Med. 1995;23:1588–95.
51. Myers JEB, Berliner L, Briere J, et al. (Eds.) The APSAC handbook on child maltreatment, 2002, 2nd edn. Newbury Park, CA: SAGE Publications.

Anaesthesia for Procedures Outside the Operating Theatre

Sona Dave

ABSTRACT

As advances in diagnostic and interventional radiological procedures increase the anaesthesiologist will have to move out of the safe confines of operation theatre and cater to the care of paediatric patients in these remote locations. Computerised tomography (CT) scan, magnetic resonance imaging (MRI) suite, positron emission tomography (PET) scan, interventional radiology suites, radiation therapy, gastrointestinal endoscopies are just a few places where these babies may need either only sedation, sedation coupled with analgesia or general anaesthesia for immobilisation and safe conduct of these procedures. General guidelines of paediatric sedation with emphasis on special requisites of individual procedures are outlined here.

The demand for sedation for paediatric procedures outside the Operating Room (OR) has increased 10% annually.[1]

Certain guidelines pertaining to safe sedation in paediatric patients will be discussed before embarking on sedation for individual procedures.

Goals for sedation in paediatric patients for diagnostic and therapeutic purposes include:[2]

- To guard the safety and welfare of the patient
- To minimise discomfort and pain to the patient
- To minimize anxiety, psychological trauma and maximise amnesia
- Movements should be minimised so as to avert complications
- Early return to awake state with fulfilment of discharge criteria should be met to allow early discharge.

To minimise complications certain principles have to be adhered to. These include:[3]

- Presedation evaluation is a must with focused airway examination
- Fasting guidelines should be properly adhered to.
- Sedative or anxiolytic drugs should be administered under strict supervision of qualified personnel.
- Equipment and skilled personnel for airway management and cardiopulmonary resuscitation should be available.
- All equipment should be checked before sedating the child. Age and size appropriate equipment should be available.
- Monitoring patient's cardiorespiratory status is vital and for deeply sedated child the concerned person should solely devote his attention to the child and vital parameters should be recorded every 5 minutes. Pulse oximeter must be used to monitor all sedated patients.

Careful history taking should include:

- History of allergies and adverse drug reactions
- History of drug ingestion
- Medical and surgical history
- History suggestive of airway obstruction such as snoring or obstructive sleep apnoea
- History of complication to sedation or anaesthesia in the past
- Family history relevant to anaesthetic complications.

There are certain *contraindications* or conditions in which sedation should be given with caution[4]

1. Conditions in which airway management is likely to be difficult
   - Airway abnormality like enlarged tonsils or anatomical abnormality of upper or lower airway
   - History of sleep apnoea
   - Nasal blockage

2. Diseases with high risk of respiratory failure
   - Neuromuscular disease
   - Altered consciousness
   - Respiratory or cardiac failure
   - Severe pulmonary hypertension
3. Conditions associated with high incidence of aspiration
   - Raised intracranial tension
   - Pneumoperitoneum
   - Bowel obstruction

Documentation before sedation

- Informed consent as per institutional protocol must be obtained.
- A brief note about the procedure and postprocedure instruction regarding the period of starvation along with a helpline contact in case of any emergencies. Any medications which have to be continued should also be mentioned for anticonvulsants.

Sedation of infants and young babies may be more difficult when they are hungry and crying. However, the risk of complications is much higher if the NPO status is not met and if inadvertently these babies slip into deep sedation.

Fasting guidelines as per American Society of Anaesthesiologist (ASA) preprocedural guidelines which were laid in 2002 and later updated in 2011 are as follows.[1]

Ingested material	Minimum fasting period (all ages)
• Clear liquids	2 hours
• Breast milk	4 hours
• Infant formula	6 hours
• Non-human milk	6 hours
• Light meal	6 hours

As approved by ASA

For emergency procedures the risk of sedating a non-fasting child must be weighed against its benefits and the lightest sedation technique must be used. In case it is imperative to deeply sedate such a child due considerations must be given to use airway protective devices especially if there are risk factors such as trauma, decreased levels of consciousness or obesity.

Sedation should be titrated to achieve optimum effect as oversedation may lead to delayed recovery, whereas undersedation may lead to increased distress. Thus continuous assessment of the level of sedation is a must.

Continuum of depth of sedation[1] as approved by ASA House of Delegates 10/13/1999 and amended 10/21/2009. Depth of sedation may vary from mild to moderate to deep[2] (Table 35.1).

As per American Academy of Paediatrics Committee on Drugs (COD), the term mild sedation is equivalent to anxiolysis and moderate sedation is equivalent to conscious sedation. The same standards for monitoring should be used for deep sedation and general anaesthesia by a dedicated personnel and time-based tracking of vital signs should be followed.[5]

In a study by Hoffman et al.[5] it was shown that planned deep sedation carried a higher risk of adverse effects than conscious sedation and the demarcation between conscious sedation and deep sedation is very grey. There is no predictability when conscious sedation may slip into deep sedation. This was especially true in cases of infants where induction of unconsciousness was required even for non-painful processes such as diagnostic imaging studies.[1]

Repeated and continuous assessment of the sedation score will prevent inadvertent risk of deep sedation.[6]

The most common side effects of sedation involves airway obstruction or depression of respiration. This may eventually result in hypoventilation, hypoxemia and apnoea. Bradycardia, hypotension and cardiorespiratory arrests are secondary consequences due to

Table 35.1 Depth of sedation may vary from mild to moderate to deep

	Minimal sedation/ anxiolysis	Moderate sedation/ "conscious sedation"	Deep sedation analgesia	General anaesthesia
Responsiveness	Normal response to verbal stimulation	Purposeful response to verbal or tactile	Purposeful response following repeated or painful stimulation	Unarousable even with painful stimuli
Airway	Unaffected	No intervention required	Intervention may be required	Intervention often required
Spontaneous ventilation	Unaffected	Adequate	May be inadequate	Frequently inadequate
Cardiovascular	Unaffected	Usually maintained	Usually maintained	May be impaired

failure of recognition of the primary respiratory compromise. Other rare complications include seizures and allergic reactions and the attending team should be prepared to deal with them.[4]

Modified Ramsey score is also used for assessment of sedation:[1, 6]

1. Patient anxious, agitated or restless awake
2. Patient cooperative, oriented and tranquil comfortable
3. Patient responds to voice commands
4. Patient responds to gentle shaking
5. Patient responds to noxious stimulus
6. Patient has no response to firm nail bed pressure or other noxious stimuli

In addition there are other scores which can also be used (Table 35.2).

Both under and oversedation may be problematic to the patient.[4]

Problems associated with undersedation include:

- Motion effect causing poor image quality
- Repeated studies may add to the radiation burden
- Repeated investigation may have a negative psychological effect on the child.
- Repeated scanning may mean additional leave for the parents which may cause additional financial burden to the parents

Oversedation carries the risk of:

- Respiratory compromise
- Cardiac depression
- Increased incidence of vomiting and aspiration

For the conduct of safe sedation, it is necessary to follow certain rules. In order not to miss anything in planning the setup, the acronym SOAP ME is useful.[2, 4]

S: Size appropriate suction catheters and suction apparatus

O: Oxygen delivery devices

A: Appropriate sized airway equipment which include nasopharyngeal and oral airways, laryngoscopes, different sized masks, stylets, endotracheal tubes and bag mask ventilating devices

P: Pharmacy: All the necessary life saving drugs and antidotes besides the anaesthetic drugs should be available.

M: Monitors which should include pulse oximeters, stethoscopes, cardioscopes, capnometer, and non-invasive blood pressure monitor.

E: Equipment such as defibrillators or drugs for specific cases.

Emergency drugs that need to be kept ready during sedation procedures [2]

- Atropine
- Albuterol
- Diphenhydramine
- Diazepam
- Epinephrine (1:1000, 1:10 000)
- Flumazenil
- Glucose (25 percent or 50 percent)
- Glycopyrrolate
- Lorazepam
- Methylprednisolone
- Naloxone
- Oxygen
- Phenytoin
- Racemic epinephrine
- Sodium bicarbonate
- Succinylcholine
- Xylocard

Drugs which can be used for sedation[4]

- *Midazolam:* It is water soluble, readily metabolised benzodiazepine drug. It has hypnotic, amnesic,

Table 35.2 Sedation agitation scale[1]

Score	Term	Description
7	Dangerously agitated	Pulling at ETT; trying to remove tubes; thrashing side to side
6	Very agitated	Does not calm despite frequent verbal reminders of limits; requires physical restraints
5	Agitated	Anxious or mildly agitated; attempting to wake up; calms to verbal instructions
4	Calm and cooperative	Calm, awakens easily, follows commands
3	Sedated	Will awaken and follow commands; required loud verbal or physical stimuli
2	Very sedated	Arouses to physical stimuli but does not awaken, communicate or follow commands
1	Unresponsive	Minimal/no response to stimuli, does not communicate or follow commands

Source: Riker 1993, Developed Maine Medical Center

anxiolytic and anticonvulsant properties. Although the degree of sedation is unpredictable, the anxiolysis and retrograde amnesia produced by it is fairly good.

The bitter taste of the drug when used by oral use can to some extent be lessened by mixing it with syrup or juice. When used for intranasal route for convenience and fast onset, the experience is unpleasant as midazolam greatly stings.

Dose: 0.05–0.15 mg/kg IV in 2–3 divided doses each bolus dose should be administered over 1–2 minutes. Its peak action is in 2–3 minutes and the action lasts approximately 45 minutes.

Oral dose is 0.5 mg/kg, 30–60 minutes before the procedure.

Metabolism: Metabolised in the liver and excreted in the urine

Mode of action: It acts on the benzodiazepine receptors in the CNS. Being water soluble it takes three times longer to produce electroencephalographic changes in the CNS compared to the fat soluble diazepam. Thus it is prudent to wait for three minutes between the IV doses to prevent the stacking of its effect.

There is a potential for respiratory depression if administered along with opioids and thus should be used with caution.

- *Chloral hydrate:* It is a sedative and hypnotic drug. Onset time after oral ingestion is 15–30 minutes and duration of action is 60–120 minutes. Dose is between 25 and 100 mg/kg. It is a safe sedative drug with a few side effects like nausea and vomiting and prolonged recovery times. However, there is a high incidence of failed sedation which may result in longer scan times. It is not available in India. Its active metabolite trichlofos is used in India.
- *Pentobarbital:* Dosing for oral or rectal use is 3–6 mg/kg. The time of onset of sedation is 15–60 minutes. Duration of action is 60–240 minutes. Cardiovascular and respiratory depression may occur. It is contraindicated in patients with porphyria.
- *Ketamine:* The intravenous dose is 1–1.5 mg/kg and 4–5 mg/kg when used intramuscularly. Onset time is 1–3 minutes and duration is 15–30 minutes. Some of its unwanted effects include hypertonicity, hypertension and re-emergence phenomenon. Mainly useful sedative in patients with respiratory problems.
- *Dexmedetomidine:* It is a selective alpha 2 agonist. Does not cause any respiratory side effects but may cause haemodynamic consequences such as low blood pressure and fall in heart rate. That is why it has to be used with caution in patients with cardiac problems. Drug is initially given by a bolus of 0.5–1 μgm/kg over 10 minutes followed by an infusion of 0.5–1 μgm/kg/hour.
- *Propofol*: It is a perfect sedative drug with short recovery times and can be easily titrated to achieve the desired sedation levels. Dose is 2–5 mg/kg/hour. However, there is a small incidence of hypotension.

In a study by Koroglu et al. it was shown that propofol and dexmedetomidine both prevented undesirable movements in children. The risk of oxygen desaturation was not there with dexmedetomidine, whereas propofol resulted in more rapid induction and recovery characteristics.[6]

- Nitrous oxide 50% mixed with oxygen is a potent anaesthetic which can significantly reduce pain. It can be used for radiological sedation in ASA I and II patients. It is contraindicated in patients with pneumothorax, pneumocephalus, pneumopericardium, otitis media or bowel obstruction.
- Sevoflurane, has been used frequently for inhalation induction of anaesthesia. Owing to its non-pungency, rapid induction and quick elimination, sevoflurane may be useful for sedation only by professionals who are skilled in general anaesthesia.
- *Reversal agents*: Naloxone an opioid antagonist is used in the dose of 0.1 mg/kg in children less than 20 kg and 2 mg for over 20 kg every 2–3 minutes. Flumazenil is the benzodiazepine antagonist which antagonises the sedation, amnesic, anticonvulsant properties. Dose is 0.01–0-0.02 mg/kg IV over 15 seconds maximum up to 1 mg. These reversal agents should be used cautiously as they may precipitate agitation in the child.

There are several advantages of anaesthesia over sedation.[1,3]

- Anaesthesiologist is always present during the procedure
- Induction and recovery are fast
- Success is reliable
- Depth of anaesthesia may be varied as per the requirement of the procedure.
- Airway and cardiovascular status are under control.

The period during which the monitoring should be stepped up include the period 5–10 minutes after IV administration of the drug and immediately after the end of the procedure when the procedural stimuli are ceased.

The level of consciousness should be assessed every 15 minutes using the sedation score. The other parameters which require continuous monitoring include:

- Ventilation should be monitored by chest auscultation and capnography.
- Oxygenation should be monitored using pulse oximetry.
- Vital signs like the pulse, BP and ECG.
- The monitored values should be recorded every 5 minutes.

There should be no difference in monitoring between deep sedation and general anaesthesia as there is a thin line of demarcation between the two and there is no boundary as to when the patient will slip from one state to another.

Discharge criteria should be met as these procedures are mostly carried out on day care basis.[1]

Postanaesthesia score (Aldrete)

Score	Criteria
Activity	
2	Able to move 4 extremities
1	Able to move 2 extremities
0	Able to move 0 extremities
Respiratory	
2	Able to breathe deep/cough
1	Dyspnoea or limited breathing
0	Apnoea
Circulation	
2	BP +/– 20% Pre-anaesthesia level
1	BP +/– 20–50% Pre-anaesthesia level
0	BP +/– 5% Pre-anaesthesia level
Awareness	
2	Fully awake
1	Arousable on calling
0	Not responding
Colour	
2	Pink
1	Pale, dusky, blotchy, jaundiced
0	Cyanotic

The following discharge criteria should be met

- Child should be conscious, intact airway reflexes, stable vital signs and no pain.
- A simple test is to let the child be in a quiet atmosphere for about 20 minutes and the child should not fall asleep.
- Aldrete score of 10, presedation ASA status and mental status.
- Should be started on orals and be able to void before discharge.

There is a risk of resedation as they are being transferred home in cosy environment and with it the attendant risk of airway obstruction. This must be borne in mind when discharging these patients and the possibility should be explained to the parents.

ANAESTHESIA FOR CT SCANS[7]

Clinical Pearls

Radiation hazard, Wide bore IV for body scans.

MRI and CT scan per se pose very little risk to the children but sedation and anaesthesia may be responsible for the complications. The principles of sedation remain the same as for other procedures. In fact CT scans are much faster today and are completed in a very short time.

Sequence of events: Registration of the patient data on the operator console by the technician should be followed by positioning of the patient. Localizing image called topogram follows this. The study is planned according to this topogram by the radiologist. Thus any craniocaudal movement after acquisition of this topogram would result in incorrect imaging.

Anaesthetic considerations: The best time to sedate the child is after registration of the data but before the topogram is acquired.

The site of the scan is also important whether it is head or body. Head scan requires taking serial tomograms, whereas body scans require acquisition of spiral data. Patient movement during any of this can degrade the image quality and require repeat scan. The total dose of contrast at a time cannot exceed 3 mL/kg. Thus a repeat scan has to be postponed to another day. This also involves repeating the radiation dose which in no way is benign for the child. Acquisition of data is over in less than 1 min after which any patient movement does not hamper the image quality. Thus it is imperative that the anaesthesiologist ensures that there is no patient movement during this brief time.

The size of IV cannula is dependent on the site to be scanned. If the pathology is inside the blood–brain barrier, then the CT scan can be done up to 10 minutes after contrast administration in which case a 24 G IV cannula will do. However in case of body scan, IV contrast has to be injected as a rapid bolus with a pressure injector in which case a larger bore IV cannula is required. Also it should be placed in the arm and not in the foot as it will lead to pooling of the contrast in the lower limb and also opacification of the inferior vena cava in abdominal CT angiograms may not be desired.

Though CT scans can now be performed within 10–40 seconds and may not require sedation there are certain situations which are of special concern. Extreme head extension may be required for scans used to visualise the sinuses, ears, inner auditory canal and the temporomandibular bones. Children with cervical instability should be screened before giving neck extension. Atlantoaxial instability is a risk in children with Down's syndrome and this history should be sought in the preprocedural evaluation. In asymptomatic child with radiological evidence of instability sedation should be given cautiously avoiding abnormal extension. However, in a symptomatic child sedation should be avoided altogether and a neurosurgical or an orthopaedic consultation should be sought.[8]

Oral gastrografin [diatrizoate meglumine/diatrizoate sodium (48.29% total iodine)] is sometimes used for evaluation of abdominal masses. The volume used may defy the NPO guidelines (60–90 mL in infant <1 month to 240–360 mL in child 1–5 years) as sedation may be required in 1–2 hour period. As full strength gastrografin (3%) is hyperosmolar, it should be diluted to 1.5% which is isotonic and isomolar and would minimise the risk to adverse sequelae to aspiration.[8]

ANAESTHESIA FOR MRI

Clinical Pearls

Exclusion of ferromagnetic objects, long scan times.

There is an increasing need for high quality imaging in modern medicine to help in diagnosis, explore treatment options and to know the response to a particular treatment. MRI is a feasible option as it is a non-invasive radiation free diagnostic procedure which is a major advantage in the paediatric population.

As the demand for anaesthesia increases, questions are raised as to how adequate sedation can be achieved without compromising on patient safety. The risk can be substantially reduced by thorough presedation assessment with proper reference to the underlying pathophysiology, close monitoring, MRI compatible equipment and trained personnel.

Principle: A magnetic field anywhere in strength between 1.5 and 7, T is used to perform the MRI. This is 140000 times the earth natural magnetic field. These magnetic forces cause all the protons in the magnetic field to be oriented in a longitudinal direction and creates a spin. A high frequency radio impulse is then applied with the same frequency as the spin which causes the protons to absorb energy. On stopping the radio frequency the protons return to the initial position and the emitted radio waves are used to create the images of MRI.[9]

Prerequisites: To obtain high quality images it is essential to alleviate any patient motion. This may take anywhere from 10 to 30 minutes. Also it is mandatory to exclude any metallic materials as they not only may act as projectile missiles but also impair the image quality and produce undesirable side effects, e.g. warming.[9]

MRI compatible equipment must be used. This equipment should present no hazard to the patient or the personnel working in the MRI suite. They should function normally in the magnetic environment and not interfere with the proper functioning of the MRI equipment.

Any ferrous objects brought to the scanning room may become dangerous missiles and may injure the personnel, patient or the equipment.

The 5 gauss line should be marked in the MRI suite for safety reasons. Beyond this line, it is safe to use ferromagnetic equipment.[4]

Advantages over CT scan: It provides excellent image quality, superior soft tissue resolution compared to CT scans, the ionising radiation.

Indications: The main indications for MRI in children are neurological disorders, vascular malformation or oncological tumour growth.

Anaesthetic concerns: These children generally present with convulsions or mental retardation and this should be borne in mind when sedating these children. These children do not need higher dose of sedation but are three times more prone to hypoventilation.[9] In newborn babies and infants bradycardia immediately follows desaturation and the anaesthesiologist should be constantly alert to avert such consequences.

In many instances the chest excursion may not be always visible and saturation may not fall for a prolonged period after cessation of respiration due to oxygen insufflations. In this context monitoring of end tidal CO_2 may be imperative.

If hypoventilation occurs it may be necessary to stop the scan and pull the scan desk outside the tube and attend to the child. Frequent stopping and interrupting the MRI scan is expensive and ineffective and thus careful titration of sedation is necessary.

Anaesthesia workstation requirements are similar to those in the OT which include an anaesthesia unit with a ventilator, anaesthetic gas monitor, capnography, pulse oximeter, ECG monitor blood pressure measurement and respiratory frequency monitor. However, all these equipment have to be MRI compatible.

MRI compatible pulse oximeters must have fiberoptic cables to avoid burns. Special electrocardiograph leads are needed and padding should be placed between the ECG cables and the patient's skin. Also loops of cables should not form within the scanner as this can induce current and burn the patient. The MRI compatible electrodes should be arranged in a narrow triangular area on the patient's chest. The leads should be short (15 cms) and braided.

ST–T complex changes mimicking hyperkalaemia may result from the artefacts produced by the currents induced by blood flowing through the transverse aorta.[10]

As most of the equipment may have to be placed away from the patient, there may be a delay of 20 seconds in obtaining the capnograph signal.

If a child is with cardiovascular catheters and accessories that have internally or externally positioned conductive wires or similar components they should be removed before the MRI because of the risk of excessive heating of wires.

Certain contraindications to MRI include presence of pacemakers, cochlear implants, certain metallic implants and devices and patients with renal impairment in whom the contrast Gadolinium is contraindicated.

Problems in the MRI Suite

Auditory considerations. MRI coils produce loud thumping noise and hence ear plugs must be placed. This is also the reason why deeper levels of sedation may be necessary. An average noise during a scan may reach 95 decibels in a 1.5 T scanner and exposure to this high noise should be restricted to 2 hours per day.

Radio frequency heating: The possibility of RF heating from induced currents is a problem with field strengths greater than 2 T. The FDA recommends limit of 0.4 Wikg. Specific absorption rates can be reduced by various methods such as changing the pulse sequence, decreasing the number of slices and switching to smaller transmitter coils.[11]

Hypothermia: Care must be taken to avoid hypothermia in all patients, especially in the paediatric population. Air flow directed through the scanner cavity increases heat loss, making hypothermia a distinct problem. Heat loss can be reduced by covering the patient, using bags of warm intravenous fluids and airway humidification. Temperature can be measured using nonferromagnetic disposable temperature strips.

In case of accidental extubation it should be possible to rapidly extricate the patient from the magnetic bore. It may sometimes be necessary to perform a laryngoscopy at the foot of the magnetic bore with a plastic laryngoscope.

In case of an arrest only basic life support can be provided as a defibrillator cannot be brought into the MRI console. Hence the child will have to be rapidly taken out for resuscitation.

Contrast agent: The most commonly used contrast agents are Gadollenium based. Used mainly for delineation of vascular structures or where tissue resolution has to be improved. It has a high therapeutic index and low incidence of side effects such as headache, nausea, vomiting, burning at the site of injection and hives. Gadollenium based contrast agents are classified as high-risk gadopentelic acids, the medium risk ones gadobenic acids and those associated with low risk—i.e. gadoteridol. The high-risk agents are contraindicated in the neonates and in the perioperative period of patients undergoing liver transplant.[12]

Sedation and Anaesthesia for MRI

Non-pharmacological methods should be tried before attempting sedation especially in infants less than 6 months where feed and wrap and prior sleep deprivation may succeed. In children above 6 years who can comprehend prior counselling may help in doing the procedure without sedation. Since dexmedetomidine does not cause respiratory depression it may be a useful drug. Also its long duration of action may be advantageous in MRI which itself may be time consuming.

The nasal vestibule airway (NVA) have been used in anaesthetised children undergoing MRI to combat the nasal obstruction that sometimes accompanies deep sedation or anaesthesia. It is a nasal tube connected to a source of oxygen for providing continuous positive airway pressure. The system is pressurised by a reservoir bag and the distending pressure of which is controlled by a valve and a pressure gauge. The breathing can be monitored by capnography and watching movement of the rebreathing bag and the pressure changes in the gauge. However, it should be remembered that nasal tube may cause bleeding and may be painful to insert.[13]

The choice between sedation and general anaesthesia for MRI procedure has to be made on case to case basis. Whatever the choice the presence of a fully equipped workstation is a pre-requisite. In children older than 3 years of age who do not have significant co-morbidities sedation may be the technique of choice, but in younger children and those with airway abnormalities or any other comorbidities a carefully planned general anaesthetic would be a safer option.[9]

GASTROINTESTINAL (GI) ENDOSCOPIES

Clinical Pearl

Upper GI scopy, colonoscopy.

GI endoscopic procedures are an essential modality for diagnosis and treatment of gastrointestinal diseases in children. These include:

- Gastrointestinal bleeding
- Unexplained iron deficiency anaemia
- Chronic diarrhoea, failure to thrive/weight loss
- Polyposis syndrome
- Foreign body removal
- Rejection of intestinal transplant
- Balloon dilatation of stenotic lesions
- Decompression of acute non-toxic megacolon

Contraindications include any coagulopathies, suspected bowel ischaemia or perforation and neutropenia.

Upper GI endoscopies can be performed by a skilled endoscopist in about 10 minutes. Adequate sedation is necessary in paediatric patients because it can elicit powerful protective reflexes. Spontaneous ventilation should be maintained during deep sedation as any airway intervention will necessitate removal of the endoscope. Topical local anaesthesia of the upper airway can help diminish the gag reflex. Transoral and transpyloric passage of the endoscope are the most stimulating events in the passage of the endoscope. Colonoscopy, on the other hand, can take a longer time and also cause discomfort and pain.[14]

The risk associated with intravenous (IV) sedation is much higher than that associated with general anaesthesia (GA) (3.7% vs 1.2%).[15]

Although GA is considered safe as it provides comfort and amnesia, it requires expertise and does not prove to be cost effective.

The aims and objectives of providing IV sedation or GA during these procedures include

- Children should allow these unpleasant procedures with amnesia
- There should be no movement to reduce the incidence of complications
- There should be safe monitoring by qualified staff to avoid complications
- High quality and cost effective standard of care must be provided
- Discharge criteria should be met with aim to early discharge.

The same guidelines for sedation and anaesthesia in these remote locations should be adhered to as laid by the American Task Force. Although GI Scopies are identified as safe procedures they are also not without any complication. Younger age, higher ASA class, female sex and IV sedation are identified as risk factors for developing complications. IV sedation has a higher incidence of cardiopulmonary complications as compared to GA.

Sedation Regimen for GI Endoscopies

A combination of benzodiazepine and opioid may be used for sedation. The attending anaesthesiologist should be continuously vigilant and extreme caution should be exercised. IV agents are reliable and can be easily titrated.

Propofol has been commonly used for sedation for these procedures because of its rapid action, short duration and favourable recovery profile. It results in mild analgesia and is associated with minimal side effects like hypotension and dose dependent respiratory depression.

In a study conducted by Hasnin et al. they compared dexmedetomidine with propofol for GI scopies. They found that dexmedetomidine was associated with more heart rate stability and respiratory safety as compared with propofol. Incidence of oxygen desaturation was higher with propofol compared with dexmedetomidine. This is a major advantage as upper GI endoscopies may sometimes result in oxygen desaturations.

The disadvantages of dexmedetomidine is the increased induction and recovery times which may influence the patient turnover rates especially in cases of upper GI scopies. However, it may be used for longer procedures like colonoscopies.[16]

During the introduction of the scope sedation score of at least 5 should be achieved to prevent any patient agitation.[17]

Sclerotherapy with alcohol may result in tissue edema particularly at the base of the tongue, neck or mediastinum. This may result in difficult extubation which may require airway support for many days.[8]

As colonoscopy is an invasive procedure it is associated with a variety of complications such as loss of protective reflexes, upper airway obstruction, respiratory disturbances, allergic reactions and cardiac arrest. The anaesthesiologist must be able to rescue the child from deeper level of sedation and provide basic life support.

INTERVENTIONAL RADIOLOGICAL PROCEDURES IN PAEDIATRIC PATIENT[18]

Keywords
Embolisations, sclerotherapy.

With the advent of sophisticated technology the radiologists have taken over many of the procedures which previously required surgical interventions. For this, the anaesthesiologist must have an understanding of the pathophysiology related to the disease process and the procedure itself, to anticipate the problems and be ready to tackle them effectively on table.

Some of the procedures that can be done by the interventional radiologist are:

- Biopsies
- Paracentesis
- Thoracocentesis
- Percutaneous drainage of abscess
- Nephrostomy tube placements
- Sclerotherapy

These are just to mention a few. Radiology is advancing in leaps and bounds and there are further advances including:

- Newer lower dose technologies allowing longer exposure times
- 3-D rotational angiography/XperCT and XperGuide
- Advanced digital imaging, etc.

These newer techniques mean it is now possible to acquire simultaneously CT, 3-D angiography and fluoroscopic images in a single room. This allows procedures which require real time imaging capability of fluoroscopy combined with 3-D spatial orientation of CT.

Anaesthetic management: The same principles that apply for anaesthetic management outside the operating room apply here. However, general anaesthetic may be required for many of these procedures as they may be long and to ensure a motionless field. Endotracheal intubation with controlled ventilation may be required in conditions which require breath holding during angiographic sequences and hypercarbia to induce vasodilation.

The scope of regional anaesthesia for paediatric patients in these situations is very limited. However, intercoastal nerve blocks can be used as an adjunct in lung or rib biopsies, chest tube insertions, biliary or subphrenic drainage procedures.

Vascular interventions may include embolisations and sclerotherapy procedures. Congenital vascular malformations may be high flow or low flow types. With large lesions there is a potential for high output cardiac failure and pulmonary oedema.

For embolisations or sclerotherapy stainless steel coils, absorbed gelatin pledges and powders, polyvinyl foams, glues, threads and ethanol may be used. Ethanol produces sclerosis by first producing a coagulum of the blood followed by endothelial necrosis. Embolizations or sclerotherapy with ethanol can produce coagulopathy and renal failure. Ethanol denatures the proteins and can result in hematuria. Thus adequate fluid replacement and frusemide (0.5–1 mg/kg) may be necessary to flush the kidneys and prevent renal failure. Alkalinisation of the urine with sodium bicarbonate (1 meq/kg) may also may necessary to prevent precipitation of haemoglobin in the renal tubules. Other potential side effects of ethanol include intoxication and cardiovascular collapse.

Ketamine is a useful anaesthetic agent for these interventional procedures. It is a useful drug which can be used for painful procedures which require immobilization without control of ventilation.

PET SCAN IN PAEDIATRIC PATIENTS

PET scan is the latest technology which has now evolved from time consuming, effort dependent procedure to the one which is routine even in paediatric patients.

Whole body imaging has now become possible and a two level emission transmission scan can now be available in 20 minutes. To obtain a high quality imaging data it is necessary to make the study as comfortable as possible for the child.[19]

Fluorodeoxyglucose or FDG is used for PET scan. It has a positron emitting radioactive isotope. It is an analogue of glucose and is taken up by living cells. There is increased glycolytic activity in the neoplastic cells which take up the tracer and help in the diagnosis of the cancer. It is excreted by the kidneys which are unable to absorb the tracer. A 50–60 minutes interval is usually needed between the administration of FDG and obtaining an image scan.

The indications for PET scan in paediatric patients include:

1. To distinguish between benign and malignant neoplasms
2. To select a site for biopsy
3. For staging of malignancy
4. To distinguish scar from residual neoplasm in children who have completed treatment.

Certain malignancies where PET scan is used for either staging or to know the response to therapy include lymphomas, sarcomas (osteosarcoma, Ewings sarcoma rhabdomyosarcoma) and neurobalstomas.

Patient consent, IV access, bladder catheterisation and sedation are the prerequisites for PET scan. A dedicated IV line is a must for injection of the tracer dye. Many of these patients are on chemotherapy and may have a central line. The line should be flushed to clear any residual tracer so that the residual activity does not interfere with the image interpretation. The line should lie on the side of the patient and not on the top also so that it lies outside the imaging area.

The fasting blood glucose levels need to be noted and have to be maintained below 120 mg/dL (6.66 mmol/L). Higher blood glucose levels may give decreased sensitivity and the patient may have to be rescheduled. Thus the child should be instructed to fast at least 4–6 hours prior to the procedure but drink water to maintain adequate hydration.[20]

FDG uptake in brown adipose tissues is noted in 15–20% during PET scans in children and this may limit the ability to detect disease in these regions. This can be reduced by increasing the ambient temperature or covering the child with a warm blanket during the tracer uptake phase. Moderate dose of oral diazepam (0.1 mg/kg) or intravenous fentanyl in the dose of 0.75–1 mcg/kg can reduce the tracer uptake by the adipose tissue. In older children propanolol (1 mg/kg) up to a maximum of 40 mg can be given 45 minutes prior to the procedure.[21]

Bladder catheterisation is essential for PET scans as:

- Activity in full bladder may interfere with the imaging in the nearby structures especially in small babies and when evaluating the pelvis.
- A distended bladder may be uncomfortable to the child.
- As anaesthesia causes smooth muscle relaxation, it can cause further distension of the bladder.

The urine collection device should also be carefully placed away from the patient so as to avoid interference by radioactive urine. A small amount of urinary FDG can contaminate a large region. Thus even drops of urine on the surrounding drapes should be avoided.

The same principles of sedation as for other procedures outside OR apply for PET scans.

Nowadays PET/CT, SPECT/CT and PET/MR are the newer hybrid techniques used in diagnosing cancers, epilepsy and even causes of back pain in children.[22]

EXTERNAL BEAM RADIATION THERAPY (XRT)[23]

It is one of the accepted modalities for treatment in paediatric oncology. Though the process is painless, there is a lot of anxiety associated with it. As with other remote locations, the anaesthesiologist will be at a distance away from the patient. However, the difference here is that there is no means of viewing the patient but one has to depend on closed circuit television monitoring.

Once a child is scheduled for XRT, he must first undergo a simulation trial which allows the oncologist to set up a proper treatment plan and also to know how well the child will cooperate for the procedure. The simulation stage may be followed by the first treatment phase. Total dose of radiation may range from 25 to 80 gray (Gy). This dose is divided into 30 equal doses which are administered once daily five times a week over 6-week period. The total procedure lasts 5–20 minutes.

Generally this can be achieved by MAC in most procedures. Though it is mandatory to leave the room during the therapy it may be possible to re-enter between doses.

Intravenous agents are the preferred drugs. Midazolam in the dose of 0.05 mg/kg is the drug of choice. If this is insufficient, this is followed by bolus dose of propofol in dose of 0.5–0.8 mg/kg followed by infusion of 7.4–10 mg/kg/hour.

Ketamine in the dose of 0.5–0.75 mg/kg can also be used. However, unlike propofol tachyphylaxis can develop with repeat doses of ketamine and by the 5th or 6th week the child may require twice the dose, though recovery time is not prolonged indicating that the metabolism of the drug is also enhanced. However, ketamine cannot be used for retinoblastomas where immobility of the globe is essential.

Fospropofol a prodrug of propofol, in the dose of 6.5 mg/kg has been approved by the US FDA for sedation. Redose is 1.5–2 mg/kg. There are minimal side effects like tingling and burning in the genital area. Incidences of hypotension, 20% from the baseline and desaturation below 92% are rare.

If GA is used, LMA should be used as repeated daily intubations may result in subglottic swellings and short acting agent should be preferred.

Ondansetron in the dose of 0.1 mg/kg should be given at the end of these procedures as these children are very prone to nausea and vomiting. Though phenothiazines and steroids have also been used, haloperidol is not helpful.

BONE MARROW ASPIRATION AND LUMBAR PUNCTURE

Multiple punctures may be required for children with leukaemia and neoplastic diseases. These painful procedures may be very distressing to the child and thus providing adequate sedation and analgesia is imperative. Sedation can be provided by oral or intranasal midazolam. However, in a study by C Crock, et al. there was a high level of pain, distress and parental concerns associated with sedation and not with GA. Advantages of GA to the medical personnel may be that procedures like bone marrow biopsy may be done quicker with adequate sample with the resultant more accurate and speedy diagnosis. Children are also not scared of repeated procedures under GA. Lesser restraint was required and at the same time there was less pain and distress.[24]

SUMMARY

As technology advances in leaps and bound, the number of radiological diagnostic and therapeutic procedures are increasing in paediatric patient. Thorough preprocedural evaluation, a well-equipped set up including emergency equipment and a well-planned backup for emergencies and complications will go long way in providing a smooth and safe anaesthesia in these remote locations. The anaesthesiologist should be well versed with the levels of sedation required for a particular procedure and be able to rescue the patient from deeper than intended levels of sedation.

FAQs

Q. Is sedation justified for an emergency procedure in a non-fasting child?

Q. In a child with difficult airway, should we secure the airway in the operation theatre prior to the procedure?

Q. How early can a child be discharged after procedural sedation? Should nausea and vomiting be considered a contraindication to discharge?

Q. Should a child be always catheterised prior to PET scan?

Q. What can be the reasons for fever after MRI?

REFERENCES

1. Jones S. Pediatric Conscious Sedation: Floating in Space. www.pedconcepts.com accessed 20 July 2014.
2. American Academy of Pediatrics and the American Academy of Pediatric Dentistry. Guideline for monitoring and management of pediatric patients during and after sedation for diagnostic and therapeutic procedures 2004.
3. Miller MGA. Anaesthesia for MRI: ...child's play? Registrar Communication Southern African Journal of Anaesthesia & Analgesia. 2005;pp 28–31.
4. Arlachov Y, Ganatra RH. Sedation/anaesthesia in paediatric radiology Br J Radiol, 2012;85(1019): e1018–e1031.
5. Hoffman GM, Nowakowski R, Troshynki TJ, et al. Risk reduction in Paediatric Procedural sedation by Application of an American Academy of Paediatric/American society of Anaesthesiologist Process model. Pediatrics. 2002; 109(2):236–243.
6. Koroglu A, Teksan H, Sagir O, et al. A Comparison of the Sedative, Hemodynamic, and Respiratory Effects of Dexmedetomidine and Propofol in Children Undergoing Magnetic Resonance Imaging. Anesth & Analg. 2006; 103:63–7.
7. Ghai B, Panda N, Makkar JK, et al. Pediatric Computed Tomographic Scan with Anaesthesia: What the Anesthesiologist Should Know. Anesth & Analg 2006;6(103):1623.
8. Mason KP, Zgleszewski SE, Holzman RS. Anesthesia and Sedation for Procedures Outside the Operating Room in Motoyama EK, Davis PJ, (Eds). Smith's Anesthesia for Infants and Children, 7th edn. Elsevier. 839–853.
9. Schulte-Uentrop L, Goepfert MS. Anaesthesia or sedation for MRI in children. Curr Opin Anaesthesiol. 2010;23: 513–517.
10. Wellis V. Paediatric Anaesthesia and pain management 'Lucile Packard Children's hospital'. Stanford University Medical Center. Department of anaesthesia and pain management. Practice Guidelines for MRT & MRI (660) 723–4728.

11. Patteson SK, Chesney JT. Anesthetic Management for Magnetic Resonance Imaging: Problems and Solutions. Anesth Analg 1992;74:121–8.
12. Farling PA, Flynn PA, Darwent G, et al. Safety in Magnetic Resonance Units: An update published by The Association of Anaesthetists of Great Britain and Ireland July 2010. Anaesthesia. Jul 2010;65(7): 766–770.
13. Arthurs OJ, Sury M. Anaesthesia or sedation for paediatric MRI: Advantages and disadvantages. Curr Opin Anesthesiol 2013;26:489–494.
14. Amornyotin S. Sedation for Colonoscopy in children: Journal of Gastroenterology and Hepatology Research. 2013;2(6):609–613.
15. Dar AQ, Shah ZA. Anesthesia and sedation in pediatric gastrointestinal endoscopic procedures: A review. World J Gastrointest Endosc. 2010, July 16;2(7):257–262.
16. Hasanin AS, Sira AM. Dexmedetomidine versus propofol for sedation during gastrointestinal endoscopy in pediatric patients. Egyptian Journal of Anaesthesia 2014;30:21–26.
17. Amornyotin S. Sedation for Colonoscopy in children: Journal of Gastroenterology and Hepatology Research. 2013;2(6):609–613.
18. Garg R, Pandey R, Darlong V, et al. Anaesthetic considerations for Interventional radiology. The internet Journal of Anaesthesiology 2008;19(1).
19. Shulkin BL. PET imaging in pediatric oncology. Pediatr Radiol 2004;34:199–204.
20. Bombardieri E, Aktolun C, Baum RP, et al. FDG-PET Procedure Guidelines For Tumour Imaging. Guidelines issued date: September 2, 2003.
21. Stauss J, Franzius C, Pfluger T, et al. Guidelines for 18F-FDG PET and PET-CT imaging in paediatric oncology. Eur J Nucl Med Mol Imaging. 2008;35(8):1581–8.
22. Treves ST, Baker A, Fahey FH, et al. Nuclear Medicine in the First Year of Life. J Nucl Med. 2011;52:905–925.
23. Harris EA. Sedation and anesthesia options for pediatric patients in the radiation oncology suite. International Journal of Pediatrics. 2010, Article ID 870921, p.9.
24. Crock C, Olsson C, Phillips R, et al. General anaesthesia or conscious sedation for painful procedures in childhood cancer: The family's perspective. Arch Dis Child 2003;88: 253–257.

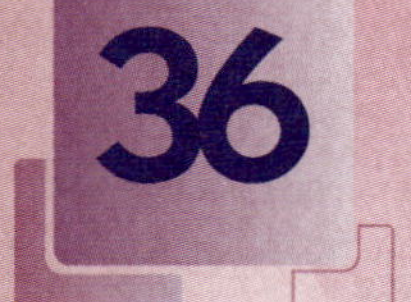

Office-based Paediatric Anaesthesia

Anita Malik and Namisha Malik

An office-based anaesthesia is performed in a location, usually an office or procedure room, that is not accredited by the state as an ambulatory surgery center (ASC) or as a hospital and where nonsurgical activities such as patient consultation and practice administration are also housed in addition.[1]

GUIDELINES FOR OFFICE-BASED ANAESTHESIA

Guidelines for office-based anaesthesia approved by the ASA House of Delegates in 1999 and last affirmed in 2009 state that since office based anaesthesia is a subset of ambulatory anaesthesia, the ASA "Guidelines for Ambulatory Anaesthesia and Surgery" should be followed in the office setting as well as all other ASA standards and guidelines that are applicable. The anaesthesiologist should adhere to the "Basic Standards for Preanaesthesia Care", "Standards for Basic Anesthetic Monitoring", "Standards for Postanaesthesia Care" and "Guidelines for Ambulatory Anaesthesia and Surgery" as currently promulgated by the American Society of Anesthesiologists. Back-up power sufficient to ensure patient protection in the event of an emergency should be available. In an office where anaesthesia services are to be provided to infants and children, the required equipment, medication and resuscitative capabilities should be appropriately sized for a paediatric population. The facility should have a written protocol in place for the safe and timely transfer of patients to a prespecified alternate care facility when extended or emergency services are needed to protect the health or well-being of the patient.[2]

Operative procedures characteristics: Various operative procedures in office-based setup are almost the same as those performed on paediatric outpatients[3] and all share several common characteristics as mentioned in Box 36.1.

Box 36.1 Operative procedures characteristics

Peripheral procedures not involving major violation of a body cavity
Usually lasting less than 2 hours
No major physiologic disturbances or blood loss
Minimal or moderate postop pain that can easily be managed at home with oral analgesics
No disturbance to oral fluids intake in the immediate postoperative period.

Paediatric Comorbidities

The paediatric comorbidities considered high risk for the office-based setup are obstructive sleep apnoea, labile asthma and other significant pulmonary disease, complex congenital heart disease, labile diabetes mellitus, significant neurologic and neuromuscular disorders, sickle cell disease, upper respiratory tract infection and increased body mass index.[4]

Important Factors

Patient's age, associated medical illnesses and ASA physical status, type of surgery, potential for blood loss, potential for significant postoperative complications, and duration of surgery are important factors to be considered while accepting the child for office-based anaesthesia.[3]

Prematurely born infants have a disturbance of breathing control, which may develop into apnoea during the first day after general anaesthesia, intravenous sedation or opioid use and may require prolonged postoperative monitoring which is not a prerequisite for office-based anaesthesia. Although no minimum age requirement for a child to undergo an office-based anaesthetic has been established, patients >6 months of age and ASA physical status 1 or 2 may be reasonable candidates.[5] Children above the age of 3–6 months are generally healthy, definitely feel happier at home than in hospital, and the surgery is usually well suited to the ambulatory setting, being superficial, short lasting, and well suited for local anaesthesia as an adjuvant per- and postoperatively.

Preanaesthetic Assessment

History and physical examination decides about laboratory tests orders on individual basis as most of the children are healthy. Infomed consent should be obtained from parents/guardians.

PREOPERATIVE FASTING GUIDELINES

Preoperative fasting guidelines (ASA task force 1999 updated in 2010)[6] recommend to fast from intake of clear liquids (e.g. water, fruit juices without pulp, carbonated beverages, clear tea, and black coffee) at least 2 hours, breast milk at least 4 hours in neonates while 4–6 hours in infants/children, infant formula at least 6 hours, a light meal or nonhuman milk 6 hours and fried or fatty foods or meat at least 8 hours before elective procedures requiring general anaesthesia, regional anaesthesia, or sedation/analgesia (i.e. monitored anaesthesia care). Same guidelines should be applicable to office-based paediatric anaesthesia.

Premedication

Prolonged sedation, postoperative nausea and vomiting and delaying discharge after office-based anaesthesia are important factors in premedication consideration. Though premedication allays anxiety and allows for easy separation in patients of >6 months, it may affect recovery after anaesthesia or produce emetic side effects,[7,8] however, in the presence of parents, children can be smoothly induced after verbal reassurance.[9,10] Children have fear of needles but for uncooperative and unmanageable children low dose ketamine (2–3 mg/kg) administered intramuscularly produces appropriate conditions for inhalational induction within 7–10 minutes.[11]

Midazolam in oral doses as low as 0.25 mg/kg have been demonstrated to be as effective as larger doses with only a slightly slower time of onset.[12] Despite having an extremely bitter, unpleasant taste, oral midazolam (0.25 to 1.0 mg/kg, maximum of 20 mg) remains the most commonly used and best tolerated method for children requiring sedation.[13–15]

EQUIPMENT AND MONITORING

According to guidelines for office-based anaesthesia approved by the ASA in any location in which anaesthesia is administered, there should be appropriate anaesthesia apparatus and equipment which allow monitoring consistent with ASA "Standards for Basic Anesthetic Monitoring" and documentation of regular preventive maintenance as recommended by the manufacturer. Back-up power sufficient to ensure patient protection in the event of an emergency should be available.[2]

A checklist of essential anaesthesia supplies for office-based setup (Box 36.2) has been proposed by Koch et al in the form of a simple mnemonic—POSEMD.

Box 36.2 POSEMD checklist

- **P:** Positive pressure ventilation (bag mask, portable ventilator)
- **O:** Oxygen in ample supply (cylinder, oxygen concentrator)
- **S:** Suction (electric, hand powered)
- **E:** Emergency equipment (airway equipment, defibrillator)
- **M:** Monitor (ECG, NIBP, SpO_2, $EtCO_2$)
- **D:** Drugs (anaesthetics, muscle relaxants, analgesics, anti-emetics, emergency drugs)

Koch ME, Gianuzzi R, Goldstein RC. Office Anesthesiology. *Anesthesiol Clini North America* 1999;17(2):395–405.

Anaesthetic Technique

All types of techniques starting from minimal sedation to general anaesthesia are used depending upon the age and cooperation level of the child, the type of procedure, the applicability of local anaesthetic administration and its efficacy in a particular surgical procedure and the available equipment. Venous access should be established in all procedures.

American Society of Anaesthesiologists has described different levels of sedation for the safe management (Table 36.1) of the patient.

Hypoxemia secondary to depressed respiratory activity is the most important risk factor for near misses and death during sedation for children undergoing procedures. Early detection may be valuable in avoiding morbidity and mortality in paediatric sedation procedures. Malviya et al. picked up desaturation in 5.5% of patients and achieved a reduction in bad outcomes.[16]

There is a high incidence of infolding of the epiglottis and malposition in children <10 kg with laryngeal

Table 36.1 Sedation levels described by American Society of Anesthesiologists (2002)

	Moderate sedation/analgesia	Deep sedation/analgesia	General anaesthesia
Drug induced depression of consciousness	+	+	Drug induced loss of consciousness
–verbal commands	+	Cannot be easily aroused	Not arousable
–purposeful stimulation response	Light touch	Repeated or painful stimulus	Not even with repeated or painful stimulus
Airway	Patent	Assistance may be required for maintenance of patent airway	Assistance often required for maintenance of patent airway
Spontaneous ventilation	Adequate	May be inadequate	Depressed spontaneous ventilation or drug-induced depression of neuro-muscular function requiring positive pressure ventilation
Cardiovascular stability	Maintained	Maintained	May not be maintained

Source: Practice Guidelines for Sedation and Analgesia by Non-anaesthesiologists: An updated report by American Society of Anesthesiologists Task Force on Sedation and Analgesia by Non-anaesthesiologist. Anesthesiology 2002;96:1004–1017.

mask airway and a significantly higher incidence of airway complications such as laryngospasm, breath-holding, obstruction, and coughing has been reported when compared with a conventional mask with oral airway.[17–19]

A carefully planned, balanced anaesthetic technique along with adequate pain control is most effective. Inhalational induction is the anaesthetic technique of choice for needlephobics or for children with difficult intravenous cannulation.[20] New agents with low blood gas partition coefficient are known to provide fast induction and rapid recovery.[21]

Sevoflurane is considered to be the agent of choice due to rapid induction and it is possible to quickly increase the inspired concentration up to 8%, while intravenous access is being attempted. As sevoflurane produces dose-related respiratory depression with decrease in both the respiratory rate and tidal volume, a respiratory assistance during this period may increase the potential for anaesthetic overdose unless the inspired concentration is markedly reduced.[22] Halothane produces a decrease in tidal volume and an increase in respiratory rate in a dose dependent manner.

Prolonged effects of neuromuscular blocking agents may lead to delayed emergence and thereby delayed discharge and turnover for subsequent cases so the use of muscle relaxants should be justified in an office-based anaesthesia.

Abu-Shawan and Mack in a study of 42 procedures used a dose of 50–80 μg/kg/min of Propofol in combination with 0.1 μg/kg/min of Remifentanil and it was found to be safe, effective and acceptable for sedation in children undergoing gastrointestinal endoscopy.[23] When compared with midazolam for sedation, Propofol provides equal or better control and more rapid recovery.[24]

A disadvantage to the use of Remifentanil is that its rapid degradation provides no postoperative analgesia.[25] It is essential, therefore, to use another agent or technique for this purpose, e.g. a regional block, or a nonsteroidal drug such as Ketorolac, and to administer it within an adequate time for action before the patient's emergence.

Even though anaesthesiologists debate the clinical (safety and outcome) and cost efficacy of relatively newer anaesthetic agents (e.g. Sevoflurane, Desflurane, Remifentanil, and Propofol) compared with some of the older agents (e.g. Halothane and Isoflurane), these newer agents offer a distinct advantage of predictability and safety.[26–29]

Motas et al. used Bispectral index (BIS) and the University of Michigan Sedation Scale to assess depth of sedation and speculated that BIS may prove to be more suitable monitor than scoring systems that require interaction with the patient for assessment during the procedure.[30]

Emergence Agitation

Another concern for the anaesthesiologist practicing in an office-based setting is **emergence agitation.** The etiology of emergence agitation appears to be multifactorial and is associated with inadequate postoperative analgesia, high preoperative anxiety levels, rapid emergence, and the newer volatile agents, and is reported to occur with both intravenous and volatile anaesthetic techniques.[31–34]

The child with emergence agitation appears wild and incoherent, inconsolable and does not appear to recognize familiar people. This phenomenon has clearly been distinguished from inadequate analgesia. The addition of midazolam reduced this problem while lengthening recovery but not discharge times. Other investigators have found that midazolam does not prevent emergence agitation, and have found better responses to opioids, dexmedetomidine, low-dose ketamine, propofol and ketorolac.[35–39] It is possible that the cause is related to the different effects of these agents on brain function that has been noted on electroencephalogram; speed of emergence does not seem to be a cause.[40–43] Aouad and colleagues found that 1 mg/kg propofol after discontinuation of sevoflurane at the end of surgery decreases the incidence without prolonging recovery.[37]

Caudal Anaesthesia

A caudal block can be used for any surgery that is performed on the lower abdomen or lower extremities (i.e. procedures involving innervations from the sacral, lumbar, and lower thoracic dermatomes). It should be remembered that, there remains a possibility of entering the dural sac in neonates because the distance from the skin to the caudal space in neonates is minimal and the dural sac may extend up to S3. Placing the caudal block at the end of the procedure does not allow the benefit of lower inhaled anesthetic agent concentrations to be used intraoperatively. If appropriate, caudal anaesthesia can be obtained using Bupivacaine or Levobupivacaine 0.125% or 0.25% with Epinephrine 1:200,000; 1 mL/kg up to 10 mL total. Test dose of 1 mL should be given after a negative aspiration through the catheter or needle. A positive test dose, in contrast to adults epidural test dose, could be indicated by an increase or decrease in heart rate, a decrease in blood pressure, or ST-T wave changes. The caudal local anaesthetic dose should be fractionated with frequent aspirations.

Perioperative Fluid Management

The child's fluid deficit is based on the fasting period and is replaced with lactated Ringer's solution. Optimum hydration status reduces incidence of drowsiness, dizziness, thirst and post-operative nausea vomiting (PONV) after surgery; this avoids delay in discharge from hospital.[44,45]

Recovery Position

The recovery position is a first aid technique recommended for assisting people who are unconscious, or nearly so, but are still breathing. This position is advantageous in recovery area.

POSTOPERATIVE PAIN

In children, role of various blocks like caudal, penile and ilioinguinal/iliohypogastric is well established.[46] Since most office-based procedures in children are minimally invasive if regional techniques are not feasible, use of nonopioid analgesics such as the nonsteroidal antiinflammatory drugs (NSAIDs) and Acetaminophen, when not contraindicated, is advocated. Ketorolac is found to be useful with an excellent safety profile for postoperative analgesia in a variety of paediatric surgical procedures, and it can be administered intravenously in a dose of 0.5 to 0.8 mg/kg (maximum dose, 30 mg).[47] Acetaminophen administration is also effective for postoperative analgesia, especially in procedures resulting in mild or moderate pain.[48] Peripheral acting parenteral analgesic like acetaminophen (15–25 mg/kg) or NSAID (diclofenac, ketorolac, COX-2 inhibitors) can be combined with smaller dose of opioids (fentanyl 1–2 µg/kg).[49,50] Rectal acetaminophen (40 mg/kg) is quite safe and effective postoperative analgesic.[51]

For PONV, combination therapy with antiemetic medications acting at different neuroreceptor sites, less emetogenic anaesthesia techniques, adequate intravenous hydration and adequate pain control are advisable.[52]

DISCHARGE CRITERIA

Time-tested objective recovery scores like Steward, Aldrete[53] should be used for assessing children before discharge. Marshall and Chung reviewed discharge[54] and complications after ambulatory surgery using modified quantitative scoring systems. Later on Patel et al.[55] suggested fast track eligibility criteria for children. Special consideration need to be given to stable haemodynamics, normal respiratory pattern, absence of excessive nausea/vomiting and dizziness, and a state of consciousness appropriate to the developmental level.

COMMON PROCEDURES PERFORMED IN OFFICE-BASED SETUP

Hydrocoele and Inguinal Hernia

Inguinal hernia in paediatric patients is mostly indirect and occurs when the processus vaginalis (a small pouch of peritoneum dragged down to the scrotum during gonadal descent) fails to obliterate. Hydrocoeles are identical to hernias in origin but have such a smaller neck that only intraperitoneal fluid, not bowel, can pass through it.

Premature infants are particularly prone to inguinal hernias. Since postoperative apnoea can occur in infants ≥ 50–60 wk postconceptual age, particularly if the infant was born premature, has neurologic disease, anaemia, or required intensive care in the early neonatal period and requires overnight admission, these patients should not be considered for office-based anaesthesia.

At times, inguinal block infiltration prior to incision distorts the anatomy and may perforate the hernia sac, thus turning a relatively simple operation into a more complex one. However, in infants, where the aponeurosis of external oblique is not well developed, it may be more effective for the surgeon to block the ilioinguinal nerve under direct vision.

General anaesthesia with ETT or LMA (± caudal or ilioinguinal/iliohypogastric block for postoperative analgesia) is the choice. Mask induction can be done in children with Sevoflurane and O_2. If child is otherwise healthy and > 18 months old, we can proceed with LMA; otherwise, tracheal intubation is preferred. Caudal anesthetic or inguinal nerve block decrease the amount of volatile anaesthetic and analgesic requirement. If LMA and spontaneous ventilation is used, deepen anaesthetic concentration at incision to minimize risk of laryngospasm. Extubate only when the child is fully awake. Inguinal block may be performed at the end of the procedure or the wound may be infiltrated with 0.25% Bupivacaine, which provides excellent postoperative analgesia and facilitates early discharge from the surgical recovery unit. If an ilioinguinal nerve block had been performed then the child should be assessed for the presence of a femoral nerve block (5%) before walking unaided. Acetaminophen (10–20 mg/kg oral, and 10 mg q6h or 30–40 mg/kg rectally on 1st dose, followed by 20 mg q6h) is advised. Optimal analgesia and presence of parents in PACU will minimize child's agitation/movement/crying.

Circumcision

Sedative premedication (oral midazolam 0.5 mg/kg; maximum 20 mg) is beneficial in older anxious boys followed by an intravenous induction and spontaneous ventilation with LMA. Inhalational induction and endotracheal intubation is preferred in infants. Maintenance is with volatile inhalational agent in oxygen and air or nitrous oxide. A combination of Acetaminophen 15 mg/kg oral 4 hourly, a NSAID, e.g. Ibuprofen 10 mg/kg oral 6 hourly and a weak opioid (such as Codeine phosphate 1 mg/kg oral 4 hourly) is prescribed. Newer considerations regarding analgesia even in the neonate recommend a penile block for this procedure. Both caudal and penile block can offer similar duration of anaesthesia (4–8 h) but leg numbness and inability to void from the caudal block should be taken into consideration in older children.

CLW Suturing (Contused Lacerated Wound Suturing)

All children with lacerations should be checked for fasting, other injuries (e.g. head/cervical spine in falls, eye in facial trauma or teeth with mouth injuries) with special attention to areas with end-arteriolar supply (extremities such as the tip of the nose, finger tips, and ear lobes) as local anaesthesia with adrenaline is avoided on such wounds.

Adequate anaesthesia is necessary for complete examination, cleansing and repair of wounds. Sedation and local anaesthesia with 1% Lignocaine with adrenaline slowly infiltrated around the wound or of nerve proximal to injury (digital ring block—use plain Lignocaine without Adrenaline).

Intravenous Ketamine is especially useful for procedures longer than 15–20 minutes in a dose of 1–1.5 mg/kg given slowly (over 1–2 min) as more rapid administration is associated with respiratory depression, with further increments of 0.5 mg/kg if sedation is inadequate or longer sedation is necessary. Intramuscular Ketamine 3–4 mg/kg can be safely used without intravenous access. Atropine 0.02 mg/kg to a maximum of 0.6 mg can be used to diminish hypersalivation. Midazolam 0.02 mg/kg may be added to ameliorate emergence phenomena in children over 5 years old.

Abscess Incision and Drainage

Nitrous oxide has both analgesia and amnestic properties. It has a quick onset of action and fast offset which makes it ideal for use in an emergency department. It has no sedative properties and thus must be used on patients who are co-operative (i.e. >4 yrs of age). Procedure is performed with patient continuing to breathe Nitrous Oxide with Oxygen for the duration of the painful part of the procedure and 1 minute after painful part of procedure is finished. Other inhalational anaesthetic agents, Ketamine or Propofol can also be used.

Tongue-Tie Surgery

Snipping the frenulum (frenotomy) of neonates and surgical revision of the frenulum ('frenectomy', 'frenulectomy', or 'frenuloplasty') which involves the release of the tissue (lingual frenulum) that attaches the tongue to the floor of the mouth and closure of the wound with stitches is performed under general anaesthesia at or after 6 months of age. TIVA with Propofol with or without Remifentanil 0.05–0.3 mcg/kg/min can be used.

However, when tongue tie (ankyloglossia) is associated with foreshortening of the genioglossus muscle, as often occurs, merely snipping the lingual frenum may not allow free and coordinated movement of the tongue sufficient for the demands of a gradually growing speech and language structure. The presence of important blood vessels in the area makes it vulnerable for the possibility of accidentally cutting these vessels and causing excessive bleeding. Endotracheal intubation is required in such cases.

Biopsy

Inhalational or IV induction is the choice depending on patient/parent preference, child's veins and likely ease of canulation. In most cases LMA is used with spontaneous ventilation and maintenance of anaesthesia with volatile inhalational agent in oxygen and air or nitrous oxide. Infiltration of local anaesthetic with adrenaline to provide analgesia and haemostasis is done by the surgeon. Acetominophen and a NSAID for post-operative analgesia is advised.

Oesophagoscopy, oesophagogastroduodenoscopy (EGD)

Therapeutic indications for rigid esophagoscopy include foreign body removal, dilation of an esophageal stricture or injection of varices and are generally performed with endotracheal intubation. Compression of the trachea distal to the endotracheal tube by the rigid oesophagoscope is a common occurrence. Diagnostic oesophagogastroduodenoscopy (EGD) is performed with a flexible oesophagoscope.

The two most stimulating portions of the EGD are transoral and transpyloric passage of the endoscope due to the large size of the endoscope and partial airway obstruction, resulting in hypoxemia and further abdominal distention as a result of air introduced into the stomach impairing diaphragmatic excursion and thus leading to hypoventilation.

Children are less resistant against hypoxemia. Infants less than seven months are at higher risk due to obligatory nasal breathing. In most cases deep sedation or general anaesthesia is necessary. Respiratory infections in children with known hyperactive airways are an absolute contraindication for elective endoscopy in sedation. All patients should be monitored for haemodynamic stability and oxygen-saturation.

If the patient is presenting for dilation alone and has no evidence to suggest reflux or retained food in the oesophagus, a standard inhalation or intravenous induction may be performed. Rapid-sequence induction is usually appropriate for foreign body removal. Atropine (0.02 mg/kg if <1 month, minimum 0.1 mg) may be administered to attenuate bradycardia from intubation. After preoxygenation for 2–3 min, anaesthesia is induced with Propofol (2–3 mg/kg) and cricoid pressure is applied, followed by administration of Rocuronium (1 mg/kg) or Succinylcholine (1–2 mg/kg) and endotracheal intubation with age-appropriate ETT is performed. Anaesthesia is maintained with volatile inhalational agent/N_2O/O_2 or Propofol (100–250 mcg/kg/min) + Remifentanil (0.05–0.2 mcg/kg/min). Movement must be avoided with rigid esophagoscopy. Neostigmine (0.05 mg/kg) and Glycopyrrolate (0.01 mg/kg) to reverse neuromuscular blockade is given and extubation is done when the child is fully awake. Complications may include esophageal perforation, aspiration, accidental extubation, stridor due to subglottic edema, esophageal perforation (more common with rigid esophagoscopy) may lead to pneumothorax. Usually postoperative pain is minimal but if the patient reports marked substernal discomfort, suspect esophageal perforation.

According to the most recent analysis and guidelines, Propofol-based sedation seems to be the safest and most convenient method of inducing a sufficient sedation.[16]

Colonoscopy

Colonoscopy in children is generally performed under moderate sedation (conscious sedation) or general anaesthesia. Advantages of moderate sedation are intact protective airway reflexes and spontaneous breathing during examination. Deep sedation can be achieved more readily, and if respiratory problems occur, airway interventions are straightforward to manage. Patients undergoing colonoscopy also experience increased stimulation during certain parts of the procedure, such as when traversing the colon to the caecum. Also, at times, abdominal pressure is applied to help guide the colonoscope. The depth of the anaesthetic should be adjusted accordingly.

Cystoscopy

The most common paediatric endoscopic procedures are: Cystoscopy and vaginoscopy, primarily as diagnostic procedures; removal of foreign bodies including indwelling ureteral stents; transurethral incision of urethral stricture, for congenital lesions or complications of urethral surgery; transurethral incision of posterior urethral valves (PUV); transurethral incision of ureterocele; subureteric injection for vesicoureteral reflux; and endoscopic injection for urinary incontinence.

If >7–9 months of age, consider oral midazolam premedication (0.5–0.75 mg/kg), or 1–2 mg IV. General anaesthesia (ETT or LMA) is provided using a paediatric circuit. A combined technique with caudal anaesthesia is often used. For patients <5–10 year, standard mask induction with Sevoflurane/O_2 is used while older patients may agree to standard IV induction, facilitated by the use of topical local anaesthetic cream.

For postoperative pain Acetaminophen is advised. Ketorolac decreases bladder spasm but may lead to renal insufficiency, so should be avoided if renal function is abnormal. As large resections are not involved and most of the procedures are short, fluid absorption toxicity is rare, however, the metabolic consequences of fluid reabsorption through catastrophic ureteral or bladder perforation during endoscopic procedures in addition to the routine water reabsorption through venous channels should be kept in mind.

The most frequent neurological complication from lithotomy position may be injury to the common peroneal nerve leading to foot drop and sensory deficit.

CORE PRINCIPLES FOR OFFICE-BASED SURGERY

To promote safety and encourage states to develop guidelines, the American Medical Association (AMA), with input from the ACS and the ASA, published a consensus list of principles.

1. Guidelines or regulations for office-based surgery should be developed by states according to levels of anaesthesia defined by the ASA.
2. Physicians should select patients for office-based anaesthesia (OBA) by specified criteria including the ASA Physical Status Classification System.
3. Where available, offices that perform surgery should be accredited by a state-recognized entity.
4. Physicians involved in office-based surgery should have admitting privileges at a nearby hospital or maintain an emergency transfer agreement with a nearby hospital.
5. Informed consent guidelines should be followed.
6. Continuous quality improvement and adverse incident-reporting programs should be kept.
7. All physicians in an office-based setting should be board certified and fully trained.
8. Physicians performing office-based surgery may show competency by maintaining privileges at an accredited hospital or ambulatory surgical centre for the procedures they perform in an office setting.
9. At least one physician who is credentialed in advanced resuscitative techniques (advanced trauma life support [ATLS], advanced cardiac life support [ACLS], or paediatric advanced life support [PALS]) must be present or immediately available with appropriate resuscitative equipment until the patient has met discharge criteria.
10. Physicians administering or supervising the anaesthetic should have appropriate education and training.

KEY POINTS

- An office-based anaesthesia is performed in a location, usually an office or procedure room, that is not accredited by the state as an ambulatory surgery centre (ASC) or as a hospital.
- Since office-based anaesthesia is a subset of ambulatory anaesthesia, the ASA "Guidelines for Ambulatory Anaesthesia and Surgery" should be followed in the office setting as well as all other ASA standards and guidelines that are applicable.
- In an office where anaesthesia services are to be provided to infants and children, the required equipment, medication and resuscitative capabilities should be appropriately sized for a paediatric population.
- Procedures for office-based anaesthesia are those not involving major violation of a body cavity, usually lasting less than 2 hours, with no major physiologic disturbances or blood loss resulting in minimal or

moderate postoperative pain that can easily be managed at home with oral analgesics, with no disturbance to oral fluids intake in the immediate postoperative period.

- All types of techniques starting from minimal sedation to general anaesthesia are used depending upon the age and cooperation level of the child, the type of procedure, the applicability of local anaesthetic administration and its efficacy in a particular surgical procedure and the available equipment.
- At the time of discharge, special consideration needs to be given to stable haemodynamics, normal respiratory pattern, absence of excessive nausea/ vomiting and dizziness, and a state of consciousness appropriate to the developmental level.

REFERENCES

1. Laurence M Hausman, Meg A Rosenblatt. Clinical Anaesthesia: Barash et al. Lippincott. 7th edn. 2013.
2. American Society of Anesthesiologists: Guidelines for office-based anaesthesia, 2009.
3. Keira P Mason, Robert S. Holzman. Anaesthesia and Sedation for Paediatric Procedures Outside the Operating Room in Smith's Anaesthesia for infants and children. In: Peter J Davis, Franklyn P Claudis, Etsuro K Motoyama (Eds) Elsevier. 8th edn. 2011.
4. Abu-Shahwan. Ambulatory anaesthesia and the lack of consensus among Canadian paediatric anaesthesiologists: A survey. Paediatr Anaesth 2007;17:223.
5. Ross AK, Eck JB. Office-based anaesthesia for children. Anesthesiol Clin North America 2002;20:195.
6. ASA fasting guidelines: ASA task force 1999 updated in 2010.
7. Ulyott SC. Paediatric Premedicaton. Can J Anaesth 1992; 39:533.
8. Jakobson H, Hertz JB, Johansen JR, et al. Premedication before day surgery. A double blind comparison of diazepam and placebo. Br J Anaesth 1985;57:300–5.
9. Kain ZN, Mayes LC, Wang SM, et al. Parental presence and sedative premedication for children undergoing surgery. A hierarchical study. Anesthesiology 2000;92: 939–46.
10. Astfalk W, Warth H, Leriche C. Day case surgery in childhood from the parent's point of view. Eur J Pediatr Surg. 1991;1:323–7.
11. Hannallah RS, Patel RI. Low dose intramuscular ketamine for anaesthesia preinduction in young children and undergoing brief outpatient procedures. Anesthesiology 1989;70:598–600.
12. Coté CJ, Cohen IT, Suresh S, et al. A comparison of three doses of a commercially prepared oral midazolam syrup in children. Anesth Analg 2002; 94(1):37–43.
13. Saint-Maurice C, Meistelman C, Rey E, et al. The pharmacokinetics of rectal midazolam for premedication in children. Anesthesiology 1986;65(5):536–538.
14. Karl HW, Rosenberger JL, Larach MG, et al. Transmucosal administration of midazolam for premedication of paediatric patients: Comparison of the nasal and sublingual routes. Anesthesiology 1993;78(5):885–891.
15. Pandit UA, Collier PJ, Malviya S, et al. Oral transmucosal midazolam premedication for preschool children. Can J Anaesth 2001;48(2):191–195.
16. Malviya S, Voepel-Lewis T, Tait AR. Adverse events and risk factors associated with the sedation of children by nonanesthesiologists. Anesth Analg. 1997;85:1207–1213.
17. Harnett M, Kinirons B, Heffernan A, et al. Airway complications in infants: Comparison of laryngeal mask airway and the facemask-oral airway. Can J Anaesth 2000;47(4):315–318.
18. Bagshaw O. The size 1.5 laryngeal mask airway (LMA) in paediatric anaesthetic practice. Paediatr Anaesth 2002; 12(5):420–423.
19. Polaner DM, Ahuja D, Zuk J, et al. Video assessment of supraglottic airway orientation through the perilaryngeal airway in paediatric patients. Anesth Analg 2006; 102(6):1685–1688.
20. Goresky GV, Muir J. Inhalational induction of anaesthesia. Can J Anaesth. 1996;43:1085.
21. Welborn LG, Hannallah RS, Norden JM, et al. Comparison of emergence and recovery characteristic of sevoflurane, desflurane, and halothane in paediatric ambulatory patients. Anesth Analg. 1996;83:917–20.
22. Morray JP, Geiduschek JM, Ramamoorthy C, et al. Anaesthesia-related cardiac arrest in children: Initial findings of the Paediatric Perioperative Cardiac Arrest (POCA) Registry. Anesthesiology. 2000;93:6–14.
23. Abu-Shahwan I, Mack D. Propofol and remifentanil for deep sedation in children undergoing gastrointestinal endoscopy. Paediatr Anaesth. 2007;17:460–463.
24. O'Hare RA, Mirakhur RK, Reid JE, et al. Recovery from propofol anaesthesia supplemented with remifentanil. Br J Anaesth. 2001;86:361–365.
25. Davis PJ, Finkel JC, Orr RJ, et al. A randomized, double-blinded study of remifentanil vs. fentanyl for tonsillectomy and adenoidectomy surgery in paediatric ambulatory surgical patients. Anesth Analg. 2000;90(4):863–871.
26. Tang J, Chen L, White PF, et al. Recovery profiles, costs, and patient satisfaction with propofol and sevoflurane for fast-track office-based anaesthesia. Anesthesiology. 1999;91:253.
27. Moore EW, Pollard BJ, Elliott RE. Anaesthetic agents in paediatric day case surgery: Do they affect outcome? Eur J Anaesthsiol. 2002;19:9.
28. Fishkin S, Litman RS. Current issues in paediatric ambulatory anaesthesia. Anesthesiol Clin North Am. 2003;21:305.

29. Bhananker SM, Ramamoorthy C, Geiduschek JM, et al. Anaesthesia-related cardiac arrest in children: update from the paediatric perioperative cardiac arrest registry. Anesth Analg 2007;105:344.
30. Motas D, McDermott NB, VanSickle T, et al. Depth of consciousness and deep sedation attained in children as administered by nonanaesthesiologists in a children's hospital. Paediatr Anaesth. 2004;14:256–260.
31. Kain ZN, Mayes LC, Caldwell-Andrews AA, et al. Preoperative anxiety, postoperative pain, and behavioral recovery in young children undergoing surgery. Paediatrics 2006;118:651.
32. Vlajkovic GP, Sindjelic RP. Emergence delirium in children: Many questions, few answers. Anesth Analg. 2007;104:84.
33. Kuratani N, Oi Y. Greater incidence of emergence agitation in children after sevoflurane anaesthesia as compared with halothane: A meta-analysis of randomized control trials. Anesthesiology. 2008;109:225.
34. König MW, Varughese AM, Brennan KA, et al. Quality of recovery from two types of general anaesthesia for ambulatory dental surgery in children: A double-blind, randomized trial. Paediatr Anaesth 2009;19:748.
35. Guler G, Akin A, Tosun Z, et al. Single-dose dexmedetomidine reduces agitation and provides smooth extubation after paediatric adenotonsillectomy. Paediatr Anaesth. 2005;15(9):762–766.
36. Hung WT, Chen CC, Liou CM, et al. The effects of low-dose fentanyl on emergence agitation and quality of life in patients with moderate developmental disabilities. J Clin Anesth 2005;17(7):494–498.
37. Aouad MT, Yazbeck-Karam VG, Nasr VG, et al. A single dose of propofol at the end of surgery for the prevention of emergence agitation in children undergoing strabismus surgery during sevoflurane anaesthesia. Anesthesiology 2007;107(5): 733–738.
38. Breschan C, Platzer M, Jost R, et al. Midazolam does not reduce emergence delirium after sevolurane anaesthesia in children. Paediatr Anaesth 2007;17(4):347–352.
39. Tsai PS, Hsu YW, Lin CS, et al. Ketamine but not propofol provides additional effects on attenuating sevoflurane-induced emergence agitation in midazolam premedicated paediatric patients. Paediatr Anaesth 2008;18(11):1114–1115.
40. Davis PJ, Greenberg JA, Gendelman M, et al. Recovery characteristics of sevoflurane and halothane in preschool aged children undergoing bilateral myringotomy and pressure equalization tube insertion. Anesth Analg 1999;88:34–38.
41. Constant I, Dubois MC, Piat V, et al. Changes in electroencephalogram and autonomic cardiovascular activity during induction of anaesthesia with sevoflurane compared with halothane in children. Anesthesiology 1999;91(6):1604–1615.
42. Cohen IT, Finkel JC, Hannallah RS, et al. Rapid emergence does not explain agitation following sevoflurane anaesthesia in infants and children: A comparison with propofol. Paediatr Anaesth 2003; 13(1):63–67.
43. Oh AY, Seo KS, Kim SD, et al. Delayed emergence process does not result in a lower incidence of emergence agitation after sevoflurane anaesthesia in children. Acta Anaesthesiol Scand 2005; 49(3):297–299.
44. Schreiner MS, Nicolson SC, Martin T, et al. Should children drink before discharge from day surgery? Anaesthesiology 1992;76:528.
45. Goodarzi M, Matar MM, Shafa M, et al. A prospective randomized blinded study of the effect of intravenous fluid therapy on postoperative nausea and vomiting in children undergoing strabismus surgery. Paediatr Anaesth 2009; 16:49.
46. Shandling B, Steward DJ. Regional analgesia for postoperative pain in paediatric outpatient surgery. J Pediatr Surg 1980;15:477–80.
47. Lynn AM, Bradford H, Kantor ED, et al. Postoperative ketorolac tromethamine use in infants aged 6–18 months: The effect on morphine usage, safety assessment, and stereo-specific pharmacokinetics. Anesth Analg. 2007; 104:1040.
48. Tobias JD. Weak analgesics and non-steroidal anti-inflammatory agents in the management of children with acute pain. Pediatr Clin North Am 2000;47:527.
49. Korpela R, Korvenoja P, Meretoja OA. Morphine sparing effect of acetaminophen in paediatric day-case surgery. Anesthesiology 1992;76:528.
50. Anderson BJ, Holford NH, Woollard GA, et al. Perioperative pharmacodynamics of acetaminophen analgesia in children. Anesthesiology 1999; 90:411.
51. Montgomery CJ, McCormack JP, Reichert CC, et al. Plasma concentrations after high dose (45 mg/kg^{-1}) rectal acetaminophen in children. Can J Anaesth. 1995;42:982.
52. Kovac AL. Prevention and treatment of postoperative nausea and vomiting. Drugs 2000;59: 213–43.
53. Aldrete JA, Kroulik D. A postanaesthetic recovery score. Anesth Analg 1970;49:924.
54. Marshall SI, Chung F. Assessment of home readiness discharge criteria and post discharge complications. Curr Opin Anaesthesiol 1997;445–450.
55. Patel RI, Verghese ST, Hannallah RS, et al. Fast-tracking children after ambulatory surgery. Anaesth Analg 2001;92:918–22.

Paediatric Intensive Care

Preetha Joshi and Vinay Joshi

TRANSPORTATION AND RECEIVING

Transport of a patient is done not only for diagnostic purpose and seeking therapeutic advice but also to provide higher level of care. However, initial resuscitation and stabilization of a critically ill child is very important for the outcome of a transport. Despite meticulous pre-planning, problems can arise during transport of a critically ill child and transport can become a challenging affair. Goals of transport are: (a) To reach the referring center as quickly as possible with trained personnel, (b) to stabilize the patient's condition and to move the child to a facility capable of providing more extensive care or additional services that will enhance patient outcome[1] and (c) to offer the level of care equal to the receiving hospital during transport.

Essential Components of Transport

1. A dedicated team skilled at providing critical care during transport,
2. Transport ambulance capabilities,
3. Communications/dispatch capabilities,
4. Clinical and operational guidelines,
5. Administrative resources,
6. Institutional endorsement and financial support.

Responsibilities of a Transport Team

Responsibilities of a transport team can be grouped into two:

1. Stabilization phase and
2. Transport phase.

Stabilization Phase includes quick assessment of patient status, stabilization of patient for transport, anticipation of problems likely to occur during transport, securing all lines and tubes and obtaining consent. Before departure, transport team should call receiving hospital with updated patient information and expected time of arrival (ETA).[2] **Transport phase** includes: Safe movement of patient in and out of ambulance, ongoing monitoring of major organ systems, prompt recognition and treatment of problems during transport and handing over a detailed report to admitting physician. During the transport, vital parameters, drug infusions, administered medications and significant events should be documented.

Legally, tertiary hospital responsibility starts when the transport team takes over the medical care at the referring institution. Every aspect of the transport event needs rigorous documentation.[3]

EMERGENCE, AGITATION AND DELIRIUM

Restless behavior upon emergence causes not only discomfort to the child, but also makes the caregivers and parents feel unhappy with the quality of recovery from anaesthesia probably as a result of introduction of a new generation of inhaled anaesthetics into paediatric clinical practice. To reduce the incidence of this adverse event, it is advisable to identify children at risk and take preventive measures, such as reducing preoperative anxiety, removing postoperative pain, and providing a quiet, stress-free environment for post-anaesthesia recovery.

History

In the early 1960s, Eckenhoff and workers[1] were the first to report the signs of hyperexcitation in patients emerging from ether, cyclopropane, or ketamine anaesthesia, particularly when administered for tonsillectomy, thyroidectomy, and circumcision. Children experience postanaesthesia agitation more often than adults (12%–13% vs 5.3%).

In children, halothane was increasingly used and was the predominant anaesthetic for decades. With the recognition of postoperative pain management in children and the increased use of analgesics, the incidence of emergence agitation (EA) was attenuated. However, with the introduction into clinical practice of the new, short-acting, volatile anaesthetics sevoflurane and desflurane, the problem of ED has reemerged.[2]

Emergence delirium is defined[3] as "a disturbance in a child's awareness of and attention to his/her environment with disorientation and perceptual alterations, including hypersensitivity to stimuli and hyperactive motor behavior in the immediate postanaesthesia period." Emergence agitation and emergence delirium have been used interchangeably in most of the literature.

Despite numerous attempts to explain the causes of emergence agitation/delirium, there is no definitive explanation. Possible causes include pain, preoperative anxiety, type of surgical procedures, personal characteristics of the patient, and type of anaesthetics, although no sole factor can explain the etiology of emergence agitation/delirium. The reported prevalence of emergence agitation/delirium varies greatly in the literature, ranging from 10% to 80%. Younger age, preoperative anxiety, and pain are all important contributory factors. Surgical procedures that involve the tonsils, thyroid, middle ear, and eye have also been reported to have higher incidences of postoperative agitation and restlessness.

Presentation

The children experience a state of dissociated state of consciousness in which the child is irritable, uncompromising, uncooperative and inconsolably crying, moaning, kicking or thrashing.[4] Restless recovery from anaesthesia may not only cause injury to the child or to the surgical site, but may also lead to the accidental removal of surgical dressings, IV catheters, and drains. This also leads to anxiety in parents.

Management

ED usually occurs within the first 30 min of recovery from anaesthesia, is self-limited (5–15 min), and often resolves spontaneously. Various attempts have been made to reduce the problem of emergence agitation/delirium. Many drugs, including propofol, fentanyl, clonidine and dexmedetomidine, have been investigated to attenuate the incidence of emergence agitation/delirium.[5] It has been known that propofol delays or modifies emergence and could decrease the incidence of emergence agitation/delirium though the effect is shortlasting at doses tried (1 mg/kg).

VASCULAR ACCESS AND PICU PROCEDURES

Indications

The indications for central lines in children[1] are similar to the indications in adults. There are various indications for central access for patients in the PICU like drug infusion, CVP measurement and sampling.

Central venous catheters (CVC) are used to deliver large volumes of irritating solutions, such as fluid boluses, antibiotics, blood products, parenteral nutrition, and sclerosing chemotherapeutic agents. Central access is also indicated when peripheral access cannot be achieved due to poor perfusion or exhausted peripheral sites. This is a common feature in children. In an emergency situation, where vascular access is unattainable after quick attempts, an intraosseous needle is the route of choice according to Paediatric Advanced Life Support (PALS) guidelines.[2]

The 4 main approaches[3] to central venous access discussed here include the internal jugular, subclavian, femoral, and peripheral intravenous central catheter (PICC) methods.

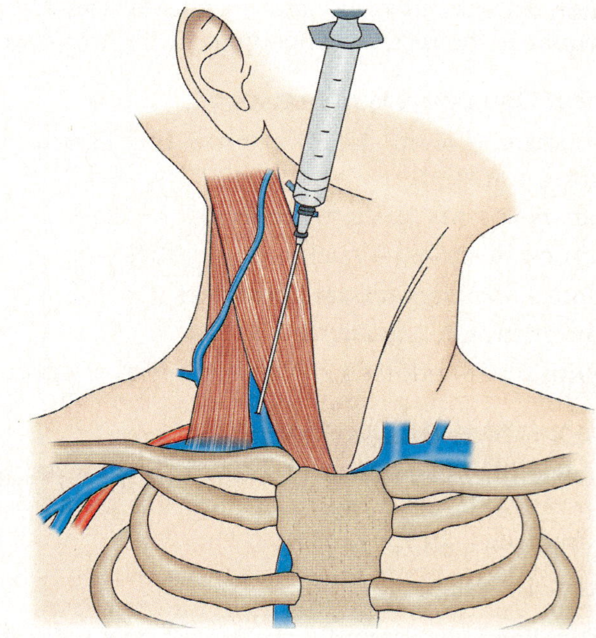

Fig. 37.1 Approach to jugular vein

Internal Jugular Approach

The internal jugular vein (IJV) is parallel and lateral to the internal carotid artery in the neck. It lies in the carotid sheath, which includes the carotid artery and vagus nerve. The IJV is a branch of the brachiocephalic vein. The approach is made through the tip of the triangle formed by the two heads of the sternocleidomastoid and base by the clavicle and aimed towards the ipsilateral nipple.

Subclavian Approach

The subclavian artery lies posterior and somewhat superior to the brachiocephalic vein. These 2 vessels are separated by the anterior scalene muscles. The subclavian vein begins distal to the branch point of the IJV. It crosses under the clavicle at the medial to proximal third of the clavicle. The subclavian artery is located deep and slightly superior to the vein.

In children, the subclavian vein is located more cephalic than it is in adults, meaning that it dives under the clavicle closer to the medial third.

Deep to the vessels lies the first rib, which is just superficial to the pleura and lung. The approach is from 1 cm below the clavicle at the junction of the proximal and lateral third of the clavicle, aiming towards the sternal notch.

Femoral Approach

The femoral vein joins the external iliac vein. It crosses deep to the medial third of the inguinal ligament. A common mnemonic for the anatomy of the femoral vessels from lateral to medial is NAVEL: Nerve, artery, vein, empty space, and lymphatics. Approach is from 1–2 cm below the inguinal ligament aiming towards the umbilicus.

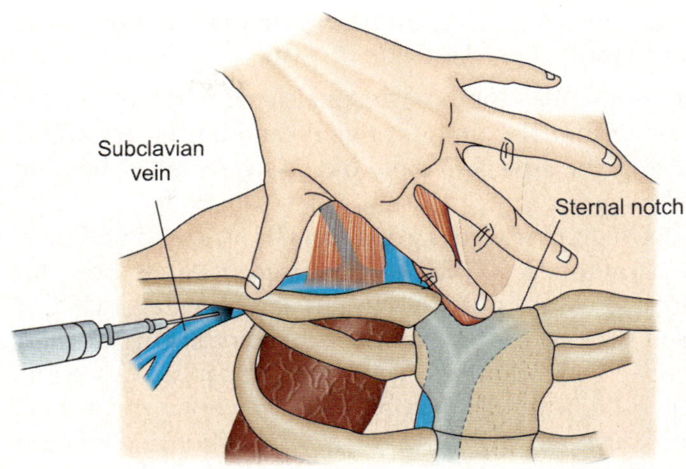

Fig. 37.2 Approach to subclavian vein cannulation

Peripheral Intravenous Central Catheters

Peripheral intravenous central catheters (PICC) lines are routinely used in neonatal intensive care units (NICUs) and are considered a mainstay of vascular access in this setting. Although the lines are placed peripherally, usually in the antecubital or saphenous vein, the line is advanced so that the distal tip remains in a large central vein. PICC lines are indicated in older children who require long term IV access for prolonged hospital therapy or even chemotherapy and parenteral nutrition.

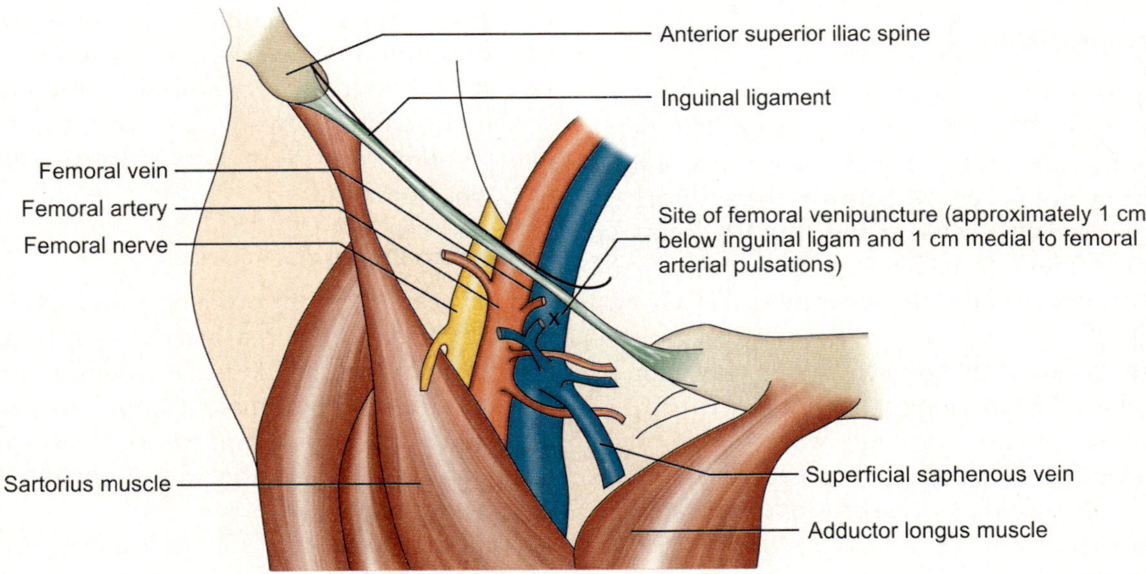

Fig. 37.3 Femoral vein access

Umbilical Artery Catheters and Umbilical Vein Catheters

Accessing the umbilical system is useful in the first few days of life. The umbilical vein can be used for access during the first 5–7 days but is rarely used beyond 7 days.

Both umbilical artery catheters (UACs) and umbilical vein catheters (UVCs) can be used: UAC is used for blood pressure monitoring and sampling, and UVC is used for central venous pressure monitoring and for similar indications as mentioned in the CVC section. The umbilical system consists of 2 arteries and 1 vein. The vein is usually at the 11 o'clock position and is larger with thinned walls. The arteries are located inferiorly with thicker walls.

Contraindications for inserting any central venous catheter (CVC) include an infection or burn over the desired insertion site, a known venous thrombosis of the vessel, an uncorrected coagulopathy, an obstruction of the vein by a tumor or mass, an abnormal vessel, and a lack of consent in a nonemergency setting.

Insertion of Intercostal Chest Drains (ICD)

Intercostal chest drains are inserted in cases of pneumothorax, bronchopleural fistula, pleural effusion and empyemas.

The drain is inserted in the 5th intercostal space in the midaxillary line. In smaller children, the spaces are very narrow and great care must be taken in inserting the drain along the upper margin of the lower rib as it can lead to haemorrhage.

MONITORING IN THE PICU

Monitoring in the PICU can be basic or advanced depending upon the severity of illness. The basic monitoring includes temperature, heart rate, blood pressure (non-invasive), respiratory rate, work of breathing and oxygen saturation (SpO_2). Invasive monitoring includes arterial blood gases, lactate, mixed venous saturations, ventilator graphics, $ETCO_2$ and cardiac output.

Heart rate varies with age and child's condition as shown in Table 37.1 (adaptation from PALS 2010).

Blood pressure varies with age, with a wide range for various ages. Table 37.2 gives cut off values for hypotension by systolic blood pressure (adaptation from PALS 2010).

Normal respiratory rate varies for various age groups as shown in Table 37.3 (adaptation from PALS 2010).

Table 37.1 Normal heart rates by age

Age	Awake rate (per min)	Mean (per min)	Sleeping rate (per min)
Newborn to 3 months	85–205	140	80–160
3 months to 2 years	100–190	130	75–160
2 to 10 years	60–140	80	60–90
>10 years	60–100	75	50–90

Table 37.2 Hypotension by systolic blood pressure (mmHg) by age

Age	Systolic blood pressure
Term Neonates (0–28 days)	<60
Infants (1 month–12 months)	<70
Children (1–10 years)	<70 + (2 × age in years)
Children (>10 years)	<90

Table 37.3 Normal respiratory rates by age

Age	Breaths per minute
Infants (<1 year)	30–60
Toddlers (1–3 years)	24–40
Preschoolers (4–5 years)	22–34
School age (6–12 years)	18–30
Adolescents (13–18 years)	12–16

Tachypnea may be associated with increased work of breathing signs of which include nasal flaring, intercostal and subcostal retractions and tracheal tug. Breathing may be associated with abnormal sounds like grunt, stridor and audible wheeze depending upon the condition and severity. A decreasing respiratory rate may herald improvement in the condition or worsening child's status with accompanying signs like deteriorating sensorium, altered breathing pattern or irregular breathing.

Monitoring Oxygen

Oxygen can be monitored non-invasively by pulse oximetry (Beer-Lambert principle) or by transcutaneous oxygen and carbon dioxide electrodes. Poor perfusion, motion artifacts and ambient light can interfere with the pulse oximeter reading. Arterial blood gas is a gold standard for the measurement of oxygen and carbon dioxide in the blood.

Mixed venous oxygen (MVO_2) is a measure of oxygen content and adequacy of oxygen supply at the tissue level. Normally the tissues utilize 20–25% of the oxygen

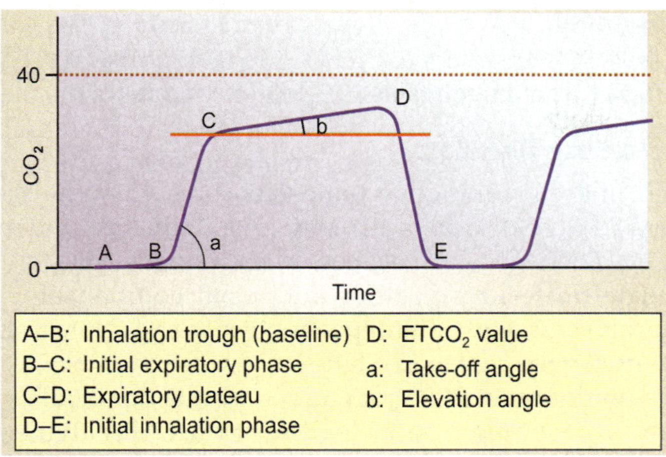

Fig. 37.4 CO_2 levels

delivered but in the diseased states the values vary with the stage and severity of the condition. Measurement of mixed venous oxygen warrants inserting central venous access, so risk-benefit ratio should be weighed.

Arterial blood gas gives the most accurate measurement of carbon dioxide in the blood (gold standard). However, end tidal CO_2 monitoring can be very useful, portable and non-invasive alternative to the blood gas measurements. $EtCO_2$ monitor displays waveform as shown in Fig. 37.4.

The changes in shape, size and contours of the waveform depict the changes in the patient's ventilation status. Under normal conditions there is a difference of 2–5 mmHg between arterial and $EtCO_2$ values ($PaO_2 > EtCO_2$) and deviation from this reflects an alteration in ventilation–perfusion ratio.

Pulmonary Graphics

Point-of-care monitoring system, ventilator waveforms help in monitoring patient's respiratory mechanics and fine-tuning ventilation parameters according to the needs. It can depict improving or worsening lung condition with respect to compliance, resistance and work of breathing. Various waveforms, which can be studied, are; scalars like pressure-time, volume-time and flow-time and loops like pressure-volume and flow-volume (Fig. 37.5).[1]

Advanced cardiovascular monitoring includes invasive blood pressure monitoring, CVP monitoring and cardiac output measurements. Blood pressure is a surrogate marker of left ventricular function. However, more accurate measure of left ventricular function will be cardiac output[2] as blood pressure varies with systemic vascular resistance, which in turn is a reflection of vasomotor tone.[4,5] Cardiac output depends upon four

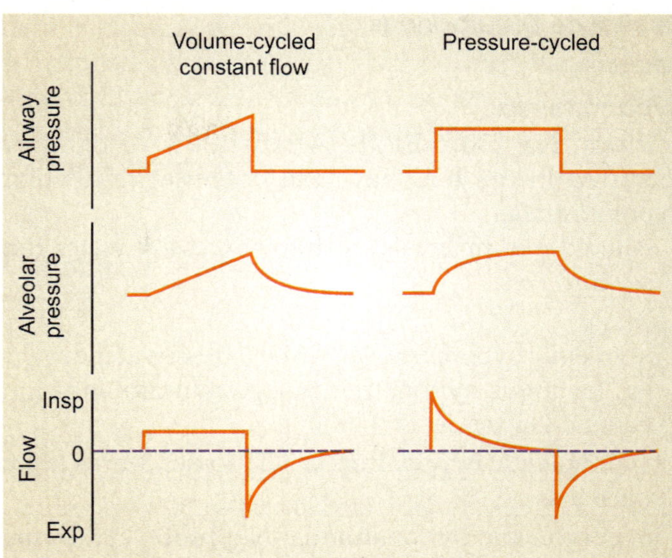

Fig. 37.5 Pressure-time, flow-time scalars in volume control and pressure control ventilation

interdependent variables; heart rate, preload, cardiac contractility and afterload.

Cardiac output can be measured by various invasive (dilution techniques) and non-invasive (pulse contour analysis, 2-D ECHO) methods. However, cardiac output directed therapeutic interventions have not shown an improvement in survival of adult patients with shock.

FLUID AND ELECTROLYTES

The main principles that govern fluid and electrolyte physiology and therapy in older children are similar to adults. There are however, some important differences in smaller children and neonates.

The total body water in the human ranges from 40 to 70%. During foetal life, this represents 90% of the body water, 75% at birth, 65% at 6 months and 60% at one year. Therefore, any significant fluid loss, represents a severe hemodynamic instability in a smaller infant.

There are 3 different situations where fluid therapy needs to be implemented in the ICU setting. It can be used as:

1. Maintenance fluid—isotonic fluids are only used in paediatrics, except in the neonate where near isotonic fluids are used or severe dyselectrolytemias.
2. Replacement fluid—isotonic fluids/near isotonic fluids are the fluids of choice.
3. Resuscitative fluids—isotonic fluids are the fluid of choice—Ringer's lactate, normal saline.

Electrolyte Disturbances

Sodium

Hyponatremia

Sodium, Na 130 mEq/L. Almost 30% of children admitted in the ICU have the potential to develop hyponatremia

Altered sodium levels are due to excessive water gain or sodium loss.

Etiology:

- Euvolemic hyponatremia: SIADH, fresh water drowning, factitious hyponatremia, e.g. mannitol infusion, diabetic ketoacidosis
- Hypovolemic hyponatremia: GIT losses, burns, third space loss
- Hypervolemic hyponatremia: Nephrotic syndrome, acute heart failure, acute kidney injury.

Management:

- Acute hyponatremia: Correction with 3% NaCl may be required as a bolus or infusion to prevent cerebral oedema.
- Chronic hyponatremia: Treated gradually over 3–5 days.

Hypernatremia

Etiology

- Water loss: GIT, burns, diabetes insipidus
- Sodium gain: Hypertonic solutions

Management

- Hypernatremic dehydration: fluid resuscitation as per guidelines followed by slow correction of hypernatremia
- Treatment of diabetes insipidus

Potassium

Potassium is a principal intracellular cation which is very important for cell membrane depolarisation and repolarisation.

Hypokalemia

- Gastroenteritis
- DKA
- Prolonged use of diuretics
- Metabolic alkalosis

Potassium supplementation is done with KCl in maintenance fluids.

Hyperkalemia

- Renal failure, burns, tumor lysis
- Excessive K supplementation

Treatment

- Bicarbonate
- Na– K exchange resins
- Glucose insulin drip
- Beta agonists

Acid-Base Disorders

All children admitted to the paediatric ICU are at risk for acid–base disorders that may complicate their underlying illness and further worsen their overall status.

The buffer, respiratory and renal compensatory mechanisms work interdependently at regular intervals to restore the acid–base status.

Rapidly progressing or sudden insults do not allow time for compensation leading to life-threatening consequences.

Analysing Acid-Base Disorders

Steps

1. What is the pH—normal, acidotic, or alkalotic?
2. What is the pCO_2—high, normal, or low?
3. What is the bicarbonate—high, normal, or low?
4. Is the primary problem respiratory or metabolic?
5. Is the problem acute, partially compensated, or compensated?

Management

After the diagnosis, the appropriate treatment is instituted based on respiratory or metabolic causes.

Metabolic: In case of metabolic acidosis, the etiology is determined from the history and clinical examination and the underlying cause is treated. In case of pH <7.1, bicarbonate may be administered to avoid ill-effects of acidosis.

Metabolic alkalosis in children is usually iatrogenic secondary to bicarbonate administration, diuretic use but can be due to compensation in chronic lung disease.

Respiratory: In case of respiratory acidosis of acute origin, immediate measures to support the lungs like ventilation must be instituted, but in case of chronic respiratory acidosis, pCO_2 levels <70 mmHg is acceptable as long as pH value is maintained.

Respiratory alkalosis is seen prior to worsening of pulmonary dysfunction, compensation for metabolic acidosis. Again, the underlying disease needs to be treated.

MECHANICAL VENTILATION

The aim of mechanical ventilation is to provide adequate gas exchange while minimizing lung injury and maximizing patient comfort. Mechanical ventilation is potentially deleterious, possibly lethal if misused. High levels of inspired O_2 (particularly more than 60%) and high tidal volume ventilation ("volutrauma") can exacerbate lung injury.[1]

Mode of ventilation can be either pressure-controlled (PC) or volume-controlled (VC). In PC ventilation, the ventilator delivers a fixed pressure for a preset inspiratory time. The advantage of PC modes is that in the presence of a leak around the ETT, gas flow will be increased in order to generate the preset pressure. The disadvantage is that as the compliance of the lung changes over time, the ventilator continues to deliver the same pressure.

In VC ventilation, the tidal volume is preset and the ventilator will use as much pressure as it needs to deliver the preset volume. This allows the ventilator to compensate for changes in lung compliance, however, has the disadvantage that it can cause excessive barotrauma (limitation-leak around ETT which is a common feature in small uncuffed tubes used in Paediatric ICU settings).[2]

AC or SIMV: There is a choice of assist controlled (PC or VC) or synchronized (SIMV-PC or SIMV-VC) modes.

Assist-controlled: In assist-controlled modes (PC or VC), the ventilator will deliver the number of breaths set on the CMV rate every minute. Additional spontaneous breaths initiated by the patient that are detected by the ventilator will be fully supported—i.e. such breaths are not limited by the effort of the patient—as soon as the patient effort meets the trigger sensitivity criteria, a full PC or CV breath will be delivered.

SIMV: In SIMV modes, patient initiated breaths are limited to the gas flow generated by patient effort (plus pressure support).

Inspiratory and expiratory times: IT ranging from 0.5 to 1.0 second—longer times for older patients, is used. Generally an I : E ratio of 1 : 2 is necessary to allow adequate exhalation, however, this may change markedly depending on the lung disease present. Patient with obstructive airway disease requires prolonged expiratory time, while patients with severe restrictive disease and short time constants will empty their lungs rapidly, allowing shorter expiratory times.

PEEP: Positive end-expiratory pressure is used in ventilated patients in order to prevent end-expiratory collapse of alveoli. PEEP also helps to overcome the increased resistance of the ETT in spontaneous breaths. Even in patients without lung disease, 3–4 cm H_2O PEEP is beneficial.

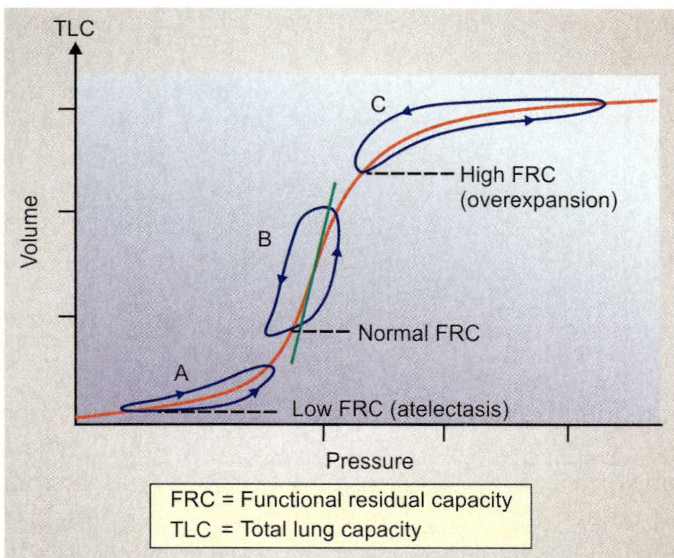

Fig. 37.6 Compliance curve of the lung and optimal recruitment

In patients with severe lung disease much higher levels of PEEP may be required. In these circumstances, PEEP is used to recruit areas of lung that would otherwise be atelectatic. It is important to maintain PEEP at a level that is above the lower inflection point of the pressure-volume curve ensuring optimal tidal volume (Fig. 37.6).[3]

The aim is to ventilate in the steeper portion of a curve-zone of maximum compliance.

Pressure Support

Pressure support provides additional pressure for each spontaneous patient-triggered breath. It can be used with CPAP to provide up to full ventilation provided the patient's respiratory drive is intact. PS can also be used to augment SIMV modes. The duration of pressure support varies with each breath. Inspiratory time is controlled by patient effort.[4]

High Frequency Ventilation

High frequency ventilation may be beneficial in infants and children with severe restrictive lung disease. It is relatively contraindicated in patients with severe obstructive airway disease. High frequency ventilation uses small tidal volumes at fast rates (generally 3–10 Hz, i.e. 180–600 breaths/min) and high mean airway pressures. The high mean pressures keep the lung "recruited" (keep the lungs open) and facilitates oxygenation. The small tidal volumes are useful in preventing shear stress to alveolar walls (barotrauma or volutrauma). Higher frequencies can be used for newborns and small infants.[5]

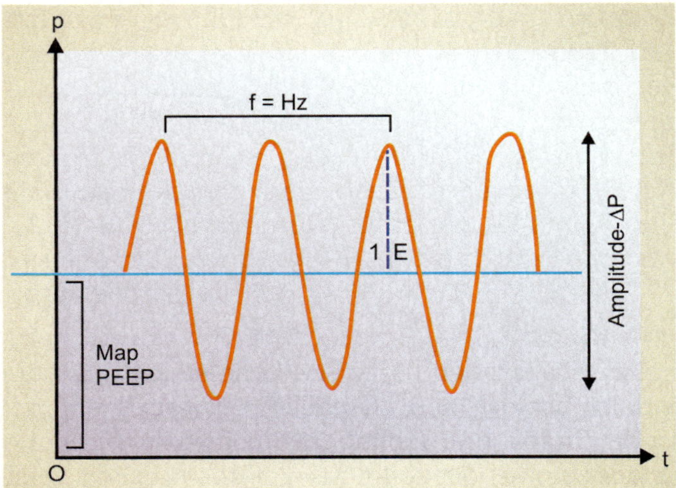

Fig. 37.7 Graphic representation of high frequency ventilation

ECMO

Extracorporeal Life Support is used in acute severe lung disease (ARDS), but may have a role in other medical conditions like septic shock, poisoning, etc. and is also used for ventricular support in postoperative cardiac patients unable to be weaned from bypass due to low cardiac output syndrome (LCOS) and as a bridge to cardiac transplant.[6]

Criteria for neonatal ECMO:

- Birth weight greater than 2000 gm
- Gestational age greater than 34 weeks
- Less than 7–10 days of positive pressure ventilation
- Reversible lung disease
- Absence of congenital heart disease
- Absence of significant intracranial haemorrhage or malformation.
- Absence of severe coagulopathy that is not reversible.
- Absence of prolonged asphyxia predicted to produce significant CNS damage.
- Failure of maximal medical treatment including surfactant, nitric oxide.

Criteria for paediatric ECMO:

- O_2 delivery insufficient to meet tissue demands despite maximal medical management.
- Life-threatening arrhythmias.
- Reversible severe low cardiac output syndrome (postoperative or postmyocarditis)
- Ability to tolerate systemic heparinisation for the duration of the procedure.
- Reasonable likelihood for 1 year survival in the absence of respiratory failure.
- Etiology of respiratory failure identified as potentially reversible.

Ventilator parameters that may be of help in determining the need for ECMO include: OI = $(MAP \times FiO_2)/(PaO_2) > 40$ for 8 hours and/or A-a $DO_2 > 610$ for > 8 hours.

POSTOPERATIVE NAUSEA AND VOMITING

Postoperative nausea and vomiting (PONV) continues to be a frequent and important cause of morbidity in children. Severe vomiting, which is much more prominent in children than in adults, can be associated with dehydration, postoperative bleeding, pulmonary aspiration, and wound dehiscence. The two most common emetogenic surgical procedures evaluated in children are strabismus repair and adenotonsillectomy.[1]

It is important to identify children at moderate-to-high risk for postoperative vomiting (POV) as prophylactic antiemetic therapy is useful in these children. Antiemetics of choice for POV in children[2] include dexamethasone, dimenhydrinate, perphenazine, ondansetron, dolasetron, granisetron, and tropisetron. The serotonin [5-hydroxytryptamine; 5-HT (3)] antagonists are the antiemetic drugs of first choice for POV prophylaxis in children because as a group they have greater efficacy for preventing vomiting than nausea. The 5-HT (3) antagonists can be effectively combined with dexamethasone with an increase in efficacy. If possible, regional anaesthesia should be considered.

CARDIAC INTENSIVE CARE

Acute Heart Failure

Acute heart failure in children is a complex condition which is managed by many with a combination of clinical experience and applications of findings from studies in adults with cardiac failure.

Definition

Acute heart failure (AHF) is a pathophysiological state in which an abnormality of cardiac function is responsible for the failure of the heart to pump blood at a level commensurate with the requirements of the metabolizing tissues, or does so only at elevated filling pressures.[1]

Factors Affecting Cardiac Output

The cardiac output (CO) is dependent on stroke volume (SV) and heart rate (HR). The SV further depends on preload, myocardial contractility and afterload.

- Preload is defined as the degree of end-diastolic fibre stretch that determines the end-diastolic volume. This is influenced by the intravascular volume status of the patient and ventricular wall thickness. For clinical purposes, central venous pressure (CVP) is a crude indicator of preload status.
- Myocardial contractility is characterized by the force and velocity of myocardial contraction and expressed as ejection fraction (EF).
- Afterload, the force resisting myocardial fibre shortening, is the amount of work that the myocardium has to do.

The heart rate and rhythm are important contributors to heart failure when abnormal.

Pathophysiology and clinical manifestations of heart failure

- **Left ventricular failure (LVF):** In LV failure, as the CO declines, the left atrial pressure rises resulting in an increase in pulmonary venous pressure. This leads to increase in work of breathing and tachypnea. When fluid extravasates into the interstitial space and alveolar space, it alters pulmonary mechanics and causes pulmonary oedema.
- **Right ventricular failure (RVF):** In RV failure, systemic venous congestion symptoms develop. Pleural effusions, hepatic dysfunction and ascites are manifestations.[2]

Etiology of AHF

LV Failure

- Congenital heart defects—large left to right shunts, e.g. atrial and ventricular septal defects, patent ductus arteriosus.
- Anomalous left coronary artery from pulmonary artery (ALCAPA)
- Left sided obstructive lesions (aortic stenosis, coarctation of aorta and interrupted arch)
- Cardiomyopathy
- Tachyarrhthmias
- Myocarditis
- Postcardiopulmonary bypass

RV Failure

- Sequelae of LV failure
- Tricuspid regurgitation
- Pulmonary hypertension
- Pulmonary stenosis

Symptoms of Acute Heart Failure

- Tachypnoea
- Dyspnoea
- Wheezing
- Feeding difficulty
- Failure to thrive
- Irritability
- Sweating
- Reduced urine output
- Tachycardia, cool extremities, feeble pulses and gallop
- Pulsus paradoxus
- Crepitations
- Hepatomegaly

Investigations

X-ray, ECG, 2D ECHO, pulse oximetry, blood gases.

Management of AHF/Low Cardiac Output Syndrome

Goals[3,4]

- Establish oxygenation and venous access.
- Positive pressure ventilation reduces afterload and work of breathing and must be instituted early in this case.
- **Optimising preload:** This requires restriction of fluids (2/3rd maintenance) and diuretics like thiazides and loop diuretics.
- **Increase myocardial performance:** Inotropes are the main stay of treatment to optimize CO. Initially precise control of blood pressure requires inotropes as continuous infusions like dopamine and dobutamine[5] and later an oral inotrope like digoxin can be used. In cases of severe low output, epinephrine is used.
- **Optimising afterload:** After the blood pressure is stabilized, inodilators form the mainstay of cardiac failure management. Milrinone, sodium nitroprusside and nitroglycerine are commonly used agents.[6] B-blockers and levosimendan is now being used in the intensive care setting.
- **Mechanical cardiac support:** In refractory heart failure, ventricular assist devices (VAD) and extracorporeal membrane oxygenation (ECMO) are the newer methods used as a bridge to transplant or spontaneous recovery.

Approach to a Cyanotic Child in Circulatory Failure

It is crucial to differentiate respiratory cause of cyanosis from cardiac cause, the latter being characterized mainly by lack of respiratory distress and a failure to improve oxygenation with a supplementation of 100% inspired O_2.

Critical cyanotic heart disease presenting in the newborn period is most commonly due to transposition of the great vessels, pulmonary or tricuspid atresia, double outlet right ventricle or total anomalous pulmonary venous drainage. In almost all circumstances, maintaining or restoring duct patency by the administration of PGE_1 will be beneficial (except obstructed TAPVC) with an infusion in a dose range of 10–100 nanograms/kg/min. A patent ductus arteriosus allows mixing of systemic and pulmonary circulations and maintains adequate oxygenation and perfusion. PGE_1 infusion is also helpful in duct dependent systemic circulation conditions like hypoplasic left heart syndrome (HLHS), interrupted aortic arch, severe coarctation of aorta and critical aortic stenosis.

Postoperative Management: General Principles

The postoperative cardiac patient is potentially among the most unstable of all patients admitted to the ICU.

Monitoring of the postoperative cardiac patient

1. Vital signs, with SpO_2
2. Cardiac rhythm (sinus), presence of residual murmurs and appearance of new murmurs.
3. Pressures-arterial and venous [(CVP, MAP), left arterial pressure (LAP) and pulmonary arterial pressure (PAP)].
4. Peripheral perfusion.
5. Bilateral air entry, note size and length of ETT.
6. Position and number of chest drains and rate of blood loss through the drains, presence of pacing wires and central venous catheters.
7. Sternum—closed or open.
8. Abdomen—liver size.
9. Vascular access and rates of various infusions (inotropes, vasopressors).
10. CXR, ABG 6 hourly, electrolytes, coagulation abnormalities, CBC at least once daily in the first 24 hrs.

Management of postoperative cardiac patient

1. Control of bleeding
2. Low cardiac output: As discussed in the previous section on AHF
3. Management of arrhythmias

RESPIRATORY FAILURE

It is important to identify the cause of respiratory failure as the management would vary.[1]

Causes of Respiratory Failure

Decreased Respiratory Drive

- Head injury
- Drug ingestion: Sedative overdose, organophosphorus poisoning, etc.
- Guillain Barré syndrome
- Intracranial bleed
- Myopathies

Increased Respiratory Drive

Upper airway obstruction

- Croup, foreign body, epiglottitis
- Congenital anomalies—laryngeal web
- Anaphylaxis

Lower airway obstruction

- Bronchiolitis
- Asthma

Parenchymal disease

- Pneumonia
- Pulmonary oedema
- ARDS
- Chronic lung disease

Manifestations of Respiratory Failure

- Tachypnoea
- Subcostal, intercostal retractions
- Head bobbing, alae nasi flaring (infants)
- Paradoxical breathing (muscle weakness)
- Cyanosis

Management

Recognition: It is important to recognise the imminent signs of failure and treat accordingly. In infants, leaving the child with the parent is of great importance.

In children, progress of respiratory distress to failure is quick.[2]

Oxygen therapy: It is instituted to maintain oxygen saturation > 95% with a non-rebreathing mask at 10–15 L/min.[3]

Ventilation: Initiation of ventilation promptly is of utmost importance before fatigue ensues. Ventilation can be initiated with any of the modes mentioned in the above section and continued with lung protective measures. Constant monitoring of clinical status, blood gases and X-rays help making timely changes.

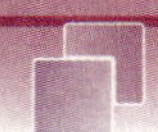

NEUROINTENSIVE CARE

Management of Traumatic Brain Injury (TBI)

Initial assessment of all trauma patients, should follow the sequence of resuscitation and stabilization, primary survey, secondary survey and definitive care.

Cervical Spine Injury

Cervical spine injury is most commonly seen in association with traumatic head injury. All patients with traumatic brain injury should be assumed to have a cervical spine injury until proven otherwise. Therefore, the neck should be immobilized in a hard collar from the time of the injury. Lateral and AP views of the entire cervical spine should be obtained. The neck should be immobilized until the patient is able to indicate whether he/she has any pain on movement of the neck.

Assessment of Conscious State

GCS/Modified GCS (in infants) helps in monitoring consciousness in patients with traumatic brain injury. Prognosis following TBI is strongly correlated with the initial GCS.

- GCS 3–5 = severe head injury with significant likelihood of neuromorbidity
- GCS 6–8 = moderately severe head injury, may have neuromorbidity
- GCS >8 = mild head injury, with good outcome.

A modified GCS is used for young infants: modified best verbal response:

5—appropriate words or social smile, fixes and follows
4—cries, but is consolable
3—persistently irritable
2—restless, agitated
1—none

While managing TBI patients, one should look for dangerous signs like unequal pupils, unequal motor response, open head injury with CSF leak (CSF rhinorrhea and CSF otorrhea) or exposed brain tissue, deterioration in the GCS by at least 2 points, established depressed skull fracture, bulging fontanelle or suture diastasis in an infant.

Principles of Management

The aim is to prevent further hypoxic insult and maintenance of adequate cerebral perfusion pressure (CPP).

$$CPP = MAP - ICP \text{ (Intracranial pressure)}$$

ICP monitoring should be an integral part of TBI management. ICP can be measured by using external ventricular drain (EVD), intraparenchymal catheters or subdural catheters.

Seizure Prophylaxis

Routine seizure prophylaxis is not generally used, however, if seizures occur phenytoin is the drug of choice.

Acute increases in ICP and neurological deterioration

Elevations in ICP can occur from a variety of causes like hypoxia, hypercapnoea, inadequate sedation and analgesia, hypotension. A decrease in BP even if the BP remains in the normal range, will result in reflex vasodilatation in the cerebral vasculature. This is a normal autoregulatory response. However, even a small amount of vasodilation can increase ICP in a tight brain. CT scan may be appropriate, particularly if there are new focal signs.

LIVER FAILURE

Liver failure is a loss of function of liver cells because of direct or indirect injury. Liver failure may be acute, chronic or "acute on chronic".

Acute liver failure is an infrequent diagnosis in children and is defined as occurrence of hepatic encephalopathy within 8 weeks of the onset of jaundice in a patient with no history of pre-existing liver disease.[1]

Etiology of Acute Liver Failure

- Infective: Hepatitis A,B, E, Herpes
- Metabolic: Galactosemia, tyrosinemia, Reye's syndrome
- Drugs: Paracetamol, valproic acid, INH
- Malignancy
- Autoimmune

Management

Investigations and monitoring: The child with fulminant hepatic failure (FHF) is best cared for in the paediatric intensive care unit due to frequent changes in haemodynamic, respiratory and neurological status. It is important to assess coagulation profile on a daily basis in addition to routine monitoring.

Aspects of Management[2,3]

- Fluid and electrolyte management
- Haemodynamic support
- Nutrition
- Infection surveillance

- Blood products
- GI prophylaxis

RENAL FAILURE

Initially any kidney dysfunction was labeled as renal failure. The terminology has changed and is labeled acute kidney injury.

Definition: Acute kidney injury (AKI) is an abrupt (within 48 hours) reduction in kidney function, defined as 50% or greater increase in serum creatinine or oliguria (<0.5 mL/kg/h or 1 mL/kg/h in a neonate[1]) for more than 6 hours.

Incidence: 1–25%

Etiology[2]

Prerenal

- Intravascular volume depletion: Dehydration, gastroenteritis, burns
- Redistribution: Sepsis, pancreatitis, nephrotic syndrome
- Decreased cardiac output: Congestive cardiac failure, Myocarditis

Renal

- Acute tubular injury: Shock, Prolonged ischaemia, NSAIDs, Heavy metals
- Acute interstitial nephritis
- Acute glomerulonephritis: Postinfectious, SLE
- Vascular pathology: Renal artery/vein thrombosis
- Congenital: Polycystic kidney disease, renal dysplasia

Postrenal

- Posterior urethral valves
- Bilateral ureteral obstruction
- Trauma

Assessment

This includes assessing the type of etiology based on clinical symptoms and signs.

Investigations: Complete blood count, CRP, blood urea, creatinine, electrolytes, blood gas, serum/urine osmolality, urine analysis, USG kidneys, renal Doppler.

Management

- Monitoring: Weight, urine output, electrolytes, renal function tests
- Fluid management
- Electrolyte management
- Hypertension control
- Nutrition
- Treatment of underlying disease
- Renal replacement therapy: May be required to give the kidney time to recover.

Prognosis

Despite all advances in renal replacement therapies, the morbidity and mortality due to AKI remains high (30–50%). The recovery and long-term outcome[3] depends on the underlying condition, need for inotropes, sepsis and multiorgan dysfunction.

NUTRITION

Enteral Nutrition

Enteral feeds are preferred whenever possible in the ICU. Infant formulae are used for patients aged 0–12 months, with paediatric formula beyond 12 months and a variety of adult formulae for older patients. For most patients nasogastric feeding is acceptable, however, if gastric feeds are poorly tolerated or there is a high risk of aspiration, then continuous naso-jejunal feeds via a transpyloric tube should be considered. Note that bolus feeds should not be given into the small bowel.

Parenteral Nutrition

TPN is a mixture of protein, carbohydrate and fat, combined with trace elements, vitamins and electrolytes. TPN is inferior to enteral nutrition, and should only be ordered if enteral nutrition is not possible and is likely not to be achieved for at least 3–5 days.

Even in patients on full TPN, a small amount of enteral feed (e.g. 1 mL/hour) should be initiated if there are no other contraindications as this will help prevent cholestasis and bacterial translocation from the gut into the circulation.

TRANSFUSION PRACTICES IN THE PAEDIATRIC INTENSIVE CARE UNIT

Blood and blood component transfusion is an integral part of managing sick children admitted to the PICU for various reasons. Major inventions in the 20th century have made blood component therapy possible.

Indications[1]

RBC Transfusion

- Acute blood loss of >15–20% blood volume with hypovolemia

- Hb < 8 gm% with
  1. Symptomatic perioperative anaemia
  2. Emergency surgery with anticipated blood loss
  3. Severe infections
  4. Septic shock (maintain Hb > 10 gm% or PCV > 30%)
- Hb < 7 gm% with chronic transfusion dependent states, e.g. haemoglobinopathies other than thalassemia major, congenital anemia.
- Paediatric oncology: When intensive chemotherapy is planned
- Patient on ventilatory support: Hb > 10 gm%

Platelet Transfusion

- Prophylactic in a non-bleeding child: < 5000–10000/cu mm
- Sick child: < 20000/cu mm especially with associated coagulopathy, severe mucositis, DIC
- Before surgery at critical sites like CNS, CVS: < 100000/cu mm
- Lumbar puncture: < 30000/cu mm

Fresh Frozen Plasma

- Inherited factor deficiency
- DIC with clinical bleeding
- Haemorrhagic disease of the newborn
- Liver disease with coagulopathy
- Plasma exchange for TTP/HUS
- Sick newborn with coagulopathy

Coagulopathy

- Hemophilia A
- Low fibrinogen levels: DIC, massive transfusion
- Factor XIII deficiency

Safety of transfusions has increased over the years with the advancement of technology. But it is very important for the clinician to use discretion at the bedside and judiciously use transfusions.

The incidence of adverse events due to human errors, ABO incompatibility, transfusion associated lung injury and bacterial contamination[2] are all a matter of concern and it is important to use strict hemovigilance.[3]

GI PROPHYLAXIS

Gastrointestinal tract is the major source of microbial invasion leading to systemic infection. Several protective mechanisms prevent the microbes invading into systemic circulation: Bactericidal action of the gastric acid, intrinsic barrier function of the mucosal lining of the bowel and reticuloendothelial system in the gut. A defect in any of the above protective mechanisms (bacterial overgrowth, mucosal disruption and impaired lymphatic clearance) leads to translocation of enteric pathogens into systemic circulation.

Indications for prophylaxis: Head injury, burns, major surgery, severe trauma, shock or multiorgan failure, mechanical ventilation, ulcerogenic medications and history of ulcer-related bleeding.

Preventive strategies include enteral nutrition, sucralfate, histamine H_2 receptor antagonists and antacids, and selective digestive decontamination.

PREVENTIVE PRACTICES AND INFECTION CONTROL

Infection Control in PICU

Incidence of nosocomial infections is around 5 to 15% of hospitalized patients and can lead to serious complications in 25–30% of those patients admitted to the intensive care unit.[1] The most common causes are pneumonia related to mechanical ventilation, catheter-related urinary tract infections, intra-abdominal infections following trauma or surgery, and bacteremia derived from intravascular devices. The policies regarding prevention and control of ventilator-associated pneumonia, catheter-related blood stream infections, urinary tract, and surgical site infections should be in place based on sound epidemiological knowledge, hospital and ICU surveillance data and hospital/ICU antibiogram. In paediatric age group, nosocomial infection attributable mortality is around 11% (NNIS data). The risk factors for nosocomial sepsis in our set up are—age, birth weight, underlying disease, immunity and invasive devices and procedures.[2] The spectrum of common organisms isolated in our PICUs is given below (NNIS data):

Blood stream infections	Pneumonia	UTI
CONS (38%)	Pseudomonas (22%)	*E. coli* (19%)
GNB (25%)	*Staph. aureus* (17%)	Candida (14%)
Enterococcus (12%)	*H. influenzae* (12%)	Pseudomonas (13%)
Staph. aureus (9%)	Enterobacter (10%)	Enterobacter (10%)

Hand hygiene

It is the most crucial step in the prevention of infection in the ICU. Steps in the hand hygiene are: (1) Remove rings, bracelets, watches, (2) Keep nails short, (3) Two to three minutes scrub of hands up to elbows with antiseptic soap on entering the PICU/and before performing invasive procedures, (4) Ten second wash/chlorhexidine based alcoholic hand rub before and after providing care to neonates and after removing gloves. Hand hygiene should be promoted with regular education, seminars and monitoring.[3]

The written waste disposal policy should be present and should be implemented strictly. It should include: (1) Avoiding handling soiled linen and dirty diapers with bare hands as it can lead to transient colonization that may not be removed with handwashing, (2) Soiled linen and soiled diapers should be packed in impervious bags and disposed 8 hourly.[4,5]

Peripheral line care bundle

- Upper extremity preferred
- Routine handwash/hand rub
- Non-sterile gloves okay if no touch method used
- Clean with alcohol
- Do not touch disinfected site
- Date lines, inspect daily
- No routine change of IV cannulas

Central line care bundle

- Hand hygiene, maximum barrier precautions
- Minimum lumens, antibiotic coated catheters
- Clean site with 2% w/v chlorhexidine
- No antibiotic ointment at exit site
- Gauze dressing 2 days, transparent 7 days
- Clean bivalves with alcohol prior to use
- Role of Clave/Smartsite/Qsyte
- Remove catheters when not needed
- No need for surveillance cultures/routine culture of tips on removal

Administration sets and tubing policy

- IV sets change every 72 hrs
- Blood sets change every 24 hrs
- Tubings for propofol every 6–12 hrs
- Transducer domes every 72 hrs
- IV lipids should be given within 24 hrs
- Use collapsible bags for IV fluids
- Use single dose vials

Prevention of UTI bundle

- If possible avoid catheterization
- Alternatives: Diaper weight, minicom
- For specimen collection: Suprapubic/minicom

If catheterized:

- Strict asepsis
- Maintain closed drainage
- Bag at lower level than catheter
- No routine change of catheter/bag
- Remove catheter when not needed

Control of VAP[6]

- Strict asepsis during intubation and suctioning
- Nurse at 45°
- Maintain good oral hygiene
- Avoid water in humidifiers
- Prefer disposable tubings
- Prevent accumulation of condensate
- Closed suction may offer some advantage
- No routine change of ventilator tubings/closed suctioning catheters (Stericath)

Antibiotic Policy

It is paramount to have an antibiotic policy to serve as a broad guideline for antibiotic use. The objective is not only to ensure appropriate treatment and improve clinical outcomes but also to prevent antibiotic misuse which is the singlemost important factor leading to antimicrobial resistance. Apart from this, antibiotic misuse also leads to increased treatment costs and adverse effects. Every PICU should have their own antibiotic policy based on the patient characteristics, organisms isolated, sensitivity pattern and surveillance data. Antibiotic policy should be adhered to in all circumstances. Use of prophylactic antibiotics (a common practice in most PICUs) should be avoided. If broad spectrum antibiotics are initiated, rapid de-escalation should be done once patient's condition improves and culture and sensitivity pattern is available.

REFERENCES AND SUGGESTED READING

Transportation and Receiving

1. Day SE. Intra-transport stabilization and management of the pediatric patient. Pediatr Clin North Am 1993;40(2): 263–274.
2. Section on Transport Medicine American Academy of Pediatrics. Transport team clinicians, health care

professionals and team composition. In: Woodward GA, Insoft RM, Kleinman ME, (Eds). Guidelines for air and ground transport of neonatal and pediatric patients. 3rd edn. Elk Grove Village (III): AAP. 2007;p. 23–9.

3. Woodward GA, Insoft RM, Pearson-Shaver AL, et al. The state of pediatric interfacility transport: Consensus of the Second National Pediatric and Neonatal Interfacility Transport Medicine Leadership Conference. Pediatr Emerg Care 2002; 18:38–43.

Emergence Agitation and Delirium

1. Eckenhoff JE, Kneale DH, Dripps RD. The incidence and etiology of postanesthetic excitement. A clinical survey. Anesthesiology. 1961;22:667–73.
2. Holzki J, Kretz FJ (Eds). Changing aspects of sevoflurane in paediatric anesthesia. 1975–99. Paediatr Anaesth. 1999;9:283–6.
3. Sikich N, Lerman J. Development and psychometric evaluation of the pediatric anesthesia emergence delirium scale. Anesthesiology. 2004; 100:1138–45.
4. Jerome EH. Recovery of the pediatric patient from anaesthesia. In: Gregory GA, (Ed). Pediatric anesthesia. 2nd edn. New York: Churchill Livingstone. 1989;629.8. Olympio MA. Postanesthetic delirium: historical perspectives. J Clin Anesth. 1991;3:60–3.
5. Lee CJ, Lee SE, Oh MK, et al. The effect of propofol on the emergence agitation in children receiving sevoflurane for adenotonsillectomy. Korean J Anesthesiol. 2010;59:75–81.

Vascular Access and PICU Procedures

1. Andropoulos DB, Bent ST, Skonsby B, et al. The optimal length of insertion of central venous catheters for pediatric patients. Anesth Analg 2001;93:883–6.
2. Keinman ME, Chameides L, Schexnayder SM, et al. Part 14: Pediatric Advanced Life Support: 2010. American Heart Association guidelines for cardiopulmonary resuscitation and emergency cardiovascular care. Circulation 2010; 122:S876.
3. Schexnayder SM, Khilnani P, Shimizu N. Invasive Procedures. In: Nichols D, et al. (Eds). Rogers textbook of Pediatric Intensive Care 2007. Williams and Wilkins (Baltimore).

Monitoring in the PICU

1. Mesiano G, Davis GM. Ventilatory strategies in neonatal and pediatric intensive care units. Pediatr Respir Rev 2008 Dec;9(4):281–8.
2. Khilnani P. Pediatric and Neonatal Mechanical ventilation 2011 2nd edn. (Jaypee Med Pub) India.
3. ARDS network: Ventilation with lower tidal volumes as compared with traditional tidal volumes of acute lung injury and the acute respiratory distress syndrome. N Eng J Med 2000;342:1301–1308.
4. Francisco R. Noninvasive ventilation in pediatric acute respiratory failure: A challenge in pediatric intensive care units. Pediatr Crit Care Med 2010; 11:750–1.
5. Clark RH, Gerstmann DL, Null DM, et al. Prospective randomized comparision of high frequency oscillatory and conventional ventilation in respiratory distress syndrome. Pediatrics 1992; 89:5–12.
6. Mugford M, Elbourne D, Field D. Extracorporeal membrane oxygenation for severe respiratory failure in newborn infants. Cochrane Database Syst Rev 2008;3:CD001340.
7. Nilsestum JO, Hargett K. Managing the patient-ventilator system using graphic analysis: An overview and introduction to Graphics corner. Resp care 1996;41:1105–22.
8. Ronco R, Riquelme C. Cardiac output measurement in children: what is lacking? Pediatr Crit Care Med 2008;9:333.
9. Tibby SM, Murdoch IA. Monitoring cardiac function in intensive care. Arch Dis Child 2001;88:46–52.
10. Tibby SM, Murdoch IA. Measurement of cardiac output and tissue perfusion. Current Opinion In Pediatrics. 2002;14:303–9.

Postoperative Nausea and Vomiting

1. Kovac AL. Management of postoperative nausea and vomiting in children. Pediatric Drugs 2007;9(1):47–69.
2. Domino KB, Anderson EA, Polissar NL, et al. Comparative efficacy and safety of ondansetron, droperidol, and metoclopramide for preventing postoperative nausea and vomiting: A meta-analysis. Anesth Analg. 1999;88:1370–9.

Cardiac Intensive Care

1. Balaguru D, Artman M, Auslender M. Management of heart failure in children. Curr Probl Pediatr 2000;30:5–30.
2. Daphne T Hsu, Gail D Pearson. Heart failure in children—Part I: History, Etiology and Pathophysiology. Circ Heart Fail 2009;2:63–70.
3. Daphne T Hsu, Gail D Pearson. Heart failure in children-Part II: Diagnosis, Treatment and Future directions. Circ Heart Fail 2009;2:490–98.
4. Paul F Kantor, Luc L Mertens. Heart failure in children. Part I: Clinical evaluation, diagnostic evaluation and initial medical management. Eur J Pediatr. 2010;169:269–79.
5. Scholz H. Inotropic drugs and their mechanism of action. J Am Coll Cardiol 1984;4:389–98.
6. Paul F Kantor, Luc L Mertens. Heart failure in children. Part II: Current maintenance therapy and new therapeutic approaches. Eur J Pediatr. 2010;169:403–10.
7. Blumberg RM, Gardiner HM. Evaluation of suspected congenital heart disease in the neonatal period. Current Paediatrics. 2000;10:229–235.

Respiratory Failure

1. Green TP, Steinhorn DM. The treatment of acute respiratory failure in children: a historical examination and landmark advances. J Pediatr. 2001; 139:604–608.
2. Hazinski MF, Zaritsky AL, Nadkarni VM, et al. (Eds). PALS Provider Manual. Dallas, Tex: American Heart Association/ American Academy of Pediatrics; 2002.

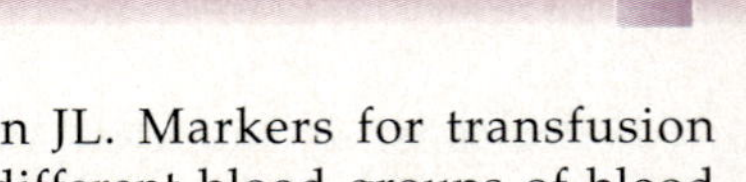

3. Matthews BD, Noviski N. Management of oxygenation in pediatric acute hypoxemic respiratory failure. Pediatr Pulmonol 2001;32:459–470.

Neurointensive Care

1. Bucuvalas MD, Nada Y, Robert H. Acute liver failure in children. Clinics in Liver Dis. 2006;10:149–68.
2. Daniel D' Agostino D, Diaz S, et al. Management and Prognosis of acute liver failure in children. Curr Gastroenterol Rep. 2012;14:262–69.
3. Steinhorn DM, Alonso EM, Bunchman TE. Acute liver failure, Liver transplantation and extracorporeal liver support. Fuhrman BP, Zimmerman JJ, (Eds). Pediatric Critical Care, 4th edn. Elseviers Saunders. 2011;p. 1248–58.

Renal Failure

1. Agras PI, Tarcan A, Saatci U. Acute renal failure in the neonatal period. Renal Fail 2004;26:305–9.
2. Andreoli SP. Acute kidney injury in children. Pediatr Nephrol 2009;24:253–263.
3. Metnitz PG, Krenn CG. Effect of acute renal failure requiring renal replacement therapy on outcome in critically ill patients. Crit Care Med. 2002;30(9):2051–8.

Nutrition

1. Practice Guidelines for blood component therapy: A report by the American Society of Anesthesiologists Task Force on Blood Component Therapy. Anesthesiology 1996;84: 732–47.
2. Starkey JM, McPherson JL. Markers for transfusion transmitted disease in different blood groups of blood donors. JAMA 1989;262:3452–54.
3. Rajesh CA, Wander GS. Blood component therapy: Which, when and how much? J Anesthesiol Clin Pharmacol 2011;27(2):278–84.

Preventive Practices and Infection Control

1. Richards MJ, Edwards JR, Culver DH, et al. Nosocomial infections in medical intensive care units in the United States. National Nosocomial Infections Surveillance System. Crit Care Med. 1999;27(5):887–92.
2. Safdar N, Maki DG. The pathogenesis of catheter-related blood stream infection with non-cuffed short term central venous catheters. Intensive Care Med 2004;30(1):62–67.
3. O'Grady NP, Barie PS, Bartlett JG, et al. Practice guidelines for evaluating new fever in critically ill adult patients. Task force of Society of Critical Care Medicine and Infectious Disease Societies of America. Cin Inf Dis. 1998;26(5): 1042–59.
4. Coffin SE, Zaoutis TE. Infection control, hospital epidemiology, and patient safety. Infect Dis Clin North Am. 2005; 19(3):647–65.
5. Costa SF, Miceli MH, Anaissie EJ. Mucosa or skin as source of coagulasenegative staphylococcal bacteremia? Lancet infect Dis. 2004;4(5):278–86.
6. Chastre J, Fagon JY. Ventilator-associated pneumonia. Am J Respir Crit Care Med. 2002;165(7):867–903.

Anaesthesia for the Patient with a Genetic Syndrome

Gayathri Bhat and Tushar Patel

Genetic disorders, as the name suggests, are conditions caused by abnormalities in the genes. Many a times the anaesthesiologists are not familiar with the genetic disorders and therefore a general approach to the patient with a genetic syndrome has to be understood. It is important to become familiar with the basic problems of the particular syndrome to devise a rational anaesthetic plan.

General considerations for anaesthetic management of these patients have been mentioned here. Also the details of a few commonly presenting syndromes are elaborated.

Airway Considerations

Many patients with genetic syndromes have an abnormal airway, and management of the airway is always a main consideration for the anaesthesiologist. Mandibular hypoplasia is the most common feature among many syndromes such as Pierre Robin, Treacher Collins and Goldenhar (hemifacial microsomia). Small mouth opening, with high arched palate, limitation of neck movement due to fusion of the cervical vertebrae macroglossia causing soft tissue obstruction, and cleft lip and palate are causes of difficult airway.

Preoperatively complete history of airway problems, like snoring, airway obstruction during sleep, and acute life-threatening events have to be noted.

Earlier anaesthetic exposures, tracheal intubations, and the data from previous anaesthesiologist, otolaryngologist or craniofacial surgeons will be useful. Airway examination consisting of mouth opening, visualization of the pharynx and soft palate if possible, along with neck movement should be done carefully. Reviewing of imaging studies of chest, neck, and facial radiographs with computed tomography (CT) or magnetic resonance imaging (MRI) scans are essential.

Cardiac Manifestations

A thorough history and physical examination of the cardiovascular system is most important. Many of the genetic syndromes have a cardiac component, often detected with systolic and/or diastolic murmurs. Echocardiography is a useful diagnostic tool.

Syndromes with frequent cardiac involvement include Vertebral anomalies, Anal atresia, Cardiac defects, Tracheoesophageal fistula, Renal and Radial anomalies and Limb defects (VACTERL), Coloboma of the eye, Heart defects, Atresia of the nasal choanae, Retardation of growth, Genital and/or urinary abnormalities, and Ear abnormalities and deafness (CHARGE) and velo-cardio-facial syndromes. When patients present for non-cardiac surgery, cardiologist consultation is desired.

Neurodevelopmental Abnormalities

Patients with genetic syndromes may present with neurodevelopmental delay with or without malformations of the central or peripheral nervous system.

There is associated general intelligence lag, gross or fine motor problems, speech and language delay, and behavioral problems. The chronological age may be very different from the developmental age and the approach to preoperative preparation, communication, premedication, and parental presence may need to be altered accordingly.

Orthopaedic Considerations

Scoliosis, hip dysplasia, and limb contractures are common in patients with genetic syndromes. Injury to the affected areas should be prevented with careful positioning during anaesthesia.

Severe scoliosis needs an evaluation of the respiratory and cardiac status, which may alter the plan for postoperative ventilation and intensive care.

Other Considerations

Limb abnormalities and multiple previous hospitalizations with procedures will pose difficulty in securing peripheral vascular access. Alternative sites like external/internal jugular veins can be used if they are not thrombosed from previous catheterizations. It is beneficial to have a reference source for the anaesthesiologists at hand because of the frequent presentation of these patients on the day of surgery. A diagnosis of the genetic disorders is done by Conventional karyotyping, chromosomal microarray (CMA) or fluorescence *in situ* hybridization (FISH), from peripheral blood lymphocytes.

Many a times the parents and other caregivers are usually extremely knowledgeable about the patient, the condition itself, and can offer valuable information about how the patient has responded to particular interventions in the past. It is important to listen to the parents and patient's requests and concerns when approaching the patient with a genetic syndrome.

DOWN SYNDROME

Down's syndrome (DS) is named after John Langdon Down, an English physician, who noted the similarities in physical characteristics. It is the most common condition of genetic mental retardation linked to trisomy of chromosome 21, occurring approximately 1 in 700 live births. Majority DS patients have an extra chromosome, trisomy 21 and others are associated with a chromosomal translocation or mosaic trisomy 21. Advanced maternal age is the most significant risk factor. Nearly 1.25% of anaesthetized cases were DS in a major US children's hospital. This series indicates the frequency with which the paediatric anaesthesiologist will encounter patients with DS, and a thorough understanding of the disease is essential to deliver appropriate anaesthetic care to these patients. Clinical features of Down's syndrome of particular importance to the anaesthesiologists are (Fig. 38.1):

1. General	Low birth weight Obesity in childhood through adult life Short stature
2. Respiratory	Obstructive sleep apnoea Subglottic and tracheal stenosis Lower respiratory tract infection
3. Cardiovascular	Congenital heart disease Pulmonary hypertension Valvular heart disease
4. Neurological	Neonatal hypotonia Intellectual impairment Alzheimer's disease Epilepsy
5. Spinal disease	Atlanto-axial instability Atlanto-occipital instability Cervical spondylitis
6. Gastrointestinal	Gastro-esophageal reflux Gastrointestinal atresia Endocrine Hypothyroidism

Preanaesthetic History/Evaluation

Patients with DS have a characteristic appearance from birth. The most common features include brachycephaly, a flat nasal bridge, epicanthic folds, upwardly slanting palpebral fissures, small mouth and ears, and relatively large tongue and a transverse (Simian) palmar crease. Neonates of DS tend to be of low birth weight, and develop obesity, at the end of infancy which continues through their adult life. Peripheral venous access is difficult because of increased adipose tissue, internal jugular access is difficult by a short webbed neck and increased adipose tissue, and radial arterial access difficult because of the small size of this artery. They also have mental retardation and hypotonia.

Airway

Anticipated difficult airway due to a narrow midface, small nasal passages, constricted_oropharyngeal space, small mouth, relative macroglossia, micrognathia, short neck and adenotonisillar hypertrophy. Despite this propensity for upper airway obstruction, the vast majority of DS patients may have a straightforward mask airway and tracheal intubation, probably because of hypotonia and ligamentous laxity around the temporomandibular joint and neck. Craniofacial anomalies lead to obstructive sleep apnoea. DS children frequently undergo adenotonsillectomy to improve the symptoms. They also have dysfunction of the central ventilatory drive. In the postoperative period, presence of central nervous system depressant drugs may worsen the upper airway obstruction causing agitation.

DS patients may have subglottic or tracheal stenosis. Severe congenital (1%) type may present at birth or may

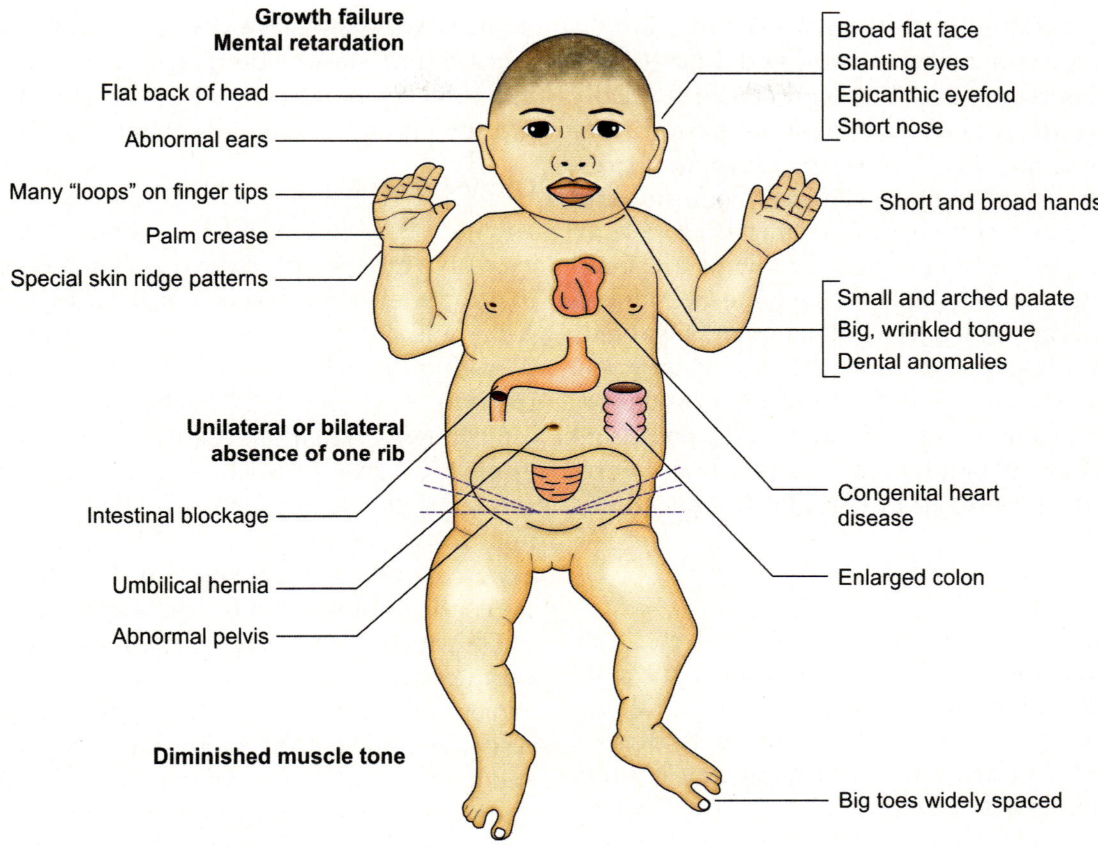

Fig. 38.1 Features of Down syndrome

remain asymptomatic for the first few months of life. DS is usually detected at the time of assessment, during intubation or during sedation for investigations. A history of stridor, wheezing, recurrent pneumonia, a previously difficult intubation, cyanotic episodes or high ventilatory pressures should arouse suspicion to select an endotracheal tube with internal diameter 1–2 mm smaller than expected for age. These patients tend to be of shorter stature and have smaller airways. A tube that is too large will cause airway oedema and obstruction. A leak-test (listen for an audible leak) with positive pressure ventilation is important in smooth conduct of the case. To prevent the postoperative chest infections, careful examination of the respiratory system prior to surgery is essential as chronic lower respiratory tract infections are frequent in DS, due to decreased immunity, gastro-esophageal reflux and hypotonia.

Cardiovascular System

Congenital heart disease (CHD) is associated with DS (16–60%). Atrioventricular canal defect is the most common. Other lesions like ventricular septal defect, patent ductus arteriosus, tetralogy of Fallot are also seen. Cardiac anomaly involving left-to-right shunt causes increased pulmonary blood flow and pulmonary vascular disease. Patients with DS develop pulmonary hypertension to a greater severity and at an earlier age than non-DS patients with similar cardiac lesions. Various mechanisms for this have been suggested, including chronic hypoxia (secondary to chronic infection, hypoventilation, obstructive sleep apnoea syndrome and pulmonary hypoplasia) and a defect of pulmonary capillaries. Pulmonary hypertension has been reported in patients with DS in the absence of cardiac disease. Therefore, an understanding of, and vigilance for, these conditions is important. Neonates with DS should be screened for congenital heart disease, and parents questioned about cardiac history. Echocardiography is the most sensitive and specific investigation for this purpose.

Nervous System

Generalized hypotonia and laxity of joint ligaments occurring in DS requires extra care while positioning patients, to avoid peripheral nerve damage. The intellectual impairment, with learning difficulty along with sensory deficits imparts difficulty in communicating. It is well known that patients with DS are generally calm and good-natured, but may become markedly agitated in the immediate postoperative period. This agitation may jeopardize intravenous lines and dressings or even spinal fixation devices. Sedation and opiates have to be used keeping in mind the risks of upper airway obstructions. These problems are familiar to paediatric anaesthetists but may be overlooked by those more accustomed to adult patients. DS patients may develop Alzheimer's dementia at a young age. Epilepsy occurs in about 10% of the DS population, patients may present for surgery taking anticonvulsant medication. These patients may require a lower minimum alveolar concentration of volatile anaesthetic agents.

Sensory System

Ocular and acoustic impairment is common and may make communication with the patient more difficult. Ocular manifestations like squints or congenital and acquired cataracts are common reasons for surgery. Severe refractive errors occur and glaucoma is more frequent. Craniofacial anomalies may lead to hearing deficits. Narrow ear canals cause accumulation of ear wax and hence increase conductive deafness. Patients have smaller Eustachian tubes which tend to collapse and cause middle ear effusions. Sixty-five percent of DS children require tympanotomy and ventilation tubes.

Gastrointestinal System

Gastrointestinal anomalies are about 10% in patients with DS. Majority of these are esophageal/duodenal atresia, annular pancreas, and tracheo-esophageal fistula. Neonate may be posted for emergency surgery to relieve bowel obstruction; a careful search for associated conditions, especially CHD, is important for the management. Hirschsprung's disease may present with intestinal obstruction, colonic perforation or enterocolitis in the neonatal period or with constipation in older children. Patients with DS may suffer from gastro-esophageal reflux, which may cause, acute and chronic respiratory disease. Reflux may also increase the risks of pre-operative aspiration of gastric contents. Therefore, appropriate precautions should be taken to prevent it.

Haematological System

Down syndrome children are at increased risk for acute leukemias, both myeloid (AML) and lymphocytic (ALL). Survival and outcome are improved in DS patients with intensive chemotherapy induction regimens which cause side effects, particularly mucositis and severe infections. The anaesthesiologist must evaluate for all of the other manifestations.

Other Systems

Atlanto-occipital instability occurs in DS patients with excessive movement of cervical flexion/extension. The incompletely ossified cervical spine vertebrae and X-ray will not give a clear picture, hence not required. A history of neck pain or neurological symptoms, and previous anaesthetics or tracheal intubations, prompts a thorough evaluation, requiring cervical spine radiography, CT scan or MRI. Very careful handling of the cervical spine during airway management and surgical positioning is indicated, which includes avoiding extremes of flexion, extension, and rotation, and holding the cervical spine in neutral position whenever possible.

DS patients may have congenital hypothyroidism or compensated hypothyroidism up to ten years of age. Screening of thyroid function before major surgery is essential. Elevated thyroid-stimulating hormone (TSH) and low-normal T4 levels should raise a suspicion which often goes undetected due to the other characteristics like, developmental delays, hypotonia, and obesity. Hypothyroidism is especially important in cardiac or other major surgery, where a subclinical state may be unmasked by the major stress in the perioperative period, which can affect myocardial function by desensitizing the heart to endogenous and exogenous catecholamines.

VACTERL Association

The VACTERL acronym comprises

V: Vertebral defects
A: Anal or other intestinal atresia
C: Cardiac defects
TE: Tracheo-esophageal fistula
R: Renal malformations
L: Limb defects

The candidate genes include:

- Defects or deletions in the sonic hedgehog gene on chromosome 7,
- FOX transcription gene cluster on chromosome 16, and
- Gli2 gene on chromosome 2.

TE fistula is often accepted as essential for the diagnosis, along with at least one of the five other major defects. Among them, cardiac lesions are the most prevalent, seen in 30–50% of patients. The common cardiac lesions include ventricular septal defect and tetralogy of Fallot. Children with CHD are usually acyanotic at presentation. The mortality after TEF repair in cases with complex CHD-like patent ductus arteriosus-dependent systemic or pulmonary circulation exceeds 50%. 25% of patients have vertebral anomalies like hemi-vertebrae, butterfly or fused vertebrae or extra vertebrae. 20% of patients have renal anomalies which include horseshoe kidney, renal agenesis, vesico-ureteral reflux, hypospadias, dysplastic kidney and cryptorchidism. 15% of patients have atresia of the gastrointestinal tract, most common being anal atresia. Limb anomalies (10%) include digital anomalies and absent radius. Preoperative evaluation includes thorough assessment of the lesions in all categories. These children are most often developmentally normal.

Preanaesthetic preparations

- Children should be kept nil per oral
- Upright position
- Upper pouch should be suctioned intermittently
- Antibiotic therapy and physiotherapy in patients with pneumonia

Intraoperative management

Gastrostomy is performed under local or general anaesthesia in infants with significant associated anomalies or sepsis as a palliative procedure. Within 24 to 72 hours, definitive repair is performed once the extent of other anomalies is defined and cardiovascular stability is established. Stomach is decompressed using gastrostomy tube thus minimizing regurgitation into lungs.

Awake intubation is generally considered safe to secure the airway in infants with TEF. It avoids positive pressure ventilation and gastric distension. Awake intubation has the potential for trauma to the airway, so intubation is done after inhalational induction with or without muscle relaxation with gentle positive-pressure ventilation. After the endotracheal tube is in place, end-tidal carbon dioxide and oxygen saturation must be monitored, and the stomach and chest should be auscultated to ensure that the lungs are adequately ventilated and the stomach is not distended with inspired gases.

Once satisfactory ventilation is ensured, the chest is opened and the lungs are retracted. Lung retraction impairs ventilation, especially in infants with respiratory dysfunction from immature lungs, pneumonia, or congenital heart disease. Intermittent release of pressure by the surgeon to allow inflation of the right lung often improves oxygenation and ventilation. Blood clots or secretions may block the endotracheal tube, and frequent endotracheal suctioning may be required. Because the trachea is a soft structure in the newborn, surgical manipulation may kink the airway and further obstruct ventilation. Thus, interference with adequate oxygenation can occur as a result of the patient's anatomy, operative positioning, and surgical manipulations.

The precordial stethoscope is repositioned after induction of anaesthesia into the left axilla. In infants with an unstable cardio-respiratory status or congenital heart disease, an arterial catheter (umbilical or right radial) should be placed. Other monitoring consists of an electrocardiogram, pulse oximetry, and end-tidal gas monitoring. In some infants, both preductal and postductal pulse oximeters are placed. The patient's temperature must be monitored, and efforts must be made to prevent hypothermia.

Postoperative management

Tracheomalacia or a defective tracheal wall at the site of the fistula can cause collapse of the airway and require reinsertion of the endotracheal tube. These specific problems with TEF, as well as the host of other cardiorespiratory problems of the newborn, generally require a period of postoperative ventilation for these infants, often for at least 24 to 48 hours. In addition, most surgeons request that ventilation with a mask and bag be avoided for at least several days postoperatively. Infants who have had repair of a "long-gap" atresia require postoperative ventilatory support for a longer (5 to 7 days) postoperative period. Neuromuscular blocking agents are administered during this time to eliminate any spontaneous ventilation. Postoperative ventilation is also planned for an infant whose lungs were contaminated, whose intraoperative course was complicated (e.g. tracheal perforation), or who has underlying lung disease associated with prematurity.

CHARGE SYNDROME

The term charge comes from the first letter of the most common features seen in this group of patients:

C: Coloboma

H: Heart defects

A: Atresia of the choanae

R: Retardation of growth and development

G: Genital and urinary abnormalities

E: Ear abnormalities or/and hearing loss.

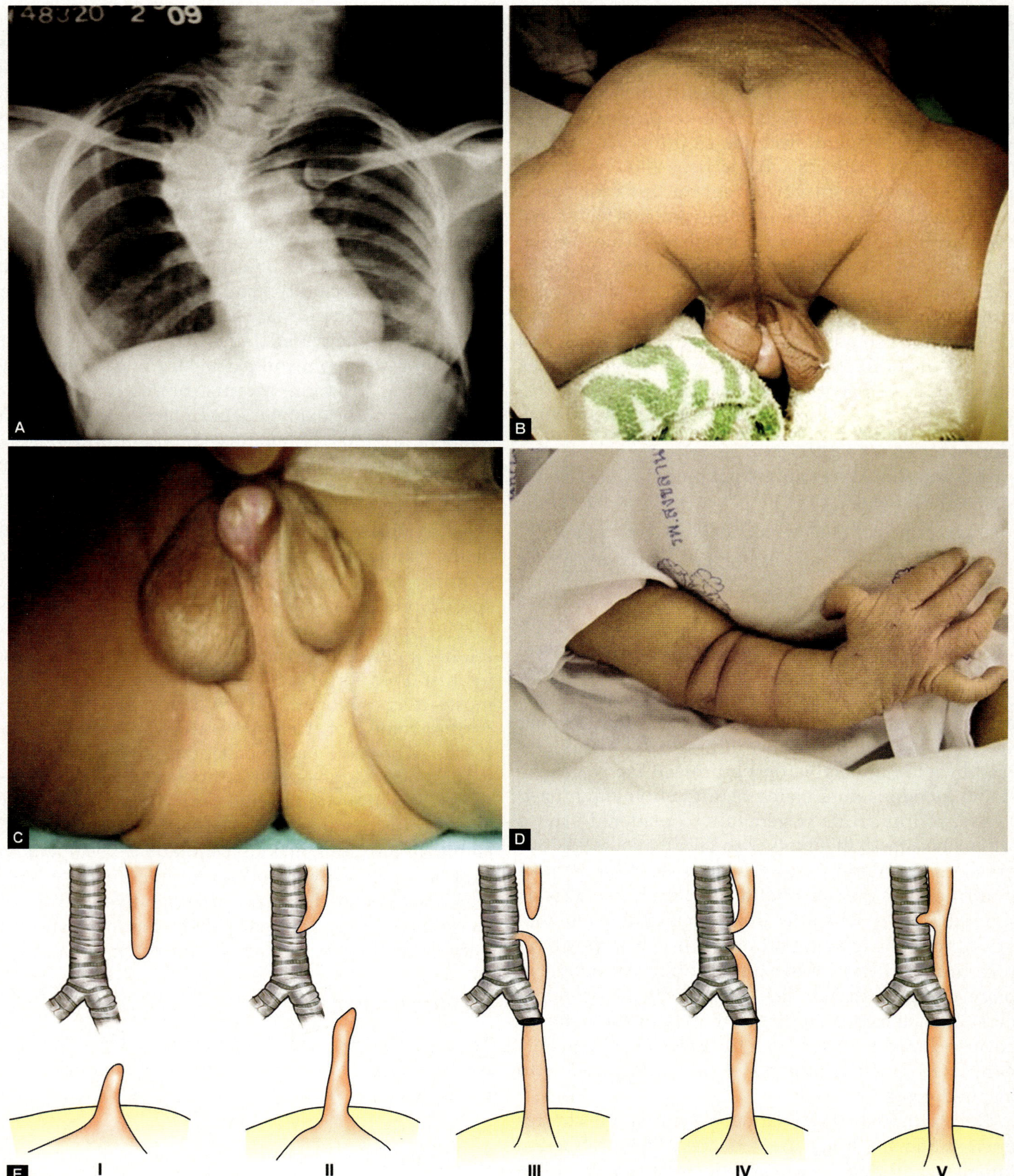

Fig. 38.2 (A) Scoliosis, (B) anorectal malformation, (C) hypospadias and bifid scrotum, (D) limb-radial hypoplasia and (E) tracheo-esophageal fistula

Several other features which may be associated are: Cleft lip and palate, tracheoesophageal fistula or atresia, facial palsy, swallowing problems, weak upper body strength, seizures, microcephaly, abnormality of the pituitary gland and poor immune system. Retardation of growth and development make pain assessment difficult in the postoperative period.

CHARGE syndrome patients are at high risk for aspiration and swallowing difficulty. Aspiration has been implicated as the most common cause of mortality and hence a challenge to the anaesthesiologist. Diagnosis of CHARGE is established based on three major and three minor criteria:

Major: Coloboma, Choanal Artesia, Ear anomalies

Minor: Heart defect, Orofacial cleft, Upper body hypotonia, Growth deficiency, Developmental delay, Scoliosis, Leg anomaly.

CHARGE syndrome affects 1:10,000 to 1:12,000 live births and occurs in, both sexes, all races and socio-economic strata. There is no cure for CHARGE syndrome but some features can be surgically corrected, such as choanal atresia, cleft lip and heart defects which can reduce the morbidity. Fitting of hearing aids, glasses and implementing appropriate educational programs have positive behavioral outcome.

Preanaesthetic Evaluation

Anaesthetist should gain the family's confidence before obtaining a more detailed history. Standard fasting guidelines are to be followed. Pre-medication must be given in order to relieve the anxiety and improve cooperation at induction. Oral midazolam (0.5 mg/kg) and oral atropine (20 μg/kg) are often preferred agents. Sedative pre-medication is best avoided in patients with pre-existing severe airway obstruction.

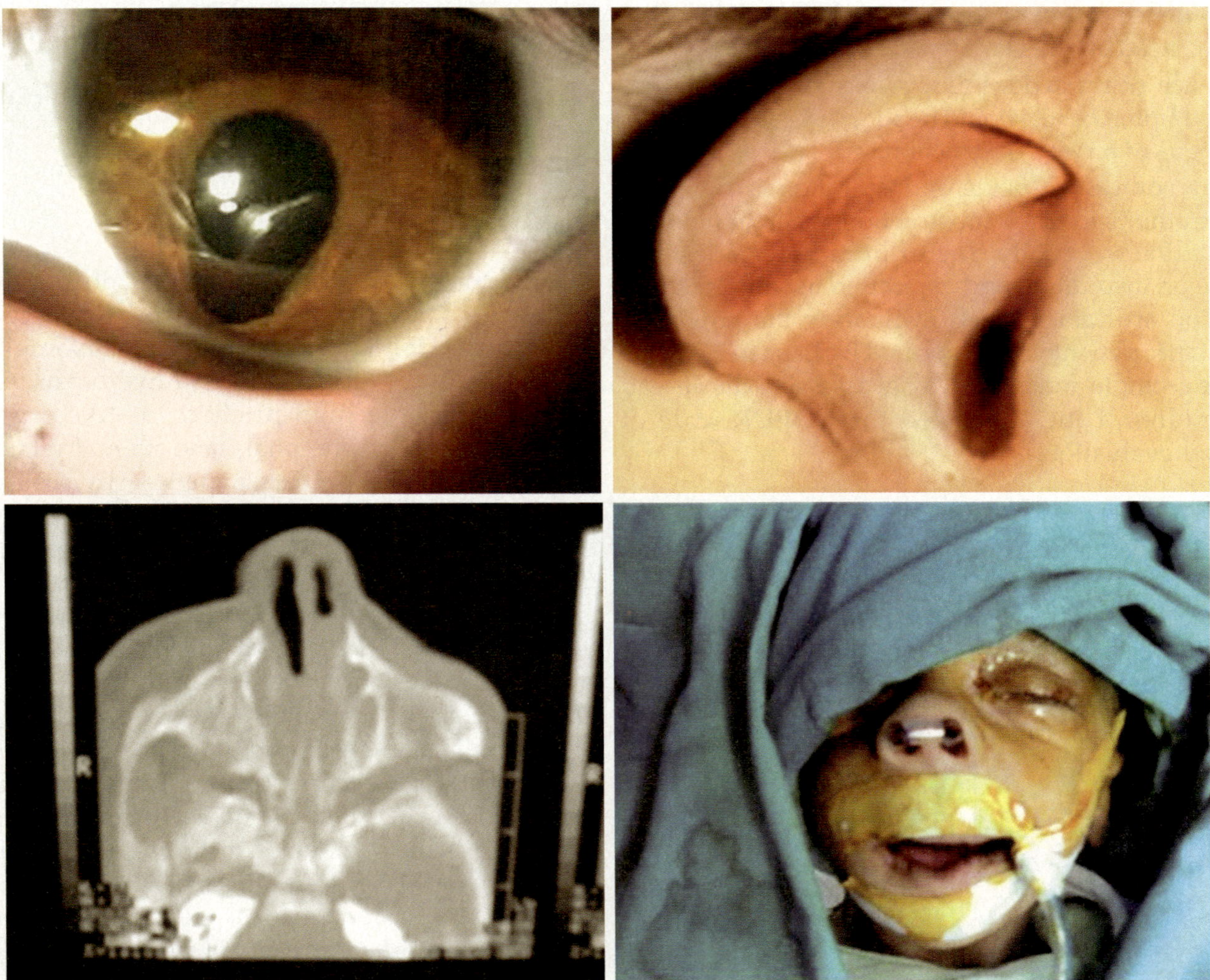

Fig. 38.3 Coloboma, ear abnormalities, choanal atresia

Airway Assessment

Airway assessment usually is difficult in children, especially those less than 3 years of age. Assessment of difficult airway in paediatric patients begins with a comprehensive history and physical examination:

- **History:** Questions to be asked regarding complaints of snoring, apnoea, stridor, hoarse voice. This information may indicate hypoxemia and pulmonary hypertension. History should also consist of a review of previous anaesthetic records with attention being paid to oropharyngeal injury, damage to teeth, awake tracheal intubation or postponement of surgery following an anaesthetic.
- **Physical examination:** It should focus on the anomalies of face, head, neck and spine. Evaluate size and shape of head, gross features of the face size and symmetry of the mandible, presence of sub-mandibular pathology, size of tongue, shape of palate, prominence of upper incisors, and range of motion of jaw, head and neck.
- Presence of retractions (suprasternal/sternal/infra-sternal/intercostal) should be sought for, they usually are signs of airway obstruction.
- **Breath sounds:** Crowing on inspiration is indicative of extrathoracic airway obstruction, whereas noise on exhalation is usually due to intrathoracic lesions. Noise on inspiration and expiration usually is due to a lesion at thoracic inlet. Evaluating the airway in paediatric patient was advocated by Lane in 2005. He made a simple and rapid way of assessing the airway in children. Lane advocated the **COPUR scale** of airway evaluation.

COPUR scale of airway evaluation:

C—CHIN From side view patient's chin is:

Normal	1
Small, moderately hypoplastic	2
Markedly recessive	3
Extremely hypoplasia	4

O—OPENING OF MOUTH (Interdental Space)

>40 mm	1
20–40 mm	2
10–20 mm	3
<10 mm	4

P—PREVIOUS INTUBATION or OSA

Previous attempt easy	1
No previous attempt, no history of OSA	2
OSA, previous history of difficult intubation	3
Extremely difficult previous intubation, tracheostomy, or patient unable to lie supine	4

U—UVULA

Whole of uvula visible	1
Uvula partially visible	2
Uvula concealed, soft palate visible	3
Soft palate not visible	4

R—RANGE (Estimate range of motion looking up and down)

>120°	1
60–120°	2
30–60°	3
<30°	4

Prediction points

5–7: Easy, normal intubation
8–10: Laryngeal pressure may help
12: Increased difficulty, fiberoptic may be preferred
14: Difficult intubation, fiberoptic or other advanced technique should be preferred
16: Dangerous airway, consider awake intubation potential tracheostomy

Scores above 10 predict difficult intubation.

CRI DU CHAT SYNDROME

Cri du chat syndrome was first described by Lejune et al. in 1963. It is a rare genetic disease resulting from a deletion of the short arm of chromosome 5. The incidence is 1:37000 to 1:50000 live births. Clinical features include high-pitched cat like cry, facial dysmorphism, microcephaly and mental retardation. Hypertelorism, low set ears, hypertonicity, scoliosis, flat foot, prominent orbital arch, dental occlusion, elongated facies, palpebral fissures, divergent strabismus and flat nasal bridge.

These patients are susceptible to recurrent respiratory tract infections. The patient can have airway abnormalities like long curved floppy epiglottis and narrowed diamond-shaped appearance of vocal cords. Congenital heart diseases are seen in 30% of the patients. These patients should receive bacterial endocarditis prophylaxis is scheduled for invasive procedures. Preoperative cardiac evaluation including a 2D echocardiography should be done. Preanaesthetic medication should be avoided in these patients as hypotonic pharyngeal muscles can cause obstruction of the airway. Endotracheal intubation can be difficult due to laryngeal abnormalities and micrognathia. Intraoperative hypothermia should be avoided in these patients.

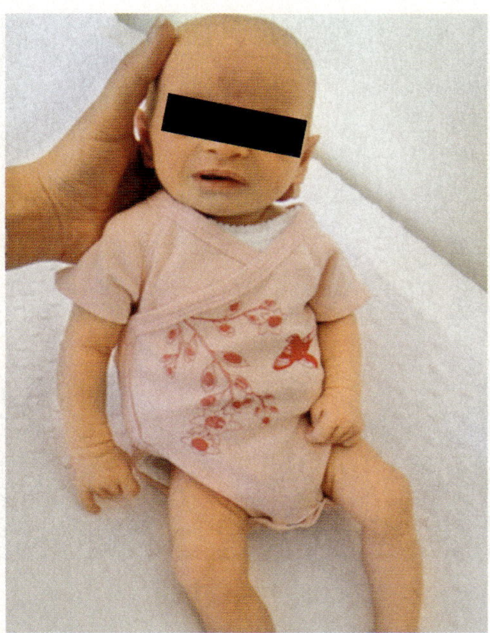

Fig. 38.4 Cri du chat syndrome showing microcephaly, hypertelorism, flat nasal bridge, small chin, skin fold over eyes

Patients should be observed for a longer period during postanaesthetic recovery till they are fully awake and free of residual anaesthetic effects.

HURLER'S SYNDROME

It is mucopolysacchridosis type 1. It is caused by deficiency of the lysosomal enzyme alpha-1 iduronidase. The airway problems in these patients are narrowed nasal passages, large tongue, adenotonsillar hypertrophy, short neck, high epiglottis, hypoplastic mandible and thickened supraglottis. The head is enlarged with coarse facial features, hypertelorism, flattened nasal dorsum and peg-like teeth. These patients can also have cervical spine instability. Facial abnormalities, stiff temporo-mandibular joint and anteriorly placed larynx can make mask ventilation and tracheal intubation difficult. These patients are at risk of respiratory sufficiency due to abnormalities of chest and spine and hepatosplenomegaly limiting the diaphragm movement. These patients can have cardiac manifestations like valvular heart disease, cardiomyopathy, congestive cardiac failure, coronary artery disease, hypertension and corpulmonale. Brain atrophy, white matter lesions and communicating hydrocephalus are common in these patients. The preoperative evaluation should include flexion and extension radiographic views of the neck for evaluation of cervical spine stability.

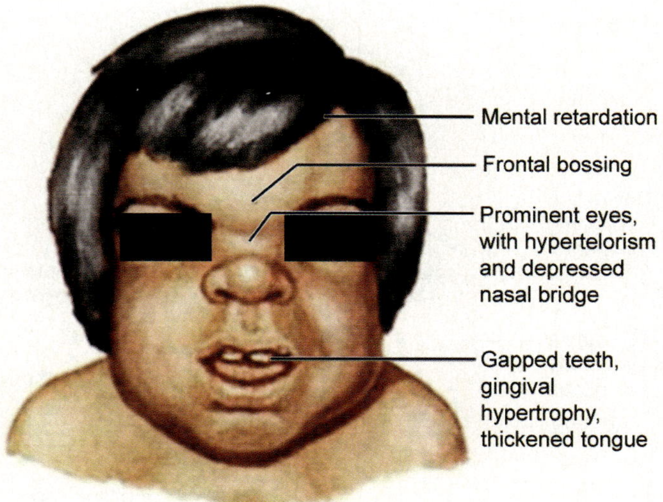

Fig. 38.5 Hurler's syndrome

Sedative premedication should be avoided. Awake fiberoptic intubation or intubation after deep inhalation induction is preferred in older patients, thereby ensuring spontaneous ventilation until the airway has been secured. Rapid sequence induction with cricoid pressure should be performed in patients with the risk of aspiration. The presence of thickened supraglottic tissue and large tongue may lead to upper airway obstruction during manual ventilation. An oropharyngeal airway may exacerbate the obstruction by displacing the epiglottis downward. Nasal airways are more effective but advancement may be difficult because of narrowed nasal passages. Laryngeal mask airway may be a better option in these patients.

Recovery after general anaesthesia in patients with MPS is slow and accompanied by periods of breath holding, apnoea, bronchospasm, negative pressure pulmonary oedema, and respiratory arrest. The child should be awake with adequate airway reflexes for extubation.

Treacher Collins Syndrome (TCS)

It is an autosomal dominant disorder affecting bilateral facial development. Incidence is 1 in 50,000 live births. TCS is a genetic developmental disorder of the first and second branchial arches, resulting in abnormal development of neural crest cells. TCS includes:

- Hypoplasia of the maxilla, zygoma, and mandible
- Lateral downward sloping of the palpebral fissures
- Coloboma of the lower eyelids
- Defects of the external and middle ears, and
- Sensorineural deafness.

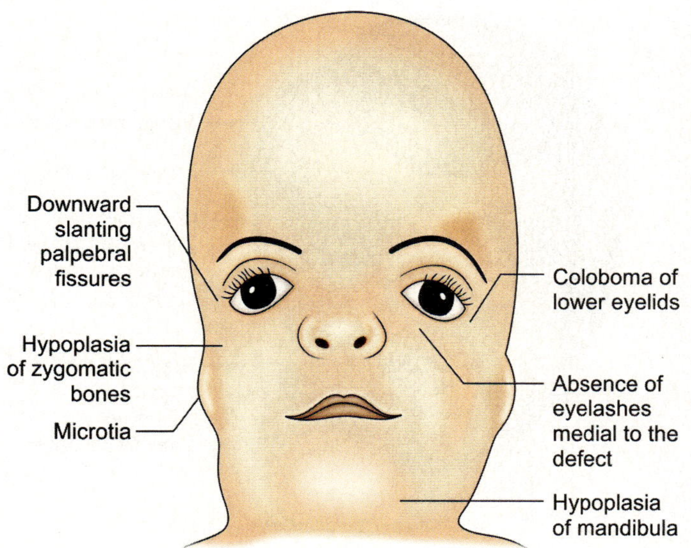

Fig. 38.6 Treacher Collins syndrome

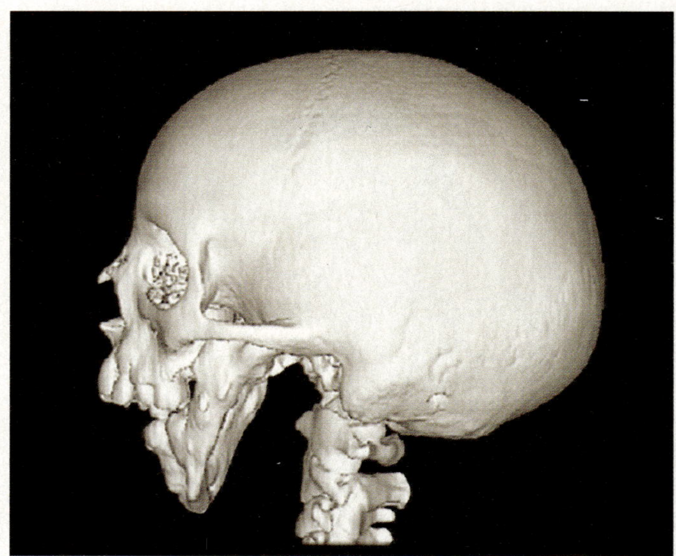

Fig. 38.7 Pierre Robin syndrome

Before 10 years of age, these patients require extensive facial reconstruction (orbital and zygomatic reconstruction) over multiple procedures. When bony growth is complete, external ear reconstruction and mandibular advancement is required. Difficulties in airway management are due to mandibular hypoplasia and high-arched palate.

Airway implications: It was recommended by Rasch and coauthors that prior to induction, laryngoscopy should be done in children with obstructive symptoms. If glotties opening is visualized, inhalational induction can be done. If glottis is not visualized, should proceed with Fibreoptic intubation. Awake oral/nasal intubation, elective tracheostomy are other options.

Pierre Robin Syndrome

The Pierre Robin Syndrome is qualified as a sequence. Association of Pierre Robin sequence with deletion 2q32.3-q33.2 has been demonstrated and mapped to a chromosome region previously shown to have a nonrandom association with cleft palate. An X-linked form and an association with trisomy 18 and other syndromes have also been advocated.

Hypoplasia of the mandibular area prior to 9 weeks in utero causes a posterior position of the tongue that prevents palatal shelves from closing on the midline. Glossoptosis, micrognathia, and cleft soft palate must evocate diagnosis. Mandible grows during the first few months so that normal mandibular profile is common at the age of 4 to 6 years old. In addition to the three classical signs that make the diagnosis, this syndrome can also include cardiovascular (cor pulmonale, vagal hyperactivity) and neuromuscular dysfunctions (brainstem dysfunction, central apnoea).

Facial abnormalities can lead to obstructive apnoea and respiratory distress in neonatal period. Prone position is often used to prevent the tongue from falling back. Nasopharyngeal airway can be useful and if necessary suture of the tongue to the lip or even tracheostomy is required to maintain patient airway. Feeding difficulties can be observed because of facial malformation and/or neurological swallowing problems.

Obtain full history of apnoea (central and/or obstructive), respiratory complications, hospital stays, protracted intubation, tracheotomy, feeding, growth, and development. Evidence of facial signs will help to precisely evaluate the airway management possibilities. Evaluate for difficult airway. These patients will have anticipated difficult face mask ventilation and intubation. Evaluate for tracheomalacia and stenosis by radiography, evaluate for cardiac defects by echocardiography. Previous surgical procedure and tracheal intubation provide precious information but cleft palate repair can provide new laryngoscopic difficulties. Obtain full personal medical history and search for existence of apnoea.

Vagal hyperreflexia is common, hence vagolytic premedication is useful both to counteract it and to avoid the presence of excessive oral secretions. The most common indication for airway intervention is endotracheal intubation for airway management during surgical correction. Some have difficulty in breathing immediately after birth and are intubated in the neonatal intensive care unit. A fibreoptic bronchoscope and an anaesthetist trained in fibreoptic intubation is the requirement when dealing with severe Pierre Robin syndrome infants.

GOLDENHAR SYNDROME

Goldenhar syndrome is also known as Oculo-auriculo-vertebral dysplasia (OAV). It was first described in 1952 by Maurice Goldenhar. It is associated with anomalous development of the first branchial arch and second branchial arch.

Etiology

Deficiency in mesodermal formation or defective interaction between neural crest and the mesoderm is causative factor. Drug ingestion (cocaine, thalidomide, retinoic acid and tamoxifen), environmental factors (insecticides and herbicides) and maternal diabetes can lead to this syndrome.

Physical Signs and Symptoms

They include unilateral or bilateral hemi facial microsomia (HFM), microlabia, chin may be closer to the affected ear, micrognathia, facial clefting, cleft lip/palate, hearing loss, missing eye or benign growths of the eye. Other unique characteristics include: Unilateral triad of craniofacial microsomia, ocular dermoid cysts and spinal abnormalities. Ocular anomalies occur in about 50% of cases (epibulbardermoid and lipodermoid are most common). Auricular defects are reported in 65% of cases, like preauricular tags, microtia, anotia, conductive hearing loss. Vertebral include absence of vertebrae, hemi vertebrae, fused ribs, kyphosis and scoliosis. Heart, kidney, and lung defects are also common in anomalies individuals with Goldenhar syndrome. These typically involve one side of the organ being underdeveloped or missing.

Preanaesthetic Evaluation

It is important that the anaesthetist should gain the family's confidence before obtaining a more detailed history. Airway examination should be undertaken along with examination of various systems. Assessment of difficult airway in paediatric patients begins with a comprehensive history and physical examination: questions to be asked regarding complaints of snoring, apnoea, stridor, hoarse voice. This information may indicate hypoxemia and pulmonary hypertension. History should also consist of a review of previous anaesthetic records with attention being paid to history of oropharyngeal injury, damage to teeth, awake tracheal intubation or postponement of surgery following an anaesthetic.

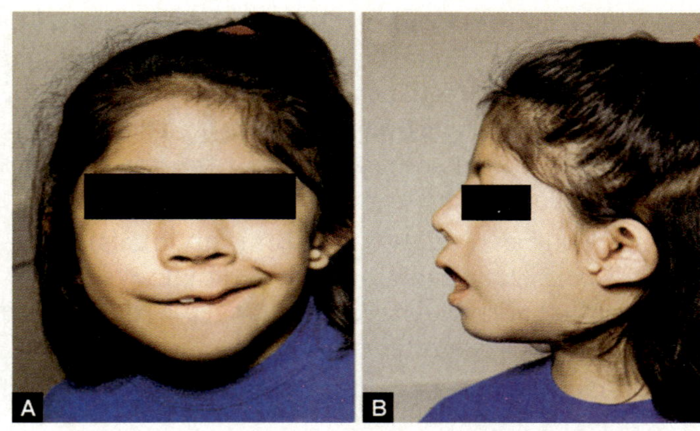

Fig. 38.8 Goldenhar syndrome: Hemi facial microsomia, ocular dermoid cyst, auricular defects

Physical examination: It should focus on the anomalies of face, head, neck and spine. Evaluation of the size and shape of head, gross features of the face size and symmetry of the mandible, presence of sub-mandibular pathology, size of tongue, shape of palate, prominence of upper incisors, and range of motion of jaw, head and neck are important. Presence of retractions (suprasternal/sternal/infrasternal/intercostal) should be sought for they usually are signs of airway obstruction. Breath sounds variety has to be considered—crowing on inspiration is indicative of extrathoracic airway obstruction whereas, noise on exhalation is usually due to intrathoracic lesions. Noise on inspiration and expiration usually is due to a lesion at thoracic inlet.

Anaesthetic Management

These patients commonly present for facial/ocular/ear reconstruction surgeries. The craniofacial abnormalities and the vertebral anomalies make the airway management difficult. Flexible fiberoptic intubation under nerve block and sedation is helpful in the management of anticipated difficult airway.

VELOCARDIOFACIAL SYNDROME

Velocardiofacial syndrome (VCFS) is a genetic condition characterized by abnormal pharyngeal arch development that results in defective development of the parathyroid glands, thymus, and conotruncal region of the heart. Shprintzen and colleagues first described the syndrome in 1978. More than 180 different clinical features are associated with velocardiofacial syndrome, with no single anomaly present in every patient. Some abnormalities are more common than others.

Affected individuals may present with structural or functional palatal abnormalities, cardiac defects, and unique facial characteristics. Individuals with a 22q11.2 deletion can suffer from many possible features, ranging in number of associated features and from the mild to the very serious. They are:

- Congenital heart disease (40% of individuals), particularly conotruncal malformations (tetralogy of Fallot, interrupted aortic arch, ventricular septal defect, and persistent truncus arteriosus)
- Cyanosis (Bluish skin due to poor circulation of oxygen-rich blood)
- Palatal abnormalities (50%), particularly velopharyngeal incompetence (VPI), submucosal cleft palate (Fig. 38.9), and cleft palate; characteristic facial features (present in the majority of Caucasian individuals) including hypertelorism.
- Learning difficulties (90%) but broad range
- Hypocalcaemia (50%) (due to hypoparathyroidism)
- Significant feeding problems (30%)
- Renal anomalies (37%)
- Hearing loss (both conductive and sensorineural) (Hearing loss with craniofacial syndromes)
- Laryngotracheoesophageal anomalies
- Growth hormone deficiency
- Autoimmune disorders
- Immune disorders due to reduced T cell numbers
- Seizures (with or without hypocalcemia)
- Skeletal abnormalities
- Psychiatric disorders

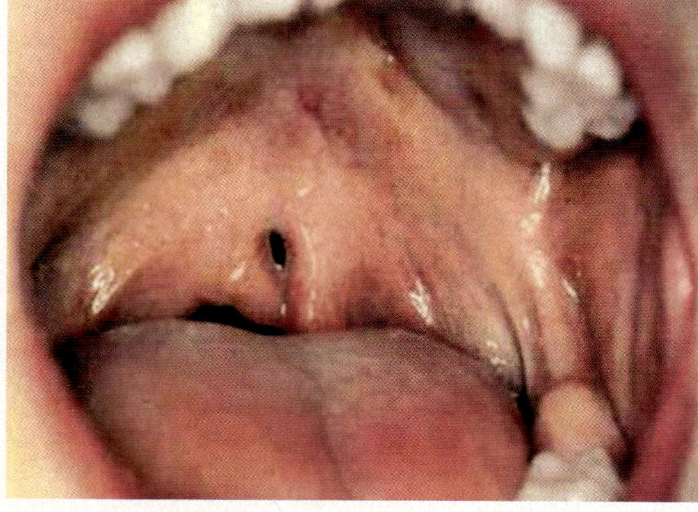

Fig. 38.9 Submucosal cleft palate

Anaesthetic Implications

These patients have craniofacial dysmorphism and may have difficult airway due to cleft palate and short trachea. Also there is risk of hypocalcaemia seizures while recovering. If serum ionized calcium levels are low, patient should be supplemented with intravenous calcium and vitamin D therapy, because hyperventilation and subsequent alkalosis further decreases serum ionized calcium resulting in seizures which may become evident during recovery. Hence, regional anaesthesia is preferred to general anaesthesia with muscle relaxants whenever feasible in these patients.

EPIDERMOLYSIS BULLOSA

Epidermolysis bullosa (EB) is a heterogeneous group of inherited rare diseases, which are characterized by trauma-induced blister formation of the skin and mucosa. The underlying cause is a functional deficiency of structural proteins of the dermo-epidermal junction. Depending on the level of the blister formation, EB is divided into EB simplex (intraepidermal), junctional EB (within the lamina lucida), dystrophic EB (below the lamina lucida) and Kindler syndrome (variable level of split formation).

Besides different distinct blister formation and pain symptoms, secondary problems like anaemia, esophageal stenosis, cardiomyopathy or squamous cell carcinoma may occur.

Shearing forces applied to the skin result in bullae formation, while compressive forces to the skin are tolerated. The challenge is to use monitoring technology without damaging the epithelial surface.

Difficult airway, positioning issues, nutritional deficiencies, poor immunity, and carcinogenic potential add to the comorbidities.

Typical surgery: Change of dressings, skin biopsy, dental surgery: Dental extraction and conservation; ophthalmic surgery; plastic surgery: Repair of pseudosyndactyly, surgery for contractures, excision of squamous cell carcinoma, skin grafting; general surgery: oesophagoscopy and dilatation, gastrostomy, fundoplication.

Necessary additional diagnostic procedures (preoperative): History taking (records of previous anaesthesia, presence of gastro-esophageal reflux, muscular dystrophy, difficult airway, steroid therapy, renal dysfunction), blood values (count, renal), echocardiogram and electrocardiogram (if cardiomyopathy is assumed).

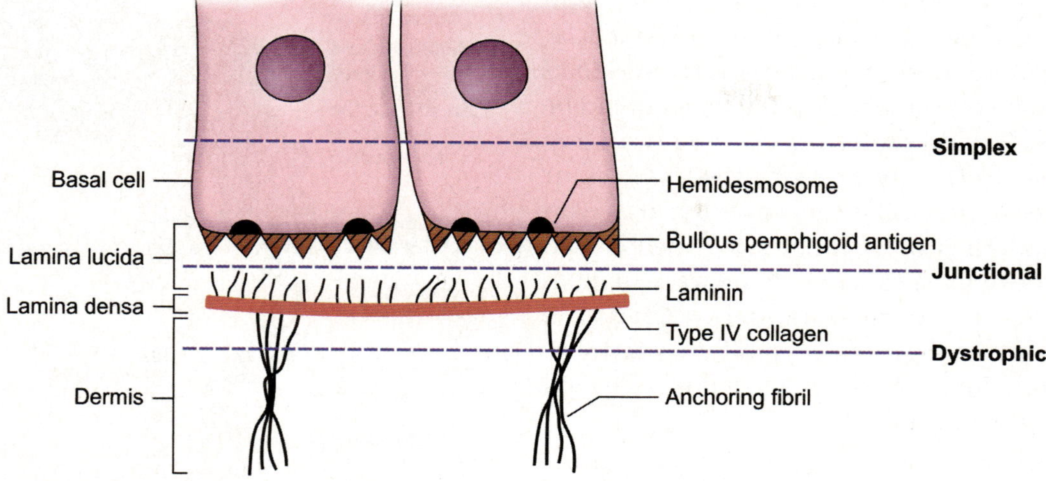

Fig. 38.10 Ultrastructure of the basement membrane zone showing the level of split in different types

Preparation for Airway Management

Evaluation of a difficult airway (history taking, records of previous anaesthesia), lubrication of face mask, laryngeal mask airway (LMA), endotracheal tube (ETT), and laryngoscope is needed. In very affected patients coverage of certain areas of the face (e.g. cheeks, chin) with special non-adhesive dressings (e.g. Mepilex transfer) is recommended LMA one size smaller than predicted by standard formulas should be inserted. Cuffed endotracheal tube (ETT) half to one size smaller than predicted by standard formula, be used. Equipment for predicted difficult airway, e.g. video laryngoscope, fiberoptic bronchoscope should be kept ready.

Preparation for transfusion or administration of blood products

Some severe forms can result in a transfusion dependent anaemia. Many factors take part in it like blood and iron loss from wounds, chronic infection, malnutrition and problems absorbing iron due to the effects EB has on the gastrointestinal tract. Oral and/or intravenous iron can be given often paired with erythropoietin shots.

Precautions for positioning, transport or mobilization

The most important task for transport or mobilization of the patient is to maintain the integrity of the skin, avoiding friction, secondary pressure and trauma. The operating table needs to be extensively padded and the patient has to be transferred very carefully.

Anaesthetic Procedure

Agitation and uncontrolled movement during induction can lead to new skin damage. A rapid and nontraumatic intravenous induction is advantageous, but inhalational induction can be considered. Intravenous access often is difficult, may need the use of ultrasound technique. Use vaseline or any lubricant for face masks, laryngoscope, endotracheal tubes and stomach tube. Endotracheal tube should be fixed with non-adhesive technique. Due to a smaller mouth opening, ankyloglossia (little tongue movement), adhered epiglottis, less reclination and possible tracheal stenosis be prepared for a difficult airway. Total intravenous anaesthesia may be useful in possibly reducing agitation and emesis in the recovery room. Succinylcholine has been used successfully. Non depolarizing muscle relaxants sometimes show prolonged duration of action due to hypoalbuminemia and low muscle mass. Very gentle and careful suctioning of the stomach and oropharynx should be done before extubating to prevent new wounds. Avoid fluid and heat loss and consider a sophisticated pain treatment.

Although general anaesthesia is mostly administered, regional anaesthesia is also possible. Single shot and continuous nerve blocks as well as central neuroaxial blocks have been performed successfully without additional risk. Subcutaneous infiltration with local anaesthetics should be minimized as new blisters can occur. For all these procedures rubbing or wiping the skin for disinfection should be avoided, whereas patting the skin with a moist wipe is usually well tolerated.

Additional monitoring

Standard monitoring is sufficient, adapted to the surgical intervention. Any adhesive is contraindicated because it may cause new blisters. ECG, intravenous catheter and any other device should be fixed with nonadhesive technique like silicon-based products. A layer of cotton-wool padding should underlay the blood pressure cuff or the tourniquet. Arterial lines should be sutured in place. For eye protection use a moisturizing ophthalmic gel, preferably free of preservatives or lanolin. After application of the gel cover the eyes with moistened gauze to protect them from mechanical trauma. Take care that the patient will not wake up with blurred vision and rub at his eyes after extubation to avoid risk of corneal abrasion. Generally consider to minimize monitoring whenever possible to avoid further harm to the patient.

Clinical Pearl

Avoid causing new blisters, especially oropharyngeal and periglottic. Difficulty in venous access is due to contracted fingers and multiple scars, difficult airway is due to small mouth opening or tracheal stenosis.

Postoperative Care

Excellent analgesia is important to prevent excessive movements and new skin trauma. A multimodal approach using nonsteroidal analgesics and opioids by the intravenous route is the most convenient method. Regional anaesthesia should be considered whenever possible. Rectal suppositories are not recommended in first line because of the risk of rectal wounds, but successful use has been reported. If used, they should be well lubricated with a jelly. Swallowing of oral medications/fluids/food can be painful after airway manipulation and due to often significant oesophageal stenosis. Many patients might not be able to swallow pills or capsules. Oxygen masks with sharp edges should be strictly avoided. In case of emergence delirium aggressive sedation is recommended.

Williams Syndrome

Williams syndrome also known as Williams-Beuren syndrome is a neurodevelopmental multisystem genetic disorder characterized by dysmorphic features and a wide range of congenital cardiac, renal, musculoskeletal anomalies.

Its inheritance is through autosomal dominant condition or has a spontaneous occurrence. Incidence is around 1:7500 to 1:20000 live births. The genetic abnormality is due to chromosomal deletion on the long arm of chromosome 7 that includes gene for the protein elastin.

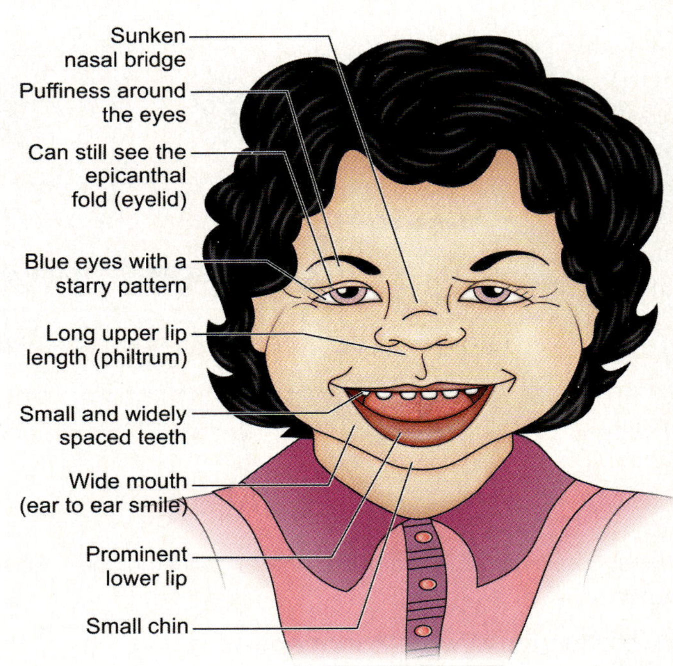

Fig. 38.11 Features of Williams syndrome

Clinical features include facial dysmorphism characterized by a distinct facial appearance with low nasal bridge, mental retardation with unusual language skills, visuospatial deficits, hypersociability, stellate iris pattern, transient hypercalcemia, genitourinary manifestations, and distinctive behavioral and emotional traits.

Cardiovascular anomalies which is seen in 50% to 80% of the cases include supravalvular or subvalvular aortic stenosis (SVAS) (72%), pulmonary stenosis (39%), hypertension (17%), mitral valve prolapse (15%), coarctation of aorta (4%). Other uncommon cardiac congenital defects are ASD, PDA, tetralogy of Fallot, coronary artery stenosis and endocardial cushion defect.

The preoperative evaluation includes thorough history and physical examination with additional noninvasive testing such as electrocardiography and transthoracic echocardiography as indicated by positive features of the preoperative exam to rule out cardiac anomalies. Hypothyroidism is a common finding associated with this disorder which raises perioperative risk considerably. So preoperative screening for thyroid function tests is necessary. Serum calcium is done to rule out hypercalcemia which is a common feature. Multiple renal problems in these patients are renovascular hypertension, hypercalcemia induced nephrocalcinosis, structural renal abnormalities like renal aplasia, horseshoe kidney and renal cyst. Hence USG abdomen to rule out renal pathologies is required.

Various anaesthetic concerns need to be addressed. There might be difficulty even for mask ventilation and these patients may require smaller endotracheal tube than expected for the age. Also there are high chances of postoperative stridor due to laryngeal edema. Anaesthesiologist has to administer titrated dosages of nondepolarising muscle relaxants with nerve stimulators due to prolonged neuromuscular blockade due to joint laxity, chronic muscle weakness and contractures. Of concern is the association of sudden death perioperatively with Williams syndrome. This is due to cardiac anomalies, mainly SVAS and acquired lesions of the coronary arteries (coronary artery stenosis). Intraoperatively avoid hypotension and hypovolemia, tachycardia. Avoid prolonged fasting and anaesthetic drugs that cause excessive veno/vasodilatation. Presence of hypothyroidism may lead to depressed myocardial function, anaemia, decreased plasma volume, hypoglycemia, and hyponatremia and decreased drug metabolism in liver and poorly controlled temperature regulation.

WILSON'S DISEASE (WD)

Wilson's disease (WD) or hepatolenticular degeneration is an autosomal recessive disorder characterized by a reduction in the synthesis of the copper transporter protein ceruloplasmin, outcome being accumulation of copper in body tissues and consequently hepatic and neurological impairment.

The clinical manifestations of WD vary amongst patients, and may be present as neurological (69%), hepatic (15%), psychiatric (2%) and osteomuscular (2%) symptoms. Osteomuscular problems are generally diagnosed during the second decade of life and are typically less severe than the other symptoms.

General anaesthetics are disadvantageous in that they may aggravate the already impaired hepatic function and may not be properly metabolized. Hypnotic and sedative drugs interfere significantly with the central nervous system and may, therefore, exacerbate neurological and psychiatric problems in the postoperative period. WD patients may be more sensitive to neuromuscular relaxants than normal patients by virtue of reduced muscle function resulting from the disease itself or from the use of D-penicillamine. Some researchers have observed that visual and auditory evoked potentials are altered in WD patients, suggesting damage of the encephalic structures and cerebral trunk. However, the peripheral nerve conduction and the somatic-sensory evoked potentials are normal. Such evidence suggests that the regional administration of local anaesthetics to WD patients may be safe, since the peripheral nerve transmission is not altered.

NOONAN SYNDROME

Noonan syndrome is a common, clinically and genetically heterogeneous condition characterized by distinctive facial features, short stature, chest deformity, congenital heart disease, and other comorbidities. It has autosomal dominant inheritance and incidence is around 1:1000 to 2500.

Characteristic features are webbed neck, low-set ears, micrognathia, flat midface with depressed nasal bridge, high-arched palate, ptosis, short stature, pectus excavatum. Congenital heart defects include pulmonary stenosis, hypertrophic cardiomyopathy and atrial septal defect. Some of the other problems include mental retardation, platelet and coagulation disorders, renal dysfunction, chylothorax, lymphedema, failure to thrive, feeding problems, developmental delay and neuropsychological/behavioral issues and visual problems.

Preoperative cardiac evaluation and preoperative renal function are required to rule out cardiac and renal anomalies. Coagulation profile and platelet count to rule out bleeding disorder is required.

In terms of anaesthetic management intravenous access may be difficult with lymphedema. Intubation may be difficult due to abnormal facies. Patient may have bleeding diathesis perioperatively.

ARTHROGRYPOSIS MULTIPLEX CONGENITAL (AMC)

Arthrogryposis is a descriptive term for the occurrence of multiple congenital joint contractures. The true etiology is unknown but is thought to relate to the effect of early fetal akinesia on joint and muscle development. Incidence is around 1:3000 to 1:10000.

Causes can be classified into external mechanical factors (oligohydramnios, twin pregnancy, amniotic bands, fibroids, uterine septi), neuropathic (disturbance of the anterior cornual cells of the spinal cord), myopathic (central core disease, myotonic dystrophy, congenital myasthenia), and abnormal connective tissue. Maternal disease like myasthenia gravis or drug consumption during pregnancy can also lead to AMC of the unborn.

The clinical classification can be performed according to the severity (Munich classification):

Type 1: Primary affection of the extremities, possibly neck and trunk muscles.

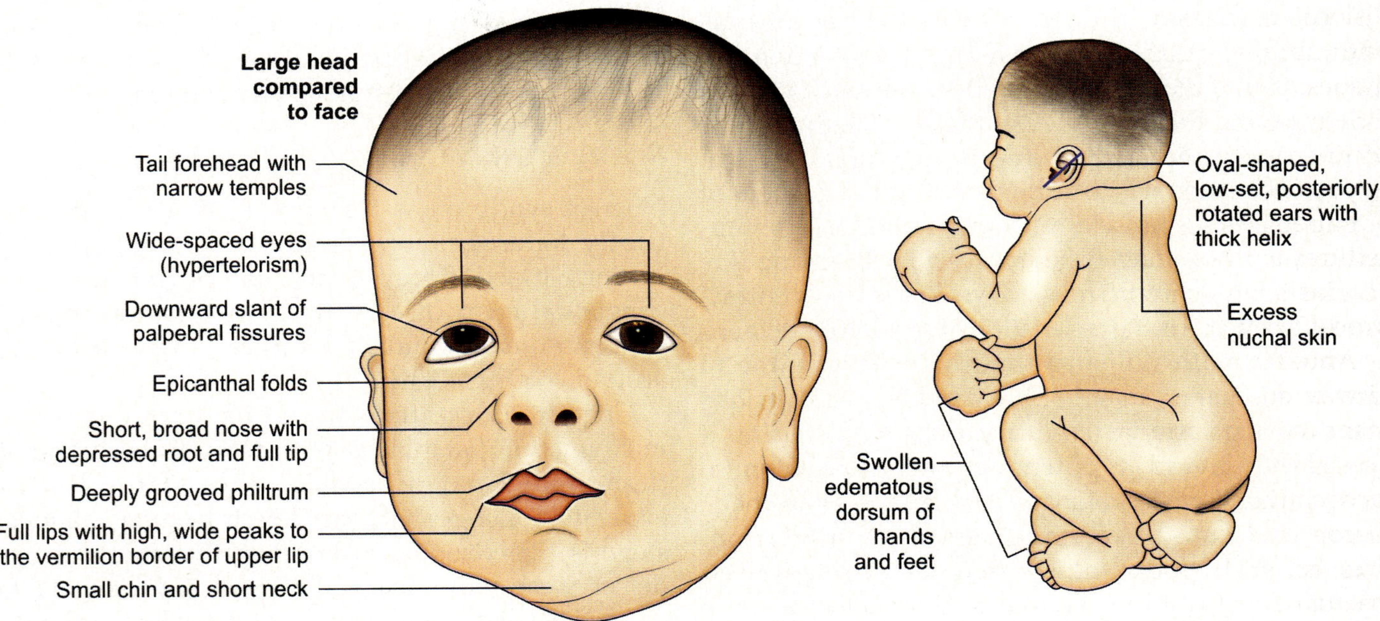

Fig. 38.12 Noonan syndrome

Type 2: Primarily midline malformations, effecting extremities as well as malformations of different organs (e.g. diaphragmatic hernia, pronounced scoliosis).

Type 3: Further dysmorphic disorders and malformations; disorders of the CNS.

Clinical features include upper limb involvement leading to internally rotated shoulders, extended elbows, flexed fingers and wrists. In the lower limbs it causes more variable features but usually severe equinovarus deformities of the feet, hips are usually flexed and dislocated and knees hyper-extended and

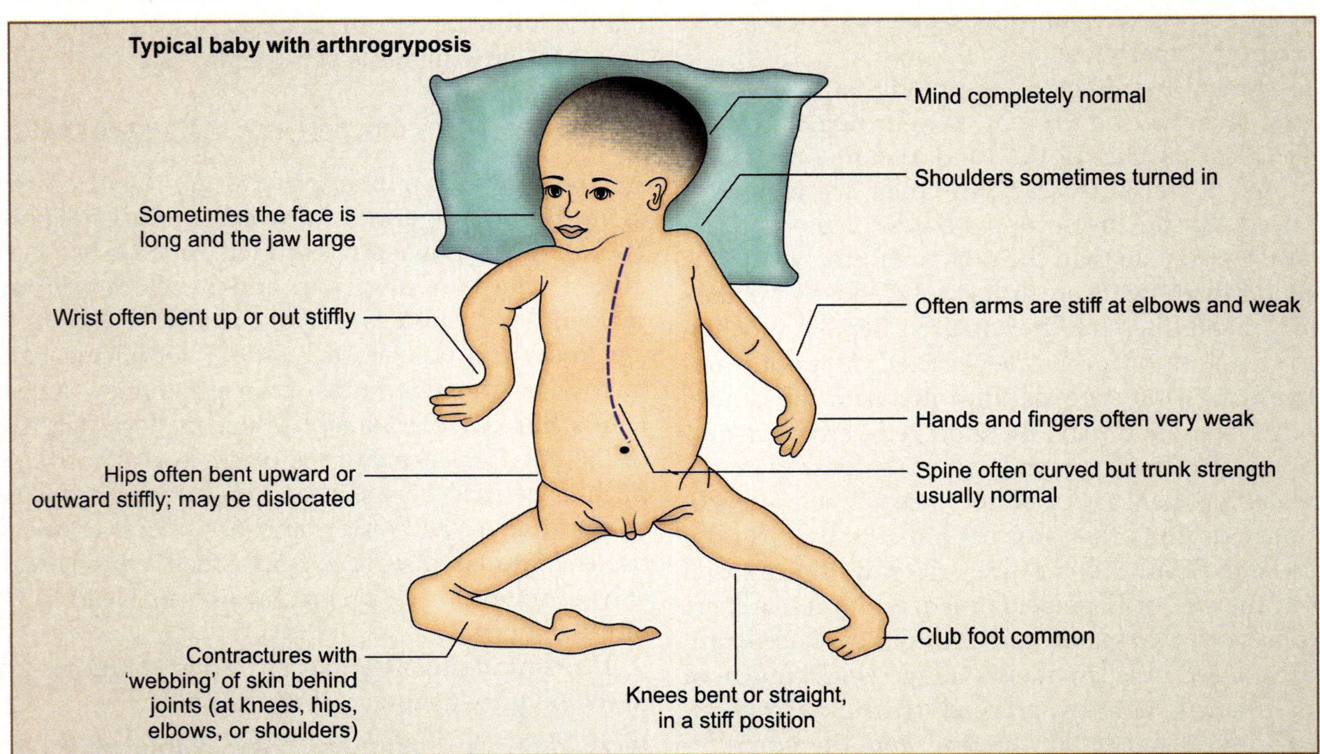

Fig. 38.13 Arthrogryposis multiplex congenital

dislocated. Distal muscles are usually small and wasted with absent reflexes. There may be webbing of soft tissues. Children with AMC have normal intelligence. Other associated features include micrognathia, congenital heart defects, scoliosis, cleft palate, and hypoplastic lungs.

Patients commonly present for orthopaedic procedures to release contractures or correct deformities, scoliosis correction surgeries, ENT, oral surgical procedures, and diagnostic muscle biopsies.

Anaesthetic management includes encountering airway difficulties because of micrognathia, temporomandibular joint involvement, trismus, cleft palate, and cervical spine involvement (scoliosis). Children may have chronic lung disease from recurrent aspiration (secondary to dysphagia) and restrictive lung disease due to scoliosis. Postoperative atelectasis and pneumonia can result because of this. Limb contractures and deficiencies of subcutaneous tissue can make IV access very difficult. Patients with an associated myopathy may be at risk of malignant hyperpyrexia. Positioning of the patient requires careful padding of pressure point areas. Regional anaesthesia can prove to be difficult due to difficulty in positioning and abnormal bony landmarks. Due to low muscle mass as well as due to the neurogenic and myopathic changes, AMC patients may show sensitive reactions to inhalational and intravenous anaesthetics, nondepolarizing muscle relaxants and to opiates. Succinylcholine should be avoided in patients with a recognized underlying myopathic cause due to high risk intraoperative hyperkalaemia. An increased sensitivity to non-depolarizing muscle relaxants may be seen.

Postoperatively, AMC patients seem to have a predisposition for respiratory problems. There can be occurrence of postextubation stridor after difficult intubation.

MARFAN SYNDROME

Marfan syndrome is an autosomal dominant, multisystem disease. The incidence ranges from 1:3000 to 1:5000 individuals. Mutations in the gene (FBN1) that encodes the extra cellular matrix protein, fibrillin-1 present on chromosome 15, cause the classical features of Marfan syndrome.

Clinical features include musculoskeletal system involvement causing a tall and thin body stature, arachnodactyly, ligamentous laxity, pectus excavatum, scoliosis with or without kyphosis, and narrow high arched palate with crowding of teeth. Ocular involvement causes subluxation of the lens (ectopialentis), myopia, increased axial globe length and retinal detachment. Cardiovascular manifestations include mitral valve prolapse, mitral regurgitation, aortic root

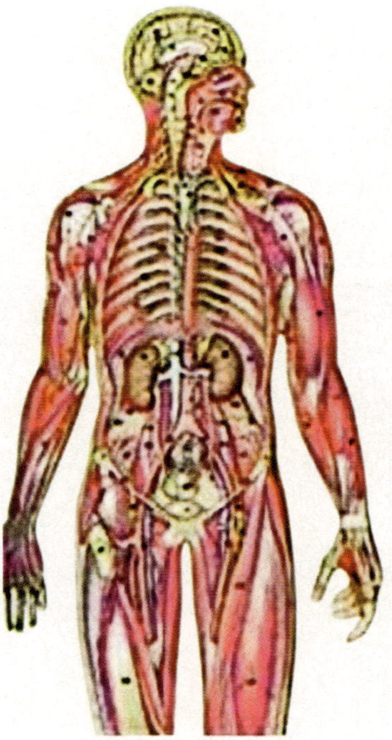

Fig. 38.14 Parts of the body affected by Marfan syndrome

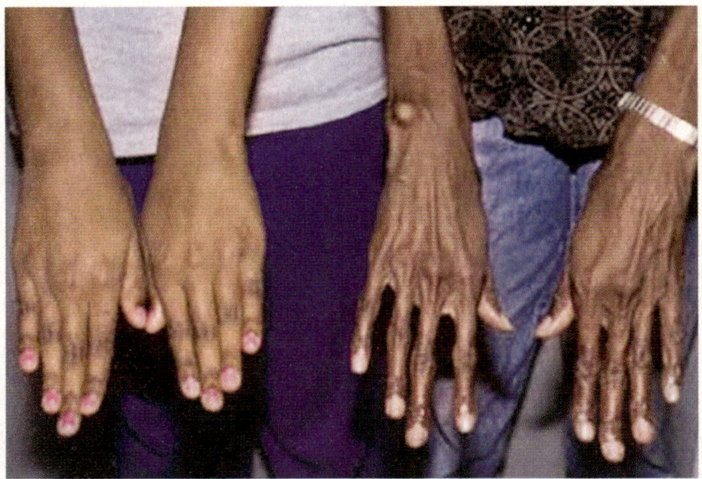

Fig. 38.15 Arachnodactyly in Marfan syndrome

dilatation, and aortic regurgitation. Echocardiograms have shown that about one-third of affected people have mitral valve prolapse, aortic root enlargement or both despite a normal clinical examination.

Other uncommon features include pulmonary blebs (predisposing to spontaneous pneumothorax), dural ectasia (widening of the spinal canal with erosion of the sacral bone), spinal arachnoid cysts or diverticula and obstructive sleep apnoea (lax pharyngeal wall).

Diagnosis is based on typical clinical features and a positive family history. In the absence of a positive family history, involvement of the skeletal and at least two other systems with a minimum of one major manifestation (ectopialentis, aortic dilatation/dissection, or dura lectasia) are required.

Cardiac investigations such as echocardiography need to be done preoperatively to rule out cardiac or aortic pathology. Patients will usually be on beta blockers prophylactically to reduce the incidence of aortic dilatation. Other investigations include chest X-ray to rule out pulmonary blebs, pulmonary function test in case with severe scoliosis, MRI of spine to rule out ductal ectasia if the procedure is planned for neuraxial blockade.

Prophylaxis against infective endocarditis in the presence of valvular abnormality is not required, unless the patient has a mechanical valve.

High-arched palate with crowded teeth poses difficulty in direct laryngoscopy. Patients must be carefully positioned and handled to avoid joint dislocations secondary to joint laxity. Pulmonary blebs increase the incidence of spontaneous pneumothorax and perioperative lung complications. Hence the peak airway pressures during anaesthesia should be minimized. Care should be taken to prevent sudden increase in myocardial contractility, producing an increase in aortic wall tension. Labetalol and nitroglycerin can be used to treat hypertensive episodes. Phenylephrine is a vasopressor of choice, because ephedrine may induce tachycardia via its beta-adrenergic effect. Adequate control of pain and anxiety will decrease the release of endogenous catecholamines. Neuraxial techniques may pose technical challenges due to kyphoscoliosis. The standard dose of local anaesthetic required for the spinal anaesthesia may be inadequate due to the presence of dural ectasia. Hence combined spinal epidural anaesthesia should be preferred.

KLIPPEL-FEIL SYNDROME

Klippel-Feil syndrome is a congenital anomaly characterized by a failure of formation or segmentation of the cervical vertebrae. Incidence is around 0.2 to 4.2 neonates out of 1000 live births. The clinical triad consists of short neck, low posterior hairline, and limited neck movement. It is divided into 3 types:

Type 1: Extensive fusions of cervical and upper thoracic vertebrae into bony blocks along with other severe syndromic abnormalities.

Type 2: Fusions occur at only one or two cervical interspaces most commonly C2/C3. It is often associated with skeletal deformities like Sprengel's deformity (congenital upward displacement of the scapula), cervical rib, hemi vertebrae and occipitoatlantal fusion.

Type 3: Fusions both at cervical and lower thoracic or lumbar spine.

Other less common associated features are spina bifida, profound deafness, cleft lip or palate, rib

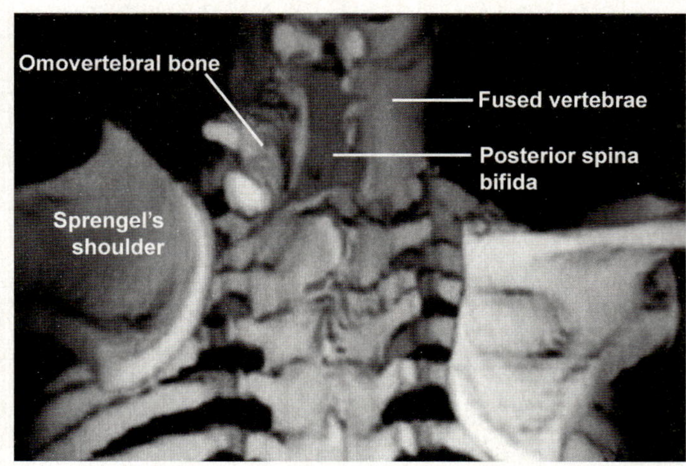

Fig. 38.16 Skeletal deformities in Klippel-Feil syndrome

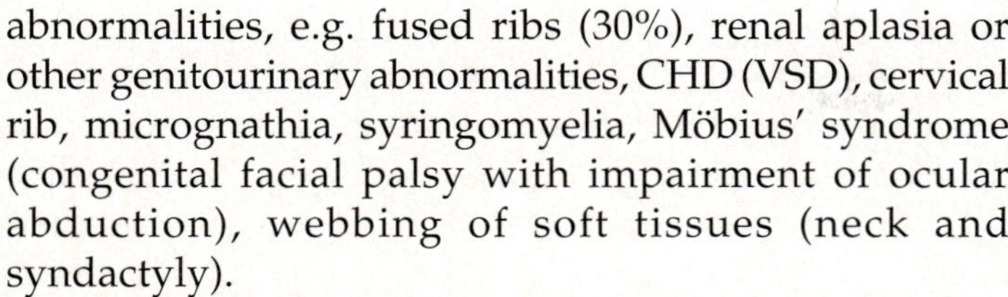

abnormalities, e.g. fused ribs (30%), renal aplasia or other genitourinary abnormalities, CHD (VSD), cervical rib, micrognathia, syringomyelia, Möbius' syndrome (congenital facial palsy with impairment of ocular abduction), webbing of soft tissues (neck and syndactyly).

Undiagnosed Klippel-Feil syndrome can present as an unexpected difficult intubation due to their short stiff neck. Preoperatively in a diagnosed case efforts should be made to identify the areas of spinal fusion and cervical stability should be assessed. Manipulation of the neck or an attempt to extend the neck during laryngoscopy and thereafter needs to be carefully controlled to avoid if neurological damage. Awake fiberoptic intubation has been used most commonly for difficult airway cases. Management of cardiovascular anomalies appropriately also decreases the risk peri-operatively.

CONCLUSION AND SUMMARY

The anaesthesiologists are usually not familiar with the genetic disorders. A general approach to the patient with a genetic syndrome has to be understood and then specific syndromes. The paediatric anaesthesiologist should have the resources of various genetic syndromes at workplace, and it is important to read beforehand and become familiar with basic problem of the specific syndrome to devise a rational anaesthetic plan for successful outcome.

FAQ with Answer

Q. Mandibular hypoplasia is common in which genetic syndrome?

A. Mandibular hypoplasia is common feature among many syndromes such as Pierre Robin, Treacher Collins and Goldenhar (hemifacialmicrosomia).

Paediatric Anaesthesia Pearls

Genetic syndromes complicate airway by presenting with small mouth opening, with high arched palate, limitation of neck movement due to fusion of the cervical vertebra, macroglossia causing soft tissue obstruction, causing difficult airway.

REFERENCES

1. Lane G. Intubation Techniques. Operative Techniques in Otolaryngology 2005;16:166–70.
2. Khan M. Airway Management.
3. The US National Institutes of Health web.nih.gov/category/Genetics Birth Defects.
4. Revista Brasileira de Anestesiologia. November–December, 2010;60(6).
5. Korean J Anaesthesiol. Nov, 2013;65(5):482–483.
6. Smith's Anaesthesia for Infants and Children, 7th edn.
7. Walker RW, Darowski P, Morris P, et al. Anaesthesia and mucopolysaccharidoses. A review of airway problems in children. Anaesthesia. 1994;49:1078–84.
8. Baum VC, O'Flaherty JE. Philadelphia: Lippincott Williams and Wilkins; Anaesthesia for genetic metabolic and dysmorphic syndromes of childhood. 2007;pp. 179–80.
9. De Beer D, Bingham R. The child with facial abnormalities. Curr Opin Anaesthesiol. 2011;24:282.
10. Taly AB, Meenaksh Sundaram S, Sinha S, et al. Wilson disease: Description of 282 patients evaluated over 3 decades. Medicine (Baltimore); 2007;86:112–21.
11. Jules EA, Charlotte JH. Down's syndrome; British Journal of Anaesthesia, CEPD Reviews, 2003; 3(3):83–86.
12. Longas Valien J, Guerrero Pardos LM, Ruiz Tramazaygues J, et al. Anaesthesia in Wilson's disease. Rev Esp Anestesiol Reanim. 2005;52:247–8.
13. Adrino Bechara DeSouza Hobaika. Anaesthesia for a patient with Wilson's disease. M E J Anaesth. 2008;19(4).
14. Rasch DK, Browder F, Barr M, et al. Anaesthesia for Treacher Collins and Pierre Robin syndromes: A report of three cases. Can Anaesth Soc J 1986; 33:364–370.

Hospital Acquired Infection in Operating Theatre

Roopali Telang and Rahul Bhamkar

ABSTRACT

Surgical Site Infection (SSI) is the commonest cause of postoperative morbidity and mortality. Paediatric population especially neonates and infants are more prone for these infections. Some simple perioperative measures and practices can significantly reduce surgical site infections. Similarly preventing hospital acquired infections in healthcare workers is equally important.

Hospital acquired infections place significant burden on healthcare system. Infections related to surgery are the secondmost common type of hospital acquired infections. They are responsible for perioperative morbidity, mortality. They increase the hospitalization stay and impose additional financial burden on the patient. Surgical site infection is still a leading complication of any surgery. Paediatric population especially neonates are more prone to these infections compared to adults as they have decrease immunity. All preventive measures effective in adult surgeries also apply to paediatric surgeries. Following some simple measures and simple protocols by healthcare workers can substantially reduce the infections related to surgery. In this chapter we will have an overview of various infections in operating theatre and their preventive strategies.

SURGICAL SITE INFECTIONS

Surgical site infections account to 14–16% of all hospital acquired infections and 38% of nosocomial infections in surgery patients.[1,2] Each SSI is associated with approximately 7–10 additional postoperative hospital days and patients with an SSI have a 2–11 times higher risk of death, compared to operative patients without an SSI.[3,4]

Surgical site infections are defined as infections occurring up to 30 days after surgery (or up to one year after surgery in patients receiving implants) and affecting either the incision or deep tissue at the operation site.[5]

The degree of surgical site contamination at the time of surgery influences the probability of surgical site infection. According to the presence and degree of contamination surgical wounds can be classified in Table 39.1.

Table 39.1 American College of Surgeons, National Surgical Quality Improvement Program (ACS-NSQIP) classification of surgical wound.[6,7]

Class I/Clean	An uninfected operative wound in which no inflammation is encountered and the respiratory, alimentary, genital, or uninfected urinary tract is not entered.
Class II/Clean-Contaminated	An operative wound in which the respiratory, alimentary, genital, or urinary tracts are entered under controlled conditions and without unusual contamination.
Class III/Contaminated	Open, fresh, accidental wounds. In addition, operations with major breaks in sterile technique (e.g. open cardiac massage) or gross spillage from the gastrointestinal tract, and incisions in which acute, non-purulent inflammation is encountered are included in this category.
Class IV/Dirty-Infected	Old traumatic wounds with retained devitalized tissue and those that involve existing clinical infection or perforated viscera. This definition suggests that the organisms causing postoperative infection were present in the operative field before the operation.

Microbiology

Pathogens causing SSI differ depending on the type of surgical procedure. Pathogens can be classified depending on their habitat as shown in Table 39.2.[8]

Classification of SSIs

Depending on the site, Centre for Disease Control (CDC) has classified SSIs into three different types as shown in Table 39.3 and Fig. 39.1.

Table 39.2 Classification of microorganism causing SSI

Exogenous flora:	These are pathogenic microorganisms acquired from exogenous source such as operating theatre environment, surgical personnel, surgical tools and instruments and other materials, e.g. *Staphylococcus aureus, Coagulase negative staphylococci, Pseudomonas aeruginosa, Escherichia coli, Staphylococci epidermidis, Enterococcus faecalis, Candida albicans*
Endogenous flora:	These are the microorganisms residing in patient's skin, mucous membranes or hollow viscera. For most of the SSIs, endogenous flora from patient is responsible. They cause infections on the breach of mucous membrane or skin. Seeding of the operative site from a distant focus of infection especially in patients with implant or prosthesis placement can be another source for SSIs. Apart from the above mentioned organisms, they include fecal flora (anaerobes and gm –ve aerobes), e.g. *E. Coli, Enterococci, Bacillus fragilis.*

Table 39.3 CDC's National Nosocomial Infection Surveillance (NNIS) system SSIs classification.[9]

Superficial Incisional SSI:

Infection occurs within 30 days after the operation and infection involves only skin or subcutaneous tissue of the incision and at least one of the following:

- Purulent drainage, with or without laboratory confirmation, from the superficial incision.
- Organisms isolated from an aseptically obtained culture of fluid or tissue from the superficial incision.
- At least one of the following signs or symptoms of infection: Pain or tenderness, localized swelling, redness, or heat and superficial incision is deliberately opened by surgeon, unless incision is culture-negative.
- Diagnosis of superficial incisional SSI by the surgeon or attending physician.

Do not report the following conditions as SSI:

- Stitch abscess (minimal inflammation and discharge confined to the points of suture penetration).
- Infection of an episiotomy or newborn circumcision site.
- Infected burn wound.
- Incisional SSI that extends into the fascial and muscle layers (see deep incisional SSI).

Note: Specific criteria are used for identifying infected episiotomy and circumcision sites and burn wounds.

Deep Incisional SSI:

Infection occurs within 30 days after the operation if no implant is left in place or within 1 year if implant is in place and the infection appears to be related to the operation and infection involves deep soft tissues (e.g. fascial and muscle layers) of the incision and at least one of the following:

- Purulent drainage from the deep incision but not from the organ/space component of the surgical site.
- A deep incision spontaneously dehisces or is deliberately opened by a surgeon when the patient has at least one of the following signs or symptoms: Fever (>38ºC), localized pain, or tenderness, unless site is culture-negative.
- An abscess or other evidence of infection involving the deep incision is found on direct examination, during reoperation, or by histopathologic or radiologic examination.
- Diagnosis of a deep incisional SSI by a surgeon or attending physician.

Notes: 1. Report infection that involves both superficial and deep incision sites as deep incisional SSI.
2. Report an organ/space SSI that drains through the incision as a deep incisional SSI.

Organ/Space SSI:

Infection occurs within 30 days after the operation if no implant is left in place or within 1 year if implant is in place and the infection appears to be related to the operation and infection involves any part of the anatomy (e.g. organs or spaces), other than the incision, which was opened or manipulated during an operation and at least one of the following:

- Purulent drainage from a drain that is placed through a stab wound into the organ/space.
- Organisms isolated from an aseptically obtained culture of fluid or tissue in the organ/space.
- An abscess or other evidence of infection involving the organ/space that is found on direct examination, during reoperation, or by histopathologic or radiologic examination.
- Diagnosis of an organ/space SSI by a surgeon or attending physician.

Risk Factors

Risk of SSI varies according to patient and operative procedure characteristics. Risk factors can be divided into two types as follows:[5]

Endogenous factors: These are the patient-related factors which include malnutrition, underlying infection, neonatal age group, prematurity, coexistent infection, immunosuppressive drugs and radiations, etc.

External factors: Type and duration of operation, surgeon's skill, quality of preoperative skin preparation, adequacy and timing of antimicrobial prophylaxis, insertion of foreign material or implants, inadequate sterilization of surgical instruments, hypothermia, hypoxemia, etc.

PREVENTIVE STRATEGIES OF SSIS

Preventive strategies of SSIs can be divided into following (Fig. 39.2).

Preoperative Strategies

Preparation of Surgical Patient

a. **Treatment of infections:** Eradicate and control all infections remote to surgical site before elective surgery whenever possible.
b. **Screening of the patients:** Preoperatively paediatric patients should be screened for presence of any congenital anomaly especially congenital cardiac disease as these patients may require special consideration for bacterial endocarditis antibiotic

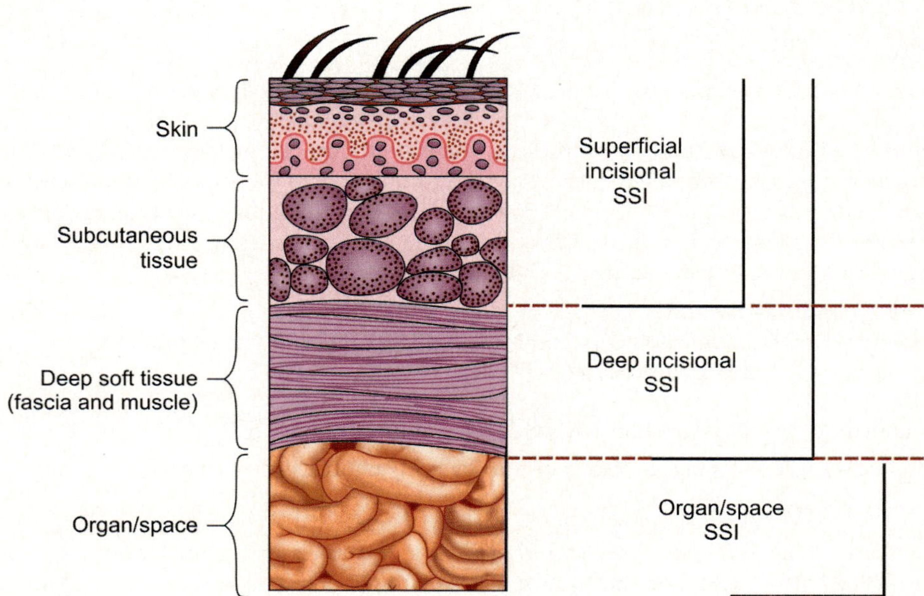

Fig. 39.1 Cross section of abdominal wall showing classification of SSI[9]

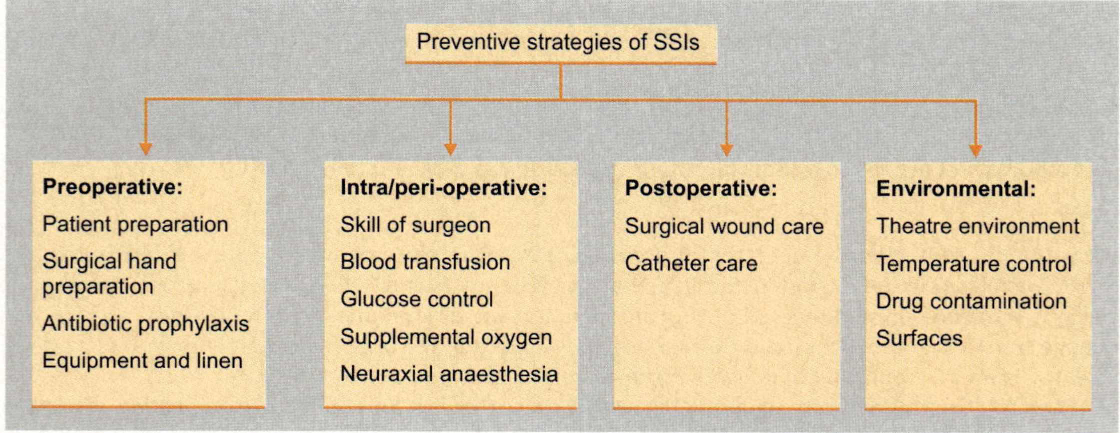

Fig. 39.2 Various preventive strategies of SSIs

prophylaxis. Patients should be screened for presence of any underlying infections by ordering some basic investigations like complete blood count, chest, X-ray, etc. if indicated. Any history of receiving chemotherapy or radiotherapy if present should be noted. Though hyperglycemia is uncommon in children, blood sugar level should always be checked preoperatively.

c. **Surgical site preparation:** Removal of hair only when needed should be done with clipper. Razors are not recommended. Microscopic cuts in the skin which occur during shaving acts as a foci for bacterial multiplication leading to increased risk of SSIs. Clipping hair immediately before surgery is associated with lower risk of SSIs than shaving or clipping a night before surgery.[10,11] Depilation though has shown to decrease risk of SSIs more than clipping or shaving, it sometimes produce hypersensitivity reactions.[12,13] Preoperative antiseptic shower or bath though have been shown to decrease the skin microbial colony counts, they have not definitely been proved to decrease the SSI rate.[14–16] Intranasal Mupirocin is recommended before surgery in known carriers of Methicillin Resistant *Staphylococcus aureus* (MRSA). Inspect and clean gross contamination of skin at and around incision site before preoperative antiseptic preparation. Antiseptic skin preparation should include surgical incision and drain site. Alcohol-chlorhexidine with 70% to 92% alcohol has been found to have greater residual antimicrobial activity than iodophors.[17–19] Also unlike iodophors, chlorhexidine is not inactivated by blood or serum proteins.[20] Skin preparation is done by applying the antiseptic solution in concentric circles beginning in the area of proposed incision. However, in neonates and preterm infants chances of systemic toxicity have been reported because of systemic absorption of these antiseptic agents as their skin is many times permeable than adult skin. Therefore, unnecessary pooling of skin disinfectant in these population should be avoided and sterile water should be used rather than alcohol to clean off the disinfectant.

Note

Preoperative shaving should not be done. Hair removal should be done only when needed that too with clipper immediately before surgery. Hair removal a night before surgery should be avoided. Although alcohol-chlorhexidine (70–92% alcohol) is considered ideal antiseptic for skin preparation, no specific agent is recommended for preterm infants and infants less than 2 months because of issues related to systemic toxicity.

Surgical Hand Preparation

Handwashing is the essence of all infection control policy. Various studies have shown that proper surgical handwashing significantly decreases the incidence of SSIs.

a. **Hand hygiene basics:** These basic principals apply to all healthcare workers (HCWs) working in operating theatre. Fingernails should be kept short (less than 0.5 cm). Artificial fingernails are strictly prohibited. Rings, wristwatch and bracelets should be removed before surgical handwash.

b. **Surgical antiseptic products:** Hands of HCWs contain two types of microbial flora: **Transient and resident flora**.[21] Transient flora is acquired during work while touching patient clothes, equipment or site. These are responsible for spreading hospital acquired infections. Examples are *staphylococci, pseudomonas, CONS, Candida albicans,* etc. Resident floras are residing in HCWs' hands. They have low pathogenicity and are sometimes responsible for infections associated with surgical implants, e.g. *Diptheroids.* It is recommended that surgical hand antiseptic product should be having residual antimicrobial activity which inhibits growth of microorganisms for six hours after handwashing.[22,23] Alcohol-based chlorhexidine antiseptic solutions are considered ideal for surgical handwashing.[24,25]

c. **Procedure surgical handwashing:** Duration for surgical handwashing should be 3–5 minutes. Recommended **steps** for surgical handwashing:
   - Scrub each side of each finger, between the fingers and back and front of the hand for 2 minutes.
   - Proceed to scrub the arms, keeping the hand higher than the arm at all times. This enables to avoid recontamination of hands from water from the elbows and prevent bacteria-laden soap and water from contaminating the hands.
   - Wash each side of the arm from wrist to the elbow for one minute.
   - Repeat the process on the other hand and arm, keeping hands above the elbow at all times. If hand touches anything at any time, the scrub must be lengthened by 1 minute.
   - Rinse hands and arms by passing them through the water in one direction only, from fingertip to elbow. Do not move the arm back and forth through the water.
   - Proceed to operating theatre holding hands above the elbow. Hands should be dried with sterile towel.

> **Note**
> At least three minute proper surgical handwashing is universally and unequivocally proved preventive measure for SSI.

Antibiotic Prophylaxis

a. **Indication:** Antimicrobial prophylaxis is defined as a brief course of antibiotic started just before the surgery.[26] It is indicated for some surgical wounds classified as clean or clean contaminated wounds (Table 39.1). Antibiotics given for treating contaminated and dirty surgical wounds prior to surgery are not considered as antimicrobial prophylaxis.

b. **Duration:** Antibiotic prophylaxis duration should not routinely exceed 24 hours (first dose at induction and two doses postoperatively). According to wide consensus in great majority single dose of intravenous antibiotic should suffice. Administration of initial dose should be 30 minutes before incision to achieve an adequate tissue concentration at the time of incision.[27]

c. **Choice of antibiotics and doses:** Antibiotic should be selected according to the most likely pathogen in the specific surgery. Cephalosporins are the most commonly used and studied antimicrobial agents for prophylaxis. They are effective against gram-negative as well as gram-positive bacteria. Cefazolin, a first generation cephalosporin, is the most widely used first choice antimicrobial agent for surgical prophylaxis.[28] It is active against Methicillin Sensitive Staph Aureus (MSSA) which is commonly responsible for causing SSI plus, it also covers gram-negative bacteria like *E. coli* and *Klebsiella.* Routine use of vancomycin is not recommended.[26] It should be used in cases of Suspected Methicillin Resistant Staph Aureus (MRSA) infection or in case of penicillin/cephalosprin allergy.[26] Metronidazole is used in combination with cephalosporin to cover anaerobes in colorectal or contaminated neck surgeries.

d. **Re-dosing:** If surgery is continuing for long duration (more than two half-lives of initial dose) or if excessive intraoperative blood loss occurs, an additional dose of antibiotic should be given. Antibiotic after wound closure is not required, on the other hand, it can lead to emergence of antibiotic resistant bacteria.

e. **Route of administration:** All prophylactic antibiotics are to be given by intravenous route to achieve desired blood concentration during incision. However, in colorectal surgeries non-absorbable oral antimicrobial agents are to be administered in divided doses for a day before surgery, in addition to, bowel preparation by enemas and cathartic agents.

> **Note**
> Antibiotic for prophylaxis should be judiciously chosen and used only when indicated. Irrational use of antibiotic should be avoided to prevent antimicrobial resistance. Vancomycin should not be routinely used for antimicrobial prophylaxis.

Antibiotic for prophylaxis should be judiciously chosen and used only when indicated. Irrational use of antibiotic should be avoided to prevent antimicrobial resistance. Vancomycin should not be routinely used for antimicrobial prophylaxis.

Equipment and Linen

Surgical Attire and Drapes: Though there is a little evidence that use of facemasks, caps decrease the

Table 39.4 Antimicrobial prophylaxis for surgery with indication, dose and re-dosing interval

Antibiotic	Dose	Indication	Redosing interval (hrs)
Cefazolin	30 mg/kg	Cardiovascular/thoracic/orthopedic surgeries	4
Cefuroxime	50 mg/kg	Cardiovascular/thoracic/orthopedic surgery	4
Amoxicillin-clavulanate	30 mg/kg of Amoxicillin	Thoracic, nasopharyngeal surgery	2
Ampicillin-sulbactam	50 mg/kg of Ampicillin	Thoracic, nasopharyngeal surgery	2
Metronidazole*	15 mg/kg Neonates <1.2 kg: 7.5 mg/kg	Colorectal, contaminated head neck surgeries	6
Vancomycin	15 mg/kg	Neurosurgeries, suspected MRSA	8
Clindamycin	10 mg/kg	Suspected MRSA	6
Gentamicin	2.5 mg/kg	Genitourinary surgeries	4
Ciprofloxacin#	10 mg/kg	Genitourinary surgeries	8

* Metronidazole given along with 3rd generation cephalosporins.

\# Though fluoroquinolones are considered to be associated with increased risk of tendon rupture in children, use of these agents for single dose prophylaxis is usually safe.

incidence of SSI, it is recommended that all personnel in OT should wear surgical mask to fully cover mouth and nose and should wear a cap to fully cover head and face hair.[26,29,30,31] If worn, mask should not be taken down to speak and should be changed in case of contamination. Scrubbed surgical team member should wear sterile gown and gloves in addition to cap, mask. Sterile surgical drapes should be used to create a barrier between the surgical field and environment. Special footwear should be worn. Shoes should be cleaned when contaminated or after every use. Shoe covers are not necessary for prevention of SSIs. Anaesthetists must wear sterile gloves for invasive procedures and contact with sterile sites. Non-sterile examination gloves should be used during contact with blood, body fluid, secretion, excretion, during contact with mucous membrane.

Surgical equipment: All surgical equipment must be clean and decontaminated before sterilization process.[32,33] Heat resistant surgical instruments should be steam sterilized. Heat sensitive instruments can be sterilized by ethylene oxide, hydrogen peroxide, peracetic acid or low temperature sterilization. Flash sterilization of surgical instruments should only be used in emergency.[34]

Anaesthetic equipment: Anaesthetic equipment may be contaminated by direct contact with patient or indirect contact with spilled fluid, secretion. Whenever possible use disposable items. All anaesthetic face mask, airways, tubes and catheter should be single use. Laryngoscope blades and handles should be properly cleaned before decontamination. Anaesthetic circuits should be routinely changed daily. If circuit is visibly contaminated or used for highly infectious patient, it should be changed in between patients.[35] If bacterial/viral filters are used between patient and circuit, routine daily sterilization of internal components of anaesthetic machine is not recommended. However, manufacturer's instructions should be followed pertaining to disinfection policy.

Intra/Perioperative Strategies

Surgical Skill

Surgical skills like gentle tissue handling to minimize trauma, minimal use of cautery, minimal blood loss, adequate debridement and removal of dead tissue are important in decreasing the risk of SSIs.[26] Use of close suction drain is advisable. Drain should be removed as soon as possible.

Blood Transfusion

Transfusion associated immunosuppression is a known entity. Immunosuppression occurs especially after transfusion of blood which was stored for long duration. Blood transfusion causes diversion of immune system response to an inappropriate focus, i.e. cleaning-up old dead white cells from circulation rather than bacteria.[36] Such immunosuppression lasts for weeks after discharge making patient susceptible to infections. To avoid this, blood transfusion should be minimized and whenever possible blood less than two weeks old should be used. Leucocyte depleted blood or leukocyte filters are also advisable.

Glucose Control

It has been proved that good perioperative glucose control improves the immune response and decreases the inflammation.[36] So glucose should be monitored perioperatively in all patients with target blood glucose level of 7—10 mmol/L. Balanced salt solution should be used for IV infusion.

Supplemental Oxygen

Augmenting tissue oxygenation to above normal partial pressure has been proved to improve host defenses against bacteria.[36] Killing of surgical pathogens by neutrophils is primarily by oxidation (superoxide radicals). It is recommended to give 80% oxygen intra-operatively and 40–80% postoperatively to all patients with risk of SSIs.

However, in premature babies excess oxygenation should be avoided at any time considering the risk of Retinopathy of Prematurity (ROP) in these patients.[37]

Temperature Control

Neonates are very prone to hypothermia because of their relatively more body surface area and absence of fat reserve.[37] Even mild hypothermia increases the risk of wound infection by three times and prolongs the hospitalization by 20%.[36] During surgery hypothermia can occur because of general anaesthesia, exposure to cold or intentional cooling which is done during cardiac surgeries to protect myocardium and central nervous system. Hypothermia triggers vasoconstriction with decreased oxygen supply to tissue ultimately affecting to immune response as mentioned above. It also increases bleeding and transfusion requirement. Therefore, core body temperature should be kept between 36 and 38°C during surgery.[36] This can be achieved by the use of warm forced air, increasing OT temperature, insulators, plastic bags or sheet and even

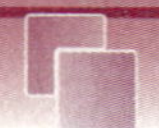

warm IV fluids. Body temperature should be routinely monitored during prolong surgery.

Neuraxial Anaesthesia

Various studies have supported decrease in the incidence of SSI with the use of neuraxial anaesthesia.[36]

The proposed mechanisms are:

- Allowing immune system to focus more on bacteria, by decreasing inflammatory response from surgery.
- Better oxidative killing by neutrophils due to increased vasodilation and improved tissue oxygenation.
- Postoperative analgesia improvement, leading to less autonomic response, which in turn causes less vasoconstriction and improved peripheral perfusion.

> **Note**
>
> Rigorous intra-operative monitoring glucose, temperature and oxygen saturation is important in preventing SSIs especially in neonates/infants. Neonates are prone for hypoglycemia and hypothermia. Hypoxemia and hyperoxemia both should be avoided in preterm neonates.

Postoperative Strategies

Postoperative Surgical Wound Care

Primarily closed clean surgical wound should be covered with sterile dressing for at least 24–48 hours postoperatively.[38] Dressing should be changed if excess oozing is seen.[39] Hand hygiene rules should be followed before and after touching the patient. Normal saline should be used to clean and remove surface bacteria and discharge from wound. Patient and caretakers should be explained about the surgical wound care.

Catheter Care

Observe insertion site of Central Venous Catheter (CVC) for any sign of local inflammation. Hands must be decontaminated using handwash/hand rub before handling catheters. CVC line should be routinely flushed with an anticoagulant when not in continuous use.[40] CVC and urinary catheters should be removed at earliest opportunity when not needed.

Environmental Factors

Theatre Environment

Unnecessary movement of people in the operating theatre should be prevented. Doors should be kept closed. Positive-pressure ventilation should be maintained for operating room. A minimum of 15 air changes per hour of which 3 of fresh air should be done.[41,42] Airflow monitoring devices with over range and under range alarms should be in place. All recirculated and fresh air should be filtered through laminar airflow high efficiency particulate air (HEPA) filters. HEPA filters remove particles ≥ 0.3 μm at 99.97% efficiency.[26] Relative humidity in operating theatre should be maintained at 30–60%.[42] Periodic checking and system maintenance is crucial to maintain OT environment as per specification. Given the standard specifications are followed, routine air microbiological sampling is not advised. Also use of tacky mats at the entrance of OT is not advisable. Temperature of OT should be maintained at 20–23°C.[42]

Drug Contamination

Multi-dose ampoules and vials should be avoided and drugs should be never shared between patients to avoid chances of contamination. All syringes, needles, infusion administration set should be single use.[36]

Surfaces

All surfaces of anaesthetic machines and monitoring equipment which are likely to be contaminated by blood or secretion should be cleaned at earliest between patients.[43] Surfaces of operating room are rarely implicated in harboring pathogens causing SSIs. However, to maintain cleanliness it is important to routinely clean them. Surfaces of the operating theatre should be smooth, easily to clean, stain resistant, impervious to moisture and suitable for wheeled traffic. There is no data to support special cleaning procedures or closing of an operating theatre after a contaminated or dirty wound surgery. However, dirty cases should preferably be scheduled as last cases and when visible soiling or contamination of surfaces occurs with blood or other body fluids, they should be cleaned by hospital disinfectant before next surgery.

> **Note**
>
> 15 changes per hour of air through HEPA filters are recommended to reduce incidence of SSIs in operating theatre. Drug ampoules/vials, infusion set should be single use and not be shared. Closing of operation theatre after a dirty wound surgery is not needed.

PREVENTION OF INFECTIONS IN HEALTHCARE WORKERS

Till now we have discussed about SSIs in patients and its preventive strategies. But another very important aspect is prevention of hospital acquired infection in HCWs. Following are the recommendations for preventing the hospital acquired infections in HCWs.

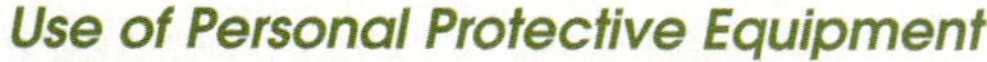

Use of Personal Protective Equipment

Disposable plastic aprons and gloves should be worn whenever there is risk of clothing becoming exposed to blood, body fluids, secretions and excretions.[43]

Disposal of Sharps

Accidental inoculation of infected blood, though small in amount, presents a definite risk to anaesthetists and other HCWs. 16% of occupational injuries in hospital are attributed to sharp injuries.[43] Some of the guidelines for sharp disposal are:

- Sharps must not be transferred between personnel and handling should be kept to a minimum.
- Needles must not be bent or broken prior to use or disposal.
- Needles should not be recapped or re-sheathed.
- Sharps and needles should be discarded in approved puncture proof container.
- Sharp container should be sealed and disposed of by incineration when two-third full or in use more than four weeks.
- Needle protection devices may reduce chances of needle stick injuries.

Vaccination

All HCWs should be vaccinated with Hepatitis B vaccine.[44]

SUMMARY

SSI is the most common cause of postoperative morbidity and mortality. All preventive measures effective in adult surgeries is applicable to paediatric surgeries. Infants and newborns are at more risk of SSIs because of their immature immune system. Preventive strategy can be classified into preoperative, intra/perioperative, postoperative and environmental measures. Risk of hospital acquired infections in healthcare worker is small but definite. Personal protective measures and proper sharp disposal is of utmost importance.

Key Learning Points

- Surgical site infections (SSIs) are defined as infections occurring up to 30 days after surgery (or up to one year after surgery in patients receiving implants) and affecting either the incision or deep tissue at the operation site.
- SSI can be divided into three types: Superficial incisional, deep incisional and organ/space SSI.
- Proper hand hygiene and surgical handwashing significantly decreases chances of SSI.
- Before surgery hair removal should be done only if necessary and clipper should be used.
- Antibiotic prophylaxis dose should be given in indicated surgery 30 minutes prior and antibiotic should be judiciously used. Antibiotic after wound closure has no role in prophylaxis.
- Blood transfusion causes diversion of immune response so should be avoided as far as possible. Using fresh or leukocyte depleted blood can be an option.
- Hypothermia, hyperglycemia increases chances of SSI and should be avoided during surgery.
- HEPA filters with laminar airflow should be used in operating theatre.
- Needles and sharp handling should be kept to minimum and should be disposed in puncture proof container.

REFERENCES

1. Weigelt JA, Lipsky BA, Tabak YP, et al. Surgical site infections: Causative pathogens and associated outcomes. Am J Infect Control 2010;38:112–20.
2. Centers for Disease Control and Prevention. National Nosocomial Infections Surveillance (NNIS) System report, data summary from January 1992 through June 2004, issued October 2004. Am J Infect Control 2004;32:470–85.
3. Anderson DJ, Kaye KS, Classen D, et al. Strategies to prevent surgical site infections in acute care hospitals. Infect Control Hosp Epidemiol. 2008;29:S51–61.
4. Engemann JJ, Carmeli Y, Cosgrove SE, et al. Adverse clinical and economic outcomes attributable to methicillin resistance among patients with *Staphylococcus aureus* surgical site infection. Clin Infect Dis. 2003;36:592–8.
5. Owens CD, Stoessel K. Surgical site infections: epidemiology, microbiology and prevention. J Hosp Infect. 2008;70: 3–10.
6. Garner JS. CDC guideline for prevention of surgical wound infections, 1985. Supercedes guideline for prevention of surgical wound infections published in 1982. (Originally published in 1995). Revised. Infect Control. 1986;7(3): 193–200.
7. Simmons BP. Guideline for prevention of surgical wound infections. Infect Control 1982;3:185–196.
8. Spagnolo AM, Ottria G, Amicizia D, et al. Operating theatre quality and prevention of surgical site infections. J Prev Med Hyg. 2013;54:131–137.
9. Horan TC, Gaynes RP, Martone WJ, et al. CDC definition of nosocomial surgical site infections, 1992: a modification of CDC definitions of surgical wound infections. Infect Control Hosp Epidemiol 1992;13(10):606–8.
10. Alexander JW, Fischer JE, Boyajian M, et al. The influence of hair-removal methods on wound infections. Arch Surg 1983;118(3):347–52.

11. Masterson TM, Rodeheaver GT, Morgan RF, et al. Bacteriologic evaluation of electric clippers for surgical hair removal. Am J Surg 1984;148:301–2.
12. Seropian R, Reynolds BM. Wound infections after preoperative depilatory versus razor preparation. Am J Surg 1971;121:251–4.
13. Hamilton HW, Hamilton KR, Lone FJ. Preoperative hair removal. Can J Surg 1977;20:269–71, 274–5.
14. Garibaldi RA. Prevention of intraoperative wound contamination with chlorhexidine shower and scrub. J Hosp Infect 1988;11(Suppl B):5–9.
15. Paulson DS. Efficacy evaluation of a 4% chlorhexidine gluconate as a full-body shower wash. Am J Infect Control 1993;21(4):205–9.
16. Hayek LJ, Emerson JM, Gardner AM. A placebo-controlled trial of the effect of two preoperative baths or showers with chlorhexidine detergent on postoperative wound infection rates. J Hosp Infect 1987;10:165–72.
17. Lowbury EJ, Lilly HA. Use of 4 percent chlorhexidine detergent solution (Hibiscrub) and other methods of skin disinfection. Br Med J 1973;1:510–5.
18. Aly R, Maibach HI. Comparative antibacterial efficacy of a 2-minute surgical scrub with chlorhexidine gluconate, povidone-iodine, and chloroxylenol sponge-brushes. Am J Infect Control 1988;16:173–7.
19. Peterson AF, Rosenberg A, Alatary SD. Comparative evaluation of surgical scrub preparations. Surg Gynecol Obstet 1978;146:63–5.
20. Brown TR, Ehrlich CE, Stehman FB, et al. A clinical evaluation of chlorhexidine gluconate spray as compared with iodophor scrub for preoperative skin preparation. Surg Gynecol Obstet 1984;158: 363–6.
21. Boyce JM, Pittet D. Guideline for hand hygiene in health-care settings: Recommendations of the Healthcare Infection Control Practices Advisory Committee and the HICPAC/ SHEA/APIC/IDSA Hand Hygiene Task Force. Am J Infect Control 2002;30(8):S1–S46.
22. Larson EL, Butz AM, Gullette DL, et al. Alcohol for surgical scrubbing? Infect Control Hosp Epidemiol 1990;11(3): 139–43.
23. Faoagali J, Fong J, George N, et al. Comparison of the immediate, residual, and cumulative antibacterial effects of Novaderm R*, Novascrub R*, Betadine Surgical Scrub, Hibiclens, and liquid soap. Am J Infect Control 1995;23(6): 337–43.
24. Nichols RL, Smith JW, Garcia RY, et al. Current practices of preoperative bowel preparation among North American colorectal surgeons. Clin Infect Dis 1997;24:609–19.
25. Wade JJ, Casewell MW. The evaluation of residual antimicrobial activity on hands and its clinical relevance. J Hosp Infect 1991;18(Suppl B):23–8.
26. Mangram AJ, Horan TC, Pearson ML, et al. The Hospital Infection Control Practices Advisory Committee. Guideline for the prevention of surgical site infection, 1999. Infect Control Hosp Epidemiol 1999;20:247–280.
27. Classen DC, Evans RS, Pestotnik SL, et al. The timing of prophylactic administration of antibiotics and the risk of surgical-wound infection. N Engl J Med 1992;326(5): 281–6.
28. Anonymous. Antimicrobial prophylaxis in surgery. Med Lett Drugs Ther 1997;39(1012):97–102.
29. Orr NW. Is a mask necessary in the operating theatre? Annals of the Royal College of Surgeons of England 1981; 63:390–2.
30. Mitchell NJ, Hunt S. Surgical face masks in modern operating rooms—a costly and unnecessary ritual? Journal of Hospital Infection. 1991;18:239–42.
31. Humphreys H, Russell AJ, Marshall RJ, et al. The effect of surgical theatre headgear on bacterial counts. Journal of Hospital Infection 1991;19:175–80.
32. Centers for Disease Control. Postsurgical infections associated with nonsterile implantable devices. MMWR Morb Mortal Wkly Rep 1992;41(15):263.
33. Soto LE, Bobadilla M, Villalobos Y, et al. Post-surgical nasal cellulitis outbreak due to Mycobacterium chelonae. J Hosp Infect 1991;19(2):99–106.
34. Association for the Advancement of Medical Instrumentation. Flash sterilization: Steam sterilization of patient care items for immediate use (ANSI/AAMI ST37-1996). Arlington (VA): Association for the Advancement of Medical Instrumentation; 1996.
35. Richard VS, Mathai E, Cherian T. Role of anaesthetic equipment in transmitting nosocomial infection. J Assoc Physicians .2001;49:454–8
36. Beck, Danchin, Durban. Infection control in theatre. South Afr J Anaesth Analg. 2011;17(1):56–64.
37. Kinouchi K. Anesthetic consideration for the management of very low and extremely low birth weight infants. Best Pract Res Clin Anaesthesiol. 2004;18:273–90.
38. Weiss Y. Simplified management of operative wounds by early exposure. Int Surg. 1983;68:237–40.
39. Chrintz H, Vibits H, Cordtz TO, et al. Need for surgical wound dressing. Br J Surg. 1989;76:204–5.
40. Department of Health 2001. Guideline for preventing infection associated with the insertion and maintenance of central venous catheters. Journal of Hospital Infection 47 (Supplement) 547–567. Available at www.epic.tvu.ac.uk
41. American Institute of Architects. Guidelines for design and construction of hospital and health care facilities. 1996 edn. Washington (DC): American Institute of Architects Press; 1996.
42. American Institute of Architects. Guidelines for design and construction of hospital and health care facilities: 2006 edition. Washington DC: American Institute of Architects Press, 2006.
43. Guidelines: Infection Control in Anaesthesia. Anaesthesia 2008;63:1027–1036.
44. Centers for Disease Control. Protection against viral hepatitis: Recommendation of Immunization Practices Advisory Committee (ACIP) MMWR 1990;39(RR-2):1.

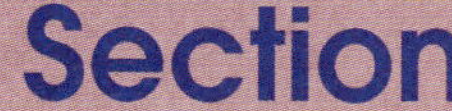

Section 4

Special Considerations: Complications of Anaesthesia, Medicolegal, Ethical Aspects of Paediatric Anaesthesia

Clinical Complications in Paediatric Anaesthesia

Pradnya Bhalerao

ABSTRACT

Difficult situations in paediatric anaesthesia are a challenge to the anaesthesiologist and include diverse respiratory, cardiac, thermoregulatory, metabolic and gastrointestinal events besides others like emergence delirium and anaphylaxis. Here an attempt has been made to highlight some important complications in paediatric patients perioperatively.

INTRODUCTION

Anaesthesiologists are faced with diverse clinical situations owing to the spectrum of patients and problems they encounter. One such group is the 'paediatric age group' where difficult situations are more common. Incidence of these complications is more in those under the age of three years.

RESPIRATORY EVENTS

Perioperative respiratory events are a major cause of morbidity and mortality in paediatric patients, commonly under five years and more so in infants and those with history of upper respiratory tract infection within two weeks of surgery.[1]

Airway Obstruction

This is one of the common problems encountered postoperatively.

Causes

The cause of obstruction includes tongue fall, laryngospasm, laryngeal oedema, incomplete reversal of neuromuscular blockade, airway surgeries or others like presence of secretions, mucous plug or even a throat pack inserted during a tonsillectomy, tongue or dental surgery.

Signs

The diagnostic signs include paradoxical see-saw breathing, intercostal indrawing, subcostal and sternal recession, tracheal tug and low oxygen saturation.

Individual Causes, Their Prevention and Treatment

Tongue fall occurs if the patient is extubated in a deeper plane due to the relaxed pharyngeal muscles. Neck extension, mouth opening and jaw-thrust alone or together might be sufficient to correct obstruction. It can also be prevented by nursing the child in lateral position with neck extended.

Presence of throat pack, mucous plug or thick secretions can be treated with throat inspection and pharyngeal suction under direct laryngoscopic vision.

Laryngospasm is one of the main causes of airway obstruction and is seen more commonly in infants than older children and those undergoing intraoral surgery.[2,3] The children anaesthetised by trainee anaesthetist have been reported to have an increased incidence by 1.7 times.[4] A recent history of upper respiratory tract infection (URTI) or asthma is associated with 2- to 7-fold increase in incidence of laryngospasm.[5] When the child is coming out of the effect of anaesthetics in the immediate postoperative period, a noxious stimulus like insertion of an airway or nasogastric tube, laryngoscope blade or even suction catheter may induce laryngospasm.

Simply extubating in a deeper plane may prevent the problem. Producing an artificial cough by applying positive pressure just before extubation to expel subglottic secretions decreases the incidence of laryngospasm possibly, because it decreases the adductor response of the laryngeal muscles.[4]

Removal of the irritant stimulus, jaw thrust and administration of 100% oxygen are the first steps in management. Oxygen therapy should be started and continuous positive airway pressure (CPAP) if given often breaks the spasm.[6] Increasing the depth using subhypnotic dose of propofol (0.8 mg/kg) helps by suppressing the laryngeal reflex. Suxamethonium 1 mg/kg with atropine 0.02 mg/kg helps counter intractable laryngospasm. If intravenous route is not available, intramuscular dose of 4 mg/kg may be considered.

Laryngeal oedema or postextubation croup is caused due to tight fitting tube with no air leak. Other causes include repeated or traumatic intubation, coughing or bucking with endotracheal tube in place, changing head position repeatedly during surgery, inappropriate anaesthetic gas humidification, presence of respiratory tract infection, children with Down's syndrome and even use of lubricating jelly. Use of endotracheal tube one size smaller, humidified gases, prophylactic steroids and less irritant tube material has definitely helped reduce the incidence.[7] Treatment includes use of humified oxygen and nebulisation with epinephrine. Role of dexamethasone is controversial. Rarely, reintubation may be needed.

Bronchospasm

Cause

Perioperative wheeze may occur in light planes of anaesthesia, kinked endotracheal tube, endobronchial intubation, secretions, foreign body, pulmonary oedema, embolus, aspiration and reactive airway.[8] Precipitants and causes for bronchospasm include lower respiratory tract infections, irritants like passive smoking, inhalational agents like isoflurane, intravenous agents like pentothal, muscle relaxants like atracurium, emotional stress, exercise, cold dry anaesthetic gases, manipulation/stimulation of pharynx and larynx and gastro-oesophageal reflux.

Treatment

Treatment includes deepening the plane of anaesthesia, inhaled beta agonists and ipatronium, lidocaine 1 mg/kg intravenously to blunt tracheal stimulation and intravenous corticosteroids.

In persistent airway obstruction neuromuscular blockade should be reassessed. Adequate reversal of neuromuscular blocking agents can be diagnosed clinically by thoraco-abdominal respiration with adequate upward movement of upper chest on inspiration, sustained eye opening, adequate muscle tone as seen in neck and abdominal muscles and by neuromuscular transmission monitor. Some children may need to be reintubated till adequate reversal is achieved.

Hypoxaemia

Cause

Infants are prone to perioperative hypoxaemia due to premature respiratory control and irregular breathing, a low functional residual capacity, high oxygen demand, tendency to airway obstruction and high oxygen affinity of the foetal haemoglobin. Hypoxaemia is more often seen in the immediate postoperative period and in the recovery (PACU).[9] Patients with residual effect of anaesthetics, sedatives and muscle relaxants and surgeries lasting more than an hour are often associated with this problem. Associated diseases respiratory or cardiac, sepsis, hypotension may all aggravate the condition.

Diagnosis and Management

Diagnosis is based on clinical signs of obstruction and respiratory distress and low oxygen saturation on pulse oximetry. Oxygen supplementation and treating the cause will prevent further damage. Giving 100% oxygen over a brief period does not pose any risk of oxygen toxicity.

Aspiration

Cause

Aspiration of secretions, blood and vomitus may occur during induction, maintenance and postoperatively. Common causes include emergency surgery, trauma, intestinal obstruction, head injury and difficult intubation. Aspiration at induction is most common.

Diagnosis and Management

The signs of laryngospasm, bronchospasm and fall in oxygen saturation are early markers. Chest X-ray may show signs of consolidation or/and atelectasis much later. Intubation, oxygenation, positive pressure ventilation, antibiotics, bronchodialators and fibreoptic bronchoscopic removal of solid particles may help.

Respiratory Depression

Cause

Postoperative respiratory depression is a common concern in this group of patients and is mainly due to the residual effect of anaesthetics, opioids, benzodiazepines or even muscle relaxants. Other factors include abdominal distension and tight abdominal bandage. When respiration is apparently normal immediately postextubation, rate and depth decrease after some time and breathing improves on stimulation, it is generally due to opioids. Children with obstructive sleep apnoea (OSA) are more prone to this opioid effect. Apnoea is common in premature babies.

Diagnosis and Management

The diagnosis is made by decrease in rate and depth of respiration, laboured breathing, tachycardia, oxygen desaturation, hypercarbia and acidosis. Treatment includes oxygenation, assisting ventilation and reversing the effect of opioids. Caffeine (10 mg/kg) has been found to be effective in treating apnoea of prematurity and nowadays is often administered in NICU to these babies.[10] Regional blocks like ilioinguinal, caudal and subarachnoid block have been reported to decrease the incidence of apnoea.[11] Providing analgesia with NSAIDs, ketamine and paracetamol infusions instead of opioids often helps in those with OSA. Postoperative monitoring in PACU is mandatory.

Pulmonary Oedema

Cause

Causes include severe airway obstruction especially laryngospasm immediate postoperatively. This occurs due to the high negative intrathoracic pressure generated by forced inspiration against a closed glottis or blocked airway which leads to increased interstitial negative pressure and increased capillary permeability.[12] Intraoperative overhydration is another important reason for this complication. Usually, it is self limiting and resolve by 24 to 48 hours.

Diagnosis and Management

Diagnosis is made by appearance of rales and wheeze in the chest, desaturation on pulse oximetry, and copious frothy pink fluid pouring out of the trachea. Once airway obstruction is relieved, child should continue to be administered CPAP (5–10 cm H_2O) with high concentration of oxygen. Diuretics and fluid restriction is helpful. If hypoxia persists, endotracheal intubation and positive pressure ventilation with positive end expiratory pressure helps.

Sore throat

An important problem due to laryngoscopy and intubation or even placing a throat pack. Dry gases are another contributing factor. Use of supraglottic airway devices and humidified gases decreases the incidence.

Key Points

1. Resistance $\propto$ 1/radius.[4] Therefore a small decrease in airway resistance causes a marked increased resistance to airflow and increased work of breathing.
2. Airway injuries of different severity after intubation, like ulcers, abrasions of the mucosa, and penetrating injuries on different anatomical levels (glottic, subglottic and tracheal) do not cause stridor as long as the lumen of the airway is not narrowed by 50%.
3. Subglottic stenosis, the worst side effect of airway injury appears late after the trauma, without the symptom of stridor in the immediate postoperative period.
4. LMA is associated with adverse respiratory events in a reactive airway.

Pearls

The children anaesthetised by trainee anaesthetist have been reported to have an increased incidence of airway related disasters.

POSTOPERATIVE NAUSEA AND VOMITING (PONV)

PONV is a very common problem in children with an incidence ranging from 8.9 to 42% in those susceptible.[4]

Cause

Nausea is the uncomfortable sensation of an impending episode of vomiting, whereas vomiting is mediated by vomiting centre in the brainstem. It receives inputs from the pharynx, GI tract, higher cortical centres (the visual, gustatory, olfactory and vestibular centres) and the Chemoreceptor Trigger Zone (CTZ). Four independent predictors of PONV, namely duration of surgery more than 30 minutes, age over 3 years, a personal or family history of PONV and strabismus surgery have been suggested.[13] PONV is commonly seen after adenotonsillectomy, strabismus surgery and orchidopexy. High incidence of vomiting in adenoidectomy and tonsillectomy is believed to be due to irritation of the pharynx and stomach by blood. In strabismus, the occuloemetic reflex via ophthalmic division of the trigeminal nerve probably causes PONV. Intraoperative use of opioids, early administration of clear fluids and early ambulation may precipitate vomiting in susceptible patients.

Treatment

Prophylactic ondensetron, a 5–HT receptor antagonist 0.1 mg/kg and/or dexamethasone 0.15 mg/kg intravenously, metaclopramide 0.25 mg/kg intravenously or use of other 5–HT antagonists like granisetron, ramosetron and even clonidine is recommended. Besides use of propofol and avoidance of precipitators like opioids and nitrous oxide helps. Treatment includes giving a head low position to prevent aspiration, drugs used in prophylaxis and intravenous fluids to avoid hypovolaemia and electrolyte imbalance.

Key Points

1. Be aware of the extrapyramidal/dystonic reactions caused by metochlopramide.
2. Dexmedetomidine infusions intraoperatively reduce incidence of PONV. However, its use in paediatric patients is not yet established.

Pearls

Emesis can be disastrous after adenotonsillectomy being the commonest cause for morbidity and readmission.

THERMOREGULATORY AND METABOLIC EVENTS

Hypothermia

Infants and neonates have been shown to be at an increased risk for perioperative hypothermia since they have a less effective thermoregulatory capacity.[14]

Cause

Children lose more heat through conduction and radiation than adults, due to less insulating subcutaneous fat, and a higher surface area to volume ratio. Besides evaporative loss is also more due to decreased keratin content in the skin. During anaesthesia, heat production through basal metabolic processes is reduced in humans of all ages by a factor of 20–30%, and in addition, neonates who are mechanically ventilated will miss heat generated through work of breathing. Inhibition of central thermoregulation also occurs, with delay of vasoconstriction to much lower core temperatures, and loss of usual heat production from non-shivering thermogenesis and shivering.

Diagnosis and Management

Hypothermia is associated with adverse clinical complications such as bradycardia, metabolic acidosis, hypoglycaemia, impaired coagulation, reduced resistance to infections, delayed wound healing, prolonged emergence, and increased time to recovery. Simple measures like warming the operation theatre up to 27–29°C, using a radiant heater at induction and recovery, covering the babies with cotton pads (especially the head), infusion of warm fluids, using warm and humidified gases and advising the surgeon to use warm irrigation fluids may prevent the occurrence of this complication. The more sophisticated warming mattress, blanket and fluid warmers and heated in circuit humidifiers are also available.

Hyperthermia

Cause

Hyperthermia may occur due to high environmental temperature, infection or life threatening conditions like malignant hyperthermia. First recognized as a cluster of anaesthetic deaths in a family, malignant hyperthermia (MH) is an inherited disorder of skeletal muscle calcium channels, which is triggered in affected individuals by exposure to inhalational anaesthetic agents, succinylcholine, or both.[15] The result is a MH crisis, which is a cascade of hypermetabolism, electrolyte derangements, arrhythmias, skeletal muscle damage, and hyperthermia, which progresses to death if untreated. The incidence of MH crisis is 1 in 5,000 to 10,000 general anaesthetics in children. The incidence increases if succinylcholine is given in addition to volatile anaesthetics. Appropriately treated, the mortality from a MH crisis is now estimated to be less than 10%.[15]

Diagnosis and Management

Most patients who are MH susceptible have normal history and physical examinations, although some association has been found with cleft palate, ptosis, clubfoot, scoliosis, strabismus, and cryptorchidism. Fifty percent of patients with MH have undergone a prior general anaesthetic without complication. The standard test to screen for MH susceptibility is the in vitro caffeine-halothane contracture test, which uses a muscle biopsy specimen. The indications for performing this test are a documented episode of hyperthermia, acidosis, and rhabdomyolysis induced by a triggering agent; an episode of masseter muscle spasm after exposure to a triggering agent; and availability of testable relatives of an MH-susceptible patient. However, this test has its limitations because it requires that the patient be at least 5 years of age and weigh 20 kg. Genetic screening, using the *RYR1* gene, has been reported. The familial mutation was found in 50% of family members, characteristic of its autosomal dominance. First and second degree family members of an MH-susceptible patient have a 50% and 25% risk, respectively, of being MH susceptible. Tachycardia, non-specific rise in $EtCO_2$, trunk/total body rigidity, masseter spasm, rapid and unexplained rise in temperature, mixed respiratory and metabolic picture on blood gases are suggestive of MH.

Treatment includes stopping all trigger agents, administering 100% oxygen and hyperventilation to treat hypercarbia. Dantrolene 2.5 mg/kg immediately followed by 1 mg/kg six hourly intravenously should be injected. For acidosis sodabicarbonate 1 mEq/kg and a drip containing glucose 0.5 gm/kg and insulin 0.15 U/kg to treat hyperkalaemia is adviced. Iced intravenous fluids and cooling blankets will help decreasing the temperature. One should ensure adequate hydration and monitor urine output. Furosemide and mannitol should be given as needed.

Key Points

1. The initial signs of MH can also occur postoperatively as fever with excessive metabolic rate and muscle injury.
2. Myoglobinuria produces renal injury in about 10% of MH cases. Renal failure is more likely when treatment with dantrolene is delayed.
3. Disseminated intravascular coagulation and cerebral edema may complicate fulminant MH.
4. After initial treatment with 2.5 to 10 mg/kg of dantrolene, at least 1 mg/kg of dantrolene should be given every 6 hours for four doses because 20% of patients experience an exacerbation or recurrence of MH within 24 hours after the acute episode.

HYPOGLYCAEMIA

Cause

Inadequate glycogen stores and deficient gluconeogenesis are important factors causing hypoglycaemia in a neonate. Thus the fasting guidelines for a paediatric patient are also different from that of adults. During surgery, there is a rise in the plasma glucose level in a normal adult, but it has been shown that children do not respond with a hyperglycaemic reaction to the same degree.

Diagnosis and Management

Hypoglycaemia is recognized as being a preoperative danger in paediatric practice predisposing to lethargy, irritability, drowsiness, hypotonia, difficulty in feeding, tachycardia and later metabolic acidosis, seizures and even coma. Mean normal fasting glucose concentration at birth is 54 mg/dL with a range of 28–96 mg/dL. The concentration increases in childhood to mean of 77 mg/dL at 2 years and 92 mg/dL at 15 years. Short-term treatment of hypoglycaemia consists of an intravenous (IV) bolus of dextrose 10% 2.5 mL/kg. The blood sample should be drawn before the glucose is administered. After the bolus is administered, an IV infusion that matches normal hepatic glucose production (approximately 5–8 mg/kg/min in an infant and about 3–5 mg/kg/min in an older child) should be continued.[16]

Key Points

1. Observe the 2–4–6 guideline for fasting to avoid hypoglycaemia.
2. Newborns of diabetic mothers may often be hypoglycaemic.

CARDIAC EVENTS

Hypotension

Cause

Hypovolaemia is a common cause of hypotension. Acute blood loss (GI bleed, trauma, and post-tonsillectomy bleed), plasma loss (burns, peritonitis, hypoproteinemia) and water loss (vomiting, diarrhoea, and diuresis) cause hypovolaemia. The signs include cold, clammy extremities, tready peripheral pulse and prolonged capillary refill. Other causes of hypotension in this group includes sepsis, anaphylaxis, spinal cord injury and vasodilatation. Cardiogenic shock is a relatively uncommon cause of hypotension seen in congenital heart disease with outflow obstruction, pneumothorax, pericardial effusion or constrictive pericarditis. Intravenous anaesthetic agents and inhalational agents are vasodilators and myocardial depressants and hence cause hypotension. Spinal anaesthesia rarely causes hypotension in children below five years.

Management

Management includes treatment of the cause and infusion of intravenous fluids like ringer lactate, colloids and blood where indicated.

Key Points

PALS guidelines for hypotension—systolic BP < 60 mmHg in a neonate, < 70 mmHg: 1 month to 12 months and <90 mmHg in >10 years.

ARRHYTHMIAS

Bradycardia

Cause

The risk of bradycardia and cardiovascular complications in children is inversely proportional to age. In children the heart rate is also a dominant factor for maintaining cardiac output, since the developing heart is less compliant and contractile and so cannot depend on stroke volume. Thus, when bradycardia occurs in children during anaesthesia, cardiac output falls and may lead to serious cardiac arrhythmias and even cardiac arrest. Causes for bradycardia can be hypoxia, hypothermia, head injury, hyperkalemia, hypercalcemia, hypoxia, hypothyroidism, and medications (digitalis and α blockers) or cardiac abnormalities like heart block and during cardiac surgeries. During general anaesthesia children are at an increased risk of bradycardia during laryngoscopy and intubation owing to vagal stimulation or even hypoxia, due to inhalational anaesthetics like halothane, intravenous agents like propofol, opioids like fentanyl or remifentanyl, muscle relaxants like suxamethonium and reversal agents like neostigmine. Clonidine, an α_2 receptor agonist which is frequently used as an additive to local anaesthesia, can also elicit bradycardia. Hypervagotonia can be evoked by oesophageal or nasal stimulation and occulocardiac reflex in ophthalmic surgery causing bradycardia.[17] OSA in patients with adenotonsillar enlargement can precipitate hypoxia and bradycardia.

Management

Premedication with vagolytics like atropine or glycopyrrolate prior intubation and laryngoscopy helps. Treatment includes atropine 0.02 mg/kg, epinephrine 0.01 mg/kg intravenous or interosseous in repeated doses, chest compression, pacing and treatment of the underlying cause.

Tachycardia

Cause

Tachycardia in this set of patients is due to anxiety, pain, hyperthermia, hypoxia, hypercarbia, hypoglycaemia, hypovolaemia and light plane of anaesthesia. Supraventricular tachycardia with a narrow QRS and regular R–R interval may be seen with a heart rate of 200–300/min in neonates and infants and 150–200/min in older children.

Treatment

Treatment includes treating the underlying cause, vagal maneuvers, adenosine 0.1–0.2 mg/kg max up to 12 mg intravenously and cardioversion (0.25–1 J/kg) in cases of SVT.

Key Points: Pulse rate/min in paediatrics

Age	Heart rate/min
0–3 months	85–205
3 months to 2 years	100–190
2–10 years	60–140
>10 years	60–100

OTHER COMPLICATIONS

Emergence Delirium

A child with emergence delirium (ED) is in a dissociated state of consciousness in which the child is irritable, uncompromising, uncooperative, incoherent, and inconsolably crying, moaning, kicking, or thrashing.[18] ED can disrupt the surgical repair and be distressing for parents and staff. Several scales have been adopted to score emergence delirium. The Watcha scale is a simpler tool to use in clinical practice and may have a higher overall sensitivity and specificity.[19]

Paediatric Emergence Delirium—Watcha Scale

Asleep	0
Calm	1
Crying but can be consoled	2
Crying but cannot be consoled	3
Agitated and thrashing around	4

There have been a wide range of reported figures for the incidence of ED in paediatric populations, ranging from 2% to 80%.

Causes

Factors associated with ED include younger age (2–5 years), no previous surgery, poor adaptability, ophthalmology and otorhinolaryngology procedures, sevoflurane, isoflurane or desflurane anaesthesia and short time to awakening. While pain is not the sole cause for ED, surgery associated with elevated postoperative pain has been thought to increase the risk of ED. Preoperative anxiety and temperament, as reflected in children who are more emotional, more impulsive, less social, and less adaptable to environmental changes, has been identified as a risk factor for ED. Sudden emergence from anaesthesia into a disordered state of consciousness or into an unfamiliar environment has been proposed as a cause of ED. However, the incidence of ED in patients receiving propofol is markedly lower than those receiving sevoflurane, despite the similar rapid emergence profile of both agents. Elevated postoperative pain has been suggested to underlie ED. But given that ED is seen in patients undergoing MRI, pain cannot be the sole factor.

Since all inhalation anaesthetics, even halothane, increase the risk of ED, while shorter-acting agents increase the incidence further, there may be an underlying mechanism of action of inhalation anaesthetics triggering ED. Volatile anaesthetics may affect brain activity by interfering with the balance between neuronal synaptic inhibition and excitation in the central nervous system.

Diagnosis

ED has been associated with adverse events like increased bleeding from surgical site, pulling out a surgical drain or an intravenous (IV) line and increased pain at the operative site. Characteristically these children do not recognize or identify familiar and known objects or people. Parents who witness this state claim the behaviour is unusual and uncustomary for the child. Although generally self-limiting (5–15 min) ED can be severe and may result in physical harm to the child and particularly the site of surgery.

Prophylaxis and Treatment

Prophylactic measures include co-administration of propofol, midazolam, or fentanyl. The efficacy of propofol is dependent on the timing of administration. Due to the rapid pharmacokinetics of propofol, a bolus of 1 mg/kg^{-1} interavenous given at the end of the procedure or continuous infusion used during maintenance of anaesthesia results in increased concentrations during emergence and thus a decreased incidence of ED. Perioperative analgesia has been shown to be effective in preventing ED. Several analgesics have been studied for the prevention of ED including: fentanyl (dose 1 μg/kg intravenous given 10 min before the end of a procedure), ketamine (0.25 μg/kg intravenously given at the end of procedure, or as a premedication 6 mg/kg orally), and α_2-adrenoreceptor agonists such as clonidine (caudally 1–3 μg/kg; intravenously 2–3 μg/kg) and dexmedetomidine (0.15–0.3 μg/kg). These preventative strategies increase sedation and therefore should be balanced against the risk of prolonging emergence or delaying discharge from the postanaesthesia care unit. Often, simply being reunited with a parent provides the quickest recovery from ED.

Anaphylaxis

Anaphylaxis is a life-threatening allergic reaction mediated by the release of histamine and other substances from mast cells after exposure to certain antigens. There is a lack of consistent clinical manifestations and hence there is a wide range of possible clinical presentations. In addition, the timing of the reaction in relation to exposure to the triggering agent can vary. Diagnosis can be difficult and a high index of suspicion is required.

Causes

Common triggering agents in anaesthesia include, muscle relaxants, latex, antibiotics and colloids. More commonly in children, anaphylaxis is caused by penicillin, contrast media or nuts. The most common presentations include: Cardiovascular collapse (88%), erythema (48%), bronchospasm (40%), angioedema (24%), cutaneous rash (13%), urticaria (8%).

Diagnosis

It has been classified clinically into 5 grades:

1. Cutaneous reaction only: Urticiaria, erythema, angioedema
2. As above but also hypotension, tachycardia or bronchospasm
3. As II but more severe: Collapse, arrhythmias
4. Cardiac and/or respiratory arrest
5. Death

Management

Immediate management includes to stop the triggering agent (if known or suspected) call for help, deliver 100% oxygen, exclude airway or breathing circuit obstruction, intubate trachea if not already done, give epinephrine, crystalloid bolus of 20 mL/kg. Consider chlorpheniramine, hydrocortisone and bronchodilators like salbutamol if persistent wheeze (Table 41.1).

Key Points

Any patient who has had a suspected anaphylactic reaction under anaesthesia should be fully investigated if possible. The patient should be made aware of the trigger agent and any hospital records should be clearly labelled with an alert.

Table 41.1 Management of anaphylaxis

Age	IV adrenaline (1:10 000) Suggested increments	IM adrenaline (1:1000)	Chlorpheniramine (IM or slow IV)	Hydrocortisone (IM or slow IV)
<6 months	5 mcg (0.05 mL)	150 mcg (0.15 mL)	250 mcg/kg	25 mg
6 months–6 years	10 mcg (0.10 mL)	150 mcg (0.15 mL)	2.5 mg if over 1 year	50 mg if over 1 year
6–12 years	25 mcg (0.25 mL)	300 mcg (0.3 mL)	5 mg	100 mg
>12 years	50 mcg (0.50 m)	500 mcg (0.5 mL)	10 mg	200 mg

Note: 10 mcg/kg = 0.1 mL/kg 1:10,000

Regional Anaesthesia

Spinal Anaesthesia

Hypotension and desaturation are rare in children. It is usually due to high block or use of sedatives. PDPH is rare in children <10 years age, because of low CSF pressure, highly elastic dura and non-ambulation. Overall incidence of 4–5% has been reported in 2–15 years age group.[20] Symptoms are generally mild. Severe PDPH is very rare (0.1%). Treatment is conservative. A crying child in upright position if becomes quiet on lying is probably having a headache. Epidural blood patch (0.2–0.3 ml/kg) should be considered if headache persists for >1 week. A lesser incidence with pencil point as against cutting tip needle has been reported (0.4% vs. 5%).[21] Backache (5–10%) is a common complaint, but its causal relationship has not been established. High or total spinal anaesthesia (0.6%) can result if infant's legs are lifted after injection of drug or with overdose and barbotage. Limited thoracic kyphosis facilitates cephalad spread and cause apnoea. Transient neurological symptoms (3–4%) are described as new onset pain and dysesthesia originating in gluteal region radiating to lower limbs. Neurological examination, imaging studies, and electro-pathological testing are usually negative. Meningitis (aseptic and septic) is rare in children. In case of post-spinal fever, LP is indicated.[22]

Local complications like inappropriate needle insertion damaging the nerve and surrounding anatomic structures, tissue coring, introduction of epithelial cells into tissues causing development of compressive tumors (especially in the spinal canal) and injection of neurotoxic solutions (syringe mismatch, epinephrine close to a terminal artery) may occur. Leakage around the puncture site where the catheter has been introduced, may cause partial block failure and favour bacterial contamination. This can be avoided by using appropriate dressing and bacterial filters. Leakage around the catheter can be reduced by tunneling the catheter and applying a slightly compressive dressing.

Systemic complications usually result from accidental intravenous (IV) injection of local anaesthetics or excessive dosing. They can be life-threatening and should be managed in the same way as in adults. The major difference between adults and children is that cardiovascular complications are not preceded by neurologic signs but are concomitant with cerebral toxicity.

Key Points

Ultrasound guided regional anaesthesia has increased the safety and efficacy in paediatric patients.

However, training is always necessary and that only experienced paediatric anaesthesiologists should perform these techniques.

CONCLUSION

Anaesthesia is a tight rope walk and thorough knowledge and vigilance is the key to balancing the act. This is even more important in the paediatric population as they respond differently to anaesthesia and the clinical complications therein.

REFERENCES

1. Paterson N, Waterhouse P. Risk in paediatric anaesthesia. Pediatr Anesth. 2011; 21:848–57.
2. Bolton CM, Myles PS, Nolan T, et al. Prophylaxis of postoperative vomiting in children undergoing tonsillectomy: A systematic review and meta-analysis. Br J Anaesth 2006;97:593–604.
3. Mamie C, Habre W, Delhumeau C, et al. Incidence and risk factors of perioperative respiratory adverse events in children undergoing elective surgery. Pediatr Anesth
4. Pawar D. Common postoperative problems in children. Indian J Anaesth. 2012;56:496–501.
5. Flick RP, Wilder RT, Pieper SF, et al. Risk factors for laryngospasm in children during general anaesthesia. Pediatr Anesth. 2008; 18:289–96.

6. Orliaguet GA, Gall O, Savoldelli GL, Couloigner V. Case Scenario: Perianesthetic Management of Laryngospasm in Children. Anesthesiology 2012;116:458–71.
7. Maloney E, Meakin G. Acute stridor in children. Br J Anaesth 2007;7(6):183–86.
8. Maxwell L, Goodwin SR, Mancuso TJ, et al. Systemic disorders in infants and children. Smith's anaesthesia for infants and children. 2006; 7:1051
9. Motoyama EK. Systemic disorders in infants and children. Smith's anaesthesia for infants and children. 2006;7: 1062–63.
10. Henderson-Smart DJ, Steer P. Postoperative caffeine for preventing apnoea in preterm infants. Cochrane Database Syst Rev. 2000;2:CD000048.
11. Thong SY, Lim SL, Ng AS. Retrospective review of ilioinguinal-iliohypogastric nerve block with general anaesthesia for herniotomy in ex-premature neonates. Pediatr Anesth. 2011;21:1109–12.
12. Thiagarajan RR, Laussen PC. Negative pressure pulmonary edema in children-pathogenesis and clinical management. Pediatr Anesth. 2007;17:307–10.
13. Tander B, Baris S, Karakaya D, et al. Risk factors influencing inadvertent hypothermia in infants and neonates during anaesthesia. Paediatr Anaesth. 2005;15:574–579.
14. Feinstein L, Miskiewicz M. Perioperative hypothermia. The Internet Journal of Anaesthesiology. 2009;27(2).
15. Hopkins PM. Malignant hyperthermia Advances in clinical management and diagnosis. Br J Anaesth. 2000;85:118–28.
16. Sharma V, Sharma R, Singh G, Qazi S. Preoperative fasting duration and incidence of hypoglycemia and hemodynamic response in children. J Chem Pharm Res. 2011;3(6): 382–391.
17. James I. Anaesthesia for paediatric eye surgery. Br J Anaesth. 2008, 8(1):5–10.
18. Vlajkovik GP, Sindjellic RP. Emergence delirium in childre: Many questions, few answers. Anaesth. Analg. 2007; 104:84–91.
19. Reduque LL, Verghese ST. Paediatric emergence delirium. Br J Anaesth. 2013;13(2):39–41.
20. Gupta A, Usha U. Spinal anaesthesia in children: A review. J Anaesthesiol Clin Pharmacol. 2014;30:10–18.
21. Apiliogullari S, Duman A, Gok F, et al. Spinal needle design and size affect the incidence of postdural puncture headache in children. Paediatr Anaesth 2010;20:177–82.
22. Pawar D. Regional anaesthesia in paediatric patients. Indian J. Anaesth. 2004;48(5):394–99.
23. Dalens BJ. Regional anaesthesia in children. Miller's anaesthesia. 2010;7:2528.

41 Evidence Based Paediatric Anaesthesia Guidelines for Practice and Psychology, Anxiety and Preoperative Preparation

Jayashree Sood, Deepanjali Pant, Archna Koul

EVIDENCE BASED MEDICINE (EBM)

Evidence based medicine is the conscientious, explicit and judicious use of current best evidence in making decisions about the care of individual patients.[1,2]

This definition was later modified as a systematic approach to clinical problem solving which allows integration of best available research evidence with clinical expertise and patient values.[3] The term was further defined as making a conscientious effort to base clinical decision on research that is most likely to be free from bias and using interventions most likely to improve how long or well patients live.[4,5] EBM is not "cookbook" medicine.

Since evidence is collected not only by research, but also by clinical expertise and patients aspirations, the term evidence 'based' medicine has shifted to evidence 'informed' healthcare, to indicate that besides research, several other parameters also contribute to 'evidence.' Other terms used are 'evidence based healthcare' or 'evidence based practice'.

One common implementation of EBM involves the use of 'clinical practice guidelines' during medical decision making to encourage effective care.

However, the EBM definition should be expanded to include not only evidence based guidelines but also evidence based individual decision making.[6]

CLINICAL GUIDELINES

Clinical guidelines are now an essential part of medicine. The Institute of Medicine (IOM) defines clinical guidelines as—systematically developed statements to assist the practitioner and patient decisions about appropriate healthcare for specific clinical circumstances.

PURPOSE OF GUIDELINES

Guidelines provide stronger scientific foundation for clinical work. They support the use of interventions that are clearly of benefit and discourage ineffective or harmful interventions.

- The purpose of the guidelines is to achieve consistency, efficiency, effectiveness, quality and safety in medical care.
- Guidelines aim to avoid over use, under use or misuse of medical care which escalates the healthcare costs.
- Practice guidelines promise to create better informed patients and clinicians by offering collectively agreed upon information about the treatment option.
- Guidelines can benefit patients by influencing public policy, particularly by highlighting areas where research is lacking and pointing out under recognized health problems and clinical services.[1,2]

GUIDELINE DEVELOPMENT PROCESS

The first step in the process of evidence based guideline development is defining the clinical question that the guideline will address. This is followed by eligibility criteria for the studies that will be included in the guideline recommendation, i.e. tracking down with maximum efficiency the best evidence to answer the clinical question. For this a systematic search of literature is conducted. Then the evidence is evaluated in terms of relevance, benefits, risks, inconvenience and cost, in addition to addressing patient's underlying values and preferences. For this, understanding of basic statistics is also required. Subsequently a grading system is developed that describes the strength of recommendation and quality of supporting evidence. Following this recommendations are formulated to be applied in clinical practice.[7,8]

GRADING OF EVIDENCE

Systematic reviews and meta-analysis of randomized control trials (RCT) are considered the highest quality of evidence. In a RCT, the quality of evidence is high but it can be downgraded if there is risk of bias, imprecision, indirectness, inconsistency or publication bias.[9]

In ascending order, the likelihood of bias influencing results increased with RCTs, non randomized intervention studies, case series, case reports and finally expert opinions.

A well done observational study demonstrating a very strong treatment may provide better evidence than an underpowered or poorly performed RCT that failed to find a significant treatment plan.[10]

LIMITATIONS OF GUIDELINES

Ideally all decisions on a practice guideline should be derived from strict scientific evidence.

- Since the "gold standard" of evidence is usually not always present, physicians often have to rely on smaller nonrandomized studies.[2]
- Guidelines can be misleading if the evidence is lacking or if the evidence was misinterpreted.
- Factors other than literature evidence can influence recommendations like author's own values, preferences or conflict of interest.
- Guidelines may not actually address patient's needs as patient preferences are difficult to capture in them.
- Guidelines are usually generalized to what is best for the average patient and are not necessarily tailored to individual needs.
- Guidelines threaten to bring stagnation and bland uniformity and are derogatorily characterized as "Cook Book Medicine."[11]
- By discouraging indiosyncrasies in clinical technique there is disincentiveness for individual innovations and may result in deskilling of practitioners.[12,13]

EVIDENCE BASED PAEDIATRIC ANAESTHESIA GUIDELINES FOR PRACTICE

Practice guidelines are systematically developed recommendations that help the physician in management of patients.

These recommendations may be practised, modified or refused.

They are not protocols and do not essentially affect outcome.

Guidelines need to be revised and updated as required.

- Anaesthesiologists practicing paediatric anaesthesia should have adequate training in this specialty.
- A thorough knowledge of paediatric anatomy, physiology and pharmacology is essential.

The American Academy of Paediatrics (AAP) has developed clinical practice guidelines for paediatric anaesthesia practice. These have been prepared internally through various entities and in collaboration with other organizations. They have described 3 sequential processes in evidence based policy setting in paediatric patients.[14]

These include

1. Determination of evidence in support (individual and aggregate) of a proposed recommendation.
2. Evaluation of balance between anticipated benefits and harms when a recommendation is carried out.
3. Designation of recommendation strength
   Evidence quality refers to the extent to which all aspects of study's design and conduct can be shown to protect against systematic bias, non-systematic bias and interferential error.

Evidence Quality

1. Well-designed RCT or diagnostic studies on relevant population
2. RCT or diagnostic studies with minor limitations, strong consistent results from observational studies
3. Observation studies

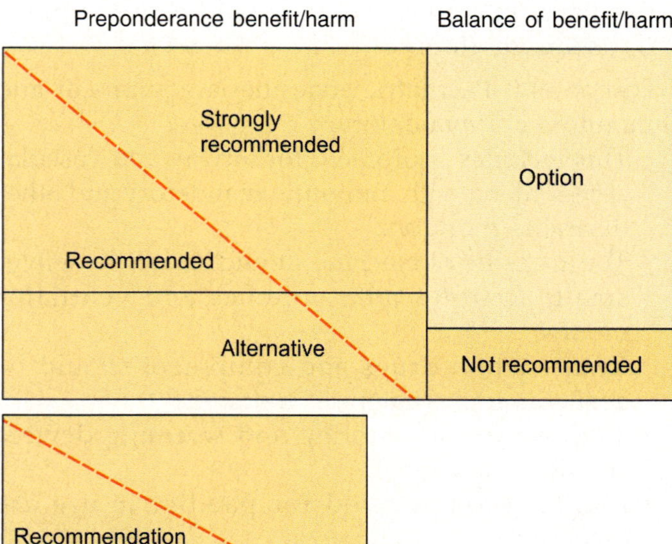

4. Expert opinion and case reports
   If validating studies cannot be performed and there is clear evidence of benefit or harm

INTERPRETING GUIDELINES RECOMMENDATIONS

The proposed classification defines 4 levels of policy

- Strong recommendation
- Recommendation
- Option
- No recommendation

Strong Recommendation

Clinicians should follow such guidelines unless a clear or compelling rationale for acting in a contrary manner is present.

Recommendation

Clinicians generally should follow such guidelines but should be alert to new information and patient preferences.

Option

If offers the most opportunity for practice variability.

No Recommendation

Clinicians should always act and make decisions on behalf of patient interests and needs. Guidelines are never intended to overrule professional judgement.

PREREQUISITES FOR SAFE PAEDIATRIC ANAESTHESIA PRACTICE[15]

1. **Staff:** All personnel (including nurses, technicians, surgeons and anaesthesiologists) working in the paediatric operating theatre should be well trained in paediatric care.
2. **Equipment:** Paediatric anaesthesia equipment and monitors are mandatory.
   - This includes equipment for airway and vascular access, along with minimum mandatory and other desirable monitors.
   - The anaesthesia machine should be able to deliver small, accurate tidal volumes and ventilator modes.
   - Resuscitation drugs and equipment should be available immediately, if required.
   - Temperature monitoring and warming devices should be available.
   - Fluids recommended for paediatric use are essential.
3. **Supportive services:**
   - As far as possible all children should have a preoperative assessment. Counselling of parents can be done simultaneously.
   - Preoperative investigations should be kept to a minimum, unless specifically indicated.[16]
   - An acute pain service (APS) should be in place.
4. **Postoperative care:**
   - All children should have a dedicated recovery area for postoperative care.
   - A neonatal and paediatric intensive care unit (PICU, NICU) is necessary for intensive care management.
   - Hospital protocols should be in place for management of critically ill children.
5. **Day care surgery and anaesthesia:**
   - Day care surgery should be encouraged.
   - The facility should be adequately equipped for day care anaesthesia.
   - Discharge criteria should be clearly followed in the recovery room.
   - Clear postoperative instructions should be given to the parents.
   - All children should be given adequate postoperative analgesia.
6. **Training and research:**
   - Training is an essential component of successful paediatric anaesthesia services.
   - Ethical research in paediatric anaesthesia should be encouraged.
   - Regular audit should be conducted.
   - Morbidity and mortality meetings should be held regularly.
7. **Administration:**
   - Any child requiring tertiary care management should be transferred accordingly to a tertiary care centre.
   - Quality commitment should be practised in the hospitals providing paediatric anaesthesia services.
8. **Informed consent:**
   - An informed consent for anaesthesia and surgery is essential.
   - Parents should be provided with full written information about the operative procedure and the anaesthesia which is going to be provided to their child.

Evidence Based Guideline for Cuffed / Non-cuffed ETT

The cuffed/non cuffed tube debate has reached a climax with the publication of the prospective randomized controlled trial by European Paediatric Endotrached Intubation Study Group.[17] This trial demonstrated that the use of microcuff tracheal tube is effective and safe in neonates and young children. A tracheal tube—microcuff paediatric *endotracheal tube* (PET), with an anatomically designed high volume, low pressure tube cuff was investigated in a large prospective randomized multicentre trial. The results indicate that cuffed tracheal tubes in small children provide a reliably sealed airway at cuff pressures ≤ 20 cm H_2O decreasing the need for tracheal tube exchanges (2.1 vs 30.8). The study, however, is only valid when the microcuff tracheal tube is used and cuff pressure is limited < 20 cm H_2O.

RECENT DEVELOPMENT IN PAEDIATRIC ANAESTHESIA EQUIPMENT [18]

Advance	Description
Airway	
Microcuff	High-volume low-pressure tube cuff
Video laryngoscope	Better view than conventional laryngoscope
Ventilation	
Ventilators	To deliver small and accurate tidal volume
Pressure/Assisted ventilation	Supraglottic airway devices
Circulation	
Safety IV cannula	To reduce needle stick injuries
Vein viewer	Assists in accessing difficult veins
Regional anaesthesia	
Ultrasound	May be helpful, however, learning curve

EVIDENCE BASED PRACTICE TO REDUCE THE RISK OF MEDICATION ERRORS

A number of evidence based recommendations for safer medication were formulated and tested against a database of incident reports involving medication errors.[19]

These Recommendations Include

- Countermeasures to be used to decrease the number of drug administration errors in anaesthesia.
- The label of any drug ampoule should be legible.
- Syringes should be correctly labeled.
- Labels should be rechecked by another individual before drawing up the drug.
- Organized and well arranged drawers where drugs are kept.
- Errors should be reported and reviewed regularly.
- Similar packaging of medicines should be avoided.[18, 20]

Evidence Based Initiatives have Reduced Drug Errors in Paediatric Practice by

- Routine measurement of weight of the child.
- Standardized concentration of continuous infusions.
- Standardized concentration of oral medications.
- Paediatric-sized packaging of drugs.
- Bar codes on medications.
- Colour coding of syringe labels.[20]

EVIDENCE BASED GUIDELINES TO MAKE PAEDIATRIC ANAESTHESIA SAFE

Certain 'key' points in the operating room are considered as high risk moments. These are departure from induction room, arrival in and departure from the OR, and arrival in the PACU. Usually the anaesthesiologist alone takes responsibility to remember these key points.

This sole responsibility of one individual may, at times, lead to errors. The introduction of ***'flow check lists'*** at each key point has increased patient safety and minimized 'errors.'[21]

The concept of using a checklist in surgical and anaesthetic practice was energized by a publication of the WHO Surgical Safety Checklist 2008.

It was believed that by routinely checking common safety issues and by better team communication and dynamics, perioperative morbidity and mortality could be improved. In fact checklists can make paediatric anaesthesia care safe and effective.[22]

The use of checklists, in particular, improves adherence to evidence based care in crisis situations, reduces blood product utilization and improves communication during the patient hand off process.[23]

Quality improvement initiatives like successful use of checklists have reduced catheter associated blood stream infections. The countermeasures used to reduce potential contamination were level 1 interventions, including education regarding intraoperative hand sanitation, and level 2 interventions like checklists for cleaning of anaesthesia workspace during OR turnover, and placing a hand sanitizer.[24]

Paediatric critic events checklists have been published by the 'Society of Paediatric Anaesthesia, Quality and Safety Committee.'

Checklist Can be

- Read and do checks or
- Challenge and response checks or
- Aide memoires or
- Combination of all three

Checklists should ideally be one page, simple, with familiar language and each element should contain no more than five to nine items. Checklists should be evidence based, should address key safety issues which if omitted would lead to serious adverse events.[25,26]

Guidelines for Placement of Central Venous Catheter

The National Institute of Clinical Excellence (NICE) in the United Kingdom advocates the use of ultrasound technology for placement of central venous cannulae where possible.[27]

However, there is currently insufficient evidence to support the use of ultrasound guidance for central venous catheterization in children.[15]

EVIDENCE BASED PRACTICE IN POSTOPERATIVE AND PROCEDURAL PAIN MANAGEMENT

Evidence based guideline for the management of postoperative and procedural pain has been developed by several associations and societies.

Pain assessment and measurement of pain intensity are vital components in pain management.[28]

The various methods which may be used to assess pain according to chronological age are:

Age	Scale
Newborn–3 years	COMFORT or FLACC
4 years	FPS–R and COMFORT and FLACC
5–7 years	FPS–R
7 years and more	VAS or NRS

Recommendations

- No individual measure can be broadly recommended for pain assessment across all children (Grade B).
- Children's self report of their pain, is the preferred approach, where possible (Grade B).
- In 3–5 years age group, along with child's self report, an observational measure should also be used, since the validity of self report in this age group is not reliable (Grade B).
- Use of physiological parameters alone, is not recommended (Grade D).

The results of pain assessment must be documented.

For brief procedures (myringotomy)

- Oral paracetamol or NSAIDs can provide adequate pain relief in the early postoperative period (Grade B).
- Opioids are effective, but not recommended routinely because of side-effects (Grade B).

Tonsillectomy

- Combination of intraoperative opioids, dexamethasone and regular perioperative mild analgesics are recommended (Grade A).
- Topical application or injection of local anaesthetic in tonsillar fossa improves early pain scores (Grade A).
- Intraoperative IV ketamine does not provide advantage over opioids (Grade B).
- Peritonsillar injection of tramadol is of no advantage over systemic injection (Grade B).

Circumcision and *orchidopexy*

Caudal epidural and dorsal nerve blocks are effective in the early postoperative period, with very few side effects and complications (Grade A).

For neonatal circumcision—a multimodal analgesic technique with local anaesthesia and paracetamol syrup should be considered.

Inguinal hernia repair

Use of an ultrasound guided method for an ilioinguinal nerve block should be encouraged.

Cleft lip and palate related surgery

Infraorbital block provides effective postoperative analgesia (Grade A).

GUIDELINES FOR USE OF IV CANNULAE

Recent introduction of 'safety' IV cannulae have the potential to reduce 'sharps' injuries. However, difficulty in inserting them has been a concern as compared to the conventional IV cannulae.

However after a short learning curve, it is believed that they are easy to insert. The current evidence is that the 'safety' IV cannulae are difficult to insert in difficult veins, and it is advisable that the standard IV cannula should also be available in difficult situations.[18]

Association of Paediatric Anaesthesia (APA) Council 2013

In an **unanticipated** 'difficult bag mask ventilation' (BMV) scenario, or a 'difficult tracheal intubation' scenario in a child aged 1 to 8 years, administer 100% oxygen and call for help. The guidelines provided by the APA should be followed.

GUIDELINES FOR THE MANAGEMENT OF POSTOPERATIVE NAUSEA AND VOMITING[29]

Postoperative nausea and vomiting (PONV) are common and distressing to patients. In children POV rate can be twice as high in adults which suggests a greater need for POV prophylaxis.[30]

The present guidelines are most recent data on PONV and an update on 2 previous sets of guidelines published in 2003 and 2007.

Guidelines: Identify children at risk of PONV.[31]

Eberhart et al. identified 4 independent predictors of POV in children.

- History of PONV in child sibling or parent.
- Age >3 years.
- Duration of surgery >30 min.
- Squint surgery.

Guidelines: Reduce baseline risk factors for PONV.

- Avoidance of GA by the use of regional anaesthesia.
- Use of propofol for induction and maintenance.
- Avoidance of N_2O and volatile anaesthetics.
- Adequate hydration.
- Minimization of intraoperative and postoperative opioids.

Guidelines: PONV prophylaxis with 1 to 2 interventions for children with medium risk.

Antiemetic doses for prophylaxis of POV in children shown in the table below.

Drug	Dose
Dexamethasone	150 mcg/kg up to 5 mg
Dimenhydrinate	0.5 mg/kg up to 25 mg
Dolasetron	350 mcg/kg up to 12.5 mg
Droperidol*	10–15 mcg/kg up to 1.25 mg
Granisetron	40 mcg/kg up to 0.6 mg
Ondansetron**	50–100 mcg/kg up to 4 mg
Tropisetron	0.1 mg/kg up to 2 mg

Evidence based recommendations and not all the drugs have an FDA indication for PONV.

*See FDA black box warning. Recommended doses 10–15 mcg/kg.

**Approved for POV in paediatric patients aged 1 month and older.

Guidelines: At increased risk of PONV, the most effective prophylactic antiemetic therapy is a combination therapy.

- Combinations in children
- Ondansetron, 0.05 mg/kg, + dexamethasone 0.015 mg/kg
- Tropisetron, 0.1 mg/kg, + dexamethasone, 0.5 mg/kg (A1) [32]

Guidelines: Provide antiemetic treatment to children with PONV who did not receive prophylaxis or in whom prophylaxis failed, use antiemetics from different class than prophylactic drug.

- Re-administer only if >6 hrs in PACU
- Do not re-administer dexamethasone.

Guidelines: Ensure PONV prophylaxis and clinical management when required.

PSYCHOLOGY, ANXIETY, AND PREOPERATIVE PREPARATION

Preoperative Preparation

Paediatric anaesthesiologists play a very challenging role in preoperative preparation for anaesthesia in children.

Most children experience significant preoperative anxiety as they cannot comprehend the need for treatment or hospitalization. In addition, they have the fear of unknown hospital environment, unprepared to encounter strangers dressed in unusual clothes, fear of separation from parents and also afraid of painful procedures like operation and anaesthesia. This issue becomes a highly challenging job when it comes to handling autistic children.[33]

To this, they not only immediately react with fear, withdrawal and struggling, but also have long-term effects on psychological and behavioural well-being.[34] The bizarre postoperative maladaptive behaviour can include general anxiety, temper tantrums, night-crying, feeding difficulties, sleep disturbance, apathy, withdrawal, fear of separation leading to clinging to mother and new-onset nocturnal enuresis. The incidence is greatest in preschoolers and sometimes it is very difficult to treat these postoperative behavioural problems. Thus alleviating preoperative anxiety is very important not only for compassionate reasons, but mainly for improving postoperative behaviour.

Almost every child is a potential difficult child, unless assessed and tackled appropriately. Preoperative anxiety is similar for elective and emergency procedures.[35] The various factors responsible for preoperative anxiety can be related to the environment, parents or the child himself.

The exclusively children hospitals are usually designed with all colorful setup and playful activities. But since most of our hospitals are not solely dedicated to children, the prevailing atmosphere is totally unsuitable for an already scared child. That is why a part of the preoperative holding area should be made child-friendly by putting colorful toys, games, etc.

Anxiety percolates to an innocent child from highly anxious parents. That is the reason parental preparation is a very important task accomplished by a detailed discussion about the risks and benefits of anaesthesia and surgery.

Age is an utmost important factor. A child with previous unpleasant experience with any medical proceedings may have significant anxiety. A shy or inhibited temperament or lack of developmental maturity and social adaptability play a very significant role. Nevertheless, a very hungry and thirsty child is also difficult to manage.

The various interventions for preventing preoperative anxiety and stress can be categorized into non-pharmacological modalities (psychological preparation) and pharmacological modalities (premedication).

Psychological development is related to the age of the child, so the interventions should be age-appropriate.[36] The medical personnel should be empathetic to both children and parents and also should be accustomed to caring for small children with good communication skill.

Prehospital programmes include tours of hospital and theatre, videos and leaflets to reduce anxiety. The effectiveness of these psychological preparation programmes in reducing anxiety in preoperative room is well established, but of questionable value during induction of anaesthesia. Extreme anxiety during induction probably inhibits processing and implementing of contents of preparation programme by children.[37,38]

Infants <8 months of age accept a parent substitute well, as separation anxiety usually starts at 8 months of age. They usually respond well to **physical contact, soothing** sound and gentle rocking and remain calm and comfortable if fasting is not prolonged.

Children of 1–3 years of age is more likely to display separation anxiety and are unable to comprehend any explanation. **Distraction technique** with toys and stories work very well when done efficiently.

Children of 3–6 years age group are still anxious about separation, but tend to respond to full explanation of what is to happen, so **reassurance** works. They mainly fear needles, torture and bodily injury, thus there is a requirement for explanation of events in a very clear and simple language as they tend to believe things literally. Use parental inputs about child's likes and dislikes and his close friend's name and birthday events which helps them to distract while putting an intravenous cannula, with prior EMLA cream application. Therapeutic play using syringes on dolls eases their anxiety too.

In age group of 7–12 years, parental separation is less of a problem and is much more amenable to reassurance. They can think logically about real objects, but have trouble understanding hypothetical concepts. So a thorough, honest and reassuring explanation regarding premedication and induction is essential. They may be given a choice of inhalation or intravenous induction and should participate in holding the mask for inhalation induction.

Adolescents have to be tackled with care as they also have fears but do not express them so easily. They may fear loss of control and death, thus need reassurance in terms of safety of modern anaesthesia practice and full control of postoperative pain management.

PARENTAL PRESENCE DURING INDUCTION OF ANAESTHESIA (PPIA)

There are varying view points about PPIA in literature. PPIA is well-established in many centres, however, there is no evidence of reduction in preoperative anxiety of child at induction or postoperative behavioural problems though it improves parental satisfaction.[39,40] However, PPIA is of enormous help during induction of children with developmental delays and behavioural problem.

In < 8 months of age group, PPIA is not indicated as separation anxiety does not exist and moreover, events like breath holding, upper airway obstruction and desaturation occur more frequently which need quick and full attention of anaesthesiologist without having to be concerned about parent's presence and emotions.[41] In children up to 3 years, the child tends to cling to the parents making inhalation induction more difficult, whereas in 4–6 years age group it is of benefit as less physical restraint is required. The parents should be mentally prepared for changes that occur during induction, like rapid loss of consciousness, incoordinated movements, upper airway obstruction, requirement of using force and restraint and should not get psychologically distressed by the experience. The contraindication to PPIA is an unwilling parent or an over-anxious parent. The benefit is measurable whenever a calm parent accompanies an anxious child and worsening effect with the reverse and no measurable benefit for both a calm parent and the child. Increase in parental satisfaction score is an advantage, whereas logistical disadvantages are of limited space, unfamiliar equipment and need to be escorted to waiting room as soon as loss of consciousness of the child occurs.

Pharmacological Intervention

Premedication is indicated in very anxious children or parents, when crying is detrimental (i.e. may deteriorate cyanosis), in pain (burns/trauma), previous negative memories, a longer waiting time and children with neurobehavioral disorders.

The various premedicants used are midazolam, dexmedetomidine, fentanyl and ketamine. The various routes used are oral, transmucosal (sublingual/ intranasal) and rectal in decreasing order of acceptability. Parenteral routes are generally avoided or used as a last resort.

The benefits of premedication are easier parental separation, no recollection of events if adequately sedated, improved co-operation and manageability, and a lower incidence of emergency delirium and haemodynamic stability. The first and foremost drawback of premedication is that timing of premedication is critical and premature separation or unanticipated delay should be avoided. Sometimes prolongs recovery phase leading to delayed discharge after minor daycare cases.

Midazolam is the most commonly used premedicant in children for its safety profile, reliability and effectiveness. Its beneficial effects are anxiolysis, sedation, anterograde amnesia, fast onset and limited duration of action, whereas its bitter taste and paradoxical excitement in some children are the demerits. A dose range of 0.2–1 mg/kg via various routes has been reported to be effective and early parental separation possible as it confers anteregrade amnesia in as little as 10 minute.[42] The dose of oral midazolam increases with decreasing age.[43,44]

Dexmedetomidine, a highly-selective α_2-adrenoreceptor agonist with a short half-life, possesses sedative, anxiolytic, sympathetic and analgesic properties without significant respiratory depression and reduces anaesthetic requirement too.[45] It is a suitable alternative to midazolam in a dose range oral of 1–2 µg/kg and provides more effective preoperative sedation as compared to midazolam across all age groups and allows a smooth induction and awakening especially in preschooler.[46–48]

For cognitively impaired children, ketamine is a suitable premedicant for its hypnotic and analgesic effect with excellent cardiovascular and respiratory stability. IM ketamine (2–5 mg/kg) has an onset time of approximately 10 minutes. Oral ketamine (5–6 mg/kg) is a suitable alternative to oral midazolam although, emesis is a problem with ketamine.

Combination premedications like oral ketamine (3 mg/kg) along with midazolam either oral (0.3 mg/kg) or intranasal (2 µg/kg) are suitable for children with increased risk for negative behavioural problems at induction of anaesthesia without the side effects of larger doses of ketamine alone.[49–50]

For a smooth recovery in postoperative period, the important factors like pain, emergence delirium, hypoxia, hypercapnia, airway obstruction, hypoglycemia, hypotension, bladder distension, PONV and hunger should be considered and prophylactically managed.

CONCLUSION

A preoperative assessment visit is a must which gives both an opportunity to assess fitness for anaesthesia and to provide reassurance to the child and his parents. To sum up, the objective is to have a calm and cooperative child up to the induction room, allow smooth induction of anaesthesia and a comfortable postoperative period. Despite increased awareness and acknowledgement of preoperative anxiety, variations in practice remain. Success is highly dependent on the skill, experience and empathy of the anaesthesiologist.

REFERENCES

1. Sackett DL, Rosenberg WM, Gray JA, et al. Evidence based medicine: What it is and what it isn't. BMJ. 1996;312:71–2.
2. Timmermans S, Mauck A. The promises and pitfalls of evidence-based medicine. Health Aff 2005;24:18–28.
3. Sackett DL, Strauss SE, Richardson NS, et al. EBM: How to practice and teach EBM 4th edn. London: Churchill Livingstone 2000.
4. Mark h, E Bell MD MS. Professor University of Georgia Editor in Chief—essential evidence plus. http://www.essentialevidenceplus.com/product/ebm_overview.cfm

5. Greenhalgh, Trisha. How to Read a Paper: The Basics of Evidence-Based Medicine 4th edn. John Wiley & Sons. 2010;p. 1.
6. Eddy DM. Evidence-based medicine: A unified approach. Health Aff. 2005;24:9–17.
7. Lim W, Arnold DM, Bachanova V, et al. Evidence-Based Guidelines—An Introduction. ASH Education Book 2008;26–30.
8. Sullivan AM, Lakoma MD, Billings JA, et al. PCEP Core Faculty. Teaching and learning end-of-life care: Evaluation of a faculty development program in palliative care. Acad Med. 2005;80:657–68.
9. Balshem H, Helfand M, Schünemann HJ, et al. GRADE guidelines: 3. Rating the quality of evidence. J Clin Epidemiol. 2011;64:401–6.
10. Kariminia A, Chamberlain ME, Keogh J, et al. Randomised controlled trial of effect of hands and knees posturing on incidence of occiput posterior position at birth. BMJ. 2004;328:490.
11. Charlton BG. Restoring the balance: Evidence-based medicine put in its place. J Eval Clin Pract 1997;3:87–98.
12. Guyatt G, Cook D, Haynes B. Evidence based medicine has come a long way. BMJ 2004;329:990–1.
13. Woolf SH, Grol R, Hutchinson A, et al. Clinical guidelines: potential benefits, limitations, and harms of clinical guidelines. BMJ 1999;318:527–30.
14. American Academy of Paediatrics. Classifying recommendations for Clinical Practice Guideline. Paediatrics 2004;114:874–877.
15. Wilkinson KA, Brennan LJ, Rollin AM. Guidelines for the provision of anaesthetic services. Paediatric anaesthesia services. www.rcoa.ac.uk/gpas2013.
16. The use of routine pre-operative tests for elective surgery (Guidance CG3) Nice, London 2008 (reviewed June 2010) www.niceorg.UK/nicemedia/pdf/preop_fuliguideline.pdf.
17. Weiss M, Dullenkopf A, Fischer JE, et al. European Paediatric Endotracheal Intubation Study Group. Prospective randomized controlled multi-centre trial of cuffed or uncuffed endotracheal tubes in small children. Br J Anaesth 2009; 103:867–73.
18. Campbell S, Wilson G, Engelhardt T. Equipment and monitoring – what is in the future to improve safety? Paediatric Anaesthesia 2011;21:815–24.
19. Jensen LS, Merry AF, Webster CS, et al. Evidence-based strategies fro preventing drug administration errors during anaesthesia. Anaesthesia 2004;59:493–504.
20. Merry AF, Anderson BJ. Medication errors—new approaches to prevention. Paediatr Anaesth. 2011; 21: 743–53.
21. Low DK, Reed MA, Geiduschek JM, et al. Striving for a zero-error patient surgical journey through adoption of aviation-style challenge and response flow checklists: A quality improvement project. Paediatr Anaesth. 2013; 23:571–8.
22. Ziewacz JE, Arriaga AF, Bader AM, et al. Crisis checklists for the operating room: Development and pilot testing. J Am Coll Surg. 2011;213:212-217.
23. Hagerman NS, Varughese AM, Kurth CD. Quality and safety in paediatric anaesthesia: How can guidelines, checklists, and initiatives improve the outcome? Curr Opin Anaesthesiol. 2014; 27:323–9.
24. Martin LD, Rampersad SE, Geiduschek JM, et al. Modification of anaesthesia practice reduces catheter-associated bloodstream infections: A quality improvement initiative. Paediatr Anaesth. 2013;23:588–96.
25. Weiser TG, Haynes AB, Lashoher A, et al. Perspectives in quality: Designing the WHO Surgical Safety Checklist. Int J Qual Health Care. 2010; 22:365–70.
26. Walker IA, Reshamwalla S, Wilson IH. Surgical safety checklists: Do they improve outcomes? Br J Anaesth. 2012;109:47–54.
27. http://www·MUE·org·UK/nicemedia/pdf/ultrasound 49 GUIDANCE
28. Association of Paediatric Anaesthetists of Great Britain and Ireland. Good practice in postoperative and procedural pain management, 2nd edition. Paediatr Anaesth. 2012; 22(Suppl 1):1–79.
29. Gan TJ, Diemunsch P, Habib AS, et al. Society for Ambulatory Anaesthesia. Consensus guidelines for the management of postoperative nausea and vomiting. Anesth Analg. 2014;118:85–113.
30. Gan TJ, Meyer T, Apfel CC, et al. Department of Anesthesiology, Duke University Medical Center. Consensus guidelines for managing postoperativenausea and vomiting. Anesth Analg 2003;97:62–71.
31. Eberhart LH, Geldner G, Kranke P, et al. The development and validation of a risk score to predict the probability of postoperative vomiting in paediatric patients. Anesth Analg 2004;99:1630–7.
32. Holt R, Rask P, Coulthard KP, et. al. Tropisetron plus dexamethasone is more effective than tropisetron alone for the prevention of postoperative nausea and vomiting in children undergoing tonsillectomy. Paediatr Anaesth 2000;10:181–8.
33. Rainey L, van der Walt JH. The anaesthetic management of autistic children. Anaesth Intensive Care. 1998;26:682–6.
34. Kain ZN, Wang SM, Mayes LC, et al. Distress during the induction of anaesthesia and postoperative behavioral outcomes. Anesth Analg. 1999;88:1042–7.
35. Holm-Knudsen RJ, Carlin JB, McKenzie IM. Distress at induction of anaesthesia in children. A survey of incidence, associated factors and recovery characteristics. Paediatr Anaesth. 1998;8:383–92.

36. McGraw T. Preparing children for the operating room: Psychological issues. Can J Anaesth. 1994;41:1094–103.

37. Kain ZN, Mayes LC, Caramico LA. Preoperative preparation in children: A cross-sectional study. J Clin Anesth. 1996;8:508–14.

38. Kain ZN, Caramico LA, Mayes LC, et al. Preoperative preparation programs in children: A comparative examination. Anesth Analg. 1998;87:1249–55.

39. Yip P, Middleton P, Cyna AM, et al. Non-pharmacological interventions for assisting the induction of anaesthesia in children. Cochrane Database Syst Rev. 2009;(3):CD006447.

40. Scully SM. Parental presence during paediatric anaesthesia induction. AORN J. 2012;96:26–33.

41. Palermo TM, Tripi PA, Burgess E. Parental presence during anaesthesia induction for outpatient surgery of the infant. Paediatr Anaesth. 2000;10:487–91.

42. Kain ZN, Hofstadter MB, Mayes LC, et al. Midazolam: Effects on amnesia and anxiety in children. Anesthesiology. 2000;93:676–84.

43. Coté CJ, Cohen IT, Suresh S, et. al. A comparison of three doses of a commercially prepared oral midazolam syrup in children. Anesth Analg. 2002; 94:37–43.

44. Kain ZN, MacLaren J, McClain BC, et al. Effects of age and emotionality on the effectiveness of midazolam administered preoperatively to children. Anesthesiology. 2007;107:545–52.

45. Yao Y, Qian B, Chen Y, et al. Intranasal dexmedetomidine premedication reduces the minimum alveolar concentration of sevoflurane for tracheal intubation in children: A randomized trial. J Clin Anesth. 2014;26:309–14.

46. Pant D, Sethi N, Sood J. Comparison of sublingual midazolam and dexmedetomidine for premedication in children. Minerva Anestesiol. 2014;80:167–75.

47. Yuen VM, Hui TW, Irwin MG, et al. A comparison of intranasal dexmedetomidine and oral midazolam for premedication in paediatric anaesthesia: A double-blinded randomized controlled trial. Anesth Analg. 2008;106: 1715–21.

48. Yuen VM, Hui TW, Irwin MG, et. al. A randomised comparison of two intranasal dexmedetomidine doses for premedication in children. Anaesthesia. 2012;67:1210–6.

49. Jia JE, Chen JY, Hu X, et al. A randomised study of intranasal dexmedetomidine and oral ketamine for premedication in children. Anaesthesia. 2013;68:944–9.

50. Funk W, Jakob W, Riedl T, et. al. Oral preanaesthetic medication for children: Double-blind randomized study of a combination of midazolam and ketamine vs midazolam or ketamine alone. Br J Anaesth. 2000;84:335–40.

42

Medicolegal and Ethical Aspects of Paediatric Anaesthesia

Mahesh Baldwa, Sushila Baldwa and Varsha Gupta

"The patient will never care how much you know, until they know how much you care."

ETHICAL ASPECTS: FOUR ETHICAL PRINCIPLES OF IMPORTANCE IN BRIEF

There are four basic ethical principles underlying good medico-ethical practice in western countries.[1] These are ***autonomy, justice, beneficence*** **and** ***non-maleficence.*** They sound tongue twisters are also of little help in day today practice yet we shall discuss the age old principles in brief to benefit our insight about ethics.

The first principle is ***autonomy:*** The right of a fully informed parent to choose out of the anaesthesia services offered to the paediatric patient.

The second principle is called ***justice:*** The right to receive what is recommended by paediatric anaesthesiologist.

The third principle is ***beneficence***, the obligation of paediatric anaesthesiologist to do good in a given situation before, during and after the administration of anaesthesia. This does *not* necessarily **imply to preserve life at all costs.** In situations, where outcome in a given situation is living a poor quality life, that it is considered less beneficial for the patient than death itself. In that case death is allowed [Euthanasia is and was illegal and unethical, immoral in India and confirmed after latest Aruna Shanbhag Supreme Court judgement].[2]

The fourth and final principle we shall discuss is ***non-maleficence***: Rhe obligation to avoid doing harm while giving anaesthesia (Latin-primum non nocere).

But we are not going to discuss these ethical principles in detail here since India has codified law on medical ethics-2002.[3] Nor are we going to discuss basic fundamentals legal principles to prove malpractice and negligence which are described in detail in Supreme Court judgement of IMA versus VP Shantha and several other Supreme Court judgements.[4,5] We briefly touch upon them to give you insight as below.

FOUR FUNDAMENTALS LEGAL PRINCIPLES TO PROVE MALPRACTICE AND MEDICAL NEGLIGENCE

1. **Duty:** The Paediatric anaesthesiologist's duty to the patient arises the moment he/she undertakes to contemplate giving anaesthesia to his patient. If there is no fiduciary Paediatric anaesthesiologist–patient relationship, there is no malpractice risk. The relationship is usually created through performance of pre-anaesthetic check up. But may be created without an actual face-to-face meeting between the anaesthesiologist and patient party in implied way through surgeon.

2. **Breach of duty:** Once the Paediatric anaesthesiologist/doctor–patient relationship has been established, then they shall conduct anaesthesia within a reasonable standard of care equivalent to ordinary specialist with that qualification in same circumstances in the same locality. Failure to meet the standard of care has been laid by Bolam's law.[6] While often difficult to define, a reasonable standard of care, which is average, not very high and not very low. Breach of such standard of duty constitutes

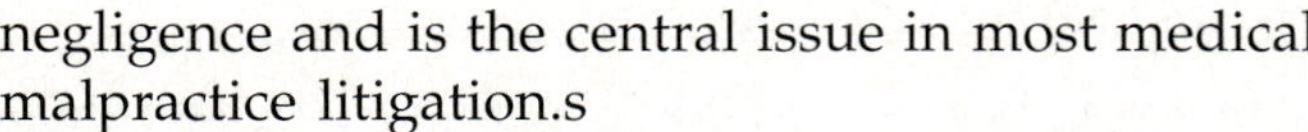

negligence and is the central issue in most medical malpractice litigation.s

3. **Proximity of causation/cause of action:** To be successful in a medical malpractice suit, the plaintiff/ patient party must prove that substandard medical care was the proximate cause of injury to the particular patient.
4. **Actual Injury/damage:** Further, to succeed, the plaintiff/patient party must establish that some type of physical or mental or psychological injury actually occurred. Having shown that a breach of duty caused an injury, one or more of three types of damages might be awarded in the form of monetary payments. These include general damages for pain and suffering; special damages for past, present and future medical expenses and for loss of income, wages, and profits. Punitive damages are generally not awarded by courts in negligence and malpractice suits. Punitive damages are usually granted for gross negligence caused by intentional harm, conscious indifference, or fraud.

DOCTOR–PATIENT RELATIONSHIP

Doctor–patient Relationship is a Pure 'Contract' in Law

So both patient as well as doctor have to agree for this relationship and that too voluntarily.

When it Starts

It arises the moment anaesthesiologist agrees to provide his or her professional services to the patient and the patient accepts this offer.

What is the Domain of Doctor-patient Relationship

Paediatric anaesthesiologist is only responsible to patients whom he undertakes to manage by written/ implied, tacit or presumed consent. Hence a consent document becomes vital piece of evidence in crystallizing doctor–patient relationship. Who are out of the domain of doctor–patient relationship?

Legally, doctor is not responsible towards all patients in general or/at large, but is responsible towards specific patients developing/establishing doctor–patient relationship.

Rights Emanating from Doctor-patient Relationship

A doctor has a right to choose his/her patient. (Regulation 2.4–ETHICS, 2002). A doctor retains the right to choose his or her patients. Ultimately, treatment today is a pure contract between two consenting adults and cannot be forced on a doctor. A doctor is therefore well within his right to refuse treatment to a patient at the outset. A doctor has a right to choose his/her patient (Regulation 2.4–ETHICS, 2002).

Duty of Particular Standard of Care Emanating from Doctor–patient Relationship

Hence next question is to whom a paediatric anaesthesiologist has duty of care? The next logical question is who amongst the patients are entitled to this standard of care. All or only some? The answer is that a doctor is under a legal obligation to provide the 'standard of care' only to those patients to whom the doctor owes the "duty of care". Doctor does not have duty of care towards anyone and everyone whom the doctor meets or speaks, even if that particular conversation is regarding medical science related to unidentified patient. The legal obligation of duty of care starts when legal doctor–patient relationship is established.

To summarize, the standard of care can be stated in simpler terms.

- A doctor must act as other doctors of the same specialty would have acted in same or similar situation.
- The fact that others would have acted differently or the majority does not subscribe to a particular course is simply irrelevant. In fact the courts have gone to the extent of accepting that doctors may even have their personal preferences.
- An injury, death, complication or unfavorable result of treatment will not necessarily mean that the doctor has deviated from the standard of care.

Two more cautions:

i. Nowadays the latest judicial trend in Indian courts is higher. Standard of care is expected from a specialist. A specialist is expected to give a higher standard of care than a non-specialist.
ii. Greater degree of care is expected for legally incompetent patients, i.e. children, lunatics, etc. Greater the disability, greater is the degree of care expected by law from doctors. Greater degree of care is expected for incompetent patients.

What is that conduct which signals doctor–patient relationship as established and when it gets terminated?

Duty of care arises in physical/telephonic/web consultations and emergencies. Duty of care may arise

- By a physical consultation
- By a telephonic conversation or web consultation or
- By legal compulsion—in case of emergencies.

Once the duty of care has arisen, it continues till the happening of any of the following contingencies:

- The patient is relieved of the ailment/anaesthesia.
- The patient is discharged or transferred
- The patient voluntarily seeks discharge from the care of the doctor The doctor terminates his treatment on valid grounds after giving proper notice.
- The patient is dead.
- In case of emergency patients, the emergency ceases to exist.

Some perfectly legal and valid reasons for termination are as follows:

- Failure of patient to pay
- Refusal by the patient to allow implementation of the anaesthesia plan
- Refusal by the patient to follow instructions
- Doctor's change of practice
- Doctor's abandonment of practice.

MEDICOLEGAL ASPECTS OF CONSENT AND RISK EXPLANATION

Informed Consent

A consent should be patient specific, procedure specific, with full disclosure about disease, its investigations and treatment without hiding anything, without misrepresentation, coercion, fraud, undue influence in writing and signed by authorized signatory which is witnessed by two adult people.

Information

Information to be given to patient party as per MCI regulation Chapter 2 which says that doctor should neither exaggerate nor minimise the gravity of the patient condition. He must ensure himself that the patient, his relatives or his responsible friends have such knowledge of patient's condition as well as serve the best interest of the patient and the family.

It is usual for a paediatric anaesthetist to explain to parents of patient and obtain their ascent procedure of anaesthesia, plan of anaesthesia, co-existing conditions influencing general medical status of child as per ASA state and also obtain ascent for further treatment in case patient deteriorates.

Reality About Informed Consent in India

It needs to be ensured that privacy will be maintained. In the context of developing countries, obtaining informed consent has been considered many times as difficult/impractical/not meeting the purpose on various grounds such as incompetence to comprehend the meaning or relevance of the consent and culturally being dependent on the decision of the head of the family. However, there is no alternative to obtaining individual's informed consent.

Who Can Consent

Any person who has completed 18 years of age as per Indian Majority Act 1975 is considered an adult. An adolescent is less than 18 years old, so legal adult status for him is a far-fetched legal dream but at the same time parents and adult relatives cannot arrogate[7] with adolescent rights.[7]

FAQ with Answer

Q. Whether the paediatric anaesthetist should also sign the consent form?

A. Not required as per any legislative act, usage and custom nor recommended by professional bodies. But as per law of contract (s.13 of ICA-1872) literally consent means consensus ad idem, hence signature of other party, i.e. doctor is preferable.

Proxy Consent (Substitute Consent)

Minors/Incompetent/ Emergency Patients—Proxy Consent

1. **Consent and Age**
   i. Child: Patient below 12 years—Take consent of the parents'/guardian only.
   ii. Emancipated child: Patient between 12 and 18 years—Take consent of the patient as well as the parents'/guardian.
   iii. Adult: Patient above 18 years—Take consent of the patient only.
2. **Proxy consent 'giver' for incompetent/ emergency patients**
   i. The lineal descendant or ascendant blood relative, or natural biological parents.
   ii. The person(s) or crowd who may have brought such a patient (e.g. in accident cases), or
   iii. Medical Superintendent or such other responsible person in institutions/hospitals.

3. **Taking proxy consent**
   i. Record specifically the name, address and telephone number of the person from whom proxy consent has been obtained.
   ii. Record specifically the reason for obtaining proxy consent.
   iii. Further, future directions/consent during the treatment may be sought from such a person.
4. Consent of any one of the parent is valid and binding even though there may be difference between both the parents.

Situations where Consent May not be Obtained

Like in medical emergencies. The well being of the patient is of paramount importance, hence medical treatment precedes legal considerations.

1. Do not wait for consent in emergencies. Proceed with oral consent or even without consent.
2. Take proxy consent, only if possible and without much effort.
3. Record specifically in the patient's medical records and/or the consent form the emergency as well as the reason(s) for not obtaining consent or for obtaining proxy consent. This exercise can be done once the emergency is over.

Duty of Care During Emergency Requires no Consent

In emergency situation, "duty of care" requires each and every doctor to attend emergency patients irrespective of specialty or whether he/she is your patient or not. This does not apply to routine and cold patients. The Supreme Court in the case of Parmanand Katara v/s Union of India wherein it was stated, "Every doctor whether at a government hospital or otherwise has the professional obligation to extend his services with due expertise for protecting life, the obligation being total, absolute and paramount."[8]

When Consent is not Valid

Consent given under fear, fraud or misrepresentation of facts, or by a person who is ignorant of the implications of the consent, or who is under 12 years of age is invalid (Sec. 90 IPC[9]).

What is implied consent

Consent that is inferred from the action of the person.

What is tacit consent

Consent can be silently or passively by omission/passage of time/ignored/waiver

What is presumed consent

Consent is presumed on the basis of knowledge, intelligence and values and beliefs of the patient.

Implied Consent (Presumed /Tacit Consent) for Paediatric Anaesthesiologists

This is by far the most common variety of consent. Paediatric anaesthesiologists in India do not obtain separate consent in practice and usually depend upon consent obtained by surgeons/hospital. The fact that a patient comes to you though indirectly for administering anaesthesia, you cannot depend on implied consent obtained by surgeons/hospital when a legal trouble arises.

Consent Form Should at Least Contain

1. Printed Consent form in English can have printed translated version in the local language appended.
2. Consent form can also be filled in the local language or the language understood by the patient.
3. Printed consent forms must have enough space to fill complete additional information.
4. Take the patient party's signature/initials on every page of the consent form.
5. Doctor-in-charge of the patient/principal surgeon/anaesthetist should also sign the consent form in whose presence parents/relatives have given consent with date and time written below signatures.
6. Consent form can have suitable directions from the patient indicating names of relatives/attendants whose directions should be followed in case the patient is not in a position to give direction, regarding what needs to be done in case patient is incapacitated to communicate. Patients can fill column/space provided for such direction with full name, address and telephone numbers of such relatives/friends and can also indicate the order of preference amongst them.

Risk Explanation/Information

1. Explain the potential risks of anaesthesia to the patient/patient's relative, especially the commonly occurring ones and enumerate such risks in the consent.

2. Risks having probability of 10% or more must be specifically spelt out to the parents and duly recorded in the consent.
3. Answer any specific question raised by the parents about risks and record the same in the consent. Risk involving loss of vision, hearing, mental function, loss of function of limbs and organs must be specified even though the risk may be rare.

Take 'High-Risk Consent'/Post-Operative Ventilatory Support Consent

1. Consent for tracheostomy
2. High risk consent for haemodynamically unstable patients/metabolically unstable patients, patient with electrolyte imbalances, surgical shock, bacteremia, toxaemia, septicemia, DIC, serious and complicated nature of surgery/latest/new surgical procedures.
3. Removing any organ, e.g. diseased organ like testes in tortion of testes, removal of kidney which is a threat to other kidney. Document reason for removal and insist on sending for histopathological examination after removing, if done under anaesthesia.
4. Removing any limb or finger, eye, hearing organ, teeth.
5. High risk patients, specify and justify medically, scientifically in consent form.
6. Proceeding with a surgery/procedure in spite of any abnormal parameter. Record both the abnormality as well as the reasons for proceeding for anaesthesia
7. Paediatric patient with syndrome pattern.

Because complications and errors are common so do not hold out any guarantee/ warranty

Do not hold out any guarantee/warranty for no mishap. Never hold out for 100% mishap freedom. Tell patient that risks exist though are rare.

Always minimize patient related mishaps to minimum by issuing written warnings and restrictions

Give warnings and restrictions regarding nil by mouth in writing, time and type of food before anaesthesia and postanaesthesia care.

Consent for Postmortem (PM)

1. Legally two types of death may need PM,
   a. PM after natural death where cause of death is not known.
   b. PM for all unnatural deaths which includes table death, postoperative death.
2. If death is natural, then the dead body is the property of relatives but if death is unnatural, then dead body becomes the property of state.
3. For PM in natural death: Consent of nearest relatives [father, mother, etc.] is required.
4. PM for unnatural death: Consent for PM is not required but information to local police is required.

Consent Key Points

1. Informed consent is the legal embodiment of the concept of the right to make decisions regarding one's well-being.
2. Informed consent should be based on the 'professional standard' or peer 'accepted risks' approach, or the 'materiality risk' or 'prudent patient' approach.
3. If the risk involved can have severe consequences, like death or serious disability, it is material and should be disclosed independent of the frequency of the occurrence.
4. Severe risks (e.g. death, paralysis, loss of eyesight or hearing and damage to any other sense organ) should always be disclosed, even when the probability of their occurrence is almost negligible.

REFERENCES

1. Gillon R, (1994). "Medical ethics: four principles plus attention to scope". British Medical Journal. 309(184). Doi:10.1136/bmj.309.6948.184.
2. Aruna Ramchandra Shanbaug vs Union of India and Ors. on 7 March, 2011, Bench: Markandey Katju, Gyan Sudha Misra.
3. The Indian Medical Council (Professional conduct, Etiquette and Ethics) Regulations, 2002.
4. Indian Medical Association vs VP Shantha and Ors on 13 November, 1995: 1996 AIR 550, 1995 SCC (6) 651.
5. Jacob Mathew vs State of Punjab & Anr on 5 August, 2005, Bench: R Lahoti, G Mathur, P.K. Balasubramanyan, CASE NO.: Appeal (crl.) 144–145 of 2004, Martin F. D'Souza vs Mohd. Ishfaq on 17 February, 2009, Bench: G Singhvi, JJ, Katju JJ, Civil Appellate Jurisdiction, Civil Appeal No. 3541 OF 2002, V. Kishan Rao vs Nikhil Super Speciality Hospital on 8 March, 2010, Bench: G.S. Singhvi, Asok Kumar Ganguly, In the supreme court of india, Civil appellate jurisdiction, Civil appeal no.2641_of 2010.
6. Bolam vs Friern Hospital Management Committee [1957] 1 WLR 582.

7. Arrogate means not undermine and prevail over welfare of adolescent, law ensures under S.125 of Criminal Procedure Code, 1973 and S. 317 of Indian Penal Code, 1860 along with S. 68 of Indian contract Act, 1872 that minors are looked after for their physical, mental, economic safety and generally and normally adults responsible are: 1. Natural parents, 2. Legally appointed guardians by court of law 3. Court itself shall ensure safety under Guardians and Wards act, 1890 their safety and security. If law enforcing authority or any person complaints welfare of adolescent legally breached, then law court shall be put in motion. If doctor or any other social spirited person or police asks for permission for benefit of such adolescent court shall be prompt to grant it for adolescent's benefit.
8. Pt. Parmanand Katara vs Union of India and Ors on 28 August, 1989: 1989 AIR 2039, 1989 SCR (3) 997.
9. Aruna Ramchandra Shanbaug vs Union of India and Ors. on 7 March, 2011, Bench: Markandey Katju, Gyan Sudha Misra

Medicolegal Aspects of Record Keeping and Operation Table Death during Anaesthesia

Mahesh Baldwa, Sushila Baldwa and Varsha Gupta

"Doctors and patients may forget but records will always remember."

RECORD KEEPING IN PAEDIATRIC ANAESTHESIOLOGY

Record Keeping as Per Ethics 2002[1]

The issue of medical record keeping has been addressed in the Medical Council of India Regulations 2002 guidelines answering many questions regarding medical records. The important issues that have been addressed are as follows:

1. Maintain indoor records along with anaesthesia records in a standard proforma for 3 years from commencement of treatment (Section 1.3.1 and Appendix 3). For anaesthesia records no particular format is prescribed. Customarily anaesthesia records should contain pre-anaesthetic check up, anaesthesia details during surgery with monitoring of vital parameters, anaesthesia reversal notes , post anaesthesia recovery room notes.
2. Request for medical records by patient or authorized attendant should be acknowledged and documents issued within 72 hours (Section 1.3.2).
3. Maintain a register of certificates with the full details of medical certificates issued with at least one identification mark of the patient and his signature (Section 1.3.3).
4. Efforts should be made to computerize medical records for quick retrieval (Section 1.3.4).

Medical Records as Evidence

Medical records are usually accepted as irrefutable piece of evidence as per Section 3 of the Indian Evidence Act[2] in a court of law established in India.

How Long to Maintain Records

1. Ideally records of adult patients are maintained for 3 years and children, for 21 years. (3 + 18 years), or till child grows up to become an adult to be able to sue. For mentally retarded children, one needs to keep records forever till the person is practicing.[3]
2. From Income tax point of view for seven years.[4]
3. As per code of medical ethics April, 2002 for 3 years.
4. As per Section 24 A of Consumer Protection Act for 3 years.[5]
5. As per Limitation Act for 2 years.[6]

How to Destroy Records

1. By giving public notice, in English as well as vernacular newspaper, with a time limit of usually one month from date of publication in which any one who wants the relevant case paper can come and take a copy of record needed.
2. After one month destroy records of everyone except,
   a. Where litigation is going on
   b. Pre-litigation process of notice exchange is going on
   c. Mentally ill or retarded patients
   d. Where you expect that there could be future trouble.

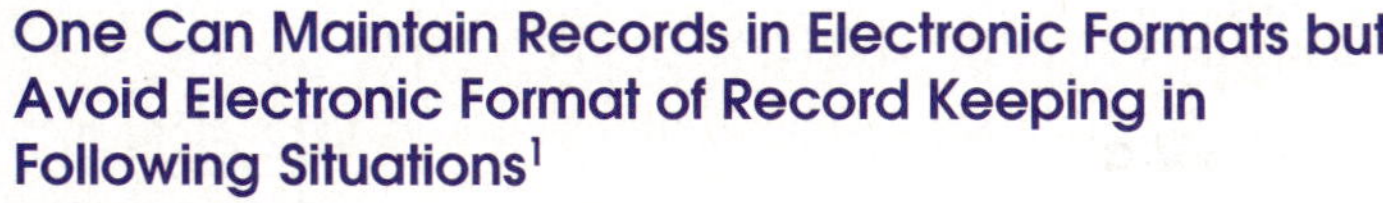

One Can Maintain Records in Electronic Formats but Avoid Electronic Format of Record Keeping in Following Situations[1]

1. They are
   a. Frequent monitoring of vitals parameters and investigations are required.
   b. Moribund patient
   c. Patient who develop complications of disease, drug, surgery, anaesthesia or procedure
   d. Patients who suddenly take a serious turn involving a lot of expenditure
   e. Patients which are transferred or referred to other hospitals/doctors
   f. Accident/suicide/attempted homicide/poisoning/burns/fracture/tetanus and cases involving violence, child abuse, child sexual abuse causing disease or injury
2. Consent needs to be on hard copy
3. Transfer to other hospital needs hard copy
4. Referral to doctor/investigations needs hard copy
5. Police cases need hard copy

Tampering/Manipulation and Alteration and keeping records blank are not permitted by law

The National Commission in another case held that the hospital was guilty of negligence on the ground that the name of the anaesthetists was not mentioned in the operation notes though anaesthesia was administered by two anaesthetists. There were two progress cards about the same patient on two separate papers that were produced in court.[2]

SUDDEN OPERATION TABLE DEATH DURING ANAESTHESIA RESORTING TO VIOLENCE /EXTORTION/ DEFAMATION BY PATIENT PARTY

Odious Situation

It is rather impossible to find a medical professional, who would say that they never faced a medico-legal situation called "Sudden unexpected death" and world at large, gazing in their face as if they were responsible for death. This type of scenario where treating team of doctors are made to feel guilty about sudden unexpected death by relatives is not uncommon[3].

A spectrum of medicolegal reactions from patient party affecting medical professional may be as below and their probable legal solutions are:

1. **Violence by patient party:** Sometimes in the event of sudden unexpected death of child occurring in front of accompanying relatives, at slightest provocation they may take law in their own hands and bash doctors and other staff members along with destroying medical equipment and hospital property. In this case file a FIR in the nearest police station under antiviolence law of respective state, like one in Maharashtra by the name of Medicare Service Persons and Medicare Service Institution (Prevention of Violence, Damage or Loss to Property) Act, 2010. The antiviolence law says anyone who attacks a doctor will be punished with a fine of ₹ 50,000 and imprisonment up to 3 years. Therefore, any attack against doctors is considered as a non-bailable offence. Similar acts are passed by your states. Insist on arresting hooligans.
2. **Arrest of doctor**: Some other times, no sooner than expected, instead relatives asking explanation about sudden unexpected death, you have policemen coming for medicolegal questioning to anaesthetist/doctor/staff as to what happened to deceased child, as they have received a medicolegal complaint from relatives. In the worst case, doctor may be arrested by police on the basis of FIR.[4] Two legal solutions come handy to the arrested doctor.
   i. Keep a copy of Jacob Mathew judgement of Supreme Court which says, without affirmative opinion of expert opining about alleged negligence, police cannot arrest the doctor [last page of judgement].[5]
   ii. Doctor can obtain regular bail Section 437(1) of Cr PC or for imminent arrest one can apply for anticipatory bail under Section 438 of Cr PC.[6]
3. **Extortion by people:** So often in the event of sudden unexpected death, you may receive a politicians telephone to resolve the issue amicably or some social worker actually walking in your office to pay for sudden unexpected death or a local goon threatening you to cough up money immediately for sudden unexpected death without asking for your explanation. The legal solution is to file a police case and move the court for being subjected to extortion under Section 383/384 of IPC.[7]
4. **Defamation:** So often in the event of sudden unexpected death, you may find media and press people gathering around you and your staff members to speak details of sudden unexpected death, which are flashed in defamatory way on TV or newspapers leaving you disgusted. The legal solution is to file a police case and move the court

for being subjected to defamation under Section 499/500 of IPC.[8]

5. **Pleader/advocate notice:** In the event of medicolegal sudden unexpected death, a legal notice might arrive weeks or months later, probing the case and asking for case papers related to medical treatment of deceased along with astronomical compensation. The legal solution is to reply to the notice through your lawyer.[9]
6. **As per the media projection:** One out of ten doctors are dragged in unnecessary prosecutions for medical negligence.[10] Court summons for sudden unexpected death and complaints narrating absurd allegations and asking astronomical sum of money as compensation is going to be on rise in coming days.

It is surprisingly true that in spite of wearing good, empathetic, sympathetic attitude and observing courteousness in communications, allegations of negligence in sudden unexpected death may put medical professionals in a medicolegal maze and leave them disgusted. Medical professionals feel they are framed in alleged medical negligence even though there is no medicolegal issue in sudden unexpected death. A new breed of legal advisors in medicolegal issues of medical negligence are on a rise on the internet who lure relatives of sudden unexpected death and show them big money in prosecuting doctors which cannot be traded off by medical professional wearing good, empathetic, sympathetic attitude and observing courteousness in communications in event of sudden unexpected death.

General solutions to odious situation

1. Membership of large professional organization like Indian Medical association.
2. Good relationship with medical fraternity.
3. Insuring oneself for professional work with professional indemnity with reputed general insurance companies every year without fail.

This subtopic is designed to reduce the trauma accompanied with alleged medical negligence in sudden unexpected death, where there is no medical negligence of doctor. Some knowledge of medicolegal aspects of sudden unexpected death may sharpen your

1. Record keeping skills
2. Communication skills while dealing with relatives, police, and politician or for that matter a goon walking in your office.

> **Medicolegal Pearl**
> In case violence breaks after death of a paediatric patient file FIR in nearest police station under antiviolence law of respective state, like one in Maharashtra by the name of Medicare Service Persons & Medicare Service Institution (Prevention of Violence, Damage or Loss to Property) Act, 2010. There are similar acts in other states also.

MEDICOLEGAL ASPECTS OF DIFFICULT SITUATIONS, DECLARATION OF DEATH AND COMMUNICATION WITH PATIENT PARTY

Most legal problems in healthcare systems arise from poor communication hence good communication can play a significant part in avoiding complaints and malpractice claims.

One big barrier to good communication

Arrogance and paternalistic attitude: Arrogance and paternalistic automatic antagonism towards patient, party is deeply ingrained into doctors. Doctors presume that they know the best about their patient, hence they always issue commands. Doctors expect patients and their parents to follow commands unquestioningly. Doctor should willingly change this situation by being more adaptive and communicating.

Delivering Bad News

Preparing to Deliver Bad News/Declaration of Death

Percepting self-reflection: Anaesthesiologist will invariably have strong negative emotions when they have to give bad news. In near death situations, anaesthesiologist should not spontaneously discuss their own emotional reaction with a preceptor; therefore they should be introducing this topic. "This is really a hard case, and everything medically possible to salvage the patient is being done, yet patient is not responding".

Create an appropriate setting: Say child is serious and every bit of best is being continuously done.

Make sure you know basic information: About the patient's disease, current situation, prognosis, and treatment options before delivering bad news.

Situations requiring extra caution: Medical professional should keep in mind certain high-risk situations, which are common causes for medical negligence actions; situations that require being extra cautions during anaesthesia, which can result in loss of sight, hearing, paralysis, vegetative life and death.

MEDICOLEGAL ASPECTS OF VICARIOUS LIABILITY

Only delegation of work is allowed by Law

Delegation of medical work to junior medical personnel, nurses, (be those qualified or unqualified staff), employed or contracted. The medical professional owes vicarious liability to patient on the basis of sound legal principle that, one can delegate medical work not responsibility.

Delegation of responsibility not allowed by Law

"Vicarious" means arising out of a vicar or a deputy or an agent. Vicarious liability indicates liability arising out of an agent's, a deputy's, or a substitute's wrongful actions or omissions of their duties, and not out of the medical professional's own wrongs. In the course of their professional duties, paediatric anaesthesiologists often have to requisite the services of nurses, technicians and paramedical staff. In hospitals there are other categories employed to assist the medical professional; in charge, of the patients, i.e. housemen and registrars, technicians, ward boys and ayahs. The vicarious civil liability is to compensate the victim monetarily for loss/damage. This liability is applicable only for civil liabilities, not criminal actions.

There is no Criminal Vicarious Liability

There is no principle of employer's liability in criminal law. There is no indirect or secondary or vicarious criminal liability.

MEDICOLEGAL ASPECTS OF EUTHANASIA, DNR, VEGETATIVE LIFE AND ACTIVE AND PASSIVE WITHDRAWAL OF LIFE SUPPORT SYSTEMS

Do-not-resuscitate Instructions by Patients (not Valid in India After SC's Aruna Shanbhag's Judgement)

1. Take a high-risk consent from the patient party for continuing neonatal resuscitation in spite of failure to resuscitate after 10 minutes explaining risks.
2. Record specifically in the consent the patient's directive/s if parents want the neonatal resuscitation to be discontinued at the end of 10 minutes.
3. Take signatures of two independent witnesses on DNR document.

Removing active life support system and passively keeping patient alive by feeding tubes etc.

1. Make sure patient is brain dead as per guidelines given in HOTA-1994.
2. Take high court order after taking consent from the patient's closest relative and caretaker that in the given circumstance it is of no use continuing active/passive life support.
3. Take signature of two independent witnesses.

Information for parents and families about ventilator withdrawal

1. The anaesthesiologist's counselling of families is a critical aspect of care for the dying patient who is to be removed from ventilator. Ideally the family will be involved in the decision to withdraw the ventilator. Before withdrawal, the following issues should be discussed.
2. **Potential outcome of ventilator withdrawal**
3. Assuming all other life-sustaining treatments have been stopped, including artificial hydration and nutrition, there are several potential outcomes: Rapid death within minutes or death within hours to days and very rarely patient may survive also.
4. **The procedure of ventilator withdrawal**
5. Never make assumptions about what the family understands; describe the procedure in clear, simple terms and answer any question. Families should be told before-hand the steps of withdrawal and whether or not it is planned/desired to remove the endotracheal tube. In addition, they should be counselled about the use of oxygen and medications for symptom control. Assure them that the patient's comfort is of primary concern. Explain that breathlessness may occur, but that it can be managed. Confirm that you will have medications available to manage any discomfort. Ensure they know that the patient will likely need to be kept asleep to control their symptoms.
6. If asked, explain that they can show love and support through touch, wiping of the patient's forehead, holding a hand and talking to him or her.
7. **Support the decision:** Even though a family is able to make a definite decision for ventilator withdrawal, such a decision is always emotionally charged. Families will constantly second-guess themselves, especially if the death appears to linger following ventilator withdrawal. Anaesthesiologist support, guidance and leadership are crucial, as the family will be looking to the anaesthesiologist to ensure them that they are "doing the right thing". Furthermore, support needs to continue following death during the bereavement period.

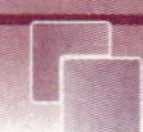

MEDICOLEGAL ASPECTS OF BLOOD TRANSFUSION

1. Blood is a FDA approved product and needs to come from registered blood bank for transfusion.
2. Counsel that transfused blood is tested for HIV, HCV, Hep B, yet no one can guarantee that these diseases will not be trasmittred to recipient. The window period of disease cannot be detected by tests done in blood banks.
3. Take separate and specific consent for blood, blood products transfusion, if transfusion is foreseeable and anticipated since bleeding might be excessive.
4. Take consent for blood transfusion for all surgeries/procedures along with consent for surgery/procedure.
5. Do not administer blood to Jehovah's witness.

MEDICOLEGAL ASPECTS OF OPERATING THEATRE MISHAPS NOT CAUSING DEATH

"Errors are an inevitable and unfortunate reality of Medical Practice"

Iatrogenic injuries caused by medical errors are moving from the realm of death conference of medical professionals to courtroom. In olden times a doctor was considered next to God and his authority and actions were rarely, if ever, questioned. But times have changed; doctors as well as patients are more aware of the inner nuances of medicine, hence one should do everything possible to reduce errors and reduce the chances of harm to the patient

Singlemost common cause of medical error

Overwork and tiredness of medical staff called on to perform extra duties. Sleep deprivation has also been cited as a contributing factor in medical errors. One study found that being awake for over 24 hours caused medical interns to double or triple the number of preventable medical errors, including those which resulted in injury or death.

Anaesthesia-related Complications

1. Misdiagnosis of an illness/condition, failure to diagnose or delay of a diagnosis
2. Oxygen deprivation is one major cause
3. Not able to read labels of injectable medicines and depend blindly on colour and size of vial/amouple
4. Use of arterial line for administration of drugs instead of venous line
5. Exchange of N_2O with O_2 gas pipes/flowmeters

MEDICAL INDEMNITY POLICY

The purpose of medical professional indemnity is to protect the medical professional persons against legal liability to pay damages to patients who have sustained loss arising from their own professional negligence.

The medical indemnity policy offers indemnity guided by law of contract and strictly covers civil legal liability/loss due to medical negligence only. The premium paid on the policy is on yearly basis and doctor has to renew every year without fail to maintain retroactive date. Retroactive date is the date of taking such policy for the first time

The rate of premium for paediatric anaesthesiologist is ₹ 3 per thousand rupees per year.

Note

Paediatric anaesthesiologist is not covered for criminal/prison sentence awarded by courts but the cost of defense can be received.

REFERENCES

1. The Indian Medical Council (Professional conduct, Etiquette and Ethics) Regulations, 2002.
2. the Indian Evidence Act, 1872 as amended up to date.
3. Section 6 in The Limitation Act, 1963.
4. Form of daily case register, Form No. 3C [See rule 6F(3)] under Section 44AA of Income Tax Act 1961.
5. Consumer Protection Act, 1986 as amended up to date.
6. The Limitation Act, 1963 as amended up to date.
7. Information Technology Act 2000 as amended up to date and the Indian Evidence Act, 1872 as amended up to date.
8. Meenakshi Mission Hospital and Research Centre V. Samuraj and Anr., I(2005) CPJ (NC).
9. Jacob Mathew vs State Of Punjab and ANR on 5 August, 2005 [Jacob Mathews case].
10. Supra at 15, Jacob Mathews case.
11. Supra at 15, Jacob Mathews case.
12. The Code of Criminal Procedure, 1973 (CrPC).
13. Indian Penal Code, 1860.
14. Indian Penal Code, 1860.
15. Advocates Act, 1961.
16. Outlook magazine April 2002 issue.

Infection Control in Operating Room and Safe Practice of Anaesthesia and Quality Management

Harshwardhan A Tikle

The awareness about transmissibility of certain diseases existed even during the era of Hippocrates and Gallen. Use of water and or wine to clean wounds and instruments was practiced even at that time. It was in 1932 that Water's first associated with anaesthesia equipments as vector for nosocomial infection. In most places the anaesthesiologist are designated OR managers and thus it is imperative that they play active role to take precautions against transmission of infection between operating room personnel's and patients, and in between the patients so as to reduce health care associated infections.

There is increasing trend in the developed as well as developing countries towards the use of disposable or single use equipment. The biggest handicaps for the most of the institutions in many part of our country and in many other places are the economic liability for the same. Thus there is lesser choice than to continue the use of reusable equipment and sticking to decontamination and sterilization practice taking appropriate infection control standards. Certain behaviors and rituals in the operating theaters can be also modified to suit infection control in the OR. Each hospital or institute should have infection control committee which should design institution specific policies for sterilization of reusable equipment and infection control in general.

INFECTION CONTROL POLICY

Every operating department should develop its own policy manual. The policy formulated should be adhered strictly to ensure that standards are maintained for safe practice. All members in the operating room should be properly trained and informed about the policies for infection control.

CURRENT RECOMMENDATIONS FOR OPERATING ROOM INFECTION CONTROL

1. The concept of universal precaution which suggests that all patients be treated with full infection control has been replaced in C.D.C. recommendations by standard precautions, with additional precautions as and when judged appropriate.
2. There is no reason for divesting patients of all their clothes. In Paediatric patients this is very important because the patients are much susceptible to hypothermia and its ill effects. If and when possible only the operating part has to exposed during the surgical procedure. The extremities and the head should always covered during the procedure. Additional warming devices can also be used to control the patient's temperature along with temperature monitoring.
3. As far as possible shaving of the operative site is to be avoided. Following are the recommendations to shaving: (a) Avoid shaving if possible, (b) Use depilatory cream a day prior, if this is not possible then use clippers immediately preoperatively and (c) shave only if no other option is available.
4. Order of patients on operating list, clean versus dirty cases: If proper diligence is applied to cleaning of the operating theater and visibly contaminated surfaces between the surgeries there is no reason to require conventionally ventilated operating room to be kept vacant room for more than 15 minutes before taking a clean case after performing a dirty case. For

operating room with vertical laminar flow only 5 minutes are required to replace the entire volume of air in the theater. Possible expectation to this may be, where there is profuse dispersion of contaminants, for example, patients with MRSA colonization or where aerosol dispersing power tools are used on infected tissues.

CLEANING AND STERILISATION OF ANAESTHESIA EQUIPMENT

With several advances in the development of anti-microbial agents and methods of sterilization several factors still influence their effectiveness. The recommendations on preferred method of cleaning and sterilization are available as evidence based guidelines. Multiuse products must be cleaned and sterilized as per the recommendation of the manufacturer.

Before we deal with topic it is important to understand definition of certain terms.

1. Disinfection describes a process that eliminates most of disease producing microorganisms except bacterial spores. For anaesthetic equipment liquid chemicals or wet pasteurization are the commonly used disinfectants.
2. Sterilization describes a process that eliminates all forms of microbial life including spores. Pressurized steam (autoclaving), dry heat, ethylene oxide gas, gamma rays and hydrogen peroxide gas plasma are some methods of equipment sterilization.
3. Decontamination describes a process wherein any multiuse equipment is properly cleaned of any visible matter that soils it. It can be done by using warm water with or without mild detergent and then air drying the equipment.

Sterilization

A particular medical device can be made sterile using physical or chemical procedure depending on the extent of its contact with the patient. Chemical sterilization is generally used for equipment that can be damaged by heat sterilization methods. Most of single use equipment are either sterilized by ethyleneoxide or gamma rays. Reusable equipment can be sterilized by either heat sterilization or chemical sterilization or both. Silicone based anaesthesia equipment, parts of anaesthesia machine, tubings are autoclavable. Plastic, polyvinyl chloride and rubber materials require chemical sterilization.

Most medical and surgical devices used in healthcare facilities are made of materials that are heat stable and therefore undergo heat, primarily steam, sterilization. However, since 1950, there has been an increase in medical devices and instruments made of materials (e.g. plastics) that require low-temperature sterilization. Ethylene oxide gas has been used since the 1950s for heat- and moisture-sensitive medical devices. Within the past 15 years, a number of new, low-temperature sterilization systems (e.g. hydrogen peroxide gas plasma, peracetic acid immersion, ozone) have been developed and are being used to sterilize medical devices. This section reviews sterilization technologies used in healthcare and makes recommendations for their optimum performance in the processing of medical devices.

Chemical Sterilization

This is fast and technically easy to carry out method of sterilization. Sterilization is achieved by completely immersing the equipment in the sterilant. This is a method of surface sterilization. The duration of immersion varies depending on the nature of equipment. Before reusing, the equipment should be thoroughly rinsed with sterile normal saline or distilled water to completely remove the chemical from the equipment.

PROPERTIES OF AN IDEAL DISINFECTANT

- Broad spectrum: Should have a wide antimicrobial spectrum
- Fast acting: Should produce a rapid kill
- Not affected by environmental factors: Should be active in the presence of organic matter (e.g. blood, sputum, faeces) and compatible with soaps, detergents, and other chemicals encountered in use
- Nontoxic: Should not be harmful to the user or patient
- Surface compatibility: Should not corrode instruments and metallic surfaces and should not cause the deterioration of cloth, rubber, plastics, and other materials
- Residual effect on treated surfaces: Should leave an antimicrobial film on the treated surface
- Easy to use with clear label directions
- Odourless: Should have a pleasant odour or no odour to facilitate its routine use
- Economical: Should not be prohibitively high in cost

- Solubility: Should be soluble in water
- Stability: Should be stable in concentrate and use-dilution
- Cleaner: Should have good cleaning properties
- Environmentally friendly: Should not damage the environment on disposal

FACTORS AFFECTING THE EFFICACY OF DISINFECTION AND STERILIZATION

The activity of germicides against microorganisms depends on a number of factors, some of which are intrinsic qualities of the organism, others of which are the chemical and external physical environment. Awareness of these factors should lead to better use of disinfection and sterilization processes and will be briefly reviewed. More extensive consideration of these and other factors is available elsewhere.

Number and Location of Microorganisms

All other conditions remaining constant, the larger the number of microbes, the more time a germicide needs to destroy all of them. Spaulding illustrated this relation when he employed identical test conditions and demonstrated that it took 30 minutes to kill 10 *B. atrophaeus* (formerly *Bacillus subtilis*) spores but 3 hours to kill 100,000 *Bacillus atrophaeus* spores. This reinforces the need for scrupulous cleaning of medical instruments before disinfection and sterilization. Reducing the number of microorganisms that must be inactivated through meticulous cleaning, increases the margin of safety when the germicide is used according to the labelling and shortens the exposure time required to kill the entire microbial load. Researchers also have shown that aggregated or clumped cells are more difficult to inactivate than monodispersed cells.

The location of microorganisms also must be considered when factors affecting the efficacy of germicides are assessed. Medical instruments with multiple pieces must be disassembled and equipment such as endoscopes that have crevices, joints, and channels are more difficult to disinfect than are flat-surface equipment because penetration of the disinfectant of all parts of the equipment is more difficult. Only surfaces that directly contact the germicide will be disinfected, so there must be no air pockets and the equipment must be completely immersed for the entire exposure period. Manufacturers should be encouraged to produce equipment engineered for ease of cleaning and disinfection.

Innate Resistance of Microorganisms

Microorganisms vary greatly in their resistance to chemical germicides and sterilization processes. Intrinsic resistance mechanisms in microorganisms to disinfectants vary. For example, spores are resistant to disinfectants because the spore coat and cortex act as a barrier, mycobacteria have a waxy cell wall that prevents disinfectant entry, and gram-negative bacteria possess an outer membrane that acts as a barrier to the uptake of disinfectants. Implicit in all disinfection strategies is the consideration that the most resistant microbial subpopulation controls the sterilization or disinfection time. That is, to destroy the most resistant types of microorganisms (i.e. bacterial spores), the user needs to employ exposure times and a concentration of germicide needed to achieve complete destruction. Except for prions, bacterial spores possess the highest innate resistance to chemical germicides, followed by coccidia (e.g. *Cryptosporidium*), mycobacteria (e.g. *M. tuberculosis*), nonlipid or small viruses (e.g. poliovirus, and coxsackievirus), fungi (e.g. *Aspergillus*, and *Candida*), vegetative bacteria (e.g. *Staphylococcus*, and *Pseudomonas*) and lipid or medium-size viruses (e.g. herpes, and HIV). The germicidal resistance exhibited by the gram-positive and gram-negative bacteria is similar with some exceptions (e.g. *P. aeruginosa* which shows greater resistance to some disinfectants). *P. aeruginosa* also is significantly more resistant to a variety of disinfectants in its "naturally occurring" state than are cells subcultured on laboratory media. *Rickettsiae*, *Chlamydiae*, and mycoplasma cannot be placed in this scale of relative resistance because information about the efficacy of germicides against these agents is limited. Because these micro-organisms contain lipid and are similar in structure and composition to other bacteria, they can be predicted to be inactivated by the same germicides that destroy lipid viruses and vegetative bacteria. A known exception to this supposition is *Coxiella burnetti*, which has demonstrated resistance to disinfectants.

Concentration and Potency of Disinfectants

With other variables constant, and with one exception (iodophors), the more concentrated the disinfectant, the greater its efficacy and the shorter the time necessary to achieve microbial kill. Generally not recognized, however, is that all disinfectants are not similarly affected by concentration adjustments. For example, quaternary ammonium compounds and phenol have a concentration exponent of 1 and 6, respectively; thus, halving the concentration of a quaternary ammonium compound requires doubling its disinfecting time, but halving the concentration of a phenol solution requires a 64-fold (i.e. 26) increase in its disinfecting time.

SUMMARY

Summary of advantages and disadvantages of chemical agents used as chemical sterilants 1 or as high-level disinfectants.

Physical and Chemical Factors

Several physical and chemical factors also influence disinfectant procedures: temperature, pH, relative humidity, and water hardness. For example, the activity of most disinfectants increases as the temperature increases, but some exceptions exist. Furthermore, too great an increase in temperature causes the disinfectant to degrade and weakens its germicidal activity and thus might produce a potential health hazard.

An increase in pH improves the antimicrobial activity of some disinfectants (e.g. glutaraldehyde, quaternary ammonium compounds) but decreases the antimicrobial activity of others (e.g. phenols, hypochlorites, and iodine). The pH influences the antimicrobial activity by altering the disinfectant molecule or the cell surface.

Relative humidity is the single most important factor influencing the activity of gaseous disinfectants/sterilants, such as ETO, chlorine dioxide, and formaldehyde.

Water hardness (i.e. high concentration of divalent cations) reduces the rate of kill of certain disinfectants because divalent cations (e.g. magnesium, calcium) in the hard water interact with the disinfectant to form insoluble precipitates.

Organic and Inorganic Matters

Organic matter in the form of serum, blood, pus, or faecal or lubricant material can interfere with the antimicrobial activity of disinfectants in at least two ways. Most commonly, interference occurs by a chemical reaction between the germicide and the organic matter resulting in a complex that is less germicidal or nongermicidal, leaving less of the active germicide available for attacking microorganisms. Chlorine and iodine disinfectants, in particular, are prone to such interaction. Alternatively, organic material can protect microorganisms from attack by acting as a physical barrier.

The effects of inorganic contaminants on the sterilization process were studied during the 1950s and 1960s. These and other studies show the protection by inorganic contaminants of microorganisms to all sterilization processes results from occlusion in salt crystals. This further emphasizes the importance of meticulous cleaning of medical devices before any sterilization or disinfection procedure because both organic and inorganic soils are easily removed by washing (Table 44.1).

Table 44.1 Summary of advantages and disadvantages of commonly used sterilization technology

Sterilization method	Advantages	Disadvantages
Peracetic Acid/Hydrogen Peroxide	No activation required • Odour or irritation not significant Limited clinical experience Potential for eye and skin damage	Materials compatibility concerns (lead, brass, copper, zinc) both cosmetic and functional
Glutaraldehyde	Numerous use studies published Relatively inexpensive Excellent materials compatibility	Respiratory irritation from glutaraldehyde vapour Pungent and irritating odour Relatively slow mycobactericidal activity Coagulates blood and fixes tissue to surfaces Allergic contact dermatitis Glutaraldehyde vapour monitoring recommended
Hydrogen Peroxide	No activation required May enhance removal of organic matter and organisms No disposal issues	Material compatibility concerns (brass, zinc, copper, and nickel/silver plating) both cosmetic and functional Serious eye damage with contact

Contd...

Table 44.1 Summary of advantages and disadvantages of commonly used sterilization technology (*Contd...*)

Sterilization method	Advantages	Disadvantages
	No odour or irritation issues Does not coagulate blood or fix tissues to surfaces Inactivates *Cryptosporidium* Use studies published	
Ortho-phthalaldehyde	Fast acting high-level disinfectant No activation required Odour not significant Excellent materials compatibility claimed Does not coagulate blood or fix tissues to surfaces claimed	Stains skin, mucous membranes, clothing, and environmental surfaces Repeated exposure may result in hypersensitivity in some patients with bladder cancer More expensive than glutaraldehyde Eye irritation with contact Slow sporicidal activity
Peracetic acid	Rapid sterilization cycle time (30–45 min.) Low temperature (50–55°C) liquid immersion sterilization Environmental friendly by-products (acetic acid, O_2, H_2O) Fully automated Single-use system eliminates need for concentration testing Standardized cycle May enhance removal of organic material and endotoxin No adverse health effects to operators under normal operating conditions Compatible with many materials and instruments Does not coagulate blood or fix tissues to surfaces Sterilant flows through scope facilitating salt, protein, and microbe removal Rapidly sporicidal Provides procedure standardization (constant dilution, perfusion of channel, temperatures, exposure)	Potential material incompatibility (e.g. aluminium anodized coating becomes dull) Used for immersible instruments only Biological indicator may not be suitable for routine monitoring One scope or a small number of instruments can be processed in a cycle More expensive (endoscope repairs, operating costs, purchase costs) than high-level disinfection Serious eye and skin damage (concentrated solution) with contact Point-of-use system, no sterile storage
Steam	• Nontoxic to patient, staff, environment • Cycle easy to control and monitor · • Rapidly microbicidal • Least affected by organic/inorganic soil among sterilization processes listed • Rapid cycle time • Penetrates medical packing, device lumens	• Deleterious for heat-sensitive instruments • Microsurgical instruments damaged by repeated exposure • May leave instruments wet, causing them to rust • Potential for burns
Hydrogen peroxide gas plasma	• Safe for the environment • Leaves no toxic residuals • Cycle time is 28–75 minutes (varies with model type) and no aeration necessary · • Used for heat- and moisture-sensitive items since process temperature < 50°C • Simple to operate, install (208 V outlet), and monitor · • Compatible with most medical devices	• Cellulose (paper), linens and liquids cannot be processed • Sterilization chamber size from 1.8 to 9.4 ft 3 total volume (varies with model type) • Some endoscopes or medical devices with long or narrow lumens cannot be processed at this time in the United States (*See* manufacturer's recommendations for internal diameter and length restrictions)

Contd...

Table 44.1 Summary of advantages and disadvantages of commonly used sterilization technology (*Contd...*)

Sterilization method	Advantages	Disadvantages
	• Only requires electrical outlet	• Requires synthetic packaging (polypropylene wraps, polyolefin pouches) and special container tray • Hydrogen peroxide may be toxic at levels greater than 1 ppmTWA
100% Ethylene Oxide (ETO)	• Penetrates packaging materials, device lumens • Single-dose cartridge and negative-pressure chamber minimizes the potential for gas leak and ETO exposure • Simple to operate and monitor • Compatible with most medical materials	• Requires aeration time to remove ETO residue • Sterilization chamber size from 4.0 to 7.9 ft 3 total volume (varies with model type) • ETO is toxic, a carcinogen, and flammable • ETO emission regulated by states but catalytic cell removes 99.9% of ETO and converts it to CO_2 and H_2O • ETO cartridges should be stored inflammable liquid storage cabinet · • Lengthy cycle/aeration time
ETO Mixtures 8.6% ETO/91.4% HCFC 10% ETO/90% HCFC 8.5% ETO/91.5% CO_2	• Penetrates medical packaging and many plastics • Compatible with most medical materials • Cycle easy to control and monitor	• Some states (e.g. CA, NY, MI) require ETO emission reduction of 90–99.9% • CFC (inert gas that eliminates explosion hazard) banned in 1995 • Potential hazards to staff and patients • Lengthy cycle/aeration time • ETO is toxic, a carcinogen, and flammable
Peracetic Acid	• Rapid cycle time (30–45 minutes) • Low temperature (50–55°C liquid immersion sterilization) • Environmental friendly by-products · • Sterilant flows through endoscope which facilitates salt, protein and microbe removal	• Point-of-use system, no sterile storage • Biological indicator may not be suitable for routine monitoring • Used for immersible instruments only • Some material incompatibility (e.g. aluminium anodized coating becomes dull) • One scope or a small number of instruments processed in a cycle • Potential for serious eye and skin damage (concentrated solution) with contact

Pasteurisation: Equipment for respiratory therapy like breathing tubes, face masks tracheal stylets, bite blocks can be sterilized by pasteurisation. In this process the decontaminated pieces of equipment are disinfected by hot water at 70° for 30 minutes. This is achieved by keeping the instrument in automated pasteurizer or washer disinfector. Following this procedure the pieces of equipment are dried in a drying cabinet with HEPA filters.

Autoclaving: It is carried out by moist heat under pressure. It is the most expensive method of sterilization. Four parameters of importance in autoclaving are steam, pressure, time and temperature. The minimum time for sterilization at 121°C is 15 minutes and 4 minutes at 132°C. Prevaccume onsite steriliser that are present in or near operation theatre have a pressure of 35 psig. Large volume off site gravity displacement autoclave system have operational pressure of approximately 85 psig at temperature of 160° with cycle time of one hour.

Ethylene oxide: Single use equipment is sterilized by ethylene oxide gas (ETO). ETO is colourless poisonous and flammable gas. The cycle time for sterilization is 3–6 hours. The main disadvantage associated with this technique are lengthy cycle time, cost and exposure hazards.

Gamma radiation: It requires a special protective environment and equipment cost are the major reasons to make this technique impracticable for everyday use. The main advantage is that once the item is sterilized, its sterility is retained indefinitely if the package is not soiled or opened. Thermo labile items can be sterilized by irradiation. This technique is non-polluting, environmentally friendly process and does not leave any harmful residue on the device.

CONSIDERATION OF INDIVIDUAL ANAESTHETIC ITEMS

1. Anaesthesia machine: All the surfaces of the anaesthesia machine should be cleaned with an appropriate intermediate or low level disinfectant on daily basis.
2. The respiratory system via the breathing circuit, ventilators and the carbon dioxide absorber can be sterilized by autoclaving according to the manufacturer's recommendations.
3. Anaesthesia face mask: The masks should be ideally for single use only as secretions from the patients can be transmitted to another patient. If it is to be reused it should be sterilized in between the patient use according to the manufacturers instruction.
4. All catheter mounts should be of single use only.
5. Suppraglottic airway device: These includes oral airways, nasal airways, LMA, etc. They should be of single use only preferably. Suppraglottic airway devices with silicone rubber should be reused only as many time as advised by the manufacturer after sterilizing it with recommendations accompanying the instruments.
6. Laryngoscopes: Current practice of decontamination and disinfection between patients are frequently ineffective. Reusable laryngoscope blades should be autoclaved in between patients. Flash sterilization can be used for them. Disposable transparent sheath covers for the laryngoscopes can also be used.
7. Fiberoptic instruments: These are expensive items which cannot be autoclaved. Decontamination is best achieved by automated system, i.e. hydrogen peroxide plasma sterilization. All lumens should be cleaned using the brush supplied by manufacturer to remove any debris in the internal ports of the scopes.
8. Instruments used for regional anaesthesia should be of single use only.

Safe practice of anaesthesia and quality management

Effective communication and team work is essential for the delivery of high quality and safe patient care. The complexity of medical care and inherent limitations of human performance warrant that the team providing care to the patient creates an environment which can deliver safe and standard care to each patient.

To provide such care it is important that care delivery to have the following elements.

1. Concept of teamwork.
2. Effective skills of communication.
3. Standard care protocols
4. Proper infection control

This part of the chapter will deal with the first three concepts for provision of safe and high quality of anaesthesia delivery services.

THE CONCEPT OF TEAM WORK

In today's practice of health care delivery much importance is being placed on patient satisfaction and quality of health care. Along with the technical knowledge about ones specialty and in present context about management of clinical scenarios in Paediatric surgery and anaesthesia, it is imperative to have good training in nontechnical or soft skills also. The non-technical skills reflect the interpersonal and cognitive skills like communication, team work, decision making and spatial awareness. Both the technical and non technical skills complement each other in daily practice. Failure in teamwork and non technical skills along with breakdown in communications within the teams and with patient and their relatives are frequently implicated in adverse events in surgical patients.

In our country and in many countries in world training modules for clinicians today severely lack the training of soft or nontechnical skills. In developed countries today the knowledge of nontechnical skills are listed as core competency skill both in training as well as in hiring health professionals. In Paediatric surgical units and in operating room these skills are very important as we have to deal with both anxious and harried patient and their parents. Failure to communicate properly with patient is the largest factor in dissatisfied patients.

Good interpersonal communications are necessary for smooth and efficient working in the operating room. It is necessary to have a cordial, friendly and hassle free environment for maximizing the work efficiency of the care giving team. Precise, accurate communication is required between all the members of team. Good teamwork and communications help in proper scheduling of surgeries and prevent unnecessary delays and cancellations of procedures. It also maximizes the rational use of theater allocations.

COMMUNICATION WITH PATIENTS AND RELATIVES

It is a well known fact that anaesthesiologist usually work in a very compressed timeframe with patients. In this time it is very necessary to have clear, succinct and respectful communication with the patients and their relatives in the paediatric patients. Mannerism, habits, general appearance and soft skills affect the impression of the attending anaesthesiologist.

Patients are generally submissive as they are in need of treatment and doctors are empowered in this situation by their knowledge in such situation. "WITH POWER COMES RESPONSIBILITY" should be our motto while dealing with patients and their relatives. While communicating with relatives and patients always show respect for them as a sensate being. Remember that communication of respect builds trust which is very important. Always speak as if the patient will remember everything. For paediatric patients always use a soft, gentle tone along with gentle touch for examination as appropriate. Respect the individuality and the socio-cultural practices of the local area.

Non-verbal signals convey our attitude and values to patient even before a single word is spoken. Observer or patients generally tend to remember and believe in non-verbal communication than in words. It is therefore important to show empathy and respect. Always start conversation by addressing the child appropriately by his name. Maintain eye contact with patient and their relatives while talking to them. Maintaining tone and volume of voice along with proper facial expressions are very reassuring to anxious patients. Whenever taking history always show intentions of sincerity. Always listen to what the patient has to say and if some point is not understood or needs clarification, check it again with the patient or informant. Accepting the patient and or informant in case of Paediatric population is an important element in creating a rapport. Reaching conclusions based on inadequate evidence is not very helpful. Allow them to ask questions freely and try to answer them in a way that they can understand.

A preoperative visit is a time for conversation with patient for specific purpose. Focusing on the purpose of this interview will be helpful in directing it properly. Remembering that we are dealing with persons in distress and that their feelings about the situation can vary. It is helpful to get proper and relevant information from patient and informants. The priority should be to remain calm and not becoming agitated due to patient's behavior. In all the patients and their relatives there are frequent and specific fears related to anaesthesia like awareness during surgery, delayed awakening and need for intensive care unit admission in postoperative period. Time should be given address these concerns of the patient. Try to give as much information as possible regarding what should be expected in perioperative time during anaesthesia. Discuss modalities of pain management strategies with the patient and relatives.

In event of any intraoperative or postoperative complication either expected or unexpected, it is the duty of the attending doctor both the surgeon and anaesthesiologist to face the patient or the relatives. We must be honest and informative towards breaking any bad news. While interacting in such situations always show genuine care for them. Always keep all channels of communication open. Show appropriate concern and sense of empathy. Expression of emotions and acknowledgement of distress should be done for comforting the patients.

REFERENCES

1. Guideline for Disinfection and Sterilization in Healthcare Facilities, 2008, CDC. Atlanta.
2. N. Sabir, V. Ramchandran; Decontamination of Anesthesia Equipments, Continuing Medical Education in Anesthesia, Critical Care and Pain; BJA. 2004;4(4).
3. Infection Control in Anesthesia, AAGBI Guidelines October 2008.
4. Juwarkar CS. Cleaning and Sterlisation of anaesthetic Equipment; IJA Sep-Oct 2013;57(5):541–50.

Index